T0212837

Register Now for Online Access to Your Book!

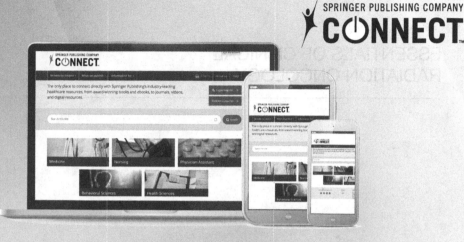

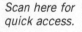

ESSENTIALS OF CLINICAL
RADIATION ONCOLOGY

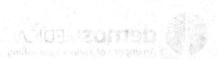

ESSENTIALS OF CLINICAL RADIATION ONCOLOGY

Editors

Matthew C. Ward, MD
Radiation Oncologist
Southeast Radiation Oncology Group
Charlotte, North Carolina

Rahul D. Tendulkar, MD
Associate Professor
Cleveland Clinic Lerner College of Medicine
Staff Physician
Department of Radiation Oncology
Cleveland Clinic
Cleveland, Ohio

Gregory M. M. Videtic, MD, CM, FRCPC, FACR
Professor of Medicine
Cleveland Clinic Lerner College of Medicine
Staff Physician
Department of Radiation Oncology
Cleveland Clinic
Cleveland, Ohio

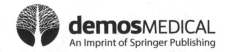

demosMEDICAL
An Imprint of Springer Publishing

Visit our website at www.springerpub.com

ISBN: 9780826168542
ebook ISBN: 9780826168559

Acquisitions Editor: David D'Addona
Compositor: Exeter Premedia Services Private Ltd.

Published by Springer Publishing Company.
Demos Medical Publishing is an imprint of Springer Publishing Company, LLC.

Library of Congress Cataloging-in-Publication Data

Names: Ward, Matthew C., 1986- editor. | Tendulkar, Rahul D. editor. |
   Videtic, Gregory M. M., editor.
Title: Essentials of clinical radiation oncology / editors, Matthew C. Ward,
   Rahul D. Tendulkar, Gregory M. M. Videtic.
Description: New York: Demos Medical, [2018] | Includes bibliographical
   references and index.
Identifiers: LCCN 2017035591 | ISBN 9780826168542 | ISBN 9780826168559 (ebook)
Subjects: | MESH: Neoplasms—radiotherapy | Handbooks
Classification: LCC RC271.R3 | NLM QZ 39 | DDC 616.99/40642—dc23
LC record available at https://lccn.loc.gov/2017035591

Printed in the United States of America by McNaughton & Gunn.
17 18 19 20 21 / 5 4 3 2 1

To the enduring commitment of past, present, and future residents in the pursuit of knowledge, without whom this work would not have been possible.

CONTENTS

IX. Hematologic

X. Sarcomas

XI. Pediatric

XII. Palliation

CONTRIBUTORS

Mohamed E. Abazeed, MD, PhD, Assistant Professor, Department of Radiation Oncology, Taussig Cancer Center, Cleveland Clinic, Cleveland, Ohio

Sudha R. Amarnath, MD, Assistant Professor, Department of Radiation Oncology, Taussig Cancer Center, Cleveland Clinic, Cleveland, Ohio

Carryn M. Anderson, MD, Clinical Associate Professor, Department of Radiation Oncology, University of Iowa Hospitals & Clinics, Iowa City, Iowa

Ehsan H. Balagamwala, MD, Resident Physician, Department of Radiation Oncology, Taussig Cancer Center, Cleveland Clinic, Cleveland, Ohio

Camille A. Berriochoa, MD, Resident Physician, Department of Radiation Oncology, Taussig Cancer Center, Cleveland Clinic, Cleveland, Ohio

Samuel T. Chao, MD, Associate Professor, Director of CNS Radiation Oncology, Department of Radiation Oncology, Taussig Cancer Center, Cleveland Clinic, Cleveland, Ohio

Sheen Cherian, MD, MSc, MRCP, FRCR, DABR, Assistant Professor, Department of Radiation Oncology, Taussig Cancer Center, Cleveland Clinic, Cleveland, Ohio

Jordan Fenner, BS, School of Medicine, Case Western Reserve University, Cleveland, Ohio

Senthilkumar Gandhidasan, MD, MPH, MHI, FRANZCR, Radiation Oncologist, Department of Radiation Oncology, Illawarra Cancer Care Center, Wollongong, NSW, Australia

Jason W. D. Hearn, MD, Assistant Professor, Department of Radiation Oncology, University of Michigan, Ann Arbor, Michigan

Nikhil P. Joshi, MD, Associate Staff, Department of Radiation Oncology, Taussig Cancer Center, Cleveland Clinic, Cleveland, Ohio

Justin J. Juliano, MD, Radiation Oncologist, Department of Radiation Oncology, New York Oncology Hematology, Clifton Park, New York

Aditya Juloori, MD, Resident Physician, Department of Radiation Oncology, Taussig Cancer Center, Cleveland Clinic, Cleveland, Ohio

Edward W. Jung, MD, Radiation Oncologist, Cranbrook Radiation Oncology Partners, Chicago, Illinois

Jeffrey Kittel, MD, Radiation Oncologist, Radiation Oncology Associates, Ltd., Department of Radiation Oncology, Aurora St. Luke's Medical Center, Milwaukee, Wisconsin

Rupesh Kotecha, MD, Radiation Oncologist, Department of Radiation Oncology, Miami Cancer Institute, Miami, Florida

Shlomo A. Koyfman, MD, Assistant Professor, Departments of Radiation Oncology and Bioethics, Taussig Cancer Center, Cleveland Clinic, Cleveland, Ohio

Aryavarta M. S. Kumar, MD, PhD, Clinical Assistant Professor, Department of Radiation Oncology, University Hospitals Cleveland; Seidman Cancer Center, Cleveland, Ohio

Nathanael J. Lee, MD, PhD Candidate, Georgetown University School of Medicine, Washington, DC

Charles Marc Leyrer, MD, Resident Physician, Department of Radiation Oncology, Taussig Cancer Center, Cleveland Clinic, Cleveland, Ohio

Bindu V. Manyam, MD, Resident Physician, Department of Radiation Oncology, Taussig Cancer Center, Cleveland Clinic, Cleveland, Ohio

Gaurav Marwaha, MD, Assistant Professor, Associate Residency Program Director, Department of Radiation Oncology, Rush University, Chicago, Illinois

Omar Y. Mian, MD, PhD, Assistant Professor, Department of Radiation Oncology, Taussig Cancer Center, Cleveland Clinic, Cleveland, Ohio

Erin S. Murphy, MD, Staff Physician, Department of Radiation Oncology, Taussig Cancer Center, Cleveland Clinic, Cleveland, Ohio

Shireen Parsai, MD, Resident Physician, Department of Radiation Oncology, Taussig Cancer Center, Cleveland Clinic, Cleveland, Ohio

Yvonne D. Pham, MD, Radiation Oncologist, Therapeutic Radiologists Inc., Kansas City, Missouri

David J. Schwartz, V, MD, Assistant Professor of Radiation Oncology, Mayo Clinic College of Medicine, Rochester, Minnesota

Jacob G. Scott, MD, DPhil, Associate Staff, Department of Radiation Oncology, Taussig Cancer Center, Cleveland Clinic, Cleveland, Ohio

Chirag Shah, MD, Staff Physician, Associate Professor, Department of Radiation Oncology, Taussig Cancer Center, Cleveland Clinic, Cleveland, Ohio

Jonathan Sharrett, DO, Resident Physician, Department of Radiation Oncology, Taussig Cancer Center, Cleveland Clinic, Cleveland, Ohio

Monica E. Shukla, MD, Assistant Professor, Department of Radiation Oncology, Medical College of Wisconsin, Milwaukee, Wisconsin

Arun D. Singh, MD, Professor of Ophthalmology, Cole Eye Institute, Cleveland Clinic, Cleveland, Ohio

Timothy D. Smile, MD, Resident Physician, Department of Internal Medicine, Kettering Medical Center, Kettering, Ohio

Kevin L. Stephans, MD, Staff Physician, Associate Professor of Medicine, Department of Radiation Oncology, Taussig Cancer Center, Cleveland Clinic, Cleveland, Ohio

Abigail L. Stockham, MD, Assistant Professor of Radiation Oncology, Mayo Clinic College of Medicine, Rochester, Minnesota

John H. Suh, MD, Chairman, Department of Radiation Oncology, Taussig Cancer Center, Cleveland Clinic, Cleveland, Ohio

Rahul D. Tendulkar, MD, Associate Professor, Cleveland Clinic Lerner College of Medicine; Staff Physician, Department of Radiation Oncology, Cleveland Clinic, Cleveland, Ohio

Martin C. Tom, MD, Resident Physician, Department of Radiation Oncology, Taussig Cancer Center, Cleveland Clinic, Cleveland, Ohio

Vamsi Varra, BS, School of Medicine, Case Western Reserve University, Cleveland, Ohio

Andrew Vassil, MD, Staff Physician, Department of Radiation Oncology, Taussig Cancer Center, Cleveland Clinic, Cleveland, Ohio

Gregory M. M. Videtic, MD, CM, FRCPC, FACR, Professor of Medicine, Cleveland Clinic Lerner College of Medicine; Staff Physician, Department of Radiation Oncology, Cleveland Clinic, Cleveland, Ohio

Matthew C. Ward, MD, Radiation Oncologist, Southeast Radiation Oncology Group, Charlotte, North Carolina

Michael A. Weller, MD, Assistant Professor, Department of Radiation Oncology, Taussig Cancer Center, Cleveland Clinic, Cleveland, Ohio

Neil McIver Woody, MD, MS, Associate Staff, Department of Radiation Oncology, Taussig Cancer Center, Cleveland Clinic, Cleveland, Ohio

Jennifer S. Yu, MD, PhD, Assistant Professor, Department of Radiation Oncology, Taussig Cancer Center, Cleveland Clinic, Cleveland, Ohio

PREFACE

Team-based learning and patient-centered care have been long-standing traditions in the Cleveland Clinic Radiation Oncology Residency program. Over the past two decades, as a complement to the formal teaching curriculum, residents have spent countless hours condensing the pertinent literature into comprehensive high-yield clinical summaries, which are bound into a study manual and updated annually. *Essentials of Clinical Radiation Oncology* is a tribute to the generations of trainees who have contributed to this ongoing process of continual learning and improvement.

In the same spirit as our first venture, *Handbook of Treatment Planning in Radiation Oncology*, we felt there was a need for a clinically oriented resource that was both succinct and comprehensive, similar to our in-house manual. Thus, we are now proud to offer *Essentials of Clinical Radiation Oncology* as our formal answer to this need. *Essentials of Clinical Radiation Oncology* has been designed to serve as the clinical companion to the more technically oriented *Handbook of Treatment Planning in Radiation Oncology*. It is intended to provide residents, students, and practicing radiation oncologists with an easy-to-access resource in the rapidly evolving field of oncology, while serving as a supplement to other currently existing resources available to radiation oncologists, such as the *AJCC Cancer Staging Manual* and published consensus guidelines from national organizations. Our intention is to update the content of this handbook regularly over time, in order to keep pace with the changing clinical environment in oncology.

Tremendous thanks must be given to our current Cleveland Clinic Radiation Oncology residents, recent graduates, and dedicated faculty who shared our vision in producing this work. The efforts of our Chief Resident, Matthew C. Ward, MD, must be particularly acknowledged, as he assumed the task of organizing the authors' efforts and serving as the lead editor. We value and appreciate suggestions from our readers on how to keep this book current, and we encourage feedback to be sent by email to RO_chiefres@ccf.org. We hope that our community of readers finds this book to be a helpful resource, and that our patients ultimately benefit from the collective wisdom reflected in it and that is brought to training each generation of oncologists.

Rahul D. Tendulkar, MD
Gregory M. M. Videtic, MD, CM, FRCPC, FACR

■ ABOUT THE FORMAT OF THIS BOOK

The intention of this book is to serve as a comprehensive resource for all levels of practitioners, from medical students to practicing physicians alike. Therefore, the reader will find clinically pertinent details starting from basic epidemiology and culminating in an evidence-based approach to important and up-to-date clinical questions. The "front matter" of each chapter contains information about the disease and its natural history. This includes a summary of the AJCC eighth edition staging system (or other relevant risk-stratification systems), printed in an abbreviated format intended for physician understanding. Next, general "treatment paradigms" are included in the midpart of each chapter to give the reader an overview of the role of each anticancer modality in the multidisciplinary care of the patient. Finally, the highlight of this resource is the "evidence-based question and answer" format of clinical studies presented to guide the reader through the most pertinent literature. Each study is block-quoted from the source with a quick-access citation to the original reference in combination with a condensed summary intended to highlight the pertinent findings. It should be noted that our intention with this book is to provide a manual of information useful to the clinician, rather than to be "prescriptive" in terms of staging, radiation delivery, or chemotherapy dosing. Our hope is that this format provides an efficient yet thorough method for practitioners to develop a deeper understanding of a disease and the current state of its treatment.

I: CENTRAL NERVOUS SYSTEM

1: GLIOBLASTOMA

Aditya Juloori, Jennifer S. Yu, and Samuel T. Chao

> **QUICK HIT:** Glioblastoma multiforme (GBM) is the most common primary brain tumor in adults. GBM has a poor prognosis with a median survival of ~14 months. Treatment is maximal safe resection with neurological preservation followed by adjuvant chemoradiation. The standard RT dose is 60 Gy with temozolomide given 75 mg/m² daily concurrently and 150 to 200 mg/m² adjuvantly for days 1 to 5 of a 28-day cycle for 6 to 12 months as tolerated. Radiation field is typically 46 Gy to T2/FLAIR edema, then additional 14 Gy boost to resection cavity and T1 contrast enhancement, generally with a 2-cm CTV expansion. The most common site of treatment failure is local progression. For elderly or frail pts, options include palliative care, short-course RT +/- temozolomide, or temozolomide alone (particularly for MGMT methylated pts).

EPIDEMIOLOGY: GBM is the most common (80%) primary malignant brain tumor in adults.[1] Incidence: three to four cases per 100,000 or about 10,000 cases/year in the United States. Median age at diagnosis is 64 and the male-to-female ratio is approximately 1.5:1.[2]

ANATOMY: Diffusely infiltrative tumor that grows along white matter tracts. Location is dependent on amount of white matter: 75% are supratentorial (31% temporal, 24% parietal, 23% frontal, 16% occipital), <20% multifocal, 2% to 7% multicentric, 10% present with positive CSF cytology.[3]

PATHOLOGY: Cell of origin is the supporting glial cells of CNS. The World Health Organization 2016 update[4] now defines three distinct types: Glioblastoma, IDH-wild-type; Glioblastoma, IDH mutant; and Glioblastoma, NOS (see the Genetics section for details on IDH1). Other rare variants include giant cell glioblastoma, gliosarcoma, or epithelioid glioblastoma. Diagnosis of a WHO grade IV glioma requires the pathognomonic finding of "pseudopalisading" necrosis OR at least three of MEAN criteria: high <u>M</u>itotic index, <u>E</u>ndothelial proliferation, nuclear <u>A</u>typia, <u>N</u>ecrosis.

GENETICS

MGMT gene methylation: O⁶-methylguanine-DNA methyltransferase is located on chromosome 10q26. Its purpose is to repair alkylation of guanine at the 0-6 position. When the promoter undergoes epigenetic silencing by methylation, the gene is downregulated. The Hegi study (see Evidence-Based Q&A) defined its prognostic and predictive value.

IDH1 mutation: Present in approximately 10% of GBM and associated with increased age and secondary tumors that developed from previous low-grade gliomas.[4] IDH1 mutation is an independent positive prognostic factor (MS 27.4 mos for IDH1-mutated vs. 14 mos for IDH1-wild-type).[5]

EGFRv3 variant: In-frame deletion of exons 2 to 7 of the EGFR gene affecting 801 base pairs and is an independent predictor of a poor prognosis with standard chemoRT.[6]

BRAF V600E mutation: Same variant as in melanoma, but seen commonly in giant cell and epithelioid glioblastomas and lower grade gliomas.[7]

ATRX: Alpha-thalassemia/mental retardation syndrome x-linked gene (ATRX) is a gene that is involved in chromatin regulation. A mutation in ATRX is frequently seen in pts with grade II/III astrocytomas as well as pts with secondary GBM.[8–10]

See Chapter 2 for discussion of 1p19q codeletion.

CLINICAL PRESENTATION: Headache, cognitive changes, seizure, motor weakness, nausea/vomiting, visual loss, sensory loss, language disturbance, dysphagia, papilledema, gait disturbance, intracranial bleed.

WORKUP: H&P with neurologic exam. Fundoscopic exam (if suspicious of increased intracranial pressure).

Labs: CBC to establish baseline for CHT.

Imaging: MRI brain with and without gadolinium (heterogeneous enhancement, central necrosis, surrounding edema; T1 hypointense and T2 edema hyperintense).

Pathology: Biopsy with genetic assessment as earlier.

PROGNOSTIC FACTORS: Clinical factors as established by Li et al[11]: KPS, age, extent of resection. MGMT status, IDH1 status. See Table 1.1 for RTOG RPA.

TABLE 1.1: RPA Classification for GBM[11]			
RPA class	Defining variables	MS (mos)	OS at 1, 3 and 5 years
III	<50 y/o and KPS ≥90	17.1	70%, 20%, 14%
IV	<50 y/o and KPS <90 ≥50 y/o, KPS ≥70, resection, and working	11.2	46%, 7%, 4%
V + VI	≥50 y/o, KPS ≥70, resection, and not working ≥50 y/o, KPS ≥70, biopsy only ≥50 y/o, KPS <70	7.5	28%, 1%, 0%

Source: Adapted from Ref. (12).

TREATMENT PARADIGM

Surgery: Primary treatment is maximal safe surgical resection with neurologic preservation. For technically unresectable tumors, a biopsy is warranted to obtain tissue. Various tools may be applied to improve safety of resection such as intraoperative ultrasound/MRI, functional mapping (phase reversal, direct brain stimulation, awake anesthesia). To evaluate the extent of resection, obtain a contrast-enhanced MRI within 72 hours of surgery (ideally 24–48 hours) to avoid confounding with subacute blood products.

Chemotherapy: As established in the Stupp trial, daily use of temozolomide (TMZ) 75 mg/m² daily concurrently during radiation course, including weekends. This is followed by the use of adjuvant TMZ for d1-5 of 28d cycle for 6 to 12 mos, starting at 150 mg/m² and escalated as tolerated to 200 mg/m². Major side effects of TMZ are constipation, thrombocytopenia, and neutropenia. Pts treated with TMZ require prophylaxis against pneumocystis pneumonia and can be given daily DS trimethoprim/sulfamethoxazole or alternatively, two pentamidine inhalation treatments during the RT course. TMZ is a prodrug converted to MTIC, which alkylates DNA. Only 5% to 10% of methylation events yield the O-6-methylguanine, but if the methyl group is not removed prior to cell division, the adducts are highly cytotoxic (see MGMT earlier).

Radiation

Indications: Adjuvant RT improves OS versus observation or CHT alone after surgery (see the following studies) and is indicated in all pts of sufficient functional status to tolerate treatment.

Dose: 60 Gy/30 fx is standard. For elderly or frail individuals, various hypofractionated schemes have been investigated (see the following studies). In the palliative setting, RT is superior to best supportive care in terms of OS.

Toxicity: Acute: Fatigue, headache, exacerbation of presenting neurologic deficits, alopecia, nausea, cerebral edema, side effects related to temozolomide.

Late: Cognitive changes, radiation necrosis, hypopituitarism, cataracts, vision loss (rare and location dependent).

Procedure: See *Treatment Planning Handbook*, Chapter 3.[13]

EVIDENCE-BASED Q&A

What is considered optimal surgery for glioblastoma?

Lacroix, MDACC (*J Neurosurg* 2001, PMID 11780887): RR showing improved OS with ≥98% resection in better prognostic pts (young, good KPS, no MRI evidence of necrosis). GTR also limits chance of cerebral edema during RT. **Conclusion: GTR improved OS in select pts compared with no clear benefit to STR.**

What are the contraindications to GTR?

Eloquent/inaccessible areas involved (brainstem, motor cortex, language centers, etc.), significant infiltration past midline, periventricular or diffuse lesions, medical comorbidities.

How did we arrive at the current standard RT dose?

The BTCG 69-01[12] and 1981 SGSG[14] studies demonstrated a doubling of survival with adjuvant RT over best supportive care. Dose escalation was beneficial to 60 Gy/30 fx but there was no benefit to escalating to 70 Gy. A subsequent University of Michigan experience[15] showed that escalating to 90 Gy still resulted in 90% in field failures and increase in toxicity. Thus 60 Gy/30 fx is considered the standard dose for GBM. A recent single-arm phase I study from the University of Michigan has shown promising median OS of 20.1 mos with safe dose escalation to 75 Gy/30 fx along with concurrent and adjuvant TMZ.[16] This has raised the question again about the potential benefit of dose escalation in the TMZ era and has in part led to the ongoing NRG BN001 trial.

What chemotherapies have been used after surgery?

Historically, nitrosoureas were utilized, until a meta-analysis of PRTs of RT versus RT+ nitrosoureas showed only modest 1-year OS benefit.[17] BCNU was the RTOG standard of care for many years. BCNU wafers (Gliadel®) were investigated in a phase III trial of RT +/- BCNU wafers: MS improved to 13.9 mos versus 11.8 mos[18] However, the survival advantage was possibly driven by grade III pts, and a subsequent 2007 meta-analysis suggested BCNU wafers are not effective or cost-effective for glioblastoma.[19]

What trial defines the current standard of care in GBM management?

RT + concurrent and adjuvant TMZ is the standard of care based on the Stupp trial.

Stupp, EORTC 26899/NCIC (*NEJM* 2005, PMID 15758009; *Lancet Oncology* 2009, PMID 19269895): PRT of 573 pts with GBM, ages 18 to 70 with ECOG PS 0-2. All pts received EBRT 60 Gy/30 fx, and were randomized to RT alone or chemoRT with concurrent TMZ 75 mg/m² d1-7 q1week then adjuvant TMZ 150 to 200 mg/m² d1-5 q4weeks x 6c. Eighty percent received the full course; 40% received full six cycles of adjuvant TMZ. OS and PFS were significantly improved (see Table 1.2) with the benefit holding across all subgroups and MGMT status as the strongest prognostic and predictive factor. **Conclusion: Concurrent chemoRT and adjuvant TMZ established as standard of care for GBM.**

TABLE 1.2: Stupp Trial Results, Including 2009 Update (All Differences Statistically Significant)				
	MS	**2-yr PFS**	**2-yr OS**	**5-yr OS**
RT	12.1 mos	1.8%	10.9%	1.9%
RT + TMZ	14.6 mos	11.2%	27.2%	9.8%

What is the impact of O⁶-methylguanine-DNA methyltransferase (MGMT) status on the prognosis for GBM and their response to TMZ?

MGMT silencing is both prognostic (better outcome regardless of treatment) and predictive (better response to a specific treatment—TMZ in this case) for GBM.

Hegi (*NEJM* 2005, PMID 15758010). Subset analysis of 206 GBM pts in the Stupp trial, 45% of whom had epigenetic silencing of MGMT by methylation. Regardless of TMZ use, MGMT methylation was associated with improved OS (MS 15.3 vs. 11.8 mos). Survival in methylated pts treated with RT + TMZ versus RT alone was 21.7 mos versus 15.3 mos (p = .007) and 2-yr OS was 46% versus 23%, p = .007. In nonmethylated pts, the MS difference between the groups was NS (12.7 vs. 11.8 mos); however, 2-yr OS was significant (13% vs. 2%). **Conclusion: MGMT methylation is both prognostic and predictive for response to TMZ.** *Comment: The use of TMZ in unmethylated pts is controversial; some feel the subset was underpowered and pts may still benefit.*

Is there any benefit to increasing the dose density of TMZ?

Gilbert, RTOG 0525 (*JCO* 2013, PMID 24101040): PRT of 833 pts treated 60 Gy/30 fx with daily TMZ (75 mg/m²) randomized to adjuvant Stupp regimen (150–200 mg/m² × 5 days) versus adjuvant TMZ 75–100 mg/m² × 21 days q4w × 6–12 cycles. Increasing the number of days that pts received TMZ did not improve OS or PFS, regardless of methylation status. However, the study did confirm the prognostic significance of MGMT methylation, with improved OS (21.2 vs. 14 mos, $p < .0001$). **Conclusion: MGMT methylation is prognostic, but dose-dense TMZ was not beneficial.**

Is there any role of hyperfractionation in GBM?

RTOG 8302[20] and RTOG 9006[21] examined this question and showed no benefit to hyperfractionated RT compared to standard fractionation in pts with malignant glioma.

Does a radiosurgery boost improve disease control for GBM pts?

Souhami, RTOG 9305 (*IJROP* 2004, PMID 15465203): PRT of GBM pts with KPS ≥70 and unifocal, enhancing, well-demarcated, ≤3 to 4 cm lesion randomized to RT + BCNU +/− upfront SRS (15–24 Gy, depending on size). MS was 13.5 mos in SRS arm versus 13.6 mos in standard arm. **Conclusion: There is no role for an upfront SRS boost in GBM.**

Is there a role for a brachytherapy boost in malignant gliomas?

Two PRTs were negative: (a) 50 Gy/25 fx +/− I-125 implant (60 Gy). MS 13.8 versus 13.2 mos[22]; (b) upfront ^{125}I seeds (60 Gy) + 60.2 Gy/35 fx EBRT with concurrent BCNU versus EBRT + BCNU alone. No difference in OS. In GBM subset, MS 64 weeks versus 58.1 weeks.[23] **Conclusion: There is no OS benefit to brachytherapy boost.**

What is the role of whole brain radiation therapy (WBRT) in GBM?

WBRT can be considered for multifocal disease/subependymal spread, or poor performance pts (KPS <60). Comparable outcomes (MS ~7 mos) to limited volume RT.[24,25]

What is the basis for the treatment volumes used during standard chemoRT?

After standard treatment, over 80% of recurrences occur within a 2-cm margin of the contrast-enhancing lesion seen on CT or MRI at original diagnosis.[26] Thus high-dose treatment volume typically includes a 2-cm CTV expansion of the resection cavity and any residual enhancing tumor, as used in RTOG protocols. Though peritumoral edema seen on T2 and FLAIR MRI sequences are typically targeted in the low-dose PTV, retrospective single institution reviews have suggested that there are no increased rates of local recurrence when peritumoral edema is not specifically targeted during radiation treatment.[27] In fact, EORTC protocols for GBM do not include targeting of edema volumes.[26]

Is there a benefit to the addition of bevacizumab to TMZ?

Gilbert, RTOG 0825 (*NEJM* 2014, PMID 24552317): PRT in 637 GBM pts treated with the Stupp regimen with or without bevacizumab 10 mg/kg q2 weeks x 12 cycles after RT. Pts were stratified by MGMT methylation status. Prespecified coprimary endpoints were OS and PFS. Use of bevacizumab did not improve MS (15.7 vs. 16.1 mos). Although PFS was increased with use of bevacizumab (10.7 vs. 7.3 mos, $p = .007$), this did not meet the prespecified endpoint of $p < .004$. Bevacizumab group also associated with increased hypertension, VTE events, intestinal perforation, neutropenia. **Conclusion: No improvement in OS with addition of bevacizumab to standard RT + TMZ; there was a modest PFS benefit but this did not reach predefined target for statistical significance.**

Chinot, AVAGLIO Study (*NEJM* 2014, PMID 24552318): PRT of 921 pts with GBM treated with Stupp regimen with or without biweekly bevacizumab 10 mg/kg q2 weeks. OS was not statistically improved 16.8 versus 16.7 mos (hazard ratio [HR 0.88], $p = .10$). PFS was statistically improved to 10.6 from 6.2 mos with addition of bevacizumab. However, higher grade III toxicity was observed in the bevacizumab arm 66.8% versus 51.3%.

What are tumor treating fields (TTF) and is there a benefit in GBM?

Polarization occurs in cells during the spindle formation process in mitosis. Alternating electric fields can be used to disrupt this normal polarization, thus inhibiting cell division. The FDA-approved NovoTTF-100A (Optune®) is a device that a pt wears on his or her head along with an attached portable battery pack that emits alternating electric fields. Despite the positive trial results as in the following, it is currently expensive and can also be difficult for pts, as it must be worn for most of the day.

Stupp (*JAMA* 2015, PMID 26670971): PRT of 695 pts with GBM treated with chemoRT (Stupp regimen) who were then randomized to either conventional adjuvant TMZ or TTF + TMZ. Preplanned interim analysis of 315 pts with a MFU of 38 mos demonstrated significantly improved OS (20.5 mos vs. 15.6 mos $p = .001$) and PFS (7.1 mos vs. 4.0 mos, $p = .001$) with use of TTF + TMZ. **Conclusion: When NovoTTF is added to adjuvant TMZ as part of Stupp protocol, it is associated with a 5-month OS benefit, though this is an interim**

analysis and further follow-up is needed. Based on interim analysis, further enrollment to the trial was discontinued (695 of planned 700 pts enrolled at time of termination).

Management of Elderly/Frail PTS with GBM

What is the role of RT over best supportive care?

Radiation therapy improves OS over best supportive care in elderly pts with good KPS.

Keime-Guibert, France (NEJM 2007, PMID 17429084): PRT of 81 pts ≥age 70 (all KPS ≥70) with newly diagnosed AA or GBM randomized to RT 50.4 Gy/28 fx versus best supportive care after biopsy/resection. MS was improved with RT (29.1 vs. 16.9 weeks, $p = .002$). There was no difference between the arms in terms of QOL or cognition. The trial was closed early after interim analysis demonstrated improved OS with use of RT. **Conclusion: RT plays an important role in improving OS in GBM pts even in the elderly pt population, without decline in QOL or measured cognitive function.**

Is hypofractionation comparable to standard fractionation for elderly/poor performance status GBM pts?

Multiple trials have demonstrated the efficacy of hypofractionated, shortened regimens for select pts who are not receiving systemic therapy. An important caveat is that these trials generally have not taken into account genetic markers and thus it is unknown what the durability of control is compared to standard therapy for those with favorable genetic profiles. Prospectively validated regimens include 40 Gy/15 fx, 34 Gy/10 fx, and 25 Gy/5 fx.

Roa, Canadian (JCO 2004, PMID 15051755): PRT of 100 pts ≥60 y/o randomized to 60 Gy/30 fx vs. 40 Gy/15 fx (no CHT), MS was 5.1 mos for standard versus 5.6 for shorter course RT ($p = NS$); shorter course arm required less steroid use (49% vs. 23% increased use of steroids at end of treatment for pts completing RT). 26% pts stopped long-course RT versus 10% in short-course arm. **Conclusion: In pts older than 60 who are not receiving systemic therapy, there is no difference in OS between 40 Gy/15 fx and standard fractionation.**

Roa, IAEA (JCO 2015, PMID 26392096): PRT of 98 elderly/frail pts (age ≥50 and KPS 50–70 or age ≥65 with KPS ≥50) with GBM randomized to 25 Gy/5 fx versus 40 Gy/15 fx. No CHT given. Pts receiving 25 Gy/5 fx had noninferior OS compared to those receiving 40 Gy/15 fx, and no difference in PFS or QOL. **Conclusion: Short-course RT delivered in 1 week (25 Gy/5 fx) is a treatment option for elderly and/or frail pts with newly diagnosed GBM.**

Can TMZ be substituted for RT in elderly pts?

TMZ alone is a noninferior option compared to standard RT in elderly pts and may be preferred over RT alone in pts with MGMT promoter methylation.

Wick, NOA-08 (Lancet Oncology 2012, PMID 22578793): PRT of 373 pts with AA (11%) or GBM (89%), age >65 and KPS ≥60 randomized to: (a) TMZ alone (100 mg/m² for 7 days, alternating with 7 days off, for as long as tolerated) versus (b) standard RT alone (60 Gy/30 fx). OS for pts receiving TMZ alone was noninferior to those receiving standard RT (8.6 mos vs. 9.6 mos). Pts who had MGMT promoter methylation had improved OS compared to unmethylated pts. Pts with MGMT methylation had significantly improved event-free survival with receipt of TMZ compared to RT. Pts without methylation had significantly improved event-free survival when receiving RT compared to TMZ. **Conclusion: TMZ alone is noninferior to standard RT alone in this elderly pt population. MGMT promoter methylation is an important prognostic factor and may be predictive for appropriate treatment regimen.**

Malmström, Nordic Trial (*Lancet* 2012, PMID 22877848): PRT of 342 pts with GBM and age >60 randomized to CHT alone (TMZ 200 mg/m^2 d1-5 of 28-day cycle for up to 6 cycles) versus 60 Gy/30 fx versus 34 Gy/10 fx. MS was significantly improved for pts receiving TMZ alone (8 mos) versus standard RT (6 mos) but not versus hypofractionated RT (7.5 mos). For pts >70, survival was improved in both the TMZ and hypofractionated arms compared to standard fractionation. **Conclusion: Elderly pts had a detriment in OS when receiving standard RT compared to TMZ alone. Use of TMZ alone or hypofractionated RT should be considered standard in the elderly population, especially if over age 70.**

Should TMZ be added to short-course RT?

Perry, EORTC 26062 (*NEJM* 2017, PMID 28296618): PRT of pts with age ≥60 with newly diagnosed GBM were treated with 40 Gy/15 fx and were randomized to no systemic therapy versus 3 weeks concurrent TMZ and monthly adjuvant TMZ up to 12 cycles. RT + TMZ significantly improved OS compared to RT alone (9.3 vs. 7.6 mos, p = .0001). PFS was improved as well (5.3 vs. 3.9 mos, p < .0001). OS improved in MGMT methylated (13.5 vs. 7.7 mos, p = .0001) but not statistically significant in unmethylated pts (10 vs. 7.9 mos, p = .055). **Conclusion: There is an OS benefit to the addition of TMZ to RT even for those receiving a hypofractionated regimen. Pts with MGMT methylation benefit most from RT + TMZ with a ~6-month improvement in OS.**

Recurrent/Progressive GBM

What are the options when there is disease recurrence?

Recurrence is common with 80% of recurrences within 2 cm of primary (26). Options include re-resection, +/– carmustine wafer placement, bevacizumab (side effects: bowel perforation, wound dehiscence, renal failure, DVT, GI bleed) and TTF (Tumor Treating Fields)—alternating electric fields to disrupt cancer cell division.

Is re-irradiation an option for progression?

Fokas (*Strahlenther Onkol* 2009, PMID 19370426): RR of 53 pts with recurrent GBM. Demonstrated MS of 9 mos after re-RT with median dose of 30 Gy in median dose/fx of 3 Gy; only KPS <70 predicted for poor survival. Well tolerated with no acute or late toxicity >2. **Conclusion: Hypofractionated, stereotactic RT is safe and feasible for re-irradiation of GBM.**

What is the role of pulsed reduced dose-rate re-irradiation to minimize toxicity?

The inverse dose-rate effect may allow for reassortment of tumor cells while the treatment is delivered, perhaps leading to increased tumor kill with decreased toxicity due to normal tissue repair.

Adkison, Wisconsin (*IJROBP* 2011, PMID 20472350): RR of 103 pts (86 with GBM) with pulsed reduced dose-rate re-RT. RT was delivered slowly at 0.0667 Gy/min to a median dose of 50 Gy. Four of 15 pts had significant RT necrosis on autopsy. MS for GBM pts after pulsed reduced dose-rate RT was 5.1 mos. **Conclusion: Pulsed reduced dose-rate RT appears safe in the re-irradiation setting in order to treat larger volumes to a higher dose.**

Is bevacizumab effective for recurrent GBM?

Bevacizumab is beneficial in improving PFS as a second-line therapy with or without re-irradiation; however, it is associated with a higher rate of toxicity.

Gutin (*IJROBP* 2009, PMID 19167838): Observational study investigating bevacizumab (10 mg/kg) + RT (30 Gy/5 fx, starting at second dose of bevacizumab, where GTV + 5 mm = PTV), MS was 12.5 mos with very minimal toxicity.

Wong (*JNCCN* 2011, PMID 21464145): 15 trial meta-analysis (mainly phase II data) with a total of 548 pts treated with bevacizumab at recurrence. MS was 9.3 mos 6% complete response, 49% partial response, and 29% stable disease.

Friedman, BRAIN Trial (*JCO* 2009, PMID 19720927): 167 pts with recurrent GBM were randomized to (a) bevacizumab or (b) bevacizumab + irinotecan. MS 9 mos in each arm, however significantly worse grade III toxicities with use of combination therapy.

REFERENCES

1. Ostrom QT, Gittleman H, Fulop J, et al. CBTRUS statistical report: primary brain and central nervous system tumors diagnosed in the United States in 2008–2012. *Neuro Oncol.* 2015;17(Suppl 4):iv1–iv62.
2. Thakkar JP, Dolecek TA, Horbinski C, et al. Epidemiologic and molecular prognostic review of glioblastoma. *Cancer Epidemiol Biomarkers Prev.* 2014;23(10):1985–1996.
3. Smith MA, Freidlin B, Ries LA, Simon R. Trends in reported incidence of primary malignant brain tumors in children in the United States. *J Natl Cancer Inst.* 1998;90(17):1269–1277.
4. Louis DN, Perry A, Reifenberger G, et al. The 2016 World Health Organization classification of tumors of the central nervous system: a summary. *Acta neuropathologica.* 2016;131(6):803–820.
5. Sanson M, Marie Y, Paris S, et al. Isocitrate dehydrogenase 1 codon 132 mutation is an important prognostic biomarker in gliomas. *J Clin Oncol.* 2009;27(25):4150–4154.
6. Pelloski CE, Ballman KV, Furth AF, et al. Epidermal growth factor receptor variant III status defines clinically distinct subtypes of glioblastoma. *J Clin Oncol.* 2007;25(16):2288–2294.
7. Kleinschmidt-DeMasters BK, Aisner DL, Birks DK, Foreman NK. Epithelioid GBMs show a high percentage of BRAF V600E mutation. *Am J Surg Pathol.* 2013;37(5):685–698.
8. Jiao Y, Killela PJ, Reitman ZJ, et al. Frequent ATRX, CIC, FUBP1 and IDH1 mutations refine the classification of malignant gliomas. *Oncotarget.* 2012;3(7):709–722.
9. Kannan K, Inagaki A, Silber J, et al. Whole-exome sequencing identifies ATRX mutation as a key molecular determinant in lower-grade glioma. *Oncotarget.* 2012;3(10):1194–1203.
10. Liu XY, Gerges N, Korshunov A, et al. Frequent ATRX mutations and loss of expression in adult diffuse astrocytic tumors carrying IDH1/IDH2 and TP53 mutations. *Acta Neuropathol.* 2012;124(5):615–625.
11. Li J, Wang M, Won M, et al. Validation and simplification of the Radiation Therapy Oncology Group recursive partitioning analysis classification for glioblastoma. *Int J Radiat Oncol Biol Phys.* 2011;81(3):623–630.
12. Walker MD, Alexander E, Jr., Hunt WE, et al. Evaluation of BCNU and/or radiotherapy in the treatment of anaplastic gliomas: a cooperative clinical trial. *J Neurosurg.* 1978;49(3):333–343.
13. Videtic GMM, Woody N, Vassil AD, ed. *Handbook of Treatment Planning in Radiation Oncology.* 2nd ed. New York, NY: Demos Medical; 2015.
14. Kristiansen K, Hagen S, Kollevold T, et al. Combined modality therapy of operated astrocytomas grade III and IV: confirmation of the value of postoperative irradiation and lack of potentiation of bleomycin on survival time: a prospective multicenter trial of the Scandinavian Glioblastoma Study Group. *Cancer.* 1981;47(4):649–652.
15. Chan JL, Lee SW, Fraass BA, et al. Survival and failure patterns of high-grade gliomas after three-dimensional conformal radiotherapy. *J Clin Oncol.* 2002;20(6):1635–1642.
16. Tsien CI, Brown D, Normolle D, et al. Concurrent temozolomide and dose-escalated intensity-modulated radiation therapy in newly diagnosed glioblastoma. *Clin Cancer Res.* 2012;18(1):273–279.
17. Fine HA, Dear KB, Loeffler JS, et al. Meta-analysis of radiation therapy with and without adjuvant chemotherapy for malignant gliomas in adults. *Cancer.* 1993;71(8):2585–2597.

18. Westphal M, Hilt DC, Bortey E, et al. A phase 3 trial of local chemotherapy with biodegradable carmustine (BCNU) wafers (Gliadel wafers) in patients with primary malignant glioma. *Neuro Oncol.* 2003;5(2):79–88.
19. Garside R, Pitt M, Anderson R, et al. The effectiveness and cost-effectiveness of carmustine implants and temozolomide for the treatment of newly diagnosed high-grade glioma: a systematic review and economic evaluation. *Health Technol Assess.* 2007;11(45):iii–iv, ix–221.
20. Werner-Wasik M, Scott CB, Nelson DF, et al. Final report of a phase I/II trial of hyperfractionated and accelerated hyperfractionated radiation therapy with carmustine for adults with supratentorial malignant gliomas. Radiation Therapy Oncology Group Study 83-02. *Cancer.* 1996;77(8):1535–1543.
21. Scott CB, Curran WJ, Yung WKA, et al. Long term results of RTOG 90-06: a randomized trial of hyperfractionated radiotherapy to 72.0 Gy and carmustine vs standard RT and carmustine for malignant glioma patients with emphasis on anaplastic astrocytoma (AA) patients. *Proc Am Soc Clin Oncol.* 1998;17(Abstract 1546):401a.
22. Laperriere NJ, Leung PM, McKenzie S, et al. Randomized study of brachytherapy in the initial management of patients with malignant astrocytoma. *Int J Radiat Oncol Biol Phys.* 1998;41(5):1005–1011.
23. Selker RG, Shapiro WR, Burger P, et al. The Brain Tumor Cooperative Group NIH Trial 87-01: a randomized comparison of surgery, external radiotherapy, and carmustine versus surgery, interstitial radiotherapy boost, external radiation therapy, and carmustine. *Neurosurgery.* 2002;51(2):343–355; discussion 355–347.
24. Kita M, Okawa T, Tanaka M, Ikeda M. [Radiotherapy of malignant glioma: prospective randomized clinical study of whole brain vs local irradiation]. *Gan no rinsho Japan J Cancer Clin.* 1989;35(11):1289–1294.
25. Shapiro WR, Green SB, Burger PC, et al. Randomized trial of three chemotherapy regimens and two radiotherapy regimens and two radiotherapy regimens in postoperative treatment of malignant glioma. Brain Tumor Cooperative Group Trial 8001. *J Neurosurg.* 1989;71(1):1–9.
26. Niyazi M, Brada M, Chalmers AJ, et al. ESTRO-ACROP guideline "target delineation of glioblastomas". *Radiother Onco.* 2016;118(1):35–42.
27. Chang EL, Akyurek S, Avalos T, et al. Evaluation of peritumoral edema in the delineation of radiotherapy clinical target volumes for glioblastoma. *Int J Radiat Oncol Biol Phys.* 2007;68(1):144–150.

2: ANAPLASTIC GLIOMAS

Shireen Parsai and Samuel T. Chao

QUICK HIT: Anaplastic gliomas are classified as WHO grade III gliomas and include anaplastic oligodendroglioma, anaplastic oligoastrocytoma, and anaplastic astrocytoma. Anaplastic astrocytomas are further characterized by IDH status (IDH mutant, IDH-wild-type, and NOS). The general treatment paradigm includes maximal safe surgical resection followed by adjuvant RT and CHT. The randomized trials that established a survival benefit in AG used neoadjuvant or adjuvant PCV. However, concurrent and adjuvant TMZ is given more often, as it is easier to administer and better tolerated. An improved understanding of genomics is rapidly informing the clinical behavior and treatment of a previously very heterogeneous entity.

EPIDEMIOLOGY: Grade III account for 25% of high-grade gliomas, majority are anaplastic astrocytomas.[1] Anaplastic oligodendrogliomas account for ~1.6% and anaplastic astrocytomas ~5.8% of newly diagnosed gliomas.[2] The peak incidence occurs around age 75 to 84. Oligodendrogliomas and oligoastrocytomas are most common in younger pts.[3]

RISK FACTORS: Previous ionizing radiation.[4] Genetic syndromes (<5% of gliomas) associated with gliomas include NF1 (17q, café au lait spots, Lisch nodules, neurofibroma, optic glioma, astrocytoma), NF2 (22q, bilateral acoustic neuroma, glioma, meningioma, ependymoma), tuberous sclerosis (ash-leaf macules, subependymal giant cell astrocytoma, gliomas), Li–Fraumeni syndrome, and von Hippel–Lindau (hemangioblastoma).[1]

ANATOMY: Most arise in the cerebral hemispheres. The frontal lobe is more common than parietal/temporal, which is more common than occipital. Cerebellar tumors are uncommon.[1,2]

PATHOLOGY: Histologic subtypes include anaplastic astrocytoma (AA), anaplastic oligoastrocytoma (AOA), and anaplastic oligodendroglioma (AO). WHO grading is classically based on the presence of two of the following criteria ("MEAN"): high mitotic index, endothelial proliferation, nuclear atypia, or necrosis.[5] WHO grade I: benign, none. Grade II: low grade, one feature. Grade III: anaplastic, two features. Grade IV: malignant, three to four features or necrosis.[1] Currently, WHO grading is now performed by integrating the phenotypic and genetic/mutational signatures.

GENETICS: See Chapter 1 for further discussion on IDH1 and ATRX. Allelic loss of the 1p and 19q chromosome arms ("1p19q codeletion") is signature of oligodendrogliomas. Oligodendrogliomas characterized by IDH mutation and 1p/19q-codeletion carry a relatively favorable prognosis. Mixed AOAs are uncommon in the molecular era. ATRX loss is characteristic of astrocytoma and is mutually exclusive with 1p19q codeletion.

CLINICAL PRESENTATION: Headache and seizures are the most common symptoms. Other symptoms may include memory loss, motor weakness, visual symptoms, language deficit, and cognitive and personality changes. In general, size and location dictate presenting symptoms.[1]

WORKUP: H&P with neurologic exam.

Labs: CBC, pregnancy test in young females, other basic labs prior to CHT.

Imaging: MRI with gadolinium contrast. Anaplastic gliomas are typically hypointense on T1 with heterogeneous enhancement with gadolinium (up to 1/3 may not enhance). In general, obtain a postoperative MRI within 72 hours (ideally 24–48 hours) to determine the extent of surgical resection and residual disease.[1]

Pathology: Must obtain tissue diagnosis by biopsy or surgical resection.

PROGNOSTIC FACTORS

Patient-related: Historically, an RPA by the RTOG classified pts based on factors such as age (<50 vs. ≥50), KPS (<90 vs. 90–100), mental status changes, and duration of symptoms (>3 mos better than ≤3 mos).[6-8] The most favorable RPA class (<50 y/o with anaplastic astrocytoma and normal mental status) demonstrated a MS of 58.6 mos.

Tumor-related: AO has a better prognosis compared to AA. The following molecular genetic alterations are positive prognostic factors: IDH1 mutations, 1p/19q codeletion, and MGMT promoter methylation.[1,9-11]

Treatment-related: Extent of surgical resection.[8]

NATURAL HISTORY: Anaplastic gliomas, like other gliomas, are locally aggressive and frequently cause symptoms related to local progression and edema of surrounding tissue by alterations in permeability of blood–brain barrier.[1,12]

TREATMENT PARADIGM

Surgery: Maximal safe resection with neurologic preservation is standard. See Chapter 1 for further details.

Chemotherapy: Randomized trials including RTOG 9402 and EORTC 26951 have established a survival benefit with PCV CHT. PCV: CCNU (i.e., lomustine, procarbazine, and vincristine). Recently, despite a lack of randomized data, temozolomide (TMZ) is given more commonly than PCV as per Stupp trial (see Chapter 1). TMZ is typically given 75 mg/m² daily with RT including weekends, followed by 150 to 200 mg/m² daily on days 1 to 5 q28 days with cycle one beginning 28 days post-RT for a total of six cycles.

Radiation

Indications: Adjuvant radiation improves overall survival compared to observation or CHT alone after surgery and is indicated for all high-grade gliomas.

Dose: The most common dose is 59.4 Gy/28 fx as per trials in the following.

Toxicity: Common acute side effects include fatigue, headache, alopecia, skin erythema, nausea, memory loss, cerebral edema. Late effects are dependent on tumor location but may include radiation necrosis, memory/cognitive changes, hearing loss, optic neuritis, cataracts, hypopituitarism.

Procedure: See *Treatment Planning Handbook*, Chapter 3.[13]

EVIDENCE-BASED Q&A

What is the role of RT in the management of anaplastic gliomas?

The role of RT was initially established in the 1970s and 1980s due to a demonstrable survival benefit.

Walker (*J Neurosurg* 1978, PMID 355604): Randomized 303 pts with anaplastic gliomas to one of four arms: (a) best supportive care, (b) BCNU alone, (c) RT alone, (d) RT + BCNU. RT was delivered as 50 to 60 Gy whole brain. MS was 14 weeks, 18.5 weeks, 35 weeks, and 34.5 weeks respectively.

What is the role of CHT in addition to RT?

Two landmark studies from RTOG and EORTC established the utility of adding CHT (PCV) to RT in anaplastic gliomas. Subsequent subset analyses have shed light on the importance of molecular markers.

Cairncross, RTOG 9402 (*JCO* 2006, PMID 16782910; Update Cairncross *JCO* 2013, PMID 23071247; Subset Cairncross *JCO* 2014, PMID 24516018): PRT of 291 pts newly diagnosed with AO/AOA randomized after surgery to (a) four cycles PCV *prior* to RT versus (b) RT alone. PCV was administered before RT every 6 weeks. RT started within 6 weeks of completion of CHT. A dose of 59.4 Gy/33 fx was given: 50.4 Gy/28 fx to the resection cavity and any T2 abnormality+2 cm then a 9 Gy/5 fx boost to the resection cavity and any T1 postcontrast enhancement plus 1 cm. Seventy-nine percent of "RT alone" pts eventually received CHT (PCV or TMZ); only 46% of PCV + RT pts received all four cycles of CHT. Original analysis in 2006 did not demonstrate a survival benefit with chemoRT as compared to RT alone for the entire cohort (4.7 years vs. 4.6 years respectively). However, on subset analysis in 2014, pts with IDH-mutated tumors lived longer after chemoRT as compared to RT alone. Also within the IDH-mutated subgroup, pts with 1p/19q codeletion lived the longest. For pts with IDH-wild-type, chemoRT did not increase survival compared to RT alone.

TABLE 2.1: Results of Cairncross RTOG 9402, 2014 Subset Analysis

	RT + PCV (MS, years)	RT alone (MS, years)	*p* value
All pts	4.6	4.7	NS
IDH-mutated, 1p19q codeleted	14.7	6.8	.01
IDH-mutated, 1p19q intact	5.5	3.3	.045
IDH-wild-type	1.8	1.3	NS

van den Bent, EORTC 26951 (*JCO* 2006, PMID 16782911; update Van de Bent *JCO* 2013, PMID 23071237): PRT of 368 pts newly diagnosed with AO/AOA randomized after surgery to (a) RT followed by PCV x6 cycles versus (b) RT alone. Pts received RT within 6 weeks of surgery. A dose of 59.4 Gy/33 fx was given: 45 Gy followed by 14.4 Gy boost. Six cycles of PCV were started within 1 month of completing RT and administered every 6 weeks. Thirty-eight percent of PCV pts discontinued CHT prematurely; 82% of RT alone pts received CHT (PCV > TMZ + others) at recurrence; 55% of RT + PCV pts received salvage CHT (TMZ > PCV + others). On post hoc path review, 1/3 of pts were found to have GBM. MFU 140 mos. OS significantly improved among the entire group with PCV: 42.3 versus 30.6 mos. Significant improvements in PFS noted in both 1p/19q codeleted (157 vs. 50 mos) and 1p/19q intact (15 vs. 9 mos). No long-term difference in QOL reported after PCV. IDH mutation and 1p/19q codeletion were independently significant on multivariate prognostic model. MGMT methylation status was not an independent prognostic factor of survival.

TABLE 2.2: 2013 Results of EORTC 26951 for Anaplastic Gliomas

	RT + PCV (MS, mos)	RT Alone (MS, mos)	*p* value
All pts	42.3	30.6	.018

(continued)

TABLE 2.2: 2013 Results of EORTC 26951 for Anaplastic Gliomas (*continued*)			
	RT + PCV (MS, mos)	RT Alone (MS, mos)	*p* value
1p19q codeleted	Not reached	112 mos	.059
1p19q intact	25	21	.185

What is the role of temozolomide (TMZ) for anaplastic gliomas?

Despite the survival advantage demonstrated with PCV in pts with AOs and AOAs, many substitute TMZ as it is easier to administer and generally better tolerated. RTOG 0131, NOA-04 and the early results of CATNON all suggest this is a reasonable substitution.

Vogelbaum, RTOG 0131 (*J Neuroncol* 2015, PMID 26088460): Phase II, single-arm trial including 48 pts undergoing TMZ x6 cycles followed by concurrent RT + TMZ (if disease progression seen on CT/MRI scans every 8 weeks while on pre-RT TMZ). RT 59.4 Gy/33 fx. MFU 8.7 years, median PFS 5.8 years, MS not reached. 1p/19q status available in 37 cases. OS and PFS not reached for codeleted pts. 4 pts (10%) achieved complete response. **Conclusion: Pre-RT TMZ followed by concurrent RT and TMZ is indirectly comparable to PCV followed by RT.**

Wick, NOA-04 (*JCO* 2009, PMID 19901110; Update Wick *Neuro Oncol* 2016, PMID 27370396): PRT of 318 pts with anaplastic glioma randomly assigned 2:1:1 (A:B1:B2) to receive (A) RT 54 to 60 Gy RT; (B1) PCV or (B2) TMZ. In Arm A, pts received CHT after progression and in arms B1 or B2, pts received RT after progression. The primary endpoint was time to treatment failure (TTF) defined as progression after RT and one CHT in either sequence. The initial results reported in 2009 did not identify any difference in TTF, PFS, or OS between primary CHT compared to RT. This was confirmed again in 2016 with report of long-term results. The study also identified IDH1 mutation as a positive prognostic factor with a stronger impact as compared to 1p/19q codeletion or MGMT methylation.

van den Bent, EORTC CATNON (*Lancet* 2017, PMID 28801186): PRT of 748 pts with newly diagnosed anaplastic glioma with *1p/19q intact*, 2x2 factorial design, randomized after surgery to (a) RT alone (CHT at progression) (b) RT and concurrent TMZ (c) RT and adjuvant TMZ (d) RT with concurrent and adjuvant TMZ. Adjuvant TMZ for 12 mos per Stupp regimen. RT is 59.4 Gy/33 fx. Stratified based on MGMT methylation and performance status. Interim analysis with MFU 27 mos. HR reduction for OS of 0.65 (99% CI 0.45–0.93) after adjuvant TMZ (5-yr OS 56% vs. 44%). MGMT prognostic of OS but not predictive of response to TMZ. **Conclusion: Adjuvant TMZ improved OS for 1p19q intact anaplastic gliomas. Further follow-up required to assess concurrent TMZ.**

What is the management of anaplastic astrocytomas (AAs)?

Though often categorized with AOs and AOAs, it is important to note that AAs were not enrolled on either RTOG 9402 or EORTC 26951. Instead, the standard of care of chemoRT is derived from historic malignant glioma trials, of which AAs constituted a minority of pts. They also made up a small minority of the pts on the Stupp trial (see Chapter 1), from which the modern treatment paradigm is generally extrapolated. The only modern prospective randomized evidence in AAs comes from RTOG 9813.

Chang, RTOG 9813 (*Neuro Oncol* 2017, PMID 27994066): PRT of 196 pts with AA or AOA (<25% oligo component) and KPS ≥60 was randomized to RT with concurrent and adjuvant TMZ versus RT and nitrosourea (either BCNU or CCNU). RT was 59.4 cGy/ 33 fx. No difference in survival between arms (3.9 vs. 3.8 years, *p* = .36). The RT + NU arm had a significantly higher rate of worse overall grade ≥3 toxicity (75.8% vs. 47.9%, *p* < .001). **Conclusion: RT + TMZ was not beneficial compared to RT + nitrosourea but was better tolerated.**

REFERENCES

1. Halperin EC, Wazer DE, Perez CA, Brady LW. *Perez and Brady's Principles and Practice of Radiation Oncology.* 6th ed. Philadelphia, PA: Lipincott Williams; 2013.
2. Ostrom QT, Gittleman H, Fulop J, et al. CBTRUS statistical report: primary brain and central nervous system tumors diagnosed in the United States in 2008–2012. *Neuro-oncol.* 2015;17 (Suppl 4):iv1–iv62.
3. Morgan LL. The epidemiology of glioma in adults: a "state of the science" review. *Neuro-oncol.* 2015;17(4):623–624.
4. Braganza MZ, Kitahara CM, Berrington de Gonzalez A, et al. Ionizing radiation and the risk of brain and central nervous system tumors: a systematic review. *Neuro-oncol.* 2012;14(11):1316–1324.
5. Marquet G, Dameron O, Saikali S, et al. Grading glioma tumors using OWL-DL and NCI Thesaurus. *AMIA Annu Symp Proc.* 2007:508–512.
6. Lamborn KR, Chang SM, Prados MD. Prognostic factors for survival of pts with glioblastoma: recursive partitioning analysis. *Neuro-oncol.* 2004;6(3):227–235.
7. Curran WJ, Jr, Scott CB, Horton J, et al. Recursive partitioning analysis of prognostic factors in three Radiation Therapy Oncology Group malignant glioma trials. *J Natl Cancer Inst.* 1993;85(9):704–710.
8. Gorlia T, Delattre JY, Brandes AA, et al. New clinical, pathological and molecular prognostic models and calculators in pts with locally diagnosed anaplastic oligodendroglioma or oligoastrocytoma: a prognostic factor analysis of European Organisation for Research and Treatment of Cancer Brain Tumour Group Study 26951. *Europ J Cancer.* 2013;49(16):3477–3485.
9. Wick W, Hartmann C, Engel C, et al. NOA-04 randomized phase III trial of sequential radiochemotherapy of anaplastic glioma with procarbazine, lomustine, and vincristine or temozolomide. *J Clin Oncol.* 2009;27(35):5874–5880.
10. van den Bent MJ, Carpentier AF, Brandes AA, et al. Adjuvant procarbazine, lomustine, and vincristine improves progression-free survival but not overall survival in newly diagnosed anaplastic oligodendrogliomas and oligoastrocytomas: a randomized European Organisation for Research and Treatment of Cancer phase III trial. *J Clin Oncol.* 2006;24(18):2715–2722.
11. Cairncross JG, Wang M, Jenkins RB, et al. Benefit from procarbazine, lomustine, and vincristine in oligodendroglial tumors is associated with mutation of IDH. *J Clin Oncol.* 2014;32(8):783–790.
12. Gramatzki D, Dehler S, Rushing EJ, et al. Glioblastoma in the Canton of Zurich, Switzerland revisited: 2005 to 2009. *Cancer.* 2016;122(14):2206–2215.
13. Videtic G, Woody, N. *Handbook of Treatment Planning in Radiation Oncology.* 2nd ed. New York, NY: Demos Medical Publishing, LLC; 2015:30–32.

3: LOW GRADE GLIOMA

Martin C. Tom and Erin S. Murphy

QUICK HIT: Low grade gliomas (LGGs) are an uncommon and heterogeneous group of primary brain tumors which present primarily in younger adults, but can also be seen in pediatric pts. Recent publications analyzing molecular and genomic factors have provided a window into prognostic stratification. Mutation in the enzyme IDH has emerged as the most informative genomic change. Despite this prognostic information, treatment paradigms remain based on clinical factors and require patient-specific decision making given the diversity of these tumors. Following surgical resection, options can include observation, RT, CHT or combined chemoRT. RT dose is typically 50.4–54 Gy. CHT often consists of either oral temozolomide or PCV (procarbazine, lomustine/CCNU, and vincristine).

TABLE 3.1: General Treatment Paradigm for Low-Grade Gliomas Based on Clinical Factors in the Pre-Genomics Era

Maximal Safe Resection	GTR	Low risk (<40 years old as per RTOG or without Pignatti risk factors as per EORTC)	Observation, CHT or chemoRT
		High Risk (≥40 years old as per RTOG or with Pignatti risk factors as per EORTC)	ChemoRT
	STR or biopsy		ChemoRT

EPIDEMIOLOGY: An estimated 64,808 new cases of primary neuroepithelial tumors are expected in the United States annually, and approximately 15% will be grade I-II tumors, 60% will be grade IV.[1] Approximately 2,600 cases are WHO grade II diffuse astrocytoma.[1,2]

RISK FACTORS: Ionizing radiation and genetic syndromes including NF-1 (17q, café au lait spots, Lisch nodules, neurofibromas, optic gliomas, & astrocytomas), NF-2 (22q, bilateral acoustic neuromas, meningiomas, ependymomas, gliomas), Tuberous sclerosis (ash-leaf macules, hamartomas, angiofibromas, periungual fibromas, subependymal giant cell astrocytoma, gliomas) or Li-Fraumeni syndrome (TP53 mutation, gliomas, sarcomas, breast cancer, leukemia, adrenocortical carcinomas).

ANATOMY: Typically LGGs arise from the supratentorial cortex. Brainstem gliomas and optic pathway gliomas, when biopsied, are often classified as low grade but are covered elsewhere.

PATHOLOGY: Gliomas represent a group of tumors with characteristics of neuroglial cells (astrocytes or oligodendrocytes). LGG represent a heterogeneous group of WHO grade I (non-infiltrative) and grade II (infiltrative/diffuse) glial neoplasms.

WHO grading: Grading is based on the presence of the following histologic features: mitoses, endothelial proliferation, nuclear atypia, and necrosis ("MEAN" mnemonic).

2016 WHO CNS classification update[3]**:** In addition to histology, the new classification includes molecular markers to better define CNS tumors (see Figure 3.1).

Oligodendroglioma, IDH-mutant and 1p19q codeleted: Median OS >10 years.[6] Favorable prognosis and response to CHT. Characterized by 1p19q codeletion. Histology shows perinuclear halos, "fried egg" with branching "chicken wire" vasculature and calcification.

Diffuse astrocytoma, IDH-mutant: Median OS typically >10 years,[4] characterized by IDH-mutation with ATRX loss, TP53 mutation, 1p19q intact.

Diffuse astrocytoma, IDH-wildtype: Median OS ~5 years,[6] less common, may act similar to WHO grade III anaplastic astrocytoma IDH-WT.[7]

Gemistocytic astrocytoma, IDH-mutant: Median OS typically <4 years,[5] high risk for malignant transformation and treated as WHO grade III glioma. Histology shows large, densely packed gemistocytes.

If molecular testing unavailable:

Diffuse astrocytoma NOS: Median OS 4-5 yrs[1]

Oligodendroglioma NOS: Historically median OS >10 yrs.[1] Of note, oligodendroglioma IDH-wildtype falls into this category (see Figure 3.1).

Oligoastrocytoma NOS: Median OS <7 yrs,[5] characteristics of both oligodendroglioma and astrocytoma, worse prognosis than pure oligodendroglioma. Can now typically be classified as oligodendroglioma or astrocytoma based on molecular markers.

Grade I tumors

Pilocytic astrocytoma: Slow growing, often cystic tumor in children and young adults demonstrating Rosenthal fibers. Enhances on MRI due to degenerative hyalinization of blood vessels. Malignant transformation rare. Common location posterior fossa.

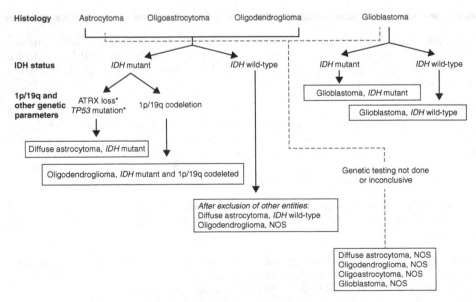

FIGURE 3.1: WHO 2016 Glioma classification.
*, characteristic but not required for diagnosis.
Source: From Ref. (3). Used with permission.

Pleomorphic xanthoastrocytoma: Large, peripheral tumor frequently with leptomeningeal involvement. Often benign despite aggressive histologic appearance.

Subependymal giant cell astrocytoma: Well-defined tumor typically along lateral ventricles.

Ganglioglioma: Composed of both neoplastic neurons and astrocytes, commonly in temporal lobe, indolent course.

Genetics

IDH1 and IDH2 mutations: Present in majority of WHO grade II gliomas, favorable prognosis compared to IDH-wildtype.[8]

1p19q codeletion: Defining feature of oligodendroglioma, favorable prognosis.[8]

TP53 mutation and/or ATRX mutation: Characteristic of IDH-mutated astrocytomas, ATRX mutation is mutually exclusive from 1p19q codeletion,[9] less favorable prognosis than 1p19q codeletion.

TERT promoter mutation: Among IDH-wild type LGG it confers a poor prognosis.[10]

MGMT methylation: Role in LGG is unclear, but has been associated with improved postrecurrence survival in presence of TMZ.[11,12]

BRAF: Mutations present in ganglioglioma, pilocytic astrocytoma, and pleomorphic xanthoastrocytoma.[13]

One analysis from the Cancer Genome Atlas ordered genomic alterations from most to least favorable: IDH-mutated and 1p19q codeleted > IDH-mutated and 1p19q intact > IDH-wildtype.[8] Another analysis from the Mayo Clinic, UCSF and MSKCC grouped from best to worst prognosis: TERT and IDH-mutation > TERT and IDH-mutation and 1p19q codeletion > IDH-mutation only > no mutations (triple-negative) > TERT only mutation.[10]

CLINICAL PRESENTATION: Depends upon location, but most commonly presents as a transient neurologic disturbance or seizure (seizure in >80% of LGG compared to 70% and 50% in anaplastic and GBM, respectively[2]). Most commonly nonenhancing hemispheric lesion (~20% do enhance[14]), rarely mass effect. Best seen on T2 MRI (hypointense on T1, nonenhancing with gadolinium). Calcifications may be present, most commonly in oligodendrogliomas, and may be more common with 1p19q codeletion.[15] Of note, pilocytic astrocytomas enhance via a different mechanism than anaplastic astrocytomas and GBM (degenerative hyalinization of blood vessels).

WORKUP: H&P, neurologic exam, neurocognitive testing, EEG if seizures. MRI with and without contrast. Functional MRI if in critical region. Establish preoperative neurocognitive baseline through testing if possible. Obtain tissue via a maximal safe resection, with biopsy-only if a resection is not possible. In general, obtain a postoperative MRI within 72 hours of surgery (ideally 24–48 hours) to determine the extent of surgical resection/residual disease and avoid confounding by blood products.

PROGNOSTIC FACTORS: There is no agreed upon definition of low-risk and high-risk pts. Various cooperative groups have defined risk factors differently. Pignatti combined EORTC trials and established five poor prognostic factors: age ≥40, astrocytoma histology, tumors ≥6 cm, tumor crossing midline, and preoperative neurologic deficits.[16] RTOG 9802 stratified pts based on age and resection status, with those <40 achieving a GTR composing the low-risk group. Seizure at presentation is a positive prognostic factor.[17] Another combined EORTC/RTOG/NCCTG analysis by Gorlia identified four externally-validated factors: neurologic deficit at presentation, <30 weeks since first symptoms, astrocyte histology, and tumor >5 cm.[18] Note that age was not prognostic in this analysis. Molecular markers have been found to be important predictors of outcome (see section on Genetics).

NATURAL HISTORY: Varies widely depending on histology, prognostic factors and molecular markers. However, most pts eventually deteriorate from tumor recurrence (typically occurring at the original site). At recurrence, up to 70% of tumors have undergone malignant transformation (i.e., WHO grade III/IV).[19]

TREATMENT PARADIGM: In general, most pts are recommended maximal safe resection followed by postoperative MRI to evaluate extent of resection. Low-risk pts may be observed, whereas high-risk pts are typically recommended adjuvant chemoRT. There is no consensus definition for low or high risk, but generally low-risk pts are <40 who achieve GTR (per RTOG 9802) or have fewer Pignatti risk factors (see section on Prognostic Factors). Current trials are also stratifying based on molecular markers (i.e., IDH mutation and 1p19q codeletion).

Surgery: Surgery is generally required to establish a diagnosis and debulk the tumor for those with extensive neurologic symptoms. There are no trials directly assessing extent of resection in LGG; however, degree of resection is a strong prognostic factor.[20] The low-risk arm from RTOG 9802 showed significant correlation between amount of residual tumor on imaging and recurrence.[21]

Observation: Following surgery, observation is an option for low-risk pts. This was supported by the "Non-Believers Trial" (as discussed in the following) and the phase II portion of RTOG 9802 which defined low-risk as those <40 years old achieving a GTR. However, close follow-up is crucial as RTOG 9802 showed a greater than 50% risk of progression at 5 years in low-risk pts undergoing adjuvant observation. RTOG 0925 will hopefully provide more insight on the role of observation for low-risk pts.

Chemotherapy: The use of adjuvant CHT (and chemoRT) in LGG continues to evolve. Pts with high-risk features may be chosen for immediate postop therapy. RTOG 9802 (phase III) investigated adjuvant RT followed by six cycles of PCV, whereas RTOG 0424 (phase II) evaluated RT with concurrent and adjuvant TMZ for 12 mos. Both regimens have activity in LGG, but level I evidence (RTOG 9802) exists only for PCV. However, many institutions favor TMZ over PCV given better tolerance and ease of administration. EORTC 22033-26033 showed no difference in PFS if treated with dose dense TMZ alone versus RT alone, however further data maturation is necessary.

Radiation

Indications: High-risk pts should undergo adjuvant chemoRT. RTOG 9802 established adjuvant chemoRT as the standard of care for high-risk pts (defined as age ≥40 or <40 years old following STR).

Dose: Doses of 45 to 54 Gy are acceptable.[22] The European trial E3F05 used 50.4 Gy/28 fx, whereas both RTOG 9802 and RTOG 0424 used 54 Gy/30 fx.

Toxicity: Acute: Fatigue, headache, exacerbation of presenting neurologic deficits, alopecia, nausea, cerebral edema, side-effects related to chemotherapy. Late: Cognitive changes, radiation necrosis, hypopituitarism, cataracts, vision loss (rare and location dependent).

EVIDENCE-BASED Q&A

Does early surgical resection improve outcomes compared to watchful waiting?

Retrospective studies favor upfront maximal safe resection, however no prospective trials are available to answer this question.

Jakola, Norwegian University Hospitals (*JAMA* 2012, PMID 23099483): Population-based study of surgical resection (and extent) compared to observation. Chosen based on patient's residential address. In hospital A, pts were biopsied and observed (50% ultimately underwent resection) but in hospital B an early resection was performed. MFU was 7 years. OS was significantly better with early surgical resection (5-yr OS 60% vs. 74%, $p = .01$) favoring early resection. Fewer pts achieved resection if delayed (89% vs. 59%). **Conclusion: Early resection is warranted if safe and feasible.**

Is it safe to observe pts after surgery and save RT for progression?

Yes, but the ideal population to observe is unclear in the genomic era and routine observation is associated with reduced PFS and increased seizure rates.

van den Bent, EORTC 22845 "Non-Believers Trial" (*Lancet* 2005, PMID 16168780): PRT of 311 pts (WHO PS 0-2) with LGG after surgery randomized to immediate RT (54 Gy/30 fx) versus observation with RT at progression. Included astrocytoma (50%), oligodendroglioma (13%), mixed (13%) and incompletely resected pilocytic astrocytomas (1%). Greater than 90% resection in 42%, 50% to 89% resection in 20%, <50% resection or biopsy in 38%. Sixty-five percent of pts in observation arm eventually received RT. Survival after first recurrence was better in pts who were observed up front (3.4 vs. 1 yr), likely due to RT salvage. Malignant transformation 70%, equal between arms. **Conclusion: Immediate (vs. delayed) RT improved PFS and decreased seizure rate, but did not improve OS.**

TABLE 3.2: Results of EORTC "Non-Believers Trial"					
	MS	5-yr OS	Med PFS	5-yr PFS	Seizures at 1 yr
Observation	7.4 yrs	65.7%	3.4 yrs	34.6%	41%
Post-op 54 Gy/30 fx	7.2 yrs	68.7%	5.3 yrs	55.0%	25%
p value	.872		<.0001		.0329

Shaw, RTOG 9802 Phase II (*J Neurosurg* 2008, PMID 18976072): Phase II portion of RTOG 9802. Postsurgery, observed 111 pts <40 y/o who achieved GTR and reported 5-yr OS of 93% and 5-yr PFS of 48%. GTR was determined by neurosurgeon at time of surgery. Review of postop MRI revealed that 59% of pts had <1 cm residual disease (26% recurrence), 32% had 1 to 2 cm residual disease (68% recurrence), 9% had >2 cm residual disease (89% recurrence). Poor prognostic factors included large tumor size (≥4 cm), astrocytoma or mixed oligoastrocytoma histology and residual disease ≥1 cm by MRI. **Conclusion: LGG in pts <40 years old following GTR have >50% risk of progression at 5 years and should be closely followed with consideration of adjuvant treatment.**

Does RT dose-escalation improve outcomes?

Despite early retrospective data supporting a benefit, two trials have failed to confirm a role for dose-escalation.[23]

Karim, EORTC 22844 "Believers Trial" (*IJROBP* 1996, PMID 8948338): PRT of 379 pts with supratentorial low-grade astrocytomas, oligodendrogliomas, and mixed oligoastrocyatoma, ages 16 to 65, KPS ≥60, randomized to 45 Gy/25 fx versus 59.4 Gy/33 fx after surgery (any degree of resection). Radiation necrosis risk 2.5% vs. 4% at 2 yrs. **Conclusion: No difference in 5-yr OS (59% vs. 58%) or PFS (50% vs. 47%) with dose escalation.**

Shaw, RTOG 9110 (*JCO* 2002, PMID 11980997): PRT of 203 pts with supratentorial grade 1 to 2 astrocytoma, oligodendroglioma, or mixed oligoastrocytoma randomized to 50.4 Gy/28 fx versus 64.8 Gy/36 fx, following surgery (any degree of resection). **Conclusion: No difference in 5-yr OS (64% vs. 72%) with higher rate of severe radiation necrosis seen with high dose arm (5% vs. 2%). Ninety-two percent of failures were in-field.**

How do tumor progression and RT affect cognition?

One reason to delay RT is to avoid the initial neurocognitive effects of treatment, but this is associated with reduced PFS ("Non-Believers Trial" previously mentioned) which may also affect cognition. Analysis of RTOG 9110 showed stable MMSE scores for most pts, and improvement in MMSE for those with lower baseline scores.[24] Analysis of RTOG 9802 showed improved MMSE scores with the addition of CHT.[25] However, MMSE may not be as reliable in evaluating neurocognitive function as more formal testing. A more extensive analysis of 20 pts in RTOG 9110 used formal cognitive testing and showed stable neurocognitive function up to 5 years out from RT.[26] RT dose-escalation may worsen QOL as analysis of the "Believers Trial" showed that pts who received dose-escalation reported worse QOL than conventional RT doses.[27]

Does adjuvant chemoRT improve outcomes compared to adjuvant RT alone?

The addition of PCV to RT nearly doubles survival in high-risk pts.

Shaw, RTOG 9802 Phase III (*JCO* 2012, PMID 22851558; Update Buckner *NEJM* 2016, PMID 27050206): Phase III component of the Phase II/III trial which randomized 251 unfavorable risk pts (age >40 or <40 y/o achieving only STR) with LGG (WHO grade II astrocytoma, oligodendroglioma, and mixed oligoastrocytoma in 26%, 42% and 32%) to RT alone versus RT followed by six cycles of PCV. RT dose was 54 Gy/30 fx to the T2 MRI signal + 2-cm block margin. The addition of PCV improved OS versus RT alone (13.3 vs. 7.8 yrs, HR 0.59, $p = .003$). Favorable prognostic variables for both OS and PFS included receipt of PCV and oligodendroglioma histology. Exploratory analysis of pts with IDH1-mutation demonstrated significantly longer OS (13.1 vs. 5.1 yrs). Power insufficient to investigate IDH1-wildtype. PCV grade 3-4 toxicity 67%. **Conclusion: The addition of PCV to RT almost doubles OS in high-risk pts.**

TABLE 3.3: Final Results of RTOG 9802 Phase III Component				
	MS	10-yr OS	Med PFS	10-yr PFS
RT alone	7.8 yr	41%	4 yr	21%
RT followed by PCV	13.3 yr	62%	10.4 yr	51%
p-value	.003		<.001	

Is treatment with temozolomide similar to PCV?

Level I data supports the addition of PCV to RT, which improves OS compared to adjuvant RT alone. However, PCV is toxic and more difficult to administer than TMZ. Many therefore give TMZ, extrapolating from high-grade glioma data. This question is being addressed in the ongoing CODEL study, a phase III trial randomizing pts with 1p19q codeletion (either LGG or AG) to adjuvant RT followed by PCV versus RT+TMZ followed by TMZ.

Fisher, RTOG 0424 (*IJROBP* 2015, PMID 25680596): Single-arm phase II of high-risk LGG (WHO grade II astrocytomas, oligodendrogliomas, and mixed oligoastrocytoma) treated with RT (54 Gy/30 fx) with concurrent daily TMZ followed by 12 cycles of monthly TMZ. Pts must have three or more of the following risk factors: age ≥40, tumor ≥6 cm, tumor crossing midline, preoperative NFS >1, astrocytoma histology. 129 pts eligible. 3-yr OS was 73.1% comparing favorably to historical rate of 54% ($p < .001$) and higher than hypothesized rate of 65%. 3-yr PFS 59% and grade 3/4 toxicity in 43%/10%. **Conclusion: Early results with TMZ are favorable, but equivalency of TMZ and PCV remains unknown.**

Are there subsets of pts who can be treated initially with CHT alone?

Given the long and variable natural history of LGG and relatively younger patient population, studies have evaluated whether RT can be deferred to avoid toxicity. EORTC 22033-26033 compared high-risk LGG treated with RT alone versus dose dense TMZ alone and found no difference in PFS, HR-QOL, or impaired cognitive dysfunction. It is important to note that the median PFS of 39 months (TMZ alone) and 46 months (RT alone) in the EORTC study was far less than the median PFS of 10.4 years (RT+PCV) in RTOG 9802.

Baumert, EORTC 22033-26033 (*Lancet Oncol* 2016, PMID 27686946): PRT of 477 pts with LGG, age ≥18, ≥1 high-risk feature (age >40, size >5 cm, progressive disease, tumor crossing midline, neurologic symptoms) randomized to RT alone (50.4 Gy/28 fx) versus dose-dense TMZ alone (75 mg/m^2 days 1–21 of a 28-day cycle, max 12 cycles). Stratified by 1p deletion, contrast enhancement, age ≥40, ECOG ≥1. Primary endpoint PFS. MFU 48 mos, mPFS 46 mos for RT alone versus 39 mos for TMZ alone ($p = .22$). OS not reached. Exploratory analysis showed IDH mutation/1p19q non-codeleted had longer PFS if treated with RT alone versus TMZ alone ($p = .0043$), but no difference for IDH mutated/1p19q codeleted or IDH wildtype. Grade 3 to 4 hematologic toxicity <1% RT versus 14% TMZ, moderate/severe fatigue 3% RT versus 7% TMZ, grade 3 to 4 infections 1% RT versus 3% TMZ. **Conclusion: No significant difference in PFS for LGG treated with RT alone versus TMZ alone. Awaiting OS endpoint and further data maturation for molecular subtypes.**

Reijneveld, EORTC 22033-26033 Health Related-QOL (*Lancet Oncol* 2016, PMID 27686943): HR QOL and global cognitive functioning evaluated in the above study (LGG treated with RT alone vs. TMZ alone) using EORTC questionnaire and MMSE. No difference in HR-QOL at 36 mos between RT alone versus TMZ alone ($p = .98$). No difference in impaired cognitive function at baseline (13% in RT vs. 14% TMZ) or at 36 mos after treatment (8% in RT vs. 6% TMZ). **Conclusion: HR QOL and global cognitive function (by MMSE) did not differ in LGG pts treated with RT alone versus TMZ alone.**

REFERENCES

1.   Ostrom QT, Gittleman H, Fulop J, et al. CBTRUS statistical report: primary brain and central nervous system tumors diagnosed in the United States in 2008–2012. *Neuro Oncol.* 2015;17(Suppl 4):iv1–iv62.
2.   Gunderson LL, Tepper JE. *Clinical Radiation Oncology, 4e.* Amsterdam, Netherlands: Elsevier; 2015.
3.   Louis DN, Perry A, Reifenberger G, et al. The 2016 World Health Organization Classification of Tumors of the Central Nervous System: a summary. *Acta Neuropathol.* 2016;131(6):803–820.
4.   Reuss DE, Mamatjan Y, Schrimpf D, et al. IDH mutant diffuse and anaplastic astrocytomas have similar age at presentation and little difference in survival: a grading problem for WHO. *Acta Neuropathol.* 2015;129(6):867–873.
5.   Okamoto Y, Di Patre PL, Burkhard C, et al. Population-based study on incidence, survival rates, and genetic alterations of low-grade diffuse astrocytomas and oligodendrogliomas. *Acta Neuropathol.* 2004;108(1):49–56.
6.   Buckner JC, Shaw EG, Pugh SL, et al. Radiation plus procarbazine, CCNU, and vincristine in low-grade glioma. *N Engl J Med.* 2016;374(14):1344–1355.
7.   Olar A, Wani KM, Alfaro-Munoz KD, et al. IDH mutation status and role of WHO grade and mitotic index in overall survival in grade II-III diffuse gliomas. *Acta Neuropathol.* 2015;129(4):585–596.
8.   Brat DJ, Verhaak RG, Aldape KD, et al. Comprehensive, integrative genomic analysis of diffuse lower-grade gliomas. *N Engl J Med.* 2015;372(26):2481–2498.
9.   Reuss DE, Sahm F, Schrimpf D, et al. ATRX and IDH1-R132H immunohistochemistry with subsequent copy number analysis and IDH sequencing as a basis for an "integrated" diagnostic approach for adult astrocytoma, oligodendroglioma and glioblastoma. *Acta Neuropathol.* 2015;129(1):133–146.

10. Eckel-Passow JE, Lachance DH, Molinaro AM, et al. Glioma groups based on 1p/19q, IDH, and TERT promoter mutations in tumors. *N Engl J Med*. 2015;372(26):2499–2508.

11. Thon N, Eigenbrod S, Kreth S, et al. IDH1 mutations in grade II astrocytomas are associated with unfavorable progression-free survival and prolonged postrecurrence survival. *Cancer*. 2012;118(2):452–460.

12. Watanabe T, Katayama Y, Yoshino A, et al. Aberrant hypermethylation of p14ARF and O6-methylguanine-DNA methyltransferase genes in astrocytoma progression. *Brain Pathol*. 2007;17(1):5–10.

13. Olar A, Sulman EP. Molecular markers in low-grade glioma-toward tumor reclassification. *Semin Radiat Oncol*. 2015;25(3):155–163.

14. Lote K, Egeland T, Hager B, et al. Prognostic significance of CT contrast enhancement within histological subgroups of intracranial glioma. *J Neurooncol*. 1998;40(2):161–170.

15. Jenkinson MD, du Plessis DG, Smith TS, et al. Histological growth patterns and genotype in oligodendroglial tumours: correlation with MRI features. *Brain*. 2006;129(Pt 7):1884–1891.

16. Pignatti F, van den Bent M, Curran D, et al. Prognostic factors for survival in adult pts with cerebral low-grade glioma. *J Clin Oncol*. 2002;20(8):2076–2084.

17. Reichenthal E, Feldman Z, Cohen ML, et al. Hemispheric supratentorial low-grade astrocytoma. *Neurochirurgia (Stuttg)*. 1992;35(1):18–22.

18. Gorlia T, Wu W, Wang M, et al. New validated prognostic models and prognostic calculators in pts with low-grade gliomas diagnosed by central pathology review: a pooled analysis of EORTC/RTOG/NCCTG phase III clinical trials. *Neuro Oncol*. 2013;15(11):1568–1579.

19. van den Bent MJ, Afra D, de Witte O, et al. Long-term efficacy of early versus delayed radiotherapy for low-grade astrocytoma and oligodendroglioma in adults: the EORTC 22845 randomised trial. *Lancet*. 2005;366(9490):985–990.

20. Aghi MK, Nahed BV, Sloan AE, et al. The role of surgery in the management of pts with diffuse low grade glioma: a systematic review and evidence-based clinical practice guideline. *J Neurooncol*. 2015;125(3):503–530.

21. Shaw EG, Berkey B, Coons SW, et al. Recurrence following neurosurgeon-determined gross-total resection of adult supratentorial low-grade glioma: results of a prospective clinical trial. *J Neurosurg*. 2008;109(5):835–841.

22. NCCN Clinical practice guidelines in oncology: central nervous system cancers. 2016; Version 1.2016. https://www.nccn.org/professionals/physician_gls/pdf/cns.pdf

23. Shaw EG, Daumas-Duport C, Scheithauer BW, et al. Radiation therapy in the management of low-grade supratentorial astrocytomas. *J Neurosurg*. 1989;70(6):853–861.

24. Brown PD, Buckner JC, O'Fallon JR, et al. Effects of radiotherapy on cognitive function in pts with low-grade glioma measured by the folstein mini-mental state examination. *J Clin Oncol*. 2003;21(13):2519–2524.

25. Prabhu RS, Won M, Shaw EG, et al. Effect of the addition of chemotherapy to radiotherapy on cognitive function in pts with low-grade glioma: secondary analysis of RTOG 98-02. *J Clin Oncol*. 2014;32(6):535–541.

26. Laack NN, Brown PD, Ivnik RJ, et al. Cognitive function after radiotherapy for supratentorial low-grade glioma: a North Central Cancer Treatment Group prospective study. *Int J Radiat Oncol Biol Phys*. 2005;63(4):1175–1183.

27. Kiebert GM, Curran D, Aaronson NK, et al. Quality of life after radiation therapy of cerebral low-grade gliomas of the adult: results of a randomised phase III trial on dose response (EORTC trial 22844). EORTC Radiotherapy Co-operative Group. *Eur J Cancer*. 1998;34(12):1902–1909.

4: MENINGIOMA

Abigail L. Stockham and David J. Schwartz, V

QUICK HIT: Meningiomas are the most primary common brain tumors in adults, representing approximately 20% to 30% of all primary brain tumors.[1,2] There is approximately a 2:1 female predominance though males are slighthy more likely to have a typical or malignant meningiomas. There is a slightly greater incidence in Black pts.[1,3] Risk factors include ionizing radiation and neurofibromatosis type 2 (NF2); less strongly associated are MEN1 and endogenous/exogenous hormones.[1,4] Maximal safe surgical resection is the standard of care for lesions that are surgically accessible. Extent of surgical resection and grade of meningioma determine initial postsurgical approach (see Simpson grading in Table 4.4). One "rule of thumb" is that recurrence rates are approximately the Simpson grade resection x 10%. Recurrent meningiomas are generally managed with re-resection followed by RT when no previous RT has been administered. Unresectable meningiomas are managed with fractionated radiotherapy or SRS, depending on size and location. Similar strategies are employed in the setting of spinal meningiomas (approximately 10% of cases). While the vast majority of meningiomas are benign, they may cause significant morbidity and mortality. Particularly in young pts, the likelihood and morbidity of recurrence must be weighed against the potential long-term sequelae of RT to the brain.

TABLE 4.1: RT Dose Guidelines for Meningioma

Extent of resection	WHO Grade I	WHO Grade II	WHO Grade III
GTR	Observe	EBRT 54 Gy/30 fx	59.4–66 Gy/30–33 fx
STR	Observe OR EBRT 54 Gy/30 fx OR SRS 12–13 Gy	59.4–60 Gy/30–33 fx	59.4–66 Gy/30–33 fx
Recurrent Disease	Consider further resection + EBRT 54 Gy/30 fx OR SRS 12–13 Gy	Consider further resection + 59.4–60 Gy/30–33 fx OR SRS 16 Gy	Consider further resection + 59.4–66 Gy/30–33 fx OR SRS 18–24 Gy (based on size)
Unresectable Disease	EBRT 54 Gy/30 fx OR SRS 12–13 Gy	59.4–60 Gy/30–33 fx OR SRS 16 Gy	59.4–66 Gy/30–33 fx OR SRS 18–24 Gy (based on size)

EPIDEMIOLOGY: 26,000 cases per year, incidence of approximately 7.8 per 100,000; approximately 80%, 65%, and 58% 1-, 5- and 10-yr survival rates (decreased survival rate with increasing age), incidence increases with age (especially >65).[3]

RISK FACTORS: Older age, ionizing radiation, NF2, MEN1, exogenous/endogenous hormones, elevated BMI, decreased physical activity, increased height (women), uterine fibroids, and breast cancer.[1,4–10] The degree to which estrogen exposure is an independent risk factor from BMI, decreased physical activity, increased height, uterine fibroids, and breast cancer is unclear.

ANATOMY: Arises from the arachnoid layer of the meninges between the dura mater and pia mater, commonly at sites of high density of arachnoid villi and associated arachnoid cap cells. Most frequently noted at supratentorial sites of dural reflection, such as at the cerebral convexity (~20%) and parafalcine/parasagittal (~25%), along the sphenoid wing (~20%) and skull base (resulting in decreased surgical accessibility), intraventricular, suprasellar region, olfactory groove (~10%), and in the posterior fossa most commonly along the petrous bone (~10%).

PATHOLOGY: Classified by the WHO into three grades: WHO grade I (benign), WHO grade II (atypical, yet still benign), and WHO grade III (malignant).

TABLE 4.2: Summary of WHO Grading for Meningiomas				
WHO Grade	Frequency	Subtypes	Characteristics/Appearance	Recurrence After GTR
Grade I	90%	Meningothelial Fibroblastic Transitional Psammomatous Angiomatous Microcystic Secretory Metaplastic Lymphoplasmacyte-rich	Psammoma bodies Cellular whorls Calcifications	7%–25%
Grade II	5%–7%	Chordoid Clear cell Atypical	≥4 mitoses/10 HPF, brain invasion OR ≥3 features below: • Hypercellularity • small cells w/ high nuclear:cytoplasm ratio • prominent nucleoli • patternless/sheet-like growth • foci of spontaneous necrosis	29%–52%
Grade III	3%–5%	Anaplastic Papillary Rhabdoid	≥20 mitoses/10 HPF and/or • carcinomatous features • sarcomatous features • melanomatous features • loss of usual growth pattern • brain invasion • abundant mitoses with atypia • multifocal necrotic foci	50%–94%

GENETICS: Genetic mutations are common but the clinical impact of mutations is evolving. *NF2* aberration (~50% of meningiomas), smoothened (*SMO*, 5%), AKT1 (~10%), *TRAF7* (~25%), PI3KA (~7%, primarily noted in skull base meningiomas), mTORC1.[11,12]

CLINICAL PRESENTATION: May be asymptomatic. If symptomatic: headaches, seizure, altered cognition, focal neurologic deficit—further detailed in Table 4.3 (data modified from Raizer, 2010).[13]

TABLE 4.3: Common Presenting Symptoms of Meningioma Based on Location
Parasagittal: Motor and/or sensory changes.
Frontal: Personality change, avolition, executive dysfunction, disinhibition, urinary incontinence, Broca's aphasia.
Temporal: Memory changes, Wernicke's aphasia (left), aprosody (right), olfactory symptoms including seizures.
Cavernous sinus: CN symptoms (nerves III, IV, V1–2, VI pass through the cavernous sinus), decreased visual acuity, impaired extra-ocular motion with resultant diplopia, numbness.
Occipital lobe: Visual field deficit.
Cerebellopontine angle (CPA): Unilateral deafness/decreased hearing, facial numbness, facial weakness.
Optic nerve sheath: Ipsilateral decreased visual acuity/blindness, exophthalmos, ipsilateral pupillary dilation nonreactive to direct light but with retained consensual contraction.
Sphenoid wing: Cranial neuropathy, seizures.
Tentorium: Extra-axial compression with associated occipital/parietal/cerebellar symptoms.
Foramen magnum: Paraparesis, urinary/anal sphincter dysfunction, tongue atrophy +/– fasciculation.
Spinal canal: Back pain, Brown-Séquard (hemispinal cord) syndrome.

WORKUP: H&P with attention to the neurologic exam, head CT, MRI brain to evaluate for a well-circumscribed, classically homogeneously enhancing extra-axial mass with a dural tail (present in more than half of meningiomas—may also be present in pts with chloroma, lymphoma, and sarcoidosis). Meningiomas are T1 isointense and CT isodense with normal brain parenchyma unless contrast is administered, underscoring the importance of IV contrast when possible. Evaluate for bone invasion and/or reactive hyperostosis. Modest perilesional edema may be present; this is more frequently encountered with rapidly enlarging atypical and/or malignant meningiomas as well as convexity or parasagittal meningiomas. Extensive perilesional edema is a relative contraindication to SRS as pts may have considerable post-treatment edema following treatment of convexity meningiomas.

PROGNOSTIC FACTORS: Poorer prognosis with increasing grade, decreasing extent of resection, proliferative index (Ki-67) >1%, brain invasion, age <45, chromosomal abnormalities involving 14 and 22, aggressive clinical behavior, p53 overexpression.[14–20]

NATURAL HISTORY: Approximately 1 to 2 mm of growth annually for grade I meningiomas. Local progression further aggravates any associated neurologic symptoms. Local failure is most common. Marginal failure around the meninges is possible, particularly with high-grade meningioma.

TREATMENT PARADIGM

Observation: Observation may be appropriate for incidentally discovered small, asymptomatic meningiomas. Observation is also appropriate for WHO grade I tumor, status post-GTR. Consider observation in pts with WHO grade I meningioma following STR. Surveillance with MRI is recommended annually for pts with WHO grade I meningiomas undergoing observation to assess for treatment.

Surgery: Standard is maximal safe surgical resection. Often requires craniotomy, but for sphenoid wing/skull base lesions, endoscopic surgery may be indicated. Simpson grade correlates with local failure (Table 4.4).

TABLE 4.4: Simpson Grading System for Meningioma	
Grade 1	GTR, including dural attachment and any abnormal bone
Grade 2	GTR, with coagulation instead of resection of dural attachment
Grade 3	GTR of meningioma without resection or coagulation of dural attachment
Grade 4	Subtotal resection
Grade 5	Tumor debulking or decompression only

Chemotherapy: No role for CHT. Agents studied include tyrosine kinase inhibitors, VEGF inhibitors, and somatostatin analogues, but medical therapy is nonstandard.[21–24]

Radiation

Dose: WHO grade I meningiomas generally are treated to 50.4 Gy/28 fx or 54 Gy/30 fx. WHO grade II meningiomas are treated to 59.4 Gy/33 fx or 60 Gy/30 fx. WHO grade III meningiomas are treated to 60–66 Gy/30–33 fx. See RTOG 0539 for common dosing strategy. SRS dose, when feasible, is 12 to 14 Gy for grade I tumors. When surrounding tissues allow, 16 Gy for grade II tumors may be considered, and RTOG 9005 dosing for grade III tumors. Brachytherapy is utilized at select institutions for multiply recurrent meningiomas.

Procedure: See *Treatment Planning Handbook*, Chapter 3.[25]

EVIDENCE-BASED Q&A

Do incidentally discovered meningiomas require aggressive intervention?

Incidentally appreciated meningiomas may not require additional intervention. In at least one study, more than half of pts' meningiomas demonstrated no growth at 5 years. These pts may be followed with imaging at 3 to 6 months and then annually thereafter if no growth is appreciated.[26]

What is the optimal first-line management in the treatment of meningiomas?

Maximal safe surgical resection provides the greatest opportunity for minimizing recurrence rates. The extent of resection is graded according to the Simpson grading system, which was the foundational study in meningioma.[27]

Mayo Clinic (*Mayo Clin Proc* 1998, PMID 9787740): RR of 581 pts treated with initial resection. GTR achieved in 80%. The 5- and 10-yr PFS was 88% and 75% for GTR, but only 61% and 39% for less than GTR. Perioperative mortality of 1.6%. A matched cohort analysis suggested nontrivial increase in morbidity and mortality from meningioma and/or treatment. Many of the risk factors for recurrence we use today were noted in this study. *Comment: Used an older data set. Surgical techniques, radiographic evaluation, and perioperative care may have improved since that time.[16]*

Kallio, Helsinki University, Finland (*Neurosurgery* 1992, PMID 1641106): RR of 935 pts from 1953 to 1980. Reported increased rates of mortality in pts with incomplete tumor removal, poor clinical condition, tumor anaplasia, and hyperostosis. Pts with less than GTR versus GTR had a 4.2 relative risk of death, and those with malignant meningiomas versus benign meningiomas had a 4.6 relative risk of death.[28]

What is the role of RT in the management of WHO grade I meningiomas?

GTR (Simpson 1–3) is generally considered definitive and pts may be followed with surveillance imaging.

However, with longer follow-up, recurrence rates as high as 20%, 40%, and 60% have been reported at 5, 10, and 15 years, likely reflecting modern imaging capabilities.[16,29–31] RT is typically reserved for salvage for these pts. For those with STR (Simpson 4–5), recurrence rates of 40% at 5 years and 60% at 10 years can be reduced to that of GTR (approximately halved) with adjuvant RT doses >50.4 Gy.[32,33]

What is the role of RT in the management of WHO grade II meningiomas?

Adjuvant RT is generally recommended after GTR and strongly recommended after STR. Adjuvant RT after GTR of a WHO grade II meningioma is 54 Gy per RTOG 0539. After STR of a WHO grade II, adjuvant RT to 59.4 Gy/33 fx or 60 Gy/30 fx is recommended to minimize risk of local recurrence based on multiple retrospective series.[34–38] Without RT, local recurrence rates of up to 60% at 5 years and CSS of only 70% at 10 years have been observed.[34,39] Following GTR (Simpson 1–2), 5-yr PFS is roughly doubled, from approximately 40% to 80% with adjuvant RT.[35,39] Following STR, adjuvant RT is strongly recommended due to high recurrence rates.

Can RT margins be reduced in pts with WHO grade II meningioma treated with IMRT?

Although RTOG 0539 used at least a 1-cm CTV expansion for WHO grade II meningiomas, retrospective data suggests a 5-mm CTV and a 3-mm PTV may be used without undue local failure.[40]

What is the role of RT in the management of WHO grade III meningiomas?

Adjuvant RT is necessary regardless of resection extent. WHO grade III meningiomas are relatively rare, with less than 300 cases per year in the United States.[3] As such, decisive data are lacking, although it is clear that OS is relatively poor with a generally accepted mean of >3 yrs.[41] A minimum dose of 60 Gy is recommended.[42–46]

Are there prospective data to guide the treatment of meningiomas in the modern era?

Rogers, RTOG 0539 (*ASTRO* 2015 Abstract 317, *ASTRO* 2016 Abstract LBA-7): RTOG 0539 is the first and only prospective trial guiding the use of RT for meningiomas. Three risk groups were defined: low, intermediate, and high (see Table 4.5). **Conclusion: This trial supports observation for low-risk pts and 54 Gy for intermediate risk pts WHO grade I pts s/p STR may warrant adjuvant RT (crude failure rate 40%).**

TABLE 4.5: RTOG 0539 Summary				
Risk Group	Definition	EBRT Dose	Target Volume	Outcomes (Preliminary)
Low	WHO grade I meningioma s/p GTR or STR	Observation	N/A	5-yr PFS: 86.1% 5-yr LF: 12.5%
Intermediate	WHO grade II meningioma s/p GTR Recurrent WHO grade I meningioma	54 Gy/30 fx	Tumor bed + 1 cm CTV, reduced to 5 mm around barriers	5-yr PFS: 83.7% 5-yr LF: 14.3%
High	WHO grade III meningioma (any resection) WHO grade II meningioma s/p STR Recurrent WHO grade II meningioma	60 Gy/30 fx (HD PTV) with simultaneous low-dose PTV 54 Gy	HD PTV: gross tumor + resection bed + 1 cm	3-yr PFS 59.2%, 3-yr LF 31.1% and 3-yr OS 78.6%
			LD PTV: gross tumor + resection bed + 2 cm	

How frequently should pts be surveyed following treatment for meningioma?

For WHO grades I and II, 2017 NCCN guidelines recommend surveillance imaging with contrast-enhanced MRI at 3, 6, and 12 months, then every 6 to 12 months for 5 years, then every 1 to 3 years thereafter. For WHO grade III meningiomas, NCCN recommends contrast-enhanced MRI every 6 to 12 months for 3 to 5 years then every 6 to 12 months.

Should pts previously treated with RT be screened for meningioma?

No. The incidence of clinically relevant meningioma in pts with history of cranial irradiation is approximately 3% at 30 years from the time of irradiation.[47] *The incidence of any meningioma in pts with no history of cranial irradiation may be as high as approximately 13% at 10 years.*[48] *The incidence may reach 20% in pts with previous cranial RT who undergo screening with MRI at 20 years following RT.*[49] *The estimated risk of neoplastic transformation from modern, highly conformal or SRS techniques is low at approximately 1 in 1,000.*[50] *Therefore, a multidisciplinary working group out of the UK has advised against screening as the risks of anxiety from serial MRI examinations and potential knowledge of an asymptomatic (and sometimes unresectable tumors) outweigh the benefits.*[51]

What dose of SRS should be used to treat meningioma and what are the outcomes?

Similar to brain metastases, SRS dose depends on the volume being treated and the dose to adjacent critical structures. Mean doses generally have ranged from 16 to 24 Gy, depending on location, with >20 Gy associated with higher rates of local control.[16,52,53] *Maximal dose for cavernous sinus meningiomas is 12 to 14 Gy, with doses >18 Gy associated with unacceptable CN toxicity.*[54–56] *Fractionated SRT with BED >50 Gy may decrease toxicity rates for pts in whom critical structures limit SRS dose.*[57] *Most SRS series report excellent local control, with 10-yr LC rates ranging from >90% for WHO grade I to >60% for WHO grades II and III.*[52,54–56]

What is meningiomatosis and how should it be managed?

Meningiomatosis is commonly associated with neurofibromatosis (NF) or multiple endocrine neoplasia (MEN) syndromes. Treatment should be coordinated in a multiple disciplinary fashion, with surgery given primary consideration due to concerns of secondary malignancy induction. RT is indicated for surgically unresectable or recurrent lesions.[58]

REFERENCES

1. Wiemels J, Wrensch M, Claus EB. Epidemiology and etiology of meningioma. *J Neurooncol.* 2010;99(3):307–314.
2. Marosi C, Hassler M, Roessler K, et al. Meningioma. *Crit Rev Oncol Hematol.* 2008;67(2):153–171.
3. Ostrom QT, Gittleman H, Fulop J, et al. CBTRUS Statistical Report: primary brain and central nervous system tumors diagnosed in the United States in 2008–2012. *Neuro-oncol.* 2015;17(Suppl 4):iv1–iv62.
4. Asgharian B, Chen YJ, Patronas NJ, et al. Meningiomas may be a component tumor of multiple endocrine neoplasia type 1. *Clin Cancer Res.* 2004;10(3):869–880.
5. Jhawar BS, Fuchs CS, Colditz GA, Stampfer MJ. Sex steroid hormone exposures and risk for meningioma. *J Neurosurg.* 2003;99(5):848–853.
6. Benson VS, Pirie K, Green J, et al. Lifestyle factors and primary glioma and meningioma tumours in the Million Women Study cohort. *Br J Cancer.* 2008;99(1):185–190.
7. Johnson DR, Olson JE, Vierkant RA, et al. Risk factors for meningioma in postmenopausal women: results from the Iowa Women's Health Study. *Neuro-oncol.* 2011;13(9):1011–1019.
8. Wiedmann M, Brunborg C, Lindemann K, et al. Body mass index and the risk of meningioma, glioma and schwannoma in a large prospective cohort study (The HUNT Study). *Br J Cancer.* 2013;109(1):289–294.

9. Niedermaier T, Behrens G, Schmid D, et al. Body mass index, physical activity, and risk of adult meningioma and glioma: a meta-analysis. *Neurology.* 2015;85(15):1342–1350.

10. Custer BS, Koepsell TD, Mueller BA. The association between breast carcinoma and meningioma in women. *Cancer.* 2002;94(6):1626–1635.

11. Brastianos PK, Horowitz PM, Santagata S, et al. Genomic sequencing of meningiomas identifies oncogenic SMO and AKT1 mutations. *Nat Genet.* 2013;45(3):285–289.

12. Clark VE, Erson-Omay EZ, Serin A, et al. Genomic analysis of non-NF2 meningiomas reveals mutations in TRAF7, KLF4, AKT1, and SMO. *Science.* 2013;339(6123):1077–1080.

13. Raizer J. Meningiomas. *Curr Treat Options Neurol.* 2010;12(4):360–368.

14. Anvari K, Hosseini S, Rahighi S, et al. Intracranial meningiomas: prognostic factors and treatment outcome in patients undergoing postoperative radiation therapy. *Adv Biomed Res.* 2016;5:83–86.

15. Durand A, Labrousse F, Jouvet A, et al. WHO grade II and III meningiomas: a study of prognostic factors. *J Neurooncol.* 2009;95(3):367–375.

16. Stafford SL, Perry A, Suman VJ, et al. Primarily resected meningiomas: outcome and prognostic factors in 581 Mayo Clinic patients, 1978 through 1988. *Mayo Clinic Proc.* 1998;73(10):936–942.

17. Pasquier D, Bijmolt S, Veninga T, et al. Atypical and malignant meningioma: outcome and prognostic factors in 119 irradiated patients: a multicenter, retrospective study of the Rare Cancer Network. *Int J Radiat Oncol Biol Phys.* 2008;71(5):1388–1393.

18. Yang SY, Park CK, Park SH, et al. Atypical and anaplastic meningiomas: prognostic implications of clinicopathological features. *J Neurol Neurosurg Psychiatry.* 2008;79(5):574–580.

19. Cai DX, Banerjee R, Scheithauer BW, et al. Chromosome 1p and 14q FISH analysis in clinico-pathologic subsets of meningioma: diagnostic and prognostic implications. *J Neuropathol Exp Neurol.* 2001;60(6):628–636.

20. Vranic A, Popovic M, Cor A, et al. Mitotic count, brain invasion, and location are independent predictors of recurrence-free survival in primary atypical and malignant meningiomas: a study of 86 patients. *Neurosurgery.* 2010;67(4):1124–1132.

21. Chamberlain MC, Glantz MJ, Fadul CE. Recurrent meningioma: salvage therapy with long-acting somatostatin analogue. *Neurology.* 2007;69(10):969–973.

22. Johnson DR, Kimmel DW, Burch PA, et al. Phase II study of subcutaneous octreotide in adults with recurrent or progressive meningioma and meningeal hemangiopericytoma. *Neuro-oncol.* 2011;13(5):530–535.

23. Chamberlain MC, Johnston SK. Hydroxyurea for recurrent surgery and radiation refractory meningioma: a retrospective case series. *J Neurooncol.* 2011;104(3):765–771.

24. Kaley TJ, Wen P, Schiff D, et al. Phase II trial of sunitinib for recurrent and progressive atypical and anaplastic meningioma. *Neuro-oncol.* 2015;17(1):116–121.

25. Videtic GMM, Woody N, Vassil AD. *Handbook of Treatment Planning in Radiation Oncology.* 2nd ed. New York, NY: Demos Medical; 2014.

26. Yano S, Kuratsu J. Indications for surgery in patients with asymptomatic meningiomas based on an extensive experience. *J Neurosurg.* 2006;105(4):538–543.

27. Simpson D. The recurrence of intracranial meningiomas after surgical treatment. *J Neurol Neurosurg Psychiatry.* 1957;20(1):22–39.

28. Kallio M, Sankila R, Hakulinen T, Jaaskelainen J. Factors affecting operative and excess long-term mortality in 935 patients with intracranial meningioma. *Neurosurgery.* 1992;31(1):2–12.

29. Mirimanoff RO, Dosoretz DE, Linggood RM, et al. Meningioma: analysis of recurrence and progression following neurosurgical resection. *J Neurosurg.* 1985;62(1):18–24.

30. Condra KS, Buatti JM, Mendenhall WM, et al. Benign meningiomas: primary treatment selection affects survival. *Int J Radiat Oncol Biol Phys.* 1997;39(2):427–436.

31. Soyuer S, Chang EL, Selek U, et al. Radiotherapy after surgery for benign cerebral meningioma. *Radiother Oncol.* 2004;71(1):85–90.

32. Miralbell R, Linggood RM, de la Monte S, et al. The role of radiotherapy in the treatment of subtotally resected benign meningiomas. *J Neurooncol.* 1992;13(2):157–164.

33. Rogers L, Barani I, Chamberlain M, et al. Meningiomas: knowledge base, treatment outcomes, and uncertainties: a RANO review. *J Neurosurg.* 2015;122(1):4–23.

34. Aghi MK, Carter BS, Cosgrove GR, et al. Long-term recurrence rates of atypical meningiomas after gross total resection with or without postoperative adjuvant radiation. *Neurosurgery.* 2009;64(1):56–60; discussion 60.

35. Park HJ, Kang HC, Kim IH, et al. The role of adjuvant radiotherapy in atypical meningioma. *J Neurooncol.* 2013;115(2):241–247.

36. Goldsmith BJ, Wara WM, Wilson CB, Larson DA. Postoperative irradiation for subtotally resected meningiomas: a retrospective analysis of 140 patients treated from 1967 to 1990. *J Neurosurg.* 1994;80(2):195–201.

37. Valent P, Ashman LK, Hinterberger W, et al. Mast cell typing: demonstration of a distinct hematopoietic cell type and evidence for immunophenotypic relationship to mononuclear phagocytes. *Blood.* 1989;73(7):1778–1785.

38. Rogers CL, Perry A, Pugh S, et al. Pathology concordance levels for meningioma classification and grading in NRG Oncology RTOG Trial 0539. *Neuro-oncol.* 2016;18(4):565–574.

39. Komotar RJ, Iorgulescu JB, Raper DM, et al. The role of radiotherapy following gross-total resection of atypical meningiomas. *J Neurosurg.* 2012;117(4):679–686.

40. Press RH, Prabhu RS, Appin CL, et al. Outcomes and patterns of failure for grade 2 meningioma treated with reduced-margin intensity modulated radiation therapy. *Int J Radiat Oncol Biol Phys.* 2014;88(5):1004–1010.

41. Perry A, Scheithauer BW, Stafford SL, et al. "Malignancy" in meningiomas: a clinicopathologic study of 116 patients, with grading implications. *Cancer.* 1999;85(9):2046–2056.

42. Dziuk TW, Woo S, Butler EB, et al. Malignant meningioma: an indication for initial aggressive surgery and adjuvant radiotherapy. *J Neurooncol.* 1998;37(2):177–188.

43. Kaur G, Sayegh ET, Larson A, et al. Adjuvant radiotherapy for atypical and malignant meningiomas: a systematic review. *Neuro-oncol.* 2014;16(5):628–636.

44. Sughrue ME, Sanai N, Shangari G, et al. Outcome and survival following primary and repeat surgery for World Health Organization Grade III meningiomas. *J Neurosurg.* 2010;113(2):202–209.

45. Boskos C, Feuvret L, Noel G, et al. Combined proton and photon conformal radiotherapy for intracranial atypical and malignant meningioma. *Int J Radiat Oncol Biol Phys.* 2009;75(2):399–406.

46. Hug EB, Devries A, Thornton AF, et al. Management of atypical and malignant meningiomas: role of high-dose, 3D-conformal radiation therapy. *J Neurooncol.* 2000;48(2):151–160.

47. Friedman DL, Whitton J, Leisenring W, et al. Subsequent neoplasms in 5-year survivors of childhood cancer: the Childhood Cancer Survivor Study. *J Natl Cancer Inst.* 2010;102(14):1083–1095.

48. Muller HL, Gebhardt U, Warmuth-Metz M, et al. Meningioma as second malignant neoplasm after oncological treatment during childhood. *Strahlenther Onkol.* 2012;188(5):438–441.

49. Banerjee J, Paakko E, Harila M, et al. Radiation-induced meningiomas: a shadow in the success story of childhood leukemia. *Neuro-oncol.* 2009;11(5):543–549.

50. Niranjan A, Kondziolka D, Lunsford LD. Neoplastic transformation after radiosurgery or radiotherapy: risk and realities. *Otolaryngol Clin North Am.* 2009;42(4):717–729.

51. Sugden E, Taylor A, Pretorius P, et al. Meningiomas occurring during long-term survival after treatment for childhood cancer. *JRSM open.* 2014;5(4):2054270414524567.

52. Kano H, Takahashi JA, Katsuki T, et al. Stereotactic radiosurgery for atypical and anaplastic meningiomas. *J Neurooncol.* 2007;84(1):41–47.

53. Choi CY, Soltys SG, Gibbs IC, et al. Cyberknife stereotactic radiosurgery for treatment of atypical (WHO grade II) cranial meningiomas. *Neurosurgery.* 2010;67(5):1180–1188.

54. Lee JY, Niranjan A, McInerney J, et al. Stereotactic radiosurgery providing long-term tumor control of cavernous sinus meningiomas. *J Neurosurg.* 2002;97(1):65–72.

55. Spiegelmann R, Cohen ZR, Nissim O, et al. Cavernous sinus meningiomas: a large LINAC radiosurgery series. *J Neurooncol.* 2010;98(2):195–202.

56. Skeie BS, Enger PO, Skeie GO, et al. Gamma knife surgery of meningiomas involving the cavernous sinus: long-term follow-up of 100 patients. *Neurosurgery.* 2010;66(4):661–668; discussion 668–669.

57. Arvold ND, Lessell S, Bussiere M, et al. Visual outcome and tumor control after conformal radiotherapy for patients with optic nerve sheath meningioma. *Int J Radiat Oncol Biol Phys.* 2009;75(4):1166–1172.

58. Wentworth S, Pinn M, Bourland JD, et al. Clinical experience with radiation therapy in the management of neurofibromatosis-associated central nervous system tumors. *Int J Radiat Oncol Biol Phys.* 2009;73(1):208–213.

5: PRIMARY CENTRAL NERVOUS SYSTEM LYMPHOMA

Jordan Fenner, Samuel T. Chao, and Erin S. Murphy

> **QUICK HIT:** PCNSL accounts for about 4% of primary brain tumors with common occurrence in the immunosuppressed population. MTX-based CHT +/– consolidation with WBRT, Ara-C +/– etoposide, or high dose CHT followed by autologous SCT are all treatment options. Careful patient selection and clinical trial availability often determine therapy.

TABLE 5.1: General Treatment Paradigm for Primary CNS Lymphoma	
Induction Phase	**Consolidation Phase After Complete Response**
MTX-based CHT	Observation
	WBRT to 23.4 Gy/13 fx (higher dose or boost if <CR)
	Ara-C +/– etoposide
	High dose CHT + ASCT

EPIDEMIOLOGY: PCNSL accounts for about 4% of primary brain tumors, with a yearly age-adjusted incidence of 4 per million.[1] In the mid-1990s the incidence rose significantly, but since then it has declined due to improvements in the management and incidence of HIV/AIDS. However, the incidence rate within immunocompetent older adults has risen in the last decade.[2] The median age of diagnosis is in the 60s.[3] It is considered an AIDS-defining illness and those with an HIV infection have a 3,600-fold increased risk of developing PCNSL.[2] In this population, EBV infection is associated with PCNSL development.

RISK FACTORS: Congenital or acquired immunodeficiency: HIV infection, iatrogenic immunosuppression, severe combined immunodeficiency, Wiskott–Aldrich syndrome, ataxia–telangiectasia, or common-variable immunodeficiency. In immunocompetent patients, the risk factors are less established. It is unclear if autoimmune disease is considered a true risk factor.[4]

ANATOMY: The majority of patients present with a single lesion (66%). Presentations include: intracranial lesions, diffuse leptomeningeal or periventricular, vitreous and spinal lesions. Location in order of decreasing frequency: frontal lobe, parietal lobe, temporal lobe, basal ganglia, corpus callosum, cerebellum, brainstem, insula, occipital lobe, and fornix.[3] 20% of cases involve the eyes (commonly bilateral) and about 1% have isolated spinal cord involvement, typically involving the lower cervical or upper thoracic regions.[5]

PATHOLOGY: The large majority (90%–95%) of PCNSL are diffuse large B-cell lymphomas with the other 5% to 10% composed of Burkitt's, lymphoblastic, marginal zone, or T cell lymphoma. Neoplastic B lymphocytes are classically described by "perivascular cuffing" with expression of CD20, CD19, CD22, BCL-6, and IRF4/MUM1; markers of: B-cells, germinal center B-cells, and late germinal center B-cell respectively.[5]

CLINICAL PRESENTATION: The clinical presentation is highly variable depending on location of disease (see Table 5.2). Nonspecific symptoms include confusion, lethargy, headaches, focal neurologic deficits, neuropsychiatric symptoms, increased intracranial pressure, or seizures.[5] In a small percentage of patients (10%–15%), gastrointestinal symptoms or respiratory illness may be seen before manifestation of neurological symptoms.[3]

TABLE 5.2: Presentation of Primary CNS Lymphoma by Location	
Primary cerebral lymphoma	Focal deficits (70%), neuropsychiatric symptoms (43%), increased intracranial pressure (33%), seizures (14%)[3]
Primary leptomeningeal lymphoma	Cranial neuropathies (58%), spinal symptoms (48%), headache (44%), leg weakness (35%), ataxia (25%), encephalopathy (25%), bowel and bladder dysfunction (21%)[6]
Primary intraocular lymphoma	Ocular complaints (62%), behavioral/cognitive changes (27%), hemiparesis (14%), headache (14%), seizures (5%), ataxia (4%), visual field deficit (2%)[7]
Primary spinal lymphoma	Myelopathies[8]
Neurolymphomatosis	Painful neuropathies including sensorimotor or pure sensory neuropathy, and pure motor neuropathy[9]

WORKUP: The International PCNSL Collaborative Group[10] recommends: H&P with complete neurologic and lymphatic exam including peripheral lymph nodes and testicular exam. Mini-Mental Status Exam. Document performance status. Ophthalmologic and slit-lamp exam.

Labs: LDH, liver function tests, renal function tests, HIV status. Lumbar puncture (at least 1 week after surgery) with assessment of CSF cytology, total protein, cell count, glucose, beta2-microglobulin, immunoglobulin heavy gene rearrangement, and flow cytometry.[6]

Imaging: Contrast-enhanced MRI brain; if spinal symptoms are present, also MRI spine. Systemic disease is discovered in 8% of patients with suspected isolated PCNSL and therefore full extent of disease should be evaluated. CT of chest, abdomen, pelvis, and/or testicular ultrasound in the elderly population or patients who have positive findings on physical exam.

Biopsy: Stereotactic needle biopsy is the standard. Needle biopsy is preferred to surgical resection due to less risk and no clinical benefit with surgical resection. An ocular biopsy or CSF cytology can also be used for diagnosis.[7] Bone marrow biopsy is also indicated.

PROGNOSTIC FACTORS: No formal staging system exists for PCNSL but multiple prognostic systems have been described as in Tables 5.3 and 5.4.

TABLE 5.3: IELSG Score for Primary CNS Lymphoma[11]			
# Risk Factors	2-yr OS: All Pts	2-yr OS (with high dose MTX)	Risk Factors: Age >60, ECOG PS >1, elevated LDH, elevated CSF protein concentration (45 mg/dL in patients ≤60 years old; 60 mg/dL in patients >60 years old), and involvement of deep structures of the brain (i.e., periventricular regions, basal ganglia, corpus callosum, brainstem, cerebellum)
0–1	80% ± 8%	85% ± 8%	
2–3	48% ± 7%	57% ± 8%	
4–5	15% ± 7%	24% ± 11%	

TABLE 5.4: MSKCC Prognostic Classification[12]		
Class 1: ≤50 years	MS 8.5 years	FFS 2 years
Class 2: >50 years, KPS ≥70	MS 3.2 years	FFS 1.8 years
Class 3: Patients ≥50 years, KPS <70	MS 1.1 years	FFS 0.6 years

TREATMENT PARADIGM

Surgery: Biopsy alone is sufficient for diagnosis. Surgical resection is not indicated. PCNSL involvement is classically widespread and involves deep brain structures. Therefore surgical resection is potentially risky and has not been shown to increase OS.[5]

Chemotherapy: CHT is considered the mainstay of treatment for PCNSL. High dose MTX (3.5–8 g/m^2) is standard. MTX can be administered as monotherapy (older adults) or more commonly as multidrug therapy. The ideal combination regimen has yet to be defined but may include MTX, rituximab, and various combinations of cytarabine, temozolomide, ifosfamide, procarbazine, or vincristine. After a complete response, consolidation therapy with Ara-C or autologous SCT are options. CHOP, which has shown success in systemic lymphoma, has thus far not been found to be as efficacious in PCNSL.[13]

Radiation

Indications: WBRT is used for consolidation after MTX-based CHT or for palliation. Historically high dose WBRT alone was the mainstay of treatment, but is no longer considered the best long-term option for disease control. The utility of low dose WBRT to 23.4 Gy/13 fx as consolidation approximately 3 to 5 weeks after CR remains controversial.[14] In patients >60 years old, WBRT in combination with MTX is concerning for neurotoxicity. It has yet to be determined if RT should be withheld in this patient population.

Dose: If WBRT is delivered after CR to CHT, standard is 23.4 Gy/13 fx. If CR is not achieved, consider 23.4 WBRT with boost to 45 Gy/25 fx.

Toxicity: Acute: fatigue, headache, nausea, alopecia, skin erythema, high frequency hearing loss, changes to hearing and taste, dry mouth. For ocular irradiation: dry eyes, less commonly retinal injury and cataracts.

Late: Neurotoxicity changes such as short-term memory loss, verbal fluency/recall, gait changes, ataxia, Parkinson-like features, behavioral changes, and leukoencephalopathy.

Procedure: See Treatment Planning Handbook, Chapter 3.[15]

MEDICAL: Traditionally, corticosteroids are held prior to biopsy unless medically necessary.[16] After biopsy, steroids can be used for quick alleviation of neurological symptoms. Radiologic regression can be transiently seen with steroids in about 40%, which is suggestive but not diagnostic of PCNSL.

EVIDENCE-BASED Q&A

What is the role for radiation therapy alone for PCNSL?

Historically, RT alone was the initial treatment for PCNSL. However, WBRT alone has shown little success in long-term disease control with high rates of local recurrence.

Nelson, RTOG 8315 (*IJROBP* 1992, PMID 1572835): Single-arm phase II of 41 pts treated with 40 Gy WBRT plus a 20 Gy boost to tumor bed plus 2-cm margin. MS 12.2 mos. 62% CR. The main location of relapse was at the local site of disease. High KPS and CR were associated with increased OS. **Conclusion: PCNSL shows a good response to WBRT alone but local recurrence is common.**

Can combination CHT with WBRT improve outcomes when compared to WBRT alone?

DeAngelis, RTOG 9310 (*JCO* 2002, PMID 12488408): Multicenter, single-arm phase II prospective study evaluating up-front MPV (methotrexate, procarbazine, vincristine) CHT combination with RT. 102 PCNSL immunocompetent pts were enrolled. 5 cycles of MTX 2.5 g/m², vincristine, intra-Ommaya MTX, procarbazine, and consolidation WBRT followed by Ara-C. WBRT was 45 Gy (1.8 Gy/fx) to 63 pts, but due to late neurotoxicity seen with this dose, 16 pts who achieved CR after induction received 36 Gy (1.2 Gy/fx BID) for 15 days instead. 34% relapsed during follow-up period. Median PFS 24 mos, MS 36.9 mos. Between the 45 Gy WBRT and the 36 Gy hyperfractionated RT (1.2 Gy BID), there was no difference noted in PFS (24.5 months vs. 23.3 months; $p = .81$) and OS (37 months vs. 47.9 months; $p = .65$). Side effects of RT included: myelosuppression (63%) and delayed neurologic toxicities classified mostly as leukoencephalopathy (15%). 8 cases of the neurologic toxicities progressed to fatalities. **Conclusion: HD-MTX in combination with other agents improved survival compared to historic rates of RT alone. This CHT combination provides a high response rate but in conjunction with WBRT it demonstrates a significant late risk of neurotoxicity.**

Is consolidation WBRT superior to CHT alone?

Thiel (*Lancet Oncol* 2010, PMID 20970380): Phase III PRT to compare HD-MTX versus HD-MTX plus WBRT. 551 pts received six cycles of HD-MTX and HD-MTX plus ifosfamide and were randomly assigned to immediate WBRT (45 Gy/30 fx of 1.5 Gy) or delayed WBRT. For pts who did not achieve CR after initial CHT, they received high dose Ara-C or WBRT. 13% died during initial CHT. In addition there was a high dropout rate, thus leaving 318 pts to be analyzed. In HD-MTX + WBRT pts, MS was 32.4 mos and median PFS was 18.3 mos. In pts who received CHT alone, the MS was 37.1 mos and median PFS was 11.9 mos. Neurotoxicity was found to be higher in the WBRT group versus the non-WBRT group in both clinical (49% vs. 26%) and neuroradiology (71% vs. 46%) assessment. **Conclusion: No statistically significant difference was found in OS or PFS between the WBRT + CHT and CHT alone, but the noninferiority endpoint of 0.9 was not met. Therefore the study was unable to conclude if WBRT has an impact on OS when added to CHT. In addition, the neurotoxicity rates were greater in the WBRT cohort.** *Comment: Small percentage of pts were treated per protocol.*

Can the dose of WBRT be reduced to avoid neurotoxicity but still maintain benefit?

Morris, MSKCC Multi-Center Trial (*JCO* 2013, PMID 24101038): Single-arm phase II trial assessing consolidation with reduced dose WBRT (rd-WBRT) 23.4 Gy and addition of rituximab to MPV. 45 Gy was delivered for those not achieving CR. Of 52 pts, 31 achieved CR postinduction. Both CR and PR received Ara-C as consolidation after RT. Of the pts who received rd-WBRT, the median PFS was 7.7 yrs, the 5-yr OS was 80%, and MS was not reached with a MFU of 5.9 yrs. For the entire cohort, the median PFS was 3.3 yrs, MS was 6.6 yrs. No evidence of cognitive decline was observed, with the exception of motor speed. **Conclusion: rd-WBRT and Ara-C following R-MPV demonstrated good control with minimal neurotoxicity.**

What is the role of temozolomide?

This is an ongoing question on the single-arm phase I/II trial RTOG 0227, which combines induction CHT (rituximab, temozolomide, and methotrexate) followed by WBRT (36 Gy/30 fx at 1.2 Gy BID) followed by adjuvant temozolomide. Results are not yet reported as of the time of publication.

Does low dose WBRT improve PFS as compared to CHT alone?

This is a question on the completed but not yet reported trial RTOG 1114. This trial delivers rituximab, methotrexate, procarbazine, vincristine, and cytarabine, randomizes to low dose WBRT (23.4 Gy/13 fx) or no RT, and then delivers two cycles of additional cytarabine. The addition of WBRT is hypothesized to improve PFS but this remains an open question.

Is there a role for stem cell transplant with high dose CHT?

High dose CHT plus autologous SCT has a role in both initial and salvage therapy for pts with PCNSL.[17,18] However, more trials are needed to fully evaluate its potential. Two randomized trials have been designed to further test HCT + ASCT, CALGB 51101, and IELSG 32. The first trial examined consolidation HCT + ASCT versus nonmyeloablative CHT. IELSG 32 is a trial with a double randomization that investigates both MTX-based initial CHT as well as rd-WBRT versus HDT + ASCT as consolidation.

How is response assessed in PCNSL?

As per International PCNSL Collaborative group guidelines,[10] in order to assess response MRI must be completed within 2 months of finishing treatment. LP and/or ophthalmologic exam must be completed if initially positive.

TABLE 5.5: Response Criteria in PCNSL as per International PCNSL Collaborative Guidelines[10]

Response	Steroid Use	Eye Exam	CSF	MRI
CR	None	Normal	Negative	No enhancement
Unconfirmed CR	Any	Normal or minor abnormality	Negative	No enhancement or minor abnormality
PR	N/A	Decrease in vitreous cells/retinal infiltrate	Persistent or suspicious	≥50% decrease in enhancement
PD	N/A	New ocular disease	Recurrent or positive	≥25% increase or new lesion/site

What is the role of WBRT in salvage therapy?

WBRT provides an adequate option as salvage therapy for recurrent or refractory PCNSL. Other options include additional CHT or HDT +ASCT.

Nguyen (*JCO* 2005, PMID 15735126): Evaluation of 27 pts with tumor relapse or progression of a refractory tumor after primary CHT of HD-MTX. Salvage WBRT plus or minus boost to tumor volume was delivered, with the majority (67%) of pts remaining on steroids. Median WBRT dose was 36 Gy (1.5 Gy/fx was most prevalent); 5 pts received a boost to a median dose of 10 Gy and two pts received SRS boost of 12 or 16 Gy, both approaches with a median base dose of 36 Gy. 74% had either a CR (10 pts) or PR (10 pts) to WBRT; eight pts later progressed or recurred at a median 18.8 mos post-WBRT. Delayed neurotoxicity was diagnosed in three pts, at a median of 25 mos, with none resulting in death. **Conclusion: WBRT is effective in the salvage setting. For older pts, withholding WBRT until the time of progression may decrease neurotoxicity rates.**

REFERENCES

1. Hoffman S, Propp JM, McCarthy BJ. Temporal trends in incidence of primary brain tumors in the United States, 1985–1999. *Neuro-Oncol.* 2006;8(1):27–37. doi:10.1215/S1522851705000323
2. Villano JL, Koshy M, Shaikh H, et al. Age, gender, and racial differences in incidence and survival in primary CNS lymphoma. *Br J Cancer.* 2011;105(9):1414–1418. doi:10.1038/bjc.2011.357
3. Bataille B, Delwail V, Menet E, et al. Primary intracerebral malignant lymphoma: report of 248 cases. *J Neurosurg.* 2000;92(2):261–266. doi:10.3171/jns.2000.92.2.0261
4. Schiff D, Suman VJ, Yang P, et al. Risk factors for primary central nervous system lymphoma. *Cancer.* 1998;82(5):975–982. doi:10.1002/(SICI)1097-0142(19980301)82:5<975::AID-CNCR25>3.0.CO;2-X
5. Ferreri AJM, Marturano E. Primary CNS lymphoma. *Best Pract Res Clin Haematol.* 2012;25(1):119–130. doi:10.1016/j.beha.2011.12.001
6. Taylor JW, Flanagan EP, O'Neill BP, et al. Primary leptomeningeal lymphoma. *Neurology.* 2013;81(19):1690–1696. doi:10.1212/01.wnl.0000435302.02895.f3
7. Grimm SA, McCannel CA, Omuro AMP, et al. Primary CNS lymphoma with intraocular involvement. *Neurology.* 2008;71(17):1355–1360. doi:10.1212/01.wnl.0000327672.04729.8c
8. Flanagan EP, O'Neill BP, Porter AB, et al. Primary intramedullary spinal cord lymphoma. *Neurology.* 2011;77(8):784–791. doi:10.1212/WNL.0b013e31822b00b9
9. Grisariu S, Avni B, Batchelor TT, et al. Neurolymphomatosis: an international primary CNS lymphoma collaborative group report. *Blood.* 2010;115(24):5005–5011. doi:10.1182/blood-2009-12-258210
10. Abrey LE, Batchelor TT, Ferreri AJM, et al. Report of an International Workshop to Standardize Baseline Evaluation and Response Criteria for Primary CNS Lymphoma. *J Clin Oncol.* 2005;23(22):5034–5043. doi:10.1200/JCO.2005.13.524
11. Ferreri AJM, Blay J-Y, Reni M, et al. Prognostic scoring system for primary CNS lymphomas: the International Extranodal Lymphoma Study Group experience. *J Clin Oncol.* 2003;21(2):266–272. doi:10.1200/JCO.2003.09.139
12. Abrey LE, Ben-Porat L, Panageas KS, et al. Primary central nervous system lymphoma: the Memorial Sloan-Kettering Cancer Center prognostic model. *J Clin Oncol.* 2006;24(36):5711–5715. doi:10.1200/JCO.2006.08.2941
13. Mead GM, Bleehen NM, Gregor A, et al. A medical research council randomized trial in pts with primary cerebral non-Hodgkin lymphoma: cerebral radiotherapy with and without cyclophosphamide, doxorubicin, vincristine, and prednisone chemotherapy. *Cancer.* 2000;89(6):1359–1370.
14. Shah GD, Yahalom J, Correa DD, et al. Combined immunochemotherapy with reduced whole-brain radiotherapy for newly diagnosed primary CNS lymphoma. *J Clin Oncol.* 2007;25(30):4730–4735. doi:10.1200/JCO.2007.12.5062
15. Videtic G, Woody N, Vassil A. *Handbook of Treatment Planning in Radiation Oncology.* Second edition. New York, NY: Demos Medical; 2015.
16. Ferreri AJM. How I treat primary CNS lymphoma. *Blood.* 2011;118(3):510–522. doi:10.1182/blood-2011-03-321349
17. Soussain C, Hoang-Xuan K, Taillandier L, et al. Intensive chemotherapy followed by hematopoietic stem-cell rescue for refractory and recurrent primary CNS and intraocular lymphoma: Société Française de Greffe de Moëlle Osseuse-Thérapie Cellulaire. *J Clin Oncol.* 2008;26(15):2512–2518. doi:10.1200/JCO.2007.13.5533
18. Illerhaus G, Marks R, Ihorst G, et al. High-dose chemotherapy with autologous stem-cell transplantation and hyperfractionated radiotherapy as first-line treatment of primary CNS lymphoma. *J Clin Oncol.* 2006;24(24):3865–3870. doi:10.1200/JCO.2006.06.2117

6: PITUITARY ADENOMA

Edward W. Jung, Nathanael J. Lee, and John H. Suh

QUICK HIT: Pituitary adenoma can be observed in up to 16% of the population but is often asymptomatic and found incidentally by MRI or autopsy.[1,2] When symptomatic, symptoms may include headache, visual impairment due to pressure on the optic chiasm or hormonal aberrations. Treatment options include surgery, medication, or SRS/fractionated RT to relieve pressure on chiasm and correct hormonal abnormalities (Figure 6.1). When defining response to treatment in the literature, LC refers to radiographic response (size criteria), whereas remission/response refers to normalization of hormone secretion (complete or partial).

EPIDEMIOLOGY: Accounts for 10% to 15% of CNS neoplasms with 10,000 cases diagnosed/year. Typically age 30 to 50 y/o, clinically apparent in 3/100,000. Male to female ratio 1:1, but females more frequently symptomatic and have higher incidence rates until 30 y/o when pattern reverses. Incidence higher in African Americans. 75% are secretory.[2-4]

RISK FACTORS: History or family history of colorectal cancer, surgically-induced menopause.[4,5] Associated syndromes: MEN1 (mnemonic: 3 Ps, pituitary (25%), parathyroid, and pancreatic islet cell tumors), isolated familial somatotropinoma, Carney complex (spotty skin pigmentation, myxomas, endocrine over activity, schwannomas).

ANATOMY: Sella turcica (sphenoid bone) borders: anterior/posterior: anterior/posterior clinoids; superior: diaphragm sella (dura); lateral: cavernous sinus (contains internal carotid arteries and CN III, IV, V1, V2, VI). Embryologically, the anterior lobe develops from Rathke's pouch, and the posterior lobe (neurohypophysis) from the third ventricle. Pituitary adenomas arise in anterior lobe, which secretes FSH, LH, ACTH, TSH, PRL, and GH (mnemonic: FLAT PiG). Posterior lobe secretes oxytocin and ADH.

PATHOLOGY: Mallory's trichrome staining can be used to identify functional adenomas. GH secreting are typically eosinophilic, ACTH secreting basophilic and nonfunctioning chromophobic.[6,7]

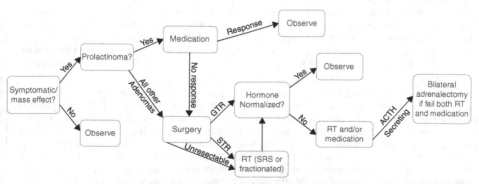

FIGURE 6.1: **General treatment paradigm for pituitary adenoma.**

CLINICAL PRESENTATION: Endocrinopathies (see Table 6.1 for specific tumors) due to hormone oversecretion and hypofunction from mass effect/apoplexy. Visual field deficits due to optic chiasm compression/involvement: bilateral hemianopsia, homonymous hemianopsia, temporal quadrantanopia (pie in the sky). Apoplexy (acute hemorrhage/infarction); treatment is emergency surgical for decompression. Cavernous sinus invasion can cause CN palsies.

WORKUP: H&P with focus on CN exam and visual field testing.

Labs: CBC, CMP, baseline endocrine function. Examine respective secretory status with TSH, T3/T4, ACTH, cortisol, PRL, IGF-1.

Normal Hormone Levels

PRL: <25 ng/mL (>100 ng/mL for macroadenoma, 30–100 ng/mL for microadenoma or loss of suppression).

GH: <10 ng/mL without elevated IGF-1. If GH and IGF-1 both elevated and GH not suppressed by hyperglycemia, >90% have tumor;

Cortisol: normal dexamethasone suppression test (cortisol <10 ng/mL); Cushing's syndrome if cortisol >10 ng/mL 8 to 9 hours after 1 mg dexamethasone administration. Cushing's syndrome has low ACTH as opposed to Cushing's disease.

TSH: 0.4 to 4.0 mIU/L. Measurable TSH in the presence of high T3/T4 is the hallmark of TSHoma.

Imaging: T1-weighted MRI with gadolinium, best seen on coronal views. Adenomas less vascular than normal pituitary, so they appear hypointense in early phase of dynamic contrast-enhanced (DCE) MRI.[1] Microadenoma <1 cm diameter, macroadenoma ≥1 cm, giant adenoma >4 cm, picoadenoma <0.3 cm. Skeletal survey if acromegaly.

Differential for Pituitary Mass

Neoplasm: pituitary tumor, craniopharyngioma, meningioma, germ cell tumor, metastatic tumor, glioma, lymphoma, chordoma.

Benign: Rathke's cleft cyst, arachnoid cyst, aneurysm, empty sella syndrome, inflammatory lesions (granuloma).

PROGNOSTIC FACTORS: Better prognosis with GTR. Worse in pts with cavernous sinus invasion.[8] *Hardy Grading:* 0: intrapituitary microadenoma with normal sella appearance; I: normal sella size with asymmetric floor; II: enlarged sella with intact floor; III: localized erosion of sella floor; IV: diffusely eroded sella floor.[9,10]

TABLE 6.1: Overview of Pituitary Adenoma Subtypes
Prolactinoma: Most common pituitary adenoma. First-line treatment is medical management with dopamine agonists (i.e., bromocriptine, cabergoline). Most pts have >50% reduction in PRL level with medication. 80% show >25% reduction in volume. Surgery is first line if visual deficit due to compression, cystic macroprolactinoma, pituitary apoplexy, or woman wishes to conceive. Lower RT remission rate when RT given alone without medical management compared to other adenoma subtypes. SRS CR is 15%–50% alone, but with medical management increases to 40%–80% at 2–8 yrs. Fractionated RT alone CR is 25%–50% and with addition of medical therapy increases to 80%–100% at 1–10 yrs.[9]
Cushing's disease (ACTH): First-line treatment is surgery. Remission rate after surgery: 89% for microadenomas, 63% for macroadenomas, and 81% for macroadenomas where GTR anticipated.[11] Tumor extension beyond sella is predictive of nonremission and late recurrence. RT is the preferred second-line treatment over medical management. Fractionated RT remission rate is 50%–80% with median time to remission 18–42 mos. SRS with medical therapy leads to remission rates of 85%–100% with median time of 7.5–33 mos for ACTH normalization.[9] Bilateral adrenalectomy, which can lead to Nelson's syndrome (rapid enlargement of pituitary adenoma, muscle weakness, and skin hyperpigmentation due to melanocyte stimulating hormone), is a final salvage approach.

(continued)

TABLE 6.1: Overview of Pituitary Adenoma Subtypes *(continued)*
Acromegaly (GH): First-line treatment is surgery. For pts failing surgery, 50%–60% show reduced GH/IGF-1 levels with somatostatin analogues (side effects: malabsorptive diarrhea, nausea/vomiting, gallbladder sludge, abdominal cramping). Remission rate of fractionated RT and SRS similar: 50%–60% at 5–10 yrs, and 65%–87% at 15 yrs.[9] GH receptor antagonist (pegvisomant) reduces IGF-1 levels (not GH) if other treatments fail. Side effects of pegvisomant: nausea/vomiting, flu syndrome, diarrhea, abnormal LFTs.
Hyperthyroidism (TSHoma): First-line treatment is surgery. Consider postoperative RT to higher dose of 54 Gy as TSHomas are locally aggressive and less responsive to RT. Medical therapy with somatostatin analogues, thyroid ablation, methimazole/propylthiouracil which inhibits thyroperoxidase (converts T3 to T4).
Pituitary carcinoma: Extremely rare (0.2% of pituitary tumors). Frequently metastatic (CSF or systemic) with mean survival 1.9 years.[1] First-line treatment is temozolomide, which is also used to treat *aggressive pituitary tumors*—not defined by histology, but rather as locally aggressive and not controlled by surgery, RT, and medication. Low MGMT (immunohistochemistry, not promoter methylation) may be a predictive marker for treatment response.[12,13]
Nonsecretory/functioning: First-line treatment is surgery to relieve compression. RT recommended for STR or recurrence.[14] At least partial reduction in size expected in two-thirds of cases. LC >90% at 10 yrs with RT.

TREATMENT PARADIGM

Observation: Most asymptomatic pituitary adenomas without lab abnormalities can be safely observed.

Surgery: Surgery is first-line treatment for all except prolactinoma and pituitary carcinoma.

Surgical technique: (a) **Transsphenoidal surgery (TSS)** performed in >95% cases. TSS has two approaches: sublabial (older technique) and transnasal (microscopic or endoscopic endonasal). Endoscopic is minimally invasive and improves surgical visualization, which may allow for more complete resection and reduced complications.[15] Complications include death (1%), meningitis, CSF leak, diabetes insipidus (6%), hemorrhage, stroke, visual deficit. (b) **Transcranial approach** for large tumors. LC approximately 95%, hormone normalization in 70% to 80% short term, 40% long term. Evolution of surgical technique over time from transcranial to microscopic TSS to endoscopic TSS has improved outcomes (lower incidence of revision surgery, postoperative hemorrhage, diabetes insipidus, and panhypopituitarism).[16] Intraoperative MRI can improve extent of surgical resection for both microscopic and endoscopic TSS.[17]

Medical Management

TABLE 6.2: Medical Management of Secretory Pituitary Adenomas			
Hormone (Frequency)	Hormone Levels	Symptoms	Medical Therapy
Prolactin (30%)	High	Female: amenorrhea, oligomenorrhea, or infertility. Male: low libido or erectile dysfunction, galactorrhea, osteoporosis.	Cabergoline, bromocriptine, quinagolide
	Low	Inability to lactate after delivery.	No treatment currently available

(continued)

TABLE 6.2: Medical Management of Secretory Pituitary Adenomas (*continued*)			
Hormone (Frequency)	Hormone Levels	Symptoms	Medical Therapy
Growth Hormone (25%)	High	Gigantism (before puberty) Acromegaly (after puberty): thickening of bones in jaw, fingers, and toes; frontal bossing; macroglossia, hyperhidrosis, muscle weakness, glucose intolerance (50%), hypogonadism, cardiomegaly, fatigue, paresthesias, arthralgias, hypothyroidism.	Octreotide, pegvisomant injection (expensive but more effective)
	Low	Infancy and childhood: growth failure. Adults: loss of strength, stamina, bone density and musculature, poor memory, depression.	Recombinant human GH preparations (i.e., somatropin)
ACTH (15%)	High	Cushing's disease (not syndrome): central obesity, hypertension, glucose intolerance, hirsutism, easy bruising, striae, osteoporosis, psychological changes, hypogonadism.	Ketoconazole, cyproheptadine, mitotane, mifepristone, metyrapone
	Low	Hypoglycemia, dehydration, weight loss, weakness, tiredness, dizziness, low blood pressure, nausea/vomiting, diarrhea.	Hydrocortisone
TSH (1%)	High	Hyperthyroidism, weight loss, anxiety, heat intolerance, palpitations, diaphoresis, irritability, muscle weakness. Graves ophthalmopathy.	Carbimazole, methimazole, propylthiouracil, somatostatin analogue (octreotide)
	Low	Cold intolerance, constipation, weight gain, fatigue, anhidrosis, dry skin, brittle hair/fingernails, infertility, hyperprolactinemia, goiter.	Levothyroxine

RADIATION

Indications: Second-line therapy if STR s/p surgery, unresectable/inoperable, recurrence after surgery, and/or refractory to medical management. Discontinue medical management 1 month prior to RT and resume after RT completed. Improved response when RT delivered off medical therapy (may alter cell cycle and radiosensitivity).[18–21] Goal is to reduce or stabilize mass effect and normalize hormone levels (takes many years). Excellent LC of 90% to 100% in most studies regardless of RT technique and adenoma subtype. Smaller tumors have improved response and lower risk of hypopituitarism. *SRS versus fractionated RT*: SRS preferred due to faster time to hormone normalization and patient convenience. Fractionated RT if tumor >3 cm or <3–5 mm from chiasm due to risk of visual deficits.[9] Risk for hypopituitarism high for both modalities (20% at 5 yrs; 80% at 10–15 years).[22] Panhypopituitarism occurs in 5% to 10% pts at 5 yrs.[9]

Dose: *SRS:* 14 to 16 Gy for nonsecretory tumors; 20 Gy or higher for secretory tumors.

Fractionated RT: 45 Gy/25 fx for nonsecretory; 50.4 to 54 Gy/28 to 30 fx for secretory.

Hypofractionated SRS: 17 to 21 Gy (3 fx), 22 to 25 Gy (5 fx) for nonsecretory; 17.4 to 26.8 Gy (3 fx), 20 to 32 Gy (5 fx) for secretory tumors.[23,24]

Re-irradiation dose: 35 Gy to 49.6 Gy, median dose 42 Gy at 1.8 to 2 Gy/fx.[25,26]

(Note: Hypofractionated SRS and re-irradiation dose requires further validation.)

Toxicity: Acute: Fatigue, headache, infection, alopecia, otitis. Late: hypopituitarism (50% at 10 yrs),[27] radionecrosis, rare vision impairment, rare hearing loss, stroke (relative risk 2–4),[28–30] second malignancy (2% at 10–20 yrs).[31]

EVIDENCE-BASED Q&A

What are the expected outcomes with SRS?

Sheehan, University of Virginia (*J Neurosurg* 2013, PMID 23621595): RR of 512 pts from nine centers treated with GKRS for nonfunctioning pituitary adenomas to a median dose of 16 Gy and treatment volume 3.3 cm³. Prior surgery in 70% of pts with cavernous sinus involvement and 33% with suprasellar extension. 3-yr LC 98%, 5-yr LC 95%, 10-yr LC 85%. Smaller target size and absence of suprasellar extension associated with improved PFS. Post-SRS complications include: CN dysfunction in 9.3% pts (CN II: 6.6%; CN III: 1.36%; CN IV: 0.23%; CN V: 0.90%; CN VI: 0.45%; CN VII: 0.23%); hypopituitarism in 21.1% (cortisol: 9.9%; thyroid: 16.3%; gonadotropin: 8.3%; GH: 8.4%); 1.4% with diabetes insipidus; 6.6% with further tumor growth; 7.7% pts requiring further surgery or RT.

Minniti (*Radiat Oncol* 2016, PMID 27729088): Review of 92 SRS publications. Biochemical remission: GH (1,802 pts) 44% at MFU 59 mos; ACTH (706 pts) 48% at 56 mos; PRL (610 pts) 44% at 49 mos. LC 95% regardless of adenoma subtype. Hypopituitarism in 24% at 5 years. Optic neuropathy 0% to 3% for Dmax <8–10 Gy optic nerves/chiasm. CN dysfunction and brain necrosis <2%.

Is there a difference between the time to endocrine response when comparing fractionated RT versus SRS?

Hormone normalization appears to occur faster after SRS in some series. Important to note that SRS cases usually have smaller volume tumors compared to fractionated RT cases, which may influence outcomes.

Kong, Korea (*Cancer* 2007, PMID 17599761): Compared outcomes of fractionated RT versus SRS in 125 pts treated at Samsung Medical Center. Median time to CR was 63 mos for fractionated RT versus 26 mos for SRS (*p* = .007). Overall CR rate was 26.2% at 2 yrs and 76.3% at 4 yrs. Similar LC in both arms.

What are the expected outcomes with proton therapy for pituitary adenoma?

Petit, Harvard (*Endocr Pract* 2007, PMID 18194929): MGH RR of 22 pts treated for GH secreting adenoma with proton SRS. All had prior TSS. Median dose to tumor margin was 20 CGE. At MFU of 6.3 yrs, PR 95%, CR 59% with median time to CR of 42 mos. Thirty-eight percent developed new pituitary deficits requiring replacement hormones and 10% developed panhypopituitarism. No visual complications or cerebral necrosis.

Petit, Harvard (*J Clin Endocrinol Metab* 2008, PMID 18029460): MGH RR of 38 pts (33 Cushing's, 5 Nelson's). All had prior TSS without biochemical cure, four pts with prior photon RT. All Nelson's syndrome pts had prior bilateral adrenalectomy. Median dose to tumor margin: 20 CGE. At MFU of 62 mos, CR 52% for Cushing's, 100% for Nelson's. Median time to CR was 18 mos. 52% developed new pituitary deficits requiring replacement hormones at a median time of 27 mos with 6% experiencing panhypopituitarism. No visual complications, CVA, or secondary tumors.

Wattson, Harvard (*IJROBP* 2014, PMID 25194666): MGH RR of 144 evaluable pts treated with three-dimensional conformal passive scattered proton therapy using two to five beams. Median dose to tumor margin: 20 CGE. LC 98% at MFU of 43 mos. New hypopituitarism developed at a median time of 40 mos with larger target volume predictive of hypopituitarism (HR 1.3, $p = .004$). 3-yr hypopituitarism rate 45%, 5-yr rate 62%. 4 pts developed temporal lobe seizures. No CVA or second malignancies at MFU 4.3 years. See Table 6.3 for biochemical CR results.

TABLE 6.3: Biochemical Outcomes After Proton Therapy for Secretory Pituitary Adenoma				
Syndrome	N	3-yr CR	5-yr CR	Median Time to CR
Cushing's	74	54%	67%	32 mos
Nelson's	8	63%	75%	27 mos
Syndrome	N	3-yr CR	5-yr CR	Median Time to CR
Acromegaly	50	26%	49%	62 mos
Prolactinoma	9	22%	38%	60 mos
TSHoma	3	0%	33%	51 mos

What is the risk of secondary malignancy with RT for pituitary adenoma?

Pollock, Mayo Clinic (*IJROBP* 2017, PMID 28333013): RR of 188 pts treated with GKRS. Median dose was 18 Gy to tumor margin. No secondary malignancy or malignant transformation reported at MFU of 8.5 years (5–22.3).

Minniti, Royal Marsden (*J Clin Endocrinol Metab* 2005, PMID 15562021): RR of 462 pts who received fractionated RT; 76% received conventional three-field RT to 45 Gy/25 fx. At MFU of 12 years, 11 pts developed secondary brain tumors (five meningioma, four highgrade astrocytoma, one meningeal sarcoma, one PNET). Cumulative risk 2% at 10 years, 2.4% at 20 years. Relative risk 10.5 compared to normal population.

REFERENCES

1. Suh JH, Chao ST, Murphy ES, Weil RJ. Pituitary tumors and craniopharyngiomas. In: Gunderson L, Tepper J, eds. *Clinical Radiation Oncology*. 4th ed. Philadelphia, PA: Elsevier; 2015: 502–520.
2. Ezzat S, Asa SL, Couldwell WT, et al. The prevalence of pituitary adenomas: a systematic review. *Cancer*. 2004;101(3):613–619.
3. McDowell BD, Wallace RB, Carnahan RM, et al. Demographic differences in incidence for pituitary adenoma. *Pituitary*. 2011;14(1):23–30.
4. Hemminki K, Försti A, Ji J. Incidence and familial risks in pituitary adenoma and associated tumors. *Endocr Relat Cancer*. 2007;14(1):103–109.
5. Schoemaker MJ, Swerdlow AJ. Risk factors for pituitary tumors: a case-control study. *Cancer Epidemiol Biomarkers Prev*. 2009;18(5):1492–1500.
6. Kovacs K, Horvath E. Tumors of the pituitary gland. In: Hartmann WH, Sobin LH, eds. *Atlas of Tumor Pathology*. Washington, DC: Armed Forces Institute of Pathology; 1986.
7. Asa SL. Tumors of the pituitary gland. In: *Atlas of Tumor Pathology*. Washington, DC: American Registry of Pathology Press; 2011.
8. Diri H, Ozaslan E, Kurtsoy A, et al. Prognostic factors obtained from long-term follow-up of pituitary adenomas and other sellar tumors. *Turk Neurosurg*. 2014;24(5):679–687.
9. Loeffler JS, Shih HA. Radiation therapy in the management of pituitary adenomas. *J Clin Endocrinol Metab*. 2011;96(7):1992–2003.
10. Di Ieva A, Rotondo F, Syro LV, et al. Aggressive pituitary adenomas: diagnosis and emerging treatments. *Nat Rev Endocrinol*. 2014;10(7):423–435.
11. Johnston PC, Kennedy L, Hamrahian AH, et al. Surgical outcomes in patients with Cushing's disease: the Cleveland clinic experience. *Pituitary*. 2017;20(4):430–440.

12. Bengtsson D, Schrøder HD, Andersen M, et al. Long-term outcome and MGMT as a predictive marker in 24 patients with atypical pituitary adenomas and pituitary carcinomas given treatment with temozolomide. *J Clin Endocrinol Metab.* 2015;100(4):1689–1698.

13. McCormack AI, Wass JA, Grossman AB. Aggressive pituitary tumours: the role of temozolomide and the assessment of MGMT status. *Eur J Clin Invest.* 2011;41(10):1133–1148.

14. Sheehan J, Lee CC, Bodach ME, et al. Congress of neurological surgeons systematic review and evidence-based guideline for the management of patients with residual or recurrent nonfunctioning pituitary adenomas. *Neurosurgery.* 2016;79(4):E539–E540.

15. Kabil MS, Eby JB, Shahinian HK. Fully endoscopic endonasal vs. transseptal transsphenoidal pituitary surgery. *Minim Invasive Neurosurg.* 2005;48(6):348–354.

16. Linsler S, Quack F, Schwerdtfeger K, Oertel J. Prognosis of pituitary adenomas in the early 1970s and today: is there a benefit of modern surgical techniques and treatment modalities? *Clin Neurol Neurosurg.* 2017;156:4–10.

17. Pala A, Brand C, Kapapa T, et al. The value of intraoperative and early postoperative magnetic resonance imaging in low-grade glioma surgery: a retrospective study. *World Neurosurg.* 2016;93:191–197.

18. Sheehan JP, Pouratian N, Steiner L, et al. Gamma knife surgery for pituitary adenomas: factors related to radiological and endocrine outcomes. *J Neurosurg.* 2011;114(2):303–309.

19. Castinetti F, Nagai M, Dufour H, et al. Gamma knife radiosurgery is a successful adjunctive treatment in Cushing's disease. *Eur J Endocrinol.* 2007;156(1):91–98.

20. Pollock BE, Jacob JT, Brown PD, Nippoldt TB. Radiosurgery of growth hormone-producing pituitary adenomas: factors associated with biochemical remission. *J Neurosurg.* 2007;106(5):833–838.

21. Pouratian N, Sheehan J, Jagannathan J, et al. Gamma knife radiosurgery for medically and surgically refractory prolactinomas. *Neurosurgery.* 2006;59(2):255–266; discussion 255–266.

22. Molitch ME. Diagnosis and treatment of pituitary adenomas: a review. *JAMA.* 2017;317(5):516–524.

23. Iwata H, Sato K, Nomura R, et al. Long-term results of hypofractionated stereotactic radiotherapy with CyberKnife for growth hormone-secreting pituitary adenoma: evaluation by the Cortina consensus. *J Neurooncol.* 2016;128(2):267–275.

24. Iwata H, Sato K, Tatewaki K, et al. Hypofractionated stereotactic radiotherapy with CyberKnife for nonfunctioning pituitary adenoma: high local control with low toxicity. *Neuro Oncol.* 2011;13(8):916–922.

25. Schoenthaler R, Albright NW, Wara WM, et al. Re-irradiation of pituitary adenoma. *Int J Radiat Oncol Biol Phys.* 1992;24(2):307–314.

26. Flickinger JC, Deutsch M, Lunsford LD. Repeat megavoltage irradiation of pituitary and suprasellar tumors. *Int J Radiat Oncol Biol Phys.* 1989;17(1):171–175.

27. Sheehan JP, Niranjan A, Sheehan JM, et al. Stereotactic radiosurgery for pituitary adenomas: an intermediate review of its safety, efficacy, and role in the neurosurgical treatment armamentarium. *J Neurosurg.* 2005;102(4):678–691.

28. Brada M, Burchell L, Ashley S, Traish D. The incidence of cerebrovascular accidents in patients with pituitary adenoma. *Int J Radiat Oncol Biol Phys.* 1999;45(3):693–698.

29. Erridge SC, Conkey DS, Stockton D, et al. Radiotherapy for pituitary adenomas: long-term efficacy and toxicity. *Radiother Oncol.* 2009;93(3):597–601.

30. Sattler MG, Vroomen PC, Sluiter WJ, et al. Incidence, causative mechanisms, and anatomic localization of stroke in pituitary adenoma patients treated with postoperative radiation therapy versus surgery alone. *Int J Radiat Oncol Biol Phys.* 2013;87(1):53–59.

31. Minniti G, Traish D, Ashley S, et al. Risk of second brain tumor after conservative surgery and radiotherapy for pituitary adenoma: update after an additional 10 years. *J Clin Endocrinol Metab.* 2005;90(2):800–804.

7: TRIGEMINAL NEURALGIA

Bindu V. Manyam, Vamsi Varra, and Samuel T. Chao

> **QUICK HIT:** Trigeminal neuralgia, also referred to as "tic douloureux," is a rare condition characterized by episodic, debilitating pain of the face. It is typically unilateral and described as an electric or shock-like sensation.[1] First-line therapy is antiepileptic medication, such as carbamazepine or oxcarbazepine.[2] Second-line therapy for pts who are refractory to medical therapy include surgical procedures such as microvascular decompression, percutaneous balloon microcompression, radiofrequency rhizotomy, and radiation therapy using stereotactic radiosurgery (SRS).[3] Long-term follow-up demonstrates good outcomes of pain relief with SRS.[2]

EPIDEMIOLOGY: Trigeminal neuralgia is the most common facial pain syndrome, with an annual incidence of 15,000 cases in the United States.[4] The male-to-female ratio is 1:1.5.[5] It usually presents in the fifth through seventh decade of life.[6]

RISK FACTORS: Trigeminal neuralgia is more common in women. Pts with multiple sclerosis are at higher risk for trigeminal neuralgia. Hypertension is a suggested risk factor due to the precipitation of tortuous vasculature, though this association is uncertain.[7]

ANATOMY: The trigeminal nerve (CN V) emerges from the midlateral surface of the pons, providing the sensory supply to the face and the motor supply to the muscles of mastication. The semilunar or Gasserian ganglion of the trigeminal nerve is located in Meckel's cave near the apex of the petrous part of the temporal bone. The three branches of the trigeminal nerve are: **ophthalmic nerve (V1)**, which exits the superior orbital fissure and supplies the cornea, ciliary body, iris, lacrimal glands, conjunctiva, and skin of the upper face; **maxillary nerve (V2)**, which exits through foramen rotundum and supplies the pterygopalatine fossa, infraorbital canal, and the skin of the external nasal/superior labial face; and **mandibular nerve (V3)**, which exits through foramen ovale and supplies the teeth and gums of the mandible, skin of the temporal region, lower lip, muscles of mastication and sensation of the anterior 2/3 of the tongue.

ETIOLOGY: Etiologies include vascular compression of the trigeminal root (most common), benign tumors, malignancy, and multiple sclerosis.[1] Compression due to an ectatic loop of artery or vein is the etiology in 80% to 90% of cases. The compression usually occurs within a few millimeters of entry into the pons (also called the "root entry zone").[8]

CLINICAL PRESENTATION: The International Classification of Headache Disorders, 3rd edition (ICHD-3), defines diagnostic criteria of classic trigeminal neuralgia as at least three attacks of unilateral facial pain occurring in one or more divisions of the trigeminal nerve without radiation beyond the trigeminal distribution and at least three of the following four characteristics: (a) recurring paroxysmal attacks lasting from a fraction of a second to 2 minutes; (b) severe intensity; (c) electric-shock-like, shooting, stabbing, or sharp in quality; and (d) at least three attacks precipitated by innocuous stimuli to the affected side of the face (some attacks may be, or appear to be, spontaneous). There must not be clinical evidence of neurologic deficit and cannot be accounted for by another ICHD-3 diagnosis.[1] Of note, pain is typically within the V2 and/or V3 distribution, with V1 the least common distribution. Unlike other facial pain syndromes, trigeminal neuralgia does not usually wake pts from sleep. Involvement of the V1 distribution can also be associated with autonomic symptoms of lacrimation, conjunctival injection, and rhinorrhea.

WORKUP: Trigeminal neuralgia can be diagnosed based on the classic clinical features described. A careful dental exam should be performed. An MRI is indicated to identify etiologies, such as demyelinating lesions, a mass in the cerebellopontine angle, or an ectatic blood vessel. The CISS sequence is especially helpful in identifying aberrant vessels. If patient is unable to get an MRI, a CT cisternogram can be obtained.

TREATMENT PARADIGM

Observation: Observation is appropriate for pts whose symptoms are tolerable and infrequent.

Medical: Antiepileptic drugs are the first-line therapy.[9] More than 25% do not respond to medical therapy or have poor tolerance secondary to the associated toxicities of dose escalation necessary for adequate pain control. Carbamazepine (600–800 mg daily) is the first-line agent and has been shown to be effective in four randomized controlled trials.[10–13] Most common side effects include drowsiness, dizziness, nausea, and vomiting.[9] Leukopenia and aplastic anemia are rare but more serious complications. Second-line agents include clonazepam, gabapentin, lamotrigine, oxcarbazepine, and topiramate.[9]

Surgery: Surgery is typically used if pts have symptoms refractory to medical therapy.[3]

- Microvascular decompression (gold standard): removal or separation of various vascular structures, usually an ectatic superior cerebellar artery, away from the trigeminal nerve.[14] About 70% of pts are pain-free at 10 yrs.[15] Risk of complications include 0.2% perioperative mortality, 0.1% brainstem infarction, and 1% ipsilateral hearing loss.[2]
- Radiofrequency rhizotomy: application of heat to the Gasserian ganglion, thought to selectively destroy pain impulses carried by unmyelinated or thinly myelinated fibers.[16] A heat probe is inserted through foramen ovale in cycles of 45 to 90 seconds at 60°C to 90°C.[17] About 75% are pain-free at 14 yrs.[18]
- Glycerol rhizolysis: injection of 0.1 to 0.4 mL of glycerol into the trigeminal cistern.[19] Provides instant pain relief; however, up to 92% have recurrence of symptoms at 6 yrs.[20]
- Balloon compression: use of a Fogarty catheter to compress the Gasserian ganglion by inflating with 0.5 to 1.0 mL of contrast dye for 1 to 6 minutes.[21]

Radiation

Indications: Stereotactic radiosurgery (SRS) is a minimally invasive option that is preferred for pts with medically refractory disease who are not good surgical candidates. Target is the proximal trigeminal root.

Dose: Typical SRS dose is 70 to 90 Gy in a single fraction prescribed to the 100% isodose line via a 4-mm shot directed at the root entry zone of the trigeminal nerve into the pons. Radiation causes axonal degeneration and necrosis.

Toxicity: Risk of complications include <10% facial numbness/paresthesia and <1% anesthesia dolorosa.[22] A nomogram developed by Lucas et al. quantifies the durability of pain relief and demonstrated that Burchiel pain type prior to treatment (defined as Type 1, in which >50% of symptoms are episodic, or Type 2, in which >50% of symptoms are constant), the BNI pain score after SRS, and post-SRS facial numbness were predictive of outcomes. Pts with type 1 Burchiel pain type, low BNI pain score after SRS, and absence of post-SRS facial numbness tend to have more durable pain relief.[23]

EVIDENCE-BASED Q&A

Medical Therapy

What are the outcomes with carbamazepine?

Wiffen (*Cochrane Database Syst Rev* 2011, PMID 21249671): Meta-analysis of 15 PRTs and 629 pts with chronic neuropathic pain of different etiologies (trigeminal neuralgia, postherpetic neuralgia, etc.). 70% of pts reported some degree of improvement in pain with a number needed to treat (NNT) of 1.7 (1.5–2.0). 66% of pts who received carbamazepine experienced at least one adverse event compared to 27% with placebo, though serious adverse events were not reported. **Conclusion: Carbamazepine is effective in the treatment of chronic neuropathic pain, but is associated with higher rate of adverse events.**

Surgery

How do microvascular decompression and partial sensory rhizotomy differ in outcomes?

Zakrzewska (*Neurosurgery* 2005, PMID 5918947): Survey of 245 pts who underwent microvascular decompression and 60 pts who underwent partial sensory rhizotomy (a procedure in which the trigeminal nerve is severed). Overall satisfaction was 89% with microvascular decompression and 72% with partial sensory rhizotomy ($p < .01$). The final outcome was reported better than expected in 80% with microvascular decompression and 54% with partial sensory rhizotomy ($p < .01$), and 22% of these felt they were worse off after partial sensory rhizotomy. **Conclusion: Patient satisfaction is higher with microvascular decompression than partial sensory rhizotomy.**

Stereotactic Radiosurgery

What is the appropriate target volume for SRS and does increasing the treatment volume improve outcomes?

Flickinger, Pittsburgh/Mayo Clinic (*IJROBP* 2001, PMID 11567820): PRT of 87 pts treated with SRS 44 were randomized to a one-isocenter and 43 were randomized to a two-isocenter technique. 75 Gy was prescribed to the max point. At a MFU of 26 mos, complete pain relief (with or without medication) was 68%. Pain relief was identical between one- and two-isocenter SRS. Improved pain relief was associated with younger age ($p = .025$) and fewer prior procedures ($p = .039$). Complications (numbness or paresthesias) correlated with the nerve length irradiated ($p = .018$). **Conclusion: Increasing the treatment volume to include longer nerve length does not significantly improve pain relief, but may increase complications.**

Does SRS dose escalation improve outcomes?

Kotecha, Cleveland Clinic/Mid-Michigan (*IJROBP* 2016, PMID 27325473): RR of 870 pts from two institutions, divided into three groups based on treatment dose using GKRS and prescribed to the 100% isodose line: ≤82 Gy (352 pts), 83 to 86 Gy (85 pts), and ≥90 Gy (433 pts). The 4-yr rate of pain response was 79%, 82%, and 92% in pts treated to ≤82 Gy, 83 to 86 Gy, and ≥90 Gy, respectively. Pts who received ≤82 Gy had an increased risk of treatment failure, compared to those who received ≥90 Gy (HR 2.0, $p = .0007$). Treatment-related facial numbness was similar among those receiving ≥83 Gy. The rate of anesthesia dolorosa was 1%. **Conclusion: Dose escalation >82 Gy to the 100% isodose line may be**

associated with increased pain relief and duration of pain relief, but at the expense of increased treatment-related facial numbness.

What are the outcomes with linear-accelerator-based radiosurgery for trigeminal neuralgia and does increasing dose in linear-accelerator-based radiosurgery improve outcomes?

Smith, UCLA (*IJROBP* 2011, PMID 21236592): RR of 179 pts treated with linear-accelerator-based radiosurgery for trigeminal neuralgia. Significant pain relief was noted at a mean of 28.8 months in 79%, with average time to pain relief of 1.92 months. 19% had recurrent pain at 13.5 months. Of the 28 pts treated with 70 Gy and 30% IDL touching brainstem, 64% had significant relief and 36% had numbness. Of the 82 pts treated with 90 Gy and 30% IDL touching brainstem, 79% had significant relief and 49% had numbness. Of the 59 pts treated with 90 Gy and the 50% IDL touching brainstem, 88% had significant relief. **Conclusion: Increased radiation dose and greater volume of brainstem irradiation may improve patient reported outcomes, but may increase numbness and trigeminal dysfunction.**

Can SRS be repeated for recurrent trigeminal neuralgia?

Herman, University of Maryland (*IJROBP* 2004, PMID 15093906): RR of 18 pts who underwent repeat SRS for recurrent trigeminal neuralgia at a median time of 8 mos after the initial procedure. Median prescription dose was 75 Gy for the first treatment and 70 Gy for the second treatment. After initial SRS, 50% excellent, 28% good, 6% fair, and 16% poor pain response was reported. After repeat SRS, 45% excellent, 33% good, 0% fair, and 22% poor pain response was reported. New or increased facial numbness was reported in 11%. Repeat SRS resulted in a median 60% improvement in quality of life and 56% of pts reported that the procedure was successful. **Conclusion: Repeat SRS provided similar rates of complete pain control as the first treatment and improvement in quality of life. However, repeat SRS was not effective for pts who had no response to the initial treatment.**

What is the more cost-effective procedure for trigeminal neuralgia?

Pollack, Mayo Clinic (*IJROBP* 2005, PMID 15951649): Prospective, cost-effectiveness study comparing microvascular decompression, glycerol rhizotomy, and SRS. The cost and outcomes of 153 procedures at a tertiary referral center were studied. Pts who underwent microvascular decompression had significantly better pain outcomes (85% and 78% at 6 and 24 mos) compared with glycerol rhizotomy (61% and 55% at 6 and 24 mos, $p = .01$) and SRS (60% and 52% at 6 and 24 mos, $p < .01$). There was no difference in outcome between glycerol rhizotomy and SRS ($p = .61$). The cost per quality-adjusted pain-free year was $6,342, $8,174, and $8,269 for glycerol rhizotomy, microvascular decompression, and SRS, respectively. The cost of glycerol rhizotomy was more than SRS due to the need for repeat procedures. **Conclusion: In pts who are medically operable, microvascular decompression may be the most efficacious and cost-effective procedure compared to glycerol rhizotomy and SRS.**

REFERENCES

1. Headache Classification Committee of the International Headache Society. The international classification of headache disorders, 3rd edition (beta version). *Cephalalgia*. 2013;33(9):629–808.
2. Gronseth G, Cruccu G, Alksne J, et al. Practice parameter: the diagnostic evaluation and treatment of trigeminal neuralgia (an evidence-based review): report of the Quality Standards Subcommittee of the American Academy of Neurology and the European Federation of Neurological Societies. *Neurology*. 2008;71(15):1183–1190.

3. Bennetto L, Patel NK, Fuller G. Trigeminal neuralgia and its management. *BMJ.* 2007;334(7586):201–205.
4. Pope JE, Narouze S. Orofacial pain. In: *Essentials of Pain Medicine.* 3rd ed. Saint Louis, MO: W.B. Saunders; 2011:283–293.
5. Maarbjerg S, Gozalov A, Olesen J, Bendtsen L. Trigeminal neuralgia: a prospective systematic study of clinical characteristics in 158 patients. *Headache.* 2014;54(10):1574–1582.
6. Ritter PM, Friedman WA, Bhasin RR. The surgical treatment of trigeminal neuralgia: overview and experience at the University of Florida. *J Neurosci Nurs.* 2009;41(4):211–214; quiz 215–216.
7. Lin KH, Chen YT, Fuh JL, Wang SJ. Increased risk of trigeminal neuralgia in patients with migraine: a nationwide population-based study. *Cephalalgia.* 2015.
8. Love S, Coakham HB. Trigeminal neuralgia: pathology and pathogenesis. *Brain.* 2001;124(Pt 12):2347–2360.
9. Attal N, Cruccu G, Haanpaa M, et al. EFNS guidelines on pharmacological treatment of neuropathic pain. *Eur J Neurol.* 2006;13(11):1153–1169.
10. Campbell FG, Graham JG, Zilkha KJ. Clinical trial of carbazepine (tegretol) in trigeminal neuralgia. *J Neurol Neurosurg Psychiatry.* 1966;29(3):265–267.
11. Killian JM, Fromm GH. Carbamazepine in the treatment of neuralgia. Use of side effects. *Arch Neurol.* 1968;19(2):129–136.
12. Nicol CF. A four year double-blind study of tegretol in facial pain. *Headache.* 1969;9(1):54–57.
13. Rockliff BW, Davis EH. Controlled sequential trials of carbamazepine in trigeminal neuralgia. *Arch Neurol.* 1966;15(2):129–136.
14. Jannetta PJ. Microsurgical management of trigeminal neuralgia. *Arch Neurol.* 1985;42(8):800.
15. Barker FG, Jannetta PJ, Bissonette DJ, et al. The long-term outcome of microvascular decompression for trigeminal neuralgia. *N Engl J Med.* 1996;334(17):1077–1084.
16. Seegenschmiedt H. *Radiotherapy for Non-Malignant Disorders: Contemporary Concepts and Clinical Results.* Berlin; London: Springer; 2008.
17. Tang Y-Z, Yang L-Q, Yue J-N, et al. The optimal radiofrequency temperature in radiofrequency thermocoagulation for idiopathic trigeminal neuralgia: a cohort study. *Medicine.* 2016;95(28):e4103–e4106.
18. Taha JM, Tew JM, Jr., Buncher CR. A prospective 15-year follow up of 154 consecutive patients with trigeminal neuralgia treated by percutaneous stereotactic radiofrequency thermal rhizotomy. *J Neurosurg.* 1995;83(6):989–993.
19. Lopez BC, Hamlyn PJ, Zakrzewska JM. Systematic review of ablative neurosurgical techniques for the treatment of trigeminal neuralgia. *Neurosurgery.* 2004;54(4):973–982; discussion 973–982.
20. Deer TR, Leong MS, Buvanendran A, American Academy of Pain Medicine. *Comprehensive Treatment of Chronic Pain by Medical, Interventional, and Integrative Approaches: The American Academy Of Pain Medicine Textbook on Patient Management.* New York, NY: Springer Publishing; 2013.
21. de Siqueira SR, da Nobrega JC, de Siqueira JT, Teixeira MJ. Frequency of postoperative complications after balloon compression for idiopathic trigeminal neuralgia: prospective study. *Oral Surg Oral Med Oral Pathol Oral Radiol Endod.* 2006;102(5):e39–e45.
22. Nurmikko TJ, Eldridge PR. Trigeminal neuralgia: pathophysiology, diagnosis and current treatment. *Br J Anaesth.* 2001;87(1):117–132.
23. Lucas JT, Jr., Nida AM, Isom S, et al. Predictive nomogram for the durability of pain relief from gamma knife radiation surgery in the treatment of trigeminal neuralgia. *Int J Radiat Oncol Biol Phys.* 2014;89(1):120–126.

8: VESTIBULAR SCHWANNOMA

Jeffrey Kittel and John H. Suh

> **QUICK HIT:** Vestibular schwannoma (VS), previously called "acoustic neuroma," is a slow-growing, benign tumor of the cerebellopontine angle that typically presents with unilateral hearing loss. Treatment options include observation, microsurgical resection and RT (SRS or fractionated). SRS is generally prescribed to 12–13 Gy and conventional fractionation to 45–54 Gy. Tumor control outcomes appear equivalent between surgery and RT, but RT may minimize impact on quality of life. Clear criteria for which pts should be treated with each modality have not been established.

EPIDEMIOLOGY: Incidence of VS is approximately 0.6–1.9/100,000, making up 8% of intracranial tumors. Incidence is increasing with increased utilization of diagnostic imaging. African Americans are approximately half as likely to be diagnosed with VS but tend to have larger tumors at diagnosis.[1] Median age at diagnosis is 50 to 55 and incidence increases with age.[1,2]

RISK FACTORS: Increasing age, NF2 (96% of pts with NF2, often bilateral), NF1 (5% of pts with NF1, unilateral), childhood exposure to RT (RR 1.14/Gy).[3] Controversial factors: cell phone use and exposure to loud noises.

ANATOMY: VS typically arises from the vestibular portion of CN VIII and is unilateral in 90% of cases. CN VIII arises from the junction of the pons and medulla, enters the internal auditory foramen along with the facial nerve (CN VII), and then divides into the vestibular and cochlear nerves. The cochlear nerve runs to the spiral ganglion and innervates the spiral organ of Corti and the cochlea. The vestibular nerve runs to the vestibular ganglion and splits into three branches. The superior branch innervates the utricle and the superior and lateral semicircular ducts. The inferior branch innervates the saccule and the posterior branch innervates the posterior semicircular duct. VS arises with equal frequency in the superior and inferior branches and rarely in the cochlear nerve. It tends to occur in the vestibular region of the foramen where the nerve acquires a Schwann cell sheath, although it can sometimes arise from or grow into the CPA.

PATHOLOGY: VS is composed of atypical proliferations of Schwann cells, which are found lining peripheral nerves. Histopathologically, they are similar to other peripheral schwannomas and are composed of alternating zones of dense and sparse cellularity, termed "Antoni A" and "Antoni B" respectively. IHC demonstrates S100 positivity.[4] Malignant degeneration is extremely rare.

GENETICS: Biallelic inactivation of NF2 on chromosome 22, which produces the tumor suppressor merlin, is common in sporadic VS and is the cause of bilateral VS in neurofibromatosis type 2.[5]

CLINICAL PRESENTATION: Hearing loss (95% but only 2/3 are aware of it, average duration ~4 years although 16% develop sudden hearing loss), tinnitus (63%, average duration ~3 years), vestibular symptoms (61%; often mild–moderate, nonspecific, and fluctuating; average duration ~2 years), headache (12%, most often occipital), trigeminal symptoms

(9%, typically facial numbness/hyperesthesia/pain, average duration ~1 year), facial nerve symptoms (6%; typically facial weakness, less commonly taste disturbance; average duration ~2 years), other symptoms from brainstem compression (ataxia, hydrocephalus, dysarthria, dysphagia, hoarseness) are uncommon.[6] The House–Brackmann and Gardner–Robertson scales are common metrics of facial paralysis and hearing loss, respectively (Tables 8.1 and 8.2).

WORKUP: H&P including Weber and Rinne tests to evoke asymmetric sensorineural hearing loss and CN exam, audiometry; consider brainstem auditory evoked response (brainstem auditory evoked response [BAER]/auditory brainstem response [ABR]; 60%–90% sensitive with lower sensitivity for small tumors, 60%–90% specific).[7] Vestibular testing uncommon.

Imaging: MRI with contrast is gold standard for diagnosis. High-resolution CT with IV contrast if unable to obtain MRI. MRI shows isointense or slightly hypointense signal to brain on T1, typically with homogeneous contrast enhancement although occasional cystic degeneration.[8] Classic finding is "ice cream cone" shape with widening of the porus acusticus.[9] Differential includes vestibular schwannoma, meningioma, glomus tumor, ependymoma, facial or trigeminal schwannoma, epidermoid cyst, metastasis.

TABLE 8.1: House–Brackmann Facial Paralysis Scale[10]	
Grade I	Normal
Grade II	Mild dysfunction (slight weakness, normal symmetry at rest)
Grade III	Moderate dysfunction (obvious but not disfiguring weakness, synkinesis) with normal symmetry at rest Complete eye closure w/ maximal effort Good forehead movement
Grade IV	Moderately severe dysfunction (obvious and disfiguring asymmetry, significant synkinesis) Incomplete eye closure Moderate forehead movement
Grade V	Severe dysfunction (barely perceptive motion)
Grade VI	Total paralysis

TABLE 8.2: Gardner–Robertson Hearing Loss Scale[11]	
Grade I	Good–excellent (70%–100% speech discrimination)
Grade II	Serviceable (50%–69%)
Grade III	Nonserviceable (5%–49%)
Grade IV	Poor (1%–4%)
Grade V	None

PROGNOSTIC FACTORS: Baseline level of hearing loss, growth rate >2.5 mm/yr, delay in diagnosis.[12–15] Initial tumor size is not prognostic.[14] Pts with growth rate >2.5 mm/yr have decreased rates of hearing preservation (32% vs. 75%, $p < .0001$)[15] and decreased median time to total hearing loss (7.0 vs. 14.8 years, $p < .0001$).[14]

NATURAL HISTORY: In a meta-analysis with 3.2 years MFU, 43% showed growth, 51% showed no growth, and 6% had spontaneous regression.[16] Mean growth rate of 1 to 3 mm per year.[12,15,16]

STAGING: Vestibular schwannomas are not staged but can be graded on the Koos grading scale (Table 8.3).[17]

TABLE 8.3: Koos Grading Scale for Vestibular Schwannoma[17]	
Grade I	Intracanalicular
Grade II	Tumor extending into the posterior fossa, with or without an intracanalicular component, without touching the brainstem
Grade III	Tumor extending into the posterior fossa, compressing the brainstem, but not shifting it from the midline
Grade IV	Tumor extending into the posterior fossa, compressing the brainstem, and shifting it from the midline

TREATMENT PARADIGM

Observation: Consider observation with MRI every 6 to 12 mos in pts without baseline hearing loss and stability or slow rate of growth. Observation is especially favored in elderly pts with significant comorbidities. Indications for treatment vary but can include >2.5 mm growth/year and onset or worsening of symptoms. Pts undergoing observation should be counseled that they have a risk of hearing loss without treatment. There is no consensus on the optimal duration of annual scans for pts managed with observation, but some suggest at least annual scans for 10 years.

Surgery: In general, surgery has excellent results for resection of the entire tumor or recurrence, but can have poor outcome with hearing preservation. Hearing preservation is most likely when the tumor is <1.5–2 cm in size.[18] Other major morbidities include CSF leaks, tinnitus, headaches, and facial paralysis.[19] Surgery is still the most common treatment for VS and is especially considered for younger pts, larger tumors, tumors causing mass effect or dizziness, cystic tumors, and small anatomically favorable tumors with good hearing.[20] There are three main surgical approaches for resection (see Table 8.4).[20–22] The goal of resection is to maximize tumor removal while minimizing morbidity.

TABLE 8.4: Surgical Techniques for Vestibular Schwannoma		
Approach	Pros	Cons
Retrosigmoid/ suboccipital	Allows for possible hearing conservation and facial nerve sparing, also provides best visualization of the posterior fossa.	Requires cerebellar retraction and intradural drilling of the IAC. Has been associated with increased risk of CSF leaks and HA. Poor visualization of lateral IAC.
Translabyrinthine	Provides excellent visualization of the facial nerve and anterior brainstem, does not require cerebellar manipulation, better at preserving facial function.	Hearing sacrifice is unavoidable, some tumors may be difficult to access, a fat graft is required, and the sigmoid sinus is more prone to injury.
Middle Fossa	Can expose the lateral third of the internal auditory canal with hearing preservation, is extradural. Recommended for smaller tumors (1.5 cm) with goal of hearing preservation.	Limited access to posterior fossa, requires temporal retraction, facial nerve more vulnerable to injury, dural lacerations likely in older pts, may cause trismus from temporalis muscle injury.

Chemotherapy: There is no role for systemic therapy with vestibular schwannoma, although bevacizumab has shown response in rare progressive situations associated with NF2.

Radiation: Several options for treatment of VS with RT exist. Stereotactic radiosurgery (SRS; with GKRS or LINAC-based radiosurgery), fractionated stereotactic radiation therapy (FSRT), and proton beam RT have been used to treat pts. RT is appropriate for pts in whom the tumor is <3 to 4 cm in size,[23] or for whom surgery is not an option or refused.

SRS: Doses above 12.5 to 13 Gy are associated with increased morbidity with regard to facial paralysis, trigeminal neuralgia, and hearing loss.[24,25] Long-term results show >95% control with minimal morbidity or impact on QOL. Impact on hearing preservation is controversial with some series showing continued long-term decline[26] and others showing no significant difference compared to pts undergoing observation.[27] In a series of 440 pts with long-term follow-up, one pt (0.3%) developed malignant transformation.[28]

FSRT: Treatments can range from 20 Gy/4 fx to 57.6 Gy/32 fx, although typical dose is 25 Gy/5 fx if hypofractionated or 45–54 Gy/25–30 fx if conventional fractionation. Controversy exists whether FSRT is superior to SRS, but it is recommended with larger tumors (>3–4 cm) and to spare normal structures (brainstem, cochlea, etc.) if close in proximity.

Procedure: See *Treatment Planning Handbook*, Chapter 3.[29]

EVIDENCE-BASED Q&A

What are the outcomes of treatment with surgical resection for pts with VS?

Surgical resection is generally technically achievable with high rates of control. The risk of significant complications is low. There may be a lower rate of complications with maximal safe resection allowing for residual tumor rather than attempted GTR in all pts. However, pts who undergo subtotal resection are at a higher risk of recurrence than pts who undergo GTR or NTR.

Gormley, George Washington University (*Neurosurgery* 1997, PMID 9218295): RR of 179 pts treated at a single institution. MFU 65 mos. Most were operated on using a retrosigmoid approach. House–Brackmann post-op facial nerve function was Grade I or II in 96% of small tumors (≤2 cm), 74% of medium tumors (2–3.9 cm), and 38% of large tumors (≥4 cm). Functional hearing preservation (Gardner–Robertson Class I or II) was achieved in 48% of small tumors and 25% of medium tumors. CSF leak was the most common complication (15%). Two pts died (1%) and one pt experienced cerebellar and brainstem injury causing permanent disability. No pts with complete resection (99%) experienced recurrence.

Samii, Hannover, Germany (*Neurosurgery* 1997, PMID 8971819): RR of 1,000 consecutive pts with VS resected by suboccipital approach between 1978 and 1993. 98% of tumors were completely removed. Anatomic preservation of the facial nerve and the cochlear nerve was achieved in 93% and 68%, respectively. Major neurologic complications included tetraparesis in one pt, hemiparesis in 1%, lower cranial nerve palsies in 5.5%, and cerebrospinal fluid fistulas in 9.2%. There were 11 deaths (1.1%) occurring at 2 to 69 days postoperatively.

Carlson, Mayo Clinic (*Laryngoscope* 2012, PMID 22252688): RR of 203 pts treated at single institution. MFU 3.5 years. Pts were classified by GTR, NTR, or STR. 144 pts underwent GTR, 32 received NTR, and 27 received STR. Twelve pts (5.9%) had a recurrence at a mean of 3.0 years after surgery. 5-yr RFS was estimated at 91.0%. Pts who received STR were 9 times more likely to fail than pts undergoing NTR or GTR. There was no significant difference between pts with NTR and GTR. Pts with nodular enhancement on initial post-op MRI had a 16-fold higher risk of recurrence compared to pts with linear patterns.

Bloch, UCSF (*Otolaryngol Head Neck Surg* 2004, PMID 14726918): RR of 79 pts treated at a single institution. In pts with adequate follow-up (mean f/u in this cohort 5 years), 1 of 33 (3%) of pts with NTR recurrence compared with 6 of 19 (32%) of pts with STR.

Which patients should undergo surgery for VS?

Sughrue, UCSF (*J Clin Neurosci* 2010, PMID 20627586): Meta-analysis of hearing outcome after microsurgery for VS, analyzing 49 articles including 998 pts. Follow-up ranged from 6 mos to 7 years. On univariate analysis, rates of hearing preservation declined with increasing age, tumor size (pts with tumors >1.5 cm had <37% hearing preservation). Pts undergoing surgery via the middle cranial fossa approach had better hearing outcomes on univariate analysis (63% vs. 47%). On multivariate analysis, tumor size >1.5 cm and the retrosigmoid approach were independent factors predicting for loss of serviceable hearing.

How does SRS compare to observation?

SRS appears to have limited impact on quality of life compared to observation.

Breivik, Norway (*Neurosurgery* 2013, PMID 23615094): Prospective cohort study of pts who underwent GKRS (113) or observation (124). Pts underwent GKRS either with small tumors (<20 mm) after growth was observed by referring physician (31 pts) or by pt choice (26 pts), or tumors >20 mm who refused surgery. Pts treated with GKRS received 12 Gy to the tumor periphery. MFU 55 mos. Serviceable hearing was lost in 76% of pts on observation and 64% of pts treated with GKRS (NS). Pts treated with GKRS had significantly less need for future treatment. Symptoms and QOL did not differ between groups. **Conclusion: GKRS prevents need for further treatment and appears not to significantly impact rates of hearing loss, symptoms, or QOL compared to observation.**

How does RT compare to microsurgical resection?

Generally, studies have shown equivalent tumor control with radiosurgery compared to microsurgical resection. Studies have generally shown better functional outcomes and less impact on quality of life with SRS. However, there is no consensus on the optimal management. The ideal population of pts for each modality overlaps (small tumors with preserved hearing) but surgery may be preferred in larger tumors, especially in pts with mass effect.

Pollock, Mayo Clinic (*Neurosurgery* 2006, PMID 16823303): Prospective cohort study of 82 pts with unilateral <3 cm VS undergoing surgical resection (n = 36) or GKRS (n = 46). GKRS mean dose 12.2 Gy to tumor margin, mean max dose 26.4 Gy. MFU 42 mos. Results: No difference in tumor control (100% vs. 96% $p = .50$). GKRS pts had better facial nerve preservation at 3 mos (100% vs. 69% $p < .001$), 1 yr (100% vs. 69%, $p < .001$) and last f/u (100% vs. 75%, $p < .01$). GKRS pts had better hearing preservation at 3 mos (77% vs. 5%, $p < .001$), 1 yr (63% vs. 5%, $p < .001$) and last f/u (63% vs. 5%, $p < .001$). GKRS pts had better physical functioning, energy, and pain at 3 mos, 1 yr and last f/u. **Conclusion: Similar tumor control with GKRS or surgery, but less morbidity with GKRS.**

Maniakas, Montreal (*Otol Neurotol* 2012, PMID 22996165): Meta-analysis of 16 studies comparing microsurgical resection and SRS. Overall, SRS showed significantly better long-term hearing preservation rates than microsurgery (70.2% vs. 50.3%, respectively, $p < .001$). Crude rates of long-term tumor progression were not significantly different between SRS and microsurgery (3.8% and 1.3%, respectively).

Régis, Marseille, France (*J Neurosurg* 2002, PMID 12450031): Prospective analysis of functional outcome and QOL of pts with 4 years of f/u after GKRS or microsurgical resection. Of pts who underwent GKRS compared to microsurgery, 100% versus 63%

had no new facial weakness, 49% versus 17% had no ocular symptoms, 91% versus 61% had no functional deterioration after treatment, 100% versus 56% kept the same professional activity after treatment, and 70% versus 37.5% of pts with preoperative Gardner–Robertson Class 1 hearing preserved Class 1 or 2 hearing after treatment. **Conclusion: Side effects occur during the first 2 years and GKRS provides better functional outcomes than microsurgery.**

What are the long-term results of SRS?

Long-term results for SRS show excellent local control. However, with longer term follow-up, it appears that rates of hearing preservation may continue to decline.

Lunsford, Pittsburgh (*J Neurosurg* 2005, PMID 15662809): RR of 829 pts treated with GKRS between 1987 and 2002. Median marginal dose was 13 Gy. 10-yr tumor control rate was 97%. Facial neuropathy was experienced by <1% of pts and trigeminal symptoms by <3%. Hearing preservation in 50% to 77%.

Hasegawa, Japan (*J Neurosurg* 2013, PMID 23140152): RR of 440 pts treated with GKRS between May 1991 and December 2000. MFU 12.5 years. Actuarial 5- and 10-year PFS was 93% and 92%, respectively. No pt failed >10 years after treatment. On multivariate analysis, significant brainstem compression, marginal dose ≤13 Gy, prior treatment, and female sex correlated with decreased PFS. Pts treated with ≤13 Gy had an increased rate of facial nerve preservation (100% vs. 97%). Ten pts (2.3%) developed delayed cyst formation. One pt (0.03%) developed malignant transformation.

Carlson, Mayo Clinic (*J Neurosurg* 2013, PMID 23101446): RR of 44 pts with long-term audiometric follow-up after SRS. SRS was given with 12 to 13 Gy to the periphery of the tumor. MFU 9.3 years. Thirty-six pts developed nonserviceable hearing at mean of 4.2 years after SRS. The Kaplan–Meier estimated rates of serviceable hearing at 1, 3, 5, 7, and 10 years following SRS were 80%, 55%, 48%, 38%, and 23%, respectively. Multivariate analysis revealed that pretreatment ipsilateral pure tone average ($p < .001$) and tumor size ($p = .009$) were statistically significantly associated with time to nonserviceable hearing.

Can SRS be used for larger tumors (>3 cm)?

Yang, Pittsburgh (*J Neurosurg* 2011, PMID 20799863): RR of 65 pts with VS between 3 and 4 cm in one extracanalicular maximum diameter (median tumor volume 9 ml) who underwent GKRS. Seventeen pts (26%) had previously undergone resection. MFU was 36 mos . Two years later, 7 tumors (11%) had grown. Eighteen (82%) of 22 pts with serviceable hearing before SRS still had serviceable hearing after SRS more than 2 years later. Three pts (5%) developed symptomatic hydrocephalus and underwent placement of a VP shunt. In four pts (6%) trigeminal sensory dysfunction developed, and in one pt (2%) mild facial weakness (House–Brackmann Grade II) developed after SRS. In univariate analysis, pts who had a previous resection ($p = .010$), those with a tumor volume exceeding 10 ml ($p = .05$), and those with Koos Grade 4 tumors ($p = .02$) had less likelihood of tumor control after SRS.

How does fractionated radiotherapy compare to SRS?

Fractionation offers a theoretical radiobiological advantage compared to single-fraction treatment, which should allow for improved sparing of normal structures. However, likely due to selection bias, evidence for differences in outcome between SRS and five-fraction or longer treatment courses is limited and possibly limited to improvement in hearing preservation.

Andrews, Thomas Jefferson (*IJROBP* 2001, PMID 11483338): RR of 125 pts with VS treated with either GKRS (n = 69) or FSRT (n = 56). Pts treated with GKRS received 12 Gy to the 50% isodose line and pts treated with FSRT were treated with 50 Gy/25 fx. MFU 119 wks for GKRS and 115 wks for FSRT. No difference in tumor control was seen between GKRS and FSRT (98% vs. 97%). At 1-year f/u, FSRT showed better hearing preservation than GK (81% vs. 33%, p = .0228). No difference was seen in any other side effect rates.

Coombs, Heidelberg (*IJROBP* 2010, PMID 19604653): Prospective cohort study of 200 pts with 202 VS treated with either LINAC-based SRS (30) or FSRT (n = 172). Pts treated with SRS received 13 Gy to 80% isodose line and pts treated with FSRT received a median of 57.6 Gy/32 fx. MFU 75 mos. No difference was seen in 5-yr tumor control (96% overall). FSRT and SRS showed equivalent hearing preservation (76% at 5 yrs) for SRS dose ≤13 Gy. For SRS dose >13 Gy (11 pts), hearing preservation was significantly worse than FSRT. Both pts who developed trigeminal neuralgia in the SRS group were treated with >13 Gy. Rate of facial nerve weakness was 17% in SRS group and 2% in FSRT group. Only one pt treated with SRS to ≤13 Gy developed facial weakness. **Conclusion: SRS with doses of ≤13 Gy is a safe and effective alternative to FSRT. FSRT should be reserved for larger lesions.**

Meijer, Netherlands (*IJROBP* 2003, PMID 12873685): RR of 129 consecutive pts treated with either single-fraction or five-fraction RT using LINAC-based SRS techniques. Pts were prospectively selected for single fraction if edentate and five fractions if dentate due to the immobilization device used. Pts in the single-fraction arm were treated with 10 to 12.5 Gy and in the five-fraction arm were treated with 20 to 25 Gy. Pts in the single-fraction arm were older (mean age 63 years vs. 49 years) but there were no other significant differences between groups. There were no significant differences in outcome between single-fraction and five-fraction treatment groups in terms of 5-year LC (100% vs. 94%), facial nerve preservation (93% vs. 97%) and hearing preservation (75% vs. 61%). Five-year trigeminal nerve preservation was significantly different (92% vs. 98%, p = .048).

REFERENCES

1. Babu R, Sharma R, Bagley JH, et al. Vestibular schwannomas in the modern era: epidemiology, treatment trends, and disparities in management. *J Neurosurg.* 2013;119(1):121–130.
2. Propp JM, McCarthy BJ, Davis FG, Preston-Martin S. Descriptive epidemiology of vestibular schwannomas. *Neuro Oncol.* 2006;8(1):1–11.
3. Shore-Freedman E, Abrahams C, Recant W, Schneider AB. Neurilemomas and salivary gland tumors of the head and neck following childhood irradiation. *Cancer.* 1983;51(12):2159–2163.
4. Sobel RA. Vestibular (acoustic) schwannomas: histologic features in neurofibromatosis 2 and in unilateral cases. *J Neuropathol Exp Neurol.* 1993;52(2):106–113.
5. Sughrue ME, Yeung AH, Rutkowski MJ, et al. Molecular biology of familial and sporadic vestibular schwannomas: implications for novel therapeutics. *J Neurosurg.* 2011;114(2):359–366.
6. Matthies C, Samii M. Management of 1,000 vestibular schwannomas (acoustic neuromas): clinical presentation. *Neurosurgery.* 1997;40(1):1–9; discussion 9–10.
7. Doyle KJ. Is there still a role for auditory brainstem response audiometry in the diagnosis of acoustic neuroma? *Arch Otolaryngol Head Neck Surg.* 1999;125(2):232–234.
8. Schmalbrock P, Chakeres DW, Monroe JW, et al. Assessment of internal auditory canal tumors: a comparison of contrast-enhanced T1-weighted and steady-state T2-weighted gradient-echo MR imaging. *AJNR.* 1999;20(7):1207–1213.
9. DeLong M, Kaylie D, Kranz PG, Adamson DC. Vestibular schwannomas: lessons for the neurosurgeon: part I: diagnosis, neuroimaging, and audiology. *Contemp Neurosurg.* 2011;33(20):1–5.
10. House JW, Brackmann DE. Facial nerve grading system. *Otolaryngol Head Neck Surg.* 1985;93(2):146–147.
11. Gardner G, Robertson JH. Hearing preservation in unilateral acoustic neuroma surgery. *Ann Otol Rhinol Laryngol.* 1988;97(1):55–66.

12. Bakkouri WE, Kania RE, Guichard JP, et al. Conservative management of 386 cases of unilateral vestibular schwannoma: tumor growth and consequences for treatment. *J Neurosurg.* 2009;110(4):662–669.

13. Stangerup SE, Tos M, Thomsen J, Caye-Thomasen P. Hearing outcomes of vestibular schwannoma patients managed with 'wait and scan': predictive value of hearing level at diagnosis. *J Laryngol Otol.* 2010;124(5):490–494.

14. Sughrue ME, Kane AJ, Kaur R, et al. A prospective study of hearing preservation in untreated vestibular schwannomas. *J Neurosurg.* 2011;114(2):381–385.

15. Sughrue ME, Yang I, Aranda D, et al. The natural history of untreated sporadic vestibular schwannomas: a comprehensive review of hearing outcomes. *J Neurol.* 2010;112(1):163–167.

16. Smouha EE, Yoo M, Mohr K, Davis RP. Conservative management of acoustic neuroma: a meta-analysis and proposed treatment algorithm. *Laryngoscope.* 2005;115(3):450–454.

17. Koos WT, Day JD, Matula C, Levy DI. Neurotopographic considerations in the microsurgical treatment of small acoustic neurinomas. *J Neurol.* 1998;88(3):506–512.

18. Gormley WB, Sekhar LN, Wright DC, et al. Acoustic neuromas: results of current surgical management. *Neurosurgery.* 1997;41(1):50–58; discussion 58–60.

19. Samii M, Matthies C. Management of 1,000 vestibular schwannomas (acoustic neuromas): surgical management and results with an emphasis on complications and how to avoid them. *Neurosurgery.* 1997;40(1):11–21; discussion 21–13.

20. Carlson ML, Link MJ, Wanna GB, Driscoll CL. Management of sporadic vestibular schwannoma. *Otolaryngol Clin North Am.* 2015;48(3):407–422.

21. Lanman TH, Brackmann DE, Hitselberger WE, Subin B. Report of 190 consecutive cases of large acoustic tumors (vestibular schwannoma) removed via the translabyrinthine approach. *J Neurosurg.* 1999;90(4):617–623.

22. Rangel-Castilla L, Russin JJ, Spetzler RF. Surgical management of skull base tumors. *Rep Pract Oncol Radiother.* 2016;21(4):325–335.

23. Yang HC, Kano H, Awan NR, et al. Gamma knife radiosurgery for larger-volume vestibular schwannomas. *J Neurosurg.* 2011;114(3):801–807.

24. Mendenhall WM, Friedman WA, Buatti JM, Bova FJ. Preliminary results of linear accelerator radiosurgery for acoustic schwannomas. *J Neurosurg.* 1996;85(6):1013–1019.

25. Combs SE, Welzel T, Schulz-Ertner D, et al. Differences in clinical results after LINAC-based single-dose radiosurgery versus fractionated stereotactic radiotherapy for patients with vestibular schwannomas. *Int J Radiat Oncol Biol Phys.* 2010;76(1):193–200.

26. Carlson ML, Jacob JT, Pollock BE, et al. Long-term hearing outcomes following stereotactic radiosurgery for vestibular schwannoma: patterns of hearing loss and variables influencing audiometric decline. *J Neurosurg.* 2013;118(3):579–587.

27. Breivik CN, Nilsen RM, Myrseth E, et al. Conservative management or gamma knife radiosurgery for vestibular schwannoma: tumor growth, symptoms, and quality of life. *Neurosurgery.* 2013;73(1):48–56; discussion 56–47.

28. Hasegawa T, Kida Y, Kato T, et al. Long-term safety and efficacy of stereotactic radiosurgery for vestibular schwannomas: evaluation of 440 patients more than 10 years after treatment with gamma knife surgery. *J Neurosurg.* 2013;118(3):557–565.

29. Videtic GMM, Woody N, Vassil AD. *Handbook of Treatment Planning in Radiation Oncology.* 2nd ed. New York, NY: Demos Medical Publishing; 2015.

9: UVEAL (CHOROIDAL) MELANOMA

Gaurav Marwaha, John H. Suh, and Arun D. Singh

QUICK HIT: Uveal melanoma (UM) is unrelated to cutaneous melanoma and was historically managed with enucleation. Now, the standard of care for small- to medium-sized tumors is episcleral plaque brachytherapy, which offers excellent tumor control and useful vision-sparing capacity. Diagnosis is often made without biopsy by a well-trained ophthalmologist at an office exam with ultrasound assistance. It is imperative to rule out distant metastases on workup, particularly liver metastases with dedicated CT/MRI.

General treatment paradigm: Very small, asymptomatic tumors (T1a) can be observed until growth/symptoms occur, at which point treatment should be offered. Small to medium-small tumors (<5 mm apical height) are probably best treated with ^{106}Ru plaque brachytherapy to 85 Gy although ^{125}I is often used. Medium-sized tumors (up to 1 cm, generally) are best treated with ^{125}I plaque brachytherapy to 85 Gy. LC for small/medium sized UM is in the 90% to 100% range, with 5-yr OS >80%. Larger tumors are best managed with enucleation. Control rates are approximately 70% with 5-yr OS approximately 60%.

EPIDEMIOLOGY: Uncommon with 1,500 to 2,000 cases/year. Most common primary eye tumor in adults, most commonly affects fair-skinned individuals with a median age of 60.

RISK FACTORS: Vast majority are sporadic. However, the following factors may increase risk: fair iris/skin color, propensity to sunburn, UV exposure (questionable), oculodermal melanocytosis.[1-3]

ANATOMY: The posterior uvea is composed of the choroid (i.e., the retina's vascular support layer), which is where light-protective melanocytes reside. The anterior uvea is the iris of the eye and ciliary body (which controls accommodation and lens movement). The entire uveal tract lies beneath the sclera (the white, fibrous protective layer of the eye).

PATHOLOGY: Uveal melanocytes arise from neural crest cells. The degree of pigmentation determines iris color. Pathologic types: spindle cell (best prognosis), mixed (majority of cases), and epithelioid (worst prognosis).

GENETICS: Unlike cutaneous melanoma, UM is not associated with BRAF or BRAS gene mutations. GNAQ and GNA11 mutations are evident early in the tumorigenesis process; also increasing evidence of families with germline BAP-1 mutations.[2] Combination of monosomy 3 and 8q gain associated with metastasis.

CLINICAL PRESENTATION: Visual symptoms (distortion, visual field loss, scotomas, floaters), retinal detachment (larger tumors), and rarely pain/eye inflammation. One-third of patients are asymptomatic.

WORKUP: Ophthalmologist can make clinical diagnosis 95% of the time.[2] Diagnostic techniques should include: slit lamp, indirect ophthalmoscopy, fundus photography, transillumination, fluorescein angiography, and ocular ultrasound (for tumor height/

diameter). Typical UMs are subretinal, brown, raised, and dome-shaped. Internal extension of tumor results in a mushroom-shaped mass apparent on ultrasonography. Biopsy is indicated in clinically atypical tumors and is also helpful for prognostication.[2] Differential diagnosis includes: metastases, benign nevus, hemangioma, retinal detachment. Metastatic evaluation: CT abdomen (MRI if highly concerned for liver metastases or if CT equivocal).

PROGNOSTIC FACTORS: Poor prognostic factors include epithelioid cell, large tumor, involvement of ciliary body, older age.

NATURAL HISTORY: The uvea lacks lymphatic channels; thus metastases from the uvea spread hematogenously to liver (90% of metastases), skin, and lungs. After RT, tumors tend to regress slowly over a few years. Useful vision (>20/200) is preserved in 50% of pts with tumor size and location being the main drivers for visual outcomes (i.e., >6 mm tumors and proximity to optic nerve/fovea predict for worse visual outcomes).

STAGING

TABLE 9.1: AJCC 8th ed. Staging (2017) for Uveal Melanoma*				
Iris Melanoma				
T1	**a** Limited to the iris, ≤3 clock hours in size	**N**	**a** Metastasis in ≥1 regional LN	
			b No regional LNs, but discrete tumor deposits in orbit, not contiguous to the eye	
	b Limited to the iris, >3 clock hours in size	**M1**	**a** Distant metastasis, all ≤3.0 cm	
	c Limited to the iris with secondary glaucoma	**M1**	**b** Distant metastasis, largest 3.1-8 cm	
T2	**a** Confluent with or extending into ciliary body without secondary glaucoma	**M1**	**c** Distant metastasis, largest ≥8.0 cm	
	b Confluent with or extending into ciliary body and choroid, without secondary glaucoma	**Group Staging**		
	c Confluent with or extending into the ciliary body, choroid or both with secondary glaucoma	I	T1aN0M0	
		IIA	T1b-dN0M0, T2aN0M0	
T3	• Confluent with or extending into the ciliary body, choroid or both with scleral extension	IIB	T2bN0M0, T3aN0M0	
T4	**a** Episcleral extension ≤5 mm in largest diameter	IIIA	T2c-dN0M0, T3b-cN0M0, T4aN0M0	
	b Episcleral extension >5 mm largest diameter	IIIB	T3dN0M0, T4b-cN0	
	Choroidal & Ciliary Body Melanoma	IIIC	T4d-eN0M0	
T1	**a** Size category 1 without ciliary body involvement and extracellular extension	IV	Any T, N1M0 or Any T, Any N, M1a-c	
	b Size category 1 with ciliary body involvement			
	c Size category 1 without ciliary body involvement but with extraocular extension ≤5 mm			
	d Size category 1 with ciliary body involvement and extraocular extension ≤5 mm			

(continued)

TABLE 9.1: AJCC 8th ed. Staging (2017) for Uveal Melanoma* (*continued*)

		Choroidal & Ciliary Body Melanoma
T2	a	Size category 2 without ciliary body involvement or extraocular extension
	b	Size category 2 with ciliary body involvement
	c	Size category 2 without ciliary body involvement, with extraocular extension ≤5 mm
	d	Size category 2 with ciliary body involvement and extraocular extension ≤5 mm
T3	a	Size category 3 without ciliary body involvement and extraocular extension
	b	Size category 3 with ciliary body involvement
	c	Size category 3 without ciliary body involvement, with extraocular extension ≤5 mm
	d	Size category 3 with ciliary body involvement and extraocular extension ≤5 mm
T4	a	Size category 4 without ciliary body involvement and extraocular extension
	b	Size category 4 with ciliary body involvement
	c	Size category 4 without ciliary body involvement but with extraocular extension ≤5 mm
	d	Size category 4 with ciliary body involvement and extraocular extension ≤5 mm
	e	Any size category with extraocular extension >5 mm

Notes: *Because of the intricacy of the above AJCC staging, in practice and in most studies, the COMS staging system is utilized. It is broken into three groups: Small—1–3 mm in apical height and 5–16 mm across (>90% 5-yr OS); Medium—3.1–8 mm in apical height and <16 mm across (80%–85% 5-yr OS); Large—>8 mm in apical height or >16 mm across (60% 5-yr OS).*

TABLE 9.2: Size Categories (Ciliary Body and Choroidal Uveal Melanoma)

Thickness (mm)							
>15					4	4	4
12.1–15.0				3	3	4	4
9.1–12.0		3	3	3	3	3	4
6.1–9.0	2	2	2	2	3	3	4
3.1–6.0	1	1	1	2	2	3	4
≤3.0	1	1	1	1	2	2	4

(continued)

TABLE 9.2: Size Categories (Ciliary Body and Choroidal Uveal Melanoma) (*continued*)							
Thickness (mm)							
	≤3.0	3.1–6.0	6.1–9.0	9.1–12.0	12.1–15.0	15.1–18.0	>18.0
	Largest Basal Diameter (mm)						

TREATMENT PARADIGM

Observation: Reasonable for asymptomatic T1a lesions, with close ophthalmic surveillance q3 to 6 months (treat for any growth or symptoms).

Surgery: Enucleation was the historic standard of care, but in the 2000s, episcleral brachytherapy became the first-line treatment for small- to medium-sized (<10 mm in apical height) tumors and offered equivalent survival with vision-sparing capability. *Enucleation* under general anesthesia, with orbital implant continues to be used when brachytherapy is not feasible (i.e., for larger tumors, poor functional outcome predicted with brachytherapy). For select larger tumors, in an effort to avoid radiation side effects, fragmentation and vitreous cutter *endoresection* can be performed a few weeks post brachytherapy.[2] Definitive, local resection (*exoresection*) may be feasible as well, in select anterior or large tumors. *Orbital exenteration* is utilized in the setting of massive orbital extension causing pain/blindness.

Chemotherapy: In stage IV disease, cytotoxic agents are of limited benefit, as is ipilimumab (anti-CTLA4), though both are still utilized. For isolated liver metastases, locally ablative therapies are employed (e.g., chemoembolization, metastectomy, RFA, internal/external radiation).

Radiation

- *Episcleral brachytherapy* typically with ^{125}I or ^{106}Ru (more common in Europe and better for smaller tumors as it offers a more rapid dose fall-off) radionuclides. The half-lives of ^{125}I and ^{106}Ru are 60 days and 374 days, respectively. Plaques are generally gold-plated, with grooves in which radiation sources are glued or molded. The plaques come in a variety of shapes/sizes to accommodate critical vision structures. The plaques contain eyelets, which the ophthalmologist will use to suture the plaque onto the episcleral surface overlying the tumor with a 2-mm margin of safety, under general anesthesia. The ophthalmologist will make a conjunctival peritomy; then the globe is transilluminated and tumor outlined. Next, a dummy plaque is used to verify the proper position. Then, the radioactive plaque is placed. Dose is 85 Gy (at a dose rate of 0.6–1.05 Gy/h) prescribed to 5 mm from inner scleral surface unless the tumor is >5 mm, in which case prescription is to apex of tumor.[4] The plaque remains in place for 3 to 7 days, during which time he or she wears a lead eye shield. The plaque is removed by the ophthalmologist and the pt returns home with bandages and pain medications.
- *Proton beam radiation* (50–70 CGE in 5 fx over 7–10 days) is utilized at some institutions with acceptable toxicity rates (difficult to administer because it requires the patient to fixate eye on a certain point in space such that the tumor is within the proton beam path).

Side Effects: Acute: pain (brachy), rarely dry eye. Late: vasculopathy (driven by disc/fovea proximity), cataract formation (especially, anterior tumors), maculopathy, retinopathy (most common side effect with brachy), optic neuropathy.

Other modalities: Transpupillary thermotherapy is associated with high risk of local recurrence alone, but can easily be combined with brachytherapy as an adjunct. For radiation failures, transpupillary thermotherapy or repeat brachytherapy can be employed.[5]

EVIDENCE-BASED Q&A

Small tumors

Is it necessary to treat all small uveal melanomas?

No, risk of death is low provided pts are serially monitored with ophthalmologic exams. Significant growth on follow-up exams is an indication for treatment.

COMS Report No. 5, "Small" Choroidal Melanoma Series (*Arch Ophthalmol* 1997, **PMID 9400787):** Nonrandomized prospective study of 204 pts with **small** choroidal melanomas (i.e., 1–3 mm height and ≥5 mm in basal diameter). MFU was 92 months. Eight percent of pts were treated at study enrollment and 33% were treated during follow-up. Tumor growth noted in 21% at 2 years and 31% at 5 years. Twenty-seven pts died, 6 from distant metastases. Five-yr OS 94% and 8-yr OS 85%. **Conclusion: Majority of pts with "small" choroidal melanomas (66%) may represent choroidal nevus and therefore can be closely monitored. Observation of small tumors may be appropriate until progression is noted.**

What factors determine the use of each isotope (^{125}I vs. ^{106}Ru)?

^{106}Ru offers a more rapid dose fall-off than ^{125}I, which may aid in sparing critical vision structures in the management of smaller tumors (<5 mm) without compromising oncologic outcomes.

Takiar, MD Anderson (*PRO 2015*, **PMID 25423888):** RR of 107 pts treated with ^{125}I (67) or ^{106}Ru (40). ^{106}Ru: 5-yr local control, PFS, and OS: 97%, 94%, and 92%, respectively. ^{125}I: 5-yr local control, PFS, and OS were 83%, 65%, and 80%, respectively. In pts with apical tumor height ≤5 mm, PFS was slightly better for ^{106}Ru ($p = .02$). Enucleation-free survival was better in ^{106}Ru pts ($p = .02$) as were radiation retinopathy ($p = .03$) and cataracts ($p < .01$). **Conclusion: Both isotopes offer excellent local control for small uveal melanomas, though ^{106}Ru does so with reduced toxicity.**

Medium tumors

How does the historic standard of enucleation compare to episcleral plaque brachytherapy?

No difference in overall survival. Eye and vision sparing with brachytherapy. In the rare event of radiation failure, pts can be salvaged effectively with enucleation.

COMS Report No.28, "I-125 vs. Enucleation" (*Arch Ophthalmol* 2006, **PMID 17159027):** PRT of 1,317 pts with medium-sized choroidal melanomas (≥2.5–10 mm height and <16 mm in largest basal diameter)—enucleation versus episcleral plaque brachytherapy with ^{125}I (85 Gy was Rx dose). Exclusions: fovea/optic disc/ciliary body involvement. Thirteen percent of episcleral plaque pts were salvaged (due to tumor progression or RT complications) with enucleation by 5 years.

TABLE 9.3: Results of COMS 28 Trial of I-125 Versus Enucleation for Choroidal Melanoma							
	5- and 12-yr OS	12-yr DMFS		I-125 arm	Median Visual Acuity	20/40 or Better	20/200 or Worse
Enucleation	81%/59%	17%		Baseline	20/32	70%	10%
I-125 plaque 85 Gy	82%/57%	21%		3 yrs after I-125	20/125	34%	45%
p value	NS	NS					

Conclusion: Episcleral plaque brachytherapy offers equivalent OS and DMFS compared to enucleation. This PRT set the precedent for plaque brachytherapy as the standard of care in this pt population.

Large tumors

Can neoadjuvant radiation improve surgical outcomes for large uveal melanoma?

Enucleation yields the best results for larger tumors, and also for pts in whom poor visual outcome would be expected with plaque brachytherapy (e.g., tumors adjacent to optic disc). Neoadjuvant EBRT did not improve outcomes on COMS 15.

COMS Report No. 15, "Large Tumors" (*Arch Ophtho* 2001, PMID 11346394): PRT of 1,003 pts with large choroidal melanomas (≥2 mm height and >16 mm in largest basal diameter or >10 mm in height regardless of diameter, or >8 mm in height if <2 mm from optic disc)—enucleation versus preoperative 20 Gy/5 fx EBRT + enucleation. Preoperative EBRT did not increase complication rate, but did have fewer local recurrences (zero vs. five). Distant metastases were most commonly seen in liver (93%), lung (24%), and bone (16%).

TABLE 9.4: Results of COMS 15 Trial of Neoadjuvant EBRT for Large Uveal Melanomas		
	5-yr OS	5-yr DSS
Enucleation alone	57%	72%
Pre-op EBRT 20 Gy + Enucleation	62%	74%
p value	.32	.64

Other radiotherapeutic options

How does plaque brachytherapy compare to external beam/heavy ion/charged particle irradiation?

Early studies suggest no difference in overall survival though with increased complications. However, some institutions are using proton beam radiation with favorable outcomes (albeit without any PRTs).

Char, UCSF (*Ophthalmology* 1993, PMID 8414414): PRT of 184 pts randomized to helium ion 70 Gy/5 fx versus episcleral plaque brachytherapy (^{125}I) for tumors <10 mm height and <15 mm diameter. Helium ion therapy had greater local control (100% vs. 83%), comparable survival, and fewer salvage enucleations (9% vs. 17%), however with more anterior complications (dry eye, neovascular glaucoma, epiphora).

Caujolle, Nice, France (*IJROBP* 2010, PMID 19910136): RR of 886 pts with UM (95% were T2-3) treated with proton beam RT. MFU 5.3 years. Five-yr/10-yr local control 94%/92%; 5-yr/10-yr OS by T stage: T1 92%/86%; T2 89%/78%; T3 67%/43%; T4 62%/41%. Eye preservation at 5-yr/10-yr was 91%/87%. Predictors for death: advanced age, greater tumor thickness and basal diameter, higher volume/eyeball ratio.

REFERENCES

1. Weis E, Shah CP, Lajous M, et al. The association between host susceptibility factors and uveal melanoma: a meta-analysis. *Arch Ophthalmol*. 2006; 124(1):54–60.
2. Seregard S, Pelayes D, Singh AD. Radiation therapy: uveal tumors. In: Singh AD. *Ophthalmic Radiation Therapy: Techniques and Application*. Basel, Switzerland: Karger; 2013; 52:36–57.

3. Singh AD, Rennie IG, Seregard S, et al. Sunlight exposure and pathogenesis of uveal melanoma. *Surv Ophthalmol.* 2004;49(4):419–428.
4. Marwaha G, Macklis R, Singh AD, Wilkinson A. Brachytherapy. In: Singh AD. *Ophthalmic Radiation Therapy: Techniques and Application.* Basel, Switzerland: Karger; 2013; 52:29–35.
5. Bellerive C, Aziz HA, Bena J, et al. Local failure after episcleral brachytherapy for posterior uveal melanoma: patterns, risk factors and management. *Am J Ophthalmol.* 2017;177:9–16.

II: HEAD AND NECK

10: OROPHARYNX CANCER

Shireen Parsai, Nikhil P. Joshi, and Shlomo A. Koyfman

> **QUICK HIT:** Squamous cell carcinoma of oropharynx is currently the most common head and neck (H&N) cancer in the United States. Its incidence continues to rise with increasing prevalence of HPV. There are two distinct etiologies: those associated with tobacco and alcohol, which are often HPV-negative, and those associated with HPV infection. These are now classified as two distinct diseases as per the AJCC 8th edition staging system. Both are currently treated with the same approach, but treatment paradigms are evolving to account for differences in natural history.

TABLE 10.1: General Treatment Paradigm for Oropharynx Cancer	
	Treatment Options
T1-2N0-1	TORS (or other function-preserving surgery), neck dissection, and risk-adapted adjuvant therapy (Chapter 18) Or Definitive IMRT
T3-4 and/or N1-3	Definitive chemoRT Or Surgery (select pts) with risk-adapted postoperative RT ± CHT

EPIDEMIOLOGY: Estimated 32,520 tongue and pharynx cases in 2016 with 5,370 deaths.[1] Male-to-female ratio approximately 4:1.[2] In the United States, incidence of HPV-associated OPC increased by 225% from 1988 to 2004 and HPV-negative cancer declined by 50% in same time frame.[3] Prevalence of HPV was quoted as 39.5% on RTOG, which increased to 68% on RTOG 0129 and further to 73% on RTOG 0522.[4-6] Peak prevalence of oral HPV DNA is bimodal: 7% for ages 30 to 34 and 11% for ages 60 to 64.[4]

RISK FACTORS: Age, high-risk sexual behavior (HPV+), tobacco, alcohol (HPV-).[4,7]

ANATOMY: Oropharynx consists of base of tongue, vallecula, palatine tonsil, soft palate, and posterior oropharyngeal wall. The superior border of the OPX is the soft palate and the inferior border is the hyoid/lingual surface of the epiglottis. The base of tongue is separated from the oral tongue by the circumvallate papillae. The base of tongue is the posterior 1/3 of the tongue and composed of lingual lymphatic tissue. The palatine tonsils sit between an arch formed by the anterior and posterior tonsillar pillars.

TABLE 10.2: Oropharynx Borders	
Site	**Boundaries**
Base of Tongue (BOT)	Anteriorly by circumvallate papillae, laterally by glossopalatine sulci, and inferiorly by vallecula. Includes pharyngoepiglottic and glossoepiglottic fold.

(continued)

TABLE 10.2: Oropharynx Borders (*continued*)	
Site	Boundaries
Tonsillar complex	Composed of anterior and posterior tonsillar pillars, true palatine tonsil, and tonsillar fossa. Tonsillar pillars are mucosal folds over glossopalatine and pharyngopalatine muscles. Tonsillar fossa is a triangular region bounded by pillars, inferiorly by glossotonsillar sulcus and pharyngoepiglottic fold and laterally by pharyngeal constrictor muscles.
Soft palate	The soft palate is defined anteriorly by hard palate, laterally by palatopharyngeal and superior pharyngeal constrictor muscles, and posteriorly by palatopharyngeal arch/uvula. Forms roof of oropharynx and floor of nasopharynx.
Posterior Pharyngeal Wall (PPW)	The PPW spans area defined by soft palate, epiglottis, posterior edge of tonsillar complexes, and lateral aspects of pyriform sinuses inferiorly. Inferior to oropharyngeal PPW is PPW of hypopharynx, one of three subsites of hypopharynx.

PATHOLOGY: Approximately 95% of OPC are squamous cell carcinomas.[8] Remaining 5% of cases consist of lymphoma, minor salivary cancers (e.g., mucoepidermoid, adenoid cystic; see Chapter 14), and rare sarcomas. HPV-positive and negative cancers appear different pathologically. HPV-positive tumors often originate from lymphoid tissue of tonsil or BOT, and are more likely to be poorly differentiated/nonkeratinizing and basaloid in appearance. HPV-negative tumors have no predilection for location and are often keratinizing. *HPV 16* serotype accounts for about 90% of HPV-associated cases. HPV viral proteins E6 and E7 bind p53 and Rb respectively with subsequent loss of tumor suppression. When E7 binds to Rb, transcription factor E2F is released and allows cyclin to bypass G1/S checkpoint. Reflexive expression of p16 protein inhibits cyclin D-CDK4 complex in an effort to prevent uncontrolled cell cycling. Overexpression of p16 protein serves as surrogate marker of HPV integration into DNA. p16 protein can be detected by immunohistochemistry. HPV DNA is detected by fluorescence in situ hybridization (FISH). p16 is more sensitive but less specific than HPV16 DNA. On RTOG 0129, 19% of HPV-negative patients were p16+ but only 3% of p16- were HPV16+. In HPV-endemic areas such as the United States, PPV of p16 status in OPC is high (~90%), but in HPV-uncommon disease sites or in the developing world, PPV of p16 status is poor (<40%). EGFR is more commonly amplified in HPV-negative tumors and is associated with poor prognosis.[2,9]

TABLE 10.3: Factors Associated With HPV Status in OPC	
HPV+	HPV–
- Younger - Non/light smoker/alcohol - Incidence increasing - Caucasian - High-risk sexual behavior - More likely tonsil/base of tongue - Poorly differentiated - Nonkeratinizing - Basaloid - p16 upregulated	- Older - Heavy smoking/drinking - Incidence decreasing - Non-Caucasian - Not related to sexual behavior - No tissue preference - Keratinizing - p53 mutation - EGFR amplified

CLINICAL PRESENTATION: Most common presentation of OPC is painless neck mass. Other symptoms related to local invasion include sore throat, dysphagia, odynophagia, or otalgia referred from cranial nerve IX via tympanic nerve of Jacobson. Oral tongue fixation (unable to protrude tongue) suggests deep musculature involvement. Trismus suggests medial pterygoid invasion.[2]

WORKUP: H&P with careful attention to H&N including palpation of BOT, dental exam, neurologic exam, mirror exam, and/or flexible laryngoscopy. CBC and BMP with attention to renal function. Initial biopsy via FNA of lymphadenopathy acceptable although confirmatory biopsy of primary via tonsillectomy or BOT biopsy with detailed exam under anesthesia is recommended. Tumor HPV testing recommended per NCCN. CT of neck with contrast is most helpful for primary tumor delineation; PET/CT is also recommended for staging and evaluation of lymphadenopathy. Consider MRI if concern for perineural or skull base invasion.[2,10] After chemoRT, it is more cost-effective to perform PET/CT at 12 weeks and proceed to neck dissection if positive than to perform planned neck dissection after chemoRT.[11] Nutrition, speech and swallowing evaluation/therapy, and audiogram as clinically indicated. EUA with endoscopy as clinically indicated.

PROGNOSTIC FACTORS: Age, smoking (both 10 and 20 pack-year cutoffs have been used for stratification), comorbidities, performance status, stage, HPV status, PET SUV.[12–14] Staging and prognostic stratification of HPV-positive pts is rapidly evolving (see Tables 10.4 and 10.5).

NATURAL HISTORY: Nodal involvement is common and initial site of drainage from oropharynx is to neck level II and subsequently down jugular chain to levels III to IV. Levels IB, V and retropharyngeal nodes can be involved but are less common.[8] Historically, locoregional recurrence responsible for majority of cancer-related morbidity and mortality.[15] While this remains true for HPV-negative disease, locoregional recurrence of HPV-positive disease is generally uncommon. Distant metastases, however, develop in both subgroups at similar rates. Most common sites of distant metastases are lung and bone.[12,16]

TABLE 10.4: AJCC 8th ed. (2017) Staging for Oropharynx (p16-)

T/M \ N		cN0	cN1	cN2a	cN2b	cN2c	cN3a	cN3b
T1	• ≤2 cm	I						
T2	• 2.1–4 cm	II	III	IVA				
T3	• >4 cm • Extension							
T4a	• Invasion[1]							
T4b	• Invasion[2]			IVB				
M1	• Distant metastasis			IVC				

Major changes from the AJCC 7th edition include incorporation of HPV-status, incorporation of ENE and definition of the pathologic staging.

Notes: Extension = Extension to lingual surface of epiglottis. Invasion[1] = invasion into larynx, extrinsic musculature of tongue, medial pterygoid muscle, hard palate, or mandible. Invasion[2] = invasion into lateral pterygoid, pterygoid plates, lateral nasopharynx, skull base, or encases carotid artery.

cN1, single ipsilateral LN (≤3 cm) and -ENE; cN2a, single ipsilateral LN (3.1–6 cm) and –ENE; cN2b, multiple ipsilateral LN (≤6 cm) and –ENE; cN2c, bilateral or contralateral LN (≤6 cm) and –ENE; cN3a, LN (>6 cm) and no ENE; cN3b, clinically overt ENE.

pN1, single LN (≤3 cm) and –ENE; pN2a, single ipsilateral or contralateral LN (≤3 cm) and + ENE or single ipsilateral LN (3.1–6 cm) and – ENE; pN2b, multiple ipsilateral LN (≤6 cm) and – ENE; pN2c, bilateral or contralateral LN (≤6 cm) and – ENE; pN3a, LN (>6 cm) and –ENE; pN3b, LN (>3 cm) and + ENE.

TABLE 10.5: AJCC 8th ed. (2017) Staging for HPV-Mediated (p16+) Oropharyngeal Cancer		cN0	cN1	cN2	cN3
T/M	N				
T1	• ≤2 cm	I		II	III
T2	• 2.1–4 cm				
T3	• >4 cm • Extension				
T4	• Invasion				
M1	• Distant metastases	IV			

Notes: Extension = Extension to lingual surface of epiglottis. Invasion= invasion into larynx, extrinsic muscles of tongue, medial pterygoid, hard palate, or beyond.

cN1, one or more ipsilateral LN (≤6 cm); cN2, contralateral or bilateral LN (≤6 cm); cN3, LN (>6 cm).

pN1, ≤4 LNs; pN2 >4 LN's.

TREATMENT PARADIGM

Surgery: Classic oncologic surgery for OPC consists of radical tonsillectomy (the simple tonsillectomy performed for biopsy is generally not sufficient for oncologic control), glossectomy (often requiring mandibulotomy), palatectomy, or pharyngectomy with ipsilateral or bilateral neck dissection depending on nodal status and laterality of primary tumor. Because of functional deficits left by these procedures, nonoperative approaches became standard in 1970s and beyond. Over the past decade, however, minimally invasive procedures such as transoral laser microsurgery (TLM) and transoral robotic surgery (TORS) have reduced morbidity of surgery and are now standard options for T1-2 and select T3 lesions (see Evidence-Based Q&A).[10] Only one trial has compared surgery with RT to definitive RT (RTOG 7303) and with small numbers found similar OS for both approaches.[17] See postoperative Chapter 16 for details on adjuvant RT. Radical neck dissection: levels IB-V with sacrifice of internal and external jugular veins, SCM, omohyoid, CN XI, and submandibular gland. Modified radical neck dissection: levels IB-V but leaves one or more of jugular veins, SCM, omohyoid, or CN XI. Selective neck dissection: modified radical but leaves one or more of levels Ib-V. Supraomohyoid neck dissection: resection of levels I-III.

Chemotherapy: Concurrent cisplatin is standard for fit pts receiving definitive RT with stage III–IV disease. Cisplatin can be given concurrently with RT as 100 mg/m² bolus weeks 1, 4, and 7 (NCCN Category 1) or 40 mg/m² weekly (NCCN Category 2B).[10] Cetuximab given concurrent with RT for nonplatinum candidates; direct comparative data between cetuximab and cisplatin is pending (see Evidence-Based Q&A). Cetuximab starts 1 week prior to RT as loading dose of 400 mg/m² followed by 250 mg/m² weekly during RT.[18] Other less common concurrent regimens include carboplatin/paclitaxel, cisplatin/5-FU, and 5-FU/hydroxyurea. Induction CHT consists of cisplatin, 5-FU, and docetaxel (TPF) every 3 weeks for four cycles completing 4 to 7 weeks prior to RT alone or with cetuximab or carboplatin (see Evidence-Based Q&A).[10,19]

Radiation

Indications: RT is indicated for definitive treatment of OPC or in postoperative setting (see postoperative Chapter 16).

Dose: In definitive setting, standard dose is 70 Gy/35 fx. Various elective nodal doses have been used including 56 Gy/35 fx, and RTOG 1016 used a third lower dose to "low-risk" neck to 50 to 52.5 Gy/35 fx. For cT1-2N0-1 OPC, 66 Gy/30 fx RT alone with elective dose of 54 Gy/30 fx is reasonable based on RTOG 0022 (see Evidence-Based Q&A). Dose reduction for HPV+ pts is the subject of clinical trial.

Toxicity: Acute: Fatigue, mucositis, dysphagia, odynophagia, xerostomia, dermatitis, aspiration. Chronic: Dysphagia, neck fibrosis, xerostomia, trismus, osteoradionecrosis, hypothyroidism, brachial plexopathy (rare but take care with gross disease in low neck).

Procedure: See *Treatment Planning Handbook,* Chapter 4.[20]

EVIDENCE-BASED Q&A

Can definitive RT lead to similar control and survival compared to radical surgeries?

This was a key question in the 1970s when surgery was the definitive therapy of choice, often requiring mandibulotomy for BOT access and subsequent functional deficits. RTOG 7303 is the only PRT addressing this question; definitive RT has become the standard option subsequently to preserve functional outcomes.

Kramer, RTOG 7303 (*Head Neck Surg* 1987, PMID 3449477): Advanced squamous carcinoma of oropharynx or oral cavity randomly assigned to preoperative RT, postoperative RT, or definitive RT (65–70 Gy). Larynx or hypopharynx cancers randomized to either preoperative (50 Gy) or postoperative RT (60 Gy). For oral cavity or OPC pts, 4-yr OS was similar between all groups: 30% preoperative, 36% postoperative, 33% definitive. 4-yr LRC was 43% preoperative, 52% postoperative, and 38% definitive. **Conclusion: Definitive RT is an ethically justified alternative compared to radical surgery.**

Can the efficacy of RT be improved by altering fractionation?

Squamous cell carcinoma is known to undergo accelerated repopulation and is sensitive to reoxygenation, so fractionation was thought to play an important role in outcomes with definitive RT. Multiple trials and meta-analysis demonstrated that when treating locoregionally advanced pts, altered fractionation appears to improve LRC and OS.

Horiot, EORTC 22791 (*Radiother Oncol* 1992, PMID 1480768): PRT of 356 pts randomized between 70 Gy/35–40 fx to hyperfractionation of 80.5 Gy/70 fx. T2-3 oropharynx (excluding base of tongue) cancers, N0-1 were included from 1980 to 1987. Hyperfractionation demonstrated LRC benefit and trend toward OS in T3N0-1 pts but not T2.

Fu, RTOG 9003 (*IJROBP* 2000, PMID 10924966; Update Beitler IJROBP 2014, PMID 24613816): PRT 1,073 pts with stages III–IV squamous carcinoma of oral cavity, oropharynx, supraglottic larynx or stage II–IV of BOT or hypopharynx were randomized to one of four arms: (1) standard fractionation to 70 Gy/ 35 fx at 2 Gy/fx, (2) hyperfractionation to 81.6 Gy/68 fx given at 1.2 Gy/fx BID with 6-hour interfraction interval, (3) split-course accelerated hyperfractionation to 67.2 Gy/42 fx given 1.6 Gy/fx BID with 6-hour interfraction interval and 2-week rest after 38.4 Gy, or (4) accelerated hyperfractionation with concomitant boost to 72 Gy/42 fx given at 1.8 Gy/fx 5 days a week with 1.5 Gy/fraction to boost field as second daily treatment given 6 hours apart for last 12 treatment days. Primary endpoint was 2-year LRC. Results at initial report: At MFU of 23 mos, both hyperfractionation (2) and concomitant boost (4) arms showed improved locoregional control but no significant difference in overall survival. All three altered fractionation arms showed increased acute effects but only concomitant boost arm showed increased late effects. In final update, hyperfractionation (2) and concomitant boost (4) decreased 5-year locoregional recurrence compared to standard fractionation, but hyperfractionation did not increase late effects.

When using only 5-year follow-up, hyperfractionation improved OS (HR 0.81, $p = .05$) but not when all follow-up data was included. **Conclusion: Altered fractionation improves disease control in locoregionally advanced squamous carcinoma of H&N.**

TABLE 10.6: Results of RTOG 9003			
	Regimen	2-yr LRC	2-yr OS
1. Standard	70 Gy/35 fx daily	46%	46%
2. Hyperfractionation	81.6 Gy/68 fx BID	54%*	54.5%[†]
3. Split course	67.2 Gy/42 fx BID with 2-week break	47.5%	46.2%
4. Concomitant boost	72 Gy/42 fx (BID final 12 days)	54.5%[‡]	50.9%
*Statistically significant difference in original and final reports. [†]Statistically significant difference (only when limited to 5-year follow-up). [‡]Statistically significant difference compared to standard arm in original report.			

Overgaard, DAHANCA 6 and 7 Combined Analysis (*Lancet* 2003, PMID 14511925): Combined analysis of two trials performed from 1992 to 1999 including 1,485 pts with stage I–IV squamous carcinoma; DAHANCA 6 of glottis carcinoma testing fractionation and DAHANCA 7 of supraglottic, pharynx, and oral cavity cancers testing fractionation and radiosensitizer nimorazole. RT given to 62–68 Gy at 2 Gy/fx and randomized to either 5 or 6 fractions per week. Overall 5-year locoregional control was improved with acceleration (70% vs. 60%, $p = .0005$). Disease-specific but not overall survival was also improved by acceleration. **Conclusion: Six fractions weekly became standard in Denmark. This result was independent of p16 status.**[21]

Bourhis, MARCH Meta-Analysis (*Lancet* 2006, PMID 16950362): Meta-analysis of 6,515 pts from 15 trials with MFU of 6 years, majority was oropharynx and larynx cancers and 74% were stage III–IV. Altered fractionation was associated with significant OS benefit of 3.4% at 5 years ($p = .003$). Hyperfractionation was significantly higher at 8% at 5 years than acceleration at 1.7% to 2% at 5 years (both $p < 0.05$). **Conclusion: Altered fractionation and particularly hyperfractionation improves OS in H&N cancer.**

Does CHT add benefit to conventionally fractionated RT?

Adelstein, H&N Intergroup (*JCO* 2003, PMID 12506176): PRT of 271 of planned 362 pts between 1992 and 1999 with stage III–IV unresectable squamous cell carcinoma (all sites except sinus, nasopharynx, or salivary) randomized to either (A) RT alone (70 Gy/35 fx), (B) cisplatin with RT (100 mg/m^2 weeks 1, 4, and 7) or (C) split-course chemoRT (cisplatin 75 mg/m^2 with 5-FU 1,000 mg/m^2 every 4 weeks with 30 Gy/15 fx first course followed by surgical evaluation and if CR or unresectable, another 30-40 Gy was given with third cycle of CHT). Trial closed early due to slow accrual. 3-yr OS for chemoRT (Arm B) was superior to arm or C. 89%of pts in arm B experienced grade 3 to 5 toxicity. **Conclusion: Bolus cisplatin when added to conventionally fractionated RT improves OS.**

TABLE 10.7: Results of H&N Intergroup			
	CR	3-yr OS	Grade 3–5 toxicity
Arm A: RT	27.4%	23%	52%
Arm B: CRT	40.2%	37%*	89%*
Arm C: Split-course CRT	49.4%*	27%	77%*
*Statistically significant relative to Arm A.			

Calais, GORTEC 94-01 (*JNCI* 1999, PMID 10601378; Denis *JCO* 2004 PMID 14657228): PRT of 226 pts with stages III–IV squamous carcinoma of oropharynx randomized to definitive RT alone (70 Gy/35 fx) with or without concurrent carboplatin and 5-FU for three cycles. OS (22% vs. 16%), DFS (27% vs. 15%), and LRC (48% vs. 25%) were all improved by statistically significant amount. Grade 3 or higher late effects occurred in 30% versus 56% (*p* = .12). **Conclusion: CHT improved survival without increasing late toxicity.**

Does CHT add benefit to hyperfractionated RT?

Although hyperfractionated RT adds benefit over conventional fractionation, CHT remains beneficial.

Brizel, Duke (*NEJM* 1998, PMID 9632446): PRT of 116 pts with T3-4 N0-3 squamous carcinoma of H&N (and T2N0 base of tongue) were treated to 75 Gy/60 fx BID and randomized to either no concurrent therapy or concurrent cisplatin (60 mg/m^2) and 5-FU (600 mg/m^2) weeks 1 and 6. At MFU of 41 mos, 3-yr OS was 55% in CHT arm compared to 34% in hyperfractionated group (*p* = .07). LRC was also improved (44% vs. 70%, *p* = .01). Toxicity was comparable. **Conclusion: CHT adds benefit to hyperfractionated RT with similar toxicity.**

Bourhis, GORTEC 99-02 (*Lancet Oncol* 2012, PMID 22261362): 3-arm PRT of stage III–IV squamous carcinoma of H&N randomized to standard chemoRT (70 Gy/35 fx with carboplatin and 5-FU), accelerated chemoRT (70 Gy in 6 weeks with carboplatin and 5-FU), or very accelerated RT alone (64.8 Gy in 36 fx BID in 3.5 weeks). Standard chemoRT and accelerated chemoRT were similar in terms of PFS (*p* = .88) Conventional chemoRT improved PFS compared with very accelerated RT (*p* = .04). **Conclusion: Acceleration alone cannot completely compensate for absence of CHT.**

Does hyperfractionated RT add benefit to chemoRT?

This question is inverse of the previous question and was partially addressed by GORTEC 99-02 earlier, but was also addressed by the RTOG (although this was not most significant finding from RTOG 0129; see HPV section later).

Nguyen-Tan, RTOG 0129 (*JCO* 2014, PMID 25366680): PRT of 721 pts with squamous carcinoma of oral cavity, oropharynx, larynx, or hypopharynx to either 70 Gy/35 fx over 7 weeks (standard fractionation) or 72 Gy/42 fx over 6 weeks with concomitant boost schedule (see RTOG 9003 earlier). Both arms received cisplatin 100 mg/m^2 every 3 weeks (two cycles for accelerated arm, three for standard arm). After MFU of 7.9 years, no differences were observed in any endpoint (OS, PFS, LRC, or DM). **Conclusion: No benefit to acceleration in presence of concurrent CHT.**

What is overall summary of chemoRT trials?

Pignon, MACH-NC Meta-analysis (*Lancet* 2000 PMID 10768432; Update *Radiother Oncol* 2009, PMID 19446902; By Disease Site: Blanchard *Radiother Oncol*, PMID 21684027): Patient-level meta-analysis of over 17,000 pts from 93 trials demonstrated OS benefit to addition of CHT of 4.5% at 5 years. Concurrent chemoRT showed absolute benefit of 6.5% at 5 years (SS); induction 2.4% at 5 years (NS). Pts above 70 years of age did not benefit in terms of OS. Both concurrent and induction CHT improved distant control (update HR 0.73 and 0.88, *p* = .0001 and .04 but not different when compared to each other).

Is cetuximab of benefit compared to RT alone?

As EGFR inhibitor, cetuximab is active against H&N cancer and improved OS compared to RT alone.

Bonner (NEJM 2006, PMID 16467544; Update Bonner Lancet Oncol 2010 PMID 19897418): PRT of 424 pts from 1999 to 2002 with stage III–IV squamous carcinomas of oropharynx, hypopharynx, or larynx randomized to either RT alone (three regimens permitted: daily, BID, and concomitant boost) or RT with cetuximab given 400 mg/m² loading dose 1 week before RT and 250 mg/m² weekly during RT. Primary endpoint was LRC. Cetuximab improved LRC and OS (MS 29 vs. 49 mos, p = .03; update also 29 vs. 49). Toxicity was not different with exception of infusion reactions and acneiform rash. Subsequent analyses did not show interaction with HPV status.[22] Survival was improved in cetuximab pts who developed grade 2 or higher acneiform rash compared to those who received cetuximab without rash. **Conclusion: Cetuximab improves OS compared to RT alone.**

Does cetuximab improve survival when added to cisplatin?

Ang, RTOG 0522 (JCO 2014, PMID 25154822): PRT of 891 pts with stage III–IV H&N cancer randomized to RT with cisplatin with or without cetuximab. Addition of cetuximab did not improve OS, DFS, LRC, or DM but did increase toxicity. EGFR expression did not predict outcome. **Conclusion: No benefit to addition of cetuximab to cisplatin.**

Is concurrent cetuximab directly comparable and less toxic than concurrent cisplatin?

RTOG 1016 is phase III randomized noninferiority trial designed to directly compare cetuximab and cisplatin with the goal of demonstrating less toxicity in cetuximab group. This trial has not yet been reported. The following Italian Phase II trial is the only available head-to-head evidence.

Magrini, Italy (JCO 2016, PMID 26644536): Randomized Phase II enrolling stage III–IVB squamous carcinoma of oral cavity, oropharynx, hypopharynx, or supraglottic larynx randomized to either weekly cisplatin or cetuximab. Primary endpoint was compliance to therapy (breaks in RT, drug reduction, drug-related adverse events, and discontinuation). Trial discontinued after 70 pts. 4 cetuximab versus 0 cisplatin pts required break in RT >10 days (p = .05). Overall grade 3 toxicity was 59% cetuximab versus 53% cisplatin. Oncologic outcomes were similar. **Conclusion: Similar efficacy, different toxicity profiles but overall similar—more study required.**

Can induction CHT improve survival by reducing rate of distant metastases?

This subject has been extensively studied and is controversial. Summary is that TPF is the preferred induction regimen but superiority of induction CHT has not been established compared to concurrent CHT.

Vermorken, TAX 323 (NEM 2007, PMID 17960012): PRT randomized 358 stage III–IV H&N cancer to four cycles of induction cisplatin/5-FU (PF) with or without docetaxel (TPF) followed by RT alone. TPF demonstrated OS benefit (MS 14.5 vs. 18.8 mos). **Conclusion: TPF is induction CHT regimen of choice.**

Posner, TAX 324 (NEJM 2007, PMID 17960013; Update Lorch Lancet Oncol 2011, PMID 21233014): PRT similar to TAX 323 above; key differences included number of cycles and addition of concurrent CHT. Randomized 501 stage III–IV H&N cancer to three cycles of induction cisplatin/5-FU (PF) with or without docetaxel (TPF) followed by RT with concurrent carboplatin. Updated results continued to show survival benefit (MS 34.8 vs. 70.6 mos). **Conclusion: TPF is induction CHT regimen of choice.**

Haddad, PARADIGM (Lancet Oncol 2013, PMID 23414589): PRT of pts with T3-4 or N2-3 squamous carcinoma comparing three cycles of TPF followed by chemoRT with either docetaxel or carboplatin vs. chemoRT with two cycles of cisplatin 100 mg/m². Trial closed early after 145 pts were enrolled. No differences were observed in terms of OS or PFS.

Induction pts experienced more febrile neutropenia. **Conclusion: No clear benefit to induction CHT compared to concurrent cisplatin.**

Cohen, DeCIDE (*JCO* 2014, PMID 25049329): PRT of pts with N2-3 H&N cancer treated with either concurrent CHT (docetaxel, 5-FU and hydroxyurea) or two cycles of TPF induction CHT with same concurrent chemoRT. RT was to 74–75 Gy given BID. Trial closed early due to slow accrual; 285 pts were included. MFU 30 mos. No difference in OS, RFS, or distant failure-free survival. **Conclusion: TPF cannot be routinely recommended for N2-3 pts.**

Which tonsil tumors can be treated with unilateral RT?

O'Sullivan published the classic series defining unilateral RT to be safe for T1-2N0 lateralized tonsil tumors with ≤1 cm of soft palate or superficial base of tongue invasion. Subsequent series have expanded indications to well-lateralized node-positive pts although this is more controversial.[23–25] Modern trials (NRG HN-002) recommend unilateral RT cT1-3 tonsil tumors, well-lateralized (<1 cm soft palate, base of tongue invasion) with minimal nodal disease (N0-2a, no ECE) with unilateral RT optional for N2b pts confined to level II without ECE.

O'Sullivan, Princess Margaret (*IJROBP* 2001, PMID 11567806): RR of 228 pts with carcinoma of tonsillar region treated with unilateral RT between 1970 and 1991. 84% were T1-2, 58% N0. Crude rate of contralateral failure was 3.5%: T1 0% (0/67), T2 1.5% (2/118), T3 10% (3/30), T4 0% (0/7). Risk was >10% if involving medial one-third of soft palate or base of tongue involved. (Generally, elective neck RT is not recommended where risk of subclinical disease is <10% due to morbidity of RT—especially salivary glands.) **Conclusion: Unilateral RT is safe in select tonsil cancers >1 cm from midline. Extension to BOT is considered relative contraindication to ipsilateral RT.**

Huang, Princess Margaret (*IJROBP* 2017, PMID 28258895): RR of 379 pts treated with unilateral RT. T1-T2N0-N2b tonsil cancer treated between 1999 and 2014 stratified by HPV status. MFU 5.03 years. Regional control was not statistically different compared between HPV+ or HPV- pts. Overall, 5-yr contralateral neck failures were 2%. **Conclusion: Ipsilateral RT to selected T1-T2N0-N2b tonsil pts results in equally excellent outcomes regardless of tumor HPV status. When considering ipsilateral RT, ≤1 cm superficial involvement of soft palate or BOT is safe, but suspicion of deeper invasion should be approached cautiously.**

When is it necessary to irradiate levels IB and V?

With modern imaging it is likely safe to spare levels IB and V for T1-2 OPC if not involved on imaging.

Sanguineti, Johns Hopkins (*IJROBP* 2009, PMID 19131181): RR of 103 pts with T1-2, clinically node-positive OPC staged with CT imaging who underwent initial neck dissection. Overall, if CT was negative, levels IB, IV, and V were involved in 3%, 6%, and 1%. Levels IB and V were <4% regardless of pathologic involvement of II to IV. Level IV was 5% if level III was not involved but 11% if level III was involved. **Conclusion: Levels IB and V are low risk and can be spared in cT1-2 OPC.**

Sanguineti, Johns Hopkins (*Acta Oncol* 2014, PMID 24274389): RR of 91 pts with HPV+ OPC and clinically positive neck nodes who underwent ipsilateral neck dissection between 1998 and 2010. Pathology was reviewed to determine risk of subclinical disease at each neck level (not evident on CT). Risk of subclinical disease in both levels IB and V is <5%, while it is 6.5% (95% CI: 3.1–9.9) for level IV. Level IB subclinical involvement >5% when 2+ ipsilateral levels besides IB are involved. Risk of occult disease in level IV is <5% when level III is not involved. Low number of events in level V did not allow analysis of predictors of involvement. **Conclusion: Consider electively covering level IB if 2+ other levels are involved. Level IV may be spared when level III is negative.**

What prospective data guided the adoption of IMRT for OPC in the United States?

Although IMRT is now standard in treatment of H&N cancer, RTOG 0022 is one of the few prospective trials investigating safety and efficacy in cooperative group setting. It is also a trial that demonstrates good outcomes for T1-2N0-1 OPC treated with RT alone.

Eisbruch, RTOG 0022 (*IJROBP* 2010, PMID 19540060): Initial RTOG multi-institutional trial demonstrating safety and efficacy of IMRT. Prospective phase II trial of 69 T1-2 N0-1 OPC treated with RT alone to 66 Gy/30 fx with IMRT. 2-yr LRF was 9%. LRF was increased in those with major deviations: 2/4 pts with deviations (50%) versus 3/49 without (6%, $p =$ .04). **Conclusion: IMRT is feasible with encouraging acute and late toxicity. Quality of IMRT is important to avoid LRF.**

What are expected outcomes with TORS? Who are ideal candidates?

Transoral robotic surgery (and transoral laser microsurgery) have transformed morbidity associated with surgical resection of OPC. FDA approval was obtained for DaVinci robot in resection of T1-2 OPC in 2009 and NCCN guidelines allow for TORS as option for select pts.[10] Series from University of Pennsylvania, Washington University, Mayo Clinic, Stanford, and Mount Sinai have established safety and efficacy of TORS.[26-33] For now, TORS remains institution and surgeon dependent as comparative data is evolving.

Do HPV-positive tumors behave differently than HPV-negative?

HPV-positive OPC is now classified as distinct disease.

Ang, RTOG 0129 (*NEJM* 2010, PMID 20530316): Retrospective analysis of RTOG 0129 (see Nguyen-Tan 2014 in the preceding) investigating role of HPV. HPV status was determined by both FISH for HPV DNA and IHC for p16. 64% of pts had HPV-positive tumors and 3-yr OS was markedly improved for these pts (82% vs. 57%, $p < .001$). 3-yr rate of local–regional disease lower for pts with HPV+ tumors than for those with HPV- tumors: 13.6% versus 35.1% ($p < .001$). Smoking and nodal stage were prognostic. RPA for OS divided pts into three classes based on HPV status, smoking, T and N stages: low risk (HPV-positive and ≤10 pack-years or HPV-positive, >10 pack-years and N0-2a), intermediate risk (HPV-positive, >10 pack-years and N2b-3 or HPV-negative, ≤10 pack-years and T2-3), or high risk (HPV-negative, ≤10 and T4 or >10 pack-years). **Conclusion: This trial defined impact of HPV status on prognosis for oropharynx pts.**

Fakhry, RTOG 2nd Analysis (*JCO* 2014, PMID 24958820): Second analysis of RTOG 0129 and 0522 including pts with initially locally advanced oropharyngeal SCC (206 HPV+, 117 HPV-) who developed recurrent disease after primary treatment. Investigated effect of HPV status on survival after disease progression. Median time to progression 8.2 mos for p16+ versus 7.3 mos for p16- (NS). 55% of pts had locoregional recurrence only, 40% had distant metastases only, 5% had both. MFU time after first event of disease progression was 4 yrs. p16+ pts had significantly improved OS after disease progression when compared to p16- pts (2.6 yrs vs. 0.8 yrs). Receipt of salvage surgery reduced risk of death after disease progression. **Conclusion: Patterns of failure do not differ based on p16 status (similar time to disease progression and anatomic site involvement) but p16+ pts have improved survival after first recurrence.**

O'Sullivan, Princess Margaret (*JCO* 2013, PMID 23295795): RR of 505 OPC pts, 382 were HPV-positive. Although OS, LC (94% vs. 80%) and regional control (95% vs. 82%) were improved in HPV-positive pts, distant control was similar (90% vs. 86%). RPA for distant control divided pts into four classes: HPV-positive low (N0-N2c and T1-3) or high risk

(N0-2c and T4 or N3) and HPV-negative low (N0-2c and T1-2) or high risk (N0-2c and T3-4 or N3). CHT seemed to reduce distant metastases for HPV-positive low-risk category pts with N2b-N2c disease. **Conclusion: HPV-positive pts with low risk of distant metastases (T1-3N0-2a) may be candidates for treatment de-intensification.**

Are there opportunities to de-intensify treatment for HPV+ pts?

No standard regimen has been identified to date but multiple trials are ongoing investigating de-intensification for low-risk HPV-positive pts, including the completed NRG HN-002.

Chera, UNC/UF/Rex Trial (*IJROBP* 2015, PMID 26581135): Prospective phase II trial of HPV-positive pts with T0-3N0-2c and ≤10 pack-years or 10 to 30 pack-years but abstinent for >5 years. Pts received 60 Gy/30 fx with weekly cisplatin 30 mg/m^2. Pts were assessed surgically within 6 to 14 weeks after completion; all pts received biopsy at primary site and if positive, transoral resection was performed. Primary endpoint was pCR and goal was to achieve pCR rate not significantly different from 87% (RTOG 0129). pCR rate was 86% and of six partial responses, all but one had pCR at primary (<1 mm focus) and others had minimal residual nodal disease. **Conclusion: De-intensification is likely safe for low-risk HPV-positive pts. Further trials are ongoing.**

Marur, ECOG 1308 (*JCO* 2017, PMID 28029303): Phase II trial involving 80 pts evaluating whether clinical complete response (cCR) to induction CHT could select pts with HPV+ OPC who could receive de-intensified therapy with goal of sparing late sequelae. Eligibility criteria: Stage III–IV, T1-3N0-N2b OPC, p16+ or HPV+, ≤10 pack-year smoking history. Treated with three cycles of induction CHT with cisplatin, paclitaxel, and cetuximab. If cCR of primary site, went on to receive IMRT to 54 Gy with weekly cetuximab. If only partial response at primary site or nodes, went on to receive 69.3 Gy to involved site and cetuximab. Primary endpoint was 2-yr PFS. 56 out of 80 pts (70%) had primary site cCR and received low dose arm; these pts had 2-yr PFS 80%. At 12 mos, pts treated with RT ≤54 Gy had less difficulty swallowing solids (40% vs. 89%, $p = .011$) or impaired nutrition (10% vs. 44%, $p = .025$). 8 of 9 failures in reduced-dose arm were locoregional. **Conclusion: For pts who respond to induction chemo, reduced-dose IMRT with concurrent cetuximab for favorable HPV-associated pts may have improved swallowing and nutritional status.**

Chen, UCLA (*Lancet Oncol* 2017, PMID 28434660): Single-arm phase II trial with biopsy-proven stage III–IV (7th edition) HPV+ OPC. Pts received carboplatin/paclitaxel x2 cycles. CR or PR received 54 Gy/27 fx, patients who developed less than a PR received 60 Gy/30 fx, both concurrent with paclitaxel. Primary endpoint PFS. 45 pts, MFU 30 mos. three LRF, one DM. Two-yr PFS 92% (95% CI: 77–97). 39% grade 3 toxicity (mostly during induction CHT). 2% feeding tube dependence at 3 mos, 0% at 6 mos. **Conclusion: Reduced-dose chemoRT associated with high PFS.**

REFERENCES

1. Siegel RL, Miller KD, Jemal A. Cancer statistics, 2016. *CA Cancer J Clin.* 2016;66(1):7–30.
2. Salama JK, Gillison ML, Brizel DM. Oropharynx. In: Halperin E, Wazer D, Perez C, Brady L, eds. *Principles and Practice of Radiation Oncology.* 6th ed. Philadelphi, PA: Lippincott Williams & Wilkins; 2013:817–832.
3. Chaturvedi AK, Engels EA, Pfeiffer RM, et al. Human papillomavirus and rising oropharyngeal cancer incidence in the United States. *J Clin Oncol.* 2011;29(32):4294–4301.
4. Gillison ML, Broutian T, Pickard RK, et al. Prevalence of oral HPV infection in the United States, 2009–2010. *JAMA.* 2012;307(7):693–703.
5. Gillison ML, Zhang Q, Jordan R, et al. Tobacco smoking and increased risk of death and progression for patients with p16-positive and p16-negative oropharyngeal cancer. *J Clin Oncol.* 2012;30(17):2102–2111.

6. Ang KK, Zhang Q, Rosenthal DI, et al. Randomized phase III trial of concurrent accelerated radiation plus cisplatin with or without cetuximab for stage III to IV head and neck carcinoma: RTOG 0522. *J Clin Oncol*. 2014;32(27):2940–2950.

7. Bagnardi V, Rota M, Botteri E, et al. Light alcohol drinking and cancer: a meta-analysis. *Ann Oncol*. 2013;24(2):301–308.

8. Cannon GM, Harari PM, Gentry LR, Avey GD, Siu LL. Oropharyngeal cancer. In: Gunderson L, Tepper J, eds. *Clinical Radiation Oncology*. 3rd ed. Philadelphia, PA: Elsevier; 2012:585–617.

9. Chung CH, Gillison ML. Human papillomavirus in head and neck cancer: its role in pathogenesis and clinical implications. *Clin Cancer Res*. 2009;15(22):6758–6762.

10. NCCN Clinical Practice Guidelines in Oncology: Head and Neck Cancers. 2015. http://www.nccn.org

11. Mehanna H, Wong WL, McConkey CC, et al. PET-CT surveillance versus neck dissection in advanced head and neck cancer. *N Engl J Med*. 2016;374(15):1444–1454.

12. Ang KK, Harris J, Wheeler R, et al. Human papillomavirus and survival of patients with oropharyngeal cancer. *N Engl J Med*. 2010;363(1):24–35.

13. Schwartz DL, Harris J, Yao M, et al. Metabolic tumor volume as a prognostic imaging-based biomarker for head-and-neck cancer: pilot results from Radiation Therapy Oncology Group protocol 0522. *Int J Radiat Oncol Biol Phys*. 2015;91(4):721–729.

14. Huang SH, Xu W, Waldron J, et al. Refining American Joint Committee on Cancer/Union for International Cancer Control TNM stage and prognostic groups for human papillomavirus-related oropharyngeal carcinomas. *J Clin Oncol*. 2015;33(8):836–845.

15. Beitler JJ, Zhang Q, Fu KK, et al. Final results of local-regional control and late toxicity of RTOG 9003: a randomized trial of altered fractionation radiation for locally advanced head and neck cancer. *Int J Radiat Oncol Biol Phys*. 2014;89(1):13–20.

16. O'Sullivan B, Huang SH, Siu LL, et al. Deintensification candidate subgroups in human papillomavirus-related oropharyngeal cancer according to minimal risk of distant metastasis. *J Clin Oncol*. 2013;31(5):543–550.

17. Kramer S, Gelber RD, Snow JB, et al. Combined radiation therapy and surgery in the management of advanced head and neck cancer: final report of study 73-03 of the Radiation Therapy Oncology Group. *Head Neck Surg*. 1987;10(1):19–30.

18. Bonner JA, Harari PM, Giralt J, et al. Radiotherapy plus cetuximab for squamous-cell carcinoma of the head and neck. *N Engl J Med*. 2006;354(6):567–578.

19. Vermorken JB, Remenar E, van Herpen C, et al. Cisplatin, fluorouracil, and docetaxel in unresectable head and neck cancer. *N Engl J Med*. 2007;357(17):1695–1704.

20. Videtic GMM, Woody N, Vassil AD. *Handbook of Treatment Planning In Radiation Oncology*. 2nd ed. New York, NY: Demos Medical; 2015.

21. Lassen P, Eriksen JG, Krogdahl A, et al. The influence of HPV-associated p16-expression on accelerated fractionated radiotherapy in head and neck cancer: evaluation of the randomised DAHANCA 6&7 trial. *Radiother Oncol*. 2011;100(1):49–55.

22. Rosenthal DI, Harari PM, Giralt J, et al. Association of Human Papillomavirus and p16 Status With Outcomes in the IMCL-9815 Phase III Registration Trial for Patients With Locoregionally Advanced Oropharyngeal Squamous Cell Carcinoma of the Head and Neck Treated With Radiotherapy With or Without Cetuximab. *J Clin Oncol*. 2015;34(12):1300–1308.

23. Chronowski GM, Garden AS, Morrison WH, et al. Unilateral radiotherapy for the treatment of tonsil cancer. *Int J Radiat Oncol Biol Phys*. 2012;83(1):204–209.

24. Al-Mamgani A, van Rooij P, Fransen D, Levendag P. Unilateral neck irradiation for well-lateralized oropharyngeal cancer. *Radiother Oncol*. 2013;106(1):69–73.

25. Liu C, Dutu G, Peters LJ, et al. Tonsillar cancer: the Peter MacCallum experience with unilateral and bilateral irradiation. *Head Neck*. 2014;36(3):317–322.

26. de Almeida JR, Li R, Magnuson JS, et al. Oncologic outcomes after transoral robotic surgery: a multi-institutional study. *JAMA Otolaryngol Head Neck Surg*. 2015;141:1043–1051.

27. Hutcheson KA, Holsinger FC, Kupferman ME, Lewin JS. Functional outcomes after TORS for oropharyngeal cancer: a systematic review. *Eur Arch Otorhinolaryngol*. 2015;272(2):463–471.

28. Leonhardt FD, Quon H, Abrahão M, et al. Transoral robotic surgery for oropharyngeal carcinoma and its impact on patient-reported quality of life and function. *Head Neck*. 2012;34(2):146–154.

29. Park YM, Kim WS, Byeon HK, et al. Oncological and functional outcomes of transoral robotic surgery for oropharyngeal cancer. *Br J Oral Maxillofac Surg*. 2013;51(5):408–412.

30. Weinstein GS, O'Malley BW, Snyder W, et al. Transoral robotic surgery: radical tonsillectomy. *Arch Otolaryngol Head Neck Surg.* 2007;133(12):1220–1226.
31. Weinstein GS, Quon H, O'Malley BW, et al. Selective neck dissection and deintensified postoperative radiation and chemotherapy for oropharyngeal cancer: a subset analysis of the University of Pennsylvania transoral robotic surgery trial. *Laryngoscope.* 2010;120(9):1749–1755.
32. Weinstein GS, O'Malley BW, Magnuson JS, et al. Transoral robotic surgery: a multicenter study to assess feasibility, safety, and surgical margins. *Laryngoscope.* 2012;122(8):1701–1707.
33. Desai SC, Sung CK, Jang DW, Genden EM. Transoral robotic surgery using a carbon dioxide flexible laser for tumors of the upper aerodigestive tract. *Laryngoscope.* 2008;118(12):2187–2189.

11: ORAL CAVITY CANCER

Bindu V. Manyam

> **QUICK HIT:** Unlike oropharyngeal squamous cell carcinoma, HPV infection is not associated with oral cavity squamous cell carcinoma. Primary management of oral cavity cancers is generally surgical resection with selective neck dissection (levels IB-III, others as indicated by primary site location and stage), followed by risk-adapted postoperative RT with or without concurrent CHT. Early stage lesions (particularly lip) may be treated with definitive RT using brachytherapy. Depth of invasion is important for decision making in oral cavity cancers.

EPIDEMIOLOGY: Oral cavity cancer: Estimated incidence of 30,000 and 5,000 deaths in the United States in 2016 and comprises 30% of all H&N malignancy. Male to female approximately 3:2.[1] Most common sites for oral cavity cancer in the United States are lip and tongue. Incidence is markedly higher internationally (20-fold increase in south Asia).[2]

RISK FACTORS: Smoking and alcohol are primary risk factors for oral cavity squamous cell carcinoma (OC-SCC). Other risk factors include chewing tobacco, poor oral hygiene, periodontal disease, chronic irritation from ill-fitting dentures, betel nut, chronic sun exposure (for lip cancer), and immune suppression (HIV or solid organ transplant). Unlike OPC, majority of OC-SCC are negative for HPV, unless near circumvallate papillae.[3] Genetic syndromes associated with OC-SCC include Fanconi's anemia and dyskeratosis congenita.[4,5]

ANATOMY: Oral cavity boundaries: anterior border junction of skin and vermilion border of lip; posterior border: junction of hard and soft palate; posterior/inferior border: circumvallate papillae of tongue; lateral border: anterior tonsillar pillars/buccal mucosa. Atlases are available for neck nodal level definition.[6]

TABLE 11.1: Oral Cavity Anatomic Definition		
Site	**Key Features**	**Pattern of Drainage**
Mucosal lip	Bordered by upper and lower lip vermillion. Upper lip innervated by infraorbital nerve (V2) and lower lip innervated by mental nerve (V3).	IA (lower lip), IB, II, III, facial lymphatics (upper lip)
Buccal mucosa	Mucosa of inner cheek and lips to attachment of mucosa of alveolar ridge and pterygomandibular raphe.	IB, II–IV
Alveolar ridges	Mucosa overlying alveolar process of maxilla (upper) and mandible (lower). Posterior margin of upper alveolar ridge is pterygopalatine arch and posterior margin of lower alveolar ridge is ascending ramus of mandible.	IB, II–IV
Retromolar trigone	Mucosa overlying ascending ramus of mandible, from posterior surface of last molar tooth to tuberosity of maxilla.	IB, II–IV

(continued)

TABLE 11.1: Oral Cavity Anatomic Definition (*continued*)		
Site	Key Features	Pattern of Drainage
Floor of mouth	Mucosa overlying mylohyoid and hyoglossus muscles, extending from inner surface of lower alveolar ridge to dorsal surface of tongue.	IA, IB, II–IV
Hard palate	Mucosa extending from inner surface of superior alveolar ridge to posterior edge of palatine bone of maxillae.	II–IV
Oral tongue (Anterior 2/3 tongue)	Mobile portion of tongue from circumvallate papillae to dorsal surface of tongue at junction of floor of mouth. Sensation is from lingual nerve (V3), taste is from chorda tympani (CN VII) and motor function is from hypoglossal nerve (CN XII).	Three routes of drainage: Tip of tongue–submental nodes Lateral tongue–IB Medial tongue–deep cervical LN II–IV 15% drain to levels III–IV skipping II

PATHOLOGY: Squamous cell carcinoma (SCC) comprises 95% of oral cavity cancers.[7] Less common histologies include minor salivary gland carcinomas, mucosal melanoma, lymphoma and sarcoma. Basal cell carcinomas can arise from vermillion border of lip. Routine HPV testing is not recommended and p16 is not specific to HPV-infection in oral cavity.

GENETICS: Mutation in p53, CDKN2A, Rb loss of function, and increased expression of EGFR are associated with worse prognosis.[4,5] Next-generation sequencing has identified subgroups of oral cavity tumors genetically distinct from other HPV-negative H&N cancers.[8]

SCREENING: Currently there is no effective screening program established for OC-SCC US. One study of 4,611 tobacco users older than 40 were screened with systematic inspection of oral mucosa, in which abnormal findings were seen in over 70% of pts, but cancer diagnosed in only 3% of pts.[9] One study in India suggested 33% reduction in risk of oral cancer death with screening by physical examination.[10]

CLINICAL PRESENTATION: Symptoms include pain, non-healing ulcer, bleeding, dysphagia, ill-fitting dentures, halitosis. Advanced lesions can present with symptoms of facial numbness, difficulty with protrusion of tongue, trismus. On examination, may present as visible or palpable mass or ulceration in oral cavity or palpable cervical lymphadenopathy.

WORKUP: H&P including of visual inspection of tumor, size and location, palpation of tumor borders, cranial nerve examination, and cervical lymph node examination. Dental evaluation is important to identify need for extraction and risk of osteoradionecrosis. Exam should include flexible nasopharyngolaryngoscopy to rule out second primary neoplasm. *Imaging:* CT neck with contrast. *Pathology:* In-office biopsy is common if safe but EUA with biopsy may be required. PET is challenging to interpret in oral cavity, but remains useful for nodal and distant staging. MRI if concern for perineural spread. Dental, nutrition, speech evaluation as indicated.

PROGNOSTIC FACTORS: Age, smoking, tumor location, stage and pathologic features (histologic grade, depth of invasion [DOI], perineural invasion, margin status, number and size of lymph nodes, extracapsular extension) have been associated with prognosis. Lymph node involvement was shown to be the most important prognostic factor for OC-SCC.[11] One study determined oral tongue to be associated with higher rate of local failure, distant metastases and lower OS compared to other oral cavity subsites, while other studies have suggested no significant difference in prognosis.[12,13]

NATURAL HISTORY: Premalignant changes (white plaques known as "leukoplakia") are often present before development of invasive carcinoma. Risk of development of leukoplakia into invasive carcinoma is estimated to be 1% to 20% in 10 years.[14] Pts with stage I-II OC-SCC have been shown to have 5-yr OS about 83% and pts with Stage III-IVa disease have been shown to have 5-yr OS of 55%.[15,16] Compared with other H&N sites, OC-SCC have higher rate of local recurrence after definitive therapy. Most frequent sites of distant metastasis are lung and bone.

STAGING:

TABLE 11.2: AJCC 8th ed. (2017) Staging for Oral Cavity		cN0	cN1	cN2a	cN2b	cN2c	cN3a	cN3b
T/M	N							
T1	• ≤2 cm • DOI ≤5 mm	I						
T2	• ≤2cm & DOI (5.1–10 mm) • 2.1–4 cm & DOI ≤10 mm	II	III		IVA			
T3	• >4 cm • DOI >10 mm							
T4a lip	• Invasion[1]							
T4a oral cavity	• Invasion[2]							
T4b oral cavity	• Invasion[3]			IVB				
M1	• Distant metastasis			IVC				

Major changes compared to 7th Edition include use of depth of invasion, removal of deep intrinsic tongue muscle invasion as T4 (included in DOI), introduction of pN classification and use of ENE in nodal classification.

Notes: Invasion[1] = invasion into cortical bone or involves inferior alveolar nerve, floor of mouth, or skin of face. Invasion[2] = invasionthrough cortical bone or mandible/maxilla, into maxillary sinus, or skin of face. Invasion[3] = invasion into masticator space, pterygoid plates, or skull base, and/or encases internal carotid artery.

cN1, single ipsilateral LN (≤3 cm) and -ENE; cN2a, single ipsilateral LN (3.1–6 cm) and –ENE; cN2b, multiple ipsilateral LN (≤6 cm) and –ENE; cN2c, bilateral or contralateral LN (≤6 cm) and –ENE; cN3a, LN (>6 cm) and –ENE; cN3b, clinically overt ENE.

pN1, single LN (≤3 cm) and –ENE; pN2a, single ipsilateral or contralateral LN (≤3 cm) and + ENE or single ipsilateral LN (3.1–6 cm) and – ENE; pN2b, multiple ipsilateral LN (≤6 cm) and – ENE; pN2c, bilateral or contralateral LN (≤6 cm) and – ENE; pN3a, LN (>6 cm) and –ENE; pN3b, LN (>3 cm) and + ENE.

TREATMENT PARADIGM

Surgery: Initial surgical resection is standard of care. Randomized trials comparing upfront surgery versus RT demonstrated significantly worse OS with RT alone.[18,19] Achieving negative surgical margins is critical, and if feasible, repeat resection of positive margin is preferred. Close surgical margin has historically been defined as within 5 mm; however, retrospective review demonstrated local recurrence-free survival was significantly higher with margins ≤2.2 mm, suggesting new definition for close margin to stratify pts for local recurrence.[20]

Early stage OC-SCC can be resected without significant functional or cosmetic deficits, though hemiglossectomy, maxillecotomy, and mandibulotomy for locally advanced disease can lead to significant speech and swallowing deficits, which can be managed with reconstruction. Standard transoral or open approaches are used for OC-SCC, and minimally invasive surgery with transoral laser or robotic surgery has not been shown to provide relative benefit in this setting.[21]

For T1 lip, upper alveolar ridge, and hard palate cancer, lymph node dissection may be able to be omitted, as risk of metastasis is low. For T1 or T2 oral tongue cancer, elective lymph node dissection of levels I-IV is typically recommended for all tumors ≥2 mm DOI. Lower alveolar ridge, floor of mouth, buccal and retromolar trigone cancers with clinically node-negative neck should undergo level I to III lymph node dissection due to high incidence of occult nodal metastases. Pts with primary tumors near or involving midline should be managed with bilateral neck dissection.

Chemotherapy: Combined analysis of two prospective randomized trials (PRT) demonstrated significant locoregional control (LRC), disease-free survival (DFS), and overall survival (OS) benefit with addition of concurrent CHT to PORT in pts with ECE and positive margin (see PORT for H&N Cancer chapter for details).[22] Two PRTs examining role of preoperative CHT demonstrated no improvement in OS with cisplatin and 5-FU or docetaxel, cisplatin, and 5-FU (TPF).[23,24]

Radiation:

Indications: Typical indications include pT3-T4a; pN2-3; pT1-2N0-1 *and* one or more of following: PNI, LVSI, close margin <5 mm or T2 oral cavity cancer with ≥5 mm DOI (can consider 4 mm based on Ganly data).[25] MSKCC and Princess Margaret Hospital (PMH) nomograms can be used to assess potential benefits of postoperative RT.[26,27] PORT should start 4 weeks after surgery.

Intraoral cone RT: Classic technique for small tumor size (<3 cm) of floor of mouth. Preserves salivary gland function and decreases risk of osteoradionecrosis. Intraoral cone RT uses 100 tos 250 kVp x-rays or 6 MeV electrons. Local control rate around 85%.[28]

Brachytherapy: Interstitial implant can be used alone or in combination with EBRT for treatment of oral tongue, floor of mouth, or buccal mucosa. Isotopes used include Ir-192, Ra-226, Cs-137, Au-198, Tantalum-182. For tumor thickness <1 cm, single-plane implant is adequate, otherwise double-plane or volumetric implant is used. Surface mold brachytherapy can be used for select superficial (<1 cm depth) initial or recurrent superficial lesions of hard palate, lower gingiva, and floor of mouth. Impression is made of surface to be irradiated with HDR catheters inserted into pre-drilled holes or grooves in mold and sealed with dental plaster.[29]

Dose: See PORT for H&N Cancer chapter for details. For T1-T2N0 lesions, interstitial LDR brachytherapy dose is 60 to 70 Gy delivered over 6 to 7 days, with minimum tumor dose rate at 30 to 60 cGy/hr. When brachytherapy used in combination with EBRT, implant dose should be at least 40 Gy.

Toxicity: Acute complications include mucositis, loss of taste, xerostomia, thrush, dermatitis, dysphagia, odynophagia. Chronic toxicity includes xerostomia, lifelong need for fluoride prophylaxis, risk for dental caries and osteoradionecrosis.

Procedure: See *Treatment Planning Handbook*, Chapter 4 for details.[30]

EVIDENCE-BASED Q&A

Why is initial surgical resection preferred over definitive RT for initial management of OC-SCC?

Two PRT, as well as several retrospective studies, suggest LRC and OS benefit for surgical resection compared to definitive RT.[18,19]

Robertson, Glasgow (*Clin Oncol* 1998, PMID 9704176): PRT of 35 pts with T2-4N0-2 OC-SCC and oropharynx randomized to surgery followed by PORT (60 Gy/30 fx) versus RT alone (66 Gy/33 fx). Trial was designed to recruit 350 pts, but was closed after only 35 pts due to significantly worse OS with RT alone. MFU was 23 months. OS significantly better with surgery and PORT (relative death rate 0.24, p = .001). Duration of LC was significantly decreased with RT alone (p = .037). **Conclusion: Definitive RT is sub-optimal for oral cavity cancer.**

Iyer, Singapore (*Cancer* 2015, PMID 25639864): PRT of 119 pts with Stage III-IV H&N squamous cell carcinoma randomized to surgery followed by PORT versus concurrent CHT and RT. MFU was 13 years. There was no significant difference in OS for entire cohort (45% vs. 35%; p = .262) and DSS (56% vs. 46%; p = .637) at 5 years for surgery versus RT alone, respectively. For pts with OC-SCC, surgery up front significantly improved 5-yr OS (68% vs. 12%; p = .038). **Conclusion: OS and DSS are significantly improved with surgery and PORT compared to RT alone for OC-SCC, but not for other sites of H&N.**

Is there benefit for elective neck dissection compared to neck dissection at nodal relapse?

Randomized data suggests survival benefit to up-front neck dissection compared to neck dissection at time of nodal relapse, though stage, pathologic features and location of primary should be considered.

D'Cruz, India (*NEJM* 2015, PMID 26027881): PRT of 596 pts with lateralized T1-2 OC-SCC randomized to elective ipsilateral neck dissection versus therapeutic neck dissection (at time of nodal relapse). MFU was 39 months. At 3 years, elective neck dissection demonstrated significantly improved OS (80% vs. 67.5%; p = .01) and DFS (69.5% vs. 45.9%; p < .001) compared to therapeutic neck dissection. Overall rate of pathologic nodal positivity in clinically node negative neck was 30%. Rates of adverse events were 6.6% and 3.6% in elective neck dissection and therapeutic neck dissection arms, respectively. **Conclusion: Ipsilateral elective neck dissection provides OS and DFS benefit in pts with early stage, well-lateralized OC-SCC, compared to therapeutic neck dissection.**

At what DOI should neck dissection be performed in early stage (cT1-2N0) oral tongue cancer?

Several retrospective studies have demonstrated DOI as significant predictor for locoregional recurrence. DOI ≥4 to 5 mm has been suggested as cutoff for neck dissection.

Huang, Princess Margaret Meta-Analysis (*Cancer* 2009, PMID: 19197973): Meta-analysis of 16 studies investigated negative-predictive value of DOI from 3 to 6 mm for cT1-2N0 oral tongue cancer. Probability of lymph node positivity at time of dissection or nodal relapse after ≥2 years follow-up increased ≥5 mm DOI. There was significant increase in nodal positivity between 4 mm and 5 mm DOI (p = .007). **Conclusion: DOI strongly predicts for cervical lymph node involvement. Elective neck dissection should be considered in pts with cN0 disease with DOI >4 mm.**

TABLE 11.3: PMH Meta-Analysis	
DOI (mm)	False Negative Rate (%)
3	5.3
4	4.5
5	16.6
6	13

Ganly, MSKCC & PMH combined analysis (*Cancer* 2013, PMID: 23184439): Combined analysis of 164 pts from MSKCC and PMH with pT1-2N0 oral tongue cancer treated with surgery alone (no postoperative RT). MFU was 66 months. Locoregional recurrence free survival at 5 years was 79.9%. Regional recurrence was ipsilateral in 61% of cases and contralateral in 39% of cases. Regional recurrence was 5.7% for tumors with < 4 mm DOI and 24% ≥4 mm DOI. Multivariate analysis demonstrated that tumor thickness ≥4 mm was significantly associated with regional recurrence free survival ($p = .02$). Pts with regional recurrence had significantly worse disease specific survival (33% vs. 97%; $p < .0001$). **Conclusion: Neck recurrence was significantly higher with DOI ≥4 mm. Contralateral neck failure was 40% in this subset of pts with early stage, cN0 disease.**

What are indications and benefit for postoperative RT for OC-SCC?

Typical indications include pT3-T4a; pN2-3; pT1-2N0-1 and one or more of following: PNI, LVSI, close margin <5 mm, or T2 oral cavity cancer with ≥5 mm DOI (can consider 4 mm based on Ganly data).[25] These are inclusion criteria for currently accruing RTOG 0920, investigating role of postoperative RT with or without cetuximab. These features have also been identified in various retrospective studies as significantly associated with inferior LRC, increased distant metastases, and inferior OS.[31,32] Many historic H&N studies included pts with OC-SCC (though lip subsite was often excluded).[22,31,33,34]

What are indications and benefit for addition of CHT to postoperative RT?

The combined analysis of Bernier and Cooper (EORTC 22931 and RTOG 9501) suggests that ECE and positive margins are indications for postoperative concurrent chemoRT (See PORT for H&N cancer for details). One recent trial at Tata Memorial in India also addressed this question.

Laskar (*ASCO* 2016, Abstract 6004): PRT of 900 pts with resectable OC-SCC who underwent surgery randomized to PORT alone (56–60 Gy in 5 fx/week) (Arm A), PORT with concurrent weekly cisplatin (30 mg/m²) (Arm B), or accelerated PORT (6 fx/week) (Arm C). MFU was 58 months. LRC at 5 years was 59.9% and 65.1% for Arm B versus Arm ($p = .203$) and 58.2% for Arm C ($p = NS$). Unplanned subset analysis demonstrated significantly improved LRC, DFS, and OS for pts with high risk features (T3-T4, N2-3, and ECE) for pts treated with standard fractionation RT and concurrent chemoRT compared to accelerated RT. **Conclusion: Intensification of therapy with concurrent CHT or accelerated RT did not improve outcomes in these pts with OC-SCC.** *Comment: Final results are pending and oral cavity cancer may have different biology in India than in the United States.*

Is there benefit to preoperative CHT, RT, or chemoRT prior to surgical resection in OC-SCC?

Several PRTs have investigated role of induction CHT with cisplatin/5-FU or TPF with no improvement in OS. Retrospective evidence suggests benefit to downstaging for pts who are unresectable.

Zhong, China (*JCO* 2013, PMID 23129742): PRT of 256 pts with Stage III-IVA resectable OC-SCC randomized to two cycles of induction TPF (docetaxel 75 mg/m² on day 1, cisplatin 75 mg/m² on day 1, and 5-FU 750 mg/m² on days 1–5) followed by surgery and PORT (54–66 Gy) versus surgery followed by PORT. MFU was 30 months. Clinical response rate to induction CHT was 80.6%. There was no significant difference in OS (HR 0.977; $p = .918$) or DFS (HR 0.974; $p = .897$) with induction TPF. Pts with clinical response or favorable pathologic response (≤10% viable tumor cells) had superior OS, LRC, and distant control with induction TPF. **Conclusion: There was no significant survival benefit with induction TPF.**

Licitra, Italy (*JCO* 2003, PMID 12525526): PRT of 195 pts with T2-4(>3 cm) N0-2 resectable OC-SCC randomized to three cycles of cisplatin and 5-FU followed by surgery versus surgery alone. PORT was included for positive margin, soft tissue invasion of face, >3 lymph nodes and/or ECE. There was no significant difference in 5-yr OS between induction CHT and surgery alone (55% vs. 55%). Fewer pts required PORT in CHT arm (33% vs. 46%). Pts who had pCR had significantly improved 10-yr OS (76% vs. 41%). **Conclusion: Induction CHT does not provide survival benefit, may decrease need for PORT.**

Patil, Tata Memorial, India (*Oral Oncol* 2014, PMID 25130412): RR of 721 pts with Stage IV unresectable OC-SCC who received two cycles of preoperative CHT. Pts either went onto surgery followed by postoperative chemoRT, definitive chemoRT, or palliative RT. Reduction in tumor size and successful resection occurred in 43% of pts. LRC at 24 months was 20.6% for entire cohort, 32% for those who underwent surgery, and 15% for those who did not (p = .0001). Median OS for pts who underwent surgery was 19.6 months and 8.16 months for those who did not (p = .0001). **Conclusion: Preoperative CHT improved rate of resection in pts with unresectable disease. Surgical resection was associated with significantly improved LRC and OS.**

Mohr, Germany (*Int J Oral Maxillofac Surg* 1994, PMID 7930766): PRT of 268 pts with T2-4N0-3 OC-SCC and oropharyngeal cancer randomized to preoperative chemoRT (36 Gy/18 fx with concurrent cisplatin) followed by surgery versus surgery alone. Surgery was completed 10 to 14 days after preoperative chemoRT. Locoregional recurrence was higher with surgery alone compared to preoperative chemoRT (31% vs. 15.6%). OS for preoperative chemoRT versus surgery alone was 19% versus 28%, respectively. **Conclusion: Induction chemoRT may provide LRC and OS benefit compared to surgery alone.**

What are patterns of failure after PORT?

Retrospective series have demonstrated that contralateral neck failure is common after ipsilateral neck RT and majority of failures are local, within high dose RT field.

Chan, Princess Margaret (*Oral Oncol* 2013, PMID 23079695): RR of 180 pts treated with PORT for Stage I-IV OC-SCC (46% oral tongue, 23% floor of mouth, 12% hard palate, 9% buccal). MFU was 34 months. LC, LRC, and OS at 2 years was 87%, 78%, and 65%, respectively. Of 38 locoregional failures, 26 were in field. Contralateral failure occurred in three of 12 pts treated to ipsilateral neck only and more common in pts with N2b disease. **Conclusion: Bilateral neck RT may be beneficial in pts with N2b disease.**

Yao, University of Iowa (*IJROBP* 2007, PMID 17276613): Retrospective review of 55 pts treated with IMRT for OC-SCC (49 pts received postoperative RT, five received definitive RT, and one received preoperative RT). OS and LRC at 2 years was 68% and 85%, respectively. All failures were in high dose RT field, except for one patient who failed in lower contralateral neck. Median time to locoregional recurrence was 4.1 months and locoregional control was significantly lower in pts with ECE. **Conclusion: Most failures after postoperative RT are in field.**

REFERENCES

1. Siegel RL, Miller KD, Jemal A. Cancer statistics, 2016. *CA Cancer J Clin.* 2016;66(s1):7–30.
2. Warnakulasuriya S. Global epidemiology of oral and oropharyngeal cancer. *Oral Oncol.* 2009;45(4–5):309–316.
3. Castellsague X, Alemany L, Quer M, et al. HPV involvement in head and neck cancers: comprehensive assessment of biomarkers in 3680 patients. *J Natl Cancer Inst.* 2016;108(6):djv403–414.

4. Kiaris H, Spandidos DA, Jones AS, et al. Mutations, expression and genomic instability of the H-ras proto-oncogene in squamous cell carcinomas of the head and neck. *Br J Cancer.* 1995;72(1):123–128.

5. Zhu X, Zhang F, Zhang W, et al. Prognostic role of epidermal growth factor receptor in head and neck cancer: a meta-analysis. *J Surg Oncol.* 2013;108(6):387–397.

6. Grégoire V, Ang K, Budach W, et al. Delineation of the neck node levels for head and neck tumors: a 2013 update. DAHANCA, EORTC, HKNPCSG, NCIC CTG, NCRI, RTOG, TROG consensus guidelines. *Radiother Oncol.* 2014;110(1):172–181.

7. Wolff KD, Follmann M, Nast A. The diagnosis and treatment of oral cavity cancer. *Dtsch Arztebl Int.* 2012;109(48):829–835.

8. Network CGA. Comprehensive genomic characterization of head and neck squamous cell carcinomas. *Nature.* 2015;517(7536):576–582.

9. Prout MN, Sidari JN, Witzburg RA, et al. Head and neck cancer screening among 4611 tobacco users older than forty years. *Otolaryngol Head Neck Surg.* 1997;116(2):201–208.

10. Sankaranarayanan R, Ramadas K, Thomas G, et al. Effect of screening on oral cancer mortality in Kerala, India: a cluster-randomised controlled trial. *Lancet.* 2005;365(9475):1927–1933.

11. Shah JP, Cendon RA, Farr HW, Strong EW. Carcinoma of the oral cavity: factors affecting treatment failure at the primary site and neck. *Am J Surg.* 1976;132(4):504–507.

12. Zelefsky MJ, Harrison LB, Fass DE, et al. Postoperative radiotherapy for oral cavity cancers: impact of anatomic subsite on treatment outcome. *Head Neck.* 1990;12(6):470–475.

13. Bell RB, Kademani D, Homer L, et al. Tongue cancer: is there a difference in survival compared with other subsites in the oral cavity? *J Oral Maxillofac Surg.* 2007;65(2):229–236.

14. Lee JJ, Hong WK, Hittelman WN, et al. Predicting cancer development in oral leukoplakia: ten years of translational research. *Clin Cancer Res.* 2000;6(5):1702–1710.

15. Luryi AL, Chen MM, Mehra S, et al. Treatment factors associated with survival in early-stage oral cavity cancer: analysis of 6830 cases from the national cancer data base. *JAMA Otolaryngol Head Neck Surg.* 2015;141(7):593–598.

16. Liao CT, Chang JT, Wang HM, et al. Survival in squamous cell carcinoma of the oral cavity: differences between pT4 N0 and other stage IVA categories. *Cancer.* 2007;110(3):564–571.

17. Cancer AJCo. *AJCC Cancer Staging Manual.* 8 th ed. Berlin, Germany: Springer Publishing; 2017.

18. Robertson AG, Soutar DS, Paul J, et al. Early closure of a randomized trial: surgery and postoperative radiotherapy versus radiotherapy in the management of intra-oral tumours. *Clin Oncol.* 1998;10(3):155–160.

19. Iyer NG, Tan DS, Tan VK, et al. Randomized trial comparing surgery and adjuvant radiotherapy versus concurrent chemoradiotherapy in patients with advanced, nonmetastatic squamous cell carcinoma of the head and neck: 10-year update and subset analysis. *Cancer.* 2015;121(10):1599–1607.

20. Zanoni DK, Migliacci JC, Xu B, et al. A proposal to redefine close surgical margins in squamous cell carcinoma of the oral tongue. *JAMA Otolaryngol Head Neck Surg.* 2017;143(6):555–560.

21. Boudreaux BA, Rosenthal EL, Magnuson JS, et al. Robot-assisted surgery for upper aerodigestive tract neoplasms. *Arch Otolaryngol Head Neck Surg.* 2009;135(4):397–401.

22. Bernier J, Cooper JS, Pajak TF, et al. Defining risk levels in locally advanced head and neck cancers: a comparative analysis of concurrent postoperative radiation plus chemotherapy trials of the EORTC (#22931) and RTOG (# 9501). *Head Neck.* 2005;27(10):843–850.

23. Bossi P, Lo Vullo S, Guzzo M, et al. Preoperative chemotherapy in advanced resectable OCSCC: long-term results of a randomized phase III trial. *Ann Oncol.* 2014;25(2):462–466.

24. Zhong LP, Zhang CP, Ren GX, et al. Randomized phase III trial of induction chemotherapy with docetaxel, cisplatin, and fluorouracil followed by surgery versus up-front surgery in locally advanced resectable oral squamous cell carcinoma. *J Clin Oncol.* 2013;31(6):744–751.

25. Ganly I, Goldstein D, Carlson DL, et al. Long-term regional control and survival in patients with "low-risk," early stage oral tongue cancer managed by partial glossectomy and neck dissection without postoperative radiation: the importance of tumor thickness. *Cancer.* 2013;119(6):1168–1176.

26. Gross ND, Patel SG, Carvalho AL, et al. Nomogram for deciding adjuvant treatment after surgery for oral cavity squamous cell carcinoma. *Head Neck.* 2008;30(10):1352–1360.

27. Wang SJ, Patel SG, Shah JP, et al. An oral cavity carcinoma nomogram to predict benefit of adjuvant radiotherapy. *JAMA Otolaryngol Head Neck Surg.* 2013;139(6):554–559.
28. Wang CC, Doppke KP, Biggs PJ. Intra-oral cone radiation therapy for selected carcinomas of the oral cavity. *Int J Radiat Oncol Biol Phys.* 1983;9(8):1185–1189.
29. Mazeron JJ, Ardiet JM, Haie-Meder C, et al. GEC-ESTRO recommendations for brachytherapy-therapy for head and neck squamous cell carcinomas. *Radiother Oncol.* 2009;91(2):150–156.
30. Videtic GMM. *Handbook of Treatment Planning in Radiation Oncology.* 2nd ed. New York City, NY: Demos Medical; 2014.
31. Ang KK, Trotti A, Brown BW, et al. Randomized trial addressing risk features and time factors of surgery plus radiotherapy in advanced head-and-neck cancer. *Int J Radiat Oncol Biol Phys.* 2001;51(3):571–578.
32. Peters LJ, Goepfert H, Ang KK, et al. Evaluation of the dose for postoperative radiation therapy of head and neck cancer: first report of a prospective randomized trial. *Int J Radiat Oncol Biol Phys.* 1993;26(1):3–11.
33. Bernier J, Domenge C, Ozsahin M, et al. Postoperative irradiation with or without concomitant chemotherapy for locally advanced head and neck cancer. *N Engl J Med.* 2004;350(19):1945–1952.
34. Cooper JS, Pajak TF, Forastiere AA, et al. Postoperative concurrent radiotherapy and chemotherapy for high-risk squamous-cell carcinoma of the head and neck. *N Engl J Med.* 2004;350(19):1937–1944.

12: NASOPHARYNGEAL CANCER

Shireen Parsai and Michael A. Weller

> **QUICK HIT:** Nasopharyngeal carcinoma (NPC) is rare in the United States, with high prevalence in endemic regions (South China, Southeast Asia, North Africa). The majority of U.S. cases (and nearly all cases in endemic areas) are related to EBV, and use of EBV DNA as a biomarker to guide therapy is under active investigation.

TABLE 12.1: General Treatment Paradigm for Nasopharyngeal Cancer[1]	
	Treatment Options
T1N0M0	Definitive IMRT (70 Gy/33–35 fx) + elective neck irradiation*
T1N1-3 and T2-4N0-3	Definitive concurrent chemoRT with adjuvant CHT
M1	CHT +/− targeted therapy with RT for palliative local control
If N0, treat RPNs and bilateral levels II–V; if node+, treat IB as well.	

EPIDEMIOLOGY: 3,200 cases per year in the United States (0.5–2 per 100,000). Endemic in South China, Hong Kong, Southeast Asia, North Africa (rates as high as 25 per 100,000). Estimated 51,000 deaths worldwide. More common in males (2.3:1 ratio).[2] In endemic areas, incidence peaks at 50 to 59 years of age; otherwise in low-risk populations incidence appears to increase with age.[3]

RISK FACTORS: EBV, salt preserved fish, preserved foods, low fruit/vegetable diet, tobacco smoke, family history, HPV.[3]

ANATOMY: Nasopharynx is cuboidal in shape and bordered anteriorly by posterior choanae (continuous with nasal cavity), posteriorly by vertebrae (C1–2), superiorly by skull base, and inferiorly by soft palate. Lateral walls are made of torus tubarius, which bounds Eustachian tube, and fossa of Rosenmüller. Most NPCs arise from fossa of Rosenmüller.[4]

PATHOLOGY: WHO classification is divided into three groups: *keratinizing* squamous cell carcinoma, *nonkeratinizing* carcinoma, which is further subdivided into differentiated and undifferentiated subgroups, and *basaloid* squamous cell carcinoma.

TABLE 12.2: WHO Classification for Nasopharyngeal Cancer			
WHO Classification[5]	**U.S. Incidence**	**Endemic Incidence[6]**	**Notes[7]**
Keratinizing	25%	1%	WHO type I (squamous cell carcinoma), associated with smoking and occasionally HPV
Nonkeratinizing • Differentiated	12%	3%	WHO type II (transitional cell carcinoma)
• Undifferentiated	63%	95%	WHO type III (lymphoepithelial carcinoma), endemic, associated with EBV, most favorable prognosis
Basaloid	–	<0.2%	Aggressive clinical course, poor survival

SCREENING: No screening protocol established. Screening methods are currently under investigation in endemic areas using EBV testing (e.g., IgA to EBV viral capsid antigen, plasma EBV DNA).

CLINICAL PRESENTATION: Most common presentations are painless neck mass, nasal or ear symptoms, headache, diplopia, or facial numbness.[1] Diplopia from local invasion, CN VI compressed first. Jacod's syndrome (cavernous sinus invasion). Dysphagia, hoarseness, Horner's syndrome, CN XI deficits can occur from lateral RPN compression on CNs IX to XII (Villaret's syndrome) or from invasion into jugular foramen (Vernet's syndrome).

WORKUP: H&P with attention to cranial nerves and neck adenopathy, nasopharyngoscopy.

Labs: Routine CBC, CMP as well as EBV DNA testing. Pretreatment plasma EBV DNA levels are prognostic.[1,8] Dental, nutritional, speech and swallowing, and audiology exam as clinically indicated. Ophthalmologic and endocrine evaluation as clinically indicated.

Imaging: MRI w/ contrast including BOS, nasopharynx, and neck to clavicles. CT of skull base/neck w/ contrast as clinically indicated. MRI is superior to CT for soft tissue/bone invasion, RPN evaluation. CT w/ contrast or PET/CT of upper mediastinum/chest as clinically indicated. Distant workup with PET/CT or CT w/ contrast especially for non-keratinizing histology, endemic phenotype, N2–N3 disease, stage III–IV disease.

PROGNOSTIC FACTORS: Stage, WHO classification (keratinizing worse, EBV-associated better), post-RT EBV DNA,[8] primary tumor volume (for LC), LDH levels (distant control).

NATURAL HISTORY: LN involvement is extremely common at diagnosis (75%–90%, bilateral in 50%). Five percent to 11% of pts have metastatic disease at time of diagnosis. Most common sites for DM are bone/lung (most common) and liver (least common).[9–11]

TABLE 12.3: AJCC 8th ed. (2017) Staging for Nasopharynx Cancer		cN0	cN1	cN2	cN3
T/M \ N					
T0	• No primary tumor, but EBV-positive cervical node				
T1	• Confined to nasopharynx or extension to oropharynx/ nasal cavity	I	II	III	IVA
T2	• Extension to parapharyngeal space and/or medial pterygoid, lateral pterygoid, prevertebral muscles				
T3	• Infiltration of bony structures[1]				
T4	• Extension[2]				
M1	• Distant metastasis		IVB		

Major changes from AJCC 7th Edition include adjacent muscle involvement (pterygoid/prevertebral) T2 classification, collapse of N3a-b into single N3 category and grouped stage IVA and IVB merged into IVA, with IVC becoming IVB.

Notes: Infiltration of bony structures[1] = Skull base, cervical vertebrae, pterygoid plates, paranasal sinuses. Extension[2] = Intracranial extension and/or involvement of cranial nerves, hypopharynx, orbit, parotid gland, soft tissue beyond lateral surface of lateral pterygoid muscle.

cN1, unilateral LNs and/or unilateral or bilateral metastasis in RPNs (≤6 cm), above caudal border of cricoid; cN2, bilateral LNs (≤6 cm), above caudal border of cricoid; cN3, unilateral or bilateral LNs (>6 cm) and/or LNs below caudal border of cricoid cartilage.

TREATMENT PARADIGM

Surgery: Surgery is not routine in up-front setting, but rather reserved as salvage option in select pts. Persistent nodal disease after primary therapy or nodal recurrence may be treated with neck dissection.

Chemotherapy: Concurrent chemoRT and adjuvant CHT is the standard of care in the United States for pts with Stage II–IVB disease. Cisplatin can be given concurrently with RT as 100 mg/m^2 bolus weeks 1, 4, and 7 or 40 mg/m^2 weekly. Adjuvant CHT consists of cisplatin (80 mg/m^2) and 5-FU (1,000 mg/m^2 for 4 days CIVI every 28 days for three cycles) beginning 4 weeks after completion of RT. Early results from NPC 0501 suggest that it may be feasible to replace 5-FU with capecitabine; however, further validation is required.[12]

Radiation

Indications: Stage I disease (T1N0M0) is generally treated with RT alone. Stage II–IVB NPC is treated with concurrent chemoRT, followed by adjuvant CHT.

Dose: Treat primary site to 70 Gy/35 fx or 69.96 Gy/33 fx (NRG HN001). Elective nodal RT (bilateral in all) to RPNs, levels II to V. Treat level IB in node-positive pts.

Toxicity: Acute: xerostomia, dysphagia, odynophagia, nausea, weight loss. *Late*: Hearing loss, dental carries, trismus, brainstem necrosis, optic neuritis, endocrinopathy.

Procedure: See *Treatment Planning Handbook*, Chapter 4.[13]

EVIDENCE-BASED Q&A

What is the role of CHT in treatment of nasopharyngeal cancer?

Concurrent chemoRT followed by adjuvant CHT is the standard of care in the United States. Historically, most pts were treated with RT alone, until intergroup Al-Sarraf trial demonstrated OS benefit to concurrent and adjuvant CHT compared to definitive RT alone in pts with stage III–IV NPC (AJCC 4th edition). These results were initially controversial, particularly in Asia. Critics argued outcomes of definitive RT alone arm were worse than historical standards. In addition, high proportion of WHO type I pts (22%) may account for poor outcomes and need for CHT. WHO type I histology is more common in the United States compared to endemic regions. Since then, multiple randomized trials have validated results of Intergroup study, and most recent update of MAC-NPC meta-analysis demonstrated absolute survival benefit of 6.3% at 5 years with concomitant CHT.[14]

Al-Sarraf, Intergroup 0099 (*JCO* 1998, PMID 9552031): PRT of 193 pts with biopsy proven stage III–IV (M0) nasopharyngeal cancer. Note that AJCC 4th edition included N1 pts in stage III (now stage II). Randomized to RT alone versus RT with concurrent bolus cisplatin and adjuvant CHT with cisplatin. Study was closed early after interim analysis of 147 pts demonstrated survival benefit in experimental arm. 63% completed all concurrent chemo, 55% completed all cycles of adjuvant. **Conclusion: Concurrent and adjuvant CHT with RT improves OS for Stage III–IV (and N1, 7/8th Edition stage II) nasopharyngeal cancer.**

TABLE 12.4: Results of Al-Sarraf INT 0099 Nasopharynx Trial		
	5-yr PFS	5-yr OS
RT	29%*	37%*
ChemoRT + Adjuvant CHT	58%*	67%*
Statistically significant.		

Blanchard, MAC-NPC Meta-analysis (*IJROBP* 2006, PMID 16377415; Update *Lancet Oncol* 2015, PMID 25957714): Update with 4,806 pts. MFU 7.7 years, addition of CHT to RT improved OS with absolute benefit of 6.3% at 5 years ($p < .0001$). Addition of CHT also improved PFS, locoregional control, distant control, and cancer mortality. Increase in OS was statistically significant for concomitant CHT (with and without adjuvant CHT), but not adjuvant CHT alone or induction CHT alone. **Conclusion: Concurrent CHT improves OS in locally advanced NPC.**

Is adjuvant CHT necessary?

This is area of active controversy. There has been one trial to directly address this question, detailed as follows. Although the trial was negative, it was heavily criticized (see the following comment). 2017 NCCN guidelines report concurrent chemoRT followed by adjuvant CHT category 2A recommendation and concurrent chemoRT alone category 2B recommendation.

Chen, Sun Yat-sen China (*Lancet Oncology* 2012, PMID 22154591): Multi-institution PRT involving institutions in China. 508 pts with stage III/IV (T3-4N0 excluded) randomized to concurrent chemoRT +/- adjuvant CHT (cisplatin 80 mg/m^2 and 5-FU 800 mg/m^2 for 120 hours q4weeks x3 cycles). Primary endpoint was failure-free survival. Two-yr FFS rate was 84% in concurrent only arm and 86% in concurrent + adjuvant arm ($p = .13$). *Comment: Did not use noninferiority design, 18% randomized to adjuvant CHT did not receive it, nearly 60% did not complete concurrent chemo, 50% required RT dose reduction, and 70% had treatment delays.*

TABLE 12.5: Pros and Cons of Adjuvant CHT for NPC	
Rationale for Eliminating Adjuvant CHT	**Rationale for Employing Adjuvant CHT**
• Historic trials investigating use of adjuvant CHT after definitive RT have been negative • PRTs evaluating RT alone vs. chemoRT (w/o adjuvant) show survival benefit to concurrent (Taiwan, Hong Kong, China). • Two meta-analyses investigating impact of CHT on outcomes have suggested that major driver of benefit is concurrent phase. Baujat analysis found 18% reduction in HR of death with CHT overall, with 40% risk reduction with concurrent and 3% risk reduction with adjuvant.[15] Langendijk analysis suggested 20% survival benefit at 5 years with concurrent CHT and no benefit to adjuvant.[16] • PRT from China randomized pts to chemoRT with weekly cisplatin +/- three cycles adjuvant cisplatin/5-FU. While there were more failures in arm without adjuvant CHT, they were not statistically different ($p = .13$).[17] • Compliance is poor, generally only 50%–60% of pts complete full course of adjuvant therapy on PRTs.	• Data from Taiwan suggest that for pts at high risk of distant failure, concurrent chemoRT is insufficient.[18] • Analysis of phase III Hong Kong data showed that concurrent cisplatin plus adjuvant cisplatin–fluorouracil was associated with improved distant control. In pts who received 0–1 cycles, 5-yr distant FFR was 68% vs. 78% for 2–3 cycles.[18] • Chinese PRT did not use noninferiority design; therefore premature to suggest it should change practice. Additionally, 18% of pts in adjuvant arm did not receive it, 50% required RT dose reduction, and 70% had treatment delays. • In modern series using IMRT, LRC is excellent, and major pattern of failure is now distant.

Which pts benefit from CHT?

Pts with stage I NPC can be treated with definitive RT alone. Majority of clinical trials demonstrating benefit with addition of CHT to RT (including INT 0099) included pts with stage III–IV disease. Pts with stage II disease have been found to have worse outcomes compared to stage I with distant failure rates as high as 10% to 15% with N1 disease. RR from Taiwan suggested that addition of CHT in stage II pts resulted in similar outcomes to those found in stage I pts treated with RT alone.[19] This led to phase III trial in China as discussed in the following.

Chen, Sun Yat-sen China (*JNCI* 2011, PMID 22056739): PRT of 230 pts with stage II NPC randomized to concurrent chemoRT with weekly cisplatin (30 mg/m^2) versus RT alone. See Table 12.6. 5-yr OS improved with CHT, at expense of worse acute toxicity. *Notes: OS* advantage driven by improvement in distant failure, LRC unchanged. Multivariate analysis showed that the number of CHT cycles delivered was the only factor associated with improved OS, PFS, and distant control.

TABLE 12.6: Sun Yat-sen Trial (China) Investigating Concurrent chemoRT for NPC

Chen	5-yr LRC	5-yr PFS	5-yr DMFS	5-yr OS	Acute G3-4	Late G3-4
RT	91%	79%	84%	86%	40%	10%
ChemoRT	93%	88%	95%	95%	64%	14%

What is the role of induction CHT?

This remains under investigation. Trials of induction CHT followed by RT alone have failed to show any survival benefit. More recently, there has been significant interest in adding neoadjuvant CHT prior to concurrent chemoRT. Rationale includes improved compliance (relative to adjuvant CHT) and potential for downstaging. Phase IIR (not powered for survival) from Hong Kong did demonstrate 26.5% absolute improvement in 3-year OS by adding induction cisplatin and docetaxel to CRT with no compromise in ability to deliver full course of chemoRT afterward.[20] However, phase IIR from Europe was negative.[21] Early results from NPC 0501 (six-arm trial investigating induction–concurrent sequence, use of capecitabine, and acceleration) were recently published, and unadjusted results also did not demonstrate improvement with induction CHT, though more follow-up is needed.[12]

Sun, China (*Lancet Oncol* 2016, PMID 27686945): Multicenter PRT involving 10 institutions in China, 480 pts, evaluating addition induction CHT (TPF: cisplatin, fluorouracil, docetaxel Q3 weeks x three cycles) to concurrent chemoRT in locally advanced NPC. Eligibility criteria included stage III–IVB (except T3-4N0). Concurrent CHT given as cisplatin 100 mg/m^2 Q3 weeks x three cycles. Primary endpoint FFS. MFU 45 months, 3-yr FFS increased from 72% to 80% (p = .034) in favor of induction chemo. Induction CHT was associated with increased grade 3/4 toxicity: 42% versus 17% neutropenia, 41% versus 17% leukopenia, 41% versus 35% stomatitis. **Conclusion: Induction CHT significantly improved 3-yr FFS compared to concurrent chemoRT alone.**

What is the role of targeted therapies?

In modern series of concurrent chemoRT using IMRT, local control is excellent (>90%), and therefore primary pattern of failure is distant metastases. Compliance with standard CHT regimens is a challenge, making the addition of further systemic therapy with the goal of addressing distant disease difficult. As such, there has been significant interest in addition of targeted therapies. Most prominent example is RTOG 0615, phase II trial of chemoRT (Al-Sarraf regimen) plus concurrent and adjuvant bevacizumab.[22] Regimen was shown to be feasible, and 2-year DM-free interval was noted to be 90.8%.

What is the role of IMRT?

IMRT is the standard of care. It has been shown in two randomized trials to improve salivary function, with multiple series suggesting rates >90%.[23,24] RTOG 0225 was designed to test feasibility of IMRT in a multi-institution setting.[24] Based on UCSF experience, 70 Gy/33 fx was delivered to gross disease, with subclinical volume receiving 59.4 Gy/33 fx. IMRT is feasible with excellent LC and very low grade 3 xerostomia.

TABLE 12.7: Results of RTOG 0225 Early IMRT for NPC

RTOG 0225	2-yr LC	2-yr LRC	2-yr DMFS	2-yr PFS	2-yr OS	Grade 3 Xerostomia
	93%	89%	85%	73%	80%	3%

What is the role of altered fractionation?

There is little data to support altered fractionation with modern treatment planning and concurrent CHT. Though NPC 9902 did show improvement in failure-free rates with accelerated RT and CHT, this was underpowered trial with older RT techniques, and majority of benefit was driven by improvement in distant metastases.[25] Most recent evidence comes from NPC 0501 (six-arm trial investigating induction–concurrent sequence, use of capecitabine, and accelerated fractionation). In this trial there was no benefit to acceleration, with increased toxicity and worse compliance with CHT. Before accrual was complete, protocol was amended to allow centers to opt out of accelerated fractionation portion of trial, and authors concluded: "Accelerated fractionation is not recommended for pts with NPC who are receiving chemoRT."[12]

What is the role of adaptive replanning?

Adaptive replanning should be strongly considered. Nasopharyngeal cancer is radiosensitive tumor, and large anatomic changes are possible during treatment. Dosimetric studies have shown that replanning can improve coverage as well as reduce dose to surrounding critical structures. In prospective study from China, 129 pts with M0 NPC were enrolled, 86 of whom were replanned before 25th fraction. Pts who were replanned were found to have superior 2-yr LRC (97% vs. 92%) and reported improved global QOL, functional QOL, and symptoms (dyspnea, appetite loss, speech problems, dry mouth, etc.).[26]

What is the role of serum EBV DNA levels?

EBV is the primary etiologic agent in pathogenesis of NPC, and EBV levels both pre- and posttreatment are prognostic for survival. Though optimal values remain to be elucidated, pts with pretreatment ranging from <1,500 copies/mL to <4,000 copies/mL tend to have improved survival. Multiple studies have shown that detectable EBV after definitive RT may serve as a poor prognostic marker.[27,28]

REFERENCES

1. NCCN Clinical Practice Guidelines in Oncology: Head and Neck Cancers (Version 2). 2017. https://www.nccn.org/professionals/physician_gls/pdf/head-and-neck.pdf
2. Ferlay J, Soerjomataram I, Dikshit R, et al. Cancer incidence and mortality worldwide: sources, methods and major patterns in GLOBOCAN 2012. *Int J Cancer.* 2015;136(5):E359–E386.
3. Chang ET, Adami HO. The enigmatic epidemiology of nasopharyngeal carcinoma. *Cancer Epidemiol Biomarkers Prev.* 2006;15(10):1765–1777.
4. Halperin E, Perez C, Brady L. *Principles and Practice of Radiation Oncology.* 6th ed. Philadelphia, PA: Lippincott Williams & Wilkins; 2013.
5. Stelow EB, Wenig BM. Update from the 4th edition of the World Health Organization classification of head and neck tumours: nasopharynx. *Head Neck Pathol.* 2017;11(1):16–22.
6. Wei WI, Sham JS. Nasopharyngeal carcinoma. *Lancet.* 2005;365(9476):2041–2054.
7. *AJCC Cancer Staging Manual.* 8th ed. New York, NY: Springer International Publishing; 2017.
8. Hui EP, Ma BB, Chan KC, et al. Clinical utility of plasma Epstein-Barr virus DNA and ERCC1 single nucleotide polymorphism in nasopharyngeal carcinoma. *Cancer.* 2015;121(16):2720–2729.
9. Vokes EE, Liebowitz DN, Weichselbaum RR. Nasopharyngeal carcinoma. *Lancet.* 1997; 350(9084):1087–1091.
10. Hsu MM, Tu SM. Nasopharyngeal carcinoma in Taiwan: clinical manifestations and results of therapy. *Cancer.* 1983;52(2):362–368.
11. Altun M, Fandi A, Dupuis O, et al. Undifferentiated nasopharyngeal cancer (UCNT): current diagnostic and therapeutic aspects. *Int J Radiat Oncol Biol Phys.* 1995;32(3):859–877.

12. Lee AW, Ngan RK, Tung SY, et al. Preliminary results of trial NPC-0501 evaluating the therapeutic gain by changing from concurrent-adjuvant to induction-concurrent chemoradiotherapy, changing from fluorouracil to capecitabine, and changing from conventional to accelerated radiotherapy fractionation in patients with locoregionally advanced nasopharyngeal carcinoma. *Cancer*. 2015;121(8):1328–1338.

13. Videtic GMM WN, Vassil AD. *Handbook of Treatment Planning in Radiation Oncology*. 2nd ed. New York, NY: Demos Medical; 2015.

14. Blanchard P, Lee A, Marguet S, et al. Chemotherapy and radiotherapy in nasopharyngeal carcinoma: an update of the MAC-NPC meta-analysis. *Lancet Oncol*. 2015;16(6):645–655.

15. Baujat B, Audry H, Bourhis J, et al. Chemotherapy in locally advanced nasopharyngeal carcinoma: an individual patient data meta-analysis of eight randomized trials and 1753 patients. *Int J Radiat Oncol Biol Phys*. 2006;64(1):47–56.

16. Langendijk JA, Leemans CR, Buter J, et al. The additional value of chemotherapy to radiotherapy in locally advanced nasopharyngeal carcinoma: a meta-analysis of the published literature. *J Clin Oncol*. 2004;22(22):4604–4612.

17. Chen L, Hu CS, Chen XZ, et al. Concurrent chemoradiotherapy plus adjuvant chemotherapy versus concurrent chemoradiotherapy alone in patients with locoregionally advanced nasopharyngeal carcinoma: a phase 3 multicentre randomised controlled trial. *Lancet Oncol*. 2012;13(2):163–171.

18. Lin JC, Liang WM, Jan JS, et al. Another way to estimate outcome of advanced nasopharyngeal carcinoma: is concurrent chemoradiotherapy adequate? *Int J Radiat Oncol Biol Phys*. 2004;60(1):156–164.

19. Cheng SH, Tsai SY, Yen KL, et al. Concomitant radiotherapy and chemotherapy for early-stage nasopharyngeal carcinoma. *J Clin Oncol*. 2000;18(10):2040–2045.

20. Hui EP, Ma BB, Leung SF, et al. Randomized phase II trial of concurrent cisplatin-radiotherapy with or without neoadjuvant docetaxel and cisplatin in advanced nasopharyngeal carcinoma. *J Clin Oncol*. 2009;27(2):242–249.

21. Fountzilas G, Ciuleanu E, Bobos M, et al. Induction chemotherapy followed by concomitant radiotherapy and weekly cisplatin versus the same concomitant chemoradiotherapy in patients with nasopharyngeal carcinoma: a randomized phase II study conducted by the Hellenic Cooperative Oncology Group (HeCOG) with biomarker evaluation. *Ann Oncol*. 2012;23(2):427–435.

22. Lee NY, Zhang Q, Pfister DG, et al. Addition of bevacizumab to standard chemoradiation for locoregionally advanced nasopharyngeal carcinoma (RTOG 0615): a phase 2 multi-institutional trial. *Lancet Oncol*. 2012;13(2):172–180.

23. Kam MK, Leung SF, Zee B, et al. Prospective randomized study of intensity-modulated radiotherapy on salivary gland function in early-stage nasopharyngeal carcinoma patients. *J Clin Oncol*. 2007;25(31):4873–4879.

24. Pow EH, Kwong DL, McMillan AS, et al. Xerostomia and quality of life after intensity-modulated radiotherapy vs. conventional radiotherapy for early-stage nasopharyngeal carcinoma: initial report on a randomized controlled clinical trial. *Int J Radiat Oncol Biol Phys*. 2006;66(4):981–991.

25. Lee AW, Tung SY, Chan AT, et al. A randomized trial on addition of concurrent-adjuvant chemotherapy and/or accelerated fractionation for locally-advanced nasopharyngeal carcinoma. *Radiother Oncol*. 2011;98(1):15–22.

26. Yang H, Hu W, Wang W, et al. Replanning during intensity modulated radiation therapy improved quality of life in patients with nasopharyngeal carcinoma. *Int J Radiat Oncol Biol Phys*. 2013;85(1):e47–e54.

27. Lin JC, Wang WY, Chen KY, et al. Quantification of plasma Epstein-Barr virus DNA in patients with advanced nasopharyngeal carcinoma. *N Engl J Med*. 2004;350(24):2461–2470.

28. Leung SF, Zee B, Ma BB, et al. Plasma Epstein-Barr viral deoxyribonucleic acid quantitation complements tumor-node-metastasis staging prognostication in nasopharyngeal carcinoma. *J Clin Oncol*. 2006;24(34):5414–5418.

13: LARYNGEAL CANCER

Aditya Juloori

> **QUICK HIT:** Laryngeal cancer includes squamous carcinoma originating from the supraglottis, glottis, or rarely the subglottis. Goal of treatment is to achieve disease control while maintaining organ function, defined as functional voice with intact swallowing. Early-stage glottic cancers can be managed with RT alone or microsurgery. Locoregionally advanced disease, defined as T3-4 or node-positive, frequently requires either total laryngectomy (with adjuvant RT as indicated) or definitive chemoRT to attempt voice preservation. For pts with T4a disease penetrating through thyroid cartilage or with significant soft-tissue extension, total laryngectomy with PORT is preferred over definitive chemoRT.

TABLE 13.1: General Treatment Paradigm for Larynx Cancer		
	Supraglottic	**Glottic**
Tis	**Endoscopic Surgery**	
T1N0	Larynx-sparing surgery OR Definitive RT (66–70 Gy) to primary tumor + elective LN levels II–IV	Definitive RT (63 Gy/28 fx at 2.25 Gy/fx) OR larynx-sparing surgery
T2N0		Definitive RT (65.25 Gy/29 fx at 2.25 Gy/fx) OR larynx-sparing surgery
T3 or node-positive	Larynx-sparing surgery w/ PORT OR definitive chemoRT (70 Gy/35 fx) to tumor + elective LN II–IV (V if LN+) w/ cisplatin	
T4a	Total laryngectomy (preferred for thyroid cartilage penetration or significant soft-tissue extension) with adjuvant RT +/− concurrent cisplatin as indicated OR Larynx preservation with concurrent chemoRT to 70 Gy/35 fx with cisplatin	

EPIDEMIOLOGY: 13,000 new diagnoses of laryngeal cancer in the United States with estimated 3,600 deaths in 2016. More common in men than women; incidence increases with age.[1]

RISK FACTORS: Smoking, alcohol, environmental exposures (asbestos, cement, wood dust, perchlorethylene).

ANATOMY: Major functions of larynx are voice production, airway patency during breathing, and airway occlusion during swallowing. It spans from C3 to C6 vertebral bodies and is bordered superiorly by hyoepiglottic ligament, inferiorly by cricoid, anteriorly by thyrohyoid membrane/thyroid cartilage, and posteriorly by arytenoid cartilage. Preepiglottic and paraglottic spaces are one continuous space anterosuperiorly. Laryngeal muscles (with exception of cricothyroid) are innervated by recurrent laryngeal nerve (branch of vagus nerve). Damage to this nerve results in a fixed, midline cord. Cricothyroid muscle is innervated by superior laryngeal nerve. Damage to this nerve results in mobile, "bowed" cords.

The larynx is divided into three segments:

1. *Supraglottis* (1/3 of all laryngeal cancers,[1] mnemonic FAVEA: false vocal cords, arytenoids, ventricles, epiglottis, aryepiglottic folds): Bordered superiorly by epiglottis, posteriorly by arytenoids, anteriorly by posterior edge of vallecula and anterior false cord, and inferiorly by epithelium of true vocal cord as it turns upward to form apex of ventricle. More than 50% of pts with supraglottic primaries present with node-positive disease due to presence of extensive lymphatics in this part of larynx. Levels II to IV are primary drainage sites for supraglottis.
2. *Glottis* (2/3 of all laryngeal cancers[2]): Consists of true vocal cords and anterior and posterior commissures. Due to sparse lymphatics, early-stage disease rarely involves regional nodes. True vocal cord is made up of the following layers: epithelial mucosa, basement membrane, superficial layer of lamina propria, and thyroarytenoid muscle.
3. *Subglottis* (1%–2% of all laryngeal cancers[3]): Starts 5 mm inferior to margin of vocal cords to inferior aspect of cricoid cartilage. Subglottic tumors can drain to pretracheal (Delphian) nodes.

PATHOLOGY: 95% of tumors are squamous cell carcinoma. Carcinoma in situ occurs in vocal cords, but is rare in supraglottis. Rare malignancies: malignant minor salivary gland, small cell, lymphoma, plasmacytoma, carcinoid, soft-tissue sarcoma, chondrosarcoma, osteosarcoma, malignant melanoma. HPV positivity has not been shown to be prognostic or predictive in laryngeal cancer.

CLINICAL PRESENTATION: Presenting clinical symptoms are classically related to site of origin. Glottic cancers often present at early stage with hoarseness but as disease progresses, pts develop otalgia, dysphagia, cough, hemoptysis, stridor. In supraglottis, cancers are often detected later and commonly present with dysphagia, globus sensation, airway obstruction, and lymphadenopathy. Otalgia is due to referred pain to auricular branch of Arnold (from vagus nerve).

WORKUP: H&P including flexible nasopharyngolaryngoscopy. Videostroboscopy can be used to evaluate mucosal wave of true cords. Pain with palpation of thyroid cartilage can be reflective of cartilage invasion.

Labs: Routine CBC and CMP. Pre-CHT audiology exam.

Imaging: CT neck with contrast and PET/CT for stage III/IV disease. CT scan has high positive-predictive value for thyroid cartilage penetration (74%) and extralaryngeal spread (81%).[4]

Pathology: EUA with triple endoscopy (~4% incidence of second primary) and biopsy. Dental, nutrition, speech and swallow evaluation as indicated.

STAGING

TABLE 13.2: AJCC 8th ed. (2017) Staging for Larynx Cancer

SUPRAGLOTTIS

T/M \\ N		cN0	cN1	cN2a	cN2b	cN2c	cN3a	cN3b
T1	• Limited to 1 subsite of supraglottis with normal vocal cord mobility	I						
T2	• Invades mucosa of >1 adjacent subsite of supraglottis or glottis, or region outside supraglottis without fixation of larynx[1]	II	III		IVA		IVB	
T3	• Limited to larynx with vocal cord fixation • Invasion[2]							
T4	a Moderately advanced local disease[3]							
	b Very advanced local disease[4]							
M1	• Distant metastasis	IVC						

Significant changes from AJCC 7th Edition include inclusion of ENE into nodal staging, refinement of pN classification and introduction of N3a/b distinction.

Notes: Larynx[1] = Regions include mucosa of BOT, vallecula, medial wall of pyriform sinus. Invades[2] = Postcricoid area, preepiglottic space, paraglottic space, and/or inner cortex of thyroid cartilage. Disease[3] = invades through thyroid cartilage outer cortex, trachea, soft tissues of neck, deep extrinsic muscles of tongue, strap muscles, thyroid, or esophagus. Disease[4] = Invades prevertebral space, encases carotid artery, or invades mediastinal structures.

cN1, single ipsilateral LN (≤3 cm) and -ENE; cN2a, single ipsilateral LN (3.1-6 cm) and –ENE; cN2b, multiple ipsilateral LN (≤6 cm) and –ENE; cN2c, bilateral or contralateral LN (≤6 cm) and –ENE; cN3a, LN (>6 cm) and –ENE; cN3b, clinically overt ENE.

pN1, single LN (≤3 cm) and – ENE; pN2a, single ipsilateral or contralateral LN (≤3 cm) and + ENE or single ipsilateral LN (3.1–6 cm) and – ENE; pN2b, multiple ipsilateral LN (≤6 cm) and – ENE; pN2c, bilateral or contralateral LN (≤6 cm) and – ENE; pN3a, LN (>6 cm) and – ENE; pN3b, LN (>3 cm) and + ENE.

GLOTTIS

T/M \\ N		cN0	cN1	cN2a	cN2b	cN2c	cN3a	cN3b
T1	a Limited to 1 vocal cord with normal mobility	I						
	b Involves 2 vocal cords with normal mobility							
T2	• Extends to supraglottis and/or subglottis and/or with impaired vocal cord mobility[1]	II	III		IVA		IVB	
T3	• Limited to larynx with vocal cord fixation • Invades[2]							
T4	a Moderately advanced local disease[3]							
	b Very advanced local disease[4]							

(continued)

GLOTTIS (continued)								
T/M N	cN0	cN1	cN2a	cN2b	cN2c	cN3a	cN3b
M1 • Distant metastasis	IVC						

Notes: Mobility[1] = Unofficially, T2 can be divided into T2a (mobile cord) and T2b (impaired cord mobility). Invades[2] = Paraglottic space and/or inner cortex of thyroid cartilage. Disease[3] = invades through thyroid cartilage outer cortex, trachea, soft tissues of neck, deep extrinsic muscles of tongue, strap muscles, thyroid, or esophagus. Disease[4] = Invades prevertebral space, encases carotid artery, or invades mediastinal structures.

Refer to supraglottic larynx for nodal staging.

SUBGLOTTIS								
T/M N	cN0	cN1	cN2a	cN2b	cN2c	cN3a	cN3b
T1 • Limited to subglottis	I					IVB	
T2 • Extends to vocal cords with normal or impaired mobility	II	III	IVA				
T3 • Limited to larynx with vocal cord fixation • Invades[1]							
T4 a Moderately advanced local disease[2]							
b Very advanced local disease[3]							
M1 • Distant metastasis	IVC						

*Significant changes from AJCC 7th Edition include inclusion of ENE into nodal staging, refinement of pN classification and introduction of N3a/b distinction.

Notes: Invades[1] = Invasion of paraglottic space and/or inner cortex of thyroid cartilage. Disease[2] = invades through thyroid cartilage outer cortex, trachea, soft tissues of neck, deep extrinsic muscles of tongue, strap muscles, thyroid, or esophagus. Disease[3] = Invades prevertebral space, encases carotid artery, or invades mediastinal structures.

Refer to supraglottic larynx for nodal staging.

TREATMENT PARADIGM

Surgery

Glottis: Modern surgical options for early glottic tumors focus on endoscopic resection with aim of preserving laryngeal function and have largely replaced external approaches. Note that at least one mobile arytenoid complex must be preserved to maintain adequate function of larynx. Endoscopic techniques can include mucosal stripping (for in situ disease), microdissection (including transoral robotic surgery [TORS]), electrocautery, CO_2 laser (transoral laser microsurgery [TLM or TOLM]), among others. Other voice-conserving options are as follows.

Vertical Hemilaryngectomy: Removes up to one true vocal cord as well as one-third of contralateral true cord. Appropriate for lesions with up to 1 cm anterior subglottic extension and 5 mm posterior subglottic extension.[5]

Supracricoid partial laryngectomy (SCPL–CHEP): Resection of true and false cords, paraglottic spaces, and entire thyroid cartilage. Arytenoids and cricoid cartilage are preserved. Cricohyoidoepiglottopexy (CHEP) is performed, which involves reconstruction by suturing cricoid to hyoid and epiglottis.

Supraglottis: Voice-preserving options include the following.

Supraglottic laryngectomy (SGL): Swallow- and voice-preserving surgery that may be used for tumors of epiglottis, single arytenoid, aryepiglottic fold, or false cord. Included in resection are hyoid bone, epiglottis, superior half of thyroid cartilage, AE folds, and false cords to arytenoids.

Supracricoid partial laryngectomy (SCPL–CHP): Resection of both true and false cords, paraglottic space, preepiglottic space, epiglottis, and thyroid cartilage. Reconstruction includes suturing of cricoid to hyoid, cricohyoidopexy. Total laryngectomy includes removal of larynx, pharynx is reconstructed (often with free flap) and permanent tracheostomy is required. For pts treated with primary surgical approach, elective neck dissection of bilateral levels II to IV is warranted for most pts with supraglottic cancer and for locally advanced glottic disease.

Chemotherapy: Concurrent CHT is not routinely given for early-stage disease, but considered by some for unfavorable T2 disease (impaired mobility). In definitive chemoRT for T2b or Stage III–IVB disease, concurrent cisplatin is the standard of care, given as 100 mg/m^2 bolus weeks 1, 4, 7 (NCCN Category 1) OR 40 mg/m^2 weekly (NCCN Category 2B). Cetuximab can be used for nonplatinum candidates, with loading dose of 400 mg/m^2 1 week prior to RT followed by 250 mg/m^2 weekly during RT. Use of induction CHT is controversial but has been used to select pts for laryngectomy versus preservation and consists of docetaxel, cisplatin, 5-fluorouracil (TPF) q3 weeks X four cycles completed 4 to 7 weeks prior to RT.

Radiation

Indications: Early-stage disease (cT1-T2N0) is typically treated with RT alone. Locally advanced disease is treated definitively (larynx preservation) or postoperatively (see PORT for Head and Neck chapter). Nodal basins are typically not electively included in RT volumes in early-stage glottic pts unless supraglottic involvement is suspected, making risk of occult nodal metastasis higher. Cervical LN levels II to IV are targeted bilaterally and level V is included for node-positive hemineck or with primary tumor extension to base of tongue. Consider inclusion of level VIa for anterior soft-tissue extension or emergency tracheostomy with tumor cut-through. Consider level VIb with subglottic extension of primary tumor.

Dose: For T1N0 glottic cancers, accelerated hypofractionation has been shown to improve LC compared to standard fractionation. Recommended dose is 63 Gy/28 fx (2.25 Gy/fx). For T2aN0 disease, common dose is 65.25 Gy/29 fx. For pts with T2bN0 disease, LC is inferior with RT alone and thus alternative approaches including addition of concurrent CHT or hyperfractionation are considered. For locally advanced disease, 70 Gy/35 fx with CHT is common.

Toxicity

Acute: Fatigue, dysphagia, mucositis, hoarseness, xerostomia, odynophagia, RT dermatitis, dysgeusia, aspiration. *Late*: Dysphagia, esophageal stricture, aspiration, hoarseness, hearing loss, renal insufficiency, neck fibrosis, stroke, hypothyroidism.

Procedure: See *Treatment Planning Handbook*, Chapter 4.[6]

EVIDENCE-BASED Q&A

Early-stage disease

What is the general treatment paradigm for early-stage disease?

Both RT and laryngeal preservation surgery provide excellent outcomes for early-stage disease.

Retrospective evidence demonstrates 5-yr DFS above 90% for stage I disease and around 80% for stage II disease with either definitive RT or surgery.[7] Randomized data is sparse, however. Small randomized trial published in 2014[8] did show less patient-reported hoarseness in those treated with RT compared to those treated with transoral laser surgery, but overall voice quality was similar. In general, voice quality is related to amount of vocal cord resected.

What is the impact of larger fraction size for early-stage disease?

Mild hypofractionation and acceleration has shown consistent improvement in local control for early disease.

Le, UCSF (*IJROBP* 1997, PMID 9300746): RR of 398 pts with T1–T2 glottic cancer (315 T1, 83 T2) treated with definitive RT to median dose of 63 Gy. Overall, 5-yr LC was 85% for T1 pts and 70% for T2 pts. Anterior commissure involvement and earlier treatment era predicted for worse LC in T1 pts. In T2 pts (but NOT T1), poor prognostic factors for LC included overall treatment time (>43 days), smaller fraction size (<1.8 Gy/fx), lower total dose (≤65 Gy) impaired VC mobility, and subglottic extension.

TABLE 13.3: UCSF Experience in Early Larynx Cancer (cT2 pts)						
	5-yr LC		**5-yr LC**			**5-yr LC**
Treatment time ≤43 days	100%	Fx ≥2.25 Gy/day	100%	>65 Gy	78%
Treatment time >43 days	84%	Fx <1.8 Gy/day	44%	≤65 Gy	60%
p value	.003	*p* value	.003	*p* value	.01
No VC mobility impaired	79%	No subglottic extension	77%		
VC mobility impaired	45%	Subglottic extension	58%		
p value	.02	*p* value	.04		

Yamazaki, Japan (*IJROBP* 2006, PMID 16169681): PRT of 180 pts with T1N0 SCC of glottis (80% T1a) treated with definitive RT and randomized to 2 Gy/fx or 2.25 Gy/fx. For standard fractionation arm, pts were treated to 60 Gy for tumor length <⅔ of glottis and to 66 Gy for ≥⅔ of glottis. In 2.25 Gy/fx arm, total dose was 56.25 and 63 Gy respectively for tumor length <⅔ of glottis and ≥⅔ of glottis respectively. 5-yr LC was 92% in hypofractionation arm compared to 77% in standard fractionation arm. Fraction size was independent predictor for LC. Acute and late toxicities were equivalent. **Conclusion: Decreasing overall treatment time with larger fraction sizes improved LC without causing increased acute or late toxicity in pts with T1N0 glottic cancer.**

What is impact of hyperfractionation for early-stage disease?

RTOG 95-12 demonstrated modest, but not statistically significant benefit in local control with use of hyperfractionated RT in pts with T2N0 glottic cancer. T2b was a negative prognostic factor.

Trotti, RTOG 9512 (*IJROBP* 2014 PMID 25035199): PRT of 250 pts with T2N0 SCC of glottis treated with definitive RT randomized to hyperfractionation (79.2 Gy/66 fx at 1.2 Gy BID) or standard fractionation (70 Gy/35 fx). Primary endpoint was LC. While there were trends toward improved outcomes with HFRT, there were no significant differences in 5-yr LC (78% vs. 70%, p = .14), 5-yr DFS (49% vs. 40%, p = .13) or 5-yr OS (72% vs. 63%, p = .29). LC in T2b pts was relatively lower (70% T2b vs. 76% T2a, p = .1). There was no difference in rates of grade 3–4 late toxicity between treatment arms. Of note, the trial was powered to detect 15% absolute difference in 5-yr LC. **Conclusion: Hyperfractionation modestly improves LC as seen in other disease sites of head and neck, though not statistically significant in this study.**

How should T2b pts be treated?

T2b glottic cancer has not been adopted by the AJCC but has been described as presence of hypo-mobile cord. Pts with T2b disease had worse local control in RTOG 9512 (63%) and in other large retrospective series[9,10] and thus may benefit from alteration from standard treatment. Options to improve local control in this unfavorable subset include hyperfractionation, hypofractionation (e.g., 65.25 Gy/29 fx), or addition of concurrent CHT.[11]

Is there any role for IMRT in early-stage population?

There is no routine role and IMRT should be considered investigational. Proposed rationale is late toxicity avoidance, particularly vascular toxicity with carotid sparing. Early series have shown that carotid sparing is feasible without detriment in local control,[12,13] but results are still immature at this time.

Locally advanced disease

What is the basis for larynx preservation for locally advanced disease?

While definitive surgery followed by PORT had been traditional paradigm, VA Laryngeal Study prospectively demonstrated equivalent survival rates with nonoperative approach and RTOG 91-11 demonstrated superior rates of larynx preservation with concurrent chemoRT compared to pts treated with either induction CHT or RT, or RT alone. T4 pts had higher rate of needing salvage laryngectomy in VA Larynx study and thus large volume T4 pts were excluded in RTOG 91-11. However, an NCDB analysis demonstrated that majority of pts with T4a disease still undergo organ preservation paradigm in clinical practice, despite general guidelines, with inferior overall survival compared to those who had TL (median survival 61 months vs. 39 months).[14] Multiple individual retrospective series have also identified tumor volume as prognostic for outcomes in addition to T stage.

Wolf, VA Larynx Study (*NEJM* 1991, PMID 2034244): PRT of 332 pts with stage III–IV locally advanced SCC of larynx (63% supraglottis, 57% vocal cord fixation) were randomized to either (a) induction CHT followed by RT or (b) total laryngectomy followed by post-op RT. Pts in larynx preservation arm received cisplatin 100 mg/m² and 5-FU 1,000 mg/m²/d x for 5 days on days 1 and 22. Tumor response was assessed by exam and indirect laryngoscopy 18 to 21 days after the second cycle. Pts w/o at least PR in larynx and those w/ any evidence of disease progression (including neck disease) underwent salvage laryngectomy. Pts w/ at least PR at primary tumor site and no progression of any neck lymphadenopathy received third cycle of CT on day 43. This was followed by definitive RT consisting of 66 to 76 Gy delivered at 1.8 to 2 Gy/fx to primary tumor site and 50 to 75 Gy to LNs. Twelve wks after completion of RT, tumor response was reassessed; pts w/ persistent disease in larynx underwent salvage laryngectomy. Pts w/ persistent neck disease alone underwent neck dissection only. All laryngectomy pts underwent post-op RT consisting of 50 to 50.4 Gy for microscopic disease, 60 to 60.4 Gy for areas felt to be at high risk for local recurrence and 65 to 74.2 Gy to areas of residual disease. MFU 33 mos. Thirty-one percent had CR and 54% had PR after two cycles of CHT. Lack of response to induction CHT, however, was not associated with reduced OS. Rate of laryngeal preservation was 64%. 56% of pts with T4 primary tumors required salvage laryngectomy (vs. 29% in remainder of study population). Rate of DM was lower in CHT arm, but LC was inferior. **Conclusion: Induction CT followed by definitive RT can be effective in preserving larynx in high percentage of pts, w/o compromising OS.**

TABLE 13.4: Results of VA Larynx Study				
	2-yr OS	2-yr LC	Recurrence at site of primary	DM
Induction CHT + Definitive RT	68%	80%	12%	11%
TL + PORT	68%	93%	2%	17%
p value	.9846	.001	.001	.001

Forastiere, RTOG 91-11 (*NEJM* 2003, PMID 14645636; Update *JCO* 2013, PMID 23182993): PRT of 518 pts with SCC of supraglottic/glottic larynx, stage III–IV (T1 or T4 with tumor extending through thyroid cartilage into neck of soft tissue or greater than 1 cm of BOT involvement were excluded) randomized to one of three arms: Arm 1 (Induction, from VA Larynx): cisplatin 100 mg/m^2 day 1 + 5-FU 1,000 mg/m^2/day for 5 days for two cycles on day 1 and day 22 followed by response evaluation. Those with less than PR or with progression proceeded to laryngectomy with PORT. Those with CR or PR continued to additional cycle of cisplatin/5-FU followed by 70 Gy/35 fx RT alone. Arm 2 (chemoRT): cisplatin 100 mg/m^2 days 1, 22, 43 concurrent with 70 Gy/35 fx. Arm 3 (RT alone): 70 Gy/35 fx. Pts with single LN ≥3 cm or multiple LNs underwent neck dissection 8 weeks after completion of therapy. Seven endpoints were reported but primary endpoint was laryngectomy-free survival (LFS). Standard arm was induction. Update published with MFU of 10.8 yrs. In update, compared to induction, chemoRT improved larynx preservation, LC, LRC but not LFS (primary endpoint) and trended to worse OS (*p* = .08) potentially suggestive of unexplained late effects. See Table 13.5. **Conclusion: Concurrent chemoRT declared "winner" due to LRC and LP benefit although LFS was similar.**

TABLE 13.5: 10-Year Results of RTOG 9111 Larynx Preservation Trial							
Arm	LFS (1°)	LP	LC	LRC	DC	DFS	OS
1. Induction	28.9%*	67.5%	53.7%	48.9%	83.4%	20.4%	38.8%
2. ChemoRT	23.5%*	81.7%*†	69.2%*†	65.3%*†	83.9%	21.6%*	27.5%
3. RT alone	17.2%†	63.8%	50.1%	47.2%	76.0%	14.8%	31.5%
Significant relative to RT alone. †Significant relative to induction (standard arm).							

What is role of cetuximab for locally advanced laryngeal cancer?

The Bonner trial[14] established survival benefit with addition of cetuximab to RT in pts with locally advanced SCCHN.

Bonner, Cetuximab Secondary Analysis (*JAMA Otolaryngol Head Neck Surg* 2016, PMID 27389475): Secondary analysis of original Bonner trial investigating role of cetuximab in larynx preservation. Arms included RT alone versus RT with concurrent cetuximab. 168 pts with larynx or hypopharynx cancers were included in this subset (90 in cetuximab, 78 in RT alone). 2-yr rates of larynx preservation were 87.9% for cetuximab and 85.7% for RT alone (HR: 0.57, 95% CI: 0.23–1.42, *p* = .22). HR for laryngectomy-free survival was 0.78 (*p* = .17). No difference in OS. **Conclusion: There was statistically nonsignificant benefit to cetuximab with regard to larynx preservation and laryngectomy-free survival.** *Comment: Conclusions are limited by lack of power and retrospective nature of subset analysis.*

REFERENCES

1. Raitiola H, Pukander J, Laippala P. Glottic and supraglottic laryngeal carcinoma: differences in epidemiology, clinical characteristics and prognosis. *Acta Otolaryngol.* 1999;119(7):847–851.
2. Hoffman HT, Porter K, Karnell LH, et al. Laryngeal cancer in United States: changes in demographics, patterns of care, and survival. *Laryngoscope.* 2006;116(9, Pt 2, Suppl 111):1–13.
3. Dahm JD, Sessions DG, Paniello RC, Harvey J. Primary subglottic cancer. *Laryngoscope.* 1998;108(5):741–746.
4. Beitler JJ, Muller S, Grist WJ, et al. Prognostic accuracy of computed tomography findings for pts with laryngeal cancer undergoing laryngectomy. *J Clin Oncol.* 2010;28(14):2318–2322.
5. Fein DA, Mendenhall WM, Parsons JT, Million RR. T1-T2 squamous cell carcinoma of glottic larynx treated with RT: multivariate analysis of variables potentially influencing local control. *Int J Radiat Oncol Biol Phys.* 1993;25(4):605–611.
6. Videtic GMM, Woody N, Vassil AD. *Handbook of Treatment Planning in RT Oncology.* 2nd ed. New York, NY: Demos Medical; 2015.
7. Tamura Y, Tanaka S, Asato R, et al. Therapeutic outcomes of laryngeal cancer at Kyoto University Hospital for 10 years. *Acta Otolaryngol Suppl.* 2007(557):62–65.
8. Aaltonen LM, Rautiainen N, Sellman J, et al. Voice quality after treatment of early vocal cord cancer: randomized trial comparing laser surgery with RT therapy. *Int J Radiat Oncol Biol Phys.* 2014;90(2):255–260.
9. Mendenhall WM, Amdur RJ, Morris CG, Hinerman RW. T1-T2N0 squamous cell carcinoma of glottic larynx treated with RT therapy. *J Clin Oncol.* 2001;19(20):4029–4036.
10. Le QT, Fu KK, Kroll S, et al. Influence of fraction size, total dose, and overall time on local control of T1-T2 glottic carcinoma. *Int J Radiat Oncol Biol Phys.* 1997;39(1):115–126.
11. Bhateja P, Ward MC, Hunter GH, et al. Impaired vocal cord mobility in T2N0 glottic carcinoma: suboptimal local control with RT alone. *Head Neck.* 2016;38(12):1832–1836.
12. Zumsteg ZS, Riaz N, Jaffery S, et al. Carotid sparing intensity-modulated RT therapy achieves comparable locoregional control to conventional RT in T1-2N0 laryngeal carcinoma. *Oral Oncol.* 2015;51(7):716–723.
13. Ward MC, Pham YD, Kotecha R, et al. Clinical and dosimetric implications of intensity-modulated RT for early-stage glottic carcinoma. *Med Dosim.* 2016;41(1):64–69.
14. Grover S, Swisher-McClure S, Mitra N, et al. Total laryngectomy versus larynx preservation for T4a larynx cancer: patterns of care and survival outcomes. *Int J Radiat Oncol Biol Phys.* 2015;92(3):594–601.

14: SALIVARY GLAND TUMORS

Martin C. Tom, Shlomo A. Koyfman, and Nikhil P. Joshi

> **QUICK HIT:** Salivary gland tumors are an uncommon group of benign and malignant tumors with natural history that varies by histology. Most common benign histology is pleomorphic adenoma. Most common malignant histology within parotid is mucoepidermoid carcinoma. Most common malignant histology within submandibular or minor salivary glands is adenoid cystic carcinoma, which uniformly demonstrates perineural invasion (PNI), high rate of indolent DM, and a long natural history. Surgery is the standard of care for all histologies and facial nerve should be preserved if possible. Postoperative RT should be considered for those with high risk of recurrence. No benefit to CHT has been demonstrated prospectively.

TABLE 14.1: General Treatment Paradigm for Malignant Salivary Cancer			
Surgical Resection With Consideration of Adjuvant RT as Follows			
Primary Site		**Ipsilateral Neck**	
Stage I–II no risk factors	Observation	cN0 or pN0 and low risk	Observation
T3-4, PNI, deep lobe involvement, bone involvement, high grade[1] or recurrent disease	60 Gy	Pathologic node-negative with risk factors (see *Terhaard and RTOG 1008*): T3-4, high grade, facial nerve deficit, recurrent disease	50–54 Gy Levels II–IV
		Node-positive, resected	60 Gy Level Ib-V
Margin-positive or close margins (<1 mm)	66 Gy	ECE	66 Gy
Gross Disease	70 Gy	Gross nodal disease	70 Gy

EPIDEMIOLOGY: Salivary gland cancers are rare tumors and represent approximately 6% of H&N cancers,[2] with roughly 2,500 cases in the United States annually.[3] Benign histologies are more common in young females (median age 46).[4,5] Malignant histologies are more common with older age (median age 54), and as age increases male predominance develops.[3,5] Histology is classified according to WHO 2005 system with over 40 different histologies defined.[3] Parotid gland is the most common site (70% of all tumors, 75% of which are benign) with 22% in minor glands and 8% in submandibular glands.[5]

RISK FACTORS: Risk factors are not clearly defined. Strongest evidence is for RT exposure as shown among Hiroshima/Nagasaki survivors.[6] Smoking is not a risk factor (except in Warthin's tumor; see Table 14.2). EBV has been implicated in lymphoepithelial carcinomas and other viruses are under investigation.[2]

ANATOMY: Major salivary glands consist of parotid, submandibular, and sublingual gland (between mylohyoid and floor of mouth mucosa). Borders of parotid are second maxillary molar (anterior), zygomatic arch (superior), internal jugular vein (deep), mastoid tip (posterior), and posterior digastric muscle (inferior). Parotid contributes primarily to stimulated serous saliva production and submandibular to unstimulated mucous/serous saliva (and therefore RT-induced xerostomia).[7] Parotid lies behind ramus of mandible and is separated into superficial and deep lobes by facial nerve. Retromandibular vein is common radiographic landmark for facial nerve. Stensen's duct drains to buccal mucosa. Facial nerve (CN VII) courses through parotid after exiting stylomastoid foramen.[8] There are five branches of CN VII: temporal, zygomatic, buccal, marginal mandibular, and cervical. CN VII controls facial muscles and taste to oral tongue. Auriculotemporal nerve originates from V3, innervates parotid (salivation/parasympathetic), and can be route of perineural spread; if damaged during surgery this can recover to innervate skin causing Frey's syndrome or gustatory sweating. Submandibular is innervated by chorda tympani and perineural spread can be to CN XII, CN V via lingual nerve, or to CN VII via chorda tympani. Minor salivary glands are distributed through aerodigestive epithelium. Multiple contouring guides are available to aid in anatomy of cranial nerves when perineural invasion is present.[9,10]

TABLE 14.2: Characteristics of Salivary Tumors

	Parotid	Submandibular	Sublingual	Minor Glands
Pathology[1,5]	75% benign, 25% malignant	50% benign, 50% malignant	>75% malignant	
Frequency[5]	70%	8%	22%	
Salivary fluid[2,7]	Serous	Mixed	Mucous	
Associated nerves	CN VII (facial) with spread to V3 via chorda tympani	V3 (lingual) and XII (hypoglossal)	V3 (lingual)	Location dependent

PATHOLOGY: There are many forms of salivary tumors, with the most common listed in Tables 14.3 and 14.4, in approximate order of decreasing incidence. Note that grade is prognostic for mucoepidermoid carcinoma, adenocarcinoma, salivary duct carcinoma, and acinic cell carcinoma.[3] Adenoid cystic carcinoma is graded by percentage of solid component (high grade if >30% solid) and is often intermediate grade.[11] Grading has less well understood significance in more rare subtypes.

TABLE 14.3: Benign Salivary Histologies

Pleomorphic adenoma	Most common salivary gland tumor, 2/3 of parotid tumors, 2/3 of pts are female in their 40s. Treatment is surgery with <5% risk of recurrence but beware of tumor spillage; recurrence can be up to 45%. Risk of second recurrence is 46%. Can degenerate into "Carcinoma ex-pleomorphic adenoma" (CExP); risk of degeneration is <1% in pts without recurrence and 4% in pts with recurrence.[4] Consider RT to 50–60 Gy for multiple recurrences, deep involvement or large tumors.[1]
Warthin's tumor	Benign tumor of parotid, often bilateral (6%).[12] Associated with smoking, more common in men.[13] Can be highly PET-avid and is often incidental finding on PET. Malignant degeneration is rare (<1%)[2] and observation is reasonable.
Godwin's tumor	Benign lymphoepithelial lesion associated with Sjögren syndrome.[14]
Basal cell adenoma	Approximately 2% of salivary tumors.[2] May be confused with basal cell of skin metastatic to parotid lymph nodes.
Oncocytoma	1% of salivary tumors. Slowly progressive parotid tumor in older patients.

TABLE 14.4: Malignant Salivary Histologies	
Mucoepidermoid	Most common parotid malignancy, grade is prognostic. Most are small and curable with surgery alone.
Adenoid cystic carcinoma	Almost always demonstrates PNI and can track along cranial nerves. Tubular pattern is most favorable, cribriform is intermediate, and solid is least favorable. Greater than 30% solid pattern is considered "high grade."[11] Long natural history. Risk of nodes is debated, classic teaching is <5% although recent data (NCDB and multi-institutional analysis) show as high as 29% (oral cavity 37%, major gland 9%–19%).[15,16] Slowly growing distant metastases in up to 50%.[2] Late recurrences (>20 years) can be seen. Most benefit from adjuvant RT.[17]
Adenocarcinoma, NOS	Grade is prognostic, nodal metastases seen in 50%–60% of high-grade lesions.[16]
Acinic cell carcinoma	Low-grade, slowly progressive tumors, 80% within parotid. Submandibular tumors are uncommon and most aggressive.[2]
Carcinoma ex-pleomorphic adenoma	4% of salivary tumors, 12% of malignancies. Degenerated pleomorphic adenoma. More than 80% of pts do not have history of known pleomorphic adenoma.
Salivary duct carcinoma	9% of salivary malignances. Males more common (4:1). Aggressive, high grade, similar to high-grade breast ductal carcinoma.[2]
Metastasis to salivary gland	5% of salivary malignancies,[2] incidence varies by region based on frequency of skin cancer. Mostly squamous cell of skin followed by melanoma.
Epithelial–myoepithelial	Only 1% of salivary tumors, twice as common in women, 60% parotid, typically slow-growing.

GENETICS: EGFR, c-kit, HER2, and androgen receptor (salivary duct cancer) have all been described but no standard role for targeted agents (see the following).[3]

CLINICAL PRESENTATION: Most tumors present initially as slowly progressive painless mass. Adenoid cystic carcinoma may present as neuropathic pain (misdiagnosis as trigeminal neuralgia) and ultimately motor deficits of facial nerve.

WORKUP: H&P including H&N exam with cranial nerve exam. Ultrasound can be helpful to delineate benign versus malignant prior to biopsy. FNA sensitivity and specificity is 80% and >95%, respectively.[1] Contrast-enhanced MRI is critical for malignant tumors to evaluate for perineural spread. CT chest for malignant histologies as indicated. PET is not standard. Dental, nutrition, speech, and swallow evaluation as indicated.

PROGNOSTIC FACTORS: Stage, grade, histology, recurrence, positive margins, bone invasion, positive lymph nodes, facial nerve palsy.[1,18,19]

TREATMENT PARADIGM

Observation: Observation may have role in select pts with benign histologies other than pleomorphic adenoma. Pleomorphic adenoma should be treated in healthy pt due to risk of malignant degeneration. Malignant histologies should be treated.

Surgery: Surgical resection of primary tumor is the standard of care for all technically resectable salivary gland tumors warranting treatment.[21] Care should be taken to minimize risk of tumor spillage; enucleation should not be performed. Preservation of functional cranial nerves should be attempted; microscopic margins should be preferred over

TABLE 14.5: AJCC 8th ed. (2017) Staging for Salivary Gland Cancer (Note that minor salivary cancers are staged according to their site of origin).

T/M \ N	cN0	cN1	cN2a	cN2b	cN2c	cN3a	cN3b
T1	• ≤2 cm	I						
T2	• 2.1–4 cm	II	III	IVA				
T3	• >4 cm and/or extraparenchymal extension							
T4a	• Invasion[1]							
T4b	• Invasion[2]	IVB						
M1	• Distant metastasis	IVC						

Major changes from AJCC 7th Edition include introduction of N3a & N3b subcategories[20].

Notes: Invasion[1] = Invasion of skin, mandible, ear canal, or facial nerve. Invasion[2] = Invasion of skull base, pterygoid plates and/or encasing carotid artery. Nodal category definition is similar to other non-HPV-associated head and neck cancers; see Table 10.4 for clinical and pathologic nodal categories.

facial nerve sacrifice although gross disease should not remain if possible.[21] Consider nerve grafting for reconstruction of sacrificed cranial nerve. For parotid tumors, elective nodal dissection of levels II to III and possibly IV is surgeon-dependent based on risk factors (size, stage, grade, histology, location). For submandibular tumors, elective dissection would include levels I to III. Clinically positive neck should be dissected. For parotid tumors, levels I and V may be at risk only if levels II to IV are involved.[1]

Chemotherapy: Addition of CHT for high-risk lesions is investigational[11] and retrospective data is inconsistent.[22–24] Inclusion criteria for RTOG 1008 are intermediate or high-grade mucoepidermoid and adenocarcinoma, high-grade acinic cell, salivary duct carcinoma, or high-grade adenoid cystic carcinoma. On this trial cisplatin 40 mg/m[2] is given weekly with RT.

Radiation

Dose and Indications: Consider RT for pT3-4 disease, close or positive margins, high-grade, recurrent disease, positive lymph nodes, perineural, lymphovascular, or bone invasion. Adenoid cystic carcinomas typically display significant PNI and are treated with RT. Role of RT for T1 lesions with risk factors is unclear (NCCN Category 2B)[21]: 60 Gy to primary site and 54 Gy to elective neck (if included) is recommended. Dose to be escalated to 66 Gy for positive margins or extracapsular extension and to 70 Gy for gross disease.[1,21] Treatment of ipsilateral neck for pathologically node-positive disease required and consideration for elective nodal coverage for pT3-4, high-grade, facial nerve deficits or recurrent disease (see the following for nodal risk factors).

Procedure: See *Treatment Planning Handbook*, Chapter 4.[25]

Complications: Oral mucositis, odynophagia, skin erythema, altered taste, partial xerostomia, trismus, hypothyroidism, and ear complications (secretory otitis media or partial hearing loss). Limit contralateral parotid to mean 26 Gy if possible. TD 5/5 of parotid is 32 Gy.

Neutrons: Higher LC but more late effects than photons. RBE is >2.6. Neutrons lack skin-sparing, are less affected by hypoxia, and are less cell-cycle-dependent than photons. Consider for unresectable or recurrent tumors (particularly adenoid cystic), since low growth fraction and long doubling time of salivary tumors (especially adenoid cystic) make them sensitive to fast neutron therapy, but at risk of higher morbidity (10% grade 3–4 toxicity in 279 pts at University of Washington[21]). Complications include osteoradionecrosis, fibrosis, cervical myelopathy, CNS necrosis, optic neuritis, palatal fistula, retinopathy, glaucoma.

Stereotactic Radiosurgery (SRS) Boost: University of Washington performed RR of 34 pts with salivary gland tumor involving BOS treated with 19.2 nGy neutrons followed by SRS boost (12 Gy), compared to historical controls of neutron therapy. Forty-mos LC was 39% versus 82% with SRS boost ($p = .04$). There was no additional toxicity.[26]

EVIDENCE-BASED Q&A

What are the indications for postoperative RT?

Because salivary cancer is relatively rare, no prospective trials have been performed. Therefore, indications for postoperative RT are based on retrospective evidence. In general, adjuvant RT indications include pT3-4 disease, close or positive margins, high-grade, recurrent disease, positive lymph nodes, PNI, LVSI, or bone invasion.

Terhaard, Netherlands (*Head & Neck* 2005, PMID 15629600): RR of 498 pts treated for salivary cancers between 1984 and 1995. 386 pts received RT to median dose of 62 Gy (60.7 Gy for negative margins, 62.4 Gy for close, and 64 Gy for positive margins). 40% received elective nodal RT. 10-yr LC improved for those with T3-4 tumors, close (<5 mm) and positive margins, PNI, and bone invasion. Unresectable pts showed dose response with LC at 5 yrs of 0% for <66 Gy and 50% for >66 Gy. **Conclusion: Postoperative RT indicated for T3-4 disease, close or positive margins, bone invasion, and PNI. Risk of nodal disease was defined using T stage and histology.**

TABLE 14.6: Terhaard Results							
			Risk of Positive Neck Nodes (%) by Score and Primary Location				
10-Year Local Control	No RT	RT	T Score + Histology Score*	Parotid	Submandibular	Oral Cavity	Other
T3-4 tumor	18%	84%	2	4%	0%	4%	0%
Close margins	55%	95%	3	12%	33%	13%	29%
Positive margins	44%	82%	4	25%	57%	19%	56%
Bone invasion	54%	86%	5	33%	60%	—	—
PNI	60%	88%	6	38%	50%	—	—
All results statistically significant.			*Scoring: T1 = 1, T2 = 2, T3-4 = 3. Acinic/adenoid cystic/CExP = 1, MucoEp = 2, Squamous/Undifferentiated = 3.				

Armstrong, Memorial Sloan Kettering (*Arch Otolaryngol Head Neck Surg* 1990, PMID 2306346): Matched-pair analysis of 46 pts treated with postoperative RT after 1966 matched to those treated with surgery alone prior to 1966. Median RT dose was 56.64 Gy. 5-yr cause-specific (determinate) survival (CSS) with RT was 68.9% versus 55% without (p = NS) and LC was 73% versus 66% (p = NS). RT improved CSS (51% vs. 10%, p = .015) and LC (73% vs. 66%, p = NS) for stage III–IV patients. Node-positive pts also demonstrated

CSS benefit (49% vs. 19%, $p = .015$) and LRC rate (69% vs. 40%, $p = .05$). **Conclusion: Stage III–IV and node-positive disease are indications for postoperative radiotherapy.**

North, Johns Hopkins (*IJROBP* 1990, PMID 2115032): RR of 87 pts with major salivary gland tumors (70 parotid and 17 submandibular) treated from 1975 to 1987 with surgery with or without RT. 34% received neck dissection and 74% received RT recommended to 60 Gy for negative margins, 66 Gy for close or positive margins, and 72 Gy for gross residual. Postoperative RT improved local recurrence for untreated and recurrent pts and improved 5-yr OS (75% vs. 59%, $p = .014$). Negative prognostic factors included facial nerve palsy, undifferentiated histology, male gender, skin involvement, and no RT. **Conclusion: RT is indicated except for low-grade T1-2 tumors with negative margins.**

Cho, Korea (*Ann Surg Oncol* 2016, PMID 27342828): RR of 179 pts with low-grade salivary gland cancer (LGSGC). 10-yr OS was 96.6% and RFS was 89.6%. Adjuvant RT improved RFS for LGSGC with node positivity, PNI, LVSI, extraparenchymal extension, positive margin, or T3-4. Close margin (<5 mm) did not increase risk of recurrence. T1-2 LGSGC without risk factors had low risk of recurrence after surgery alone. **Conclusion: Adjuvant RT improves RFS for high-risk LGSGC. Low-risk LGSGCs (T1-2 without risk factors) have good outcomes after surgery alone.**

Which pts have high incidence of nodal metastases?

High-grade, vascular invasion, facial nerve palsy, histology, and higher T stage appear to predict for nodal metastases.

Xiao, Nodal Metastasis in Parotid Cancer NCDB (*Arch Otol H&N Surg* 2016, PMID 26419838): NCDB analysis of 22,653 cases of primary parotid cancer with pathologic LN evaluation. N0 pts had improved 5-year OS versus N+ (79% vs. 40%, $p < .001$). Low grade had improved 5-yr OS versus high grade (88% vs. 69%, $p < .001$). Incidence of N+ independently predicted by high grade (50.9% vs. 9.3% in low grade) and high T stage. **Conclusion: Occult N+ varies by histology. High T stage and grade predict for N+ in most histologies of primary parotid cancer.**

TABLE 14.7: Incidence of Nodal Metastases in NCDB (Xiao)			
Primary Parotid Cancer Histology	cN+ (%)	Occult N+ (%)	Occult N+ (High Grade % N+/T4 % N+)
Salivary ductal carcinoma	53.5	23.6	36/40
Adenocarcinoma NOS	45.2	19.9	31.6/31.6
Carcinoma ex-pleomorphic adenoma	23.9	11.8	19.2/35.5
Mucoepidermoid carcinoma	20.2	9.3	21.8/21.6
Adenoid cystic carcinoma	14.2	7.0	9.6/13
Acinar cell carcinoma	10	4.4	24.5/11.5
Basal cell adenocarcinoma	9.4	6.3	6.7/22.2
Epithelial–myoepithelial carcinoma	4.8	1.5	0/0
Total	24.4	10.2	

Stennert, Cologne, Germany (*Arch Otol H&N Surg* 2003, PMID 12874071): RR of 160 pts with salivary cancer treated with neck dissection. 53% of pts were confirmed node-positive and 13% were clinically node-positive and 45% of clinically node-negative pts were pathologically node-positive. **Conclusion: T stage and high-grade histology predicted for occult node involvement.**

Yoo, Korea (*J Surg Oncol* 2015, PMID 25976866): RR of 363 patients, 51 of whom underwent therapeutic neck dissection, 110 who underwent elective neck dissection, and 202 who did not have neck dissection. 15% of elective neck dissections were positive and 2.5% of pts without neck dissection recurred. **Conclusion: Grade, site, and lymphovascular invasion predicted for nodal metastases.**

Can salivary cancer be treated with RT alone?

Based on retrospective evidence, it appears surgery plays a significant role in local-control and is the accepted standard of care for medically operable and technically resectable pts with salivary cancer.

Mendenhall, University of Florida (*Cancer* 2005, PMID 15880750): RR of 224 pts treated between 1964 and 2003 with RT alone (n = 64) or surgery with RT (n = 160). Median dose for RT alone was 74 Gy versus 66 Gy for postoperative patients. LRC was significantly worse in RT alone cohort (stages I–III 89% vs. 70%, p = .01, stage IV 66% vs. 24%, p = .002, overall 81% vs. 40%, p < .0001). **Conclusion: RT alone controlled approximately 20% of technically unresectable pts but was inferior to surgery combined with RT.**

Can we improve LC of salivary tumors with neutron therapy?

Local control is improved without survival benefit. Cost and toxicity are significant.

Laramore, RTOG 80-01-MRC Trial (*IJROBP* 1993, PMID 8407397): PRT in England and the United States of 32 pts (25 evaluable) with inoperable or unresectable salivary cancer randomized to photon/electron therapy or neutron therapy. Complete responses were more common in neutron arm leading to significantly improved LC (56% vs. 17%, p = .009) and early closure of trial. Overall survival was not significantly different (15% vs. 25%, p = NS). Severe late complications were seen in 69% of neutron pts and 15% of photon pts (p = .07). **Conclusion: Neutron RT improves local control but does not improve survival and carries higher rate of long-term toxicity.**

Douglas, University of Washington (*Arch Otolaryngol Head Neck Surg* 2003, PMID 12975266): RR of 279 pts treated with fast neutrons at University of Washington, 263 of which had evidence of gross disease at time of treatment. MFU of 36 months. Total dose delivered was between 17.4 and 20.7 nGy with fractions given three to four times per week. CSS and LRC was 67% and 59% at 6 years, respectively. Grade 3–4 RTOG toxicity at 6 years was 10%. **Conclusion: Neutrons are effective with gross residual disease.**

Is modern RT as effective as neutron therapy with less toxicity?

This was suggested by a small RR from MSKCC, though data is limited.

Spratt, MSKCC (*Radiol Oncol* 2014, PMID 24587780): RR of 27 pts for unresectable salivary cancer treated with photons to median dose of 70 Gy with IMRT or 3D-CRT. CHT (mostly platinum) was used for 18 patients. MFU 52 months, 5-yr LRC of 47%, which compared favorably to neutron arm of RTOG/MRC trial. **Conclusion: Modern photon therapy with or without CHT may be reasonable alternative to neutrons with less toxicity.**

Is there another type of particle therapy being explored to treat malignant salivary gland tumors?

Germany is exploring adding carbon ion boost to IMRT. Phase II study showed moderate toxicity with promising local control.[27]

Does addition of adjuvant chemoRT improve outcomes compared to adjuvant RT alone?

Several small retrospective analyses have demonstrated promising control rates.[22-24] Conversely, NCDB analysis revealed inferior survival with adjuvant chemoRT compared to RT alone.[28] RTOG 1008 is phase II/III RCT that aims to answer this question in high-risk salivary gland cancer.

Amini, NCDB (*JAMA Otolaryngol Head Neck Surg* 2016, PMID: 27541166): NCDB analysis of salivary gland cancer s/p resection comparing adjuvant chemoRT to adjuvant RT alone. Included grade 2 or 3 with ≥1 adverse feature (T3-4, N+, or margin+). 2,210 patients, RT alone (83.3%) and chemoRT (16.7%). MFU 39 mos. Unadjusted 5-yr OS was inferior to chemoRT (38.5% vs. 54.2%). OS with chemoRT was inferior on MVA (HR: 1.22, 95% CI: 1.03–1.44, p = .02) and trended to inferiority on propensity score matched analysis (HR: 1.20, 95% CI: 0.98–1.47, p = .08). **Conclusion: In high-risk salivary gland cancer, adjuvant chemoRT did not improve OS compared to adjuvant RT alone.**

Is targeted therapy effective for pts with actionable mutations?

Early studies with targeted agents (imatinib,[29] lapatinib,[30] and dasatinib[31]) for salivary tumors have had disappointing results.

REFERENCES

1. Terhaard CH. *Principles and Practice of RT Oncology*. 6th ed. Philadelphia, PA: Wolters Kluwer; 2013.
2. Eveson J, Auclair P, Gnepp D, El-Naggar A. Pathology & genetics: H&N tumors. In: Barnes L, Eveson JW, Reichart P, eds. *WHO Classification of Tumors*.2005. https://www.iarc.fr/en/publications/pdfs-online/pat-gen/bb9/BB9.pdf
3. Guzzo M, Locati LD, Prott FJ, et al. Major and minor salivary gland tumors. *Crit Rev Oncol Hematol*. 2010;74(2):134–148.
4. Andreasen S, Therkildsen MH, Bjørndal K, Homøe P. Pleomorphic adenoma of parotid gland 1985–2010: Danish nationwide study of incidence, recurrence rate, and malignant transformation. *Head Neck*. 2015;38(S1):E1364–E1369.
5. Spiro RH. Salivary neoplasms: overview of 35-year experience with 2,807 patients. *Head Neck Surg*. 1986;8(3):177–184.
6. Saku T, Hayashi Y, Takahara O, et al. Salivary gland tumors among atomic bomb survivors, 1950–1987. *Cancer*. 1997;79(8):1465–1475.
7. Paulsen D. Glands associated with digestive tract. In: Paulsen DF, ed. *Histology and Cell Biology: Examination & Board Review*. 5th ed. New York, NY: McGraw-Hill; 2010:229–246.
8. Skandalakis JE, Carlson GW, Colborn GL, et al. Neck. In: Skandalakis JE, Colburn GL, Weidman TA, et al., eds. *Skandalakis' Surgical Anatomy*. New York, NY: McGraw-Hill; 2004.
9. Gluck I, Ibrahim M, Popovtzer A, et al. Skin cancer of H&N with perineural invasion: defining clinical target volumes based on pattern of failure. *Int J Radiat Oncol Biol Phys*. 2009;74(1):38–46.
10. Ko HC, Gupta V, Mourad WF, et al. Contouring guide for H&N cancers with perineural invasion. *Pract Radiat Oncol*. 2014;4(6):e247–e258.
11. RTOG 1008: randomized Phase II study of adjuvant concurrent RT and CHTversus RT alone in high-risk malignant salivary gland tumors. 2010. https://www.rtog.org/ClinicalTrials/ProtocolTable/StudyDetails.aspx?study=1008
12. Maiorano E, Lo Muzio L, Favia G, Piattelli A. Warthin's tumour: study of 78 cases with emphasis on bilaterality, multifocality and association with other malignancies. *Oral Oncol*. 2002;38(1):35–40.
13. Pinkston JA, Cole P. Cigarette smoking and Warthin's tumor. *Am J Epidemiol*. 1996;144(2):183–187.
14. Laudenbach P, Leygue MC, Bertrand JC, Deboise A, Vieillefond A. [Godwin's tumor and Gougerot-Sjögren syndrome. Apropos of 2 cases]. *Rev Stomatol Chir Maxillofac*. 1985;86(4):248–254.

15. Amit M, Binenbaum Y, Sharma K, et al. Incidence of cervical lymph node metastasis and its association with outcomes in pts with adenoid cystic carcinoma. international collaborative study. *Head Neck*. 2015;37(7):1032–1037.

16. Xiao CC, Zhan KY, White-Gilbertson SJ, Day TA. Predictors of nodal metastasis in parotid malignancies: national cancer data base study of 22,653 patients. *Otolaryngol Head Neck Surg*. 2016;154(1):121–130.

17. Lee A, Givi B, Osborn VW, et al. Patterns of care and survival of adjuvant RT for major salivary adenoid cystic carcinoma. *Laryngoscope*. 2017;127(9):2057–2062.

18. Carrillo JF, Vázquez R, Ramírez-Ortega MC, et al. Multivariate prediction of probability of recurrence in pts with carcinoma of parotid gland. *Cancer*. 2007;109(10):2043–2051.

19. Storey MR, Garden AS, Morrison WH, et al. Postoperative RT for malignant tumors of submandibular gland. *Int J Radiat Oncol Biol Phys*. 2001;51(4):952–958.

20. Edge S, Byrd DR, Compton CC, et al. *AJCC Cancer Staging Manual*. New York, NY: Springer Publishing; 2011.

21. Douglas JG, Koh WJ, Austin-Seymour M, Laramore GE. Treatment of salivary gland neoplasms with fast neutron radiotherapy. *Arch Otolaryngol Head Neck Surg*. 2003;129(9):944–948.

22. Pederson AW, Salama JK, Haraf DJ, et al. Adjuvant chemoRTfor locoregionally advanced and high-risk salivary gland malignancies. *Head Neck Oncol*. 2011;3:31.

23. Schoenfeld JD, Sher DJ, Norris CM, et al. Salivary gland tumors treated with adjuvant intensity-modulated RTwith or without concurrent chemotherapy. *Int J Radiat Oncol Biol Phys*. 2012;82(1):308–314.

24. Tanvetyanon T, Qin D, Padhya T, et al. Outcomes of postoperative concurrent chemoRT for locally advanced major salivary gland carcinoma. *Arch Otolaryngol Head Neck Surg*. 2009;135(7):687–692.

25. Videtic GMM, Woody N, Vassil AD. *Handbook of Treatment Planning in RT Oncology*. 2nd ed. New York, NY: Demos Medical; 2015.

26. Douglas JG, Goodkin R, Laramore GE. Gamma knife stereotactic radiosurgery for salivary gland neoplasms with base of skull invasion following neutron radiotherapy. *Head Neck*. 2008;30(4):492–496.

27. Jensen AD, Nikoghosyan AV, Lossner K, et al. COSMIC: regimen of intensity modulated RT therapy plus dose-escalated, raster-scanned carbon ion boost for malignant salivary gland tumors: results of prospective Phase 2 trial. *Int J Radiat Oncol Biol Phys*. 2015;93(1):37–46.

28. Amini A, Waxweiler TV, Brower JV, et al. Association of adjuvant ChemoRTvs RTAlone with survival in pts with resected major salivary gland carcinoma: data from National Cancer Data Base. *JAMA Otolaryngol Head Neck Surg*. 2016;142(11):1100–1110.

29. Hotte SJ, Winquist EW, Lamont E, et al. Imatinib mesylate in pts with adenoid cystic cancers of salivary glands expressing c-kit: Princess Margaret Hospital Phase II consortium study. *J Clin Oncol*. 2005;23(3):585–590.

30. Agulnik M, Cohen EW, Cohen RB, et al. Phase II study of lapatinib in recurrent or metastatic epidermal growth factor receptor and/or erbB2 expressing adenoid cystic carcinoma and non-adenoid cystic carcinoma malignant tumors of salivary glands. *J Clin Oncol*. 2007;25(25):3978–3984.

31. Wong SJ, Karrison T, Hayes DN, et al. Phase II trial of dasatinib for recurrent or metastatic c-KIT expressing adenoid cystic carcinoma and for nonadenoid cystic malignant salivary tumors. *Ann Oncol*. 2016;27(2):318–323.

15: CARCINOMA OF UNKNOWN PRIMARY OF THE HEAD AND NECK

Senthilkumar Gandhidasan and Jeffrey Kittel

> **QUICK HIT:** Cancer of unknown primary (CUP) represents ~3% of H&N cancers. Detailed diagnostic workup is required to identify a primary source for malignancy: must include comprehensive physical exam, analyzing anatomic disease distribution (nodal levels), also advanced imaging (e.g., PET/CT), and guidance by pathologic findings. Biopsy showing adenocarcinoma in the low neck should prompt evaluation for salivary gland tumors, thoracic, gynecologic, or gastrointestinal primaries. Squamous cancers remaining as "unknown primary" despite thorough workup are assumed to arise from H&N sites (mucosal or skin) and treated based on probability of primary site given anatomic location of nodal involvement. Two broad treatment approaches exist: primary surgery (with risk-adapted adjuvant RT or chemoRT) and definitive RT (with or without CHT).

TABLE 15.1: General Treatment Paradigm for Unknown Primary Presenting as Squamous Carcinoma of H&N Lymph Nodes

	Treatment Options
cT0N1	Option 1: Neck dissection • Add PORT for pN2/3 (see PORT for Head & Neck Cancer Chapter) • Add chemoRT for ECE+ Option 2: RT alone Option 3: TORS lingual tonsillectomy, neck dissection, and risk-adapted PORT
cT0N2-3	Option 1: Definitive chemoRT Option 2: Neck dissection • Add PORT for pN2/3 (see PORT for Head & Neck Cancer Chapter) • Add chemoRT for ECE+ Option 3: TORS lingual tonsillectomy, neck dissection, and risk-adapted PORT
Treat gross disease to 66–70 Gy, uninvolved neck to 54–56 Gy, and potential mucosal sites to 54–66 Gy.	

EPIDEMIOLOGY: CUP represents 2% to 3% of all H&N carcinomas. Median age at diagnosis is 50 to 70, male prevalence with male-to-female ratio of 4:1. Majority (74%) of squamous pts in modern era present with HPV-associated disease.[1]

RISK FACTORS: Risk factors for H&N cancer apply as do other primaries that spread to cervical neck nodes.

General: Alcohol, tobacco, betel and areca nuts, Plummer–Vinson syndrome, HPV.

Nasopharyngeal: EBV, dimethylnitrosamine (salted fish), occupational smoke/dust exposure.

Sinonasal: Nickel, wood dust, leather tanning agents.

Cutaneous: UV exposure.

ANATOMY: Pattern of nodal involvement helps direct exam toward potential sites of the occult primary.

TABLE 15.2: Lymph Node Levels and Correlation With Possible Primary Site		
Level	**Anatomic Correlation**	**Possible Primary Site**
Ia	Submental	Anterior oral cavity/lower lip
Ib	Submandibular	Oral cavity (upper and lower lip, cheek, nose) and skin (lip, nose, medial canthus)
II	Upper jugular	Oropharynx, hypopharynx, oral cavity, larynx
III	Middle jugular	Oropharynx, larynx, hypopharynx, thyroid
IV	Inferior jugular	Larynx, hypopharynx, thyroid, cervical esophagus, trachea
V	Posterior cervical triangle	Nasopharynx, skin of postneck, scalp, hypopharynx
VI	Prelaryngeal (Delphian), pre/paratracheal, tracheoesophageal	Larynx, thyroid
Retropharyngeal (RPN)	Rouviere's	Nasopharynx, oropharyngeal wall, hypopharynx, paranasal sinuses
Supraclavicular	Also level IVB (medial SCV) and level Vc (lateral SCV)	Thyroid, cervical esophagus, infraclavicular primary (i.e., lung)
Parotid		Skin

PATHOLOGY: Most common presenting pathology of CUPs of H&N is squamous cell carcinoma. Adenocarcinoma, neuroendocrine carcinoma, and poorly differentiated tumors are less common. Lymphoma, sarcoma, thyroid, melanoma, and germ cell tumor are other potential diseases.

CLINICAL PRESENTATION: Classic presentation is unilateral painless neck mass. Level II (~50%), followed by level III are involved most commonly. Unilateral LN is common and ~25% present as N1. Anatomic location of node and histology provides clues to search for primary lesion. For example, adenocarcinoma in lower neck nodes is commonly metastatic but one must rule out salivary, thyroid, or parathyroid tumors. In cases of SCC/undifferentiated carcinoma, occult primary typically resides in skin or upper aerodigestive tract with most likely primary sites including tonsil, BOT, and pyriform sinus.

WORKUP: Comprehensive H&P with attention to past history of malignancy (including skin) or risk factors. Exam should focus particular attention on skin (scalp), inspection and palpation of mucosa, and flexible nasopharyngolaryngoscopy (specifically evaluating sinonasal cavity, nasopharynx, pharyngeal walls, BOT, larynx, and hypopharynx).

Labs: CBC, CMP (thyroglobulin and calcitonin if adenocarcinoma).

Biopsy: FNA of LN for initial biopsy (unless suspicious of lymphoma). If FNA was non-diagnostic, proceed to core needle biopsy. Excisional biopsy is alternative. Testing of viral markers from biopsy specimen helps direct search for primary tumor: EBV suggests nasopharynx and HPV+ and/or p16+ suggests oropharyngeal primary. p63 positivity is marker for squamous cell carcinoma. p16 positive but high-risk HPV negative suggests skin primary.[2] Test adenocarcinoma for TTF-1 (thyroid or lung).

Imaging: Contrast-enhanced CT head/neck; consider MRI when needed. PET/CT should be performed prior to panendoscopy with biopsies, if possible, to guide selection of biopsy sites and to avoid uncertainties of interpretation due to false-positive FDG avidity at sites manipulated during endoscopy. PET detection rate of primary tumor is approximately 30% in pts with CUP after standard workup.[3]

Procedures: Following PET/CT, next step is EUA w/ panendoscopy with directed biopsies of any suspicious areas seen on imaging or EUA and ipsilateral/bilateral tonsillectomies. Tonsillectomy increases detection of primary tumor by about 10-fold as compared to tonsillar biopsy (3% vs. 30%).[4] Utility of random biopsies in absence of PET/CT or exam suspicion is very low and is not necessary. If no primary is identified, consider blind biopsies of NPX, BOT, both pyriform sinuses, hypopharyngeal wall, and postcricoid region. In studies of diagnostic value of panendoscopy, primary site could be identified by panendoscopy in 50% to 65% of pts with suspicious radiographic or physical findings and in 15% to 29% of pts without suspicious findings.[5,6]

PROGNOSTIC FACTORS: Histology, number of LNs, LN level (upper vs. lower/SCV), KPS, extracapsular extension, and grade among others.

NATURAL HISTORY: Mucosal emergence rates, historically, are low after comprehensive RT. One series suggested rates of 25% after neck dissection alone and rates from 8% to 14% with RT. These rates may be lower in modern era with improved imaging. Regional failure in neck and distant metastases are more common at 20% to 35%.[7]

STAGING: T classification for cancer of unknown primary is T0 (not TX, which implies incomplete workup). Lymph node staging is per standard H&N staging (see Chapter 10 for details). EBV-associated unknown primary is a defined entity under nasopharynx staging.

TREATMENT PARADIGM

Surgery: Surgery can be either primary treatment or reserved for salvage setting. Results have generally been comparable with either approach and institutional bias often determines treatment algorithm.[8–10] Treatment strategy should take into account analysis of toxicities of each therapy.[11] NCCN guidelines suggest surgery as primary therapy for N1 disease where there may not be firm indication for chemoRT.[12] With modern staging, outcomes after surgery alone for N1 disease are excellent with 90% control above clavicles.[11] If neck dissection is performed, typically selective dissection is performed with levels I to V dissected based on anatomic location of involved nodes and potential primary site (e.g., for potential oropharynx primary, consider II–IV or IB–V). Potential complications of neck dissection include: hematoma, seroma, lymphedema, wound infection/dehiscence, fistula, cranial nerve damage (e.g., CN XI) and carotid rupture. Minimally invasive procedures such as transoral laser microsurgery (TLM) and transoral robotic surgery (TORS) are emerging techniques for lingual and palatine tonsillectomy for diagnosis.

Chemotherapy: CHT is recommended for occult primary squamous cancers for pts with either (a) ECE/residual disease after neck dissection or (b) cN2-3 disease treated nonoperatively. These concepts are largely extrapolated from major definitive and post-op studies in setting of known H&N primaries (see Chapters 10–14 and 16). There have been small observational studies in setting of unknown primary that have shown good outcomes with chemoRT for pts with N2–N3 nodal disease.[13–16] If delivered, CHT dosing strategy is similar to other H&N sites and most commonly includes bolus cisplatin 100 mg/m^2 on days 1, 22, and 43 or cisplatin 40 mg/m^2 weekly.

Radiation

Indications: RT can be employed in either (a) high-risk postoperative setting or (b) nonoperative setting. Following neck dissection, RT indications include more than one involved node (N2-3), ECE, or residual disease (observation appropriate for pN1 pts without ECE). In definitive setting, RT can be delivered alone or with concurrent CHT (cN2-3; see the preceding text). Most commonly, RT is delivered to putative mucosal sites along with bilateral neck. Potential gain w/ comprehensive RT in controlling primary should be weighed against its effects on QOL/toxicity. Classically, comprehensive RT included nasopharynx, oropharynx, and hypopharynx with exclusion of oral cavity and larynx (sites that can be easily visualized). Target volumes are evolving in modern era, with some targeting only oropharynx for HPV+ disease (ipsilateral tonsil/BOT), only nasopharynx for EBV+ disease, although there exists spectrum and significant heterogeneity in practice. If treating, most treat bilateral neck including levels II to IV and others (IB, V) as indicated by concern for occult primary location.

Dose: As in target delineation, practice in dosing is heterogeneous. Acceptable RT approach is 70 Gy/35 fx to gross nodal disease and 56 Gy/35 fx to uninvolved neck and mucosal sites at risk of harboring occult primary.

Toxicity: Acute: Mucositis, erythema/desquamation, odynophagia, fatigue, aspiration, xerostomia, taste alterations. Chronic: xerostomia, taste alteration, fibrosis, trismus, decreased hearing, hypothyroidism, submental lymphedema, dysphagia, esophageal strictures.

EVIDENCE-BASED Q&A

Does association with HPV carry same implications in CUP as it does in oropharyngeal cancer?

Much like in cancer of oropharynx, HPV-associated CUP appears to portend improved prognosis relative to p16-negative CUP, independent of nodal status.[17] In one study, 5-yr OS was 92% if p16+ versus 30% if p16 negative.[1] As incidence of HPV-related oropharyngeal cancers rises, some institutions have seen increase in CUP.[18] HPV positivity also leads practitioners to target only likely primary sites (i.e., oropharynx).

What is role of transoral lingual tonsillectomy in workup of CUP?

Recently, transoral robotic surgery (TORS) has been used to perform lingual tonsillectomy in search of occult primary.

Mehta, Pittsburgh (*Laryngoscope* 2013, PMID 23154813): 10 pts with squamous carcinoma of unknown primary underwent transoral robotic base of tongue resection. In 9 of 10 pts (90%), primary was detected with mean diameter of 0.9 cm.

Patel, Multi-Institution (*JAMA Otolaryngol Head Neck Surg* 2013, PMID 24136446): Retrospective multi-institution series of pts treated with TORS to identify primary site in pts with squamous cell unknown primary of head and neck. Six institutions enrolled a total of 47 pts. Primary site was found in 72%. Primary was in BOT in 59% and in tonsil in 38%. In 18 pts without suspicious radiographic or examination findings, 72% of primaries were identified with TORS. **Conclusion: TORS is helpful to identify primary site in squamous carcinoma of unknown primary.**

Does bilateral neck RT improve outcomes as compared to unilateral treatment?

Unilateral treatment is controversial considering that occult primary tumors likely reside in the base of tongue, which is a midline structure. Table 15.3 provides a summary of various series investigating unilateral treatment. Although failure rate appears low (approximately 10%), this remains controversial. Of note, most of the historic papers compared ipsilateral RT without mucosal coverage to comprehensive RT.

TABLE 15.3: Studies Investigating Unilateral Neck Treatment					
Author	Institution	Year	Ipsilateral LN Treated, N	Contralateral Failure, N (%)	Comment
Carlson et al.[19]	MDACC	1986	13	2 (15.6%)	2D fields, no CT imaging
Colletier et al.[20]	MDACC	1998	14	1 (7.1%)	May overlap with Carlson; unclear if one contralateral failure was in ipsilateral only treated pt
Reddy et al.[21]	U Chicago	1997	16	9 (56%)	All nodes treated ipsilaterally with electron beam only; five of nine recurrences were primary and contralateral nodes synchronously
Grau et al.[22]	Denmark	2000	26	1 (4%)	Pts treated with bilateral RT on study had 2% contralateral failure
Beldi et al.[23]	Milan	2007	33	Not Reported	Report worse survival in unilateral pts but many were treated palliatively
Ligey et al.[24]	Dijon	2009	59	6 (10.2%)	Seven primary tumors emerged in unilateral group
Fakhrian et al.[25]	Munich	2012	17	1 (5.9%)	
Cuaron et al.[26]	MSKCC	2015	6	0 (0%)	Small but all CT imaging
Perkins et al.[27]	Wash U	2012	21	1 (5%)	All treated postneck dissection
Overall Approximate Crude Rate			**172**	**21 (12.2%)**	**Excluding Reddy: 12/156 = 7.7%**

REFERENCES

1. Keller LM, Galloway TJ, Holdbrook T, et al. p16 status, pathologic and clinical characteristics, biomolecular signature, and long-term outcomes in head and neck squamous cell carcinomas of unknown primary. *Head Neck.* 2014;36(12):1677–1684.
2. McDowell LJ, Young RJ, Johnston ML, et al. p16-positive lymph node metastases from cutaneous head and neck squamous cell carcinoma: no association with high-risk human papillomavirus or prognosis and implications for the workup of the unknown primary. *Cancer.* 2016;122(8):1201–1208.
3. Johansen J, Buus S, Loft A, et al. Prospective study of 18FDG-PET in the detection and management of patients with lymph node metastases to the neck from an unknown primary tumor: results from the DAHANCA-13 study. *Head Neck.* 2008;30(4):471–478.
4. Waltonen JD, Ozer E, Schuller DE, Agrawal A. Tonsillectomy vs. deep tonsil biopsies in detecting occult tonsil tumors. *Laryngoscope.* 2009;119(1):102–106.
5. Cianchetti M, Mancuso AA, Amdur RJ, et al. Diagnostic evaluation of squamous cell carcinoma metastatic to cervical lymph nodes from an unknown head and neck primary site. *Laryngoscope.* 2009;119(12):2348–2354.

6.   Mendenhall WM, Mancuso AA, Parsons JT, et al. Diagnostic evaluation of squamous cell carcinoma metastatic to cervical lymph nodes from an unknown head and neck primary site. *Head Neck*. 1998;20(8):739–744.

7.   Nieder C, Ang KK. Cervical lymph node metastases from occult squamous cell carcinoma. *Curr Treat Options Oncol*. 2002;3(1):33–40.

8.   Christiansen H, Hermann RM, Martin A, et al. Neck lymph node metastases from an unknown primary tumor. *Strahlenther Onkol*. 2005;181(6):355–362.

9.   Demiroz C, Vainshtein JM, Koukourakis GV, et al. Head and neck squamous cell carcinoma of unknown primary: neck dissection and radiotherapy or definitive radiotherapy. *Head Neck*. 2014;36(11):1589–1595.

10. Balaker AE, Abemayor E, Elashoff D, St John MA. Cancer of unknown primary: does treatment modality make a difference? *Laryngoscope*. 2012;122(6):1279–1282.

11. Galloway TJ, Ridge JA. Management of squamous cancer metastatic to cervical nodes with an unknown primary site. *J Clin Oncol*. 2015;33(29):3328–3337.

12. NCCN Clinical Practice Guidelines in Oncology: Head and Neck Cancers. 2017. https://www.nccn.org

13. Sher DJ, Balboni TA, Haddad RI, et al. Efficacy and toxicity of chemoradiotherapy using intensity-modulated radiotherapy for unknown primary of head and neck. *Int J Radiat Oncol Biol Phys*. 2011;80(5):1405–1411.

14. Argiris A, Smith S, Stenson K, et al. Concurrent chemoradiotherapy for N2 or N3 squamous cell carcinoma of the head and neck from an occult primary. *Ann Oncol*. 2003;14(8):1306–1311.

15. Shehadeh NJ, Ensley JF, Kucuk O, et al. Benefit of postoperative chemoradiotherapy for patients with unknown primary squamous cell carcinoma of the head and neck. *Head Neck*. 2006;28(12):1090–1098.

16. Chen AM, Farwell DG, Lau DH, et al. Radiation therapy in the management of head-and-neck cancer of unknown primary origin: how does the addition of concurrent chemotherapy affect the therapeutic ratio? *Int J Radiat Oncol Biol Phys*. 2011;81(2):346–352.

17. Dixon PR, Au M, Hosni A, et al. Impact of p16 expression, nodal status, and smoking on oncologic outcomes of patients with head and neck unknown primary squamous cell carcinoma. *Head Neck*. 2016;38(9):1347–1353.

18. Motz K, Qualliotine JR, Rettig E, et al. Changes in unknown primary squamous cell carcinoma of the head and neck at initial presentation in the era of human papillomavirus. *JAMA Otolaryngol Head Neck Surg*. 2016;142(3):223–228.

19. Carlson LS, Fletcher GH, Oswald MJ. Guidelines for radiotherapeutic techniques for cervical metastases from an unknown primary. *Int J Radiat Oncol Biol Phys*. 1986;12(12):2101–2110.

20. Colletier PJ, Garden AS, Morrison WH, et al. Postoperative radiation for squamous cell carcinoma metastatic to cervical lymph nodes from an unknown primary site: outcomes and patterns of failure. *Head Neck*. 1998;20(8):674–681.

21. Reddy SP, Marks JE. Metastatic carcinoma in the cervical lymph nodes from an unknown primary site: results of bilateral neck plus mucosal irradiation vs. ipsilateral neck irradiation. *Int J Radiat Oncol Biol Phys*. 1997;37(4):797–802.

22. Grau C, Johansen LV, Jakobsen J, et al. Cervical lymph node metastases from unknown primary tumours: results from a national survey by the Danish Society for Head and Neck Oncology. *Radiother Oncol*. 2000;55(2):121–129.

23. Beldì D, Jereczek-Fossa BA, D'Onofrio A, et al. Role of radiotherapy in the treatment of cervical lymph node metastases from an unknown primary site: retrospective analysis of 113 patients. *Int J Radiat Oncol Biol Phys*. 2007;69(4):1051–1058.

24. Ligey A, Gentil J, Créhange G, et al. Impact of target volumes and radiation technique on loco-regional control and survival for patients with unilateral cervical lymph node metastases from an unknown primary. *Radiother Oncol*. 2009;93(3):483–487.

25. Fakhrian K, Thamm R, Knapp S, et al. Radio(chemo)therapy in the management of squamous cell carcinoma of cervical lymph nodes from an unknown primary site: a retrospective analysis. *Strahlenther Onkol*. 2012;188(1):56–61.

26. Cuaron J, Rao S, Wolden S, et al. Patterns of failure in patients with head and neck carcinoma of unknown primary treated with radiation therapy. *Head Neck*. 2016;38(Suppl 1):E426–E431.

27. Perkins SM, Spencer CR, Chernock RD, et al. Radiotherapeutic management of cervical lymph node metastases from an unknown primary site. *Arch Otolaryngol Head Neck Surg*. 2012;138(7):656–661.

16: POSTOPERATIVE RADIATION FOR HEAD AND NECK CANCER

Carryn M. Anderson

> **QUICK HIT:** Surgery is the preferred initial management of resectable H&N cancers of oral cavity, salivary gland, nasal cavity/paranasal sinuses, thyroid, and some oropharynx and larynx cancers. Organ preservation is utilized in nasopharynx cancer and many oropharynx, larynx, and hypopharynx cancers. Oncologic surgery alone is often sufficient treatment for T1-T2N0-1 tumors when resected with negative margins. Adjuvant RT (PORT) is recommended for specific pathologic risk factors and with concurrent CHT given for positive margins and extracapsular extension (ECE) in mucosal H&N squamous cell carcinoma (HNSCC).

TABLE 16.1: PORT Indications and Dosing Summary

Risk Group	Treatment	Patient Characteristics
Low Risk	Observation	pT1-T2, pN0-1, -PNI, +/−LVSI, -margins, -ECE
Intermediate risk	60 Gy	pT3-T4, pN2-3 disease, PNI, LVSI, close margins (<5 mm), pT1-2N0-1 with multiple minor risk factors or depth of invasion >4 mm in oral tongue[1]
	66 Gy	Multiple of above risk factors
High risk	66 Gy+CHT	+ECE, microscopic positive margins[2]
	70 Gy+CHT	Gross disease

EPIDEMIOLOGY: Worldwide incidence of >550,000 (fifth most common cancer), male-to-female ratio 3:1, 2016 estimated U.S. incidence of 48,330 cases and 9,570 deaths.[3]

RISK FACTORS: Tobacco (cigarettes and chew, 5–25x increased risk), alcohol (dose dependent and synergistic with tobacco), HPV infection (oropharyngeal), EBV infection (nasopharyngeal), HIV, immunosuppressed from transplant drugs or autoimmune diseases, HSV, betel nut chewing (oral cavity), sun exposure (skin), previous radiation, occupational/environmental exposures.

ANATOMY: See Chapters 10–15 for site-specific anatomy. For maxillary sinus tumors, one important landmark is Ohngren's line: extends from medial canthus of eye to angle of mandible. Anteroinferior/infrastructures have good prognosis whereas superoposterior/suprastructures have poor prognosis and have early extension into eye, skull base, pterygoids, and infratemporal fossa.

PATHOLOGY: Most common histology is squamous cell carcinoma: "keratin pearls" are seen in well-differentiated SCC, often associated with classic HNSCC related to smoking/alcohol abuse; nonkeratinizing poorly differentiated "basaloid" squamous cancer often associated with HPV-associated p16+ oropharyngeal SCC. Other histologies include mucoepidermoid carcinoma, adenoid cystic carcinoma, adenosquamous, adenocarcinoma, acinic cell, lymphoma, lymphoepithelial carcinoma, melanoma.

CLINICAL PRESENTATION: Dependent on primary site. Paranasal sinus/nasal cavity/nasopharynx: nasal obstruction, epistaxis, lateral gaze palsy, unilateral hearing loss, epiphora. Oropharynx: dysphagia, trismus, otalgia, odynophagia. Oral cavity: nonhealing ulceration, dysarthria, loose teeth. Larynx: hoarseness, stridor, dysphagia, odynophagia, otalgia. Hypopharynx: dysphagia, hoarseness, weight loss. Many pts are asymptomatic from their primary disease and present with adenopathy, most commonly level II jugulodigastric node.

WORKUP: H&P including flexible nasopharyngolaryngoscopy or mirror examination.

Labs: Routine labs including CBC, CMP, audiology if platinum CHT.

Imaging: CT neck with contrast, PET/CT for stage III/IV patients, CT chest to screen for metastasis or second primary in smokers if PET/CT not obtained. If unknown primary by office exam and imaging, obtain PET/CT prior to panendoscopy/exam under anesthesia.[4]

Pathology: FNA biopsy of neck node and/or biopsy of primary site. See Chapters 10–15 for site-specific workup. Optimally multidisciplinary consult should be performed prior to resection.

PROGNOSTIC FACTORS: Positive margins and ECE are most important pathologic prognostic factors. Other negative pathologic factors include close margins, PNI, LVSI, tumor size, depth of invasion (oral tongue in particular). HPV-associated cancers have better prognosis overall, and ECE and advanced nodal stage do not have same negative impact on survival, as reflected in AJCC 8th edition Staging Manual. *Extracapsular extension* ranges from microscopic (small break in capsule, desmoplastic stromal reaction) to macroscopic (visible to eye at surgery) to gross soft tissue deposits (no evidence of LN architecture, which likely represents complete LN replacement).[5] Recurrence rate doubles when ECE is present. CT can predict ECE with frequent false negatives but uncommon false positives (Sens/Spec/PPV/NPV 43%, 97%, 82%, and 87%).[6] Nodes <2.5 cm on CT imaging have approximately 6% rate of pathologic ECE as compared to larger nodes with 32% rate.[6]

NATURAL HISTORY: Vast majority of disease-related recurrences will occur within first 2 years of treatment completion. Most common site of distant metastasis is lung with bone second most common. HPV-associated cancers have been known to spread to less common sites such as liver, skin, soft tissues, brain, and leptomeninges.[7]

STAGING: AJCC 8th edition has significant changes to H&N staging, separating HPV-associated oropharynx cancer from others.[8] See Chapters 10–15 for staging details.

TREATMENT PARADIGM

Observation: Observation is appropriate following surgery for low-risk patients, loosely defined as pT1-2N0-1 without LVSI, PNI, ECE, shallow depth of invasion (especially oral tongue, <4 mm) and with negative margins (>5 mm ideally).

Surgery: Resection of primary should be performed with least morbidity possible. Free flap reconstruction may be necessary for larger tumors (hemiglossectomy, total glossectomy, mandibular reconstruction, laryngopharyngectomy, etc.). Free flaps typically include radial forearm, anterolateral thigh or fibula (when bone is required). Minimally invasive techniques such as TORS and TLM are evolving. For sinonasal tumors, endoscopic surgery is preferred, performed in piecemeal way. Transoral robotic surgery (TORS) is performed using robotic platform, suggested for oropharynx and possibly larynx/hypopharynx primaries. TORS is FDA approved for cT1-2 tumors.[9]

Transoral laser microsurgery (TLMS) is piecemeal removal of tumor through laryngoscope using CO_2 laser aimed via micromanipulator attached to microscope (only available at few specialized centers). Both are suggested as a possible method to improve toxicity through lower RT doses (70 Gy+cisplatin needed for definitive vs. 60–66 Gy±CHT post-op) and as a way to intensify treatment for advanced disease (see ongoing RTOG 1221). See review for issues specific to TORS/TLM.[10,11] Neck dissection typically performed at time of surgery (see Table 16.2).

TABLE 16.2: Neck Dissection Types for H&N Cancer	
Radical neck dissection	All LN groups I–V, CN XI, IJ vein, SCM
Modified radical neck dissection	All LN groups I–V, preserves ≥1 of CN XI, IJ, SCM
Selective neck dissection (SND)	Preservation of ≥1 LN group
Supraomohyoid	SND of only I–III, considered for oral cavity cases
Lateral neck dissection (thyroid cancer)	SND II–IV (oropharynx, hypopharynx, larynx)
Central neck dissection (thyroid cancer)	SND VI

Chemotherapy: CHT can be added concurrently with RT in postoperative setting to escalation treatment for high-risk cancers. Bolus cisplatin is most common, given at 100 mg/m^2 days 1, 22, 43. Weekly cisplatin 40 mg/m^2 is an acceptable alternative. Ongoing trials are investigating role of cetuximab (RTOG 0920) for intermediate risk and alternative multiagent regimens for high-risk pts (RTOG 1216).

Radiation

Indications: Risk-adapted approach to RT is used to escalate therapy in postoperative setting. Indications for PORT are described (Table 16.1) by loosely defined risk groups of low (observation), intermediate (RT alone), and high (chemoRT). For sinonasal tumors, PORT is almost always recommended (except for T1 ethmoid). RT should be initiated within 6 weeks of surgery for optimal LRC and OS.[12]

Dose: In era of IMRT SIB technique, University of Iowa uses doses of 66 Gy, 59.4 Gy, and 56.1 Gy in 33 fx to areas of high risk (microscopic margin positive, ECE, or multiple primary site risk factors), intermediate risk (post-op bed or undissected neck at risk), and low risk (elective lower risk nodal areas) respectively. In cases without high-risk features, 60 Gy/30 fx is delivered to post-op bed simultaneously with 54 Gy to high-risk undissected neck/low-risk neck.

EVIDENCE-BASED Q&A

What evidence suggests that PORT is effective?

Most evidence is retrospective although there are two older randomized trials demonstrating improved LRF with PORT compared to observation.[13,14]

Historically, what evidence suggests postoperative RT is superior to preoperative radiation?

Tupchong, RTOG 7303 (*IJROBP* 1991, PMID 1993628): Phase III PRT of preoperative RT versus PORT for supraglottic larynx and hypopharynx cancer. Preoperative RT was 50 Gy, PORT was 60 Gy. 277 pts, follow-up from 9 to 15 years. LRC improved in PORT group compared to preoperative (70% vs. 58%, $p = .04$). No difference in OS ($p = .15$). **Conclusion:** PORT improves LRC compared to preoperative RT. Because of this trial, PORT has become standard in pts managed with primary surgery.

What data supports current standard dosing for PORT?

All pts require minimum dose of 57.6 Gy at 1.8 Gy/fx to whole operative bed. High-risk areas of ≥2 adverse factors or ECE require 63 Gy at 1.8 Gy/fx.

Peters, MD Anderson (*IJROBP* 1993, PMID 8482629): PRT of stage III/IV SCC of oral cavity, oropharynx, hypopharynx, and larynx stratified by risk factors. Lower risk pts randomized to 52.2 to 57.6 Gy vs 63 Gy and higher risk pts randomized to 63 Gy vs 68.4 Gy, all in 1.8 Gy fractions. On interim analysis, pts who received dose of ≤54 Gy had significantly higher primary failure rate and dose group was increased to 57.6 Gy, improving LRF (p = .02). Overall, no dose–response was demonstrated. However, if ECE was present, recurrence was significantly higher at 57.6 Gy than at ≥63 Gy. ECE was the only independent variable prognostic of LRR. Having two or more of following were progressively prognostic: oral cavity primary, mucosal margins close or positive, nerve invasion, ≥2 positive lymph nodes, largest node >3 cm, treatment delay greater than 6 weeks, and Zubrod performance status ≥2. **Conclusion: Minimum dose of 57.6 Gy to whole operative bed should be delivered with boost of 63 Gy to sites of increased risk (e.g., ECE). Treatment should be started as soon as possible after surgery. Dose escalation above 63 Gy at 1.8 Gy per day does not appear to improve therapeutic ratio. This trial defined most common dosing regimens used today (60–66 Gy).**

What data supports risk-adapted approach to PORT?

Ang, MD Anderson (*IJROBP* 2001, PMID 11597795): Multi-institutional PRT of 213 pts with advanced HNSCC of oral cavity, oropharynx, larynx, and hypopharynx assessing role of risk stratification and PORT scheduling (concomitant boost vs. standard). Pts received therapy predicated on set of pathologic risk features: oral cavity site, mucosal margin status, nerve invasion, >1 positive node, >1 positive nodal group, largest node >3 cm, ECE, and treatment delay of >6 weeks. See Table 16.3. **Conclusion: Dosing based on risk stratification is legitimate approach to PORT for H&N cancer.** *(See altered fractionation in the following for the second conclusion.)*

TABLE 16.3: Results of MD Anderson Risk-Adapted PORT for H&N Cancer			
Risk Group	**PORT**	**5-yr LRC**	**5-yr OS**
Low Risk: no adverse factors	None	90%	83%
Intermediate Risk: One adverse factor other than ECE	57.6 Gy/6.5 weeks	94%	66%
High Risk: ≥2 adverse factors or ECE	63 Gy/5 or 7 weeks (±conc. boost)	68%	42%

With definitive RT, altered fractionation improves control (RTOG 9003), so should we accelerate pts receiving PORT?

No benefit for most patients; however, acceleration may account for delay in PORT after surgery beyond 6 weeks.

Sanguineti, Italy (*IJROBP* 2005, PMID 15708255): Phase III trial of PORT 60 Gy/6 weeks (conventional fractionation, [CF]) or altered fractionation (AF) with "biphasic concomitant boost" schedule, with boost delivered during first and last weeks of treatment (64 Gy/5 weeks). 2-yr LRC CF 80% versus AF 78% (p = .52), trend to benefit for pts with RT delay >7 weeks. 2-yr OS 67% versus 64% (p = .84). Toxicity: Confluent mucositis CF 27% versus AF 50% (p = .006), duration same. Late toxicity 18% versus 27% (NS). **Conclusion: Accelerated fractionation not beneficial overall, might be option for pts who delay starting RT.**

Ang, MD Anderson (*IJROBP* 2001, PMID 11597795): Same trial as detailed earlier. Regarding hyperfractionation, only "trend" to benefit when comparing 5 weeks versus 7 weeks in high-risk pts (LRC $p = .11$, OS $p = .08$). However, when looking at interval from surgery to PORT initiation for high-risk pts, acceleration seemed to make up for delay.

Chemotherapy

Which pts benefit from treatment escalation with concurrent chemoRT?

In high-risk patients, pts with ECE or positive margins seem to benefit based on combined RTOG 9501/EORTC 22931 analysis.

Bernier, EORTC 22931 (*NEJM* 2004, PMID 15128894): PRT of 334 pts w/ HNSCC (oral cavity, oropharynx, hypopharynx or larynx) s/p primary surgical resection w/ high-risk features comparing postop RT alone (66 Gy/33 fx) versus chemoRT (cisplatin 100 mg/ m^2 on days 1, 22, 43 w/ same RT). Eligible pts included pT3-4 and N_{any} (except pT3N0 of larynx w/ negative margins); or T1-2 and N2-3; or T1-2N0-1 w/ unfavorable pathologic findings (ENE, + margins, PNI or vascular tumor embolism); or oral cavity/oropharynx tumors w/ level IV-V LNs. Overall, 67% had pT3-4, 57% had pN2-3, 28% had +margins, 54% had ≥2 positive LNs. MFU 60 mos. See Table 16.4. Acute Gr 3-4 mucosal adverse effects were worse w/ chemoRT (41% vs. 21%, $p = .001$), while cumulative incidence of late effects was not. **Conclusion: Post-op chemoRT improves survival over RT alone for pts w/ locally advanced HNSCC (and w/ unfavorable clinical + pathologic factors) w/o high incidence of late effects.**

TABLE 16.4: Results of Bernier EORTC CHT Trial						
	Median PFS	**5-yr PFS**	**MS**	**5-yr OS**	**5-yr LRR**	**5-yr DM**
Post-op RT	23 mos	36%	32 mos	40%	31%	25%
Post-op chemoRT	55 mos	47%	72 mos	53%	18%	21%
p value	.04		.02		.007	.61

Cooper, RTOG 9501 (*NEJM* 2004, PMID 15128893, Update Cooper *IJROBP* 2012, PMID 2274963): PRT of 416 pts (update 410 pts) w/ HNSCC (oral cavity, oropharynx, hypopharynx, or larynx) s/p macroscopic complete resection w/ high-risk features (any or all of: histologic invasion of ≥2 LNs, ECE or +margins), comparing RT alone (60–66 Gy/30–33 fx) versus chemoRT (cisplatin 100 mg/m^2 on days 1, 22, 43). Overall, 18% had positive margins, 82% had ≥2 LNs or ECE. MFU 6.1 yrs, update 9.4 yrs for survivors. See Table 16.5. Incidence of acute adverse effects ≥grade 3 was 34% and 77% in RT and chemoRT arms, respectively ($p < .001$). In the first report, CHT improved LRF and DFS but not OS. With long-term follow-up CHT improved LRF in pts with ECE or +margins. **Conclusion: ECE and +margins remain indications for concurrent CHT and PORT.**

TABLE 16.5: Results of RTOG 9501 Postoperative CHT Trial						
	Original Report (2004)			**Long-term Update (2012)**		
	2-yr LRC (2004)	**2-yr DFS (2004)**	**2-yr OS (2004)**	**10-yr LRF, All (2012)**	**10-yr LRF, ECE or +margins (2012)**	**10-yr OS, ECE or +margins (2012)**
PORT	72%	HR 0.78	HR 0.84	28.8%	33.1%	19.6
Postop chemoRT	82%			22.3%	21.0%	27.1
p value	.01	.04	.19	.10	.02	.07

Bernier, Pooled Analysis EORTC and RTOG (*Head Neck* 2005, PMID 16161069): Data from EORTC 22931 and RTOG 95-01 were pooled for comparative analysis. ECE and/or microscopically +margins were only risk factors with significant impact of chemoRT in both trials. **Conclusion: +margins and ECE are most significant prognostic factors for poor outcome, and postop chemoRT improves outcome in pts w/ one or both of these risk factors.**

Laskar, Tata Memorial (*ASCO* 2016, Abstract 6004): PRT of 900 pts with resectable OC-SCC who underwent surgery randomized to PORT alone (56–60 Gy in 5 fx/week, Arm A), PORT with concurrent weekly cisplatin (30 mg/m^2, Arm B), or accelerated PORT (6 fx/week, Arm C). MFU was 58 months. LRC at 5 years was 59.9% and 65.1% for Arm B versus Arm A (*p* = .203) and 58.2% for Arm C. Unplanned subset analysis demonstrated significant improvement LRC, DFS, and OS for pts with high-risk features (T3-T4, N2-3, and ECE) for pts treated with standard fractionation RT and concurrent chemoRT compared to accelerated RT. **Conclusion: Intensification of therapy with concurrent CHT or accelerated RT did not improve outcomes in these pts with OC-SCC, but concurrent chemoRT and standard fractionation RT may be beneficial in pts with high-risk features.** *Comment: Oral cavity squamous carcinoma in India may be different from that in the United States.*

How much ECE triggers addition of CHT?

Randomized data included any ECE. Recent data shows survival detriment proportional to amount of ECE.[15,16] There does not appear to be level of ECE low enough to omit CHT and those with gross ECE have inferior survival even with chemotherapy. In HPV era, this is evolving with multiple trials investigating omission of CHT for those with minor ECE ≤1 mm.

Management of lower risk patients

Is PORT necessary in N1 pt?

A microscopic single node without other risk factors was not sufficient to receive PORT in the preceding Ang trial. It is likely that these pts, in absence of other risk factors and after adequate neck dissection, can be observed although this is controversial.

Schmitz, Belgium (*Eur Arch Otorhinolaryngol* 2009, PMID 18648835): RR of 146 pts and 249 neck dissections. 25% cN0 pts were pN+ with 3% regional recurrence overall, 2% in dissected neck and 1% in undissected neck. pN0 failure rate of 1%. pN1 failure rate without PORT 9% versus with PORT 5%. **Conclusion: Selective node dissection reliable to stage cN0 neck, and as definitive operation for pN0, most pN1 and pN2b necks. PORT not justified for pN1 but justified for pN2b and ECE.**

Jäckel, Germany (*Head Neck* 2008, PMID 18302275): RR of 118 pts with curative surgery, pN1 disease without ECE. Majority had selective neck dissection (level II-III 63%, level I-III 19%, level II-IV 15%). PORT in 20%, post-op chemoRT in 19%. Isolated nodal failure 7% (surgery 10% vs. PORT 2%), all nodal failures 16% (21% vs. 9%). 3-year neck recurrence rate 11% versus 3% (*p* = .09). **Conclusion: Data suggest trend to improved regional control for pN1 with PORT.**

REFERENCES

1. Ganly I, Goldstein D, Carlson DL, et al. Long-term regional control and survival in pts with "low-risk," early stage oral tongue cancer managed by partial glossectomy and neck dissection without postoperative radiation: importance of tumor thickness. *Cancer.* 2013;119(6):1168–1176.

2. Bernier J, Cooper JS, Pajak TF, et al. Defining risk levels in locally advanced H&Ncancers: comparative analysis of concurrent postoperative RT plus CHT trials of EORTC (#22931) and RTOG (#9501). *Head Neck.* 2005;27(10):843–850.

3. Siegel RL, Miller KD, Jemal A. Cancer statistics, 2016. *CA Cancer J Clin.* 2016;66(1):7–30.

4. Mani N, George MM, Nash L, et al. Role of 18-Fludeoxyglucose positron emission tomography-computed tomography and subsequent panendoscopy in H&N squamous cell carcinoma of unknown primary. *Laryngoscope.* 2016;126(6):1354–1358.

5. Lewis JS, Jr., Carpenter DH, Thorstad WL, et al. Extracapsular extension is poor predictor of disease recurrence in surgically treated oropharyngeal squamous cell carcinoma. *Mod Pathol.* 2011;24(11):1413–1420.

6. Prabhu RS, Magliocca KR, Hanasoge S, et al. Accuracy of computed tomography for predicting pathologic nodal extracapsular extension in pts with head-and-neck cancer undergoing initial surgical resection. *Int J Radiat Oncol Biol Phys.* 2014;88(1):122–129.

7. Trosman SJ, Koyfman SA, Ward MC, et al. Effect of human papillomavirus on patterns of distant metastatic failure in oropharyngeal squamous cell carcinoma treated with chemoradiotherapy. *JAMA Otolaryngol Head Neck Surg.* 2015;141(5):457–462.

8. Lydiatt WM, Patel SG, O'Sullivan B, et al. Head and neck cancers: major changes in American Joint Committee on cancer eighth edition cancer staging manual. *CA Cancer J Clin.* 2017;67(2):122–137.

9. FDA 510(k) summary. 2009; http://www.accessdata.fda.gov/cdrh_docs/pdf9/K090993.pdf

10. Ward MC, Koyfman SA. Transoral robotic surgery: RT oncologist's perspective. *Oral Oncol.* 2016;60:96–102.

11. Huang SH, Hansen A, Rathod S, O'Sullivan B. Primary surgery versus (chemo)RT in oropharyngeal cancer: RT oncologist's and medical oncologist's perspectives. *Curr Opin Otolaryngol Head Neck Surg.* 2015;23(2):139–147.

12. Tribius S, Donner J, Pazdyka H, et al. Survival and overall treatment time after postoperative radio(chemo)therapy in pts with H&Ncancer. *Head Neck.* 2016;38(7):1058–1065.

13. Kokal WA, Neifeld JP, Eisert D, et al. Postoperative RT as adjuvant treatment for carcinoma of oral cavity, larynx, and pharynx: preliminary report of prospective randomized trial. *J Surg Oncol.* 1988;38(2):71–76.

14. Mishra RC, Singh DN, Mishra TK. Post-operative RT in carcinoma of buccal mucosa, prospective randomized trial. *Eur J Surg Oncol.* 1996;22(5):502–504.

15. Prabhu RS, Hanasoge S, Magliocca KR, et al. Extent of pathologic extracapsular extension and outcomes in pts with nonoropharyngeal H&N cancer treated with initial surgical resection. *Cancer.* 2014;120(10):1499–1506.

16. Greenberg JS, Fowler R, Gomez J, et al. Extent of extracapsular spread: critical prognosticator in oral tongue cancer. *Cancer.* 2003;97(6):1464–1470.

III: **SKIN**

17: NONMELANOMA SKIN CANCER

Neil McIver Woody and Jonathan Sharrett

> **QUICK HIT:** Nonmelanomatous skin cancer is the most common cancer. Basal cell carcinoma (BCC) and squamous cell carcinoma (SCC) represent the majority of cases. Vast majority of pts are classified as low risk and effectively treated with surgical excision or other focal therapy. Infrequently, lesions may act aggressively and require aggressive surgical resection with adjuvant RT or definitive RT.

TABLE 17.1: General Treatment Paradigm for Nonmelanoma Skin Cancer		
SCC or BCC	Low risk	Surgical resection (Mohs, WLE for noncosmetic areas), electrodissection, curettage, definitive RT (nonsurgical)
	High risk	Surgery (WLE or Mohs) + adjuvant RT (indications: +PNI, +margins, bone invasion, multiple recurrences, node-positive) Or Definitive RT (nonsurgical candidates)
	Node-positive	Nodal dissection followed by adjuvant RT (pN2 or greater, pN1 controversial) Rare for BCC
	Metastatic	Platinum-based CHT (SCC) Vismodigib (BCC, although mets are rare)

EPIDEMIOLOGY: Nonmelanomatous skin cancer includes cutaneous squamous cell carcinoma (SCC), basal cell carcinoma (BCC), and Merkel cell carcinoma. Prevalence in the United States was estimated to be 5.4 million cases in 2012. BCC accounts for 65% to 70% of cases while SCC accounts for 30% with adnexal and Merkel cell carcinomas representing small percentage of cases.[1]

RISK FACTORS: Risk factors for SCC and BCC include: older age, higher UV exposure (UV-B 290–320 nm is higher risk than UV-A), fair complexion, prior RT exposure (e.g., uranium miners, prior RT, tinea capitis, acne, enlarged thymus, childhood cancer survivors), chemical exposure (arsenic, coal tar), prior phototherapy, steroid use, and chronic ulcers/scars/inflammation. Of note, chronic inflammation increases risk of SCC significantly more than risk of BCC. SCC is a major contributor to morbidity and mortality in immune-suppressed pts (x65 risk,[2] organ-transplant pts on calcineurin inhibitors have higher risk than mTOR inhibitor sirolimus; see the following for details).

Genetic syndromes: Basal cell nevus syndrome (Gorlin syndrome) is disorder of patched tumor suppressor gene (PTCH), which results in macrocephaly, frontal bossing, bifid ribs, palmar and plantar pitting, medulloblastoma, and bone cysts. PTCH is in sonic hedgehog (SHH) signaling pathway. BCC also associated with Bazex–Dupre–Christol syndrome, which is X-linked dominant syndrome characterized by multiple BCC and pitting or "ice pick" scars of skin (follicular atrophoderma). Others: xeroderma pigmentosum (XP) with 57% lifetime incidence of skin cancer (autosomal recessive [AR] disorder associated with mutations in seven identified genes [XPA to XPG] resulting in impaired ability to correct UV-related DNA damage due to nucleotide excision repair), albinism with 35% lifetime incidence of skin cancer, Bloom's syndrome, epidermolysis bullosa, Fanconi's anemia, and Muir–Torre syndrome (autosomal dominant [AD] disorder characterized by sebaceous skin tumors [eyelid] +/− keratoachanthoma and internal malignancies [GI/GU]). Associated with germline mutation of DNA mismatch repair genes: MSH-1 and MLH-1 exhibiting microsatellite instability.

ANATOMY: Skin is the largest organ in the body and composed of two primary layers: epidermis superficially (devoid of lymphatics) and dermis, which contains superficial lymphatic plexus. Dermis is composed of papillary region superficially connecting with epidermis and reticular region below. Beneath the dermis is the subdermis (or hypodermis), composed primarily of fat and connective tissue. Basement membrane separates epidermis from dermis. Tumors of epidermis may be characterized by Clark's levels: level 1: tumor confined to epidermis (in situ); level 2: invasion into papillary dermis; level 3: invasion to junction of papillary and reticular dermis; level 4: invasion into reticular dermis; and level 5: invasion into subcutaneous fat.

PATHOLOGY

BCC: Arises from basal layer of epidermis and has three presentations. Nodular subtype accounts for 60% of cases and presents with pink- or flesh-colored papule. These may become ulcerated and hence term noduloulcerative ("rodent ulcer"). Superficial subtype accounts for 30% of cases and demonstrates red, scaly macule. Morpheaform subtype accounts for 5% to 10% of cases and presents as light-colored macules, or shiny, atrophic lesions w/ indistinct margins; morpheaform subtype is more likely to have infiltrating growth. Rare subtypes include infiltrative and basosquamous subtypes, which are more aggressive with basosquamous behaving similarly to SCC.

SCC: Clinically, often begin as round to irregular, plaque-like or nodular, and overlaid with warty keratotic scale or conical keratinized protrusion ("cutaneous horn"). May also see as ulcer or induration and propensity to bleed. Histology demonstrates pleomorphism, numerous and atypical mitoses, dyskeratosis, and "horn pearl" formation. Bowen's disease: SCC in situ; red-brown epidermal plaque is in sun-exposed sites. Known as "erythroplasia of Queyrat" if on glans penis.

SCREENING: Pts with prior diagnosis of BCC or SCC should be screened by dermatologist at regular intervals to detect new skin cancers. American Academy of Dermatology provides guidelines for patient self-surveillance while USPSTF suggests there is insufficient evidence to recommend routine screening of asymptomatic patients. Two PRTs confirm that application of sun screen reduces incidence of actinic keratosis (AK), BCC, and SCC.[3,4]

CLINICAL PRESENTATION: Appearance of primary BCC and SCC described earlier under pathology.

WORKUP: H&P including complete skin examination and history of prior operations, procedures, or prior RT to involved area or other history of skin cancers or premalignant lesions. Review for any neurologic symptoms suggestive of PNI. In cases of SCC, additional emphasis on regional lymph node (LN) exam. Biopsy confirmation of nonmelanoma skin cancer is recommended as amelanotic melanoma can mimic BCC appearance.

Pathology: Biopsy approaches include punch, shave, or excisional biopsy.

Imaging: CT/MRI should be considered with lesions involving medial/lateral canthi, positive PNI or suspicious symptoms, lymphadenopathy, or fixed lesion to underlying muscle, bone or fascia.

PROGNOSTIC FACTORS: Prognostic factors include tumor size, depth of invasion, immunosuppression, location, chronic inflammation, prior RT, neurologic symptoms, recurrent tumor, and poor differentiation. NCCN defines high-risk factors, which can be used to stratify pts.

TABLE 17.2: NCCN Definition of High Risk for Nonmelanoma Skin Cancers[5,6]		
	SCC	BCC
Location/Size	• Trunk or extremities and size ≥20 mm • Cheeks, forehead, scalp, neck and pre-tibia and ≥10 mm • "Mask" area (central face, eyelids, eyebrows, periorbital, nose, lips, chin, mandible, pre/postauricular, temple, ear), genitalia, hands and feet, and ≥6 mm	
Borders	Poorly defined	
Recurrent	Yes	
Immunosuppression	Present	
Subtype	Adenoid, adenosquamous, desmoplastic, or metaplastic	Aggressive growth pattern (morpheaform, basosquamous, sclerosing, mixed infiltrative, or micronodular features)
Perineural, lymphatic or vascular involvement	Yes	Yes
Prior RT to site	Yes, or site of chronic inflammation	Yes
Differentiation	Poorly differentiated	
Depth	Clark's level IV-V or depth ≥2mm	
Symptoms	Neurologic symptoms, rapid growth	

STAGING: BCC and SCC of skin are staged according to AJCC 8th edition staging system. The exception is SCC of eyelid, which is staged separately.[2]

TABLE 17.3: AJCC 8th ed. (2017) Staging System for Cutaneous Squamous Cell Carcinoma								
T/M \ N		cN0	cN1	cN2a	cN2b	cN2c	cN3a	cN3b
T1	• <2 cm	I						
T2	• 2.1–4 cm	II	III		IVA			
T3	• >4 cm • 1 high risk feature[1]							
T4a	• Gross cortical bone							
T4b	• Invasion into skull base				IVB			
M1	• Distant metastasis				IVC			

Notes: 1 high risk feature[1] = Minor bone erosion, PNI (nerve measuring ≥0.1 mm), or deep invasion (beyond subcutaneous fat or >6 mm depth). Nodal category definition is similar to other non-HPV-associated head and neck cancers; see Table 10.4 for clinical and pathologic nodal categories.

A second Brigham and Women's Hospital staging system has been proposed for SCC. This T-staging system was found to better discriminate prognosis of pts in internal cohort than AJCC staging system.[7]

TABLE 17.4: Brigham and Women's Hospital Staging System for Cutaneous Squamous Cell Carcinoma

		10-yr LR	High-Risk Factors
T1	0 High-risk factors	0.6%	Tumor ≥ 2 cm
T2a	1 High-risk factor	5%	Poor differentiation
T2b	2–3 High-risk factors	21%	PNI ≥ 0.1 mm
T3	≥ 4 High-risk factors	67%	Tumor beyond fat (bone invasion automatically T3)

TREATMENT PARADIGM: General treatment paradigm for early-stage low-risk lesions is surgical excision or alternative focal therapy. For high-risk lesions, or LN involvement, resection followed by adjuvant therapy where indicated.

Surgery: Surgical resection has two forms: wide local excision and Mohs surgery. Local excision is efficient as surgical procedure but involves resecting wider margin of tissue to achieve negative margin. Wide local excision is appropriate for small BCC and SCC in noncritical areas. Surgical margin (SM) should be 3 to 5 mm w/ BCC, 4 to 6 mm w/ SCC. Alternatively, Mohs surgery provides on-site margin assessment and is preferred for lesions located in critical areas for which larger surgery would be disfiguring. During surgery, horizontal layers of tissue are serially excised at oblique angle and systematically mapped w/ particular attention to peripheral and deep margins. Map of resection is typically created to guide this process, and location of positive margins during excision process is generated and can help inform planning of adjuvant RT. Goal of Mohs resection is to obtain negative margins with maximal sparing of normal tissue. Mohs surgery is associated with cure rates for BCC around 99% for primary and 95% for recurrent tumors.

Other local therapies: Local therapies are appropriate for small low-risk lesions: Cryotherapy with liquid nitrogen for two to three applications can be employed for low-risk lesions with cell kill resulting from hypertonic damage. Cryotherapy is both convenient and inexpensive but provides no histologic diagnosis, no margin assessment, and is associated with subsequent hypopigmentation. Curettage and electrodessication is similar to cryotherapy where tumor is scraped with curette and base electrodesiccated. Procedure is guided by "feel" of tumor versus dermis with the goal of achieving 3 to 4 mm margin on curetting. It may have superior cosmetic outcomes to cryotherapy, but is contraindicated in patients with pacemakers or other electronic implants and is not recommended in hair-bearing areas where feel of tumor versus normal tissue is more difficult due to hair follicles. Topical CHT: Active agents include 5-FU and cisplatin. Topical therapy is applied twice daily for 5 to 6, or sometimes up to 10 weeks depending upon clinical response. Topical 5-FU is often employed for preinvasive lesions including Bowen's disease, AKs, and cases of Gorlin's syndrome (basal cell nevus syndrome). Imiquimod is immune response modifier thought to promote apoptosis and/or stimulate release of tumoricidal mediated immunity factors from monocytes/macrophages. Cure rates are as high as 90% for low-risk BCC, but only 75% for nodular BCC.

Systemic therapy: For SCC, anti-EGFR therapy has shown good response rates in advanced or metastatic SCC. Phase II study of cetuximab in 36 pts with unresectable or metastatic SCC with EGFR expression revealed 69% disease control rate at 6 months.[8] Acneiform rash was associated with more prolonged response. Other active CHT agents include platinum agents and antimetabolite 5-FU. Limited data is presently available on efficacy of immunotherapy in SCC.[9]

For BCC, disruption of SHH pathway with vismodegib 150 mg daily is systemic therapy of choice. Open label STEVIE study of 499 pts with locally advanced (inoperable/multiply recurrent) or metastatic BCC demonstrated 66.7% overall response rate and 30.7%

complete response rate. 22% of pts developed serious AEs and 21 deaths (4.2%) were attributable to AEs.[10] Sonidegib (a second-generation SHH inhibitor) and itraconazole (anti-SHH signaling activity) have also both been employed in BCC.[11]

Radiation

Indications: RT is indicated as definitive therapy for unresectable, inoperable, or cosmetically unacceptable cases.[12] For lesions of eyelid, external ear, or nose, RT is often preferred. In adjuvant setting RT is employed for positive margins or positive LNs. In cases of PNI (particularly clinically symptomatic PNI), multiply recurrent tumor, or bone/cartilage invasion, consider treating entire nerves up to base of skull (BOS) and certainly if major named nerves are clinically/radiographically involved. Ipsilateral LNs should be treated in cases of parotid LN involvement, or N2/3 disease.[13] RT has advantages of being noninvasive, painless, and relatively less expensive than Mohs followed by reconstruction. RT cosmesis outcomes worsen with time and are increased with use of larger fx sizes.

Dose: ACR appropriateness criteria[14] recommend the following as curative regimens for nonmelanomatous skin cancer: 60–70 Gy/30–35 fx, 50–55 Gy/17–20 fx, 40–44 Gy/10 fx, 40 Gy/5 fxs (twice weekly), 30 Gy/3 fx (once weekly), or 20–25 Gy/1 fx. In areas where target volumes exist in close proximity to critical structures or cosmetically sensitive areas, more protracted RT courses are recommended. For adjuvant therapy to primary site, NCCN guidelines recommend 64–66 Gy/32–33 fx, 55 Gy/20 fx or others. For adjuvant therapy to lymph nodes, consider standard head and neck dosing schemes at 2 Gy/fx.

Toxicity: Acute: Fatigue, erythema, RT dermatitis, hypo/hyperpigmentation, alopecia/epilation, others location dependent. Late: Hypo/hyperpigmentation, fibrosis, ulceration, alopecia/epilation, lymphedema, others location dependent.

EVIDENCE-BASED Q&A

What are outcomes of definitive RT for BCC and SCC?

Locke, Washington University (*IJROBP* 2001, PMID 11697321): RR of 531 lesions (BCC-389, SCC-142) treated with superficial RT (60%), electrons (19%), combination (20%), or MV photons (<2%). At MFU of 5.8 yr, LC rates were marginally better for BCC than SCC in both primary (94% vs. 89%) and recurrent setting (86% vs. 68%). T4 tumors with cartilage and bone invasion had reduced LC: 75% and 67%, respectively. Outcomes for LN + pts were: LC of 81%, LN control of 86%, and 5-yr DFS of 53%. BCC of 1 to 5 cm had better LC with larger fx sizes (>2 Gy/fx). Cosmesis was good with 92% of pts experiencing excellent or good outcome.

Schulte, Germany (*J Am Acad Dermatol* 2005, PMID 16310060): RR of 1,113 pts treated with "soft" x-rays (<100 kVp) for epithelial skin cancers. MFU of 82 mos. Used 5 Gy/fx for most tumors, and two to three times weekly for outpatients; 6 days weekly for inpatients. Target dose was 45 Gy for BCC and 60 Gy for SCC—however, tx was continued until involution of tumor and subsequent ulceration was seen (often with cone down midway through tx), up to 85 Gy. Average total dose of 61 Gy for BCC and 63 Gy for SCC. LC was 95% for both; 6.3% soft-tissue necrosis; 83% healed w/ conservative tx. After 4 yrs of follow-up, rate of hypopigmentation was 91.8%, and telangiectasia incidence was 82.2%. Pts reporting "visual irritation" of their appearance was 12% for women and 4% for men.

Kwan, British Columbia (*IJROBP* 2004, PMID 15380573): RR of 182 pts (121 SCC and 61 BCC) treated with RT for primary or recurrent tumor. RT dose ranged from 35 Gy/7 fx, 45 Gy/10 fx, 55 Gy/20 fx, and 60 to 70 Gy in 30 to 35 fx. At MFU of 42 mos, 37 pts, all with SCC had died with 81% experiencing LF prior to distant failure (DF). LN failure was correlated with T stage: T2 (1/7, 14%), T3 (7/24, 29%), T4 (3/6, 50%). **Conclusion: Definitive RT can provide excellent LC with good cosmetic outcome.**

What is importance of clinical and microscopic PNI in SCC?

Garcia-Serra, University of Florida (*Head Neck* 2003, PMID 14648861): RR of 135 pts with PNI (microscopic in 59, clinical in 76) treated with surgery and RT or RT alone. 5-yr LC was 87% in cases of microscopic PNI and 55% in cases of clinical PNI. Positive SM on initial resection was present in 88% of cases experiencing LF.

Jackson, Australia (*Head Neck* 2009, PMID 19132719): RR of 118 pts with cutaneous H&N cancer with PNI treated with surgery and post-op RT (median dose 55 Gy). At MFU of 84 mos, 5-yr LC was 90% for microscopic PNI compared to 57% for pts with clinical/symptomatic PNI ($p < .0001$). DFS and OS were inferior for clinical PNI. **Conclusion: It is important to identify clinical PNI to determine risk of recurrence with treatment.**

Gluck, Michigan (*IJROBP* 2009, PMID 18938044): Patterns of failure study of 11 pts with cPNI tx with 3DCRT or IMRT who recurred. Most pts had single nerve involved initially, while all pts recurred with involvement of multiple nerves, indicating substantial cross communication between nerve branches of cranial nerve V and VII. **Conclusion: In cases of perineural involvement, it is crucial to cover involved nerve proximally to cavernous sinus.** For CN VII, cover nerve to brainstem and distally, skin innervated by nerve, major communicating branches, and compartment in which it is embedded/innervates (e.g., orbit for V1 or V2 involvement; masticator space for V3 involvement; parotid gland for VII involvement).

What studies have compared definitive RT to surgical resection?

Avril, Institut Gustave Roussy (*Br J Cancer* 1997, PMID 9218740): PRT of 347 pts with primary BCC of face <4 cm in maximal diameter randomized to Mohs resection versus definitive RT. RT techniques included Ir[192] brachytherapy to 65–70 Gy over 5 to 7 days (55%), contact therapy with two fractions of 18 to 20 Gy spaced 2 weeks apart (33%), and orthovoltage RT with 2 to 4 Gy per day to total dose of up to 60 Gy (12%). Mohs surgery was associated with significantly improved 4-yr failure rate of 0.7% versus 7.5%. Cosmetic results were good for 87% of surgical pts and 69% of RT pts. **Conclusion: Mohs surgery offers improved control and cosmesis of facial BCC compared to RT although comparison is not with electron or modern photon RT.**

What studies have defined worse prognosis of immunosuppressed SCC pts?

Manyam, Multi-Institution (*Cancer* 2017, PMID 28171708): Multi-institutional RR of 205 pts from three institutions investigating effect of immune status on disease outcomes in patients with primary or recurrent stage I-IV SCC of H&N who underwent surgery and received post-op RT between 1995 and 2015. 138 pts (67.3%) were immunocompetent and 67 (32.7%) were immunosuppressed (chronic hematologic malignancy, human immunodeficiency/acquired immunodeficiency syndrome, or had received immunosuppressive therapy for organ transplantation ≥6 months before diagnosis). Locoregional RFS (47.3% vs. 86.1%; $p < .0001$) and PFS (38.7% vs. 71.6%; $p = .002$) were significantly lower in immunosuppressed pts at 2 yrs. 2-yr OS rate in immunosuppressed pts demonstrated similar trend (60.9% vs. 78.1%; $p = .135$) but did not meet significance. On MVA, immunosuppressed status (HR 3.79; $p < .0001$), recurrent disease (HR 2.67; $p = .001$), poor differentiation (HR 2.08; $p = .006$), and PNI (HR 2.05; $p = .009$) were significantly associated with LRR. **Conclusion: Immunosuppression led to dramatically inferior outcomes compared with immunocompetent status, despite receiving bimodality therapy.**

Is there data suggesting alteration of specific immunosuppressive agents can prevent recurrent SCC?

mTOR inhibitors (sirolimus) improve outcomes in immunosuppressed pts compared to calcineurin inhibitors (tacrolimus, cyclosporine).

Euvrard, TUMORAPA (*NEJM* 2012, PMID 22830463): Multicenter PRT in kidney-transplant pts with hx of at least one SCC while on calcineurin inhibitors randomized to either same therapy (56 pts) versus switching to sirolimus (64 pts). Primary end point was survival free of SCC at 2 yrs. Secondary end points included time until onset of new SCC, occurrence of other skin tumors, graft function, and problems with sirolimus. Survival free of SCC was significantly longer in sirolimus group than in calcineurin-inhibitor group. Overall, new SCC developed in 14 pts (22%) in sirolimus group (six after withdrawal of sirolimus) and in 22 (39%) in calcineurin-inhibitor group (median time until onset, 15 vs. 7 mos, $p = .02$), with relative risk reduction in sirolimus group of 0.56 (95% CI: 0.32–0.98). There were 60 serious adverse events in sirolimus group, as compared with 14 such events in calcineurin-inhibitor group (average, 0.938 vs. 0.250). **Conclusion: Switching from calcineurin inhibitors to sirolimus had antitumoral effect among kidney-transplant pts with previous SCC. These observations may have implications concerning immunosuppressive treatment of pts with SCC.**

What is data supporting advantages of Mohs surgery over conventional excision?

Smeets, Netherlands (*Lancet* 2004, PMID 15541449): PRT of 612 BCCs (408 primary, 204 recurrent) of Mohs versus wide excision. Mohs trended to better 2-yr LC at 2% versus 3% for primary and 2% versus 8% for recurrent. Excision with worse cosmesis and more likely to have +margins (in 18% of primary and 32% of recurrent), especially with aggressive histology, high-risk location (except lips and preauricular), and recurrent tumor. **Conclusion: Mohs surgery may permit better cosmesis and reduce +margin rate for tumors in difficult locations or recurrent tumors.**

What data guides treatment of pts with node-positive SCC or those at risk of node-positive disease?

Veness, Australia (*Laryngoscope* 2005, PMID 15867656): RR of 167 pts with SCC with parotid or LN metastasis (50% parotid only) with 87% receiving adjuvant RT to median dose was 60 Gy/30 fx to dissected necks and 50 Gy to sites of subclinical disease. LF was 20% for treated versus 43% for untreated necks. Seventy-three percent of pts who experienced LF died of disease.

Moore, MDACC (*Laryngoscope* 2005, PMID 16148695): Prospective cohort evaluation of 193 pts with SCC in H&N skin cancer. 40 pts (21%) were found to have LN or parotid metastases at presentation. 37 of these pts received adjuvant RT to median dose of 60 Gy. Recurrent tumor, poorly differentiated histology, LVSI, inflammatory associated, and invasion beyond subcutaneous fat were all associated with nodal metastases. 37% of lesions >4 cm and 31% of lesions invading more than 8 mm were LN positive. **Conclusion: Pts with ipsilateral neck or parotid LN metastasis from SCC should receive adjuvant RT regardless of clinical nodal status.** Exception may be single node <3 cm without ECE/PNI. Pts with direct invasion of parotid, tumor >2 cm, PNI, or recurrence in tissue adjacent to parotid or immune compromise should be considered for LN dissection and may also benefit from adjuvant RT.

REFERENCES

1. Rogers HW, Weinstock MA, Feldman SR, Coldiron BM. Incidence estimate of nonmelanoma skin cancer (keratinocyte carcinomas) in U.S. population, 2012. *JAMA Dermatol.* 2015;151(10):1081–1086.
2. *AJCC Cancer Staging Manual, Eighth Edition.* 8th ed. New York, NY: Springer Publishing; 2017.
3. Thompson SC, Jolley D, Marks R. Reduction of solar keratoses by regular sunscreen use. *N Engl J Med.* 1993;329(16):1147–1151.
4. Green A, Williams G, Neale R, et al. Daily sunscreen application and betacarotene supplementation in prevention of basal-cell and squamous-cell carcinomas of skin: randomised controlled trial. *Lancet.* 1999;354(9180):723–729.
5. NCCN Clinical Practice Guidelines in Oncology: Basal Cell Skin Cancer. 2017; I.2017. https://www.nccn.org
6. NCCN Practice Clinical Guidelines in Oncology: Squamous Cell Skin Cancer. 2017; I.2017. https://www.nccn.org
7. Karia PS, Jambusaria-Pahlajani A, Harrington DP, et al. Evaluation of American Joint Committee on Cancer, International Union Against Cancer, and Brigham and Women's Hospital tumor staging for cutaneous squamous cell carcinoma. *J Clin Oncol.* 2014;32(4):327–334.
8. Maubec E, Petrow P, Scheer-Senyarich I, et al. Phase II study of cetuximab as first-line single-drug therapy in patients with unresectable squamous cell carcinoma of skin. *J Clin Oncol.* 2011;29(25):3419–3426.
9. Borradori L, Sutton B, Shayesteh P, Daniels GA. Rescue therapy with anti-programmed cell death protein 1 inhibitors of advanced cutaneous squamous cell carcinoma and basosquamous carcinoma: preliminary experience in five cases. *Br J Dermatol.* 2016;175(6):1382–1386.
10. Basset-Seguin N, Hauschild A, Grob JJ, et al. Vismodegib in patients with advanced basal cell carcinoma (STEVIE): pre-planned interim analysis of international, open-label trial. *Lancet Oncol.* 2015;16(6):729–736.
11. Dummer R, Guminski A, Gutzmer R, et al. 12-month analysis from basal cell carcinoma outcomes with LDE225 treatment (BOLT): phase II, randomized, double-blind study of sonidegib in patients with advanced basal cell carcinoma. *J Am Acad Dermatol.* 2016;75(1):113–125.e115.
12. Mendenhall WM, Amdur RJ, Hinerman RW, et al. RT for cutaneous squamous and basal cell carcinomas of head and neck. *Laryngoscope.* 2009;119(10):1994–1999.
13. Veness MJ, Morgan GJ, Palme CE, Gebski V. Surgery and adjuvant RT in patients with cutaneous head and neck squamous cell carcinoma metastatic to lymph nodes: combined treatment should be considered best practice. *Laryngoscope.* 2005;115(5):870–875.
14. Koyfman SA, Cooper JS, Beitler JJ, et al. ACR Appropriateness Criteria(®): aggressive nonmelanomatous skin cancer of head and neck. *Head Neck.* 2016;38(2):175–182.

18: MALIGNANT CUTANEOUS MELANOMA

Aditya Juloori and Nikhil P. Joshi

> **QUICK HIT:** Melanoma is increasing in incidence. Primary treatment is surgical excision with lymph node evaluation (sentinel lymph node biopsy [SLNB] with completion dissection if positive). Historically, adjuvant high-dose interferon was routinely recommended in pts with stage III disease. Adjuvant treatment is evolving in the immunotherapy era with ipilimumab used more commonly today. Role for adjuvant RT is controversial but may be considered in pts with multiple risk factors to improve local and/or regional control. Definitive RT can be used for lentigo maligna or lentigo maligna melanoma when surgery would be disfiguring.

TABLE 18.1: General Indications for Adjuvant RT of Malignant Melanoma After Resection

Primary site	Desmoplastic neurotrophic histology Ulceration Satellitosis Breslow >4 mm Positive margins Locally recurrent disease
Regional lymph nodes	ECE Multiple positive LNs (see trial by Burmeister et al; criteria vary by site) Size ≥3–4 cm

EPIDEMIOLOGY: Roughly 87,000 new diagnoses of melanoma and 9,700 melanoma-related deaths expected in 2017. Melanoma incidence has been rising for the past 30 years and risk increases with age (median age at diagnosis 63). In patients younger than 45, melanoma more commonly diagnosed in females—however by age 65, incidence of melanoma is twice as high in men compared to women. Melanoma is 20 times more common in Caucasians than African Americans.[1] Roughly 84% will present with localized disease, 9% with regional disease, and 4% with distant metastatic disease.[2]

RISK FACTORS: Fair skin, red/blond hair, high-density freckling, light eyes (green/hazel/blue); increased lifetime exposure to sunlight (natural or artificial), family history of melanoma or dysplastic nevi, immunosuppression (congenital or acquired). UVB (intermittent exposure/sunburn during early ages) is more significant risk factor than UVA (tanning beds, PUVA therapy). 10% of melanoma cases are familial with mutations in CDKN2A, CDK4, XP, BRCA2 genes.[1]

ANATOMY: Melanocyte is of neural crest in origin, migrating to basal layer of epidermis/hair follicle during development. Melanocytes are present in all areas of skin, eye, upper respiratory, GI and GU tracts. There are three layers of skin: epidermis, dermis, and subcutis. Epidermis is made up of three subsections, from superficial to deep—protective stratum corneum, keratinocytes (squamous cells), and basal layer, which contains basal cells which develop into keratinocytes. 5% to 10% of basal layer is also made up of melanocytes, which produce melanin and can develop into melanoma. Dermis layer contains sweat glands, vessels, lymphatics, pain/touch receptors, and hair follicles. It is also composed of collagen, which provides strength and resilience. Subcutis is the deepest layer and contains collagen and fat cells, which help to conserve body heat.

PATHOLOGY: Most common subtype of melanoma is superficial spreading, which makes up 70% of malignant melanoma cases.[3] These usually occur in trunk/extremities and are usually related to sun exposure. Nodular melanoma subtype makes up 15% to 30% of cases.[3] Lentigo maligna subtype commonly occurs in older patients in areas of skin with history of sun damage, commonly arises as macule, similar in appearance to freckle.[4] Least commonly occurring melanoma subtype is acral lentiginous melanoma, which makes up less than 5% of cases.[3] It is most common type among patients of Asian origin and in those with dark skin; this subtype most commonly arises in palms of hand and soles of feet. Mucosal melanoma is rare, and makes up approximately 1% of all melanoma cases.[5] These most commonly occur in head and neck, anorectum, vagina, and vulva.[6] V600 or BRAF mutation status can help guide systemic therapy.

SCREENING: Clinician skin exams may reduce risk of advanced melanoma, but no prospective randomized evidence exists to suggest decreased mortality/morbidity with clinical exams. USPSTF found insufficient evidence to recommend either for or against routine screening for general population. American Academy of Dermatology (AAD) recommends that those at high risk (strong family history of melanoma or personal history of multiple clinically atypical moles) undergo frequent self-examination with at least annual physician exam. In general ABCDE system is important for screening—asymmetry, border irregularities, color variegation (different colors in same region), diameter >6 mm, enlargement or evolution of color change, shape, or symptoms. Genetic counseling should be considered for those with strong family history.

WORKUP: H&P with thorough full body skin exam and thorough lymph node evaluation. 20% of clinically node-negative patients have metastatic involvement, while 20% of clinically node-positive patients are pathologically negative.

Pathology: Excisional biopsy of lesion with at least 1- to 3-mm margins. Alternatively can consider full-thickness punch or incisional biopsy depending on location of tumor (palm/sole, digit, face, ear) or for larger tumors. Shave biopsy can be used if clinical suspicion is low but may complicate depth assessment. Thus, per NCCN guidelines, sentinel lymph node biopsy is routinely recommended for patients with ≥0.75-mm thickness or those patients with <0.75-mm thickness but with ≥1 risk factor for nodal involvement—primary tumor ulceration, LVSI, or mitotic rate ≥1/mm².[7]

Imaging: Cross-sectional imaging (CT, PET, MRI brain) to rule out distant metastasis if symptoms or for stage III or higher disease, per NCCN (consideration for stage III with SLN+ and recommended for stage III with clinically positive node).[7]

PROGNOSTIC FACTORS: SLNB status is the most important predictor for local recurrence and DSS. ECE, number of lymph nodes, lymph node size, anatomic region, pathologic factures, margins are used to determine whether patient will benefit from adjuvant primary or nodal RT. Breslow thickness is more prognostic than Clark's level.

STAGING

N / T/N		cN0	cN1a	cN1b	cN1c	cN2a	cN2b	cN2c	cN3a	cN3b	cN3c
T1a	• <0.8 mm thick with no ulceration	IA									
T1b	• <0.8 mm thick with ulceration • 0.8–1.0 mm thick	IB					III				
T2a	• 1–2 mm with no ulceration	IB									
T2b	• 1–2 mm with ulceration	IIA									
T3a	• 2–4 mm with no ulceration	IIA									
T3b	• 2–4 mm with ulceration	IIB									
T4a	• >4 mm with no ulceration	IIB									
T4b	• >4 mm with ulceration	IIC									
M1a	• Skin, muscle, non-regional LN's						IV				
M1b	• Lung										
M1c	• Non-CNS visceral										
M1d	• CNS										

Major changes in 8th Edition include removal of mitotic rate in T-classification, use of T0 for unknown primary, clarification of "microscopic" which is now "clinically occult", stratification in N and M classifications among others.

cN1a, 1 clinically occult LN (detected by SLN biopsy); cN1b, 1 clinically detected LN; cN1c, negative regional LN, with in-transit, satellite or microsatellite metastasis; cN2a, 2–3 clinically occult LN; cN2b, 2–3 LN, at least one of which clinically detected; cN2c, 1 clinically occult or clinically detected LN with in-transit, satellite, or microsatellite metastasis; cN3a, ≥4 clinically occult LN; cN3b, ≥4 LN, at least one of which was clinically detected or presence of any number of matted nodes without in-transit, satellite, or microsatellite metastasis; cN3c, ≥2 clinically occult or clinically detected LN and/or presence of any number of matted nodes with presence of in-transit, satellite, or microsatellite metastasis.

TREATMENT PARADIGM

Surgery: Surgical excision is primary treatment for melanoma. Wide local excision is recommended, with margin requirement based on thickness of tumor. NCCN guidelines outline the following margin requirement based on findings from multiple randomized surgical trials, though these can be modified for individual anatomic or functional needs.

TABLE 18.3: NCCN Recommended Clinical Margins for Malignant Melanoma	
Tumor Thickness	**NCCN Recommended Clinical Margins**
In situ	0.5–1.0 cm
≤1.0 mm	1.0 cm
1–2 mm	1–2 cm
2.01–4 mm	2.0 cm
>4 mm	2.0 cm

Sentinel lymph node status is the most important prognostic factor for recurrence in patients with melanoma. SLNB is recommended for patients with ≥0.75 mm or those with <0.75-mm thickness with any high-risk feature (ulceration, LVSI, or mitotic rate greater than or equal to $1/mm^2$). Completion lymphadenectomy is recommended for patients with positive SLNB as ~18% of those with +SLN will have additional regional LN.[9,10] However, there has been no prospective evidence establishing impact of completion dissection on recurrence and survival for this population; this is being studied in MSLT-II trial. Lymph node dissection is also required for those with clinically node-positive patients (stage III). Adequate dissections require >10 LNs in groin, >15 LNs in axilla and neck.

Systemic therapy

Adjuvant: Multiple randomized trials have demonstrated improved DFS with use of adjuvant high-dose interferon for patients with high-risk melanoma after complete resection. High-dose IFNα continued for 1 year has historically been the standard of care for patients with resected node-positive melanoma (stage III) and should be considered for patients with negative nodes and increased risk of recurrence (stage IIB and IIC). Side effects include fatigue, headache, nausea, weight loss, myelosuppression, and depression. Role of immunotherapy in adjuvant setting is evolving. NCCN now has ipilimumab (see the following for details) use as category 1 treatment option in adjuvant setting after resection of clinical stage III disease, based on results of EORTC 18071, which demonstrated RFS benefit with use of adjuvant ipilimumab compared to placebo.[11]

Metastatic disease: In patients with metastatic disease, first-line treatment options include immunotherapy, BRAF-targeted therapy for those with targetable mutations, or enrollment on clinical trial. Ipilimumab—monoclonal antibody acts by blocking cytotoxic T-lymphocyte antigen-4 (CTLA-4) receptor present on T-lymphocytes. CTLA-4 downregulates T-cell activation and thus ipilimumab stimulates T-cell activity. Multiple PRTs have demonstrated improvement in OS in metastatic setting with use of this drug.[12,13]

Vemurafenib—specific inhibitor of V600 mutation of BRAF (seen in 40%–60% of advanced melanoma patients).[14–16] PRT demonstrated improved OS and PFS in patients with BRAF mutations compared to dacarbazine.[17,18] Dabrafenib and trametinib (MEK inhibitor) are also approved for use in BRAF-mutated metastatic melanoma.[19,20]

Pembrolizumab/Nivolumab are anti-PD-1 inhibitors with evolving use in melanoma. PD-1 receptor is inhibitory receptor present on activated T-cells. When checkpoint inhibitors like pembrolizumab/nivolumab are used, result is restoration of immune response with potential for antitumor activity. In multiple PRTs, pembrolizumab improves PFS in patients with metastatic disease compared to standard CHT[21] and improves OS compared to ipilimumab.[22] Nivolumab has been shown to improve PFS and OS compared with CHT[23]; it improves PFS compared to ipilimumab with lower toxicity.[24]

Radiation

Definitive: For lentigo maligna melanoma, definitive RT used when surgery would be disfiguring. No standard dose, but 50 Gy/20 fx using appropriate energy electrons is reasonable. For more deeply invasive tumors, data is sparse, though there have been reports of effective local control with much higher doses (100+ Gy) delivered with 60 kVp x-rays.

Adjuvant: Indications for treating primary tumor bed including melanomas with desmoplastic or neurotropic features, thick lesions (>4 mm) particularly if ulcerated or associated with satellitosis. Can also be used for +margins, but re-resection preferred. See Table 18.1. Indications for RT are stronger if multiple risk factors are present. Potential indications for treating regional LNs include: multiple positive LNs, ECE, lymph node size ≥3 to 4 cm, sentinel lymph node involvement but without complete or inadequate lymph node dissection and recurrent disease. NCCN suggests that patients who meet Burmeister criteria may be considered for adjuvant RT.

Dose: Most common dose/fx including 48 Gy/20 fx over 4 weeks (Burmeister) or 30 Gy/5 fx over 2.5 weeks (MDACC, Ang in the following).

Toxicity: Acute: fatigue, RT dermatitis, others location dependent. Late: fibrosis, hypo/hyperpigmentation, lymphedema, others location dependent.

EVIDENCE-BASED Q&A

Which patients benefit from adjuvant RT to regional nodal basin?

Even with adequate lymphadenectomy, recurrence in nodal basin can be relatively common and quite morbid, negatively impacting quality of life. This led to multiple prospective studies evaluating nodal RT.

Ang, MDACC (*IJROBP* 1994, PMID 7960981): Phase II study of 174 patients (and later 2003 updated RR).[25] Inclusion criteria (three groups of H&N pts): (a) elective RT after WLE of lesions >1.5-mm thick/Clark's level IV/V (b) adjuvant RT after WLE/LND with pN+ (stage II/III) (c) RT for nodal only relapse s/p nodal dissection. Treatment: adjuvant RT 30 Gy/5 fx over 2.5 weeks. MFU 78 mos. 10-yr local and locoregional control of 94% and 91%. **Conclusion: Hypofractionated RT (30 Gy/5 fx) is safe and effective for adjuvant treatment of melanoma with excellent 10-year LRC and rare toxicity.** Authors recommended adjuvant RT for ECE, LN ≥3 cm (in axilla or inguinal region), LN ≥2 cm (cervical), involvement of multiple lymph nodes (≥4 nodes in axilla or inguinal region, 2 or more if cervical), recurrent disease, or selective LND (rather than modified radical or radical LND).

Burmeister, ANZMTG 01.02/TROG 02.01 (*Lancet* 2012, PMID 22575589; Update *Lancet* 2015, PMID 26206146) PRT including 250 patients with clinically node-positive melanoma after LND with specific high-risk features: ≥1 parotid, ≥2 cervical or axillary or ≥3 groin nodes, extra nodal spread of tumor, maximum metastatic node diameter ≥3 cm in neck or ≥4 cm in groin/axilla. Randomization was to adjuvant RT 48 Gy/20 fx over 4 weeks or observation. Of note, if there were positive resection margins, dose used in study was 51 Gy/21 fx. Previous phase II study described the regional fields used in detail.[26] Patients in observation group who recurred received resection and RT at that time. At 6 years, lymph node field relapse significantly improved with RT (21% vs. 36%). OS and RFS not different between groups. There was 22% rate of grade 3 to 4 toxicity, mostly skin/subcutaneous. Constraints: cord ≤40 Gy, bowel/plexus/larynx ≤45 Gy, femoral neck, bowel V1000 cc ≤35 Gy. **Conclusion: Adjuvant nodal RT reduces nodal recurrence in select patients with high-risk features after nodal dissection.**

Comment: Trial was performed prior to systemic therapy/immunotherapy era (<5% received inter-feron).[27] *23 of 26 pts in observation group with regional failure in observation group underwent salvage surgery with similar 5-yr OS to overall cohort.*

Agrawal, Roswell Park/MDACC (*Cancer* 2009, PMID 19701906): Multi-institution RR of 615 patients with high-risk features after therapeutic LND who had been treated with or without RT. Largest published retrospective experience of adjuvant nodal RT. MFU 5 years. 5-yr regional control 81%. Nodal recurrence rate improved with adjuvant RT (10% vs. 40%). On MVA, number of positive lymph nodes and receipt of adjuvant RT predicted for better regional control. DSS significantly improved with adjuvant RT.

What should the field extent be for patients treated with axillary nodal RT?

In patients with axillary metastasis, limiting RT field to axillae rather than extending it to supr-aclavicular region provided equivalent local control rates, while extended field RT was associated with significantly higher rate of treatment-related complications.

Beadle, MDACC (*Cancer* 2009, PMID 18774657): RR of 200 pts with melanoma meta-static to axillary lymph node region who had high-risk features and received postopera-tive RT. High risk was defined as: LN ≥3 cm in size, ≥4 positive lymph nodes, presence of ECE, recurrent disease after initial resection. 48% of patients were treated to axilla only and 52% were treated to axilla and supraclavicular fossa. Patients were treated with 30 Gy/5 fx MDACC regimen. MFU 59 mos. 5-yr axillary control was 89% (axilla) versus 84%, no significant difference. OS, DSS, and DMFS were not significantly different. On MVA, extended field RT was associated with increased risk of complications. **Conclusion: Limiting RT field to axilla rather than extending to adjacent SCV nodal area provides equivalent control with decreased toxicity.**

Which patients need adjuvant RT to primary site?

The data for primary site RT is sparse. Certain risk factors associated with higher risk of local recurrence have been demonstrated in surgical series such as increased tumor thickness, ulceration, head and neck location, and desmoplastic/neurotropic features. Desmoplastic melanoma is rare subtype of melanoma which tends to be locally aggressive with increased chance of LR rather than distant or LN metastasis. It tends to spread along path of large named nerves (neurotropic), espe-cially in head and neck–region where wide surgical margins are difficult to achieve. Retrospective evidence from MDACC suggests that use of postoperative RT significantly reduces local recur-rence in patients with desmoplastic melanoma.[28] *TROG (TROG 08.09)/ANZ Melanoma Trials Group (ANZMTG 01.09) is randomized trial currently under way to prospectively determine impact of adjuvant RT in this population.*

What is role of sentinel lymph node biopsy in surgical management of melanoma?

Morton, Multi-Institutional Selective Lymphadenectomy (MSLT-I) Trial (*NEJM* 2014, PMID 24521106): 2,000 patients with clinically node-negative melanoma were rand-omized to SLNB or observation. Those with positive lymph node biopsy underwent com-pletion lymphadenectomy, while those with negative SLNB or in observation arm had therapeutic lymph node dissection at time of nodal recurrence. 16% of patients in SLNB arm had positive lymph node, 17% of patients in observation arm had eventual nodal recurrence. 10-year report demonstrated that in patients with intermediate (1.2–3.5 mm) or thick (>3.5 mm) tumors, melanoma-specific survival was significantly lower at 10 years in those with positive SLNB (intermediate: 62% vs. 85%; thick: 48% vs. 65.6%) compared to those who had negative biopsy. There was no difference in 10-year DSS between patients who underwent SLNB compared to those in observation arm. However, in patients with intermediate thickness tumors, those with positive SLNB did have improved survival compared to subgroup of those initially observed who later on developed nodal metastases. **Conclusion: SLNB is important staging and prognostic test for recurrence and DSS; however, there is no evidence that SLNB improves DSS.**

Can RT replace neck dissection?

Single-institution retrospective data from MDACC suggests that patients with stage I/II cutaneous melanoma who did not have SLNB or LND who went on to have subsequent adjuvant treatment with hypofractionated regional nodal RT had good outcomes (89% 5- and 10-yr actuarial regional control and 10-yr symptomatic complication rate of 6%).[29] This is not standard of care and is limited by retrospective analysis and selection bias.

Is adjuvant ipilimumab safe and effective?

Eggermont, EORTC 18071 (*Lancet* 2015, PMID 25840693): Prospective phase III randomized trial including 951 patients with stage III cutaneous melanoma (excluding lymph node metastasis ≤1 mm or in-transit metastasis) after complete surgical excision. Randomization to ipilimumab (10 mg/kg) every 3 weeks for four doses, then every 3 months for up to 3 years or placebo. MFU 2.74 years. RFS was 26.1 versus 17.1 mos ($p = .0013$). 52% of patients randomized to ipilimumab had discontinuation of therapy due to adverse events during initial four cycles. **Conclusion: Ipilimumab improves RFS in adjuvant setting though there is concern for toxicity profile. Further study needed to determine impact on OS and DMFS as well as comparison to interferon.**

When do we consider the use of definitive RT?

In general, RT alone is considered in patients with superficial lentigo maligna (confined to epidermis) and lentigo maligna melanoma (invasive into dermis). These patients are often elderly and can present with large superficial lesions on face; nonsurgical options can offer better function and cosmesis. Recurrence rates vary by series (as did RT technique), but pooled estimates suggest reasonable outcomes.

REFERENCES

1. American Cancer Society—Melanoma. 2017. http://old.cancer.org/cancer/analcancer/detailedguide/anal-cancer-what-is-anal-cancer, 2017.
2. Siegel RL, Miller KD, Jemal A. Cancer statistics, 2015. *CA Cancer J Clin.* 2015;65(1):5–29.
3. Wolff K, Goldsmith L, Katz S, et al. *Fitzpatrick's Dermatology in General Medicine.* 7th ed. New York, NY: McGraw-Hill; 2008:1134.
4. Clark WH, Jr., Mihm MC, Jr. Lentigo maligna and lentigo-maligna melanoma. *Am J Pathol.* 1969;55(1):39–67.
5. Chang AE, Karnell LH, Menck HR. The National Cancer Data Base report on cutaneous and noncutaneous melanoma: a summary of 84,836 cases from the past decade. The American College of Surgeons Commission on Cancer and the American Cancer Society. *Cancer.* 1998;83(8):1664–1678.
6. Mihajlovic M, Vlajkovic S, Jovanovic P, Stefanovic V. Primary mucosal melanomas: a comprehensive review. *Int J Clin Exp Pathol.* 2012;5(8):739–753.
7. NCCN Clinical Practice Guidelines in Oncology: Melanoma. 2017. https://www.nccn.org
8. Amin MB, Edge S, Greene F, et al. *AJCC Cancer Staging Manual,* 8th ed. New York, NY: Springer Publishing; 2017.
9. Cascinelli N, Bombardieri E, Bufalino R, et al. Sentinel and nonsentinel node status in Stage IB and II melanoma patients: two-step prognostic indicators of survival. *J Clin Oncol.* 2006;24(27):4464–4471.
10. Lee JH, Essner R, Torisu-Itakura H, Wanek L, et al. Factors predictive of tumor-positive nonsentinel lymph nodes after tumor-positive sentinel lymph node dissection for melanoma. *J Clin Oncol.* 2004;22(18):3677–3684.

11. Eggermont AM, Chiarion-Sileni V, Grob JJ, et al. Adjuvant ipilimumab versus placebo after complete resection of high-risk stage III melanoma (EORTC 18071): a randomised, double-blind, phase 3 trial. *Lancet Oncol.* 2015;16(5):522–530.

12. Hodi FS, O'Day SJ, McDermott DF, et al. Improved survival with ipilimumab in patients with metastatic melanoma. *N Engl J Med.* 2010;363(8):711–723.

13. Robert C, Thomas L, Bondarenko I, et al. Ipilimumab plus dacarbazine for previously untreated metastatic melanoma. *N Engl J Med.* 2011;364(26):2517–2526.

14. Wellbrock C, Hurlstone A. BRAF as therapeutic target in melanoma. *Biochem Pharmacol.* 2010;80(5):561–567.

15. Smalley KS, Sondak VK. Melanoma: an unlikely poster child for personalized cancer therapy. *N Engl J Med.* 2010;363(9):876–878.

16. Long GV, Menzies AM, Nagrial AM, et al. Prognostic and clinicopathologic associations of oncogenic BRAF in metastatic melanoma. *J Clin Oncol.* 2011;29(10):1239–1246.

17. Chapman PB, Hauschild A, Robert C, et al. Improved survival with vemurafenib in melanoma with BRAF V600E mutation. *N Engl J Med.* 2011;364(26):2507–2516.

18. McArthur GA, Chapman PB, Robert C, et al. Safety and efficacy of vemurafenib in BRAF(V600E) and BRAF(V600K) mutation-positive melanoma (BRIM-3): extended follow-up of a phase 3, randomised, open-label study. *Lancet Oncol.* 2014;15(3):323–332.

19. Robert C, Karaszewska B, Schachter J, et al. Improved overall survival in melanoma with combined dabrafenib and trametinib. *N Engl J Med.* 2015;372(1):30–39.

20. Long GV, Stroyakovskiy D, Gogas H, et al. Combined BRAF and MEK inhibition versus BRAF inhibition alone in melanoma. *N Engl J Med.* 2014;371(20):1877–1888.

21. Ribas A, Puzanov I, Dummer R, et al. Pembrolizumab versus investigator-choice chemotherapy for ipilimumab-refractory melanoma (KEYNOTE-002): a randomised, controlled, phase 2 trial. *Lancet Oncol.* 2015;16(8):908–918.

22. Robert C, Schachter J, Long GV, et al. Pembrolizumab versus ipilimumab in advanced melanoma. *N Engl J Med.* 2015;372(26):2521–2532.

23. Robert C, Long GV, Brady B, et al. Nivolumab in previously untreated melanoma without BRAF mutation. *N Engl J Med.* 2015;372(4):320–330.

24. Larkin J, Chiarion-Sileni V, Gonzalez R, et al. Combined nivolumab and ipilimumab or monotherapy in untreated melanoma. *N Engl J Med.* 2015;373(1):23–34.

25. Ballo MT, Bonnen MD, Garden AS, et al. Adjuvant irradiation for cervical lymph node metastases from melanoma. *Cancer.* 2003;97(7):1789–1796.

26. Burmeister BH, Mark Smithers B, Burmeister E, et al. A prospective phase II study of adjuvant postoperative radiation therapy following nodal surgery in malignant melanoma: Trans Tasman Radiation Oncology Group (TROG) Study 96.06. *Radiother Oncol.* 2006;81(2):136–142.

27. Brady MS. Adjuvant radiation for patients with melanoma. *Lancet Oncol.* 2015;16(9):1003–1004.

28. Guadagnolo BA, Prieto V, Weber R, et al. The role of adjuvant radiotherapy in the local management of desmoplastic melanoma. *Cancer.* 2014;120(9):1361–1368.

29. Bonnen MD, Ballo MT, Myers JN, et al. Elective radiotherapy provides regional control for patients with cutaneous melanoma of the head and neck. *Cancer.* 2004;100(2):383–389.

19: MERKEL CELL CARCINOMA

Matthew C. Ward and Nikhil P. Joshi

QUICK HIT: Merkel cell carcinoma (MCC): rare primary neuroendocrine malignancy of skin. MCC can be aggressive with rapid regional, in transit, marginal and distant recurrence. Management is primarily surgical with WLE + SLNB standard (depending on site and nodal drainage) followed by wide-field adjuvant RT. MCC is radiosensitive, and definitive RT is an option for unresectable lesions. In most cases, there is no clear role for systemic therapy except in metastatic setting, although investigations with PD-1 inhibitors are ongoing.

TABLE 19.1: Adjuvant RT Dosing for Postoperative Treatment of Merkel Cell Carcinoma[1]			
Primary Lesion		**Regional Lymph Nodes**	
Negative margins	50–56 Gy/25–28 fx	**Negative SLNB**	Observe (*unless accuracy of SLNB is in question, such as head and neck*)
Microscopic margins	56–60 Gy/28–30 fx	**Microscopic node-positive**	50–56 Gy (*or observation after full dissection with only one positive node*)
Gross residual or definitive RT	60–66 Gy/30–33 fx	**Extracapsular extension**	56–60 Gy

EPIDEMIOLOGY: Rare primary neuroendocrine malignancy of skin, incidence of 0.6 per 100,000.[2] Occurs mostly in older adults (average age 74–76) with fair skin. Male-to-female ratio approximately 2:1.

RISK FACTORS: Light skin, older age, UV exposure, immune suppression, organ transplant (x24 risk),[3] CLL, melanoma, myeloma.[4] Merkel cell polyomavirus is ubiquitous and can be detected in normal skin flora as well as other tumors, but clonal integration of viral DNA provides evidence of causal relationship.[5]

ANATOMY: Normal Merkel cells exist in basal epidermis and around hair follicles and act as mechanoreceptors. Merkel cell carcinoma is most common in sun-exposed areas (42.6% head and neck, 23.6% upper limb, 15.3% lower limb per NCDB).[6]

PATHOLOGY: Small round blue cell tumor of uncertain origin. Merkel cell polyomavirus detected in >80% of MCC.[7,8] Theories of origin include sensory cells in skin mechanoreceptors or skin stem cells that undergo malignant differentiation.[9,10] Three subtypes exist (small cell type, trabecular type, and intermediate type) but these are not thought to be prognostic.

CLINICAL PRESENTATION: MCCs typically present as firm, painless, rapidly growing, single red or purple cutaneous dome-shaped nodule. 65% present with localized disease.[6]

WORKUP: H&P including physical exam of area and total skin, investigation for skip lesions, and regional nodal examination. Biopsy of primary lesion. PET/CT recommended for regional and distant staging (rule out small cell of lung). MRI with contrast of primary tumor as clinically indicated to assess for deep/adjacent structure invasion. MRI brain recommended for clinical suspicion (not required in all cases). Sentinel node biopsy is generally recommended. Differential includes other small round blue cell tumors such as small cell of lung, Ewing's sarcoma, etc. Immunostaining includes CK20 and cytokeratin (typically positive) as well as TTF1 and CK7 (negative in Merkel cell, positive in small cell carcinoma of lung).

PROGNOSTIC FACTORS: Presence of nodal disease is the most important prognostic factor. Merkel cell virus antigen expression and presence of tumor-infiltrating lymphocytes[11] are associated with favorable prognosis. LVSI, large tumor size, infiltrating pattern, deep invasion, extracapsular extension, and older age are associated with unfavorable prognosis.[12] Anti-VP1 (Merkel polyomavirus) antibody titer >10,000 copies are associated with favorable prognosis.[13]

NATURAL HISTORY: Local and nodal failure is common. Recurrences can occur early (start RT early if concerned), with median time to recurrence of 9 months.[14] Nodal failure is the most common site of first failure (55% of failures), followed by distant (29% of failures), local (15% of failures), and in transit (9% of failures).[14]

STAGING

TABLE 19.2: AJCC 8th ed. (2017) Staging for Merkel Cell Carcinoma[6]									
T/M \ N		cN0	cN1	pN1a(sn)	pN1a	pN1b	c/pN2	c/pN3
T1	• ≤2 cm	I							
T2	• 2.1–5 cm	IIA		IIIA			IIIB		
T3	• >5 cm								
T4	• Invasion[1]	IIB							
M1a	• Distant skin • Subcutaneous tissue • Distant LN			IV					
M1b	• Lung								
M1c	• Any other visceral sites								

Major changes in the AJCC 8th Edition include delineation between clinical & pathologic N categories, new N2-N3 categories and updates to the prognostic staging groups.

Notes: Invasion[1] = Invasion into fascia, cartilage, bone, or muscle.

cN1, metastasis in regional LN(s); pN1a(sn), clinically occult regional LN identified by sentinel lymph node biopsy only; pN1a, clinically occult regional LN following lymph node dissection; pN1b, clinically and/or radiologically detected regional LN with microscopic confirmation; c/pN2, in-transit metastasis (discontinuous from primary tumor, located between primary tumor and draining lymph node basin), without LN metastasis; c/pN3, in-transit metastasis with LN metastasis.

TREATMENT PARADIGM

Surgery: Surgery is the mainstay of therapy for locoregionally confined MCC. For clinically node-negative patients, perform wide local excision with 1- to 2-cm margins (or Mohs in cosmetically sensitive areas) with sentinel lymph node biopsy (SLNB controversial in head & neck locations). If lymph nodes are clinically positive, either regional lymph node dissection should be performed or biopsy should be obtained (FNA appropriate) with subsequent regional nodal RT (see RT in the following). If surgery to primary would be disfiguring or otherwise morbid, definitive RT may be appropriate (see RT in the following).

Chemotherapy: Although CHT is highly effective for small cell carcinoma of lung, for MCC, there is no clear role for concurrent or adjuvant CHT for locoregionally confined disease. The most common regimen used is either cisplatin/etoposide or carboplatin/etoposide. There is no clear data for benefit to concurrent chemoRT although phase II data does exist with concurrent cisplatin/etoposide.[15] In metastatic setting, phase II data suggests response rates of >50% to PD-1 or PD-L1 (avelumab) inhibition.[16–18]

Radiation

Indications: Limited evidence available suggests that RT reduces locoregional recurrence. Risk factors, which some consider indications for PORT after definitive surgery, include LVSI, immune suppression, positive margins (further resection not possible).[1,19] PORT should be initiated without delay (approximately 4 weeks) as rapid recurrences can occur. For small tumors (<1 cm) without risk factors, observation may be reasonable. Regional nodal RT is indicated for SLNB-positive patients, but if full node dissection is performed and there are no adverse features (multiple nodes positive or ECE), consider observation. After negative SLNB, it is reasonable to observe regional nodes unless patient is at high risk for false-negative SLNB.

Dose: For margin-negative resection, consider 50–56 Gy/25–28 fx. For microscopically positive margins, consider 56 to 60 Gy. For gross residual disease or for definitive treatment, consider 60 to 66 Gy. For microscopically positive nodal disease (+SLNB or node dissection), consider 50 to 56 Gy to regional nodes. Consider up to 60 Gy to regional nodes for extracapsular extension.

Toxicity: Acute: skin erythema, fatigue, others based on location of treatment. Late: lymphedema, fibrosis, others as indicated by location.

Procedure: See *Treatment Planning Handbook*, Chapter 4.[20]

EVIDENCE-BASED Q&A

Does RT improve survival for early-stage MCC?

Mojica, SEER (*JCO* 2007, PMID 17369567): SEER analysis of 1,665 pts with Merkel cell investigating role of adjuvant RT. 89% were treated with surgery and 40% of these with adjuvant RT. Adjuvant RT was associated with improved OS (MS 63 vs. 45 months, $p = .0002$). This association was true for all primary tumor sizes, but particularly those over 2 cm. *Comment: Did not use propensity matching methods, only Cox multivariate to adjust for confounders and did not investigate MCC-specific survival.*

Kim, SEER (*JAMA* Dermatol 2013, PMID 23864085): SEER analysis of 747 pts (eliminated pts with survival <4 months arguing this biased the Mojica analysis). Performed propensity-matched analysis comparing surgery alone to surgery with adjuvant RT. Age and stage correlated with OS and MCC-specific survival. Matched analysis demonstrated improved OS but not MCC-specific survival in group receiving adjuvant RT. **Conclusion: Survival differences observed in adjuvant RT group are related to selection bias.** *Comment Analysis may be underpowered.*

Bhatia, NCDB (*JNCI* 2016, PMID 2725173): NCDB analysis of 6,908 pts with stage I-III MCC investigating role of adjuvant RT. After adjustment, adjuvant RT was associated with improved OS in stage I-II MCC but not in stage III pts (HRs stage I 0.71, $p < .001$;

stage II HR 0.77 p < .001; stage III HR 0.98, p = .80). Less than 5% of stage I, ~10% of stage II, and 29% of stage III pts received CHT. CHT was not associated with improved OS in any stage. **Conclusion: Adjuvant RT is associated with improved OS in stage I-II MCC.**

Vargo, NCDB Re-analysis (*JNCI* 2016, PMID 28423400): Extended Bhatia NCDB analysis to include variables previously omitted including type of primary surgery. Also performed propensity matching, which confirmed association with RT and improved OS (HR 0.76, p<0.001). Best OS was demonstrated in WLE plus RT group. **Conclusion: Adjuvant RT remains associated with improved OS.**

Is RT to lymph nodes indicated in stage I patients?

In pre-SLNB and pre-PET/CT era, RT improved nodal recurrence rates. In modern era, omission of nodal RT is recommended for patients with negative SLNB. For patients with positive SLNB but no nodal dissection, RT is recommended. For patients with complete nodal dissection, RT is recommended for multiple positive nodes or ECE.[1]

Jouary, France (*Ann Oncol* 2012, PMID 21750118): PRT (first PRT in Merkel cell) from 1993 to 2005 including patients with stage I Merkel carcinoma. Pts were treated with WLE and RT to primary tumor bed, then randomized to observation of regional nodes versus prophylactic RT. Notably excluded pts with unclear nodal drainage (median head and trunk), immune suppression, and for delay in RT initiation over 6 weeks. RT consisted of 50 Gy to primary bed and nodal region (if randomized to nodal RT) with 3-cm margin. Powered to detect 20% gain in OS (N = 105). Study stopped early after 83 pts accrued as SLNB became common in France and this was not permitted on protocol. No difference in OS. Regional recurrence 16.7% versus 0% favoring nodal RT (p = .007). PFS 89.7% versus 81.2% favoring nodal RT (p = .4). **Conclusion: In pre-SLNB, pre-PET/CT era, nodal RT improved rate of nodal recurrence but trial did not accrue sufficiently to detect impact on OS.**

What is optimal dose for definitive treatment of MCC?

Retrospective evidence suggests that doses >50 Gy are necessary to achieve locoregional control.[21] NCDB supports dose ranging from 50 to 55 Gy, although selection bias may factor into higher doses above 55 Gy.[22] Furthermore, impressive results have been observed in metastatic setting from 8 Gy/1 fx, with complete response rates of up to 45%.[23] This suggests that there may be immune–system interaction. Further work is ongoing.

What treatment margins should be used around tumor bed?

Given proclivity for in-transit recurrences and lymphovascular spread, wide margins of 3 to 4 cm are generally recommended.[21] Treat regional lymphatics in continuity (same field) with primary lesion if tolerable (the TROG 9607 trial defined "tolerable" as less than 20 cm with cone down).[15]

Is there benefit to addition of concurrent CHT with RT?

Concurrent chemoRT has been studied but is not standard given good responses seen with RT alone and of unclear benefit with CHT.

Poulsen, TROG 9607 (*JCO* 2003, PMID 14645427): Single-arm phase II of 53 nonmetastatic Merkel cell carcinoma pts with either high-risk postoperative (gross residual, tumor >1 cm, involved nodes), occult primary with positive nodes or recurrent disease. 28% were treated definitively, 72% adjuvantly. Pts treated to 50 Gy/25 fx. 45 Gy with boost to 50 Gy (shrinking field) was possible for large fields and 45 Gy alone was recommended if 50 Gy was felt to be intolerable. Four cycles of concurrent and adjuvant carboplatin AUC 4.5 and etoposide (80 mg/m^2/day for 3 days) were delivered on weeks 1, 4, 7, and 10. 3-yr

OS, LRC, and DC were 76%, 75%, and 76%, respectively. Tumor location and presence of nodes were associated with LC and OS. **Conclusion: High levels of LC and OS were achieved compared to historical controls; further study is warranted.**

REFERENCES

1. NCCN Clinical Practice Guidelines in Oncology: Merkel Cell Carcinoma. 2017; https://www.nccn.org

2. Albores-Saavedra J, Batich K, Chable-Montero F, et al. Merkel cell carcinoma demographics, morphology, and survival based on 3870 cases: a population-based study. *J Cutan Pathol.* 2010;37(1):20–27.

3. Clarke CA, Robbins HA, Tatalovich Z, et al. Risk of Merkel cell carcinoma after solid organ transplantation. *J Natl Cancer Inst.* 2015;107(2). doi:10.1093/jnci/dju382

4. Howard RA, Dores GM, Curtis RE, et al. Merkel cell carcinoma and multiple primary cancers. *Cancer Epidemiol Biomarkers Prev.* 2006;15(8):1545–1549.

5. Feng H, Shuda M, Chang Y, Moore PS. Clonal integration of a polyomavirus in human Merkel cell carcinoma. *Science.* 2008;319(5866):1096–1100.

6. Harms KL, Healy MA, Nghiem P, et al. Analysis of prognostic factors from 9387 Merkel cell carcinoma cases forms the basis for the new 8th Edition AJCC staging system. *Ann Surg Oncol.* 2016;23(11):3564–3571.

7. Santos-Juanes J, Fernández-Vega I, Fuentes N, et al. Merkel cell carcinoma and Merkel cell polyomavirus: a systematic review and meta-analysis. *Br J Dermatol.* 2015;173(1):42–49.

8. Rodig SJ, Cheng J, Wardzala J, et al. Improved detection suggests all Merkel cell carcinomas harbor Merkel polyomavirus. *J Clin Invest.* 2012;122(12):4645–4653.

9. Tilling T, Moll I. Which are the cells of origin in Merkel cell carcinoma? *J Skin Cancer.* 2012;2012:680410. doi:10.1155/2012/680410

10. Ratner D, Nelson BR, Brown MD, Johnson TM. Merkel cell carcinoma. *J Am Acad Dermatol.* 1993;29(2 Pt 1):143–156.

11. Paulson KG, Iyer JG, Tegeder AR, et al. Transcriptome-wide studies of Merkel cell carcinoma and validation of intratumoral CD8+ lymphocyte invasion as an independent predictor of survival. *J Clin Oncol.* 2011;29(12):1539–1546.

12. Sihto H, Kukko H, Koljonen V, et al. Merkel cell polyomavirus infection, large T antigen, retinoblastoma protein and outcome in Merkel cell carcinoma. *Clin Cancer Res.* 2011;17(14):4806–4813.

13. Touzé A, Le Bidre E, Laude H, et al. High levels of antibodies against Merkel cell polyomavirus identify a subset of patients with Merkel cell carcinoma with better clinical outcome. *J Clin Oncol.* 2011;29(12):1612–1619.

14. Allen PJ, Bowne WB, Jaques DP, et al. Merkel cell carcinoma: prognosis and treatment of patients from a single institution. *J Clin Oncol.* 2005;23(10):2300–2309.

15. Poulsen M, Rischin D, Walpole E, et al. High-risk Merkel cell carcinoma of the skin treated with synchronous carboplatin/etoposide and radiation: a Trans-Tasman Radiation Oncology Group Study–TROG 96:07. *J Clin Oncol.* 2003;21(23):4371–4376.

16. Winkler JK, Bender C, Kratochwil C, et al. PD-1 blockade: a therapeutic option for treatment of metastatic Merkel cell carcinoma. *Br J Dermatol.* 2017;176(1):216–219.

17. Nghiem PT, Bhatia S, Lipson EJ, et al. PD-1 Blockade with pembrolizumab in advanced Merkel-cell carcinoma. *N Engl J Med.* 2016;374(26):2542–2552.

18. Kaufman HL, Russell J, Hamid O, et al. Avelumab in patients with chemotherapy-refractory metastatic Merkel cell carcinoma: a multicentre, single-group, open-label, phase 2 trial. *Lancet Oncol.* 2016;17(10):1374–1385.

19. Decker RH, Wilson LD. Role of radiotherapy in the management of Merkel cell carcinoma of the skin. *J Natl Compr Canc Netw.* 2006;4(7):713–718.

20. Videtic GMM, Woody N, Vassil AD. *Handbook of Treatment Planning in Radiation Oncology.* 2nd ed. New York, NY: Demos Medical; 2015.

21. Veness M, Foote M, Gebski V, Poulsen M. The role of radiotherapy alone in patients with Merkel cell carcinoma: reporting the Australian experience of 43 patients. *Int J Radiat Oncol Biol Phys.* 2010;78(3):703–709.
22. Patel SA, Qureshi MM, Mak KS, et al. Impact of total radiotherapy dose on survival for head and neck Merkel cell carcinoma after resection. *Head Neck.* 2017;39(7):1371–1377.
23. Iyer JG, Parvathaneni U, Gooley T, et al. Single-fraction radiation therapy in patients with metastatic Merkel cell carcinoma. *Cancer Med.* 2015;4(8):1161–1170.

20: MYCOSIS FUNGOIDES

Vamsi Varra, Matthew C. Ward, and Gregory M. M. Videtic

> **QUICK HIT:** Mycosis fungoides (MF): most *common* cutaneous lymphoma in the United States and originates from the T cell. Final diagnosis often revealed by skin biopsies since it is often confused with other entities. Appropriate imaging and lymph node biopsies are utilized to evaluate for extracutaneous disease. Treatments tend to be localized (skin-directed therapy, phototherapy, and localized superficial irradiation) for early stages of disease and systemic for more advanced or refractory disease.

TABLE 20.1: General Treatment Paradigm for Mycosis Fungoides[1]	
Stage I	Observation, skin-directed therapy, phototherapy, TSEBT
Stage II	Observation, skin-directed therapy, phototherapy, TSEBT, interferon alpha
Stage III	TSEBT, photophoresis, interferon alpha, phototherapy, methotrexate
Stage IV	CHT, TSEBT, oral bexarotene, interferon alpha, vorinostat, romidepsin, low dose methotrexate, clinical trials

EPIDEMIOLOGY: In America and Europe, six cases of mycosis fungoides are diagnosed annually per million people. Disease accounts for approximately 4% of all non-Hodgkin's lymphoma diagnoses. It affects men almost twice as often as women and has higher prevalence in Black population.[2] Median age at diagnosis is 55 to 60.[3]

RISK FACTORS: Risk factors for MF are unclear. Although human T-lymphotropic virus type 1 (HTLV1) has been found in skin lesions of pts with mycosis fungoides, there are also studies providing evidence against role of HTLV1 as risk factor.[4]

ANATOMY: Although lesions can present anywhere on the body, they are most commonly seen over a truncal distribution.[5] In rare cases, malignant T cells can be found in peripheral blood and in advanced stages, disease may present in regional or distant lymph nodes, or other organ systems, most commonly including lungs, oral cavity, pharynx, or central nervous system.[3,6]

PATHOLOGY: Pathogenesis of MF is currently unclear. On histology, skin biopsies show Pautrier's abscesses (pathognomonic, present in 38% of cases), haloed lymphocytes, exocytosis, disproportionate epidermotropism, epidermal lymphocytes larger than dermal lymphocytes, hyperconvoluted intraepidermal lymphocytes, and lymphocytes aligned within basal layer.[7] Disease can also present with circulating malignant T cells (Sézary cells) that usually possess CD4+/CD7- or CD4+/CD26- immunophenotype.[8]

CLINICAL PRESENTATION: Typical clinical presentation of MF is preceded by a premycotic period, defined by nonspecific, slightly scaling lesions, accompanied by nondiagnostic skin biopsies. As deposition of malignant T cells becomes more persistent, disease presents with heterogeneous patches that may evolve into plaques, and then finally cutaneous tumors. MF commonly presents with debilitating pruritus.[9]

WORKUP: H&P including percentage of body surface area affected by patches, plaques, or tumor lesions. Laboratory studies should include CBC, CMP, LFTs, and serum LDH, as well as evaluation for Sézary cells (PCR/flow cytometry). Skin biopsies should be taken from at least two sites, and should be assessed with H&E staining, immunostaining for surface marker expression profiles, and PCR for clonal TCR rearrangement. If only one biopsy can be obtained, lesion with greatest induration should be chosen.[8] Chest x-ray or nodal ultrasound is sufficient for pts with early-stage disease. However, CT scan of chest, abdomen, and pelvis, or whole-body integrated PET/CT should be performed for pts with T2b disease or greater in order to rule out any lymphadenopathy or visceral involvement.[10]

PROGNOSTIC FACTORS: Current standard for staging MF utilizes TNMB system proposed by ISCL/EORTC. Specific prognostic factors for poor outcomes are presence of cutaneous plaques as opposed to patches, lymph node involvement, and peripheral blood T-cell clones in pts with less than 5% Sézary cells detected.[11]

More specifically, pts with limited patches, papules, and/or plaques that cover <10% of the skin are classified as T1. Pts with lesions covering ≥10% of the skin surface are classified T2. If ≥1 tumor ≥1 cm in diameter, classified as T3. If with erythema covering ≥80% of the body surface, classified as T4.[8]

Pts without clinically abnormal peripheral lymph nodes are N0. Disease with clinically abnormal peripheral lymph nodes with a histopathology Dutch grade of 1 or NCI LN0-2 are N1. Nodal disease with a histopathology Dutch grade of 2 or NCI LN3 are N2. Nodal disease with a histopathology Dutch grade of 3–4 or NCI LN4 are N3. Clinically abnormal peripheral lymph nodes without histologic confirmation are NX.[8]

Pts without visceral organ involvement are classified as M0 and with visceral organ involvement are M1.

A peripheral blood involvement classification of B0 is defined by absence of significant blood involvement (≤5% of peripheral blood lymphocytes as atypical Sézary cells). B1 disease is defined by a low blood-tumor burden: >5% of peripheral blood lymphocytes as Sézary cells, but still less than the B2 criteria, which is greater than 1,000 Sézary cells/μL with positive clone.[8]

Note that N1a/b, N2a/b, B0a/b, B1a/b subclassifications are defined but not included here for brevity, and can be found in the original definition by Olsen et al.[8] Grouped stage provided in Table 20.2.

TABLE 20.2: TNMB Clinical Staging System[8]				
N T/B/M	N0	N1	N2	N3
T1	IA	IIA		IVA2
T2	IB			
T3	IIB			
T4	IIIA (if B0) or IIIB (if B1)			
B2	IVA1			
M1	IVB			

TREATMENT PARADIGM

Observation: Expectant observation is recommended for informed pts with stage 1A disease, but requires attentive monitoring and proper patient education.[1]

Medical: Various skin-directed therapies should be considered as first-line treatment in early disease and supplemental treatment in more advanced disease. Preferred initial skin-directed therapies are topical corticosteroids, topical nitrogen mustard (e.g., carmustine) and topical retinoids.[1] Pruritus is highly prevalent in pts with MF and should be treated according to general guidelines for managing pruritus.

Surgery: There is no clear role for surgical resection in MF.

Chemotherapy: Although skin-directed therapies should be attempted initially in pts with early disease, CHT should be considered early in pts with extensive, advanced, or refractory disease. Common CHT regimens include low dose methotrexate, pegylated liposomal doxorubicin, gemcitabine, pralatrexate, fludarabine with cyclophosphamides, fludarabine with interferon alpha, CHOP (cyclophosphamide, doxorubicin, vincristine, and prednisolone), and EPOCH (etoposide, vincristine, doxorubicin, cyclophosphamide, and prednisolone).[12] Other systemic therapies include retinoids and histone deacetylase inhibitors.[1]

Radiation: Localized RT is indicated for pts with stage IA disease presenting with one to three lesions that are in close enough proximity to be targeted by single or abutting RT fields.[13] It is also indicated as palliative treatment for pts with advanced disease. Photons as well as electron beam may be used. Local superficial irradiation for curative treatment of unilesional stage IA disease should be dosed at least 20 to 30 Gy at 2 Gy per fraction with five fractions per week, and palliative treatment for advanced disease can be dosed at 8 to 20 Gy given in one to five fractions.[14,15] Adverse effects include mild dermatitis, local alopecia, and pigmentation changes.[13]

TSEBT: In total skin electron beam therapy (TSEBT), electrons are calibrated to penetrate skin to limited depth, targeting epidermis, adnexal structures, and dermis. It can be considered in all stages of disease. Historically treatment dosed to 26–36 Gy to 4- to 6-mm depth (surface dose 31–36 Gy), given in 30 to 36 treatments (2 days per fraction) over 9 weeks, 4 days per week. Recent evidence suggests short course of 12 Gy may be effective, for shorter duration of control. During treatment, some of symptoms of MF, such as pruritus and cutaneous erythema, may be exacerbated. In addition, alopecia, temporary nail stasis, peripheral edema, epistaxis, blisters to fingers and feet, anhidrosis, parotiditis, gynecomastia, corneal tears, chronic nail dystrophy, chronic xerosis, and fingertip dysesthesias may occur.[16] For technical details regarding both local superficial irradiation and TSEBT, see *Treatment Planning Handbook*, Chapter 10.[17]

Other modalities: Phototherapy may be used in treatment of MF, including ultraviolet B (UVB) and psoralen plus ultraviolet photo-CHT (PUVA). More recently, treatments also include UVA1 and excimer laser.[18] In case of MF that is refractory to other modalities, transplantation of allogenic hematopoietic stem cells may be considered.[19]

EVIDENCE-BASED Q&A

Do patients benefit from early aggressive therapy?

While CR is higher in those undergoing aggressive therapy with TSEBT and CHT, there is no benefit in DFS or OS with significantly increased toxicity rate.

Kaye (*NEJM* 1989, PMID 2594037): RCT of 103 PTS w/ MF randomized to 30 Gy TSEBT w/ CHT (cyclophosphamide, doxorubicin, etoposide, and vincristine) or sequential topical treatment. Higher rate of CR in pts treated w/ combination therapy (38% vs. 18%, p = .032) but no difference in DFS or OS after 75 months of FU. Increased toxicity in combination therapy group including hospitalization for fever/neutropenia, and CHF. **Conclusion: Early aggressive therapy with RT and CHT does not improve prognosis for pts with MF as compared with conservative treatment beginning with sequential topical therapies.**

What dose should be used for localized disease?

When using standard fractionation, dose of 20 to 30 Gy is necessary for durable response/control. However, recently, doses as low as 7 Gy have been shown to be effective.

Cotter (*IJROBP* 1983, PMID 6195138): RR of 110 lesions from 14 pts with MF who underwent RT with Co-60 or electors. Doses ranged from 6 to 40 Gy. 53% of lesions were plaques, 20% were tumors ≤3 cm in diameter, 27% were tumors >3 cm in diameter. CR in 95% of plaques, 95% of tumors ≤3 cm, and 93% in tumors >3 cm in diameter. CR in all tumors receiving >20 Gy. In lesions having CR, 42% had infield recurrence if they received <10 Gy, 32% for 10 to 20 Gy, 21% for 20 to 30 Gy, and 0% for >30 Gy with mean time to first recurrence 5 months, 10 months, and 16 months respectively for each dose range. 83% of 30 recurrences were within 1 year while 100% were within 2 years of treatment. **Conclusion: Tumor doses equivalent to at least 30 Gy at 2 Gy per fraction, five fractions per week (TDF greater than or equal to 49) are suggested for adequate local control of cutaneous mycosis fungoides lesions.**

Thomas, Northwestern University (*IJROBP* 2013, PMID 22818412): RR of 270 pts treated with single fraction RT dosed to 7 Gy or more. MFU 41.3 mos. CR in 94.4% of pts, PR in 3.7%, conversion to CR after second treatment in 1.5%, and no response in 0.4%. Problem with localized RT is that new lesions can develop outside of field. **Conclusion: Single fraction of 7 to 8 Gy is sufficient to provide palliation for CTCL lesions.**

Wilson, Yale (*IJROBP* 1998, PMID 9422565): RR of 21 pts with 32 lesions receiving curative local superficial RT for stage IA MF. 9 pts received prior focal therapy (steroids, PUVA, BCNU, UVB) and 6 received adjuvant therapy after local RT (PUVA, steroids). Median FU was 36 months. Median surface dose was 20 Gy (6–40 Gy) with median fraction number of 5. For fields receiving >20 Gy, median fraction number was 10. CR was 97% overall with one pt having PR, treated with 6 Gy. 3 pts had LR at 52 months (8 Gy), 16 months (20 Gy), and 4 months (20 Gy). 10-year DFS of 91% for those receiving ≥20 Gy with 91% LC. **Conclusion: Pts should be offered choice of LSR alone, without adjuvant therapies, to dose of 20 Gy or greater with minimum margin of 1 to 2 cm around target.**

What dose should be used for TSEBT?

TSEBT is conventionally dosed to at least 30 Gy, yielding greater CR rates and lower rates of disease recurrence. However, recent phase II studies suggest 12 Gy can provide rapid reduction of disease burden for a sustained period of time and reduce toxicity.

Hoppe (*IJROBP* 1977, PMID 591404): 176 pts with MF treated with TSEBT at Stanford University from 1958 to 1975 with varying doses. CR rates increased with decreased skin involvement, ranging from 86% in limited plaques to 44% in tumors. Survival also related to extent of disease with 10-year OS of 76%, 44%, and 6% in those with limited plaques, generalized plaques, and tumors respectively. Stage also correlated with survival, exemplified by 5-year OS of 80% and 51% for stage I and II pts respectively, along with lack of stage III/IV long-term survivors. CR was directly related to initial dose of TSEBT with 18% CR for 8 to 9.9 Gy, 55% for 10 to 19.9 Gy, 66% for 20 to 24.9 Gy, 75% for 25 to 29.9 Gy, and 94% for 30 to 36 Gy. 39% (20 pts) of 51 who had CR after TSEBT >30 Gy remained without disease 3 to 14 years after completion. **Conclusion: Pts with total TSEBT dose of at least 30 Gy experienced greatest rates of CR and had lower rates of disease recurrence.**

Hoppe, Stanford (*J Am Acad Dermatol* 2015, PMID 25476993): Pooled data from three clinical trials using low dose (12 Gy) TSEBT. All trials involved TSEBT-naïve pts with stage IB to IIIA MF. Treatment was 12 Gy, 1 Gy per fraction over 3 weeks. Primary end point was clinical response rate. 33 pts enrolled; 18 males. Stages were 22 IB, 2 IIA, 7 IIB, and 2 IIIA. Overall response rate was 88% (29/33), including nine pts with complete response. Median time to response was 7.6 weeks (3–12.4 weeks). Median duration of clinical benefit was 70.7 weeks (95% CI: 41.8–133.8). **Conclusion: Low dose TSEBT provides reliable and rapid reduction of MF, can be administered safely multiple times during the course of a pt's disease, and has acceptable toxicity profile.**

REFERENCES

1. Trautinger F, Eder J, Assaf C, et al. European Organisation for Research and Treatment of Cancer consensus recommendations for the treatment of mycosis fungoides/Sezary syndrome: update 2017. *Eur J Cancer*. 2017;77:57–74.
2. Criscione VD, Weinstock MA. Incidence of cutaneous T-cell lymphoma in the United States, 1973–2002. *Arch Dermatol*. 2007;143(7):854–859.
3. Willemze R, Jaffe ES, Burg G, et al. WHO-EORTC classification for cutaneous lymphomas. *Blood*. 2005;105(10):3768–3785.
4. Wood GS, Salvekar A, Schaffer J, et al. Evidence against a role for human T-cell lymphotrophic virus type I (HTLV-I) in the pathogenesis of American cutaneous T-cell lymphoma. *J Invest Dermatol*. 1996;107(3):301–307.
5. Pimpinelli N, Olsen EA, Santucci M, et al. Defining early mycosis fungoides. *J Am Acad Dermatol*. 2005;53(6):1053–1063.
6. Kim YH, Liu HL, Mraz-Gernhard S, et al. Long-term outcome of 525 patients with mycosis fungoides and Sezary syndrome: clinical prognostic factors and risk for disease progression. *Arch Dermatol*. 2003;139(7):857–866.
7. Smoller BR, Bishop K, Glusac E, et al. Reassessment of histologic parameters in the diagnosis of mycosis fungoides. *Am J Surg Pathol*. 1995;19(12):1423–1430.
8. Olsen E, Vonderheid E, Pimpinelli N, et al. Revisions to the staging and classification of mycosis fungoides and Sezary syndrome: a proposal of the International Society for Cutaneous Lymphomas (ISCL) and the cutaneous lymphoma task force of the European Organization of Research and Treatment of Cancer (EORTC). *Blood*. 2007;110(6):1713–1722.
9. Olsen EA, Whittaker S, Kim YH, et al. Clinical end points and response criteria in mycosis fungoides and Sezary syndrome: a consensus statement of the International Society for Cutaneous Lymphomas, the United States Cutaneous Lymphoma Consortium, and the Cutaneous Lymphoma Task Force of the European Organisation for Research and Treatment of Cancer. *J Clin Oncol*. 2011;29(18):2598–2607.
10. Tsai EY, Taur A, Espinosa L, et al. Staging accuracy in mycosis fungoides and sezary syndrome using integrated positron emission tomography and computed tomography. *Arch Dermatol*. 2006;142(5):577–584.
11. Agar NS, Wedgeworth E, Crichton S, et al. Survival outcomes and prognostic factors in mycosis fungoides/Sezary syndrome: validation of the revised International Society for Cutaneous Lymphomas/European Organisation for Research and Treatment of Cancer staging proposal. *J Clin Oncol*. 2010;28(31):4730–4739.
12. Hughes CF, Khot A, McCormack C, et al. Lack of durable disease control with chemotherapy for mycosis fungoides and Sezary syndrome: a comparative study of systemic therapy. *Blood*. 2015;125(1):71–81.
13. Wilson LD, Kacinski BM, Jones GW. Local superficial radiotherapy in the management of minimal stage IA cutaneous T-cell lymphoma (mycosis fungoides). *Int J Radiat Oncol Biol Phys*. 1998;40(1):109–115.
14. Cotter GW, Baglan RJ, Wasserman TH, Mill W. Palliative radiation treatment of cutaneous mycosis fungoides: a dose response. *Int J Radiat Oncol Biol Phys*. 1983;9(10):1477–1480.
15. Neelis KJ, Schimmel EC, Vermeer MH, et al. Low-dose palliative radiotherapy for cutaneous B- and T-cell lymphomas. *Int J Radiat Oncol Biol Phys*. 2009;74(1):154–158.

16. Jones GW, Kacinski BM, Wilson LD, et al. Total skin electron radiation in the management of mycosis fungoides: consensus of the European Organization for Research and Treatment of Cancer (EORTC) Cutaneous Lymphoma Project Group. *J Am Acad Dermatol*. 2002;47(3):364–370.
17. Videtic GMM, Woody N, Vassil AD. *Handbook of Treatment Planning in Radiation Oncology*. 2nd ed. New York, NY: Demos Medical; 2015.
18. Olsen EA, Hodak E, Anderson T, et al. Guidelines for phototherapy of mycosis fungoides and Sezary syndrome: a consensus statement of the United States Cutaneous Lymphoma Consortium. *J Am Acad Dermatol*. 2016;74(1):27–58.
19. Duarte RF, Boumendil A, Onida F, et al. Long-term outcome of allogeneic hematopoietic cell transplantation for patients with mycosis fungoides and Sezary syndrome: a European society for blood and marrow transplantation lymphoma working party extended analysis. *J Clin Oncol*. 2014;32(29):3347–3348.

IV: BREAST

21: EARLY-STAGE BREAST CANCER

Rahul D. Tendulkar and Chirag Shah

QUICK HIT: For early-stage breast cancer, treatment typically involves surgical resection followed by adjuvant therapy (CHT, RT, and/or endocrine therapy) depending on pathologic features. Breast-conserving surgery (BCS) + adjuvant RT is an equivalent alternative to mastectomy for most pts with unifocal cancers who desire organ preservation. Whole breast irradiation (WBI) after BCS improves local recurrence rates (from 26% to 7% at 5 years) and OS by 5% at 15 years.[1] Conventional WBI dose is 45 to 50 Gy, followed by a tumor bed boost of 10 to 16 Gy, which further improves LC. Hypofractionated WBI regimens (40–42.5 Gy/15–16 fx) are acceptable alternatives for most pts, particularly in those not requiring elective nodal irradiation. In pts with limited axillary nodal involvement on sentinel lymph node biopsy, a completion axillary lymph node dissection is not necessary, provided that the pt undergoes WBI. Lower risk pts (e.g., older age, T1N0, ER+, negative margins) may be eligible for partial breast RT, intraoperative RT, or endocrine therapy alone after lumpectomy.

EPIDEMIOLOGY: Worldwide, breast cancer is the most frequently diagnosed and leading cause of cancer death in women. In the United States, >250,000 new diagnoses in 2017 and >40,000 deaths.[2] Lifetime risk is one in eight women (approximately 1 in 50 by age 50). Median age at diagnosis is 61. About two-thirds have no significant risk factors. Males account for 1% (a/w Klinefelter syndrome and BRCA2; 90% are ER+).

RISK FACTORS

Estrogen exposure: Female gender, older age, early menarche, nulliparity, older age at first birth (>30 years), lack of breast feeding, late menopause (>55 years), hormone replacement therapy.

Family history: Risk increases with more first-degree relatives.

Genetics (5%–10% hereditary): BRCA1—AD (17q21), 60% to 80% lifetime risk of breast cancer, 30% to 50% lifetime risk ovarian cancer, higher risk of triple negative (ER-/PR-/HER2-); BRCA2—AD (13q12), 50% to 60% lifetime risk of breast cancer, 10% to 20% lifetime risk of ovarian cancer, male breast cancer, prostate, bladder, endometrial, and pancreatic CA; Li–Fraumeni—AD (17p), p53, a/w sarcoma, leukemia, brain, adrenocortical carcinoma; Cowden syndrome—AD (10q23), PTEN, a/w hamartomas of skin and oral cavity; ataxia–telangiectasia—AR (11q22), ATM; Peutz–Jeghers.

Personal history of breast disease: Prior breast cancer, DCIS, LCIS, atypical ductal hyperplasia, dense breast tissue, history of radiation treatment during youth (age <30 years).

Lifestyle/exposure: High-fat diet, postmenopausal obesity, sedentary lifestyle.

ANATOMY: The breast overlies the pectoralis major muscle, extends from ~2nd to 6th rib and from the lateral sternum to anterior axillary fold. The axillary tail of Spence extends laterally into the low axilla. Glandular tissue is arranged in 15 to 20 lobes with a system of lactiferous ducts that open at the nipple. UOQ contains greatest volume of glandular tissue (most common location of breast cancers). Least common location is lower inner quadrant. Breast is supported by Cooper's ligaments, which are fibrous septae joining the superficial fascia (skin) and deep fascia covering the pectoralis major muscle. Lymphatic drainage is primarily to the axilla. Axillary lymph node (ALN) levels I, II, III are respectively located inferolateral, deep and superomedial to pectoralis minor, which inserts on coracoid process of the scapula. Rotter's nodes are located between pectoralis major and minor (anterior to level II). Internal mammary nodes (IMN) are situated along IM vessels adjacent to sternum in the first three intercostal spaces, about 2- to 3-cm lateral to midline, and 2- to 3-cm deep. Approximately 30% of medial tumors and 15% of lateral tumors drain to the IMN.

PATHOLOGY: Breast carcinomas arise from epithelial elements and comprise a diverse group of lesions with differing biologic behavior, although often discussed as a single disease. Estrogen receptor (ER) and/or progesterone receptor (PR) are expressed in 70% of tumors (more common in postmenopausal pts). HER2/neu (c-ERbB-2 or human epidermal growth factor receptor 2) is a receptor tyrosine kinase, with HER2 amplification seen in 25% to 30% of invasive cancers. Triple negative breast cancer (TNBC) is an aggressive entity in which tumors do not express ER, PR, or HER2, accounting for ~15% of cases and more commonly found in BRCA mutation carriers.

Invasive ductal carcinoma: 80% of cases, firm mass with desmoplastic reaction, solid cords of cells.

Invasive lobular carcinoma: 5% to 10% of cases, rubbery texture, less visible on mammogram (better imaged with MRI), "Indian filing" histology, often bilateral/multicentric, >80% are ER+, spreads to unusual locations such as meninges, serosal surfaces, BM, ovary, and RP.

Rarer subtypes (need >90% predominant pattern): *Tubular*—small, well-differentiated variant of IDC, >75% tubules, usually ER+/PR+. *Medullary*—a/w BRCA1, presents at younger age (<50 years), LNs are large/hyperplastic, most are triple negative. *Mucinous/colloid*—older pts, favorable. *Papillary*—older pts, often multifocal/diffuse, often LN+ even when small size. *Cribriform*—ER+/PR+. *Other uncommon variants* include metaplastic (poor prognosis), squamous cell, invasive micropapillary, adenoid cystic, mucoepidermoid, secretory, apocrine, spindle cell, lymphoma, neuroendocrine small cell, and clear cell. Mammary carcinoma is a mixture of invasive ductal and lobular carcinoma.

Extensive intraductal component (EIC): EIC is defined as ≥25% DCIS within the invasive carcinoma specimen and extending beyond edges of tumor. EIC was originally identified as a risk factor for LR after BCT, but no longer considered the case provided margins are negative.

Paget's disease: Chronic eczematous changes of the nipple–areolar complex, with an underlying intraepidermal adenocarcinoma of the nipple (in 95%). About 50% have a palpable mass (>90% are invasive cancer) and 50% have no mass (typically DCIS). Low risk of axillary nodal mets.

Cystosarcoma phyllodes: Fibroepithelial, "leaf-like," large, encapsulated tumors, usually benign w/o invasion. Can grow slowly then have sudden rapid increase in size. Uncommonly malignant and nodal mets are rare.

GENETICS: A number of gene expression profiling (GEP) models exist, including the Amsterdam 70-gene good-versus-poor outcome model (low signature vs. high signature),[3] the 21-gene recurrence score model,[4] and the intrinsic subtype model.[5] The

21-gene recurrence score (Oncotype DX®) was developed for pts w/ LN-negative, ER+ breast cancers, receiving tamoxifen +/− CHT on NSABP B-14, and is stratified into low risk (<18 score), intermediate risk (18–30), and high risk (>30) of recurrence in order to estimate the relative benefit of CHT in addition to hormonal therapy.[4] Rates of distant recurrence in the low-risk, intermediate-risk, and high-risk groups were 6.8%, 14.3%, and 30.5% at 10 years. There are four main intrinsic subtypes: luminal A (best prognosis), luminal B, HER2 enriched (HER2+), and basal-like (worst prognosis).[5] Note that the luminal A and B clinicopathologic surrogate definitions have been updated: *luminal A-like*: ER+/HER2- with either low Ki-67 (<14%) or the combination of PR+ (≥20%) and intermediate Ki-67 (14-19%); *luminal B-like (HER2-)*: ER+/HER2- with either high Ki-67 (≥20%) or the combination of intermediate Ki-67 (14-19%) with PR- or low (<20%), or ER+/PR+ with HER2+; *basal-like*: usually triple negative (~70%–80% correlation), high prevalence in young African American women and BRCA mutation carriers; *HER2 enriched*: usually ER-/PR-, HER2+, high Ki-67.[6] The luminal subtypes, while usually HER2-, can be HER2+. Higher response rates to neoadjuvant CHT are seen with basal-like and HER2 enriched cancers.

SCREENING: Screening mammograms (90% sensitive/specific) reduce mortality by 35% (relative risk) in women 50 to 74 years of age. 40% of breast lesions are detected by mammogram only, but 10% have palpable tumors that are not visualized.

- *ACR Appropriateness Guidelines*[7]: Begin annual screening at 45 y/o (opportunity at 40–44 y/o appropriate); biennial screening after 55 y/o (until poor health or <10 yrs life expectancy); screen at 25 to 30 y/o for BRCA1 carriers and untested relatives of carriers; screen at 25 to 30 y/o or 10 years earlier than first-degree relatives (whichever is later) with lifetime risk for breast cancer ≥20%. Screen 8 years after or 25 years of age (whichever is later) for women <30 years of age who received mantle RT/thoracic RT. Screen at any age for women with biopsy-proven lobular neoplasia, atypical ductal hyperplasia, DCIS or invasive breast cancer. Supplemental screening may be necessary in women with genetic predisposition to disease and/or dense breasts. Clinical breast examination not recommended in average risk women.
- *U.S. Preventative Services Task Force*[8]: Recommends biennial screening for ages 50 to 74, no routine screening for 40 to 49 (self-exams controversial). High-risk women should begin screening 10 yrs before age of youngest first-degree relative diagnosed. Insufficient evidence for benefit/harm of clinical exam; however, recommended against teaching breast self-examination.

CLINICAL PRESENTATION: Typically detected by screening mammogram (~90%), self-breast exam, and/or clinical exam (~10%).[9] Most common presentation is as a painless mass, but can occasionally present with pain (~5%), nipple discharge (though usually benign), nipple retraction or axillary lymphadenopathy with occult primary. A mass is less concerning for malignancy if associated with changes in menstrual cycle. Most common location is in UOQ (40%), followed by central area (30%), UIQ (15%), LOQ (10%), and LIQ (5%). Bilateral disease occurs in 1% to 3% of cases. Risk of developing contralateral cancer after primary diagnosis is 0.75% per year. *Multifocal* defined as ≥2 cancer foci in same quadrant (typically eligible for breast conservation). *Multicentric:* ≥2 foci in different quadrants or >5 cm apart (typically not eligible for breast conservation). *Differential Diagnosis:* Fibroadenoma (solitary mass, well-defined, mobile); cysts (more diffuse and less firm, suspicious if blood in aspirate or contents reaccumulate quickly); infection (mastitis or abscess); Mondor's disease (thrombophlebitis of superficial breast veins); fat necrosis; intraductal papilloma (common cause of bloody discharge); sclerosing adenosis (nodular benign condition consisting of hyperplastic lobules of acinar tissue); lactocele.

TABLE 21.1: BI-RADS Classification[10]			
BI-RADS	Description	Malignancy %	Follow-up
0	Incomplete	1%	Completion of imaging or review of previous imaging not previously available
1	Negative	<1%	Routine annual screening
2	Benign lesion	<1%	Routine annual screening
3	Probably benign	<2%	Short interval f/u (6 months)
4a	Low suspicion for malignancy	2%–10%	Biopsy
4b	Mod suspicion for malignancy	10%–50%	Biopsy
4c	High suspicion for malignancy	50%–95%	Biopsy
5	Highly suggestive of malignancy	>95%	Biopsy
6	Biopsy proven malignancy	100%	Appropriate treatment per stage

WORKUP

H&P: Full H&P with attention to breast and LN exam

Imaging: mammogram and ultrasound are typical first steps. Systemic staging workup not routinely indicated per NCCN for stage I-II pts in the absence of suspicious symptoms, physical exam findings or lab abnormalities (e.g., elevated alk phos or LFTs). If suspicious, studies may include PET/CT or CT chest/abdomen/pelvis and bone scan, +/− MRI brain.

- *Mammography*: On craniocaudal (CC) view, the lateral edge of the film is typically marked by "CC" marker. On mediolateral oblique (MLO) view, assess for image quality by ensuring pectoralis muscle is included. Concerning mammographic findings: calcifications 100 to 300 microns, >10 clustered linear calcifications, spiculated lesions. Spot compression views are useful for suspicious masses (vs. disappearance of dense breast tissue on compression), and magnification views are used for evaluation of calcifications.
- *Ultrasound*: Helps to distinguish solid from cystic masses (but not useful for calcifications) and to evaluate nonpalpable masses identified on mammogram.
- *MRI*: Higher sensitivity (>90%) than mammography, but lower specificity (39%–95%) due to false positives. Suspicious features for malignancy: strong, rapid contrast enhancement, spiculated margins, rim enhancement, heterogeneous appearance. ACS guidelines recommend screening MRI for women with 20% to 25% or greater lifetime risk of breast cancer, including women with hereditary mutations (BRCA, Li–Fraumeni, Cowden), strong family history of breast/ovarian cancer, and women who received prior thoracic RT for Hodgkin's disease before 30 years of age.[11] Other potential indications for MRI include an obscured breast (silicone implants), suspicious masses with negative mammogram and ultrasound, evaluation of poorly imaged tumors such as ILC or DCIS without microcalcifications, or pts presenting with positive axillary nodes of unknown primary (MRI detects primary tumor in breast 80%–90% of the time). MRI can change surgical management in 25% of cases but does not reduce positive margins, re-excision rates, or LR rates.[12–14]

Procedures: Core biopsy, needle aspirate (if cystic on ultrasound). FNA may detect abnormal cells, but cannot distinguish DCIS from IDC and cannot identify ER/PR/HER2 status—thus core biopsy is preferred. US-core biopsy for palpable masses. Stereotactic core biopsy or needle localization if nonpalpable lesion with suspicious calcifications. Punch biopsy for Paget's or if suspicious of dermal involvement (e.g., suspected inflammatory breast cancer).

PROGNOSTIC FACTORS: Poor prognostic factors include LN+ (strongest factor), young age, ER/PR-negativity, HER2/neu amplification (in the absence of HER2-directed therapy), high grade, LVSI+, basal-like subtype.[15]

STAGING

TABLE 21.2: AJCC 8th ed. (2017) Staging for Breast Cancer					
cT/pT		**cN**		**pN**	
Tis	• Carcinoma in situ	N0	• No palpable LNs	N0	**(i-)** negative IHC
					(i+) positive IHC (≤0.2 mm)
					(mol-) negative RT-PCR
					(mol+) positive RT-PCR
T1mic	• ≤0.1 cm	N1	• Mobile ipsilateral level I/II axillary LNs	N1	**mi** >0.2 mm and/or >200 cells, but ≤2 mm
					a 1-3 axillary LNs
					b IM LN+ pathologically, but not clinically
					c pN1a + pN1b
T1	**a** >0.1 cm and ≤0.5 cm	N2a	• Fixed/matted ipsilateral axillary LNs	N2	**a** 4-9 axillary LNs
	b >0.5 cm and ≤1 cm				
	c >1 cm and ≤2 cm				**b** IM LNs+ pathologically and clinically, but with negative axillary LNs
T2	• >2 cm and ≤5 cm	N2b	• Clinically detected ipsilateral IM LNs, without axillary LNs	N3	**a** ≥10 axillary LNs or + infraclavicular LNs
					b Pathologically and clinically + IM LNs with + axillary LNs; or pathologically, but not clinically + IM LN's with >3 axillary LNs
					c Ipsilateral SCV LNs
T3	• >5 cm	N3a	• Ipsilateral infraclavicular LNs	**Group Staging**	

(continued)

TABLE 21.2: AJCC 8th ed. (2017) Staging for Breast Cancer (*continued*)

T4	a Extension to chest wall (except pectoralis major)	N3b	• Ipsilateral IM and axillary LNs	0	Tis
				IA	T1N0M0
	b Peau d'orange, ulcer, or satellite skin nodules			IB	T0-1N1miM0
				IIA	T0-1N1M0, T2N0M0
	c Both T4a and T4b			IIB	T2N1M0, T3N0M0
	d Inflammatory carcinoma			IIIA	T2N1M0, T3N0M0
cT/pT		**cN**		**pN**	
M0(i+)	• Circulating tumor cells in bone marrow	N3c	• Ipsilateral supraclavicular LNs	IIIB	T4N0-2M0
				IIIC	Any T, N3M0
M1	• Distant metastasis			IV	M0(i+), M1

Major changes in the 8th edition from the 7th edition: In addition to anatomic staging, prognostic group staging has been developed to include grade and ER/PR/HER2 status and is preferred over the historic "anatomic" stage groups listed above (included for context of interpreting trials below). Additionally, LCIS is considered benign and no longer as stage Tis.

TREATMENT PARADIGM: Local therapy options include modified radical mastectomy (MRM) versus breast conservation therapy (BCT) composed of lumpectomy + RT. There are no significant differences in LR (with negative margins), distant DFS, or OS between MRM and BCT at extended follow-up in at least six prospective trials. CHT, if needed, is delivered either neoadjuvantly or postoperatively, but generally before RT (the Recht trial initially demonstrated reduced recurrences rates in pts treated with CHT prior to radiation, although the curves converged at later follow-up).[16,17] Hormonal therapy is indicated for hormone receptor-positive cancers, and usually follows all other therapies. Breast cancer is both a local and distant disease. Halsted theorized that breast cancer spreads with orderly anatomic progression of disease, such that aggressive local treatment should improve survival. Fisher theorized that intrinsic tumor factors dictate patterns of spread, such that systemic therapy should improve outcomes. Hellman merged the two theories, recognizing that breast cancers fall under a heterogeneous spectrum, and that optimizing both LC and systemic therapy can provide the best outcomes.[18]

Prevention: Tamoxifen as chemoprevention reduces the risk of noninvasive and invasive cancers in high-risk women by up to 50% (NSABP-P1).[19] Raloxifene is as effective as tamoxifen and with lower rate of thromboembolic events (NSABP P-2 "STAR").[20] Vitamin D and calcium may decrease risk in premenopausal pts. Prophylactic mastectomy reduces breast cancer risk by >90% in those with a strong family history and may improve survival in BRCA carriers.[21] Prophylactic oophorectomy decreases risk in BRCA carriers by 50% if before 40 years of age.[22] No conclusive evidence of a benefit from special dietary changes; however, alcohol/obesity is associated with increased risk of developing breast cancer.

Surgery

TABLE 21.3: Surgical Options for Breast Cancer

| Radical mastectomy (RM) | Popularized by Halsted starting in 1894. Involves en bloc removal of the breast, overlying skin, pectoralis major, pectoralis minor, and level I, II, and III lymph nodes; there are currently no absolute indications for this procedure. |

(*continued*)

TABLE 21.3: Surgical Options for Breast Cancer (*continued*)	
Modified radical mastectomy (MRM)	Complete removal of breast tissue, pectoralis fascia, and level I and II lymph nodes (preserves pectoralis major, lateral pectoral nerve, and level III nodes).
Total mastectomy (TM)	Removal of breast tissue only (preservation of both pectoralis muscles and axillary lymph nodes).
Skin-sparing mastectomy (SSM)	Resection of biopsy scar and/or skin immediately overlying the tumor, and removal of breast parenchyma. Preservation of majority of breast skin for reconstruction.
Nipple-sparing mastectomy (NSM)	Skin-sparing mastectomy with preservation of the nipple–areolar complex.
Lumpectomy or partial mastectomy (PM)	Removal of only part of the breast containing the cancer (i.e., breast conservation surgery). Margins are considered negative if there is "no tumor on ink."[23]
Axillary lymph node dissection (ALND)	In cN0, ~30% are positive on dissection (false negatives). In cN+, ~25% negative on dissection (false positives). A complete ALND can yield up to 20–25 LNs, while a typical level I and II ALND yields ~15 LN. Removal of level III nodes is generally unnecessary unless grossly positive. Incidence of skip metastases to level III nodes without involved level I nodes is <3%.
Sentinel lymph node biopsy (SLNB)	Tc-99m sulfur colloid and/or isosulfan blue dye are injected at tumor site for 3–7 minutes, and gamma camera identifies SLNs. False negative rate is 8%–10% after negative SLNB.[24] SLNB results in less lymphedema, less pain, and better arm mobility compared to ALND.

Chemotherapy

Adjuvant: Typically given post-op to LN+ pts, ER-negative, HER2+, and women with multiple adverse features (e.g., young age or high Oncotype DX® scores). Virtually all subgroups of women have a benefit in DFS from adjuvant CHT, though benefit is more pronounced in younger women, LN+, and ER-negative pts. *Neoadjuvant*: Equivalent survival as adjuvant (NSABP B-18) but may allow for less extensive surgery. Note: Role of CHT is unclear in women >70 y/o because this age group was excluded from early clinical trials. *Trastuzumab* for 1 yr has OS advantage for HER2+ pts in addition to cytotoxic CHT.[25] Trastuzumab is not given concurrently with adriamycin because of cardiotoxicity concerns, but is safe to give with RT. Trastuzumab-related cardiac effects are reversible, so obtain cardiac echo q3 mos to monitor. Pertuzumab has been added to trastuzumab to provide dual anti-HER2 therapy, which results in pCR rates of 50% to 60% in the neoadjuvant setting. Common CHT regimens include:

- AC: Adriamycin 60 mg/m^2 + cyclophosphamide 600 mg/m^2 q3weeks x four cycles.
- AC→T: Adriamycin 60 mg/m^2 + cyclophosphamide 600 mg/m^2 q3weeks x four cycles followed by paclitaxel 175 mg/m^2 q3weeks x four cycles or 80 mg/m^2 q1weeks x 12 weeks (dose-dense regimen is q2weeks w/ filgrastim or pegfilgrastim for support).
- AC→TH: Same as AC→T, with the addition of trastuzumab 4 mg/kg loading dose followed by 2 mg/kg per week concurrently with paclitaxel, then trastuzumab monotherapy (6 mg/kg q3weeks) for 1 year.
- TC: docetaxel 75 mg/m^2 and cyclophosphamide 600 mg/m^2.
- TCH: nonanthracycline regimen consisting of docetaxel 75 mg/m^2 + carboplatin (C; AUC 6 mg/mL/min) q3weeks x six cycles + trastuzumab (4 mg/kg loading dose followed by 2 mg/kg per week concurrently with TC) and then trastuzumab monotherapy (6 mg/kg q3weeks) for 1 year.

Anthracycline-based CHT is superior to nonanthracycline based regimens, and may especially benefit HER2 amplified pts. The addition of a taxane has OS benefit for LN+

pts compared to AC alone.[26,27] Dose-dense regimens (q2weeks instead of q3weeks) offer OS advantage for high-risk pts as well.[28] Other CHT regimens include: TAC: docetaxel, Adriamycin and cyclophosphamide q3weeks x six cycles; CMF: cyclophosphamide, methotrexate, fluorouracil; FAC: fluorouracil, doxorubicin, cyclophosphamide; FEC: fluorouracil, epirubicin, cyclophosphamide.

Hormone therapy: Indicated for essentially all ER+ or PR+ pts, unless a specific contraindication exists. *Tamoxifen* is a partial estrogen agonist which functions as a competitive inhibitor. Premenopausal women are typically treated with tamoxifen 20 mg daily for 5 yrs, though 10 yrs of therapy was recently found to further reduce recurrence and reduce breast cancer mortality by ~1/3 in the first 10 yrs following diagnosis and by ~1/2 subsequently.[29] Side effects include hot flashes, vaginal discharge/bleeding, cataracts, retinopathy, thromboembolic events (1%), endometrial cancer (RR 2-7), and uterine sarcomas. Aromatase inhibitors (AIs) such as anastrozole or letrozole block conversion of androgens to estrogen in fat, liver, and muscle and are ineffective in premenopausal women (due to ovarian production of estrogen). Postmenopausal women are typically treated with anastrozole 1 mg daily for 5 yrs. Compared to tamoxifen in postmenopausal women, AIs improve DFS and have higher rates of myalgias, arthralgias, and osteoporosis, but less risk of endometrial cancer and DVTs.[30,31]

Radiation: Whole breast irradiation (WBI) after lumpectomy significantly lowers risk of LRR when compared to lumpectomy alone, and improves 15-yr OS by reducing mortality from breast cancer.[1]

Indications: WBI is indicated in most pts following breast-conserving surgery. Favorable subgroups (e.g., older pts with T1N0 ER+ breast cancers) may be treated with APBI, IORT, or adjuvant endocrine therapy alone.

Absolute contraindications to BCS: Persistently positive resection margins after re-excision attempts, multicentric tumors, diffuse malignant-appearing mammographic microcalcifications, prior RT to the breast or chest wall, inflammatory breast cancer.

Relative contraindications to BCS: Pregnancy (can perform BCS in third trimester and defer RT until after delivery), active lupus/scleroderma, large tumor in a small breast (cosmetic outcome may not be satisfactory). BRCA mutation carriers are not contraindicated to receive RT. However their risk of developing new primary cancers will remain high after BCT, so bilateral mastectomies are commonly performed.

Dose: Conventional WBI is 45 to 50.4 Gy in 1.8 to 2 Gy/fx, typically with a boost of 10 to 16 Gy. Hypofractionated regimens are typically 40 to 42.5 Gy at 2.66 Gy/fx with consideration of boost.

Timing: RT usually starts within 4 to 6 weeks of completion of surgery or CHT; delaying RT for longer than 16 weeks after surgery a/w higher breast relapse rates.[32]

Procedure: See *Treatment Planning Handbook*, Chapter 5.[33]

Toxicity: Acute effects: erythema, pruritus, tenderness, desquamation. Late effects: hyperpigmentation, volume loss, fibrosis, rib fracture, lymphedema, pulmonary fibrosis, secondary malignancies (<1% at 10 yrs, with angiosarcoma being most common) and cardiac effects.[34]

EVIDENCE-BASED Q&A

Is there a role for radical mastectomy in the modern era?

NSABP B-04 established that there is no advantage to radical mastectomy versus total mastectomy with or without RT.

Fisher, NSABP B-04 (*NEJM* 2002, PMID 12192016): PRT of nonfixed, operable tumors confined to breast/axilla (n = 1079 LN- and n = 586 LN+). Randomization of cN0 pts to RM versus TM + RT (50 Gy/25 fx tangents + PAB; 45 Gy/25 fx IM + SCV; boost if LN+) versus TM alone; cN+ pts were randomized to RM versus TM + RT. No significant differences between the three arms of LN- pts or between the two arms of LN+ pts for DFS, RFS, DDFS, or OS. Among cN0 pts, no difference in survival between RM versus TM +/- RT, and no survival benefit to RT (after TM in cN0). ALN status is a strong prognostic indicator, but no survival advantage to removing occult positive nodes at surgery. 40% of cN0 women had pathologically positive nodes; 17.8% of TM alone pts needed delayed ALND for axillary failure, usually within first 2 years. **Conclusion: RM not necessary for operable breast cancer.**

TABLE 21.4: NSABP B-04 Results										
	25-yr DFS		25-yr RFS		25-yr DDFS		25-yr OS		25-yr LR	
	LN-	LN+	LN-	LN+	LN-	LN+	LN-	LN+	LN-	LN+
RM	19%	11%	53%	36%	46%	32%	25%	14%	5%	8%
TM + RT	13%	10%	52%	33%	38%	29%	19%	14%	1%	3%
TM	19%	-	50%	-	43%	-	26%		7%	

How does mastectomy compare to breast conservation?

At least six randomized trials have demonstrated no significant differences in OS between BCT and mastectomy. Two trials, which did not require negative margin lumpectomies (e.g., 48% in the EORTC trial had positive margins), found higher LR rates with BCT, likely due to inadequate surgery.[35,36] At 20-yr follow up in the Milan trial, there were higher rates of LR in the BCT arm (8.8% after quadrantectomy vs. 2.3% after radical mastectomy), likely due to new primary tumors (as 2/3 of recurrences were in other quadrants and only 1/3 occurred in the index quadrant scar).[37] A 1992 NCI consensus statement declared both mastectomy and BCT to be acceptable standards of care for operable breast cancer.

TABLE 21.5: Prospective Randomized Trials of BCT vs. M/RM									
Trial	Years	N	Stage	Surgery	Adjuvant	F/U	OS % (p)	DFS % (p)	LR % (p)
Milan[37]	1973–80	701	I	Q/RM	CMF	20 yrs	58/59 (NS)		9/2 (<.001)
Gustave-Roussy[38]	1972–80	179	I	WE/MRM	None	15 yrs	73/65 (.19)		9/14 (NS)
NSABP B-06[39]	1976–84	1,219	I–II	WE/MRM	MF	12 yrs	63/59 (.12)	50/49 (.21)	10/8
NCI[35]	1979–87	237	I–II	WE/MRM	AC	10 yrs	77/75 (.89)	72/69 (.93)	19/6 (.01)
EORTC 10801[36]	1980–86	868	I–II	LE/MRM	CMF	10 yrs	65/66 (NS)		20/12 (.01)
Danish[40]	1983–89	904	I–III	Q, WE/ MRM	CMF, Tam	6 yrs	79/82 (NS)	70/66 (NS)	3/4 (NS)

A, Adriamycin; C, cyclophosphamide; F, 5-FU; LE, local excision; M, melphalan; Q, quadrantectomy; Tam, tamoxifen; WE, wide excision.

What is the role of adjuvant RT after breast-conserving surgery?

Up to 40% of women after surgical resection of gross tumor will have residual microscopic disease that can develop into recurrence. The Holland study demonstrated that 43% of unifocal cancers in mastectomy specimens had tumor foci located >2 cm from the index lesion.[41] NSABP B-06 showed that 20-yr LR rates were reduced from 39% to 14% with the addition of RT.[39] The EBCTCG meta-analysis was the first study large enough to demonstrate that adjuvant WBI improves survival—the individual trials were not sufficiently powered. RT decreased 15-yr risk of death from breast cancer from 31% to 26% for LN-pts and 55 to 48% for LN+.[1] The EBCTCG meta-analysis suggested a "4:1 ratio"—one breast cancer death was avoided by year 15 for every four local recurrences prevented by year 5 and for every four any-recurrences prevented by year 10.[42] There has been no subgroup (age, grade, size, hormone status), which has not been shown to benefit from RT.

Fisher, NSABP B-06 (*NEJM* 2002, PMID 12393820): PRT of 1,843 pts from 1976 to 1978 with stage I-II, mobile tumor ≤4 cm, mobile axillary LNs and negative margins randomized to MRM versus lumpectomy versus lumpectomy + WBI 50 Gy/25 fx. ALND was level I-II. Pts with +LNs received CHT (5-FU and melphalan). Similar DFS and OS observed between MRM and BCT. The 20-yr IBTR rate was 39% after lumpectomy alone and 14% after lumpectomy + RT, with significant benefit to RT in both LN+ and LN-. **Conclusion: Mastectomy and BCT have similar long-term outcomes. Adjuvant WBI after lumpectomy reduces IBTR by ~2/3.**

TABLE 21.6: Results of NSABP B-06						
NSABP B-06	5-yr IBTR	5-yr DFS	5-yr OS	20-yr IBTR	20-yr DFS	20-yr OS
MRM (TM + ALND)		67%	82%		36%	47%
Lumpectomy	28%	64%	83%	39%	35%	46%
Lumpectomy + RT	8%	71%	84%	14%	35%	46%

EBCTCG 2005 Meta-analysis (*Lancet* 2005, PMID 15894097): Meta-analysis of 42,080 women with breast cancer treated on 78 randomized trials that began by 1995. Studies included RT versus no RT (N ~23,500), more versus less surgery (N ~9,300), and more surgery versus RT (N ~9,300). In 10 trials 7,311 pts were treated with BCS + RT versus BCS alone. Overall, RT reduces the RR of 5-yr LR by 70%. The absolute 19% reduction in LR at 5-yr translated to a 5% reduction in breast cancer mortality at 15-yr—hence for every four LR prevented, one death was avoided.

TABLE 21.7: 2005 EBCTCG Meta-Analysis							
	All pts (N = 7,311)			LN− (N = 6,097)		LN+ (N = 1,214)	
	5-yr LR	15-yr BCM	15-yr OS	5-yr LR	15-yr BCM	5-yr LR	15-yr BCM
BCS + RT	7%	31%	65%	7%	26%	11%	48%
BCS alone	26%	36%	60%	23%	31%	41%	55%
p value	<.00001	.0002	.005	sig	.006	sig	.01

EBCTCG 2011 Meta-analysis (*Lancet* 2011, PMID 22019144): Meta-analysis of 10,801 early-stage breast cancer pts s/p BCS from 17 PRTs, 77% of whom were pN0. RT reduced the 10-yr risk of any recurrence by approximately half. With addition of RT to BCS, about one breast cancer death was avoided by year 15 for every four overall recurrences avoided at 10 yrs, another 4:1 ratio.

TABLE 21.8: 2011 EBCTCG Meta-Analysis						
	10-yr Recurrence (Any)			15-yr BCM		
	All	pN0	pN+	All	pN0	pN+
BCS + RT	19%	16%	43%	21%	17%	43%
BCS alone	35%	31%	64%	25%	21%	51%

Does completion ALND after a positive SLNB benefit cN0 patients? Can RT replace ALND in select cN0 patients?

NSABP B-04 demonstrated that not all undissected nodal disease results in clinical recurrence. Several randomized trials have since shown similar rates of axillary recurrence and DFS between SLNB and ALND among clinically node-negative pts, most of whom received adjuvant RT. ACOSOG Z0011 and IBCSG 23-01 showed that completion ALND after SLNB offered no difference than SLNB alone in SLN+ pts, for both macrometastases and micrometastases. The AMAROS trial evaluated ALND versus axillary RT after a positive SLNB, and found no difference in recurrence rates, but ALND had twice the rate of lymphedema (28% vs. 14%). Pts undergoing mastectomy were not well represented in AMAROS, and so completion ALND remains appropriate after for SLN+ pts after mastectomy. Select pts in whom PMRT is already planned may be spared ALND, provided there are no grossly enlarged LNs on exam or imaging.

Guiliano, ACOSOG Z0011 (*JAMA* 2011, PMID 21304082; Lucci *JCO* 2007, PMID 17485711; Jagsi *JCO* 2014 PMID 25135994; Update *Ann Surg* 2016, PMID 27513155): PRT of 891 pts with cT1-T2 N0 who underwent lumpectomy and SLNB with 1 to 2 LN+, randomized to completion ALND or not. All pts received WBI, without node-directed RT (per protocol). Pts were excluded for >2 LN+, matted LNs, gross ENE, received neoadjuvant CHT, or underwent mastectomy. Study target enrollment was 1,900 but closed early due to very low mortality rate. Primary end point of OS was similar in both arms. 96% to 97% received systemic therapy. Median 17 ALNs removed in ALND arm and 2 in SLNB arm ($p < .001$). In ALND arm, 27% had additional metastases in dissected LNs, and 14% had ≥ 4 LN+. ALND arm had higher rates of subjective lymphedema (13% vs. 2% at 1 yr, $p < .0001$), wound infections, axillary seromas, and paresthesias than SLNB alone. While standard tangent fields were specified by protocol, ~50% utilized high tangents (defined as ≤ 2 cm from humeral head), and 19% received regional nodal RT to include at least SCV nodes. At 10-yr update, nodal recurrences were 0.5% in ALND arm versus 1.5% in SLNB arm, and 10-yr IBTR were 6.2% versus 5.3% ($p = $ NS). **Conclusion: Completion ALND is not necessary in pts with 1 to 2 SLN metastases who receive WBI and systemic therapy.**

TABLE 21.9: ACOSOG Z0011 Results					
	5-yr IBTR	Nodal Recurrence	Lymphedema	5-yr DFS	5-yr OS
BCS + ALND +RT	3.1%	0.6%	13%	82%	92%
BCS + SLNB + RT	1.6%	1.3%	2%	84%	93%

Galimberti, *IBCSG* 23-01 (*Lancet Oncol* 2013, PMID 23491275): PRT of 931 pts with cT1-2N0 who underwent SLNB and had ≥ 1 micrometastatic (≤ 2 mm) SLNs w/o ECE, randomized to completion ALND or not (noninferiority design). 91% underwent BCT, 9% had mastectomy. Median 21 LNs removed at ALND, and 13% had additional nodal metastases. 5-yr DFS 87.8% in SLNB arm versus 84.4% in ALND arm ($p = .16$); 5-yr OS was also similar and >97%. **Conclusion: Supports ACOSOG Z-11 trial in omission of completion ALND for low-volume SLN metastases.**

Donker, AMAROS/EORTC 10981/22023 (*Lancet* 2014, PMID 25439688): There were 4,806 pts with cT1-2N0 breast cancer registered and randomized preoperatively prior to SLNB; 1,425 pts (30% of initial cohort) with SLN+ received axillary RT (n = 681) versus completion ALND (n = 744) in a noninferiority design. Axillary RT was to levels I-III and SCV fossa to 50 Gy/25 fx. 82% underwent BCT and 18% mastectomy. 33% of those undergoing ALND had additional LN+. Primary end point was 5-yr axillary recurrence rate, which was 0.43% after ALND versus 1.19% with axillary RT (p = NS). In comparison, nonrandomized pts with negative SLNB had similar axillary recurrence rate of 0.8%. OS and DFS rates similar between ALND and RT; however, lymphedema more frequent after ALND (28% vs. 14%). **Conclusion: For SLN+ pts, axillary RT provides similar control with less risk of lymphedema compared to ALND.**

TABLE 21.10: AMAROS Trial Results			
	Lymphedema	5-yr DFS	5-yr OS
BCT + ALND	28%	87%	93%
BCT + RT	14%	83%	93%
p value	<.001	.18	.34

Wong, Harvard (*IJROBP* 2008, PMID 18394815): Prospective, single-arm trial of 74 pts >55 y/o with stage I/II, cN0, ER+ breast cancer treated with lumpectomy (negative margins) without ALND or SLNB and WBI with high tangents (blocked humeral head) + tumor bed boost + 5 yrs hormonal therapy. Median age 74.5, median tumor size 1.2 cm. MFU 52 months. No pt had local or axillary recurrence. **Conclusion: High tangential RT and hormonal therapy w/o ALND is a reasonable option in older pts with early-stage ER/PR+ cN0 breast cancer.**

What is the role of regional nodal irradiation in breast conservation patients?

After lumpectomy, RNI is indicated for certain high-risk patients, such as those with LN+ and/or ER-negative disease. The NCIC MA.20 and EORTC 22922/10925 trials showed an improvement in LRR, DM, DFS and a trend toward OS with the use of comprehensive nodal radiation.[43,44] It remains an area of controversy which pts may be adequately treated with high tangents versus comprehensive RNI. See Locally Advanced Breast Cancer (Chapter 22) for additional details.

For pts with early breast cancer, can the duration of treatment be reduced via hypofractionation?

At least four randomized trials from the UK and Canada have demonstrated similar outcomes between conventionally fractionated and hypofractionated WBI with respect to IBTR, cosmesis, toxicity, and OS (some trials demonstrated less toxicity with hypofractionation). Hypofractionation is generally acceptable for early-stage (pT1-2N0) breast cancer in older pts (>50 y/o) not receiving regional nodal irradiation; limited data exist in those receiving CHT (as these pts were not well represented in the early trials) though hypofractionation can be considered in these patients.[45]

TABLE 21.11: Summary of Hhypofractionated WBI Trials			
	Dose	% Boost	10-yr LRR
RMH/GOC[46]*	50 Gy/25 fx	74%	12.1%
	42.9 Gy/13 fx QOD	75%	9.6%
	39 Gy/13 fx QOD	74%	14.8%
START A[47]*	50 Gy/25 fx	60%	7.4%
	41.6 Gy/13 fx QOD	61%	6.3%
	39 Gy/13 fx QOD	61%	8.8%
START B[47]	50 Gy/25 fx	41%	5.5%
	40 Gy/15 fx	44%	4.3%
Whelan, Canadian OCOG 93-010[48]	50 Gy/25 fx	0%	6.7%
	42.56 Gy/16 fx	0%	6.2%
OCOG, Ontario Cooperative Oncology Group; RMH/GOC, UK Royal Marsden Hospital/Gloucestershire Oncology Centre; START, Standardisation of Breast Radiotherapy.			
All schedules in RMH/GOC and START-A trials delivered over 5 weeks.			

Haviland, START A&B (*Lancet Oncol* 2013, PMID 24055415): Two UK PRTs enrolled women with pT1-T3 N0-1 s/p complete excision, no immediate breast reconstruction from 1999 to 2002. **START A:** 2,236 pts randomized to 50 Gy/25 fx over 5 weeks versus 41.6 Gy (3.2 Gy/fx) or 39 Gy (3.0 Gy/fx) in 13 fx QOD over 5 weeks. 85% underwent BCT (of whom 61% received RT boost); 29% LN+; 14% underwent regional nodal RT. MFU 9.3 years. No difference in 10-yr LRR between 41.6 Gy and 50 Gy (6.3% vs. 7.4%; HR 0.91, p = .65) or 39 Gy and 50 Gy (8.8% vs. 7.4%; HR 1.18, p = .41). **START B:** 2,215 pts randomized to 50 Gy/25 fx over 5 weeks versus 40 Gy/15 fx over 3 weeks. 92% underwent BCT; 23% LN+; 7% underwent regional nodal RT. MFU 9.9 years. No difference in 10-yr LRR between 40 Gy and 50 Gy (4.3% vs. 5.5%; HR 0.77, p = .21). Breast shrinkage, telangiectasia, and breast edema were significantly less common with 40 Gy than with 50 Gy. **Conclusion: Hypofractionated WBI is safe and effective for pts with early breast cancer. Based on START-B, 40 Gy/15 fx is the current UK standard of care.**

Whelan, Canadian OCOG 93-010 (*NEJM* 2010, PMID 20147717; Update Bane, *Annals Oncol* 2014, PMID 24562444): PRT of 1,234 pts with pT1-2 pN0 breast cancer, negative margins, separation <25 cm, s/p lumpectomy/ALND randomized to 42.5 Gy/16 fx (2.66 Gy/fx) versus 50 Gy/25 fx. RT was by two opposed tangents with 2D planning and wedges; no boost, no regional nodal RT. MFU 12 years. 25%were <50 y/o, 33% T2, 26% ER-. Chemo used in only 11%, tamoxifen in 41%. Grade 3 skin toxicity or fibrosis at 10-yr was 3% to 4% in both arms. No grade 4 ulceration or necrosis. No difference in outcomes between arms, including LR, OS, and cosmesis. On subgroup analysis, LR of high-grade tumors in hypofractionation arm was 15.6% versus 4.7% in conventional arm (p = .01). An updated subgroup analysis found HER2+ was most significant predictor of IBTR, regardless of fractionation. **Conclusion: Accelerated, hypofractionated WBI is similar to conventionally fractionated RT for women with negative-margin BCS, pN0, breast separation <25 cm.**

TABLE 21.12: OCOG 93-010 Hypofractionation Trial Results					
	10-yr LR	Excellent/Good Cosmesis	Grade 3 Skin Toxicity	10-yr DSS	10-yr OS
42.5 Gy/16 fx	6.2%	70%	2.5%	87%	84%
50 Gy/25 fx	6.7%	71%	2.7%	87%	84%

Which patients benefit from a tumor bed boost?

The EORTC 22881 and Lyon trials demonstrated that a tumor bed boost reduces IBTR compared to WBI alone. The relative risk reduction was observed in all age subsets proportionally, although the absolute risk reduction was greatest in younger women.[49,50] A boost does not improve DFS or OS, and is associated with an increase in fibrosis and telangiectasia rates.[51] Predictive factors of IBTR include younger age, high grade, and associated DCIS.[52]

Bartelink, EORTC 22881 (*NEJM* 2001, PMID 11794170; Update *JCO* 2007, PMID 17577015; Update *Lancet Oncol* 2015, PMID 25500422; Update Vrieling *JAMA Oncol* 2017, PMID 27607734): PRT of 5,569 pts with stage I-II (T1-2, N0-1), age ≤70, treated with lumpectomy + RT (50 Gy). For negative margins (95% of pts), pts randomized to either no boost or 16 Gy boost to tumor bed + 1.5-cm margin (by electrons, tangential photons or Ir-192 implant). For positive margins (5%), pts randomized to low dose boost (10 Gy) or high dose boost (26 Gy); however, these pts were excluded from this analysis. 90% cN0, 78% pN0. Pts with negative margins treated with a boost had a significantly lower rate of LR (4% vs. 7% at 5-yr, p < .0001; 6% vs. 10% at 10-yr, p < .0001). A boost reduced the number of salvage mastectomies by 41%. DMFS and OS were similar in both groups. All age subsets benefited proportionally from a boost, although the absolute risk reduction was greatest in younger women.

TABLE 21.13: EORTC Boost Trial Results						
10-yr LR rates	Overall	Age ≤40	41–50	51–60	61–70	Fibrosis
No boost	10.2%	23.9%	12.5%	7.8%	7.3%	1.6%
16 Gy boost	6.2%	13.5%	8.7%	4.9%	3.8%	4.4%
p value	<.0001	.0014	.0099	.0157	.0008	<.0001

Romestaing, Lyon Trial (JCO 1997, PMID 9060534): PRT of 1,024 pts <70 y/o with breast cancers ≤3 cm, treated with lumpectomy (1 cm surgical margin) + WBI (50 Gy/20 fx) and randomized to electron boost (10 Gy/4 fx). 98% had negative margins. Pts treated with boost had significantly lower LR at 3.3 yrs (3.6% vs. 4.5%, p = .044). There was no difference in self-reported cosmetic outcomes (>90% good/excellent), but higher rates of telangiectasias.

What is the role of IMRT in early-stage breast cancer?

Compared to older 2D techniques, IMRT improved dosimetry and was associated with lower acute toxicity. A randomized trial showed negative change in breast appearance by photographs in 58% of pts randomized to 2D versus 40% for those randomized to IMRT.[53] Another randomized trial of IMRT versus 2D showed improved dose homogeneity and reduced moist desquamation with IMRT.[54] IMRT has been studied as a technique to deliver a simultaneous integrated boost, 45 Gy/25 fx with SIB to 56 Gy, with 5-yr LR of 2.7%.[55] However, no trial has compared IMRT to 3D-CRT techniques, and 3D-CRT is likely sufficient to provide adequate dose homogeneity in most patients.

What is the role of cardiac-sparing RT techniques?

Darby et al. found that rates of major coronary events (MI, coronary revascularization, or death from ischemic heart disease) after breast RT increased linearly with mean heart dose by a relative risk of 7.4% per Gy (p < .001) with no apparent threshold.[56] Cardiac-sparing techniques for left-sided breast RT include selective use of a heart block (as long as target coverage is not compromised), deep inspiration breath hold (DIBH), and prone positioning. In current trials (RTOG 1005, NSABP B-51) mean heart dose <4 Gy is ideal (<5 Gy acceptable), although "ALARA" principles apply. In series using older RT techniques, left-sided breast cancer pts had higher risk of cardiac mortality.[57] Using modern RT techniques, laterality does not appear to influence survival.[58]

Darby (NEJM 2013, PMID 23484825): Population-based case-control study of 2,168 women undergoing RT in Sweden & Denmark from 1958 to 2001. Primary end point was major coronary events (MCE: myocardial infarction, coronary revascularization, or death from ischemic heart disease). Mean heart dose (MHD) was 4.9 Gy (6.6 Gy for left-sided, 2.9 Gy for right-sided). MCE rates increased linearly with MHD by a relative risk of 7.4% per Gy (p < .001) with no apparent threshold; but did not correlate with mean dose to left anterior descending artery. The increase in MCE started within 5 yrs of RT and continued >20 yrs. However, absolute event rates remain low: for an average 50 y/o woman without baseline cardiac risk factors, a MHD of 3 Gy would increase absolute risk of cardiac death before age 80 above baseline by 0.5% (from 1.9% to 2.4%) and risk of acute coronary event by 0.9% (from 4.5% to 5.4%). Women with pre-existing cardiac disease have higher *absolute* risk of MCE, but RT had similar *relative* effects in women with or without pre-existing cardiac risk factors. *Comment: Examined outdated RT techniques; cardiac doses were estimated by "virtual simulation" onto a woman with "typical anatomy."*

What is the role of endocrine therapy in BCT? Are there some patients in whom RT may be omitted after lumpectomy?

NSABP B-21 showed that adjuvant tamoxifen alone is inferior to RT alone, but together they act synergistically to reduce IBTR in low-risk pts undergoing BCT. Omission of RT may be considered in carefully selected pts with T1N0, ER/PR+, HER2-, negative margins, who are older (>65–70 y/o) or with reduced life expectancy, and who are committed to taking 5 years of endocrine therapy (~30%–40% stop endocrine therapy before completion of 5 years). Multiple trials (Table 21.17) have studied omission of RT in pts low at low risk for recurrence—none were powered to observe a difference in DFS or OS, and there remains an increased risk of IBTR in the absence of RT.[59-64] Overall, careful consideration of risks/benefits and life expectancy are required, and pts who decline adjuvant RT must be willing to accept a higher risk of IBTR and commit to taking endocrine therapy for at least 5 years.

Fisher, NSABP B-21 (*JCO* 2002, PMID 12377957): PRT of 1,009 pts (54%–59% ER+) with ≤1 cm, N0 breast cancer, randomized after WLE to post-op tamoxifen alone, WBI alone, or WBI + tamoxifen (20 mg QD x 5 yrs). No ER testing was performed. RT was 50 Gy/25 fx; 25% received 10 Gy boost at clinician discretion.

TABLE 21.14: NSABP B-21 Results			
	8-yr IBTR	8-yr CBC	8-yr OS
WLE + Tamoxifen	16.5%	2.2%	93%
WLE + WBI	9.3%	5.4%	94%
WLE + WBI + Tamoxifen	2.8%	2.2%	93%

Fyles, PMH (*NEJM* 2004, PMID 15342804; Update Liu *JCO* 2015, PMID 25964246): PRT of 769 pts age ≥50 y/o with T1-2N0 (>80% ER+), treated with lumpectomy + tamoxifen ± WBI (40 Gy/16 fx + 12.5 Gy/5 fx boost). At 5 yrs, tamoxifen + WBI arm had better LR (0.6% vs. 7.7%), axillary recurrence (0.5% vs. 2.5%), and DFS (91% vs. 85%), but no difference in DM or OS. For subset of T1 and ER+ pts, LR rates were 0.4% vs. 5.9%. At *ASTRO* 2006 update, the 8-yr IBTR was 4.1% versus 12.2% ($p < .0001$) and 8-yr DFS was 82% versus 76% ($p = .05$) in favor of WBI. 8-yr OS was same at 89%. On MVA after stratifying by IHC biomarkers, RT use, clinical risk group, and luminal A subtype were associated with IBTR. **Conclusion: Lumpectomy followed by WBI + tamoxifen is superior to tamoxifen alone for women over age 50.**

Hughes, CALGB 9343 (*NEJM* 2004, 351:971 PMID 15342805; Update *JCO* 2013, PMID 23690420): PRT of 636 pts age ≥70 with cT1N0, ER+, treated with lumpectomy (axillary staging not performed on all patients) + tamoxifen ± RT (45 Gy/25 fx + 14 Gy/7 fx boost). RT arm had significantly lower LRR (1% vs. 4% at 5-yr, $p < .001$), but no difference in rates of mastectomy, DM, or OS (87% vs. 86%) compared to tamoxifen alone. Of the 334 deaths, only 21 were due to breast cancer. **Conclusion: Lumpectomy followed by tamoxifen alone may be an option for T1N0, ER+ pts over 70 y/o, but have higher LR rate by the omission of RT.**

TABLE 21.15: CALGB 9343 Hughes Trial Results				
	10-yr LRR	Mastectomy-Free	10-yr DM-Free	10-yr OS
BCS + tamoxifen + WBI	2%	98%	95%	67%
BCS + tamoxifen	10%	96%	95%	66%
p value	<.001	.17	.50	.64

Kunkler, PRIME II (*Lancet Oncol* 2015, PMID 25637340): PRT of 1,326 pts with age ≥65, T1-2 (≤3 cm), negative margins (≥1 mm), s/p ALND or SLNB, randomized to tamoxifen +/− RT (WBI 40–50 Gy/15–25 fx +/− boost 10–20 Gy). Pts could have G3 or LVSI+ but not both. MFU 5 years. 5-yr IBTR rates were 1% versus 4% in favor of RT arm, but no difference in DM or OS. Unplanned subgroup analysis by ER score showed a decrease in LR in ER rich versus ER poor (1.2% vs. 10.3%) without RT and with RT (3.3% vs. 0%). **Conclusion: Supports CALGB**

9343 in considering adjuvant endocrine therapy alone for low-risk patients; longer follow-up will be important to assess the impact on DM and OS.

TABLE 21.16: PRIME II Trial Results

	5-yr IBTR	5-yr DM	5-yr OS
BCS + tamoxifen + WBI	1.3%	0.5%	93.9%
BCS + tamoxifen	4.1%	1.0%	93.9%
p value	.0002		.34

What is the role of intraoperative radiation (IORT) in early breast cancer?

Two large prospective randomized trials have demonstrated higher rates of LR following IORT compared to WBI. Advantages to IORT include improved patient convenience, less absolute cost, and less acute skin erythema due to rapid dose falloff. Disadvantages to IORT include lack of long-term efficacy data, no pathology information available at the time of treatment, inability to visualize dose to normal structures, longer anesthesia time, and limited availability. Some are concerned that the dose falloff may be too steep, as evidenced by the increased risk of LR.

Vaidya, TARGIT-A (*Lancet* 2010, PMID 20570343; Update *Lancet* 2014, PMID 24224997): Phase III noninferiority trial of WBI versus IORT in 3,451 pts ≥45 y/o with clinically unifocal IDC. Pts stratified by timing: some pts randomized before surgery (prepathology) and others after final pathology, in which case IORT was given in a second procedure (postpathology). For prepathology pts who already received IORT, if final pathology revealed high-risk disease (ILC, EIC, or a site-specific criterion such as grade III, LN+, or LVI+), WBI was given, omitting the tumor bed boost (after re-excision to achieve negative margins if applicable). For postpathology pts, these high-risk pathologic features were excluded, and thus only lower risk women were randomized. WBI varied by center (typically 40–56 Gy +/– boost of 10–16 Gy). IORT was 20 Gy to cavity surface (~5–7 Gy at 1 cm) with 50 kV photons via Intrabeam®. 15% of pts randomized to IORT received WBI (21.6% prepathology, 3.6% postpathology). At MFU 2.4 yrs, 5-yr IBTR was 1.3% in WBI arm and 3.3% in IORT arm (*p* = .04, within noninferiority design). IBTR was higher with IORT in postpathology pts 5.4% versus 1.7% (*p* = .069) but not in prepathology pts. **Conclusion: For selected low-risk pts with early-stage breast cancer, IORT may be considered as an alternative to standard WBI, although IBTR rates were higher and MFU remains short (2.4 yrs).**

Veronesi, ELIOT Trial (*Lancet Oncol* 2013, PMID 24225155): 1,305 pts age 48 to 75 y/o with unicentric tumors <2.5 cm s/p quadrantectomy, randomized to WBI (50 Gy/25 fx + 10 Gy boost) versus ELIOT (21 Gy/1 fx prescribed to 90% IDL using 3–12 MeV electrons). Equivalence trial design with primary end point of IBTR. 89% received endocrine therapy. 5-yr LR was 0.4% with WBI and 4.4% with ELIOT (*p* < .0001). 5-yr OS same at >96%. Overall toxicity favored the ELIOT group (*p* = .0002), due to lower incidence of skin erythema (*p* < .0001), dry skin (*p* = .04), hyperpigmentation (*p* = .0004), breast edema (*p* = .004), and breast itching (*p* = .002). However, ELIOT had higher fat tissue necrosis. **Conclusion: ELIOT has higher rate of IBTR than WBI.**

TABLE 21.17: Select Prospective Trials of WBI Versus no WBI (Either Hormonal Therapy Alone or With Intraoperative Radiotherapy) for Low-Risk Pts

IBTR	N/FU	Eligibility	% Hormone Therapy	WBI	IORT	HT only	*p*
PRIME II Kunkler 2015[61]	N = 1,326 5 yrs	Age ≥65 ≤3 cm	100%	1.3% (5-yr)		4.1% (5-yr)	.0002

(continued)

IBTR	N/FU	Eligibility	% Hormone Therapy	WBI	IORT	HT only	p
TABLE 21.17: Select Prospective Trials of WBI Versus no WBI (Either Hormonal Therapy Alone or With Intraoperative Radiotherapy) for Low-Risk Pts (*continued*)							
CALGB 9343 Hughes 2013[60]	N = 636 12.6 yrs	Age ≥70 ≤2 cm, ER+	100%	1% (5-yr) 2% (10-yr)		4% (5-yr) 10% (10-yr)	<.001
NSABP B-21 Fisher 2002[59]	N = 1,009 8 yrs	≤1 cm	100% (+tam) 0% (−tam)	2.8% (+tam) 9.3% (−tam)		16.5% (8-yr)	<.0001
TARGIT-A Vaidya 2014[65]	N = 3,451 2.5 yrs	Age ≥45 87% ≤2 cm	NR (93% ER+)	1.3% (5-yr)	3.3% (5-yr) *15% received WBI		.042
ELIOT Veronesi 2013[66]	N = 1,305 5.8 yrs	Age 48–75 ≤2.5 cm	89%	0.4% (5-yr)	4.4% (5-yr)		<.0001

In whom is accelerated partial breast irradiation (APBI) acceptable?

The rationale for APBI is that the majority of recurrences after BCT are seen at or near the tumor bed (~80%), and irradiation of this region alone instead of the entire breast may eradicate residual disease while maintaining acceptable cosmesis and toxicity outcomes.[67–69] *In addition, the prolonged course of conventional WBI has been an obstacle in the wider use of BCT.*[70] *Advantages of PBI include: shorter treatment time of ~5 to 15 days, potentially less tumor repopulation between surgery and RT, and potentially better cosmesis (depending on technique).*[69] *Disadvantages of PBI include: lack of long-term data with some APBI techniques (and outstanding long-term outcomes with the alternative hypofractionated WBI), potential for unknown late effects with high fractional doses, twice daily treatment with many of the techniques (which may not be convenient for some pts), and more intensive physicist/physician time. Accepted APBI selection criteria are listed in Tables 21.18 and 21.19.*[71,72]

TABLE 21.18: Eligibility Criteria for APBI Based on Professional Society Recommendations			
	ABS	ASBS	NSABP B-39/ RTOG 0413
Age	50 yrs	Invasive 45 yrs; DCIS 50 yrs	18 yrs
Histology	Invasive or DCIS	IDC, DCIS	Unifocal IDC, DCIS
Size	≤3 cm	≤3 cm	≤3 cm
Margins	Negative	Negative	Negative
Nodes	N0	N0	0-3+ LN
LVSI	No	-	-
Estrogen Receptor	Positive or Negative	-	-

TABLE 21.19: 2017 ASTRO Consensus Guidelines for APBI Suitability[72]		
Suitable	**Cautionary**	**Unsuitable**
Age ≥50 yrs Margins ≥2 mm T1 Tis (DCIS), if: screen-detected, low–intermediate grade, ≤2.5 cm, AND margins ≥3 mm	Age 40–49 if all other suitable criteria met. Age ≥50 yrs if at least one pathologic factor in the following and no unsuitable factors: • Clinically unifocal with total size 2.1–3.0 cm • Margins <2 mm • Limited/focal LVSI • ER-negative • Invasive lobular histology • Pure DCIS ≤3 cm if suitable criteria not met • EIC ≤3 cm	Age <40 yrs Margins positive Size >3 cm (invasive or DCIS) Age 40–49 and does not meet cautionary criteria Node positive

Is APBI safe and effective compared to standard WBI?

To date, seven modern randomized trials evaluating various techniques of APBI as compared to WBI have been published in either abstract or manuscript form (Table 21.19), and all have demonstrated similar rates of IBTR between APBI and WBI. The most mature trial utilized primarily interstitial brachytherapy, and demonstrated no difference in clinical outcomes with improved cosmesis noted with brachytherapy compared to WBI.[73] The GEC-ESTRO trial found no difference in IBTR rates or cosmetic outcomes, with reduced late grade 2-3 skin toxicity with APBI.[73–75] Several prospective trials have evaluated external beam based APBI. The RAPID trial utilized APBI by 3D-CRT (38.5 Gy/10 fx BID), and found increased grade 1–2 toxicity and worse cosmetic outcomes with APBI compared to WBI.[76] Concerns regarding toxicity outcomes from 3D-CRT APBI using similar dose fractionation were noted in other institutional series as well but not an interim analysis of NSABP B-39.[77–79] APBI by IMRT with or without altered fractionation (daily RT as in IMPORT LOW, or every other day RT as in University of Florence trial) may improve outcomes further.[80]

NSABP B-39/RTOG 0413 is the largest PRT completed to date, with over 4,300 pts with stage 0-II (≤3 cm) breast cancer or DCIS s/p lumpectomy with negative margins and 0-3 LN+ randomized to WBI (50 Gy with optional 10 Gy boost) versus APBI via either multicatheter brachytherapy (34 Gy/10 fx BID), intracavity brachytherapy (MammoSite® 34 Gy/10 fx BID), or 3D-CRT (38.5 Gy/10 fx BID). An interim analysis of 3D-CRT APBI pts found low rates of grade 3 fibrosis and no grade 4/5 fibrosis.[81]

TABLE 21.20: Randomized Trials of APBI Versus WBI						
	N/FU	**Eligibility**	**Technique**	**Dose**	**IBTR**	**Toxicity**
Hungary[73] Polgar 2013	258 10.2 yrs	pT1, pN0-1mi, Gr 1–2, nonlobular, neg margins, age >40	Interstitial or electrons	36.4 Gy/7 fx (IB) 50 Gy/25 fx (e-)	5.9% vs. 5.1%	PBI improved cosmesis (81% vs. 63%)
GEC-ESTRO[75] Strnad 2016	1,184 6.6 yrs	pT1-2 (<3 cm), pN0-1mi, IDC/ILC/DCIS, margins >2 mm, no LVSI, age >40	Interstitial	32 Gy/8 fx or 30.2 Gy/7 fx (HDR), 50 Gy (PDR)	1.4% vs. 0.9%	APBI reduced breast pain, less late gr 2–3 skin toxicity

(continued)

TABLE 21.20: Randomized Trials of APBI Versus WBI (continued)

	N/FU	Eligibility	Technique	Dose	IBTR	Toxicity
Florence[80] Livi 2015	520 5.0 yrs	pT1-2 (<2.5 cm), Neg margins, clips in cavity, age >40	IMRT	30 Gy/5 fx QOD	1.5% vs. 1.5%	APBI less toxicity
Barcelona[82] Rodriguez 2013	102 5.0 yrs	pT1-2 (<3 cm), N0, gr 1–2, IDC, neg margins, age >60	3D-CRT	37.5 Gy/10 fx	0%	Lower rates of late toxicity with APBI, no difference in cosmesis
RAPID[76] Olivotto 2013	2,135 3.0 yrs	pT1-2 (<2 cm), pN0, IDC/DCIS, neg margins, age >40	3D-CRT	38.5 Gy/10 fx BID	NR	APBI increased gr 1–2 toxicity, adverse cosmesis
NSABP B-39 Closed/NR	4,300 3.5 yrs	pT1-2 (<3 cm), pN0-1 (no ECE, cN0), invasive or DCIS, neg margins, age >18	3D-CRT or brachy (interstitial/ applicator)	38.5 Gy/10 fx BID (3D), 34 Gy/10 fx BID (brachy)	NR	3D subset: gr 2 fibrosis 12%, gr 3 3%, no gr 4–5
IMPORT LOW[83] Coles 2017	2,018 6.0 yrs	pT1-2 (<3 cm), N0-1, Invasive adenocarcinoma, margins ≥2 mm, age ≥50	IMRT	40 Gy/15 fx WBRT vs. 36 Gy WBRT+40 Gy APBI vs. 40 Gy/15 APBI	1.1% vs. 0.2% vs. 0.5%	Reduced toxicity in both experimental arms

What APBI techniques are available and how do they differ?

APBI can be delivered via interstitial brachytherapy, intracavitary brachytherapy, or EBRT. See Table 21.21 for details.

TABLE 21.21: Techniques of APBI

Interstitial brachytherapy	APBI technique with longest follow-up.[84,85] Catheters are placed through the breast tissue in 1.0- to 1.5-cm intervals. Primary limitation is technical complexity with few practitioners having expertise. *Dose:* 34 Gy/10 fx, 32 Gy/8 fx, 30.2 Gy, or 36.4 Gy/7 fx, usually delivered BID with 6-hour interfraction interval. *Target:* PTV = tumor cavity + 15 mm and limited by 5 mm from skin and posterior breast tissue.
Intracavity brachytherapy	MammoSite® was the first intracavitary device approved by the FDA in May 2002.[86] Advantages of this technique include ease of use and reproducibility. A silicone balloon is connected to a double-lumen catheter with an inflation channel and port for passage of the HDR source. A cavity evaluation device can be placed in the cavity at the time of surgery, which is replaced by the treatment device postoperatively (after pathology confirmation) under ultrasound guidance. The balloon is filled with saline (30–70 cc) and mixed with a small amount of contrast (1–2 cc) to achieve a diameter of 4–6 cm.

(continued)

TABLE 21.21: Techniques of APBI (*continued*)	
	This allows visualization of the device for treatment planning and opposes the balloon wall to the tumor bed. At the completion of treatment, the catheter is removed in an outpatient setting. The most robust data with applicator APBI comes from the MammoSite® registry, which demonstrated a 5-yr LR rate of 3.8% with low toxicity.[87,88] Though population-based data have suggested higher rates of toxicity and subsequent mastectomy, this has not been validated prospectively.[89,90] More recently, multilumen and strut applicators have been developed, which can improve target coverage and allow for smaller skin spacing. Initial studies evaluating these options have demonstrated good clinical outcomes and low toxicity rates.[91,92] *Dose*: 34 Gy/10 fx BID with 6-hour interfraction interval. *Target*: PTV = tumor cavity + 10 mm, and limited by 5 mm from skin and posterior breast tissue. *Exclusion criteria*: Air/fluid >10% PTV_EVAL, skin spacing or chest wall spacing <3–5 mm (ideally want ≥7 mm with single-lumen devices), poor cavity delineation.
EBRT	Noninvasive technique, with advantages including widespread availability, fewer technical/QA demands, and potentially better dose homogeneity. *Dose*: 38.5 Gy/10 fx BID, 40 Gy/15 fx QD, or 30 Gy/5 fx QOD (IMRT). *Target*: CTV = tumor cavity + 1.5 cm (limited by 5 mm from skin posterior breast tissue); PTV = CTV + 10 mm, excluding volume outside breast and 5 mm from skin, and beyond posterior breast.

REFERENCES

1. Clarke M, Collins R, Darby S, et al. Effects of radiotherapy and of differences in the extent of surgery for early breast cancer on local recurrence and 15-year survival: an overview of the randomised trials. *Lancet*. 2005;366(9503):2087–2106.
2. Siegel RL, Miller KD, Jemal A. Cancer Statistics, 2017. *Cancer J Clin*. 2017;67(1):7–30.
3. van de Vijver MJ, He YD, van't Veer LJ, et al. A gene-expression signature as a predictor of survival in breast cancer. *N Engl J Med*. 2002;347(25):1999–2009.
4. Paik S, Shak S, Tang G, et al. A multigene assay to predict recurrence of tamoxifen-treated, node-negative breast cancer. *N Engl J Med*. 2004;351(27):2817–2826.
5. Perou CM, Sorlie T, Eisen MB, et al. Molecular portraits of human breast tumours. *Nature*. 2000;406(6797):747–752.
6. Maisonneuve P, Disalvatore D, Rotmensz N, et al. Proposed new clinicopathological surrogate definitions of luminal A and luminal B (HER2-negative) intrinsic breast cancer subtypes. *Breast Cancer Res*. 2014;16(3):R65.
7. Mainiero MB, Lourenco A, Mahoney MC, et al. ACR Appropriateness criteria breast cancer screening. *J Am Coll Radiol*. 2016;13(11S):R45–R49.
8. U.S. Preventive Services Task Force. Screening for breast cancer: U.S. Preventive Services Task Force recommendation statement. *Ann Intern Med*. 2009;151(10):716–726, W-236.
9. Smart CR, Hartmann WH, Beahrs OH, Garfinkel L. Insights into breast cancer screening of younger women: evidence from the 14-year follow-up of the Breast Cancer Detection Demonstration Project. *Cancer*. 1993;72(4 Suppl):1449–1456.
10. Vanel D. The American College of Radiology (ACR) Breast Imaging and Reporting Data System (BI-RADS): a step towards a universal radiological language? *Eur J Radiol*. 2007;61(2):183.
11. Saslow D, Boetes C, Burke W, et al. American Cancer Society guidelines for breast screening with MRI as an adjunct to mammography. *CA Cancer J Clin*. 2007;57(2):75–89.
12. Tillman GF, Orel SG, Schnall MD, et al. Effect of breast magnetic resonance imaging on the clinical management of women with early-stage breast carcinoma. *J Clin Oncol*. 2002;20(16):3413–3423.
13. Houssami N, Turner R, Morrow M. Preoperative magnetic resonance imaging in breast cancer: meta-analysis of surgical outcomes. *Ann Surg*. 2013;257(2):249–255.
14. Houssami N, Turner R, Macaskill P, et al. An individual person data meta-analysis of preoperative magnetic resonance imaging and breast cancer recurrence. *J Clin Oncol*. 2014;32(5):392–401.

15. Hattangadi-Gluth JA, Wo JY, Nguyen PL, et al. Basal subtype of invasive breast cancer is associated with a higher risk of true recurrence after conventional breast-conserving therapy. *Int J Radiat Oncol Biol Phys*. 2012;82(3):1185–1191.

16. Recht A, Come SE, Henderson IC, et al. The sequencing of chemotherapy and radiation therapy after conservative surgery for early-stage breast cancer. *N Engl J Med*. 1996;334(21):1356–1361.

17. Bellon JR, Come SE, Gelman RS, et al. Sequencing of chemotherapy and radiation therapy in early-stage breast cancer: updated results of a prospective randomized trial. *J Clin Oncol* 2005;23(9):1934–1940.

18. Punglia RS, Morrow M, Winer EP, Harris JR. Local therapy and survival in breast cancer. *N Engl J Med*. 2007;356(23):2399–2405.

19. Fisher B, Costantino JP, Wickerham DL, et al. Tamoxifen for the prevention of breast cancer: current status of the National Surgical Adjuvant Breast and Bowel Project P-1 study. *J Natl Cancer Inst*. 2005;97(22):1652–1662.

20. Vogel VG, Costantino JP, Wickerham DL, et al. Update of the National Surgical Adjuvant Breast and Bowel Project Study of Tamoxifen and Raloxifene (STAR) P-2 Trial: preventing breast cancer. *Cancer Prev Res (Phila)*. 2010;3(6):696–706.

21. Hartmann LC, Schaid DJ, Woods JE, et al. Efficacy of bilateral prophylactic mastectomy in women with a family history of breast cancer. *N Engl J Med*. 1999;340(2):77–84.

22. Eisen A, Lubinski J, Klijn J, et al. Breast cancer risk following bilateral oophorectomy in BRCA1 and BRCA2 mutation carriers: an international case-control study. *J Clin Oncol*. 2005;23(30):7491–7496.

23. Moran MS, Schnitt SJ, Giuliano AE, et al. Society of Surgical Oncology-American Society for Radiation Oncology consensus guideline on margins for breast-conserving surgery with whole-breast irradiation in stages I and II invasive breast cancer. *Int J Radiat Oncol Biol Phys*. 2014;88(3):553–564.

24. Veronesi U, Paganelli G, Viale G, et al. Sentinel-lymph-node biopsy as a staging procedure in breast cancer: update of a randomised controlled study. *Lancet Oncol*. 2006;7(12):983–990.

25. Smith I, Procter M, Gelber RD, et al. Two-year follow-up of trastuzumab after adjuvant chemotherapy in HER2-positive breast cancer: a randomised controlled trial. *Lancet*. 2007;369(9555):29–36.

26. Henderson IC, Berry DA, Demetri GD, et al. Improved outcomes from adding sequential Paclitaxel but not from escalating Doxorubicin dose in an adjuvant chemotherapy regimen for patients with node-positive primary breast cancer. *J Clin Oncol*. 2003;21(6):976–983.

27. Martin M, Pienkowski T, Mackey J, et al. Adjuvant docetaxel for node-positive breast cancer. *N Engl J Med*. 2005;352(22):2302–2313.

28. Citron ML, Berry DA, Cirrincione C, et al. Randomized trial of dose-dense versus conventionally scheduled and sequential versus concurrent combination chemotherapy as postoperative adjuvant treatment of node-positive primary breast cancer: first report of Intergroup Trial C9741/ Cancer and Leukemia Group B Trial 9741. *J Clin Oncol*. 2003;21(8):1431–1439.

29. Davies C, Pan H, Godwin J, et al. Long-term effects of continuing adjuvant tamoxifen to 10 years versus stopping at 5 years after diagnosis of oestrogen receptor-positive breast cancer: ATLAS, a randomised trial. *Lancet*. 2013;381(9869):805–816.

30. Baum M, Budzar AU, Cuzick J, et al. Anastrozole alone or in combination with tamoxifen versus tamoxifen alone for adjuvant treatment of postmenopausal women with early breast cancer: first results of the ATAC randomised trial. *Lancet*. 2002;359(9324):2131–2139.

31. Dowsett M, Forbes JF, Bradley R, et al. Aromatase inhibitors versus tamoxifen in early breast cancer: patient-level meta-analysis of the randomised trials. *Lancet*. 2015;386(10001):1341–1352.

32. Recht A, Come SE, Gelman RS, et al. Integration of conservative surgery, radiotherapy, and chemotherapy for the treatment of early-stage, node-positive breast cancer: sequencing, timing, and outcome. *J Clin Oncol*. 1991;9(9):1662–1667.

33. Videtic GMM, Woody N, Vassil AD. *Handbook of Treatment Planning in Radiation Oncology*. 2nd ed. New York, NY: Demos Medical; 2015.

34. Buchholz TA. Radiation therapy for early-stage breast cancer after breast-conserving surgery. *N Engl J Med*. 2009;360(1):63–70.

35. Jacobson JA, Danforth DN, Cowan KH, et al. Ten-year results of a comparison of conservation with mastectomy in the treatment of stage I and II breast cancer. *N Engl J Med*. 1995;332(14):907–911.

36. van Dongen JA, Voogd AC, Fentiman IS, et al. Long-term results of a randomized trial comparing breast-conserving therapy with mastectomy: European Organization for Research and Treatment of Cancer 10801 trial. *J Natl Cancer Inst.* 2000;92(14):1143–1150.

37. Veronesi U, Cascinelli N, Mariani L, et al. Twenty-year follow-up of a randomized study comparing breast-conserving surgery with radical mastectomy for early breast cancer. *N Engl J Med.* 2002;347(16):1227–1232.

38. Arriagada R, Le MG, Rochard F, Contesso G. Conservative treatment versus mastectomy in early breast cancer: patterns of failure with 15 years of follow-up data. Institut Gustave-Roussy Breast Cancer Group. *J Clin Oncol.* 1996;14(5):1558–1564.

39. Fisher B, Anderson S, Bryant J, et al. Twenty-year follow-up of a randomized trial comparing total mastectomy, lumpectomy, and lumpectomy plus irradiation for the treatment of invasive breast cancer. *N Engl J Med.* 2002;347(16):1233–1241.

40. Blichert-Toft M, Rose C, Andersen JA, et al. Danish randomized trial comparing breast conservation therapy with mastectomy: six years of life-table analysis. Danish Breast Cancer Cooperative Group. *J Natl Cancer Inst Monogr.* 1992;(11):19–25.

41. Holland R, Veling SH, Mravunac M, Hendriks JH. Histologic multifocality of Tis, T1-2 breast carcinomas: implications for clinical trials of breast-conserving surgery. *Cancer.* 1985;56(5):979–990.

42. Darby S, McGale P, Correa C, et al. Effect of radiotherapy after breast-conserving surgery on 10-year recurrence and 15-year breast cancer death: meta-analysis of individual patient data for 10,801 women in 17 randomised trials. *Lancet.* 2011;378(9804):1707–1716.

43. Whelan TJ, Olivotto IA, Parulekar WR, et al. Regional nodal irradiation in early-stage breast cancer. *N Engl J Med.* 2015;373(4):307–316.

44. Poortmans PM, Collette S, Kirkove C, et al. Internal mammary and medial supraclavicular irradiation in breast cancer. *N Engl J Med.* 2015;373(4):317–327.

45. Smith BD, Bentzen SM, Correa CR, et al. Fractionation for whole breast irradiation: an American Society for Radiation Oncology (ASTRO) evidence-based guideline. *Int J Radiat Oncol Biol Phys.* 2011;81(1):59–68.

46. Yarnold J, Ashton A, Bliss J, et al. Fractionation sensitivity and dose response of late adverse effects in the breast after radiotherapy for early breast cancer: long-term results of a randomised trial. *Radiother Oncol.* 2005;75(1):9–17.

47. Haviland JS, Owen JR, Dewar JA, et al. The UK Standardisation of Breast Radiotherapy (START) trials of radiotherapy hypofractionation for treatment of early breast cancer: 10-year follow-up results of two randomised controlled trials. *Lancet Oncol.* 2013;14(11):1086–1094.

48. Whelan TJ, Pignol JP, Levine MN, et al. Long-term results of hypofractionated radiation therapy for breast cancer. *N Engl J Med.* 2010;362(6):513–520.

49. Bartelink H, Horiot JC, Poortmans PM, et al. Impact of a higher radiation dose on local control and survival in breast-conserving therapy of early breast cancer: 10-year results of the randomized boost versus no boost EORTC 22881-10882 trial. *J Clin Oncol.* 2007;25(22):3259–3265.

50. Romestaing P, Lehingue Y, Carrie C, et al. Role of a 10-Gy boost in the conservative treatment of early breast cancer: results of a randomized clinical trial in Lyon, France. *J Clin Oncol.* 1997;15(3):963–968.

51. Bartelink H, Maingon P, Poortmans P, et al. Whole-breast irradiation with or without a boost for patients treated with breast-conserving surgery for early breast cancer: 20-year follow-up of a randomised phase 3 trial. *Lancet Oncol.* 2015;16(1):47–56.

52. Vrieling C, van Werkhoven E, Maingon P, et al. Prognostic factors for local control in breast cancer after long-term follow-up in the EORTC Boost vs No Boost Trial: a randomized clinical trial. *JAMA Oncol.* 2017;3(1):42–48.

53. Donovan E, Bleakley N, Denholm E, et al. Randomised trial of standard 2D radiotherapy (RT) versus intensity modulated radiotherapy (IMRT) in patients prescribed breast radiotherapy. *Radiother Oncol.* 2007;82(3):254–264.

54. Pignol JP, Olivotto I, Rakovitch E, et al. A multicenter randomized trial of breast intensity-modulated radiation therapy to reduce acute radiation dermatitis. *J Clin Oncol.* 2008;26(13):2085–2092.

55. Freedman GM, Anderson PR, Bleicher RJ, et al. Five-year local control in a phase II study of hypofractionated intensity modulated radiation therapy with an incorporated boost for early stage breast cancer. *Int J Radiat Oncol Biol Phys.* 2012;84(4):888–893.

56. Darby SC, Ewertz M, McGale P, et al. Risk of ischemic heart disease in women after radiotherapy for breast cancer. *N Engl J Med.* 2013;368(11):987–998.

57. Darby SC, McGale P, Taylor CW, Peto R. Long-term mortality from heart disease and lung cancer after radiotherapy for early breast cancer: prospective cohort study of about 300,000 women in US SEER cancer registries. *Lancet Oncol.* 2005;6(8):557–565.

58. Rutter CE, Chagpar AB, Evans SB. Breast cancer laterality does not influence survival in a large modern cohort: implications for radiation-related cardiac mortality. *Int J Radiat Oncol Biol Phys.* 2014;90(2):329–334.

59. Fisher B, Bryant J, Dignam JJ, et al. Tamoxifen, radiation therapy, or both for prevention of ipsilateral breast tumor recurrence after lumpectomy in women with invasive breast cancers of one centimeter or less. *J Clin Oncol.* 2002;20(20):4141–4149.

60. Hughes KS, Schnaper LA, Bellon JR, et al. Lumpectomy plus tamoxifen with or without irradiation in women age 70 years or older with early breast cancer: long-term follow-up of CALGB 9343. *J Clin Oncol.* 2013;31(19):2382–2387.

61. Kunkler IH, Williams LJ, Jack WJ, Cameron DA, Dixon JM. Breast-conserving surgery with or without irradiation in women aged 65 years or older with early breast cancer (PRIME II): a randomised controlled trial. *Lancet Oncol.* 2015;16(3):266–273.

62. Fyles AW, McCready DR, Manchul LA, et al. Tamoxifen with or without breast irradiation in women 50 years of age or older with early breast cancer. *N Engl J Med.* 2004;351(10):963–970.

63. Winzer KJ, Sauerbrei W, Braun M, et al. Radiation therapy and tamoxifen after breast-conserving surgery: updated results of a 2 x 2 randomised clinical trial in patients with low risk of recurrence. *Eur J Cancer.* 2010;46(1):95–101.

64. Potter R, Gnant M, Kwasny W, et al. Lumpectomy plus tamoxifen or anastrozole with or without whole breast irradiation in women with favorable early breast cancer. *Int J Radiat Oncol Biol Phys.* 2007;68(2):334–340.

65. Vaidya JS, Wenz F, Bulsara M, et al. Risk-adapted targeted intraoperative radiotherapy versus whole-breast radiotherapy for breast cancer: 5-year results for local control and overall survival from the TARGIT-A randomised trial. *Lancet.* 2014;383(9917):603–613.

66. Veronesi U, Orecchia R, Maisonneuve P, et al. Intraoperative radiotherapy versus external radiotherapy for early breast cancer (ELIOT): a randomised controlled equivalence trial. *Lancet Oncol.* 2013;14(13):1269–1277.

67. Gage I, Recht A, Gelman R, et al. Long-term outcome following breast-conserving surgery and radiation therapy. *Int J Radiat Oncol Biol Phys.* 1995;33(2):245–251.

68. Vicini FA, Kestin LL, Goldstein NS. Defining the clinical target volume for patients with early-stage breast cancer treated with lumpectomy and accelerated partial breast irradiation: a pathologic analysis. *Int J Radiat Oncol Biol Phys.* 2004;60(3):722–730.

69. Vicini F, Shah C, Tendulkar R, et al. Accelerated partial breast irradiation: An update on published level I evidence. *Brachytherapy.* 2016;15(5):607–615.

70. Morrow M, White J, Moughan J, et al. Factors predicting the use of breast-conserving therapy in stage I and II breast carcinoma. *J Clin Oncol.* 2001;19(8):2254–2262.

71. Shah C, Vicini F, Wazer DE, et al. The American Brachytherapy Society consensus statement for accelerated partial breast irradiation. *Brachytherapy.* 2013;12(4):267–277.

72. Correa C, Harris EE, Leonardi MC, et al. Accelerated partial breast irradiation: executive summary for the update of an ASTRO Evidence-Based Consensus Statement. *Pract Radiat Oncol.* 2017;7(2):73–79.

73. Polgar C, Fodor J, Major T, et al. Breast-conserving therapy with partial or whole breast irradiation: ten-year results of the Budapest randomized trial. *Radiother Oncol.* 2013;108(2):197–202.

74. Polgar C, Ott OJ, Hildebrandt G, et al. Late side-effects and cosmetic results of accelerated partial breast irradiation with interstitial brachytherapy versus whole-breast irradiation after breast-conserving surgery for low-risk invasive and in-situ carcinoma of the female breast: 5-year results of a randomised, controlled, phase 3 trial. *Lancet Oncol.* 2017;18(2):259–268.

75. Strnad V, Ott OJ, Hildebrandt G, et al. Five-year results of accelerated partial breast irradiation using sole interstitial multicatheter brachytherapy versus whole-breast irradiation with boost after breast-conserving surgery for low-risk invasive and in-situ carcinoma of the female breast: a randomised, phase 3, non-inferiority trial. *Lancet.* 2016;387(10015):229–238.

76. Olivotto IA, Whelan TJ, Parpia S, et al. Interim cosmetic and toxicity results from RAPID: a randomized trial of accelerated partial breast irradiation using three-dimensional conformal external beam radiation therapy. *J Clin Oncol.* 2013;31(32):4038–4045.

77. Liss AL, Ben-David MA, Jagsi R, et al. Decline of cosmetic outcomes following accelerated partial breast irradiation using intensity modulated radiation therapy: results of a single-institution prospective clinical trial. *Int J Radiat Oncol Biol Phys.* 2014;89(1):96–102.

78. Hepel JT, Tokita M, MacAusland SG, et al. Toxicity of three-dimensional conformal radiotherapy for accelerated partial breast irradiation. *Int J Radiat Oncol Biol Phys.* 2009;75(5):1290–1296.

79. Chafe S, Moughan J, McCormick B, et al. Late toxicity and patient self-assessment of breast appearance/satisfaction on RTOG 0319: a phase 2 trial of 3-dimensional conformal radiation therapy-accelerated partial breast irradiation following lumpectomy for stages I and II breast cancer. *Int J Radiat Oncol Biol Phys.* 2013;86(5):854–859.

80. Livi L, Meattini I, Marrazzo L, et al. Accelerated partial breast irradiation using intensity-modulated radiotherapy versus whole breast irradiation: 5-year survival analysis of a phase 3 randomised controlled trial. *Eur J Cancer.* 2015;51(4):451–463.

81. Julian T, Constantino J, Vicini F. Early toxicity results with 3D conformal external beam (CEBT) from the NSABP B-39/RTOG 0413 accelerated partial breast irradiation (APBI) trial. *J Clin Oncol.* 2011;29:suppl; abstr 1011.

82. Rodriguez N, Sanz X, Dengra J, et al. Five-year outcomes, cosmesis, and toxicity with 3-dimensional conformal external beam radiation therapy to deliver accelerated partial breast irradiation. *Int J Radiat Oncol Biol Phys.* 2013;87(5):1051–1057.

83. Coles C, Agarwal R, Ah-See M. Partial-breast radiotherapy after breast conservation surgery for patients with early breast cancer (UK IMPORT LOW trial): 5-year results from a multicentre, randomised, controlled, phase 3 non-inferiority trial. *Lancet.* 2017;390:1048–1060.

84. Polgar C, Major T, Fodor J, et al. Accelerated partial-breast irradiation using high-dose-rate interstitial brachytherapy: 12-year update of a prospective clinical study. *Radiother Oncol.* 2010;94(3):274–279.

85. Shah C, Antonucci JV, Wilkinson JB, et al. Twelve-year clinical outcomes and patterns of failure with accelerated partial breast irradiation versus whole-breast irradiation: results of a matched-pair analysis. *Radiother Oncol.* 2011;100(2):210–214.

86. Benitez PR, Keisch ME, Vicini F, et al. Five-year results: the initial clinical trial of MammoSite balloon brachytherapy for partial breast irradiation in early-stage breast cancer. *Am J Surg.* 2007;194(4):456–462.

87. Shah C, Badiyan S, Ben Wilkinson J, et al. Treatment efficacy with accelerated partial breast irradiation (APBI): final analysis of the American Society of Breast Surgeons MammoSite® breast brachytherapy registry trial. *Ann Surg Oncol.* 2013;20(10):3279–3285.

88. Shah C, Khwaja S, Badiyan S, et al. Brachytherapy-based partial breast irradiation is associated with low rates of complications and excellent cosmesis. *Brachytherapy.* 2013;12(4):278–284.

89. Smith GL, Xu Y, Buchholz TA, et al. Association between treatment with brachytherapy vs whole-breast irradiation and subsequent mastectomy, complications, and survival among older women with invasive breast cancer. *JAMA.* 2012;307(17):1827–1837.

90. Presley CJ, Soulos PR, Herrin J, et al. Patterns of use and short-term complications of breast brachytherapy in the national Medicare population from 2008-2009. *J Clin Oncol.* 2012;30(35):4302–4307.

91. Cuttino LW, Arthur DW, Vicini F, et al. Long-term results from the Contura multilumen balloon breast brachytherapy catheter phase 4 registry trial. *Int J Radiat Oncol Biol Phys.* 2014;90(5):1025–1029.

92. Yashar C, Attai D, Butler E, et al. Strut-based accelerated partial breast irradiation: report of treatment results for 250 consecutive patients at 5 years from a multicenter retrospective study. *Brachytherapy.* 2016;15(6):780–787.

22: LOCALLY ADVANCED BREAST CANCER

Yvonne D. Pham and Rahul D. Tendulkar

QUICK HIT: Locally advanced breast cancer (LABC) generally includes clinical stage IIB (T3N0) to stage III, including inflammatory breast cancer (IBC), which represents a subset of LABC.

TABLE 22.1: General Treatment Paradigm	
Neoadjuvant Chemotherapy (NACT)	Associated with high rates (15%–20%) of pCR and allows for cosmetically acceptable surgery, but does not improve DFS or OS compared to adjuvant CHT. For HER2+ disease, add trastuzumab and pertuzumab neoadjuvantly (w/ CHT).
Surgery	Performed 3 to 6 weeks after completing NACT. Usually MRM w/ ALND, although LABC is not a contraindication to BCT.
RT	Initiated about 4 weeks following surgery (or CHT if given adjuvantly). Indications after NACT: initially clinical stage III (regardless of response to CHT) or residual LN+. Indications after adjuvant CHT: any pathologic stage III pts (controversial for stage II).

EPIDEMIOLOGY: The incidence of stage III disease in 2014 was 7.3% per NCDB, which has been steadily decreasing over time from 9.6% in 2004.[1] LABC represents a heterogeneous class of tumors. Some LABC cases present between routine screening mammograms and represent disease with a rapid growth rate. This is particularly true for inflammatory breast cancer (IBC), which accounts for ~2% of all new breast malignancies, and is slightly more common in African Americans than in Caucasians.[2] LABC also includes pts with slow-growing, neglected tumors that have become extensive over time. With this heterogeneous group, there are no clear risk factors unique to pts presenting with advanced disease. However, young/premenopausal women and African Americans are more likely to present with LABC.[3]

RISK FACTORS, ANATOMY, PATHOLOGY, GENETICS, SCREENING: See Chapter 21 for details.

CLINICAL PRESENTATION: Breast masses are typically found by self-breast exam, mammogram, or clinical exam, and are rarely painful (~5%). Lesions present late (T3/T4) usually as a result of lack of screening, delay due to patient neglect or misdiagnosis, or aggressive tumor biology. Other LABC signs may include axillary adenopathy, skin erythema, dimpling, nipple retraction, bloody discharge, or change in size or shape of the breast. IBC is a clinical diagnosis that requires erythema and dermal edema (peau d'orange) of ≥1/3 of the breast, which develops in ≤6 mos and includes rapid enlargement of the breast, generalized induration in the presence or absence of a distinct breast mass, and a biopsy-proven carcinoma. The pathologic hallmark for IBC is tumor emboli within the dermal lymphatics (present in 50%–75% of cases), but is neither sufficient nor required for diagnosis of IBC. Occult dermal lymphatic invasion w/o clinical signs of IBC is unusual (<2% of cases).[4] Pts with IBC are more frequently hormone receptor negative and HER2+ than other breast cancers; most are LN-positive and ~30% present with distant metastases.

WORKUP: H&P with attention to extent of disease, especially the extent of skin involvement if IBC (photo documentation), assess mobility/fixation of the tumor and LNs. As many pts will receive NACT, it is important to assess and document extent of disease prior to therapy.

Labs: CBC, CMP, alkaline phosphatase.

Imaging: Bilateral mammograms and ultrasound as necessary. For clinical stage IIIA and higher (T3N1 or any N2), order CT chest/abdomen/pelvis and bone scan or PET/CT for identifying unsuspected regional nodal disease and/or distant metastases.[5] Additional imaging may include an MRI brain if neurologic symptoms are present, and plain films of areas of increased uptake on bone scan.

Procedures: Core needle biopsy (full thickness of skin for IBC) rather than FNA for determination of ER/PR and HER2 status.

Other: MUGA scan prior to anthracycline CHT (adriamycin contraindicated w/ LVEF <30%–35%; cardiotoxicity seen after cumulative dose of 450–500 mg/m^2).

PROGNOSTIC FACTORS

Favorable: pCR following induction CHT, negative margins following MRM, use of taxane-based CHT.

Poor: LN involvement (most important), IBC, African American race, ER-negative, extensive erythema, presence of microcalcifications, mutation of p53, presentation in pregnancy.

STAGING: See Chapter 21 for AJCC staging system.

TREATMENT PARADIGM

In general, use NACT followed by surgery or surgery followed by adjuvant CHT with RT as indicated.

Chemotherapy: No difference in DFS or OS between NACT or adjuvant CHT,[6,7] but NACT may help make upfront inoperable disease more amenable to surgery, improve cosmetic outcomes following surgery, and assess effectiveness of neoadjuvant systemic therapy. Some subtypes of breast cancer (HER2+ or TNBC) have a better response to NACT. Pts who are diagnosed during pregnancy and unable to have surgery may also benefit from NACT. Pts <60 years of age, African American, and those treated in academic centers are more likely to receive NACT.[8] The choice of a specific NACT regimen should be based on tumor biology and the cancer subset type. In general, use an anthracycline-containing regimen and taxane; subsitute docetaxel for doxorubicin if a contraindication exists. NACT regimens that have been tested in large multicenter phase III trials and yielded pCR rates of 15% to 20% are doxorubicin/cyclosphosphamide/docetaxel (AC/T); epirubicin/paclitaxel; cyclophosphamide/methotrexate/5-FU (CMF).[9] NSABP B-27 demonstrated that pre-op AC+docetaxel had a higher overall clinical response rate (91% vs. 86%; $p < .001$) and higher pCR (26% vs. 14%; $p < .001$) compared to pre-op AC alone, but no difference in DFS or OS.[10] A common regimen is dose-dense AC for four cycles followed by weekly paclitaxel for 12 weeks. Pts with a pCR at surgery have significant improvements in DFS (HR 0.48) and OS (HR 0.48) compared to those with residual disease.[11]

For HER2+ pts, adding trastuzumab to neoadjuvant anthracycline and taxane-based CHT improves rates of pCR and risk of relapse in a pooled analysis of two randomized studies.[12] The long-term outcomes from one of these trials (NOAH) showed a benefit in EFS at 5 yrs compared to CHT alone.[13] For pts with HER2+ disease who receive trastuzumab as part of their neoadjuvant therapy, pCR is associated with improvements in DFS and OS.[14] Additional HER2+ directed agents include lapatanib (orally available, tyrosine kinase inhibitor of HER2 pathways) and pertuzumab (humanized monoclonocal antibody that blocks the dimerization domain of HER2, preventing the formation of HER2 heterodimers). Based on results from two randomized phase II studies in which higher pCR rates (46%–66%) were seen with the addition of pertuzumab to NACT and trastuzumab, the FDA granted expedited approval for pertuzumab in the neoadjuvant setting.[15,16] A common regimen is TCHP.

Surgery: Prior to the start of NACT, evaluation of the tumor and lymph nodes should be performed. Radio-opaque clips should be placed in the tumor to aid in planning of locoregional treatment and subsequent pathologic assessment (facilitates locoregional treatment should a CR to CHT occur). The tumor size should also be documented for staging (using ultrasound or breast MRI). For suspicion of an involved axilla, perform FNA and/or core needle biopsy with placement of a radio-opaque clip in the suspicious lymph node. If the FNA is negative, then perform a SLNB to stage the axilla. If the axilla is clinically benign, can consider pre-NACT SLNB (institutional preference) or wait until the time of surgery; if negative, no further evaluation.

Surgery is typically performed 3 to 6 weeks after completing NACT and usually involves a MRM w/ ALND. ALND involves levels I and II axillary dissections; level III may be dissected if disease is apparent in level I or II. In the setting of NACT for LABC pts, the use of SLNB rather than ALND is controversial given possible changes in lymphatics; a meta-analysis revealed a false negative rate of 14.2% (95% CI: 12.5–16) with the use of SLNB in this setting.[17] LABC is not a contraindication to BCT but must be undertaken with caution; at least one PRT has shown BCT after NACT does not decrease OS, but IBTR is higher in pts who were downstaged to be eligible for BCT.[18] At the time of mastectomy, axillary dissection should be performed if SLNB is positive, particularly if PMRT is to be omitted (see ASCO guidelines for use of SLNB).

Radiation

Indications: Indications for PMRT generally include clinical stage III (regardless of response to NACT), residual LN-positive after NACT, or pathologic stage III. PMRT is controversial for stage II disease. As per the ongoing NSABP B-51, comprehensive nodal radiation includes the axilla, supraclavicular lymph nodes, and internal mammary nodes. Historical indications for treating the full axilla with a posterior axillary boost (PAB) are based on risk factors for subsequent axillary recurrence: gross extranodal extension, ≥10 +LNs, >50% +LN nodal ratio, or undissected axilla. IM nodal RT has been controversial over the rarity of documented IM nodal failures and concerns about cardiotoxicity, but was performed in all the classic PMRT trials. Indications for IM nodal RT may include clinically positive IM nodes, central/medial tumor location, or axillary LN-positive disease. RT usually initiated about 4 weeks following surgery or CHT (whichever is last) provided adequate healing has taken place.

Dose: General dose to chest wall and regional lymph nodes is 50 Gy/25 fx; however, there is insufficient evidence as per PMRT guideline to recommend a total dose, fraction size, use of scar boosts or bolus.[19] If margins are close or positive consider boost to 60 Gy, and boost gross residual (unresectable) disease to ≥66 Gy. For inflammatory breast cancer, treat with tri-modality including CHT, mastectomy, and PMRT (regardless of response to NACT).

Procedure: See *Treatment Planning Handbook*, Chapter 5.[20]

EVIDENCE-BASED Q&A

What are the classic data on recurrence patterns after mastectomy and adjuvant CHT?

Fowble, ECOG Pooled Analysis (*JCO* 1988, PMID 3292711): RR of 627 women treated on ECOG adjuvant CHT trials from 1978 to 1982 without RT. Pre- and postmenopausal pts undergoing mastectomy included. Eligibility criteria: age <66, primary tumor confined to breast and ipsilateral axilla w/o fixation, arm edema, inflammatory changes, ulceration, satellite skin nodules, peau d'orange >1/3 of the breast, or skin infiltration >2 cm. All pts had positive LNs. MFU 4.5 yrs. On MVA, the following factors were significant for LRR within 3 years: tumor size >5 cm, ≥4 LN+, ER-negative, tumor necrosis, and pectoral fascia involvement. **Conclusion: Consider PMRT for LN+ pts with high-risk features.**

TABLE 22.2: Factors Associated With LRR in ECOG Trials								
	LRR	*p value*		LRR	*p value*		LRR	*p value*
Tumor Size		.004	ER Status		.02	Pectoral Fascia Involvement		.007
≤2 cm	9%		Positive	8%				
2–5 cm	9%							
>5 cm	19%		Negative	14%		Absent	10%	
LNs		.006	Tumor Necrosis		.002	Present	29%	
1–3 +	7%		Absent	8%				
4–7 +	15%		Present	17%				
≥8 +	15%							

Taghian, NSABP Pooled Analysis (*JCO* 2004, PMID 15452182): Pooled analysis from multiple NSABP trials (B-15, B-16, B-18, B-22 and B-25) of LN+ pts treated with mastectomy and adjuvant CHT (90% received doxorubicin-based CHT) +/− tamoxifen and without PMRT. At 10 yrs, 12.2% had isolated LRF, 19.8% had LRF with or without DF, and 43.3% had DF alone as a first event. LRF (+/− DF) as a first event was 13% for one to three +LN, 24.4% for four to nine +LN, and 31.9% for ≥10 +LN (*p* < .0001). LRF was 14.9% for tumors ≤2 cm, 21.3% for 2.1 to 5.0 cm, and 24.6% for >5 cm (*p* < .0001). The majority of recurrences occurred in the chest wall and around the mastectomy scar (56.9% of pts), followed by supraclavicular LN recurrence (22.6% of all LRF), and axillary failure (11.7%). Parasternal and subclavicular failures were less than 1% of the total LRF. Age, tumor size, premenopausal status, number of LN+, and number of dissected LN were significant predictors on MVA for LRF as first event. **Conclusion: LRF as first event is high for pts with large tumors and ≥4 positive LNs, and therefore, recommend PMRT to those groups. Axillary LN status is the most important predictor for LRR, of which the majority occur in the chest wall.**

What randomized evidence demonstrates the benefit of PMRT after adjuvant CHT?

At least three randomized trials have demonstrated a survival benefit to PMRT for high-risk patients, particularly those with LN+ disease. In the modern era, the risk of LRR in pT1-2N1 pts without PMRT is less (<10%) compared to historical series (20%–30%), and so this remains a controversial subgroup.

Ragaz, British Columbia (*NEJM* 1997, PMID 9309100; Update *JNCI* 2005, PMID 15657341): PRT of 318 premenopausal women with stage I or II breast cancer, enrolled if pathologically node-positive after receiving an MRM + ALND (levels I and II) comparing adjuvant CHT with CMF + PMRT versus CMF alone. The median number of LNs removed was 11. CMF was given for 6 to 12 months. PMRT was delivered between the fourth and fifth cycle of CHT. The chest wall was treated to 37.5 Gy/16 fx w/ opposed tangents. The mid-axilla received 35 Gy/16 fx through an AP SCV field and PAB. A direct IM field treating both IM chains received 37.5 Gy/16 fx. All fields were treated w/ Co-60. MFU 150 mo. **Conclusion: PMRT improves long-term LRC, DFS, and OS.**

TABLE 22.3: Results of British Columbia PMRT Trial						
	15-yr LRC	15-yr DFS	15-yr OS	20-yr LRC	20-yr DFS	20-yr OS
CMF + PMRT	87%	50%	54%	90%	48%	47%
CMF alone	67%	33%	46%	74%	30%	37%
p value	.003	.007	.07	.002	.001	.03

Overgaard, Danish Breast Cancer Cooperative Group 82b (*NEJM* 1997, PMID 9395428): PRT of 1,708 premenopausal high-risk women who had undergone a total mastectomy w/ ALND for stage II or III breast cancer comparing adjuvant CHT with CMF + PMRT versus CMF alone. High risk was defined as +axillary LNs, tumor >5 cm, and/or invasion of the skin or pectoral fascia. Premenopausal defined as amenorrhea for <5 yrs or hysterectomy before the age of 55. Median of seven LNs removed. CHT consisted of eight cycles of CMF in pts receiving RT and nine cycles in those treated w/ CHT alone. RT was given after the first cycle of CHT. CHT then resumed 1 to 2 weeks after RT. RT delivered in five-field arrangement to an intended median dose of 50 Gy/25 fx in 35 days or 48 Gy/22 fx in 38 days to axilla, SCV, ICV, chest wall, and IM nodes (upper four intercostal spaces). Posterior axillary fields also recommended if AP diameter too large to limit max dose to 55 Gy/25 fx or 52.8 Gy/22 fx. Most were treated w/ linac. MFU 114 mo. **Conclusion: Statistically significant survival benefit with PMRT for all T stages, N stages (even N0), and histopathologic grades.** *Comment: Median of seven LNs dissected was low for this era, likely understaging many pts.*

TABLE 22.4: Results of Danish 82b PMRT Trial			
	10-yr LRC	10-yr DFS	10-yr OS
CMF + RT	91%	48%	54%
CMF alone	68%	34%	45%
p value	<.001	<.001	<.001

Overgaard, Danish Breast Cancer Cooperative Group 82c (*Lancet* 1999, PMID 10335782): PRT of 1,375 postmenopausal high-risk women <70 yrs s/p total mastectomy w/ ALND for stage II or III breast CA. Randomized to PMRT + tamoxifen versus tamoxifen alone versus CMF + tamoxifen (arm not reported). High risk defined as in 82b trial. Postmenopausal: ≥5 yrs of amenorrhea, or hysterectomy after the age of 55. 58% of pts had one to three LN+. All pts received tamoxifen 30 mg/day for 1 year. Median of seven LNs removed. PMRT same as 82b. All but 69 pts were treated with linacs. MFU 123 mo. **Conclusion: The addition of PMRT to adjuvant tamoxifen reduces LRR and prolongs OS in high-risk postmenopausal women with breast cancer.** *Comment: Only 1 year of tamoxifen is insufficient systemic therapy.*

TABLE 22.5: Results of Danish 82b PMRT Trial

	LRR as First Site of Recurrence	DM First Recurrence	10-yr DFS	5-yr OS	10-yr OS
Tam + PMRT	8%	39%	36%	63%	45%
Tam alone	35%	25%	24%	62%	36%
p value	<.001		<.001		.03

Overgaard, 82b and 82c Combined Analysis (*Radiother Oncol* 2007, PMID 17306393): Because many women on 82b and 82c had limited ALNDs, a subgroup analysis was done for 1,152 pts with ≥8 LNs removed, which showed that PMRT significantly improved LRC and OS in all LN+ pts, with the magnitude of improvement similar in one to three versus ≥4 LN+ pts. Overall, this indicated that PMRT is beneficial and unrelated to the absolute number of positive LNs.

TABLE 22.6: Combined 82b and 82c Analysis in Patients With 1-3 LN+

	15-yr OS All pts	15-yr LRF 1-3 LN+	15-yr OS 1-3 LN+	15-yr LRF 4+ LN+	15-yr OS 4+ LN+
No PMRT	29%	27%	48%	51%	12%
PMRT	39%	4%	57%	10%	21%
p value	.015	<.001	.03	<.001	.03

Clarke, EBCTCG Meta-analysis (*Lancet* 2005, PMID 16360786; Update *Lancet* 2014, PMID 24656685): Meta-analysis of individual data for 8,135 women in 22 RCT from 1964 to 1986 who underwent mastectomy and ALND +/− PMRT; 3,786 women had ALND of levels I and II; median of 10 LNs removed. All pts were enrolled onto trials in which RT included the chest wall, SCV or axilla fossa (or both), and IM chain. For 3,131 pN+ pts, PMRT improved 10-year risk of LRR and any recurrence (AR) as well as 20-year risk of breast cancer mortality (BCM). There was no benefit to PMRT for pts who were node-negative. For 1,772 women with ≥4 LN+, PMRT significantly improved outcomes. For subset of 1,314 pts with one to three LN+, PMRT significantly reduced LRR, AR, and BCM.

TABLE 22.7: Early Breast Cancer Trialists' Collaborative Group Meta-Analysis (2014 Update)

	10-yr LRR	10-yr Any First Rec.	20-yr BCM
pN1-3 (1314)			
RT	3.8%	34.2%	42.3%
No RT	20.3%	45.7%	50.2%
p value	2p < .00001	2p = .00006	2p = .01
pN4+ (1772)			
RT	13.0%	66.3%	70.7%
No RT	32.1%	75.1%	80.0%
p value	2p < .00001	2p = .0003	2p = .04
pN0 (700)			
RT	3.0%	22.4%	28.8%
No RT	1.6%	21.1%	26.6%

(continued)

TABLE 22.7: Early Breast Cancer Trialists' Collaborative Group Meta-Analysis (2014 Update) (*continued*)

	10-yr LRR	10-yr Any First Rec.	20-yr BCM
p value	*p* > .1	RR 1.06, *p* > .1	RR 1.18, *p* > .1
pN+ (3,131)			
RT	8.1%	51.9%	58.3%
No RT	26.0%	62.5%	66.4%
p value	2*p* < .00001	2*p* < .00001	2*p* = .001

TABLE 22.8: EBCTCG Subset of 1,133 Pts With 1-3 LN+ Who Received Systemic Therapy

	10-yr LRR	10-yr Any Recurrence	20-yr BCM
pN1-3+ (1,133)			
RT	4.3%	33.8%	41.5%
No RT	21.0%	45.5%	49.4%
p value	2*p* = .00001	2*p* = .00009	2*p* = .01

Are T3N0 tumors at high risk for recurrence?

The utility of PMRT for pT3N0 patients is controversial. At least two large RRs show low LF rates <10% for mastectomy + systemic therapy alone for pT3N0. Conversely, a 2014 SEER analysis and single-institution data suggest a benefit with PMRT for T3N0 pts.

Taghian, NSABP Pooled Analysis (*JCO* 2006, PMID 16921044): RR of 313 pts from five NSABP PRTs (B-13, B-14, B-19, B-20, B-23) for pN0, ≥5 cm (pT3N0) breast cancers treated with mastectomy without PMRT. MFU 15 yrs. 34% received adjuvant CHT, 21% adjuvant tamoxifen, 19% both, and 26% no systemic tx. 28 pts experienced LRF. Only 7% of pts with tumors = 5 cm and 7.2% of pts with >5 cm had LRF. The overall 10-year cumulative incidences of isolated LRF, LRF with and w/o distant failure (DF), and DF alone as first event were 7.1%, 10.0%, and 23.6%, respectively. 24 of 28 failures occurred on chest wall. Pts with >10 LNs removed had 7.3% LRF versus one to five LNs removed had 16.7% LRF (*p* = .21). For pts who underwent no systemic treatment, CHT alone, tamoxifen alone, or CHT plus tamoxifen, the LRF incidences were 12.6%, 5.6%, 4.6%, and 5.3%, respectively (*p* = .2). **Conclusion: Pts who are pT3N0 treated by mastectomy w/ adjuvant systemic therapy and no PMRT have low rates of LRF. PMRT is not routinely indicated for these pts.**

Floyd, Multi-institutional T3N0 Analysis (*IJROBP* 2006, PMID 16887288): RR of 70 pts from three institutions (Yale, MGH, MDACC) with pT3N0 (5 cm+) from 1981 to 2002. 5-yr OS 83%, 5-yr DFS 86%, 5-yr LRF 7.6%. 5 LRFs: four chest wall and one axilla. Only prognostic marker was LVI; LRF for +LVI was 21% versus -LVI 4% (*p* = .017). **Conclusion: Can likely omit PMRT for T3N0 without +LVI.**

Johnson, SEER Analysis (*Cancer* 2014, PMID 24985911): RR of 2,525 T3N0 pts dx from 2000 to 2010 who underwent MRM, 1,063 received PMRT. On UVA at 8 years, PMRT was associated with improved OS (76.5% vs. 61.8%, *p* < .01) and CSS (85.0% vs. 82.4%, *p* < .01). Use of PMRT remained significant on MVA for OS (HR 0.63, *p* < .001) and CSS (hazard ratio 0.77, *p* = .045). **Conclusion: PMRT should be considered in T3N0M0 pts, and is associated with improvement in OS and CSS, although selection bias remains a potential confounder.**

Nagar, MDACC (*IJROBP* 2011, PMID 21885207): RR of 162 pts with cT3N0 who received NACT and underwent mastectomy. Median number of LN dissected was 15. 45% of pts were ypN+ after NACT. 119 pts (73%) received PMRT and 43 pts did not. MFU 75 mos. For all pts, 5-year LRR rate was 9%. 5-year LRR rate after PMRT was 4% versus 24% for those who did not receive PMRT ($p < .001$). CW was most common site of LR, then axilla and SCV (equally). A significantly higher proportion of irradiated pts had ypLN+ and were ≤40 years of age. **Conclusion: Consider PMRT for pts with cT3N0 as LRR risk is still >10%.** *Comment: Clinical understaging of axillary lymph nodes is common, as 45% of cT3N0 pts were found to have residual ypN+ disease after NACT.*

What is the role of PMRT for pts with a TNBC molecular subtype?

Women with TNBC have an aggressive clinical course (early relapse, higher incidence of visceral and brain metastases, and relatively poor prognosis compared to other subtypes), so some consider PMRT in these pts even with earlier stage disease.

Wang, Chinese Randomized Trial (*Radiother Oncol* 2011, PMID 21852010): Multicenter PRT of 681 women with TNBC stage I-II (82% LN-negative) s/p mastectomy, randomized to systemic CHT +/− PMRT (50 Gy/25 fx +/− RNI as clinically indicated). At a MFU of 7.2 years, PMRT improved the 5-year RFS (74.6% to 88.3%, $p = .02$) and 5-year OS (78.7% vs. 90.4%, $p = .03$). *Comment: Independent confirmation would be valuable to confirm the role of PMRT in LN-negative TNBC.*

Should the SCV and/or IM nodes be included in the radiation field?

IMNs were included in the three randomized PMRT trials (British Columbia, DBCCG 82b/82c), although isolated recurrence in the IMN is low (~1% or less). The incidence of IMN involvement in extended radical mastectomy series was based on the location and size of the primary tumor along with the extent of axillary involvement. Hennequin et al. showed no OS benefit (though underpowered), while a Danish prospective nonrandomized cohort study suggested an OS benefit. The EORTC 22922 trial demonstrated a DFS benefit to including IMN-SCV fields over omitting them, although it remains unclear whether the benefit was achieved by inclusion of the IMN or SCV fields (or both).

Hennequin, French Trial (*IJROBP* 2013, PMID 23664327): PRT of 1,334 pts w/ axillary LN+ or central/medial tumors (irrespective of axillary involvement). All pts underwent MRM with ALND of Levels I and II. No IMN dissection allowed. PMRT delivered to chest wall + SCV. For pN+ cases, levels I + II covered, mainly 50 Gy/25 fx. Randomized between +/− IMNI (included first five intercostal spaces) to a dose of 45 Gy/18 fx (2.5 Gy/fx) using mixed photon and electron fields. MFU 11.3 yrs. 10-year OS 59.3% without IMNI versus 62.6% with IMNI ($p = .8$). IMNI did not significantly improve OS for any subgroup. **Conclusion: No benefit to IMNI.** *Comment: included node-negative pts (25%) who have lower risk for IMN involvement; used 2D planning, which may have underestimated the coverage of IMNs; study was powered for a 10% survival benefit, which is likely optimistic given that the British Columbia/Danish trials of PMRT versus no RT showed a ~10% OS benefit.*

Poortman, EORTC 22922-10925 (*NEJM* 2015, PMID 26200978): PRT of 4,004 pts with axillary LN+ and/or a medially located primary tumor (irrespective of axillary involvement), randomized to +/− RNI to include IMNs (first three intercostal spaces or up to first five for LIQ tumors) + medial SCV (50 Gy/25 fx); 7.4% of control versus 8.3% in RNI group received axillary RT. BCT in 76%; mastectomy in 24%. After mastectomy, chest wall RT was given to 73% in both arms (not all). 44% were node-negative. MFU 10.9 years. **Conclusion: RNI improved DFS, distant DFS, and BCM with**

minimal increase in acute side effects. However, an OS difference was not statistically significant.

TABLE 22.9: EORTC 22922 Results							
10-yr Results	DFS	Distant DFS	BCM	OS	Pulmonary Fibrosis	Cardiac Disease	Lymphedema
Surgery+ RNI	72.1%	78%	12.5%	82.3%	4.4%	6.5%	12%
Surgery	69.1%	75%	14.4%	80.7%	1.7%	5.6%	10.5%
p value	$p = .04$	$p = .02$	$p = .02$	$p = .06$	$p < .001$	$p = .25$	

Whelan, MA.20/NCIC-CTG (*NEJM* 2015, PMID 26200977): PRT of 1,832 pts who underwent BCT and SLNB or ALND with LN+ or LN-negative with high-risk features (tumor ≥5 cm or tumor ≥2 cm with fewer than 10 ALNs removed and at least one of the following: grade 3, ER-, LVSI). Exclusion: T4, cN2-3, M1. Pts randomized to WBI only (50 Gy/25 fx +/– boost) +/– RNI. RNI included IM nodes in first three intercostal spaces + SCV + axilla (covered levels I+II if <10 axillary nodes removed or >3 LN+) with optional PAB. Primary endpoint was OS. MFU 9.5 yrs. 85% had one to three positive LNs, 5% had ≥4 positive LNs, and 10% were LN-. Absolute magnitude of benefit is variable across the population and suggests need for risk stratified approach to these pts. In subgroup of ER-negative pts, DFS was significantly improved with RNI (82% vs. 71%, $p = .04$) and OS approached significance (81.3% vs. 73.9%, HR: 0.69, 95% CI: 0.47–1.00, $p = .05$). **Conclusion: RNI improved DFS, locoregional DFS, and distant DFS, but no OS benefit was observed.**

TABLE 22.10: NCIC MA.20 Results							
10-yr Results	DFS	Locoregional DFS	Distant DFS	BCM	OS	Pneumonitis	Lymphedema
Lump + CHT + WBI + RNI	82%	95.2%	86.3%	10.3%	82.8%	1.2%	8.4%
Lump + CHT + WBI	77%	92.2%	82.4%	12.3%	81.8%	0.2%	4.5%
p-value	$p = .01$	$p = .009$	$p = .03$	$p = .11$	$p = .38$	$p < .001$	$p < .001$

Thorsen, DBCG-IMN (*JCO* 2015, PMID 26598752): Prospective population-based cohort study of 3,089 pts with unilateral LN+ breast cancer underwent mastectomy or BCS with ALND (levels I–II). Included pT1-T3 and pN1-3. Pts with right-sided disease received IMNI while left-sided disease did not receive IMNI (due to concerns of RT-induced heart disease). RT to breast/chest wall, scar, SCV, infraclavicular (level III), and axillary levels I-II to 48 Gy/24 fx. IMNI in R-sided cancer included intercostal spaces 1 to 4 treated with anterior electron field or included in tangential photon fields. Primary endpoint was OS. MFU 8.9 years. 3% OS benefit with IMNI (75.9% vs. 72.2%, $p = .005$). 3% of right-sided did not receive IMNI, while 10% of left-sided received IMNI. Equal number of cardiac deaths in two groups. Subgroup analysis showed lateral tumors with ≥4 LNs had OS benefit with IMNI, HR 0.71 (95% CI: 0.57–0.89). **Conclusion: IMNI may improve OS in LN+ breast cancer.** *Comment: Not a randomized trial and excluded pts unfit for standard RT, which may potentially lead to overestimation of IMNI effect.*

TABLE 22.11: DBCG-IMN Results			
DBCG-IMN 8-yr Results	OS	BCM	DM
With IMNI	75.9%	20.9%	27.4%
Without IMNI	72.2%	23.4%	29.7%
p value	$p = .005$	$p = .03$	$p = .07$

What are the current indications for PMRT after neoadjuvant CHT?

Typical indications for PMRT include positive margins and pathologic stage III disease—stage IIB is controversial. In those undergoing neoadjuvant CHT, indications include either clinical stage III (regardless of response to CHT) or those with residual nodal positivity.

Recht, ASCO Guidelines (*JCO* 2001, PMID 11230499): In the setting of adjuvant CHT, give PMRT for pathologic stage III pts: T3N1, N2-N3, T4. There is insufficient evidence to recommend PMRT for or against pts with close/positive margins.

Recht, ASCO/ASTRO/SSO Guidelines (*JCO* 2016, 27646947): PMRT for pts with T1-2N1 reduces LRF, any recurrence, and BCM, but PMRT should be used only if expected benefits outweigh potential toxicity risks. PMRT indicated for pts who are ypN+ (any T) after NACT. For pts who are cN0 before NACT or have a complete pathologic response in the axilla, there is insufficient evidence to recommend for or against PMRT for these pts, and it is recommended to enroll these pts into clinical trials (such as NSABP B-51). When PMRT is used, it should routinely include the chest wall/reconstructed breast, supraclavicular-axillary apical nodes, and internal mammary nodes, although there are subgroups that may not derive benefit from treating all nodal regions.

Which pts are at increased risk for LRR after NACT alone (and therefore should consider additional therapy)?

Based on retrospective reviews from MDACC and a combined analysis of NSABP B-18 and B-27, pts with clinical stage III disease (T1-2N2 or T3N1 or higher) are at increased risk for LRR after NACT alone.

Buchholz, MDACC (*IJROBP* 2002, PMID 12095553): RR of 150 pts who received NACT and 1,031 pts who received adjuvant CHT; all underwent MRM but no PMRT. 55% of NACT group had clinical stage IIIA or higher disease versus 9% in adjuvant group. 5-yr LRR was higher in the NACT group versus adjuvant group (27% vs. 15%, $p = .001$). Pts with ≥4+ LNs had higher LRR in the NACT versus adjuvant group (53% vs. 23%, $p < .001$). Pathologic size of tumor and number of +LNs were less in NACT group ($p < .001$). Matched subset analysis showed no difference in LRR by tumor size or LNs except for 2.1 to 5 cm and 1-3+LNs (5-yr LRR 32% NACT group vs. 8% adjuvant group, $p = .03$). **Conclusion: Pts with ≥4+ LNs, tumor size >5 cm, or clinical stage IIIA or greater disease should receive PMRT regardless of whether they receive neoadjuvant or adjuvant CHT.**

Mamounas, Combined NSABP B-18 and B-27 (*JCO* 2012, PMID 23032615): Combined analysis of NSABP B-18 and B-27, included cT1-3, N0-N1 pts. NACT was either doxorubicin/cyclophosphamide (AC) alone or AC followed by neoadjuvant/adjuvant docetaxel. Lumpectomy pts received breast RT alone while mastectomy pts received no PMRT. The 10-year cumulative LRR rate in mastectomy pts was 12.3% (8.9% local; 3.4% regional); predictors of LRR on MVA included clinical tumor size (before NACT), clinical nodal status (before NACT), and pathologic nodal status/breast tumor response. For lumpectomy pts, the LRR was 10.3% (8.1% local; 2.2% regional); predictors of LRR included age, clinical nodal status (before NACT), pathologic nodal status/ breast tumor response.

Conclusion: The 10-year risk of LRR is significant after NACT (>10%) and certain clinical and pathologic features may portend a higher risk of LRR.

Which is preferred, neoadjuvant CHT or adjuvant CHT?

There is no difference in DFS or OS between neoadjuvant or adjuvant CHT. NACT is associated with high rates of pathologic response and a higher likelihood for allowing a cosmetically acceptable surgery. With NACT, there is downstaging of the tumor and involved axillary LNs with an increased rate of BCT.

Fisher, NSABP B-18 (*JCO* 1997, PMID 9215816; Update Fisher *JCO* 1998, PMID 9704717; Wolmark *J Natl Cancer Inst Monogr* 2001, PMID 11773300; Rastogi *JCO* 2008, PMID 18258986): PRT of 1,523 pts with operable breast cancer (T1-3N0-1M0) randomized to pre-op AC x 4 versus post-op AC x 4. CHT was q21 days, doxorubicin 60 mg/m^2 and cyclophosphamide 600 mg/m^2. Tamoxifen (10 mg bid x 5 yrs) was given to all pts ≥50 y/o regardless of ER status (status unknown for many pts). All pts who had a lumpectomy received RT to 50 Gy. Breast tumor size decreased by ≥50% in 80% of pts. Pts in the preoperative AC group had 36% clinical CR, 43% clinical PR, and 13% pCR. Pts with a pCR had significantly improved DFS (HR 0.47, $p < .0001$) and OS (HR 0.32, $p < .0001$) versus pts who did not have a pCR. MVA showed that post-treatment pathologic nodal status was also a strong predictor of OS and DFS ($p < .0001$). IBTR was greater in the pre-op group who had BCT due to downstaging versus pts who were planned to have BCT (14.5% vs. 6.9%, $p = .04$).[18] **Conclusion: Preoperative CHT is equivalent to adjuvant CHT in regard to OS and DFS.**

TABLE 22.12: NSABP B-18 Results					
16-yr data	pN+	BCS Rate	IBTR	DFS	OS
Pre-op CHT	42%	68%	13%	42%	55%
Post-op CHT	58%	60%	10%	39%	55%
p value	.001	.001	.21	.27	.90

Van Der Hage, EORTC 10902 (*JCO* 2001, PMID 11709566; Update Van Nes, *Breast Cancer Res Treat* 2009, PMID 18484198): PRT of 698 pts with operable breast cancer (T1c-3,T4b, N0-1M0) comparing pre-op FEC (5-FU, epirubicin, cyclophosphamide) x 4 versus post-op FEC. All pts who had BCT received RT to 50 Gy to breast and 45 Gy to IM nodes and SCV. Tamoxifen 20 mg QD was given to all pts ≥50 regardless of ER status. Tumors were assessed by clinical and mammographic evaluation. MFU 10 yrs. No difference in OS, DFS, or LRR between groups. NACT improves the rate of BCT compared to adjuvant CHT (35% vs. 22%, respectively). Pts who received BCT due to tumor downsizing did not have an increase in LRR or worse OS compared to pts who had BCT without downsizing of the tumor. **Conclusion: NACT does not lead to a detriment in OS or DFS compared to adjuvant CHT.**

In those groups with an increased risk for LRR after NACT, which studies show a benefit to adding radiation therapy?

Huang, MDACC (*JCO* 2004, PMID 15570071): RR of 542 pts treated on six consecutive prospective trials with NACT followed by mastectomy and PMRT compared to 134 pts on same trials who did not receive PMRT. PMRT significantly reduced 10-yr LRR rate (11% vs. 22%, $p = .0001$) and increased CSS in pts with stage IIIB or worse, clinical T4 or ≥4+ LNs. For stage III or IV pts who achieved a pCR, the LRR for those treated with and without PMRT was 3% versus 33% ($p = .006$), respectively. **Conclusion: PMRT improves 10-yr LRR and CSS in IIIB, T4, or N2 pts as well as LRR in stage III/IV pts who achieve a pCR after NACT.**

Krug, Meta-analysis of Gepar trials (*ASCO* 2015, Abstract 1008): Pooled analysis of the randomized NACT trials GeparTrio, GeparQuattro, and GeparQuinto; included 3,481 pts with operable and nonoperable breast cancer. 94% received RT. Found a significant benefit for 5-yr LRFS with RT versus w/o RT (90% vs. 81.5%, $p < .001$) and 5-yr DFS (75.4% vs. 67.4%, $p < .001$), respectively. The absolute advantage of RT for both LRFS and DFS was highest among pts with clinically LN+ at first diagnosis (LRFS: HR: 2.32, 95% CI: 1.54–3.50; $p < .001$; DFS: HR: 1.97, 95% CI 1.48–2.62; $p < .001$). For pts with pCR, 5-yr LRFS with and without RT was 95.7% versus 86.6% (HR: 3.32, 95% CI 1.00–11.08; $p = .051$) and 5-yr DFS was 86.9% and 56.1% (HR: 3.52, 95% CI: 1.82–6.83, $p < .001$), respectively. **Conclusion: Pts managed without RT after NACT have a significantly worse outcome even if they achieve a pCR.**

REFERENCES

1. National Cancer Database—American College of Surgeons. Site by stage of top 14 (out of 14) sites cancers diagnosed in 2004 to 2014: all diagnosis types, all types hospitals in all states - data from 1493 hospitals. https://oliver.facs.org/BMPub/Docs. Published 2016.
2. Levine PH, Steinhorn SC, Ries LG, Aron JL. Inflammatory breast cancer: the experience of the surveillance, epidemiology, and end results (SEER) program. *J Natl Cancer Inst.* 1985;74(2):291–297.
3. Li CI, Malone KE, Daling JR. Differences in breast cancer hormone receptor status and histology by race and ethnicity among women 50 years of age and older. *Cancer Epidemiol Biomarkers Prev.* 2002;11(7):601–607.
4. Gruber G, Ciriolo M, Altermatt HJ, et al. Prognosis of dermal lymphatic invasion with or without clinical signs of inflammatory breast cancer. *Int J Cancer.* 2004;109(1):144–148.
5. Sandhu A, Sethi R, Rice R, et al. Prostate bed localization with image-guided approach using on-board imaging: reporting acute toxicity and implications for radiation therapy planning following prostatectomy. *Radiother Oncol.* 2008;88(1):20–25.
6. Fisher B, Brown A, Mamounas E, et al. Effect of preoperative chemotherapy on local-regional disease in women with operable breast cancer: findings from National Surgical Adjuvant Breast and Bowel Project B-18. *J Clin Oncol.* 1997;15(7):2483–2493.
7. van der Hage JA, van de Velde CJ, Julien JP, et al. Preoperative chemotherapy in primary operable breast cancer: results from the European Organization for Research and Treatment of Cancer trial 10902. *J Clin Oncol.* 2001;19(22):4224–4237.
8. Mougalian SS, Soulos PR, Killelea BK, et al. Use of neoadjuvant chemotherapy for patients with stage I to III breast cancer in the United States. *Cancer.* 2015;121(15):2544–2552.
9. Kaufmann M, Hortobagyi GN, Goldhirsch A, et al. Recommendations from an international expert panel on the use of neoadjuvant (primary) systemic treatment of operable breast cancer: an update. *J Clin Oncol.* 2006;24(12):1940–1949.
10. Bear HD, Anderson S, Brown A, et al. The effect on tumor response of adding sequential preoperative docetaxel to preoperative doxorubicin and cyclophosphamide: preliminary results from National Surgical Adjuvant Breast and Bowel Project Protocol B-27. *J Clin Oncol.* 2003;21(22):4165–4174.
11. Mieog JS, van der Hage JA, van de Velde CJ. Preoperative chemotherapy for women with operable breast cancer. *Cochrane Database Syst Rev.* 2007(2):CD005002.
12. Petrelli F, Borgonovo K, Cabiddu M, et al. Neoadjuvant chemotherapy and concomitant trastuzumab in breast cancer: a pooled analysis of two randomized trials. *Anti-cancer drugs.* 2011;22(2):128–135.
13. Gianni L, Eiermann W, Semiglazov V, et al. Neoadjuvant and adjuvant trastuzumab in patients with HER2-positive locally advanced breast cancer (NOAH): follow-up of a randomised controlled superiority trial with a parallel HER2-negative cohort. *Lancet Oncol.* 2014;15(6):640–647.
14. Untch M, Fasching PA, Konecny GE, et al. Pathologic complete response after neoadjuvant chemotherapy plus trastuzumab predicts favorable survival in human epidermal growth factor receptor 2-overexpressing breast cancer: results from the TECHNO trial of the AGO and GBG study groups. *J Clin Oncol.* 2011;29(25):3351–3357.

15. Gianni L, Pienkowski T, Im YH, et al. Efficacy and safety of neoadjuvant pertuzumab and tras-tuzumab in women with locally advanced, inflammatory, or early HER2-positive breast cancer (NeoSphere): a randomised multicentre, open-label, phase 2 trial. *Lancet Oncol.* 2012;13(1):25–32.

16. Schneeweiss A, Chia S, Hickish T, et al. Pertuzumab plus trastuzumab in combination with standard neoadjuvant anthracycline-containing and anthracycline-free chemotherapy regimens in patients with HER2-positive early breast cancer: a randomized phase II cardiac safety study (TRYPHAENA). *Ann Oncol.* 2013;24(9):2278–2284.

17. Mocellin S, Goldin E, Marchet A, Nitti D. Sentinel node biopsy performance after neoadjuvant chemotherapy in locally advanced breast cancer: a systematic review and meta-analysis. *Int J Cancer.* 2016;138(2):472–480.

18. Fisher B, Bryant J, Wolmark N, et al. Effect of preoperative chemotherapy on the outcome of women with operable breast cancer. *J Clin Oncol.* 1998;16(8):2672–2685.

19. Recht A, Edge SB, Solin LJ, et al. Postmastectomy radiotherapy: clinical practice guidelines of the American Society of Clinical Oncology. *J Clin Oncol.* 2001;19(5):1539–1569.

20. Videtic GMM, Woody N, Vassil AD. *Handbook of Treatment Planning in Radiation Oncology.* 2nd ed. New York, NY: Demos Medical; 2015.

23: DUCTAL CARCINOMA IN SITU

Jonathan Sharrett, Chirag Shah, and Rahul D. Tendulkar

QUICK HIT: DCIS (i.e., intraductal carcinoma) represents ~20% of all breast cancers. Without treatment, up to 25% to 30% of DCIS cases can progress to invasive breast cancer over 30 yrs. Standard treatment involves either breast conservation therapy (lumpectomy plus adjuvant RT) or mastectomy. After lumpectomy, adjuvant RT results in 50% relative risk reduction in local recurrence but no improvement a in overall survival. Absolute risk of local recurrence depends on grade, histologic subtype, size, estrogen receptor status, and margin status. Lobular carcinoma in situ is a distinct entity from DCIS, which is mammographically undetectable and does not require a negative margin excision (except possibly pleomorphic subtype) or adjuvant RT.

EPIDEMIOLOGY: Over 60,000 cases of in situ breast cancers are diagnosed in the United States annually, of which 80% are ductal carcinoma in situ (DCIS) and 20% are lobular carcinoma in situ (LCIS).[1] Incidence increased fivefold with the introduction of mammography. DCIS is less common than invasive BC (~200,000 per year). Left untreated, ~25% to 30% of pts with DCIS develop into invasive cancer over 30 yrs.[2-4]

RISK FACTORS: Similar to invasive BC[1]: female gender, older age, BRCA status, family history (first-degree relative), unopposed estrogen (includes early menarche, late menopause, nulliparity, late age at first birth), obesity, alcohol (dose-dependent), prior RT, atypical ductal hyperplasia.

PATHOLOGY: DCIS implies that the basement membrane is preserved despite malignant cells arising from the ductal epithelium. Typically grows toward nipple. Five histologic subtypes (mnemonic: C^2PMS): Cribriform, Comedo (worst prognosis), Papillary, Micropapillary, Solid (second worst prognosis). Overall three main categories of grading:

- *Grade 1 (low grade):* Monomorphous nuclei with inconspicuous nucleoli and diffuse chromatin. Typically estrogen receptor (ER) and progesterone receptor (PR)-positive, have a low proliferative rate and rarely (if ever) show abnormalities of the HER2/neu or p53 oncogenes.
- *Grade 2 (intermediate grade):* Nuclei are neither grade 1 nor 3.
- *Grade 3 (high grade):* Nuclei are large and pleomorphic, >1 nucleolus per cell, irregular chromatin. Typically exhibit aneuploidy, ER and PR-negative and have a high proliferative rate, overexpression of the HER2 oncogene, mutations of the p53 tumor suppressor, and angiogenesis in the surrounding stroma.

LCIS can be commonly associated with or without atypical ductal hyperplasia or atypical lobular hyperplasia and is not considered a malignancy. However, pleomorphic LCIS is considered to have similar biological behavior as DCIS, and clinicians may consider complete excision with negative margins, albeit data is lacking. Furthermore, multifocal/extensive LCIS involving >4 terminal ductal lobular units on core biopsy is thought to increase chances of finding invasive cancer on surgical excision.

Hormone receptor status: 75% to 80% of DCIS cases are ER-positive. Up to 35% are HER2/neu amplified, and the clinical significance is under investigation.[5]

SCREENING: Mammographic screening reduces BC mortality by 20% (relative risk).[6] ACS, ACR, AMA, NCI, NCCN recommend routine screening initiated at age 40. See Chapter 21 for additional details. Risk-prediction models may help with pt-specific decisions. MRI screening recommended by the NCI/ACS for pts with a 20% to 25% lifetime risk of BC (BRCA mutation, first-degree relative with BRCA mutation, history of thoracic RT, Li–Fraumeni/Cowden syndrome or based on family history calculator).[7,8] MRI screening is not recommended for <15% risk (prior BC, atypical ductal hyperplasia, DCIS, ALH, LCIS, dense breasts).

CLINICAL PRESENTATION: *In situ* breast disease is generally asymptomatic and usually detected mammographically. On occasion, DCIS may be palpable. It may also be discovered incidentally during investigation of a nearby breast mass (benign or malignant).

WORKUP: H&P with breast and lymph node exam.

Imaging: bilateral diagnostic mammograms with spot compression views (to evaluate masses) and magnification (to evaluate calcifications) as necessary. Concerning findings on mammography: include 100 to 300 μm clustered or linear calcifications, spiculated or new lesions. Linear/branching calcifications are associated with high-grade DCIS and necrosis whereas fine/granular calcifications are associated with low-grade DCIS.[9] 90% of DCIS present with calcifications and 80% of lesions with calcifications contain DCIS.[9,10] Breast Imaging Reporting and Data System (BI-RADS) is the standard mammographic terminology. MRI may be superior to mammography for detecting DCIS (especially high-grade or multicentric disease) but has a high rate of false positives.[11] Concerning MRI findings include non-mass-like enhancement with segmental or ductal distribution and granular internal enhancement (BI-RADS 5), or enhancement in late postcontrast phase, or enhancement not following milk ducts, or asymmetric (BIRADS 4).

Biopsy technique: Fine needle aspiration (FNA) inadequate to distinguish DCIS from invasive cancer, and therefore stereotactic core or excisional biopsy recommended. Stereotactic guided "bracketing" of the suspicious areas to help facilitate excision. Use ultrasound guidance for masses. Atypical ductal hyperplasia on core biopsy requires complete excision as 20% of pts are upstaged.[12]

PROGNOSTIC FACTORS: Higher risk of recurrence[13] for: young age, high grade, comedonecrosis, multifocality, large tumor size, positive surgical margins, ER negativity, HER2/neu amplification.

TABLE 23.1: Updated VNPI			
Score	1	2	3
Size	≤15 mm	16–40	>40
Margin	≥10 mm	1–9	<1
Grade	Grade 1/2 without Necrosis	Grade 1/2 with necrosis	Grade 3
Age	>60	40–60	<40

Van Nuys Prognostic Index (VNPI)[14,15]: Quantifies prognostic factors for local recurrence (LR) in pts with DCIS (tumor size, margin width, grade, age). Note that VNPI has not been prospectively validated.[16,17]

STAGING: T classification is Tis and stage is 0 for all DCIS/LCIS.

TREATMENT PARADIGM: Options include observation if short life expectancy due to comorbidities, lumpectomy alone, lumpectomy with adjuvant RT +/– tamoxifen/

anastrozole (based on menopausal status and if ER-positive) or mastectomy. A risk-based pt-specific assessment is necessary.

Prevention: Tamoxifen and raloxifene both reduce the risk of BC (invasive and noninvasive) by ~50% in high-risk populations. ER-positive tumors are reduced by 69% but no difference in ER-negative tumors.

Surgery: Either lumpectomy (LR higher without RT)[13] or simple mastectomy (LR 1%–2% without RT).[18] No trials have compared breast conserving therapy (lumpectomy + RT; BCT) to mastectomy. Data from the Netherlands shows only 8% of DCIS is present beyond 1 cm from the initial focus.[19] According to NCCN guidelines, sentinel node dissection should not be performed in the absence of invasive cancer but may be considered for microinvasion or for large tumors >4 cm. Sentinel lymph node biopsy (SLNB) should be considered in those undergoing mastectomy given the limitation of future sampling if invasion is demonstrated on final pathology. 10% to 20% [20,21] of pts diagnosed as having DCIS only on biopsy will have invasive cancer identified at surgery. Follow-up specimen radiograph prior to RT useful to confirm complete excision of the suspicious calcifications.

Chemotherapy: No indication in DCIS/LCIS. Trials are ongoing investigating the role of trastuzumab for HER2/neu amplified cases.

Hormonal therapy: Consider adjuvant tamoxifen given 20 mg/day or anastrozole 1 mg/day for 5 yrs after excision of ER-positive DCIS. NCCN recommends tamoxifen for pts with ER-positive tumors treated with excision alone or lumpectomy and RT.[22]

Radiation

Indications: Whole breast irradiation (WBI) after surgery is indicated for pts choosing BCT. Five randomized controlled trials have demonstrated a LC benefit to RT, although CSS and OS are similar to lumpectomy alone. NCCN guidelines suggest either mastectomy or BCT as level treatment options and lumpectomy alone as IIB.[22]

Dose: Treat whole breast using opposed tangents to 50 Gy/25 fx (standard) or 42.5 Gy/16 fx (hypofractionated). No prospective randomized data exists for hypofractionation in DCIS although 42.5 Gy/16 fx was used in MDACC trial and reported in a large Canadian series showing similar outcomes. Although no randomized data exists, consider adding a boost of 10 to 16 Gy in 5 to 8 fractions.

Accelerated partial breast irradiation (APBI): Rationale: 80% to 90% of LR occur at/near lumpectomy site, underutilization of BCT due to treatment duration, transportation. Modalities: Applicator brachytherapy, multicatheter interstitial, EBRT.

Intraoperative radiation therapy (IORT): Higher rates of LR in two randomized trials for invasive BC; however, limited data in DCIS. IORT not recommended for DCIS off-protocol.

BCT contraindications: Absolute: persistently positive surgical margins despite maximal re-excision, multicentric tumors (unless resected as single specimen), diffuse malignant-appearing calcifications, inability to receive post-op RT (prior chest/breast irradiation, pregnancy). *Relative:* active connective tissue disease (scleroderma, active lupus), ataxia telangiectasia, poor cosmesis (large tumor [>4–5 cm] in small breast).

Toxicity: Acute effects: erythema, pruritus, tenderness, desquamation. Late effects: hyper/hypo pigmentation, volume loss, fibrosis, rib fracture, lymphedema, pulmonary fibrosis, secondary malignancies, and cardiac toxicity.

EVIDENCE-BASED Q&A

Can RT reduce the risk of recurrence after lumpectomy?

Yes, RT has consistently demonstrated an approximately 50% relative reduction in the risk of recurrence of both DCIS and invasive recurrence across all trials and in a meta-analysis.

EBCTCG Meta-analysis (*JNCI* Monographs 2010, PMID 20956824): Individual pt data from four PRTs of lumpectomy with or without RT; 3,729 pts. RT reduced 10-yr risk of IBTR by 54% relative risk reduction (RR) and 15% absolute RR (NNT 6.7), with a greater proportional reduction in older women. No difference by subgroup when divided by age, extent of resection, tamoxifen, method of detection, margins, focality, grade, necrosis, architecture, or size. Even in small, low-grade tumors resected with negative margins, RT still reduced 10-yr in-breast tumor recurrence (IBTR) risk by 18% absolute and 52% relative risk. There was no effect on mortality (breast-cancer specific mortality [BCSM], non-BC, or all cause). 10-yr BCSM was 4.1% versus 3.7% with and without RT, respectively. **Conclusion: RT reduced 10-year risk of invasive and noninvasive IBTR after lumpectomy irrespective of risk factors, but no effect was seen on mortality.**

Fisher, NSABP B-17 (*NEJM* 1993, PMID 8292119; *JCO* 1998, PMID 9469327; *Semin Oncol* 2001, PMID 11498833; *JNCI* 2011, PMID 21398619): PRT of 818 DCIS pts randomized to excision with or without WBI. Stratified by age ($\leq$49 or >49 yrs), tumor type (DCIS or DCIS + LCIS), detection (mammography, clinical exam, or both) or axillary dissection (performed or not). All margins were tumor-free and RT was initiated within 8 weeks of lumpectomy to a dose of 50 Gy/25 fx. 9% of pts received a tumor bed boost. RT reduced the risk of recurrence by 58%. Comedonecrosis was an independent predictor IBTR. **Conclusion: Lumpectomy with RT reduces LR over lumpectomy alone.**

Holmberg, SweDCIS (*JCO* 2008, PMID 18250350; *JCO* 2014, PMID 25311220): PRT of 1,067 pts with DCIS treated with lumpectomy and randomized to RT or observation. RT was given to the whole breast 50 Gy/25 fx with no boost. Stratified by age, size, focality, detection mode, and margins. 20-year absolute risk reduction of ipsilateral breast events (IBE) of 12% and a 37% relative risk reduction with the addition of RT; 59.4% and 45.4% of IBE were invasive in the RT and control arms, respectively. No effect on survival. Increasing effect of RT with age (8-yr IBTR rates: 24% vs. 8% in >60 years of age and 31% vs. 20% in <50 years of age). No group was identified with an acceptably low risk of recurrence without RT. All women had at least a 1% per year incidence of recurrence in absence of RT. **Conclusion: All women benefit from RT and "further search for clinical variables predictive of a low-risk group that does not need RT does not seem fruitful."** *Comment: No formal histopathologic protocol, ~10% margin status unknown.*

Julien, EORTC 10853 (*Lancet* 2000, PMID 10683002; *JCO* 2006, PMID 16801628; *JCO* 2013, PMID 24043739): PRT of 1,002 pts (<70 y/o, DCIS $\leq$5 cm) treated with lumpectomy and randomized to observation or RT. Margins must have no DCIS at the sample margin. Post-op mammograms or specimen radiographs were not required. RT given <12 weeks post-op, using opposed tangents 50 Gy/25 fx with no boost recommended (although 5% received a tumor bed boost with median 10 Gy). LR-free rate at 15 yrs was 69% versus 82% in favor of RT. **Conclusion: RT after local excision of DCIS reduced overall number of invasive and noninvasive recurrences in ipsilateral breast.**

Wapnir, NSABP-B17/24 Long Term Outcomes (*JNCI* 2011, PMID 21398619): Long-term outcomes of invasive IBTR after lumpectomy for DCIS. RT reduced invasive IBTR by 52%. Invasive IBTR was associated with increased mortality risk (hazard ratio [HR] of death 1.75, 95% CI: 1.45–2.96, p < .001). After invasive IBTR, 22/39 deaths were attributed to BC.

TABLE 23.2: Summary of DCIS Trials Evaluating RT Versus no RT									
	EBCTG 10-yr		NSABP-B17 15-yr		SweDCIS 20-yr		EORTC 10853 15-yr		UK/ANZ RT Arm 12.7-yr	
	RT	No RT	RT	No RT	RT	No RT	RT	No RT	RT	No RT
IBTR	12.9*	28.1	19.8*	35	20.0*	32.0	18*	31	7.1*	19.4
Invasive ecurrence	NR	NR	10.7*	19.6	15.1	20.1	10*	16	3.3*	9.1
CSS	95.9	96.3	95.3	96.9	95.9	95.8	96	95	NR	NR
OS	91.6	91.8	82.9	84.2	77.2	73.0	88	90	NR	NR
*Statistically significant difference.									

Is there a subset of patients at a low enough absolute risk of recurrence that radiation can be omitted?

Although there are women with a low risk of recurrence, this subset has not been clearly defined and remains a pt-specific decision based on life expectancy and pt wishes. See the preceding Van Nuys Prognostic Index and the following prospective data.

Wong, Dana Farber/Harvard (*JCO* 2006, PMID 16461781; Wong *BCRT* 2014, PMID 24346130): Prospective single-arm study enrolling "low-risk" women with DCIS defined as: predominantly grade 1-2, ≤2.5 cm mammographically with margins ≥1 cm or re-excision without residual DCIS and no tamoxifen. Accrued 158/200 pts (stopped early). At 8 yrs the incidence of LR was 13%, and 32% of recurrences were invasive. **Conclusion: Despite margins of ≥1 cm, LR is substantial in pts with small low-grade DCIS treated by excision alone. The estimated annual risk of LR in this group of pts is 1.9% per year.**

Solin, ECOG 5194 (*JCO* 2009, PMID 19826126; *JCO* 2015, PMID 26371148): Single-arm trial of 711 DCIS pts (grades 1–2 and ≤2.5 cm OR grade 3 and ≤1 cm) treated with local excision only (margins ≥3 mm, 30% received tamoxifen). Median tumor sizes were 7 mm and 6 mm respectively. 12-year IBE was 14.4% for grade 1–2 and 24.6% for grade 3. The 12-yr IBR was 7.5% for grades 1–2 and 13.4% for grade 3. **Conclusion: Rate of recurrence increases without plateau (~1% per year for grades 1–2 and 2% per year for grade 3).**

McCormick, RTOG 9804 (*JCO* 2015, PMID 25605856): PRT of "low-risk" DCIS (Grades 1–2, size <2.5 cm, mammographically detected with margins ≥3 mm) randomized to WBI 50 Gy/25 fx versus observation. 636 pts enrolled of a planned 1,790. MFU 7.2 yrs. 62% received tamoxifen (optional). Primary endpoint was ipsilateral LR. At 7 yrs, LR was 0.9% RT versus 6.7% observation (*p* < .001). **Conclusion: RT reduces LR even in a very low-risk cohort.**

Is adjuvant tamoxifen beneficial? Who should receive it?

Tamoxifen lowers the incidence of any breast event (B24 and UK/ANZ) and contralateral breast events but does not affect ipsilateral invasive recurrences and therefore is not a substitute for RT (UK/ANZ). Tamoxifen benefits only ER-positive pts (B-24).

Fisher, NSABP B-24 (*Lancet* 1999, PMID 10376613; *JNCI* 2011, PMID 21398619): PRT of 1,798 DCIS pts comparing BCS with RT with or without tamoxifen. Stratified by age (≤49 or >49 yrs), tumor type (DCIS or DCIS + LCIS) and detection method (mammography, clinical exam, or both). Pts with a positive margin postlumpectomy or residual scattered calcifications were eligible. RT given within 8 weeks of lumpectomy with tangents to 50 Gy/25 fx. Placebo or tamoxifen 10 mg BID given within 56 days of lumpectomy for 5 yrs.

31% stopped tamoxifen due to side effects, personal reasons, or unspecified reasons. Any BC event decreased by 37% (13% vs. 8% at 5 yrs, $p = .0009$) as was the rate of invasive breast (7% vs. 4%, $p = .004$). Note that ER status was initially unknown (see Allred).

Allred, NSABP B-24 subgroup (*JCO* 2012, PMID 22393101): 732 pts evaluated from B-24 for ER status. 76% were ER+ and in these pts, tamoxifen decreased the 10-yr incidence of BC (HR 0.49, $p <. 001$) but showed no benefit with ER-negative pts.

Houghton, UK/ANZ Trial (*Lancet* 2003, PMID 12867108; *Lancet Oncol* 2011, PMID 21145284): Four-arm PRT of 1,694 DCIS pts after lumpectomy randomized using a 2 × 2 design: +/− RT and +/− tamoxifen. Surgery was a resection with specimen radiograph and negative margins; microinvasion was allowed. RT: 50 Gy/25 fx without a boost. Tamoxifen: 20 mg QD for 5 yrs. Pts could choose the 4-way randomization or one of the 2-way randomizations. Only pts randomized to a treatment were analyzed for that arm. At 10 yrs, risk of any breast event was no adjuvant treatment (32%), tamoxifen alone (24%), RT alone (13%), RT and tamoxifen (10%). Both tamoxifen and RT significantly decreased the risk of IBTR. Tamoxifen did not affect invasive recurrences and therefore is not a substitute for RT.

TABLE 23.3: Summary of DCIS Trials Evaluating Tamoxifen Versus no Tamoxifen						
	NSABP B24 10 yrs			UK/ANZ Tamoxifen Randomization 12.7 yrs		
	Tam	No Tam	HR	Tam	No Tam	HR
IBTR	13.2	16.6	0.68*	15.7	19.6	0.78*
Invasive Recur	6.6	9	NR	6.8	6.9	0.95
CBTR	4.9	8.1	0.68*	1.9	4.2	0.44*
OS	82.9	85.6	NR	NR	NR	NR
*Statistically significant difference.						

Is anastrozole superior to tamoxifen for DCIS?

Margolese, NSABP B-35 (*ASCO* 2015 Abstract LBA500): Phase III PRT of 3,104 postmenopausal women with ER or PR-positive DCIS comparing 1 mg/day anastrozole to 20 mg/day tamoxifen for 5 yrs. The primary endpoint was breast cancer-free interval (BCFI), defined as the time from randomization to any BCE including local, regional, distant recurrence or contralateral disease, invasive or DCIS. MFU 8.6 yrs. BCFI at 10 yrs was 89% versus 93% (HR 0.73) in favor of anastrozole ($p = .03$). Benefit was primarily in women <60 yrs of age. There was a nonsignificant (NS) trend for a reduction in breast second primary cancers with anastrozole (HR 0.68; $p = .07$). 10-yr estimates for OS were 92.1% for tamoxifen, 92.5% for anastrozole (NS).

Since tamoxifen prevents contralateral recurrences in the preceding trials, can we use it to prevent breast cancer in high-risk pts?

Yes, although often the side effects make this less frequently used.

Fisher, NSABP P-1 (*JNCI* 1998, PMID 9747868): 13,388 women with risk factors (≥60 y/o or with risk ≥1.66% or with a history of LCIS) randomized to placebo or tamoxifen for 5 yrs. Tamoxifen reduced the risk of invasive BC by 49% with older women benefiting more. All subgroups benefited. ER-positive tumors were reduced by 69% but no difference was seen in ER-negative.

Vogel, NSABP P-2 "STAR" (*JAMA* 2006, PMID 16754727): PRT comparing tamoxifen to raloxifene with the goal of reducing side effects of tamoxifen and testing efficacy of raloxifene. Overall raloxifene appeared similar in efficacy with a lower rate of thromboembolic events.

What is the optimal dose and fractionation for DCIS? Is hypofractionation appropriate?

Nearly all prospective DCIS trials used 50 Gy/25 fx with or without a boost. Hypofractionation has been studied prospectively (NYU trial and MD Anderson trial with oncologic outcomes pending[23]). However, given the efficacy and safety in invasive breast cancer, most consider hypofractionation to be appropriate for DCIS.

Lalani, Ontario Series (*IJROBP* 2014, PMID 25220719): RR of 1,609 pts treated in Ontario from 1994 to 2003. 60% treated with conventional RT, 40% with hypofractionation (42.4 Gy/16 fx). 15% of conventional pts received a boost whereas 54% of the hypofractionated pts received a boost. MFU 9.2 yrs. 10-yr local recurrence free survival (LRFS) 86% versus 89% for hypofractionated (p = .03). Hypofractionation was not associated with recurrence on multivariate analysis. **Conclusion: Hypofractionation was of similar efficacy to conventional schedules.**

Williamson, Princess Margaret Hospital (*R&O* 2010, PMID 20400190): RR of 266 pts with conventional 50 Gy in 25 fx (39%) versus hypofractionated 42.4 Gy in 16 fx or 40 in 16 fx+12.5 Gy boost (61%). MFU 3.76 yrs. No difference in LR. 4-yr recurrence 6% versus 6.7% for hypofractionation. High grade increased risk of LR (11% for Gr3 vs. 4% Gr1/2).

Hathout, Quebec (*IJROBP* 2013, PMID 24113057): 440 pts treated with hypofractionation, 28% with a boost. MFU 4.4 yrs. LRFS at 5 yrs was 3%.

Ciervide, NYU (*IJROBP* 2012, PMID 22579378): Pooled analysis of two institutional trials of hypofractionated WBI (42 Gy or 40.5 Gy in 15 fx) in DCIS. 145 pts, MFU 60 months. LR of DCIS 4.1% at 5 yrs; none were invasive recurrences.

Is it necessary to boost the tumor bed for DCIS patients?

This is controversial as there is no prospective randomized evidence directly comparing (trials ongoing). Note that a boost was performed in a small minority of pts on prospective trials (5%–9% NSABP B-17/EORTC, not recommended on SweDCIS/UK/ANZ/RTOG 9804). Retrospective series are noted in the following.

Omlin, Switzerland (*Lancet Oncol* 2006, PMID 16887482): RR of 373 pts from 18 institutions, all ≤45 yrs of age. Fifteen percent had no RT after surgery, 45% had RT without boost, 40% had RT with a 10 Gy boost. LRFS at 10 yrs improved for those given a boost (no RT 46%, RT no boost 72%, RT with boost 86%). **Conclusion: Boost should be considered in young pts.**

Wai, British Columbia (*Cancer* 2011, PMID 20803608): RR of 957 pts between 1985 and 1999 with MFU 9.3 yrs. 50% had no RT, 35% RT no boost, and 15% had RT with a boost. While RT was associated with improved LC, no difference between those with or without a boost.

Wong, McGill (*IJROBP* 2012, PMID 21664063): RR of 220 pts all with lumpectomy+RT, 36% received a boost, MFU 46 months. Boosted pts were higher risk but had lower LR (p = .03). **Conclusion: Consider a boost to offset risk factors for LR.**

Julian, NSABP B-24 (*ASCO* 2008 Abstract 537). RR of NSABP B-24; 1,569 analyzed, 692 underwent optional boost from 1 to 20 Gy (82% received 10 Gy) along with 50 Gy to whole breast. MFU 14 yrs. Although boosted pts were at higher risk, there was no impact on LR.

Rakovitch, Toronto (*IJROBP* 2013, PMID 23708085): RR of Ontario Registry; 1,895 pts w/ DCIS tx w/ BCS and RT. 70% with hypofractionation (40–44 Gy in 16 fxs), 561 w/ boost. Ten-yr LR 13% w/ boost, 12% w/ out; 10-yr invasive LR 6% versus 7% without. 10-yr DCIS LR 5% versus 7%. No significant benefit of boost for LR.

Moran, Multi-Institutional (*JAMA Oncol* 2017, PMID 28358936): RR of pooled patient-level data from 10 institutions including 4,131 patients treated between 1980 and 2010. Boost associated with significantly lower rate of ipsilateral breast tumor recurrence with benefit of 0.8% at 5 years, 1.6% at 10 years and 3.6% at 15 years. **Conclusion: Boost reduced rate of ipsilateral breast tumor recurrence across all age groups, similar to findings with invasive breast cancers.**

What factors predict for recurrence?

Beyond the Van Nuys Prognostic Index, other studies have discussed predictive factors that can aid in pt selection. A combined analysis of B-17 and B-24 demonstrated younger age, clinically detected DCIS, comedonecrosis, and positive margins to be associated with a higher risk of recurrence.[24]

Ringberg, SweDCIS (*Eur J Cancer* 2007, PMID 17118648): Factors for recurrence after BCT from SweDCIS Trial: Grade III histology and necrosis were predictors for higher likelihood of recurrence—all pts benefited from RT.

Vicini, Beaumont (*JCO* 2002, PMID 12039936): RR showing younger age is predictive of failure.

Rakovitch, Ontario (*JCO* 2007, PMID 17984181): RR showing that multifocality is a risk factor for recurrence but can be accounted for with RT (LR 20% vs. 40% if no RT given for multifocality).

What surgical margins are necessary?

Dunne, Ireland (*JCO* 2009, PMID 19255332). Study-level meta-analysis of 4,660 pts on 22 trials of BCS w/ adjuvant RT in DCIS looking at IBTR and margin status. Median time to IBTR 5 yrs. Negative margins had lower IBTR than positive (64% less), close or unknown margins after RT. No significant difference in IBTR with 2-mm versus >5-mm margins. **Conclusion: Margins of 2 mm or more are sufficient when RT is used.**

Morrow, SSO/ASTRO/ASCO Consensus Guideline (*JCO* 2016, PMID 2758719): No prior consensus regarding the optimal margin width for DCIS treated with BCS and WBI. Multidisciplinary consensus panel used a meta-analysis of margin width and IBTR rates from a systematic review of 20 studies including 7,883 pts and other published literature to obtain guidelines. Negative margins (no ink on DCIS) halves the risk of IBTR compared with positive margins. When WBI is given, a 2-mm margin minimizes the risk of IBTR compared with smaller negative margins with statistically significant odds ratio (OR) of 0.51. Margins greater than 2 mm and up to 10 mm do not significantly decrease IBTR compared with 2-mm margins (with WBI). Clinical judgment should be used in determining the need for further surgery in pts with negative margins <2 mm.

Are there any patients who require radiation after a mastectomy for DCIS?

Childs, Harvard (*IJROBP* 2012, PMID 22975615): RR of 142 pts with mastectomy without post-op RT with pure DCIS (no microinvasion). 15% with positive margin, 16% with margin ≤2 mm. One pt with positive margin and one pt with close margins experienced chest wall recurrence. **Conclusion: Postmastectomy radiation therapy (PMRT) not likely warranted even with positive margins.**

Chan, UCSF (*IJROBP* 2010, PMID 20646871): RR of 193 pts with mastectomy: 55 with close margin, 4 with positive margin. Risk of chest wall recurrence 1.7% for all, and 3.4% for high-grade pts.

Carlson, Emory (*JACS* 2007, PMID 17481544): RR of 223 pts with skin-sparing mastectomy and reconstruction without RT. LR 3.3%, regional recurrence 0.9%, distant recurrence 0.9%. If margin <1 mm LR 10%.

Can we use Oncotype® for DCIS?

It may be an independent prognostic tool for the risk of recurrence. However, the test may not be cost-effective,[25] the low-risk subset has a risk of 10%, and many women may choose RT anyway in this situation.

Solin, ECOG E5194 (*JNCI* 2013, PMID 23641039): Molecular profiling of pts with negative margins treated without RT on the ECOG E5194 study. Oncotype DX® performed on subset of 327 pts. Identified three groups (70% low risk, 16% intermediate, and 14% high) with IBTR risks of 10.6%, 26.7%, and 25.9% at 10 yrs, for low, intermediate, and high risk, respectively. Invasive recurrence risks were 3.7%, 12.3%, and 19.2% for the three groups. Prognostic value persisted on multivariate analysis.

Rakovitch, DCIS Oncotype® (*Breast Cancer Res Treat* 2015, PMID 26119102): Validated Oncotype DX® in a retrospective population-based cohort of 718 cases treated with surgery alone with negative margins. MFU 9.6 yrs. Oncotype DX® independently predicted the risk of recurrence on multivariate analysis. The 10-yr LR risk for low, intermediate & high-risk groups was 12.7%, 33% and 27.8% respectively. **Conclusion: Oncotype for DCIS adds independent value in an external subset; however, even in the low-risk group the LR risk may be high enough to offer RT.**

Is accelerated partial breast irradiation (APBI) feasible in DCIS?

Multiple studies support the use of APBI in appropriately selected pts. Current ASTRO, ABS, and ASBS guidelines support the use of APBI for selected pts with DCIS.

Jeruss, MammoSite® Registry (*Ann Surg Oncol* 2011, PMID 20577822): 194 pts with DCIS underwent APBI via MammoSite®. 46% developed seroma. 92% with favorable cosmetic outcome at follow-up; 3.1% with IBTR; 5-yr LR of 3.39%.

Shah, Beaumont (*Clin Breast Cancer* 2012, PMID 22658839): 99 pts treated with APBI with MFU of 3 yrs. At 5 yrs IBTR was 1.4%, CSS was 100%, and OS was 94%.

Shah, MammoSite® Registry (*Ann Surg Oncol* 2013, PMID 23975302): 194 pts with DCIS who underwent APBI with MammoSite® (34 Gy in 10 fx). Median follow-up 63 months. 5-yr actuarial IBTR rate of 4.1%. Tumor size (OR = 1.1, $p = .03$) and ER negativity (OR = 3.0, $p = .0009$) were associated with IBTR, while a trend was noted for positive margins (OR = 2.0, $p = .06$) and cautionary/unsuitable status compared with suitable status (OR = 1.8, $p = .07$).

Vicini, ASBS/WBH Pooled Analysis (*Ann Surg Oncol* 2013, PMID 23054123): Pooled analysis from American Society of Breast Surgeons (ASBS) MammoSite Registry Trial and William Beaumont Hospital of 300 women with DCIS who underwent APBI over 17-year period. Rate of IBTR was 2.6% at 5 yrs with no regional recurrences, with CSS 99.5% and OS of 99.5%. When comparing the cautionary DCIS group to the invasive suitable/cautionary group, no difference in IBTR was noted (2.6 vs. 3.1 %, $p = .90$) with significant improvements in distant metastases (DM; 0 vs. 2.5 %, $p = .05$), disease-free survival (98.5 vs. 94.4 %, $p = .05$), and OS (95.7 vs. 90.8 %, $p = .03$) noted for DCIS pts. When comparing cautionary DCIS pts to invasive suitable pts, no difference in IBTR were noted (2.6 vs. 2.4 %, $p = .76$), while improved OS for DCIS pts was noted (95.7 vs. 90.9 %, $p = .02$).

Strnad, GEC-ESTRO Multicatheter Trial (*Lancet* 2015, PMID 26494415): PRT of 1,184 women randomized to multicatheter brachytherapy versus WBI (50 Gy + 10 Gy boost). Included women with stage 0-IIA tumors ≤3 cm, pN0/Nmi, no LVSI and clear margins ≥2 mm (≥5 mm for DCIS). For DCIS, only Van Nuys low or intermediate scores (<8) included (n = 60 or 5%). APBI performed to the tumor bed with ≥2-cm margins to 32 Gy in 8 fx or 30.3 Gy in 7 fx BID or pulsed-dose brachytherapy to 50 Gy. APBI was considered noninferior if the 5-yr LR rate in the APBI arm did not exceed 3% more than the WBI arm. 5-yr LR rate was 0.92% in the WBI arm versus 1.44% in the APBI arm.

Is there a role for intraoperative radiation therapy (IORT) in the treatment of DCIS?

Intraoperative radiation therapy has been shown to have higher rates of local recurrence in two randomized trials (TARGIT and ELIOT). Limited data are available for pts with DCIS and thus IORT is not recommended off-protocol at this time.

Rivera, IORT for DCIS (*Breast* 2016, PMID 26534876): Prospective nonrandomized trial of 30 women with pure DCIS considered eligible for IORT based on preoperative mammography and contrast-enhanced magnetic resonance imaging (CE-MRI). Inclusion: lesion was ≤4 cm in maximal diameter on both digital mammography and CE-MRI, pure DCIS on biopsy or wide local excision, and considered resectable with clear surgical margins (2 mm) using BCS. Median pt age was 57 yrs (range 42–79 yrs) and median histologic lesion size was 15.6 mm (2–40 mm). A total of 14.3% (5/35) of pts required some form of additional therapy. At 36 months MFU (range of 2–83 months), only two pts experienced LR of cancer (DCIS only), yielding a 5.7% LR rate. No deaths or DM were observed.

Is there a survival benefit to radiation after DCIS?

None of the prospective trials or the meta-analysis mentioned earlier demonstrated a survival benefit (although women on NSABP B-24 who developed an invasive recurrence demonstrated inferior survival).

Narod, SEER (*JAMA* Oncol 2015, PMID 26291673): SEER analysis of 108,196 DCIS pts with an MFU of 7.5 yrs. 20-year BCSM was 3.3% and was higher in women <35 yrs of age and black women. RT reduced the risk of invasive recurrence at 10 yrs (2.5% vs. 4.9%) but did not improve BCSM. **Conclusion: Prevention of IBTR did not alter BC mortality at 10 yrs.**

With long-term follow-up, do the outcomes for DCIS change?

Solin, multi-institutional (*Cancer* 2005, PMID 15674853): 1,003 women treated at 10 North American centers with BCS+RT. 15-yr rate of any LF was 19%. Older pts (≥50) and negative margins experienced fewer failures. CSS was 98%.

Wilkinson, Beaumont (*Ann Surg Onc* 2012, PMID 22644510): Long-term outcomes of 129 pts treated between 1980 and 1993 with a median follow-up of 19 yrs. 20-year rate of IBTR was 16%.

What is LCIS and how does it differ from DCIS?

Lobular carcinoma in situ (LCIS) is asymptomatic and is not considered a premalignant condition but rather a risk factor for developing invasive breast cancer.[1] The exception is pleomorphic

LCIS, which may be treated surgically with excellent outcomes based on small retrospective data if negative margins are obtained.[26] The risk of developing breast cancer is approximately 7% at 10 yrs with an equal chance of developing a malignancy in either breast.[27] If a suspicious lesion is detected on mammography and only LCIS is discovered on excision, it is important to repeat imaging/excision to ensure the entire area was removed. There is no role for radiation therapy in the treatment of LCIS.

REFERENCES

1. Cancer Facts & Figures 2015. 2015. http://www.cancer.org/acs/groups/content/@editorial/documents/document/acspc-044552.pdf
2. Collins LC, Tamimi RM, Baer HJ, et al. Outcome of patients with ductal carcinoma in situ untreated after diagnostic biopsy: results from the Nurses' Health Study. *Cancer*. 2005;103(9):1778–1784.
3. Eusebi V, Feudale E, Foschini MP, et al. Long-term follow-up of in situ carcinoma of the breast. *Semin Diagn Pathol*. 1994;11(3):223–235.
4. Sanders ME, Schuyler PA, Dupont WD, Page DL. The natural history of low-grade ductal carcinoma in situ of the breast in women treated by biopsy only revealed over 30 years of long-term follow-up. *Cancer*. 2005;103(12):2481–2484.
5. Siziopikou KP, Anderson SJ, Cobleigh MA, et al. Preliminary results of centralized HER2 testing in ductal carcinoma in situ (DCIS): NSABP B-43. *Breast Cancer Res Treat*. 2013;142(2):415–421.
6. Screening IUPoBC. The benefits and harms of breast cancer screening: an independent review. *Lancet*. 2012;380(9855):1778–1786.
7. Bevers TB, Anderson BO, Bonaccio E, et al. NCCN clinical practice guidelines in oncology: breast cancer screening and diagnosis. *J Natl Compr Canc Netw*. 2009;7(10):1060–1096.
8. Saslow D, Boetes C, Burke W, et al. American Cancer Society guidelines for breast screening with MRI as an adjunct to mammography. *CA Cancer J Clin*. 2007;57(2):75–89.
9. Holland R, Hendriks JH, Vebeek AL, et al. Extent, distribution, and mammographic/histological correlations of breast ductal carcinoma in situ. *Lancet*. 1990;335(8688):519–522.
10. Dershaw DD, Abramson A, Kinne DW. Ductal carcinoma in situ: mammographic findings and clinical implications. *Radiology*. 1989;170(2):411–415.
11. Kuhl CK, Schrading S, Bieling HB, et al. MRI for diagnosis of pure ductal carcinoma in situ: a prospective observational study. *Lancet*. 2007;370(9586):485–492.
12. McGhan LJ, Pockaj BA, Wasif N, et al. Atypical ductal hyperplasia on core biopsy: an automatic trigger for excisional biopsy? *Ann Surg Oncol*. 2012;19(10):3264–3269.
13. Correa C, McGale P, Taylor C, et al. Overview of the randomized trials of radiotherapy in ductal carcinoma in situ of the breast. *J Natl Cancer Inst Monogr*. 2010;2010(41):162–177.
14. Silverstein MJ. An argument against routine use of radiotherapy for ductal carcinoma in situ. *Oncology (Williston Park)*. 2003;17(11):1511–1533; discussion 1533–1514, 1539, 1542 passim.
15. Silverstein MJ, Lagios MD. Choosing treatment for patients with ductal carcinoma in situ: fine tuning the University of Southern California/Van Nuys Prognostic Index. *J Natl Cancer Inst Monogr*. 2010;2010(41):193–196.
16. Whitfield R, Kollias J, de Silva P, et al. Management of ductal carcinoma in situ according to Van Nuys Prognostic Index in Australia and New Zealand. *ANZ J Surg*. 2012;82(7–8):518–523.
17. MacAusland SG, Hepel JT, Chong FK, et al. An attempt to independently verify the utility of the Van Nuys Prognostic Index for ductal carcinoma in situ. *Cancer*. 2007;110(12):2648–2653.
18. Hwang ES. The impact of surgery on ductal carcinoma in situ outcomes: the use of mastectomy. *J Natl Cancer Inst Monogr*. 2010;2010(41):197–199.
19. Faverly DR, Burgers L, Bult P, Holland R. Three dimensional imaging of mammary ductal carcinoma in situ: clinical implications. *Semin Diagn Pathol*. 1994;11(3):193–198.
20. Kurniawan ED, Rose A, Mou A, et al. Risk factors for invasive breast cancer when core needle biopsy shows ductal carcinoma in situ. *Arch Surg*. 2010;145(11):1098–1104.
21. Yen TW, Hunt KK, Ross MI, et al. Predictors of invasive breast cancer in patients with an initial diagnosis of ductal carcinoma in situ: a guide to selective use of sentinel lymph node biopsy in management of ductal carcinoma in situ. *J Am Coll Surg*. 2005;200(4):516–526.
22. Gradishar WJ, Anderson BO, Balassanian R, et al.; NCCN Clinical Practice Guidelines in Oncology. Breast cancer version 2.2015. *J Natl Compr Canc Netw*. 2015;13(4):448–475.

23. Shaitelman SF, Schlembach PJ, Arzu I, et al. Acute and short-term toxic effects of conventionally fractionated vs hypofractionated whole-breast irradiation: a randomized clinical trial. *JAMA Oncol.* 2015;1(7):931–941.

24. Wapnir IL, Dignam JJ, Fisher B, et al. Long-term outcomes of invasive ipsilateral breast tumor recurrences after lumpectomy in NSABP B-17 and B-24 randomized clinical trials for DCIS. *J Clin Oncol.* 2016;34(33):3963–3968.

25. Raldow AC, Sher D, Chen AB, et al. Cost effectiveness of the oncotype DX DCIS score for guiding treatment of patients with ductal carcinoma in situ. *J Clin Oncol.* 2016.

26. Flanagan MR, Rendi MH, Calhoun KE, et al. Pleomorphic lobular carcinoma in situ: radiologic-pathologic features and clinical management. *Ann Surg Oncol.* 2015;22(13):4263–4269.

27. Chuba PJ, Hamre MR, Yap J, et al. Bilateral risk for subsequent breast cancer after lobular carcinoma-in-situ: analysis of surveillance, epidemiology, and end results data. *J Clin Oncol.* 2005;23(24):5534–5541.

24: RECURRENT BREAST CANCER

Martin C. Tom, Camille A. Berriochoa, and Chirag Shah

QUICK HIT: Locoregional recurrence (LRR) of breast cancer is associated with an increased risk of distant metastases and mortality. The majority of recurrences occur in the ipsilateral breast or chest wall within 5 years of initial treatment. Treatment is dependent upon the pt's initial management and the location of recurrence, often utilizing surgery and/or RT, with consideration of CHT or endocrine therapy. RT may also be given with concurrent hyperthermia or CHT.

TABLE 24.1: General Treatment Paradigm for Locoregionally Recurrent Breast Cancer[1]

Local recurrence only:	Initial BCS+RT	Total mastectomy + ALN staging (if level I/II dissection not previously done), then consider CHT
	Initial mastectomy only	Surgery if possible + RT, then consider CHT either pre-op or post-op
	Initial mastectomy + ALN I/II dissection + RT	Consider CHT, then surgery if possible, then consider re-irradiation
Regional ± local recurrence:	ALN recurrence	CHT, then surgery + RT if possible (consider re-irradiation)
	SCV or IMN recurrence	CHT, then RT if possible

EPIDEMIOLOGY: There are ~3.5 million breast cancer survivors in the United States.[2] LRR occurs in approximately 5% to 15%.[3–6] Most recur within 5 years of diagnosis, with recurrences after mastectomy occurring earlier than after BCT (1.2 years earlier).[7] Following LRR, 5-yr OS varies widely, ranging from 25% to 75%.[7–10]

RISK FACTORS: Younger age, premenopausal status, larger tumor size, higher BMI, increasing number of LN+, decreased number of dissected LN, ER-negative, HER2+ not treated with trastuzumab, high grade, lymphovascular invasion, no tamoxifen, margin positivity, BCS without RT, mastectomy without RT when indicated.[11–16] Genetic susceptibility (BRCA1 or BRCA2) increases the risk of a new primary.

ANATOMY: Following BCT, LRR occurs most commonly in the ipsilateral breast. Following mastectomy, LRR occurs in the CW (~60%) > SCV (~20%) > ALN (~10%).[11]

CLINICAL PRESENTATION: Usually detected via mammography (following BCT), physical exam, or other imaging. Symptoms include palpable mass, new-onset lymphedema, palpable LN, skin changes, or brachial plexopathy.[17–19]

WORKUP: H&P, labs (CBC, LFT, alkaline phosphatase, creatinine to evaluate renal function in anticipation of contrast-enhanced imaging), CT chest, CT (or MRI) abdomen/pelvis, MRI brain if symptomatic, bone scan, PET/CT, x-rays of symptomatic bones or suspicious areas noted on bone scan, biopsy with comparison to original pathology, receptor status evaluation, genetic counseling (if high risk).[1] Consider breast MRI for those with intact breast.

PROGNOSTIC FACTORS: Prognosis is better if LRR is isolated in the CW/axilla/IM nodes alone (5-yr OS 44%–49%) versus SCV/multiple sites (5-yr OS 21%–24%).[20] Worse prognosis if LRR within 2 years of initial treatment, following mastectomy (vs. following BCT), skin involvement, larger primary tumor, initial multiple LN+, older age, African American, or higher BMI.[9,14,20,21]

STAGING: Assign a recurrent TNM (rTNM) stage per AJCC (see Chapter 21 for staging).

TREATMENT PARADIGM

Surgery: Surgical options are dependent on the location of the recurrence, previous surgery performed, and feasibility of resection. In general, in-breast recurrences after previous lumpectomy may be salvaged with mastectomy. CW recurrences and nodal recurrences should be excised if feasible, sometimes after cytoreductive systemic therapy.

Chemotherapy: Choices of systemic therapy are determined by the tumor receptor status (ER, PR, HER2) and previous therapy received. CHT concurrent with RT may be considered in select pts typically with gross residual disease. For all recurrences consider CHT after maximum local control achieved, especially if ER-negative (per the CALOR trial).

Radiation: For the adjuvant treatment of a radiation-naïve pt, doses of 50 to 60 Gy are appropriate. For margin-positive disease in the radiation-naïve pt, doses of 60 to 64 Gy or higher are recommended. For definitive treatment of unresected gross disease in the radiation-naïve pt, doses of 66 to 70 Gy are recommended. Many different regimens have been used for re-irradiation. One option includes 45 Gy at 1.5 Gy/fx given BID to the partial breast (RTOG 1014). For re-irradiation of gross disease, consider concurrent hyperthermia to improve LC. Sequelae can include fatigue, radiation dermatitis, fibrosis, lymphedema, brachial plexopathy, chest wall pain, rib fracture, pneumonitis, and cardiotoxicity.

Hyperthermia (HT): Typically given to superficial CW recurrences concurrent with re-irradiation to temperatures of 43°C. HT is utilized to increase tumor cell kill in conjunction with other therapies. At 43°C there is a dramatic decrease in the cell survival slope (Arrhenius plot). HT dosing is frequently described in terms of CEM43°C T90, which represents the number of cumulative equivalent minutes at 43°C exceeded by 90% of the monitored points within the tumor. HT-related damage is cell cycle nonspecific (as opposed to RT, which is most damaging during G2/M and least effective in S). When used in conjunction with RT, HT impairs the cell's ability to repair RT-induced DNA damage, resulting in more effective tumor cell kill. However, cells may develop thermotolerance (resistance to subsequent HT), which is a phenomenon thought to be due to the production of heat shock proteins. A commonly used treatment regimen is 32 Gy in eight fractions delivered twice weekly with weekly HT as per the ESHO 5-88 trial published in 1996 (see Vernon et al. later), with more recent data using this regimen published by Dutch investigators in 2015. HT techniques include microwave heating, regional perfusional HT, ultrasound, and pt wrapping.

EVIDENCE-BASED Q&A

How are true recurrences (TR) and new primaries (NP) differentiated? How does this change prognosis?

Characteristics of a NP include different histology, change in receptor status, different location, loss of heterozygosity (LOH), and change from aneuploid to diploid compared to the original tumor.

NP and TR occur at a similar rate until 8 years; subsequently NP occurs more frequently. A NP has a more favorable prognosis compared to a TR (10-yr OS 75% vs. 55%).[22-24]

Can a sentinel lymph node biopsy be repeated for LRR breast cancer?

Yes. A 2013 meta-analysis found repeat SLNB was feasible, accurate, spared pts from unnecessary ALND, and provided information that can alter management. It included 692 pts who had prior SLNB or ALND who underwent repeat SLNB. There was successful SLN identification in 65% (more successful if no prior ALND) with 19% node positive. Aberrant drainage was seen more frequently in those with prior ALND. SLNB findings changed management in 18%. The false negative rate was 0.2%.[25] Previous RT may worsen repeat SLN identification.[26]

Local Recurrence After BCT

What is the preferred treatment for LRR after initial BCT?

Mastectomy is preferred; ~80% to 95% of pts with LRR after BCT are suitable mastectomy candidates.[27,28] After salvage mastectomy, second LRR ranges from 4% to 25%, with 5-yr OS ranging from 57% to 100%, and 10-yr OS ~66% (see Table 24.2).[29]

After initial BCT, is salvage BCS an option?

Many clinicians prefer salvage mastectomy given the higher observed LR rates following salvage BCS (4%–25% vs. 7%–49%).[29] However, no prospective trials have compared the two strategies. Two retrospective studies showed that following primary BCT with a subsequent IBTR, salvage mastectomy versus salvage BCS had no difference in OS.

Alpert, Yale (*IJROBP* 2005, PMID 16199315): RR of 146 pts s/p BCT with IBTR. 30 had salvage breast-conserving surgery (SBCS), 116 underwent salvage mastectomy. MFU 13.8 yrs. OS similar (SBCS 58.0% vs. salvage mastectomy 65.7%, *p* = NS). LR and DM rate similar between groups, both about 7%. **Conclusion: Salvage BCS is feasible with comparable outcomes to salvage mastectomy, but pts remain at risk for further IBTR.**

Salvadori, Milan (*Br J Surg* 1999, PMID 10027366): RR of 209 pts s/p quadrantectomy, ALND and RT with IBTR. 57 had local excision and 134 had total mastectomy. MFU 73 mos. 5 yr OS with local excision 85% versus TM 70%. LR at 5 years with local excision 19% versus TM 4%. **Conclusion: Breast conservation surgery can be considered for IBTR.**

TABLE 24.2: Outcomes After Salvage Mastectomy for IBTR After BCT				
Series	N	MFU (mos)	LR (%)	5-yr OS (%)
Alpert et al[28]	116	166	**6.9**	
Shah et al[29]	18	49	**10**	100
Dalberg et al[30]	65	156	**12**	
Kurtz et al[31]	43	53	**12**	
Jacobson et al[32]	18	120	**17**	
Voogd et al[33]	208	52	**25**	
Salvadori et al[34]	134	60	**4**	70
Ofuchi et al[35]	51	53	**11**	57–100
Kurtz et al[36]	66	84	**12.1**	68
Chen et al[37]	568			78

TABLE 24.3: Outcomes After Excision Alone for IBTR After BCT				
Series	N	MFU (mos)	LR (%)	5-yr OS (%)
Alpert et al[28]	30	116	6.7	
Shah et al[29]	18	49	0	100
Dalberg et al[30]	14	13	33	
Kurtz et al[31]	46	53	36	
Voogd et al[33]	16	52	38	
Salvadori et al[34]	57	60	14	85
Ofuchi et al[35]	73	53	49	89–94
Kurtz et al[36]	52	84	23	79
Chen et al[37]	179			67

After initial BCT, is re-irradiation safe and feasible?

Yes, however data is limited. Retrospective data suggest re-irradiation is feasible with acceptable acute/late toxicity. RTOG 1014 (repeat BCT with 3D partial breast re-irradiation) 3-year data shows acceptable toxicity and promising control rates; however, one must consider its stringent entrance criteria and the need for longer follow-up. Consider HT, especially for superficial tumors.

Wahl, Multi-institutional (*IJROBP* 2008, PMID 17869019): RR of 81 pts with LRR who underwent repeat RT to breast or chest wall. Median first course RT was 60 Gy and second course was 48 Gy, with median total dose 106 Gy. 20% received BID RT, 54% received concurrent HT, and 54% concurrent CHT. MFU from second RT was 1 year. 4 pts had late grade 3/4 toxicity. CR in 57%, with trend to improved CR with HT (67% vs. 39%, $p = .08$). 1-yr local DFS 100% if no gross disease versus 53% with gross disease. No treatment-related mortality. **Conclusion: Repeat RT is feasible with acceptable toxicity.**

Arthur, RTOG 1014 (*ASTRO* 2016, Late-breaking Abstract #10): Phase II, 3D conformal partial breast re-irradiation (PBrI) following repeat lumpectomy for IBTR after previous BCS+WBI. Included IBTR>1 year following BCT, <3 cm, unifocal and negative margins, ≤3 LN+ without ECE. PBrI to surgical cavity + 1.5 cm CTV, +1 cm PTV. 45 Gy, 1.5 Gy BID in 30 fx with 3DCRT. 58 pts (23 DCIS, 35 invasive, median age 67.5 years). MFU 3.6 years; 6.9% late grade 3 AE, no grade 4. 3-yr IBTR 3.7%, DMFS 95%, OS 95%. **Conclusion: Supports concept of repeat lumpectomy with PBrI as an alternative to mastectomy.**

Is interstitial brachytherapy after LRR safe and feasible?

Yes, though data is still limited. The largest retrospective study suggests outcomes are comparable to mastectomy with promising cosmetic results and limited toxicity.

Hannoun-Levi, GEC-ESTRO (*Radiother Oncol* 2013, PMID 23647758): RR of 217 pts with IBTR following primary BCT (surgery + whole breast with or without regional nodes) retreated with lumpectomy followed by interstitial multicatheter brachytherapy (MCB; LDR, PDR, or HDR). MFU 3.9 years. 10-yr actuarial second LR, DM, and OS rates were 7%, 19%, and 76%, respectively. Excellent/good cosmetic result achieved in 85%. **Conclusion: With IBTR, lumpectomy plus MCB is feasible and effective in preventing second LR with an OS rate at least equivalent to those achieved with salvage mastectomy.**

Local recurrence after mastectomy

How should local/CW recurrences after mastectomy be treated?

Excision (rather than incisional biopsy) improves outcomes. If possible, aggressive RT after resection is preferred (see Halverson) with consideration of CHT afterwards as per the CALOR study.

Schwaibold, U. Pennsylvania (*IJROBP*** 1991, PMID 2061107):** RR of 128 pts with LRR after mastectomy (most commonly CW, then SCV). 78 pts had excisional biopsy and 49 had incisional biopsy; followed by RT. 5-yr LRC was 43%. On MVA, excisional biopsy was prognostic for improved 5-yr OS and 5-yr RFS. **Conclusion: Excision of gross disease improves outcomes.**

Halverson, Washington U. (*IJROBP*** 1990, PMID 2211253):** RR of 244 pts with LRR following mastectomy alone. Based on findings, they had four recommendations: (a) Large field RT (i.e., entire CW) improved control compared to localized RT (i.e., lesion +1–2-cm margin). 10-yr control 63% versus 18%, $p < .01$. (b) Elective RT to SCV nodes 46 to 50 Gy reduced SCV failure from 16% to 6%, $p = .049$. (c) Elective RT to uninvolved CW to >50 Gy. Pts with SCV or ALN disease failed in CW 29% and 21%, respectively. RT to uninvolved CW decreased recurrence from 27% versus 17%, $p = .32$. (d) Treatment to >50 Gy for completely excised recurrences and >60 Gy for incompletely excised <3-cm recurrences (tumors <3-cm control with ≥60 Gy vs. <60 Gy was 100% vs. 76%). Tumor control for >3-cm lesions was only 50% despite doses of 70 Gy.

Is re-irradiation in the postmastectomy setting safe and feasible?

Wahl's study (described earlier) included 31 pts s/p mastectomy and demonstrated that re-irradiation to the CW appears safe. Acute/late toxicity occurred at acceptable rates and were most commonly skin related (e.g., dermatitis, fibrosis, skin infection) or the development of lymphedema. However, one must account for the risk of brachial plexopathy and pneumonitis.

Regional Recurrence To Axillary Lymph Nodes Or Supraclavicular Lymph Nodes

Following mastectomy, LRR occurs in the chest wall (~60%) > SCV (~20%) > ALN (~10%).[11] Prognosis is better if LRR is isolated to CW/ALNs/IMNs alone (5-yr OS 44%–49%) versus SCV/ multiple sites (5-yr OS 21%–24%).[20]

What series demonstrates outcomes after treatment for supraclavicular recurrence?

SCV recurrence (SCVr) is associated with a poor prognosis. However, long-term survival is possible with SCVr and aggressive treatment may benefit these pts.

Reddy, MD Anderson (*IJROBP*** 2011, PMID 21168284):** RR of 140 pts with LRR following initial MRM and CHT, 47 pts involving SCV (23 isolated SCVr). Pts with SCVr had worse DMFS and OS than those without SCV involvement. However, those with isolated SCVr did similar to those with isolated CW LRR with 5-yr OS of 25%. **Conclusion: SCVr carries a poor prognosis, but those with isolated SCVr can achieve long-term OS.**

What series demonstrates outcomes after treatment for axillary recurrence?

de Boer, Netherlands (*Br J Surg*** 2001, PMID 11136323).** RR of 59 pts with axillary recurrence (ALNr). Median time to ALNr 2.6 yrs. 41 pts had resection and 25 pts achieved complete resection. 5-yr OS 39%. Complete resection improved LRC and OS. **Conclusion: Pts with ALNr had a poor prognosis, but complete excision associated with improved outcomes.**

Newman, MD Anderson (*Am J Surg* 2000, PMID 11113430). RR of 44 ALNr. Median time to ALNr was 19.8 months and was isolated in 68% of cases. Most presented with a palpable mass (93%). ALNr was completely controlled in 71% with most being treated with multimodality therapy of surgery followed by RT and/or systemic therapy. 50% developed DM at median of 23 months from ALNr, which was more common if ALNr was not controlled (77% vs. 39%, *p* = .02). Pts who received trimodality therapy had improved control over those with single- or dual-modality treatment (94% vs. 69% vs. 36%, *p* = .005). **Conclusion: Half of pts with ALNr develop DM. Durable control is best accomplished with multimodality therapy consisting of surgery plus RT and/or systemic therapy.**

What is the role of locoregional recurrence?

For all recurrences consider CHT after maximum local control achieved, particularly if ER-negative.

Aebi, CALOR Trial (*Lancet Oncol* 2014, PMID 24439313): PRT of 162 pts with isolated LRR s/p radical resection (R0 or R1) randomized to adjuvant multiagent CHT or observation. All could receive hormone/HER2 therapy or RT. Excluded SCVr. The CHT used was not standardized but rather was left to clinician discretion. MFU 4.9 yrs. 5-yr DFS better in the chemo arm (69% vs. 57%, HR 0.59, *p* = .046). 5-yr OS also improved in CHT arm (88% vs. 76%, HR 0.41, *p* = .024). CHT was significantly more effective in ER-negative (*p* = .046). CHT had 15% grade ≥3 AE. **Conclusion: Following complete resection for isolated LRR, adjuvant CHT should be recommended, especially for those who are ER-negative.**

Does RT with hyperthermia (HT) improve complete response (CR) rates compared to RT alone?

Yes. Two prospective studies and a meta-analysis show significantly improved CR rates with RT and HT compared to RT alone (~40% vs. ~60%), and favorable CR rates (~66%) for re-irradiation with HT.

Datta, Hyperthermia Meta-analysis (*IJROBP* 2016, PMID 26899950): Meta-analysis of RT+HT in locally recurrent breast cancers. 34 studies (8 two-arm, 26 single-arm). Treatment was median of seven HT sessions at an average of 42.5°C, mean RT dose 38.2 Gy (26–60 Gy). In the two-arm studies (627 pts) RT+HT had CR in 60% versus RT alone 38% (SS). In the single-arm studies, RT+HT had CR rate of 63%. Among the 779 pts with previous RT, RT+HT had CR of 67%. Mean acute and late grade 3/4 toxicities with RT + HT were 14% and 5%, respectively. **Conclusion: In LRBC, RT+HT improves CR rates compared to RT alone. For reirradiation + HT, CR was achieved in 67% of patients.**

Linthorst, Re-irradiation + Hyperthermia (*Radiother Oncol* 2015, PMID 26002305): RR of 248 pts with breast cancer recurrence treated with re-irradiation (32 Gy/8 fx, twice weekly) and HT (once weekly after RT). MFU 32 mo. CR 70%. LC and OS at 1, 3, and 5 yrs was 53%, 40%, and 39%, and 66%, 32%, and 18% respectively. 10-yr OS was 10%. Thermal burns in 23%, but healed with conservative tx. 5-yr late G3 toxicity 1%. **Conclusion: Re-irradiation has high rate of LC with acceptable late toxicity. Many pts achieved LC during survival period.**

Jones, Duke (*JCO* 2005, PMID 15860867): PRT of 109 pts with superficial tumors (≤3-cm depth) comparing RT±HT. CR 66.1% in RT+HT arm and 42.4% in RT alone arm. Pts with prior RT had most benefit (68% vs. 23%, SS). No OS benefit was seen. Toxicity well tolerated, one grade III thermal burn. **Conclusion: Adjuvant HT with a thermal dose >10 CEM 43°C T(90) significantly improves LC in pts with superficial tumors receiving RT.**

Vernon, International Collaborative Hyperthermia Group (*IJROBP* 1996, PMID 8690639): Merged five PRTs (including the ESHO 5-88 PRT from the Netherlands) due to slow accrual. 306 pts with advanced primary or recurrent breast cancer. Target 43°C with RT given in various fractionations. Primary endpoint was local CR. Overall CR for RT alone 41% versus RT+HT 59% (p = SS). Greatest effect of HT in recurrent lesions in previous RT, where re-irradiation dose was low. 2-yr OS ~40% (p = NS), 74% pts progressed outside HT area during follow-up. **Conclusion: There *seems* to be a benefit to HT, but well-designed, prospective trials with appropriate criteria are warranted.**

REFERENCES

1. NCCN Clinical Practice Guidelines in Oncology: Breast Cancer. 2016; 2.2016. https://www.nccn.org/professionals/physician_gls/pdf/breast_blocks.pdf
2. Miller KD, Siegel RL, Lin CC, et al. Cancer treatment and survivorship statistics, 2016. *CA Cancer J Clin.* 2016;66(4):271–289.
3. Fisher B, Anderson S, Bryant J, et al. Twenty-year follow-up of a randomized trial comparing total mastectomy, lumpectomy, and lumpectomy plus irradiation for the treatment of invasive breast cancer. *N Engl J Med.* 2002;347(16):1233–1241.
4. Ragaz J, Jackson SM, Le N, et al. Adjuvant radiotherapy and chemotherapy in node-positive premenopausal women with breast cancer. *N Engl J Med.* 1997;337(14):956–962.
5. Overgaard M, Nielsen HM, Overgaard J. Is the benefit of postmastectomy irradiation limited to patients with four or more positive nodes, as recommended in international consensus reports? A subgroup analysis of the DBCG 82 b&c randomized trials. *Radiother Oncol.* 2007;82(3):247–253.
6. Overgaard M, Jensen MB, Overgaard J, et al. Postoperative radiotherapy in high-risk postmenopausal breast-cancer patients given adjuvant tamoxifen: Danish Breast Cancer Cooperative Group DBCG 82c randomised trial. *Lancet.* 1999;353(9165):1641–1648.
7. van Tienhoven G, Voogd AC, Peterse JL, et al. Prognosis after treatment for loco-regional recurrence after mastectomy or breast conserving therapy in two randomised trials (EORTC 10801 and DBCG-82TM). EORTC Breast Cancer Cooperative Group and the Danish Breast Cancer Cooperative Group. *Eur J Cancer.* 1999;35(1):32–38.
8. Wapnir IL, Anderson SJ, Mamounas EP, et al. Prognosis after ipsilateral breast tumor recurrence and locoregional recurrences in five National Surgical Adjuvant Breast and Bowel Project node-positive adjuvant breast cancer trials. *J Clin Oncol.* 2006;24(13):2028–2037.
9. Anderson SJ, Wapnir I, Dignam JJ, et al. Prognosis after ipsilateral breast tumor recurrence and locoregional recurrences in patients treated by breast-conserving therapy in five National Surgical Adjuvant Breast and Bowel Project protocols of node-negative breast cancer. *J Clin Oncol.* 2009;27(15):2466–2473.
10. Reddy JP, Levy L, Oh JL, et al. Long-term outcomes in patients with isolated supraclavicular nodal recurrence after mastectomy and doxorubicin-based chemotherapy for breast cancer. *Int J Radiat Oncol Biol Phys.* 2011;80(5):1453–1457.
11. Taghian A, Jeong JH, Mamounas E, et al. Patterns of locoregional failure in patients with operable breast cancer treated by mastectomy and adjuvant chemotherapy with or without tamoxifen and without radiotherapy: results from five National Surgical Adjuvant Breast and Bowel Project randomized clinical trials. *J Clin Oncol.* 2004;22(21):4247–4254.
12. Recht A, Gray R, Davidson NE, et al. Locoregional failure 10 years after mastectomy and adjuvant chemotherapy with or without tamoxifen without irradiation: experience of the Eastern Cooperative Oncology Group. *J Clin Oncol.* 1999;17(6):1689–1700.
13. Cheng SH, Horng CF, Clarke JL, et al. Prognostic index score and clinical prediction model of local regional recurrence after mastectomy in breast cancer patients. *Int J Radiat Oncol Biol Phys.* 2006;64(5):1401–1409.
14. Nielsen HM, Overgaard M, Grau C, et al. Loco-regional recurrence after mastectomy in high-risk breast cancer–risk and prognosis: an analysis of patients from the DBCG 82 b&c randomization trials. *Radiother Oncol.* 2006;79(2):147–155.
15. Wo JY, Taghian AG, Nguyen PL, et al. The association between biological subtype and isolated regional nodal failure after breast-conserving therapy. *Int J Radiat Oncol Biol Phys.* 2010;77(1):188–196.

16. Warren LE, Ligibel JA, Chen YH, et al. Body mass index and locoregional recurrence in women with early-stage breast cancer. *Ann Surg Oncol.* 2016;23(12):3870–3879.

17. Dershaw DD, McCormick B, Osborne MP. Detection of local recurrence after conservative therapy for breast carcinoma. *Cancer.* 1992;70(2):493–496.

18. Montgomery DA, Krupa K, Jack WJ, et al. Changing pattern of the detection of locoregional relapse in breast cancer: the Edinburgh experience. *Br J Cancer.* 2007;96(12):1802–1807.

19. Montgomery DA, Krupa K, Cooke TG. Follow-up in breast cancer: does routine clinical examination improve outcome? A systematic review of the literature. *Br J Cancer.* 2007;97(12):1632–1641.

20. Halverson KJ, Perez CA, Kuske RR, et al. Survival following locoregional recurrence of breast cancer: univariate and multivariate analysis. *Int J Radiat Oncol Biol Phys.* 1992;23(2):285–291.

21. Gage I, Schnitt SJ, Recht A, et al. Skin recurrences after breast-conserving therapy for early-stage breast cancer. *J Clin Oncol.* 1998;16(2):480–486.

22. Smith TE, Lee D, Turner BC, et al. True recurrence vs. new primary ipsilateral breast tumor relapse: an analysis of clinical and pathologic differences and their implications in natural history, prognoses, and therapeutic management. *Int J Radiat Oncol Biol Phys.* 2000;48(5):1281–1289.

23. Huang E, Buchholz TA, Meric F, et al. Classifying local disease recurrences after breast conservation therapy based on location and histology: new primary tumors have more favorable outcomes than true local disease recurrences. *Cancer.* 2002;95(10):2059–2067.

24. McGrath S, Antonucci J, Goldstein N, et al. Long-term patterns of in-breast failure in patients with early stage breast cancer treated with breast-conserving therapy: a molecular based clonality evaluation. *Am J Clin Oncol.* 2010;33(1):17–22.

25. Maaskant-Braat AJ, Voogd AC, Roumen RM, Nieuwenhuijzen GA. Repeat sentinel node biopsy in patients with locally recurrent breast cancer: a systematic review and meta-analysis of the literature. *Breast Cancer Res Treat.* 2013;138(1):13–20.

26. Vugts G, Maaskant-Braat AJ, Voogd AC, et al. Improving the success rate of repeat sentinel node biopsy in recurrent breast cancer. *Ann Surg Oncol.* 2015;22(Suppl 3):S529–S535.

27. Kurtz JM, Jacquemier J, Amalric R, et al. Is breast conservation after local recurrence feasible? *Eur J Cancer.* 1991;27(3):240–244.

28. Alpert TE, Kuerer HM, Arthur DW, et al. Ipsilateral breast tumor recurrence after breast conservation therapy: outcomes of salvage mastectomy vs. salvage breast-conserving surgery and prognostic factors for salvage breast preservation. *Int J Radiat Oncol Biol Phys.* 2005;63(3):845–851.

29. Shah C, Wilkinson JB, Jawad M, et al. Outcome after ipsilateral breast tumor recurrence in patients with early-stage breast cancer treated with accelerated partial breast irradiation. *Clin Breast Cancer.* 2012;12(6):392–397.

30. Dalberg K, Mattsson A, Sandelin K, Rutqvist LE. Outcome of treatment for ipsilateral breast tumor recurrence in early-stage breast cancer. *Breast Cancer Res Treat.* 1998;49(1):69–78.

31. Kurtz JM, Amalric R, Brandone H, et al. Local recurrence after breast-conserving surgery and radiotherapy. Frequency, time course, and prognosis. *Cancer.* 1989;63(10):1912–1917.

32. Jacobson JA, Danforth DN, Cowan KH, et al. Ten-year results of a comparison of conservation with mastectomy in the treatment of stage I and II breast cancer. *N Engl J Med.* 1995;332(14):907–911.

33. Voogd AC, van Tienhoven G, Peterse HL, et al. Local recurrence after breast conservation therapy for early stage breast carcinoma: detection, treatment, and outcome in 266 patients. Dutch Study Group on Local Recurrence after Breast Conservation (BORST). *Cancer.* 1999;85(2):437–446.

34. Salvadori B, Marubini E, Miceli R, et al. Reoperation for locally recurrent breast cancer in patients previously treated with conservative surgery. *Br J Surg.* 1999;86(1):84–87.

35. Ofuchi T, Amemiya A, Hatayama J. [Salvage surgery for patients with ipsilateral breast tumor recurrence after breast-conserving treatment]. *Nihon Rinsho.* 2007;65(Suppl 6):439–444.

36. Kurtz JM, Amalric R, Brandone H, et al. Results of salvage surgery for mammary recurrence following breast-conserving therapy. *Ann Surg.* 1988;207(3):347–351.

37. Chen SL, Martinez SR. The survival impact of the choice of surgical procedure after ipsilateral breast cancer recurrence. *Am J Surg.* 2008;196(4):495–499.

V: **THORACIC**

25: EARLY-STAGE NON–SMALL-CELL LUNG CANCER

Gaurav Marwaha, Matthew C. Ward, Kevin L. Stephans, and Gregory M. M. Videtic

> **QUICK HIT:** Surgical resection is the standard of care for operable early-stage non–small-cell lung cancer (NSCLC). For medically inoperable pts, SBRT is the standard of care. For high-risk operable pts, in absence of randomized trials, there is controversy as to which is most appropriate, surgery or SBRT, if long-term survival is primary endpoint for these pts.

TABLE 25.1: General Treatment Paradigm for Early-Stage NSCLC

	Operable			Medically Inoperable *(FEV1 <40%, DLCO <40%)*
	Surgery	**CHT**	**RT**	
Stage IA (*cT1a-bN0*)	Lobectomy + mediastinal LND	No	No PORT (except possibly for +margins if not re-resectable)	SBRT *Peripheral—Range of schedules, e.g., 54 Gy/3 fx (with heterogeneity correction) per RTOG 0236; 34/1 fx or 48/4 fx per RTOG 0915 Central—50 Gy/5 fx per RTOG 0813*
Stage IB (*cT2aN0*)		Debatable (LACE meta-analysis)		
IIA and select IIB (*cT2bN0, cT3N0*)		Yes (LACE meta-analysis)		

EPIDEMIOLOGY: Lung cancer: most common noncutaneous cancer worldwide, second most common in the United States (second to breast and prostate) and leading cause of cancer mortality in the United States. Estimated 224,390 new cases and 158,080 deaths in the United States.[1] NSCLC comprises ~80% of all lung cancer; 15% to 20% of NSCLC pts present with early-stage disease.

RISK FACTORS: Smoking, radon, asbestos, family history, pulmonary fibrosis, occupational (silica, cadmium, arsenic, beryllium, diesel exhaust, coal soot).

ANATOMY: Lobes in both lungs separated by oblique fissure, right lung also separated by horizontal fissure. Trachea starts at C3/4, carina at T5. Nodal stations range from 1 to 14; see atlas by Lynch.[2]

PATHOLOGY

- ADENOCARCINOMA: Most common histology, 38% of all lung cancers. Majority are peripheral. Bronchoalveolar carcinomas (subtype of adenocarcinoma) arise from type II pneumocytes and grow along alveolar septa with long natural history.

- SQUAMOUS: ~20% of all lung cancers. Majority are centrally located.
- SMALL CELL CARCINOMA: 13% of all lung cancers, almost always associated with smoking (see Chapter 27).
- OTHER: Consists of other rare histologies and other neuroendocrine carcinomas such as large cell or carcinoid.

GENETICS: >95% clinically relevant mutations are found in adenocarcinomas. Epidermal growth factor receptor (EGFR) is transmembrane tyrosine kinase. Mutations found in about 17% of NSCLC and are sensitive to drugs like erlotinib, gefitinib, afatinib. Anaplastic lymphoma kinase (ALK) rearrangements have prevalence of ~5% in NSCLC. It is associated with younger age, never smokers; tumors respond to TKIs like crizotinib, alectinib, ceritinib. *ROS-1* is seen in 1% to 2% of pts and can respond to crizotinib.[3] *BRAF V600E*, *MET*, and *RET* are emerging driver mutations that are thought to respond to vemurafenib, crizotinib, and cabozantinib, respectively.

SCREENING: Screen with low dose CT for pts aged 55 to 74 and ≥30 pack-year smokers and cessation <15 yrs ago. Also screen if age ≥50, ≥20 pack-years, and one additional NCCN risk factor for lung cancer (see the preceding text).[4]

CLINICAL PRESENTATION: Cough, dyspnea, wheeze, stridor, hemoptysis, anorexia, weight loss, decline in performance status, paraneoplastic syndromes such as hypercalcemia from PTHrP (squamous cell carcinoma) or hypertrophic pulmonary osteoarthropathy.

WORKUP: H&P

Labs: CBC, CMP. PFT: See ACCP guidelines for details.[7] Medical inoperability used on trials to define criteria for SBRT (Indiana University criteria): baseline FEV1 <40% predicted, predicted post-op FEV1 <30% predicted, DLCO <40% predicted, pO_2 <70 mmHg, pCO_2 >50 mmHg, exercise oxygen consumption <50% predicted. Note these are different than advanced resections and definitive therapy used in Chapter 26. Preoperative cardiac workup if necessary.

Imaging: CT chest (with contrast if evaluating nodes, consider CT abdomen for metastatic workup but at least review liver and adrenal), PET scan. "Pathologic" lymph nodes defined as short-axis diameter >1.0 cm and "bulky" lymphadenopathy as short axis >3.0 cm, multiple matted nodes, radiographic ECE or ≥3 stations involved. Brain imaging: MRI brain for stage II or higher (NCCN 2017); consider MRI brain for central stage IB (NCCN optional recommendation); otherwise brain imaging unnecessary unless neurological symptoms are present. CT brain with contrast sufficient if MRI is too difficult.[5]

Pathology: Biopsy indicated (EBUS, CT-guided, or thoracentesis depending on location/presence of effusion; sputum pathology is unreliable but at least three needed to be negative), EBUS/mediastinoscopy to confirm positive LN on CT or PET and for all T3 or central T1-2 tumors (EBUS/mediastinoscopy reaches stations 2, 4, 7. EBUS also reaches station 10). Chamberlain procedure or VATS required to reach stations 5 to 6, EUS for stations 8 to 9. MRI of thoracic inlet for superior sulcus tumors and octreotide scan for carcinoid.

PROGNOSTIC FACTORS: Stage, weight loss >5% in 3 mos, KPS <90, age >70, +LVSI, marital status.

STAGING

TABLE 25.2: AJCC 8th ed. (2017) Staging for Lung Cancer						
T/M	N	cN0	cN1	cN2	cN3
T1	a ≤1 cm[1]	IA1				
	b 1.1–2 cm	IA2				
	c 2.1–3 cm	IA3	IIB	IIIA	IIIB
T2[2]	a 3.1–4 cm	IB				
	b 4.1–5 cm	IIA				
T3	• 5.1–7 cm • Invasion[3] • Same lobe nodules	IIB				
T4	• >7 cm • Invasion[4] • Separate lobe nodules		IIIA	IIIB	IIIC
M1a	• Separate nodules in contralateral lobe • Pleural nodules • Malignant pleural/pericardial effusion	IVA			
M1b	• Single extrathoracic metastasis in single organ • Single non-regional lymph node	IVA			
M1c	• Multiple extrathoracic metastasis	IVB			

Notes: ≤1 cm[1] = or rare superficial spreading tumor with invasive component limited to bronchial wall. T2[2] = or involves main bronchus, but not carina, invades visceral pleura, or atelectasis or obstructive pneumonitis extending to hilar region. Invasion[3] = Invasion of parietal pleura, chest wall, phrenic nerve, or parietal pericardium. Invasion[4] = Invasion of diaphragm, mediastinum, great vessels, trachea, carina, recurrent laryngeal nerve, esophagus, or vertebral body.

cN1, Ipsilateral peribronchial and/or ipsilateral hilar LNs (stations 10–14); cN2, ipsilateral mediastinal and/or subcarinal LNs (stations 2–9); cN3, contralateral mediastinal, hilar, or any scalene or supraclavicular LNs (station 1).

TREATMENT PARADIGM

Observation: "Active surveillance" is not an established option for diagnosed invasive NSCLC because even in medically inoperable pts, lung cancer specific mortality is 53%.[6] Since majority of these pts will die of their disease if not treated, active surveillance/ watchful waiting is generally inappropriate unless lesion is too small to diagnose (see following Solitary Pulmonary Nodule).

Solitary pulmonary nodule: Discrete opacity in lung parenchyma ≤3 cm (>3 cm is "mass" and malignancy until proven otherwise). Differential includes granuloma, abscess, fungal infection, hamartoma, tuberculosis, metastasis, lymphoma, carcinoid. Factors associated with malignancy: faster growth rate, lack of calcification, greater size (<4 mm 0%, 4–7 mm 1%, >2 cm 75%), spiculated (vs. smooth or lobulated margins), air bronchogram, solid (vs. ground glass), contrast enhancement, high SUV. If ≥8 mm consider PET/CT or biopsy, see NCCN for additional size-specific follow-up guidelines. LU-RADS is evolving standardization system for follow-up of indeterminate nodules.

Surgery: Standard treatment for medically operable pts. Lobectomy superior to wedge/ segmentectomy. VATS lobectomy comparable to open lobectomy.[8] For accurate staging, mediastinal LN dissection should be performed. Preoperative medical workup including PFTs (see Workup) and cardiac clearance necessary.

Chemotherapy: See LACE pooled analysis later. Generally no role for stage I. Note also that uracil–tegafur has been shown to be beneficial in Japanese population but is not used in the United States due to nonreproducible results.[9]

Radiofrequency Ablation (RFA): Placement of electrode in tumor and uses RF ablative heating. Retrospective series have reported complete radiographic responses from 38% to 93% with treated tumor relapse rates from 8% to 43%. Factors associated with CR include smaller tumors, metastases, and ablation zone 4x tumor diameter. Pneumothorax is risk associated with procedure.

Radiation:

Indications: Historically, fractionated RT was standard treatment for medically inoperable pts, with results inferior to surgery. SBRT, however, may be comparable to surgery and it is considered standard (rather than wedge or RFA) for medically inoperable pts. Adjuvant RT is not indicated in completely resected stage I/II pts (although Italian trial by Trodella et al. does show benefit; other trials have not).

Dose: Post-op dose is 54 to 60 Gy for microscopically (R1) positive margins and ≥60 Gy for macroscopically (R2) positive margins.[9] SBRT given in 1 to 5 fx of 10 to 34 Gy per fx; see the following data. Most common dosing schemes include 50 Gy/5 fx, 60 Gy/3 fx over minimum 8 days (without heterogeneity per RTOG 0236), 48 Gy/4 fx, 34 Gy/1 fx (with heterogeneity corrections).

Toxicity: Acute: Toxicity with SBRT is minimal; expect some fatigue but most pts will not experience significant acute effects. Rarely: cough, pneumonitis, esophagitis, subacute chest wall pain. Late: Radiation pneumonitis, chest wall pain. On average, PFTs remain stable (some improve, some decrease, often related to baseline comorbidity).

Procedure: See Treatment Planning Handbook, Chapter 6.

EVIDENCE-BASED Q&A

Screening and staging

Is there benefit to routine radiographic screening for lung cancer? Which pts should be screened?

Previously, routine screening with CXR or sputum cytology had not been shown to reduce mortality. This paradigm was changed by NLST and NCCN revised guidelines in response to this trial.

National Lung Screening Trial (*NEJM* 2011, PMID 21714641): PRT of 54,454 pts at high risk for lung cancer to three annual screenings with either low dose CT or single-view PA CXR. There were 247 versus 309 deaths from lung cancer per 100,000 person-yrs in low dose CT group versus CXR group, representing relative reduction in mortality from lung cancer of 20.0% ($p = .004$). Rate of death from any cause was also reduced in low dose CT group, as compared with CXR group, by 6.7% ($p = .02$). Notably, false positive rate was 96.4% in low dose CT group and 94.5% in CXR group, but majority of false positives (>90%) were observed with scans and did not result in unnecessary procedures. Number needed to screen with low dose CT to prevent one lung cancer death was 320. **Conclusion: Low dose CT screening reduces mortality from lung cancer.**

What defines "early-stage" lung cancer? Why is it important to investigate mediastinum?

Early stage is typically defined as stage I or II, but from treatment standpoint, pts are differentiated as node-negative or node-positive. For example, T1N1 pt is stage II but would be treated differently than T2N0 pt. Therefore, careful staging of mediastinum is necessary. PET/CT has sensitivity of 79% (CT staging 60%),[11] but investigation of mediastinum via either mediastinoscopy or endobronchial ultrasound (EBUS) can improve this.

What is difference between mediastinoscopy and EBUS? What is sensitivity and specificity of either approach or combination?

Mediastinoscopy is historical standard for evaluation of regional lymph nodes but EBUS has advantage of being "minimally invasive" and can reach station 10 (hilar lymph nodes). Clinical staging is important to avoid unnecessary thoracotomies: that is, those who will need CHT and/ or RT anyway and did not benefit from surgery. Historically, 25% to 30% of thoracotomies were unnecessary due to incomplete clinical staging.

Annema, ASTER Trial (*JAMA* 2010, PMID 21098770): PRT trial in 241 pts with resectable NSCLC either underwent mediastinoscopy or EBUS followed by mediastinoscopy at time of surgery. Primary outcome was sensitivity for N2/N3 metastases. All received PET/CT up-front, known N2-3 pts excluded. Sensitivity of mediastinoscopy: 79%, EBUS: 85%, EBUS followed by mediastinoscopy: 94%. Unnecessary thoracotomies: 18% (mediastinoscopy) versus 7% (EBUS). **Conclusion: EBUS plus mediastinoscopy resulted in fewer unnecessary thoracotomies and increased sensitivity compared to mediastinoscopy or EBUS alone.**

Medically operable patients

What is the surgery of choice? Is wedge resection sufficient?

Ginsberg (following) showed that wedge is inferior local therapy to lobectomy and that distant metastases are driving factor for cancer-related death.

Ginsberg (*Ann Thorac Surg* 1995, PMID 7677489): PRT of 247 pts comparing limited resection (segmentectomy or wedge resection) versus lobectomy in peripheral T1N0 NSCLC. RML tumors were excluded due to small size of lobe. At least 2 cm of normal lung tissue was required to be resected. Note: Pts randomized intraoperatively. 40% of pts who were registered (but ultimately not enrolled) had benign disease. **Conclusion: Lobectomy is surgery of choice.**

TABLE 25.3: Results of Ginsberg Trial of Limited Versus Lobar Surgery for Early-Stage Lung Cancer				
	LRR	**Nonlocal Recurrence**	**Death With Cancer**	**Death From All Causes**
Limited Resection	17%	14%	25%	39%
Lobectomy	6%	12%	17%	30%
p value	.008	.672	.094	.088

Can we improve surgical outcomes with sublobar resection + brachytherapy?

Although the following ACOSOG trial was negative study, it is useful to note that "modern" wedge resection is better than wedge resection in era of Ginsberg.

Fernando, ACOSOG Z4032 (*JCO* 2014, PMID 24982457): PRT of wedge resection ± I-125 mesh brachytherapy for medically high-risk pts. Note that this can be quoted as modern surgical outcomes in addition to older Ginsberg data showing 17% LRR. Crude LF rate, defined by staple-line, lobar or hilar nodal failure was 7.7%. There were no differences in time to local recurrence or types of local recurrence between arms. Moreover, in pts with potentially compromised margin (margin <1 cm, margin-to-tumor ratio <1, positive staple-line cytology, wedge resection nodule size >2.0 cm), brachytherapy did not reduce LF. 3-yr OS was 71% in both arms. **Conclusion: Brachytherapy does not reduce local recurrence after sublobar resection but risk of recurrence is low in current era.**

Which pts with early-stage lung cancer may benefit from adjuvant postoperative RT?

PORT is not indicated in completely resected stage I/II pts. Refer to PORT meta-analysis in locally advanced lung cancer chapter. PORT meta-analysis showed detriment to routine PORT for pts without N2 node. The following study should be noted because it did show benefit in stage I, but this is not routine, as it has not been reproduced.

Trodella, Italian Trial (*Radiother Oncol* 2002; PMID 11830308): PRT of adjuvant RT versus observation in 104 pts with completely resected (R0) pathologic stage I NSCLC. RT was to 50.4 Gy/28 fx. Target volume included bronchial stump and ipsilateral hilum. No treatment-related deaths. 5-yr DFS favored RT arm (71% vs. 60%, *p* = .039). 5-yr OS favored RT arm as well (67% vs. 58%, *p* = .048). **Conclusion: Adjuvant RT may be safe and beneficial in terms of DFS and OS in select stage I pts.**

Which pts benefit from adjuvant CHT?

Consideration for stage II based on LACE meta-analysis. Stage IB is debatable—CALGB study suggested benefit for tumors ≥4 cm (included in LACE analysis). Note, Japanese study showed uracil–tegafur's benefit, but is not used in the United States.[8]

Pignon, LACE Pooled Analysis (*JCO* 2008, PMID 18506026): Pooled individual data from 4,584 pts included on five PRTs of adjuvant CHT in NSCLC. MFU 5.2 years. Overall HR of death was 0.89 (*p* = .005), corresponding to 5-yr absolute benefit of 5.4%. Benefit varied with stage: detrimental for stage IA (HR 1.4), nonsignificant for IB (HR 0.93), and beneficial for stage II (HR 0.83) and III (HR 0.8). Benefit was higher in pts with better performance status. Type of CHT, sex, age, histology, type of surgery, planned RT, and dose of cisplatin were not associated with outcome. **Conclusion: CHT confers survival advantage in stage II/III NSCLC. IB controversial—there may be subset whose benefit based on size of primary (CALGB 9633). IA not indicated (except in Japan[8]).**

Strauss, CALGB 9633 (*JCO* 2008, PMID 18809614): PRT of four cycles of adjuvant paclitaxel (200 mg/m[2]) and carboplatin (AUC 6) day 1 q3 weeks x four cycles versus observation in completely resected IB NSCLC. 384 pts randomized. 3-yr OS was 79% versus 70% favoring CHT (*p* = .045). 5-yr OS no different (60% vs. 57%, *p* = .32). **Conclusion: Although trial initially closed early after planned interim analysis, 5-yr data showed insignificant OS benefit. Subgroup analysis showed that for tumors ≥4 cm there was improved DFS (median DFS 96 vs. 63 mos) and OS (MS 99 vs. 77 mos) with CHT.**

Medically inoperable

What are the outcomes with conventional RT for early NSCLC?

Historically, medically inoperable pts received conventionally fractionated definitive RT to 50–60 Gy or supportive care only. Conventional RT provided LC in the range of 40% to 60% with about 30% to 40% of pts dying of lung cancer within 2 years.[12] There was some evidence for benefit of dose escalation to 70.2 Gy[13] and hypofractionation (60 Gy/15 fx),[14] but ultimately as technology improved, SBRT rendered previous forms of definitive RT obsolete in most cases. Two recent trials to know follow.

Cheung, NCIC CTG BR.25 (*JNCI* 2014, PMID 25074417): Multi-institution phase II trial of 80 pts with T1-T3N0 NSCLC treated to 60 Gy/15 fx on consecutive days using 3D-CRT technique (no IMRT) without inhomogeneity correction. GTV was tumor only; PTV was

1.5 cm margin (could be decreased to 1.0 cm in transverse plane if close to critical structures). Primary endpoint was 2-yr tumor control. MFU of 49 mos. 2-yr primary tumor control rate was 87.4% and 2-yr OS was 68.7%. 2-yr regional relapse rate 8.8% and distant relapse 21.6%. Most common grade 3+ toxicities were fatigue (6.3%), cough (7.5%), dyspnea (13.8%), and pneumonitis (10.0%). **Conclusion: Conformal RT to 60 Gy/15 fx using 3D-CRT technique results in favorable tumor control rates and OS without severe toxicities.**

Nyman, SPACE Trial (*Radiother Oncol* 2016, PMID 27600155): Randomized phase II trial of 102 medically inoperable pts with Stage I NSCLC comparing SBRT (66 Gy/3 fx over 1 week) and 3D-CRT (70 Gy/35 fx over 7 weeks). MFU of 37 mos. No difference between 1-, 2-, and 3-yr PFS of: SBRT: 76%, 53%, 42% and 3D-CRT: 87%, 54%, 42%. By end of study, 70% of SBRT pts had not progressed compared to 59% (3D-CRT, $p = .26$). Toxicity was lower in SBRT pts (pneumonitis: 19% [SBRT] and 34% [3DCRT, $p = .26$]; esophagitis: 8% [SBRT] and 30% [3DCRT, $p = .006$]). **Conclusion: No difference in PFS or OS between two but trend to improvement disease control rate in SBRT group with better quality of life and lower toxicity, so SBRT should be standard.**

What trials defined the role of stereotactic body RT therapy (SBRT)?

SBRT, formally defined as high dose per fraction delivered in ≤5 fractions, was first developed in Sweden. Dr. Timmerman at Indiana University led dose-escalation trial in 2003, which then led to phase II discovering high rate of central toxicity for 60 Gy/3 fx. In 2002, RTOG 0236 (JAMA 2010) opened, which defined role of SBRT for early peripheral lesions. Since there is debate on value of surgery, RTOG 0618 investigated SBRT for operable pts, reserving surgery for salvage if needed. Since central tumors are considered high risk using 60 Gy/3 fx (but not with 50 Gy/5 fx), RTOG 0813 studied safety and dose escalation for central tumors starting at 50 Gy/5 fx and going to 60 Gy/5 fx. RTOG 0915 investigated single-fraction SBRT for peripheral lesions.

Timmerman, Indiana (*Chest* 2003, PMID 14605072): Phase I dose-escalation trial of extracranial stereotactic radioablation (ESR) in 37 pts with T1-2N0 biopsy-confirmed NSCLC. Initial dose was 24 Gy/3 fx and increased to tolerated dose 60 Gy/3 fx. Abdominal compression was used to decrease respiratory motion. MFU 15.2 mos. 87% response rate (27% CR). 6 pts experienced LF, all receiving doses <18 Gy/fx x3. One patient (treated at 14 Gy per fx x3) developed symptomatic pneumonitis. **Conclusion: ESR is feasible and results in good response rates.**

Timmerman, Central Toxicity (*JCO* 2006, PMID 17050868): Phase II, cT1-2N0M0 medically inoperable, N = 70. SBRT 60 to 66 Gy/3 fx 1 to 2 weeks. MFU was 17.5 mos. 2-yr LC was 95%. Treatment-related death 6/70 pts. MS 32.6 mos and 2-yr OS was 54.7%. Grade 3 to 5 toxicity in 14 pts. Median time to toxicity was 10.5 mos. Pts with peripheral tumors had 2-yr freedom from severe toxicity of 83% compared with 54% for central tumors. **Conclusion: High rates of LC with this regimen, but high toxicity for central tumors.**

Fakiris, Indiana Phase II Update (*IJROBP* 2009, PMID 11773176): MFU of 50.2 mos. 3-yr LC of 88%. Nodal and distant recurrence was 8.5% and 13%, respectively. MS was 32.4 mos. 3-yr CSS 82%, 3-yr OS was 43%. MS for T1 versus T2 tumors was 39 versus 24.5 mos, respectively ($p = .019$). Tumor size or location did not impact control outcomes. Grades 3–5 toxicity occurred in 10% of pts with peripheral lesions and 27% of pts with central tumors.

Onishi, Japan (*JTO* 2007, PMID 17603311): RR of 14 institutions: 257 pts from April 1993 to February 2003; 164 T1N0, 93 T2N0 tumors. Median age 74. MFU 38 mos. Dose of 18 to 75 Gy in 1 to 22 fx. Median BED10 was 111 Gy. Tumors <6 cm. No restrictions on location except to keep cord dose tolerable. Included either medically inoperable or pts refusing surgery. Grade >2 pulmonary toxicity in 14 pts (5.4%). Local progression in 36 pts (14%). LR 8% versus 43% for BED >100 Gy or <100 Gy, respectively ($p < .001$). 5-yr OS for <u>medically operable</u> pts refusing surgery was 71% versus 30% for BED ≥100 Gy and <100 Gy, respectively ($p < .05$). **Conclusion: SBRT is safe and effective for stage I lung cancer. When BED ≥100 Gy used, LC is excellent and 5-yr OS for** *medically operable* **pts is similar to surgical series (compare with 70% OS in Ginsburg for lobectomy of only stage IA pts).**

All of the preceding trials come from single institutions. Are there any cooperative group data?

RTOG 0236 is probably most important SBRT trial to know, which showed it could be effective in cooperative group setting.

Timmerman, RTOG 0236 (*JAMA*** 2010, PMID 20233825; Update *ASTRO* 2014, Abstract #56):** Phase II multi-institution study of SBRT for medically inoperable stage I/II NSCLC (peripheral location, T1T2N0 <5 cm). Prescription was 60 Gy/3 fx, though later analysis showed dose equivalent to 54 Gy/3 fx after accounting for heterogeneity. Treatment duration was ≥8 and <14 days. 55 evaluable pts. Grade 3 adverse events 12.7%, grade 4 adverse events 3.6%. No grade 5 adverse events.

TABLE 25.4: Outcomes from RTOG 0236		
	Initial Results (3 yrs)	**Long-term Results (5 yrs)**
OS	56%	40%
MS	48 mos	48 mos
LC	98%	93%
Lobar Control	91%	80%
LRC	87%	62%
Distant Failure	22%	31%

Note: No EBUS was required in RTOG 0236. Lobar failure is a bigger problem in comparison to lobectomy and would require EBRT-alone salvage as many of these pts are not CHT candidates up-front or in salvage setting. Lobar recurrence is more easily salvaged with SBRT. **Conclusion: Pts with medically inoperable NSCLC treated with SBRT had modest survival, high rates of local tumor control, and moderate treatment-related morbidity. Longer-term follow-up has shown increased lobar and regional failures.**

Is SBRT an appropriate option for medically operable pts?

No, SBRT is not standard and multiple trials that have tried to answer this question have closed early due to poor accrual. Nevertheless, multiple analyses attempt to answer this question while we await additional randomized data.

Chang, Pooled Analysis of STARS & ROSEL (*Lancet Onc*** 2015, PMID 25981812):** Pooled analysis of two independent phase III PRT of SBRT versus lobectomy and mediastinal lymph node dissection (VU University Medical Center and MDACC), which closed early due to slow accrual. 58 pts were included. Six surgery pts died compared to one in SBRT group, leading to 3-yr OS of 95% in SBRT group versus 79% in surgery group (HR 0.14, $p = .037$). RFS was similar: 86% (SBRT) versus 80% (surgery, $p = .54$). Grade 3+ events were 10% (SBRT) compared to 44% (surgery) with one postoperative death (4%). **Conclusion: SBRT appears viable in medically operable pts but additional PRTs are warranted.**

Onishi, Japan (*IJROBP* 2011, PMID 20638194): Review of outcomes for *medically operable subset*, MFU of 55 mos. Cumulative LC rates for T1 and T2 tumors at 5 yrs after SBRT were 92% and 73%, respectively. Pulmonary complications above grade 2 arose in one patient (1.1%, in this case it was grade 3). 5-yr OS for stage IA and IB was 72% and 62%, respectively. One patient who developed local recurrence safely underwent salvage surgery. **Conclusion: SBRT is safe and promising for operable stage I NSCLC with survival rate approximating that for surgery.**

Zheng, Meta-Analysis (*IJROBP* 2014, PMID 25052562): Study-level (not patient-level) meta-analysis of 7,071 pts treated with surgery or SBRT (BED ≥100). Median age for SBRT and surgery was 74 and 66, MFU of 28 mos and 37 mos. OS at 1, 3, and 5 yrs for SBRT versus lobectomy was 83% vs. 92%, 56% vs. 77%, 41% vs. 66%. After adjustment for proportion of operable pts and age, SBRT and surgery have comparable DFS and OS. **Conclusion: Randomized trial needed because SBRT appears comparable to surgery for medically operable pts.**

Timmerman, RTOG 0618 (*ASCO* 2013, Abstract 7523): Single-arm phase II study of SBRT in pts with operable stage I/II NSCLC (peripheral location, T1-3N0 <5 cm) treated with 60 Gy/3 fx. Primary endpoint was tumor control with early surgical salvage as part of protocol design in event of LR. 33 pts with MFU of 25 mos. 2-yr LF (primary tumor plus involved lobe) was 19.2%, regional failure was 11.7%, and distant failure was 15.4%. 2-yr PFS was 65.4% and OS was 84.4%. **Conclusion: SBRT appears to be associated with high tumor control rates and infrequent need for surgical salvage.**

Can SBRT be safely delivered in a single fraction?

While not standard yet, Phase II data does demonstrate safety and efficacy.

Videtic, RTOG 0915 (*IJROBP* 2015, PMID 26530743): Randomized phase II study of 94 medically inoperable T1-2N0 by PET comparing 34 Gy/1 fx (arm 1) to 48 Gy/4 fx (arm 2). Powered to detect adverse event (AE) rate >17%. Secondary endpoints: LC, OS, and PFS. MFU: 30.2 mos. AEs experienced by 10.3% of pts in arm 1 and 13.3% in arm 2. LC at 1 yr: 97.0% for arm 1 and 92.7% for arm 2. 2-yr OS rate: 61.3% for arm 1 and 77.7% for arm 2. 2-yr DFS: 56.4% for arm 1 and 71.1% for arm 2. **Conclusion: 34 Gy/1 fx yielded lower toxicity rate for comparable LC; 34 Gy/1 fx deserves further study.**

Videtic, Roswell Park 1509 (*ASTRO* 2016, Abstract 17): Randomized phase II study of 98 medically inoperable cT1-T2N0 by PET comparing 30 Gy/1 fx (arm 1) to 60 Gy/3 fx (arm 2). Powered to detect AE >17%. Secondary endpoints: LC, 1-yr toxicity, OS, PFS. MFU 24 mos. AEs experienced by 27% of pts in arm 1 and 33% in arm 2. PFS at 1 yr: 63% for arm 1 and 50% for arm 2. 2-yr OS rate: 70% for arm 1 and 77.7% for arm 2. **Conclusion: 30 Gy/1 fx was equivalent to 60 Gy/3 fx in terms of OS, PFS, and toxicity.**

What data is there for safety of SBRT for central lung tumors?

Central tumors are high risk based on the "no fly zone" (2 cm around the proximal bronchial tree) defined by Timmerman (JCO 2006).

Bezjak, RTOG 0813 (*ASTRO* 2015, Abstract LBA10; *ASTRO* 2016, Abstract 16): Phase I/ II study designed to determine maximum tolerated dose (MTD) and efficacy of SBRT for cT1-2 (<5 cm). Central tumors were defined as tumors within 2 cm of tracheal–bronchial tree or immediately adjacent to mediastinal or pericardial pleura (where PTV would touch pleura). SBRT dose schedule started at 10 Gy/fx to 50 Gy and was escalated by 0.5 Gy/fx increments to 12 Gy/fx (60 Gy) every other day over 1.5 to 2 weeks. 120 pts treated with MFU of 26.6 mos. MTD was 12 Gy/fx and dose-limiting toxicity on this arm was 7.2%. Update at ASTRO 2016 included MFU of 33 mos in pts treated to two highest dose cohorts

(11.5 Gy/fx and 12 Gy/fx). 2-yr LC (~88%), PFS (~53%), and OS (~70%) with 7/33 pts with grade 3+ toxicity. **Conclusion: Low but significant toxicity with dose escalation to 60 Gy/5 fx.** *Comment: Many ways to qualify as "central" on this trial besides original Timmerman definition.*

REFERENCES

1. *Cancer Facts & Figures 2014.* Atlanta, GA: American Cancer Society; 2014.
2. Lynch R, Pitson G, Ball D, et al. Computed tomographic atlas for the new international lymph node map for lung cancer: a radiation oncologist perspective. *Pract Radiat Oncol.* 2013;3(1):54–66.
3. Shaw AT, Ou SH, Bang YJ, et al. Crizotinib in ROS1-rearranged non–small-cell lung cancer. *N Engl J Med.* 2014;371(21):1963–1971.
4. *NCCN Clinical Practice Guidelines in Oncology, Lung Cancer Screening.* https://www.nccn.org/professionals/physician_gls/pdf/lung_screening.pdf. Published 2016.
5. Yokoi K, Kamiya N, Matsuguma H, et al. Detection of brain metastasis in potentially operable non–small-cell lung cancer: a comparison of CT and MRI. *Chest.* 1999;115(3):714–719.
6. McGarry RC, Song G, des Rosiers P, Timmerman R. Observation-only management of early stage, medically inoperable lung cancer: poor outcome. *Chest.* 2002;121(4):1155–1158.
7. Brunelli A, Kim AW, Berger KI, Addrizzo-Harris DJ. Physiologic evaluation of the patient with lung cancer being considered for resectional surgery: diagnosis and management of lung cancer, 3rd ed: American College of Chest Physicians evidence-based clinical practice guidelines. *Chest.* 2013;143(5 Suppl):e166S–e190S.
8. Yan TD, Black D, Bannon PG, McCaughan BC. Systematic review and meta-analysis of randomized and nonrandomized trials on safety and efficacy of video-assisted thoracic surgery lobectomy for early-stage non–small-cell lung cancer. *J Clin Oncol.* 2009;27(15):2553–2562.
9. Kato H, Ichinose Y, Ohta M, et al. A randomized trial of adjuvant chemotherapy with uracil-tegafur for adenocarcinoma of the lung. *N Engl J Med.* 2004;350(17):1713–1721.

26: STAGE III NON–SMALL-CELL LUNG CANCER

Matthew C. Ward and Gregory M. M. Videtic

> **QUICK HIT:** Stage III NSCLC is heterogeneous due to a wide range of local and nodal presentations. Given smoking association, stage III treatment is frequently impacted by patient performance and medical comorbidities. Treatment options involve appropriate selection of CHT, RT, and surgery, alone or in combination.

TABLE 26.1: General Treatment Paradigm for Stage III Lung Cancer		
Treatment Option	**Ideal Candidate**	**Treatment Details**
Neoadjuvant chemoRT followed by resection (trimodality)	Good performance, lobectomy-appropriate, nonbulky single station mediastinal node	45 Gy/25 fx with concurrent cisplatin 50 mg/m² and etoposide 50 mg/m²
Initial surgery	Good performance cT1-3N0-1	Adjuvant CHT for ≥stage II PORT following CHT for N2 nodes (50–54 Gy) or chemoRT for positive margins or ECE (54–60 Gy)
Definitive concurrent chemoRT	Good performance status, stage III, acceptable baseline pulmonary function	60 Gy/30 fx with concurrent cisplatin/etoposide or carboplatin AUC 2/paclitaxel 45 mg/m²
Sequential chemoRT	Impaired performance status OR stage III (any T/N), impaired baseline pulmonary function	CHT (e.g., carboplatin AUC 6/ paclitaxel 200 mg/m²) followed by 60 Gy/30 fx
RT alone	Marginal performance status	60 Gy/30 fx, 45 Gy/15 fx, 30 Gy/10 fx
Palliative care alone	Poor performance, poor risk IIIB NSCLC	

EPIDEMIOLOGY, RISK FACTORS, ANATOMY, PATHOLOGY, GENETICS, SCREENING: See Chapter 25.

CLINICAL PRESENTATION: Cough, dyspnea, wheeze, stridor, hemoptysis, anorexia, weight loss, decline in performance status, paraneoplastic syndromes such as hypercalcemia from PTHrP (squamous cell carcinoma) or hypertrophic pulmonary osteoarthropathy. Hoarseness from recurrent laryngeal (left-sided more common), Horner's syndrome (ptosis, miosis, anhydrosis). Pancoast syndrome (Horner's, brachial plexopathy, shoulder pain). SVC syndrome.

WORKUP: H&P

Labs: CBC, CMP, PFTs.

Imaging: CT chest (with contrast if evaluating nodes, consider CT abdomen for metastatic workup but at least review liver and adrenal), PET/CT. "Pathologic" lymph nodes defined as short-axis diameter >1.0 cm and "bulky" lymphadenopathy as short-axis >3.0 cm, multiple matted nodes, radiographic ECE or ≥3 stations involved. *Brain imaging:* MRI brain for stage II or higher[1]; consider MRI brain for central stage IB (NCCN optional recommendation), otherwise brain imaging unnecessary unless neurological symptoms are present. CT brain with contrast sufficient if MRI is too difficult.[2] *PFT:* ACCP guidelines define standard for PFT evaluation.[3] For any surgery, preoperative FEV_1 >2 L (or 80% predicted) and DLCO >80% predicted are generally safe. For stage III pts undergoing neoadjuvant therapy followed by surgery, if preoperative FEV_1 is <2 L, recommended preresection DLCO is ≥50% and predicted postresection FEV_1 is ≥0.8 L.[4] For pneumonectomy, current ACCP guidelines recommend predicted postoperative FEV_1 and DLCO to both be >60% predicted.[3] For definitive chemoRT, pretreatment FEV_1 ≥1–1.2 L has been used as criteria for clinical trials.[5,6] Note that these are different than criteria for early-stage lung undergoing lobectomy (see Chapter 25).

Pathology: Biopsy indicated (EBUS, CT-guided or thoracentesis depending on location/presence of effusion; sputum pathology is unreliable but at least three needed to be negative), PET scan (upstages ~20%, prevents unnecessary thoracotomies but no improvement in survival).[7] For T4 and/or superior sulcus tumors, obtain MRI to investigate degree of local invasion. EBUS/mediastinoscopy to confirm positive LN on CT or PET and for all T3 or central T1-2 tumors (EBUS/mediastinoscopy reaches stations 2, 4, 7; EBUS also reaches station 10). Chamberlain procedure (anterior mediastinotomy) or VATS is required to reach stations 5 and 6, EUS for stations 8 and 9. MRI of thoracic inlet for superior sulcus tumors and octreotide scan for carcinoid.

PROGNOSTIC FACTORS: Stage, weight loss >5% in 3 mos, KPS <90, age >70, LVSI, marital status.

STAGING: See Chapter 25 for AJCC 8th edition staging.

TREATMENT PARADIGM

Surgery: Surgery is the standard local therapy modality.[1] Sublobar resections are not recommended for stage III disease due to need for mediastinal lymphadenectomy. Surgical plan should be decided prior to initiation of treatment. Role of surgery in N2 disease is controversial (see the following). N3 disease, bulky N2 disease (>3 cm) or multiple N2 nodes are relative contraindications to surgery. Pneumonectomy carries increased risk of operative mortality.

Chemotherapy: CHT is indicated in essentially all stage III pts who are fit enough to tolerate treatment. CHT can be delivered in preoperative, postoperative, or sequenced along with RT either concurrently or sequentially. Common concurrent regimens with RT include cisplatin 50 mg/m² on days 1, 8, 29, and 36 and etoposide 50 mg/m² 1–5 and 29–33 or carboplatin AUC 2 and paclitaxel 50 mg/m² weekly (with or without additional two adjuvant cycles). No consensus on optimal regimen (see the following data). For definitive sequential chemoRT, give carboplatin AUC 6 and paclitaxel 200 mg/m² every 3 weeks for two cycles followed by RT. Cisplatin and pemetrexed (multitarget antimetabolite) is an option for nonsquamous histologies.

Radiation

Indications: RT is an option for definitive local therapy when surgery is not recommended or as adjunct delivered either before or after surgery; 45 Gy/25 fx is given for neoadjuvant chemoRT followed by resection. Postoperatively, for negative margins deliver 50–54 Gy/25–30 fx, for microscopic positive margins or ECE give 54 to 60 Gy and for gross residual give 60 Gy. In postoperative setting, give CHT first followed by RT, although for gross residual consider concurrent chemoRT. For definitive chemoRT, concurrent RT provides survival benefit compared to sequential chemoRT; giving 60 Gy/30 fx as dose escalation is potentially harmful and does not provide benefit. For poor performance pts not candidates for combined chemoRT, options include 60 Gy/30 fx, 45 Gy/15 fx, or palliative treatment alone.

Toxicity: Acute: Fatigue, cough, shortness of breath, pneumonitis, esophagitis. Late: Pneumonitis, cardiac toxicity, brachial plexopathy.

Procedure: See *Treatment Planning Handbook*, Chapter 6.[8]

EVIDENCE-BASED Q&A

Medically operable stage IIIA with negative mediastinal nodes (T3-4N1, T4N0)

Which stage III pts are optimal candidates for initial surgery?

Pts with resectable and medically operable T3-4N1 or T4N0 may be candidates for initial surgery, particularly if T category is due to multiple nodules in the same lobe or invasion of chest wall, mediastinum or mainstem bronchus <2 cm from carina. Induction therapy may also be feasible for these pts to facilitate surgery. Pts felt not to be good candidates for surgery should be treated with definitive chemoRT as follows if tolerable.

Which pts should be offered postoperative RT (PORT)?

pN2 disease and positive margins are indications for PORT. Recent ASTRO and ACR guidelines suggest consideration for pN2 pts following CHT but omission in routine pN0-1 patient.[9,10]

PORT Meta-analysis (*Lancet* 1998, PMID 9690404; Update Burdett *Lung Cancer* 2005, PMID 15603857): Meta-analysis of nine PRTs between 1965 and 1995 consisting of 2,128 pts treated postoperatively to doses between 40 Gy and 60 Gy . Results demonstrated detrimental effect overall (7% absolute reduction in 2-yr OS). On subset analysis, this was limited to stage I-II pts but for those with stage III (N2) disease, no clear detriment was identified. Most recent update demonstrated benefit in LC for N2 pts. **Conclusion: PORT recommended in pN2 pts but not in others after negative-margin resection.** *Comment: RT was with older regimens and techniques.*

Lally, SEER (*JCO* 2006, PMID 16769986): SEER analysis of 7,645 stage II-III pts treated with lobectomy or pneumonectomy. Overall there was no effect of PORT on survival, but in pN2 group there was benefit, whereas there was detriment to survival in pN0-1 groups.

Douillard, ANITA Second Analysis (*IJROBP* 2008, PMID 18439766): ANITA (Adjuvant Navelbine International Trialist Association) was PRT of 799 pts with resected stage IB-IIIA NSCLC (39% stage IIIA) randomized to four cycles of vinorelbine and cisplatin versus observation. PORT was recommended but optional for pN-positive disease. 24% of CHT pts and 33% of observation pts received PORT. Overall, trial improved OS by 8.6% at 5 yrs, mostly in stage IIA-IIIA pts. This unplanned subset analysis investigated the role of PORT and found that pN1 pts that received CHT had deleterious effect, pN1 that did not receive CHT had beneficial effect, and those with pN2 disease had improved OS with PORT in both arms. **Conclusion: Consider PORT for pN2 disease.**

Robinson, NCDB pN2 Analysis (*JCO* 2015, PMID 25667283): RR of NCDB including 4,483 pN2 pts from 2006 to 2010 stratified by use of PORT (1,850 PORT, 2,633 no PORT). MFU 22 mos. On multivariable analysis, PORT was associated with improved OS (MS 40.7 vs. 45.2 mos).

Does CHT in addition to surgery improve survival?

Adjuvant CHT following surgery consistently provides 5% to 8% absolute benefit to 5-yr OS. Many trials exist but few to be familiar with include IALT (cisplatin doublet vs. observation, 4% OS benefit at 5 years), ANITA (see the preceding text), and LACE meta-analysis (see Chapter 25).[11]

Medically operable with positive N2/mediastinal lymph node(s)

What is the rationale for multimodality therapy?

From the preceding trials we know that CHT in addition to surgery improves survival (LACE, ANITA, IALT) and that RT in addition to surgery improves LC for N2 pts and may improve survival.

Does trimodality therapy improve survival compared to chemoRT for pts with N2 disease?

If each modality alone improves outcomes, perhaps a combination of all three may give best outcomes. INT 0139 (Albain) did not show this overall, but trimodality may still be treatment of choice for select pts (controversial).

Albain, Intergroup 0139 (*Lancet* 2009, PMID 19632716): PRT of 429 potentially resectable NSCLC pts with biopsy-proven N2 disease randomized to either induction chemoRT followed by surgery 3 to 5 weeks later or to definitive chemoRT. Induction therapy for both arms was cisplatin 50 mg/m^2 and etoposide 50 mg/m^2 for two cycles (weeks 1 and 5) concurrent with 45 Gy/25 fx; those on definitive arm continued RT to 61 Gy without interruption (CT and PFTs were performed midtreatment in both arms to assess for progression). Two cycles of consolidation cisplatin/etoposide were given after local therapy. No significant difference in MS between groups (23.6 vs. 22.2 mos), 5-year OS was 27% for surgery and 20% for chemoRT. PFS was improved in surgery arm (median 12.8 vs. 10.5 mos). Treatment-related death rate was 8% for surgery and 2% for chemoRT. Exploratory analysis demonstrated that lobectomy pts showed improved OS compared to chemoRT but pneumonectomy pts did not. **Conclusion: No OS difference was demonstrated between approaches, so definitive chemoRT often favored although for healthy lobectomy pts, trimodality may be considered.** *Comment: Pneumonectomy mortality rate was higher than expected at 26%.*

For those who respond to CHT, is surgery superior to RT?

Van Meerbeeck, EORTC 08941 (*JNCI* 2007, PMID 17374834): PRT of pts with N2 NSCLC treated with three cycles of platinum-doublet induction CHT and then randomized to surgery versus 60 to 62.5 Gy. PORT (56 Gy) only delivered for positive margins. 61% responded and were randomized. In surgery arm, 42% showed nodal downstaging, 25% nodal clearance, and 5% pCR. Only 50% achieved complete resection. MS was no different: 16.4 mos surgery versus 17.5 mos for RT. **Conclusion: Sequential chemoRT is reasonable treatment option but induction CHT alone may not provide optimal surgical outcomes (in comparison to induction chemoRT).**

Is induction chemoRT superior to induction CHT followed by PORT?

Likely not, provided adjuvant RT is delivered postoperatively. Caution is warranted for pneumonectomy pts.

Thomas, German Lung Cancer Cooperative Group (*Lancet Oncol* 2008, PMID 18583190): Phase III PRT randomizing 524 pts with stage IIIA-B NSCLC after invasive mediastinal staging to either cisplatin/etoposide for three cycles, then surgery, then RT (54 Gy) or cisplatin/etoposide (3 cycles), then concurrent RT (45 Gy/30 fx BID) with carboplatin/vindesine, and then surgery. Primary endpoint PFS. ChemoRT improved mediastinal downstaging (46% vs. 29%, $p = .02$) and pathologic response (60% vs. 20%, $p < .0001$) but no difference in PFS (9.5 vs. 10 mos). Pneumonectomy was required in 35% for both groups but mortality after chemoRT was higher (14% vs. 6%). **Conclusion: Neoadjuvant chemoRT improved response rates but not OS.**

Nonoperative management

Is RT alone an optimal strategy for stage III NSCLC?

RT alone is an option for pts unable to tolerate multimodality therapy. Previous dose-escalation studies demonstrated inferior outcomes despite high dose treatment. This study clarified 60 Gy/30 fx as standard regimen for NSCLC. In modern era, RT alone is option for poor performance pts, and 45 Gy/15 fx was alternative biologically equivalent regimen allowed on RTOG 0213 (see the following).

Perez, RTOG 7301 (*IJROBP*** 1980, PMID 6998937):** Four-arm PRT of definitive RT dose escalation for stage III NSCLC: 40 Gy split course (20 Gy/5 fx, 2-week break, then another 20 Gy/5 fx) or 40 Gy, 50 Gy, or 60 Gy given five fractions per week. OS at 2 years was 10% to 18% with split course giving worst rates. Response was better in 50 and 60 Gy arms. **Conclusion: 60 Gy is standard dose.**

Gore, RTOG 0213 (*Clin Lung Cancer*** 2011, PMID 21550559):** Phase I/II trial of celecoxib concurrent with 60 Gy/30 fx or 45 Gy/15 fx for stage IIB-IIIB lung cancer pts with "intermediate" prognosis (PS 2 or weight loss >5%). Closed early after 13 pts. MS 10 mos. **Conclusion: Although underpowered, this gives one reference for management of "intermediate prognosis" pts.**

Does CHT followed by RT improve survival?

Multiple trials have demonstrated improved survival with sequential chemoRT, selected studies follow.

Dillman, CALGB 8433 (*NEJM*** 1990, PMID 2169587; Update Dillman ***JNCI*** 1996, PMID 8780630):** PRT of 155 pts with stage III NSCLC randomized to cisplatin with vinblastine followed by 60 Gy/30 fx versus immediate identical RT. Long-term results reported 5-yr OS rate of 17% versus 6% in favor of CHT arm and confirmed initial results. **Conclusion: Sequential chemoRT is superior to RT alone.**

Sause, RTOG 8808/ECOG 4588 (*JNCI*** 1995, PMID 7707407):** Three-arm PRT of 452 pts with stage II-IIIB unresectable NSCLC randomized to either 60 Gy/30 fx alone, induction cisplatin/vinblastine followed by 60 Gy/30 fx or hyperfractionated RT: 69.6 Gy/58 fx at 1.2 Gy/fx BID. MS in each arm was 11.4, 13.8, and 12.3 months, respectively, with statistically significant improvement in CHT arm. **Conclusion: Sequential chemoRT is superior to standard and hyperfractionated RT alone.**

Does CHT concurrent with RT improve survival?

Multiple trials have demonstrated improved survival with concurrent compared to sequential chemoRT at expense of increased acute toxicity. Selected studies follow.

Curran, RTOG 9410 (*JNCI*** 2011, PMID 21903745):** Three-arm PRT of 610 pts with unresectable stage III NSCLC. See Table 26.2. Statistical significance was demonstrated between sequential and concurrent daily arms. **Conclusion: Concurrent CHT is superior to sequential.**

TABLE 26.2: RTOG 9410 Stage III Lung Trial		
Arm	5-yr OS	MS (mos)
Sequential cisplatin/vinblastine x2c then 63 Gy/34 fx	10%	14.6
Concurrent cisplatin/vinblastine x2c with 63 Gy/34 fx	16%	17
Concurrent cisplatin/etoposide with 69.6 Gy at 1.2 Gy/fx delivered BID	13%	15.6

Note: 63 Gy delivered 45 Gy/25 fx followed by 18 Gy/9 fx boost without heterogeneity corrections is comparable to 60 Gy/30 fx

Aupérin, NSCLC Collaborative Group Meta-Analysis (*JCO* 2010, PMID 20351327): Individual patient data meta-analysis of six of seven eligible trials, 1,205 pts. Concurrent chemoRT demonstrated 4.5% absolute survival benefit at 5 yrs compared to sequential chemoRT. Concurrent therapy decreased locoregional but not distant progression and increased esophageal but not pulmonary toxicity. **Conclusion: Concurrent chemoRT improves survival at cost of manageable but increased esophageal toxicity.**

What is the optimal CHT regimen when given concurrently with RT?

Many regimens have been used but cisplatin/etoposide and carboplatin/paclitaxel are the most common regimens used in the United States. Carboplatin/paclitaxel and cisplatin/pemetrexed (for nonsquamous cancers) may have similar efficacy with reduced toxicity. Retrospective data suggests that carboplatin/paclitaxel is associated with increased radiation pneumonitis, which was confirmed by Liang as follows.[12] However, others feel cisplatin/etoposide is more difficult to tolerate.

Liang, China (*Ann Oncol* 2017, PMID 28137739): PRT comparing cisplatin/etoposide to carboplatin/paclitaxel both with concurrent RT to 60–66 Gy. Primary endpoint OS, powered for 17% improvement in 3-yr OS. 200 pts, MFU 73 mos. 3-yr OS improved in cisplatin/etoposide arm by 15% (p = .024), MS 23.3 versus 20.7 mos favoring cisplatin/etoposide. Grade ≥2 pneumonitis increased in the carboplatin/paclitaxel arm (33.3% vs. 18.9%, p = .036), esophagitis increased in the cisplatin/etoposide arm (20.0% vs. 6.3%, p = .009). **Conclusion: Cisplatin/etoposide may be superior to carboplatin/etoposide.**

Senan, PROCLAIM (*JCO* 2016, PMID 26811519): PRT of 555 pts with unresectable stage IIIA/B nonsquamous NSCLC randomized to receive either (a) pemetrexed 500 mg/m^2 and cisplatin 75 mg/m^2 every 3 weeks for three cycles plus 60 to 66 Gy followed by consolidation pemetrexed every 3 weeks for four cycles or (b) cisplatin 50 mg/m^2 with etoposide 50 mg/m^2 every 4 weeks for two cycles plus same RT with consolidation platinum doublet. Trial stopped early due to futility. Pemetrexed was not superior but was associated with less grade 3-4 adverse events. **Conclusion: Pemetrexed is not superior but may be associated with fewer adverse events.**

Santana-Davila, VA Health Data (*JCO* 2015, PMID 25422491): RR of 1,842 pts from Veterans Health Administration data comparing cisplatin/etoposide with carboplatin/paclitaxel from 2001 to 2010. After adjustment methods, there was no survival advantage to cisplatin/etoposide but was associated with more hospitalizations.

Does RT dose escalation improve outcomes when given with concurrent CHT?

Dating back to the 1970s, RTOG 7301 demonstrated 60 Gy/30 fx to be standard regimen. RTOG 9311 was phase I/II dose-escalation trial that delivered escalated doses based on achieved V20 with doses ranging from 70.9 Gy to 90.3 Gy without concurrent CHT. This led to RTOG 0617 as follows.

Bradley, RTOG 0617 (*Lancet Oncol* 2015, PMID 25601342): 2x2 PRT of 544 pts randomized to either 60 Gy/30 fx or 74 Gy/37 fx with concurrent carboplatin AUC 2/paclitaxel 45 mg/m² weekly. Adjuvant CHT was given 2 weeks after RT with carboplatin AUC 6/paclitaxel 200 mg/m² with second randomization to addition of cetuximab during adjuvant phase. 47% treated with IMRT. See Table 26.3. Overall, no difference in toxicity rates between 60 Gy and 74 Gy, but grade ≥3 esophagitis was increased in 74 Gy arm. Noncompliance was higher in 74 Gy arm. Cetuximab increased grade ≥3 toxicity but did not improve OS, PFS, or DM. **Conclusion: 60 Gy is standard of care. 74 Gy is harmful and not superior. No benefit to cetuximab.** *Comment: Hypotheses as to why 74 Gy survival was inferior: Treatment-related deaths were highest in 74 Gy+cetuximab arm, effect of RT on heart, PTV coverage was sacrificed in 74 Gy arm for safety thus leading to failures. Second analysis demonstrated dosimetric benefits to IMRT, reduced lung dosimetry, and correlation of heart V40 with survival.*[13]

TABLE 26.3: Results of RTOG 0617 for Stage III NSCLC						
<u>Arms</u>	MS (mos)	OS (1 yr)	PFS (median, mos)	PFS (1 yr)	LF (1 yr)	DM (1 yr)
60 Gy/30 fx	28.7	80%	11.8	49.2%	16.3%	32.2%
74 Gy/37 fx	20.3	69.8%	9.8	41.2%	24.8%	35.1%
p value	.004	.004	.12	.12	.13	.48

Is there benefit to adding induction CHT prior to concurrent chemoRT or additional consolidation CHT after concurrent chemoRT?

The use of consolidation CHT after definitive chemoRT was given in RTOG 0617 and is optional as per NCCN guidelines but is not standard and may increase toxicity without benefit. Induction provides no benefit.

Belani, LAMP (*JCO* 2005, PMID 16087941): Phase II PRT of 276 pts with stage IIIA/B NSCLC randomized to induction carboplatin/paclitaxel followed by 63 Gy RT alone; induction carboplatin/paclitaxel followed by 63 Gy RT with concurrent carboplatin/paclitaxel or 63 Gy RT with concurrent carboplatin/paclitaxel followed by consolidation carboplatin/paclitaxel. MFU 39.6 mos, MS 13.0, 12.7, and 16.3 mos in favor of consolidation. Grade 3/4 esophageal toxicity was worse with concurrent arms. **Conclusion: RT with concurrent and adjuvant carboplatin/paclitaxel is associated with improved OS in this phase II study.**

Hanna, Hoosier Oncology Group (*JCO* 2008, PMID 19001323; Update Jalal, *Ann Oncol* 2012, PMID 22156624): Phase III PRT of 203 pts with stage IIIA/B NSCLC treated with cisplatin/etoposide concurrent with RT to 59.4 Gy, then randomized to adjuvant docetaxel versus observation. Closed early due to futility. MS not significantly different (initial publication 21.7 vs. 21.2 mos, no difference on update). Toxicity was increased in docetaxel arm. **Conclusion: Consolidation docetaxel increases toxicity but not survival.**

Vokes, CALGB 39801 (*JCO* 2007, PMID 17404369): PRT comparing induction CHT followed by chemoRT versus chemoRT alone. No statistically significant difference in OS. **Conclusion: No benefit to induction CHT prior to chemoRT.**

Ahn, Korean KCSG-LU05-04 (*JCO* 2015, PMID 26150444): PRT of 437 pts with stage III NSCLC treated to 66 Gy with cisplatin/docetaxel, then randomized to receive either three additional cycles of docetaxel/cisplatin or no further treatment. 62% in consolidation arm completed. PFS was 8.1 mos in observation versus 9.1 mos in consolidation arm (*p* = .36).

MS was also not different (20.6 vs. 21.8 mos, $p = .44$). **Conclusion: Additional CHT did not improve outcomes after chemoRT.**

Superior sulcus tumors

Superior sulcus tumors were classically associated with poor rates of complete resection. SWOG 9416 changed paradigm and these tumors are recommended to undergo induction chemoRT to facilitate resection.

Rusch, SWOG 9416/Intergroup 0160 (*J Thorac Cardiovasc Surg* **2001, PMID 11241082; Update** *JCO* **2007, PMID 17235046):** Single-arm phase II trial of 111 pts with mediastinoscopy-negative and supraclavicular node-negative T3-4N0-1 superior sulcus tumors treated with two cycles of cisplatin/etoposide with concurrent 45 Gy/25 fx. If disease was stable or responding on reassessment, thoracotomy was performed 3 to 5 weeks later. Thereafter, two more cycles of CHT was delivered. 111 enrolled, 95 were eligible for surgery and 83 underwent thoracotomy, 72 had complete resection (92%). 65% of thoracotomy specimens demonstrated CR. On update, 5-yr OS was 44% overall and 56% after complete resection. **Conclusion: Induction combined modality therapy became standard for superior sulcus tumors after this trial.**

REFERENCES

1. NCCN Clinical Practice Guidelines in Oncology: Non-small Cell Lung Cancer. 2017(4.2017). https://www.nccn.org/professionals/physician_gls/pdf/nscl.pdf
2. Yokoi K, Kamiya N, Matsuguma H, et al. Detection of brain metastasis in potentially operable non-small cell lung cancer: a comparison of CT and MRI. *Chest.* 1999;115(3):714–719.
3. Brunelli A, Kim AW, Berger KI, Addrizzo-Harris DJ. Physiologic evaluation of the patient with lung cancer being considered for resectional surgery: diagnosis and management of lung cancer, 3rd ed: American College of Chest Physicians evidence-based clinical practice guidelines. *Chest.* 2013;143(5, Suppl):e166S–e190S.
4. Edelman MJ. NRG Oncology RTOG 0839 Randomized Phase II Study of Pre-Operative Chemoradiotherapy +/– Panitumumab (IND#110152) Followed by Consolidation Chemotherapy in Potentially Operable Locally Advanced (Stage IIIA, N2+ Non-Small Cell Lung Cancer). 2014. https://www.rtog.org/ClinicalTrials/ProtocolTable/StudyDetails.aspx?study=0839
5. Bradley JD, Bae K, Graham MV, et al. Primary analysis of the phase II component of a phase I/II dose intensification study using three-dimensional conformal radiation therapy and concurrent chemotherapy for patients with inoperable non-small-cell lung cancer: RTOG 0117. *J Clin Oncol.* 2010;28(14):2475–2480.
6. Bradley JD, Paulus R, Komaki R, et al. Standard-dose versus high-dose conformal radiotherapy with concurrent and consolidation carboplatin plus paclitaxel with or without cetuximab for patients with stage IIIA or IIIB non-small-cell lung cancer (RTOG 0617): a randomised, two-by-two factorial phase 3 study. *Lancet Oncol.* 2015;16(2):187–199.
7. Fischer B, Lassen U, Mortensen J, et al. Preoperative staging of lung cancer with combined PET-CT. *N Engl J Med.* 2009;361(1):32–39.
8. Videtic GMM, Woody N, Vassil AD. *Handbook of Treatment Planning in Radiation Oncology.* 2nd ed. New York, NY: Demos Medical; 2015.
9. Rodrigues G, Choy H, Bradley J, et al. Adjuvant radiation therapy in locally advanced non-small cell lung cancer: executive summary of an American Society for Radiation Oncology (ASTRO) evidence-based clinical practice guideline. *Pract Radiat Oncol.* 2015;5(3):149–155.
10. Willers H, Stinchcombe TE, Barriger RB, et al. ACR Appropriateness Criteria(®) induction and adjuvant therapy for N2 non-small-cell lung cancer. *Am J Clin Oncol.* 2015;38(2):197–205.
11. Arriagada R, Bergman B, Dunant A, et al. Cisplatin-based adjuvant chemotherapy in patients with completely resected non-small-cell lung cancer. *N Engl J Med.* 2004;350(4):351–360.

12. Palma DA, Senan S, Tsujino K, et al. Predicting radiation pneumonitis after chemoradiation therapy for lung cancer: an international individual patient data meta-analysis. *Int J Radiat Oncol Biol Phys*. 2013;85(2):444–450.

13. Chun SG, Hu C, Choy H, et al. Impact of intensity-modulated radiation therapy technique for locally advanced non-small-cell lung cancer: a secondary analysis of the NRG Oncology RTOG 0617 randomized clinical trial. *J Clin Oncol*. 2017;35(1):56–62.

27: SMALL-CELL LUNG CANCER

Camille A. Berriochoa and Gregory M. M. Videtic

QUICK HIT: SCLC is classically described as either limited (fits within one radiation portal; LS-SCLC) or extensive (metastatic; ES-SCLC). Treatment for LS-SCLC consists of concurrent chemoRT with platinum-based regimens followed by CHT, with PCI offered for those with response to therapy. Treatment for ES-SCLC consists of (typically six) cycles of CHT, with many arguing that partial and complete responders receive post-CHT thoracic RT and PCI should brain remain free of metastases. Outcomes are generally poor, with MS 20 to 30 mos for LS-SCLC and 9 to 12 mos for ES-SCLC.

TABLE 27.1: General Treatment Paradigm for Small-Cell Lung Carcinoma	
Disease Extent	**General Treatment Paradigm**
Limited stage (30% of SCLC)	• Concurrent ChemoRT w/ EP CHT x 4 cycles delivering CHT w/ either cycle 1 or 2 start. • CHT: cisplatin 60 mg/m² d1 and etoposide 120 mg/m² d1-3 q3w x 4c. • RT standard: 45 Gy/30 fx in 3w at 1.5 Gy/fx BID. Alternatives include 40 Gy/15 fx at 2.67 Gy/fx, 66–70 Gy/33–35 fx. • Prophylactic cranial irradiation (PCI): 25 Gy/10 fx for responders.
	• T1-T2N0M0 disease (5% of cases). Assessment by thoracic surgeon, resection with adjuvant CHT + PCI. Medically inoperable cases: consider SBRT as surgical surrogate.

Extensive stage (70% SCLC)	• Cisplatin-based CHT (4–6 cycles).
	• Palliative RT to symptomatic sites.
	• Areas of controversy:
	  1. In pts w/o brain metastases, PCI (25 Gy/10 fx) for those w/ *any* response to CHT
	  2. In selected pts, consolidative thoracic RT: consider concurrent CHT and chest RT (54 Gy in 36 fx BID w/ cycle 4) or post 4–6 cycles CHT (30 Gy/10 fx)

EPIDEMIOLOGY: SCLC represents ~15% of all lung cancer diagnoses with decreasing incidence.[1] Approximately 30,000 people are diagnosed in the United States each year.[2] More common in men although gender difference is narrowing.[1]

RISK FACTORS: Occurs almost exclusively in smokers (>98%)—typically heavy smokers.[3] Uranium mining is another risk factor (radon exposure from uranium decay).[4]

ANATOMY: See Chapter 25.

PATHOLOGY[5,6]**:** SCLC is of neuroendocrine origin and lies along spectrum of other lung neuroendocrine tumors including low-grade neuroendocrine carcinoma (typical carcinoid), intermediate grade (atypical carcinoid), and high grade (large-cell neuroendocrine carcinoma [LCNEC], and SCLC). Light microscopy classically reveals clusters or sheets of small round blue cells, twice the size of normal lymphocytes. Cytoplasm is sparse and nucleus manifests finely dispersed chromatin without distinct nucleoli. Mitotic rates are high and necrosis is common. Specimen processing often creates characteristic *crush artifact* (diagnostic). Up to 30% of SCLC autopsy specimens have areas of differentiation into NSCLC, suggestive that carcinogenesis occurs in pluripotent stem cells capable of varied differentiation. Three groups of antigen clusters have been identified: neural, epithelial, and neuroendocrine. Epithelial markers include keratin, epithelial membrane antigen, and TTF1. Neuroendocrine and neural markers include DOPA decarboxylase, calcitonin, neuron specific enolase (NSE), synaptophysin, chromogranin A, CD56 (neural cell adhesion molecule, NCAM), gastrin releasing peptide, and IGF-1. Though these are common in SCLC, they are not specific, with about 10% of NSCLCs being positive for these classic neuroendocrine markers.[7] 75% of SCLC will manifest at least one neural/neuroendocrine marker.

GENETICS: In contrast to NSCLC, driving alterations in EGFR, K-ras, ALK, and p16 are rarely seen.

CLINICAL PRESENTATION: SCLC arises sub-mucosally in central airways, often obstructing bronchial lumen. Commonly appears on imaging as large hilar mass with bulky mediastinal adenopathy.[8] Two-thirds present with extensive stage disease, one-third present with limited stage disease. Common symptoms include new or worsening cough, dyspnea, chest pain, hoarseness, hemoptysis, malaise, anorexia, and weight loss. If other thoracic structures are compromised by enlarging mass, dysphagia or SVC syndrome (facial edema/plethora, distention of superficial veins, laryngeal edema, altered mental status) may be present. Most common sites of distant spread are liver, adrenals, bone, and brain. Brain mets incidence: 10% to 20% at diagnosis, 50% to 80% at 2 yrs.[9,10] As detailed in Table 27.2, pts may present with paraneoplastic syndromes (SCLC is most common solid tumor associated with paraneoplastic syndromes).[11] Fundamentally, treatment of underlying malignancy is necessary to manage these syndromes, but temporizing management steps are described as follows.

TABLE 27.2: Paraneoplastic Syndromes Commonly Diagnosed in SCLC	
SIADH	Overproduction of ADH with euvolemic hyponatremia. May present with altered mental status, seizures. Treat with water restriction, hypertonic saline, demeclocycline, vasopressin inhibitors, and/or lithium.
Cushing syndrome	Ectopic production of ACTH. Treat with ketoconazole.
Lambert–Eaton	Auto-antibodies to presynaptic calcium channels. Proximal muscle weakness that improves later in day. Treat with pyridostigmine, prednisone, IVIG and by treating cancer.
Others (rare)	Subacute cerebellar degeneration, subacute sensory neuropathy, limbic encephalopathy, encephalomyelitis (anti-Hu antibodies)

WORKUP[6]: H&P. Encourage smoking cessation.[12]

Labs: CBC, BMP, LFTs, LDH, alkaline phosphatase, PFTs.

Imaging: CT chest with contrast (including liver and adrenals) and PET/CT (nearly 100% sensitive for SCLC; note that PET upstages 19% of pts initially diagnosed with LS disease).[13] Forego bone scan if PET obtained. Contrast-enhanced brain MRI (preferred) or CT brain (CT brain positive in 10%; MRI brain positive in 20%).[10]

Pathology: For tissue diagnosis: sputum, bronchoscopy with biopsy/FNA (though note that FNA may not always adequately differentiate SCLC from carcinoid tumors), CT-guided biopsy or thoracentesis for pleural effusion. Consider bone marrow biopsy if neutropenia/thrombocytopenia/nucleated RBCs on peripheral smear. About 5% of pts present with cT1-2N0 disease. In this setting, mediastinal staging is useful (see Chapter 25). If LNs are uninvolved, up-front resection (or SBRT in medically inoperable pts) can be considered.

PROGNOSTIC FACTORS: Favorable: limited stage, female gender, performance status (0–1), absence of weight loss, absence of paraneoplastic syndromes, normal labs (LDH, sodium, albumin), smoking cessation.[12,14,15] Hyponatremia (MS 9 mos if Na <135, 13 mos if Na ≥135, p < .001).[16] LDH has been shown to correspond with disease burden, can raise concern for bone marrow involvement, and may be risk factor for early death.[17] More than 5% weight loss is poor prognostic factor.[18]

NATURAL HISTORY: Distant failure is common with brain metastases in up to 80%.[9,10] Although distant failure is predominant driver of mortality, local failure is also common (36%–52% per Turrisi). Untreated, MS for LS-SCLC is 12 weeks and for ES-SCLC is 6 weeks.[19]

STAGING: The VA system (Table 27.3) is relevant historically but AJCC staging now standard; see Chapter 25.

TABLE 27.3: VA Lung Cancer Study Group[20]				
Limited stage	Tumor confined to one hemithorax (including both ipsi and contralateral mediastinum) and ipsilateral SCV nodes	MS: 20–30 mos	2-yr OS: 40%	5-yr OS: 20% to 30%
Extensive stage	Tumor beyond boundaries of limited disease, including distant metastases, malignant pericardial/pleural effusions, and contralateral SCV/hilar LN involvement	MS: 12 mos	2-yr OS: 5%	5-yr OS: <5%

TREATMENT PARADIGM

Surgery: Surgery is not standard for most LS-SCLC based on historic MRC trial published in 1973 randomizing SCLC pts to either surgery or RT, with improved survival observed in those who received RT (mean OS improved from ~7 to 10 mos, p = .04).[21] However, ~4% to 5% of SCLC diagnoses present as solitary pulmonary nodules (SPN). For T1-2 SPN SCLC tumors, lobectomy with mediastinal LN dissection is recommended, followed by CHT and/or radiation depending on pathologic nodal status. Note that adjuvant CHT is indicated even if pN0.[6] A 2017 NCDB analysis showed increasing use of definitive surgical management in clinical stage I disease from 15% in 2004 to almost 30% in 2013 (the use of SBRT also increased from 0.4% to 6% in this time frame).[22]

Chemotherapy: Compared with no therapy, CHT improves MS fivefold. Cisplatin and etoposide (EP) are standard and found to be equally effective and less toxic than older regimens.[23,24] Current standard is four cycles of EP with concurrent RT. Dose of cisplatin is 60 to 100 mg/m² on day 1, and etoposide 120 mg/m² on days 1 to 3, every 3 weeks. Japanese data showed improved survival with irinotecan + cisplatin versus EP for ES-SCLC (2-yr OS: 19.5% vs. 5.2%); however, this was not reproduced by randomized studies in the United States, Canada, or Australia, potentially due to biological differences in Japanese study population.[25,26] Additional CHT strategies such as dose intensification, triplet therapy, high dose consolidation, alternating/sequential regimens, and maintenance therapy all have not demonstrated improvements in OS. Some substitute cisplatin with carboplatin for more favorable side effect profile, with the 2012 COCIS meta-analysis of four randomized trials (including both LS and ES disease) showing no difference in response rate (about 70% for both groups), PFS (about 5 months for both), or OS (about 9 mos for both) between two platinum-based regimens.[27]

Radiation

Indications: Radiation, when added to CHT, was found to reduce intrathoracic failures by 50% (from 75%–90% to 30%–60%). RT also improves survival by 5.4% at 2 to 3 yrs (see *Warde* and *Pignon* in the following). For regimens using EP, concurrent chemoRT appears superior to sequential. Advantages of concurrent chemoRT: early use of both treatment modalities, more accurate RT planning, high-intensity treatment in short time, and radio-sensitization of tumor. Main disadvantage is higher tissue toxicity (esophagitis, pneumonitis, myelosuppression), potentially leading to treatment breaks or discontinuation. Most studies have demonstrated benefit to early RT with CHT cycles 1 and 2. LS-SCLC pts who have complete response or good partial response to primary therapy (and ES-SCLC with any response to CHT) should be treated with PCI to 25 Gy/10 fx, as this reduces incidence of brain metastases and improves OS (see Auperin meta-analysis). Of note, SBRT may have a role similar to surgery in well-selected early-stage pts. A 2017 multi-institution RR demonstrated excellent 3-yr LC (≥95%) for 74 T1-2N0 pts treated with SBRT.[28] This series also showed improved OS in those who also received subsequent CHT (31 vs. 14 mos, *p* = .02). Following thoracic treatment, PCI 25 Gy/10 fx should be given to all LS-SCLC pts who respond to chemoRT with many also advocating delivery of PCI to those with ES-SCLC without brain mets at diagnosis who respond to initial CHT.

Dose: Standard accelerated dose is 45 Gy/30 fx at 1.5 Gy/fx BID in 3 weeks with concurrent EP CHT based on results from the landmark Turrisi trial.[29] Proposed radiobiological advantages of BID fx in SCLC include high growth fraction, short cell cycle time and small/absent shoulder on cell survival curve. Cycle 2 start RT dose can be utilized when delivering 40 Gy/15 fx at 2.67 Gy/fx.[30] Although many argue that BID fractionation is standard of care based on Turrisi's findings (supported by CONVERT trial below), a 2003 patterns of care practice survey found that fewer than 10% of clinicians employ BID RT approach, with >80% of pts receiving daily RT to a median dose of 50.4 Gy.[31] NCCN states that if daily fractionation is used, 60 to 70 Gy should be given (not based on level 1 evidence). Once complete, results from RTOG 0538 will provide additional data regarding outcomes of BID versus daily—albeit using higher dose RT (70 Gy/35 fx per RTOG 0538; 66 Gy/33 fx per CONVERT).

Toxicity

Acute: Fatigue, esophagitis, pneumonitis, nausea. Chronic: Pneumonitis, cardiac injury, dysphagia.

EVIDENCE-BASED Q&A

Limited stage small-cell lung cancer

Is there a benefit to RT in addition to CHT?

Multiple RCTs compared CHT alone to chemoRT, which formed the basis of the seminal Warde and Pignon meta-analyses, both of which showed 5% benefit in OS with addition of thoracic RT to CHT. [32,33]

Warde, Ontario Meta-Analysis (*JCO* 1992, PMID 1316951): Meta-analysis of 11 randomized trials of LS-SCLC pts treated with CHT alone versus chemoRT. Demonstrated significant 25.3% improvement in LC (47% vs. 24%) and 5.4% improvement in 2-yr OS (20% vs. 15%) with addition of RT, with pts under age 60 deriving greatest benefit. There was no significant difference in treatment-related death.

Pignon, French Meta-Analysis (*NEJM* 1992, PMID 1331787): Meta-analysis of 13 randomized trials of 2,140 pts with LS-SCLC treated with CHT alone versus chemoRT.

Addition of thoracic RT improved 3-yr OS by 5.4% (14.3% vs. 8.9%) over CHT alone, with 14% relative reduction in mortality rate. Younger pts (age <55) had greater benefit from addition of radiation to CHT compared to pts over age 70.

What is the ideal dose and fractionation for LS-SCLC?

There are varying practices, but 45 Gy BID regimen defined by Turrisi's Intergroup trial is the current standard of care.[29] *A more recent trial, RTOG 0239, was phase II whose goal was to determine whether 61.2 Gy/34 fx delivered via daily fractionation for first 22 days followed by BID treatments for last 9 days would improve outcomes. Given ongoing controversy, however, there are two recent phase III trials (EORTC CONVERT trial and RTOG 0538) investigating optimal dose and fractionation. CONVERT is completed with results as follows; RTOG 0538 is still enrolling.*

Turrisi, RTOG 88-15/INT 0096 (*NEJM*** 1999, PMID 9920950):** Phase III PRT of 417 pts treated with concurrent CHT and either daily or BID radiation. CHT was 60 mg/m² cisplatin on day 1 and 120 mg/m² etoposide on days 1 to 3 every 3 weeks for four cycles. RT was started on day 1 of CHT and was based on University of Pennsylvania RT technique reported in 1988.[34] RT dose was 45 Gy/25 fx in 5 weeks at 1.8 Gy/fx daily versus 45 Gy/30 fx in 3 weeks at 1.5 Gy/fx BID. Fields taken off cord at 36 Gy. Pts with CR received PCI 25 Gy/10 fx. Note that there was 60% to 70% risk of esophagitis in the subgroup of pts age >70 so altering dose for elderly pts may be important. **Conclusion: BID fractionation significantly improved OS, though with higher acute grade 3 esophageal toxicity but not late toxicity.** *Comment: Employing 45 Gy/25 fx as standard arm may represent suboptimal dose given that this represents low BED for pts with gross disease. Also, experimental arm tested two additional variables: (a) decreased time between doses; and (b) finishing treatment in shorter period of time—both of which may have independently improved outcomes.*

TABLE 27.4: Results of Turrisi RTOG 8815/INT 0096, Hyperfractionation for SCLC

Turrisi	MS (mos)	5-yr OS	Local Failure (Thoracic Relapse)	Acute Grade 3 Esophagitis
45 Gy QD	19	16%	52%	11%
45 Gy BID	23	26%	36%	27%
p value	.04	.04	.06	<.001

Faivre-Finn, CONVERT (*Lancet Oncol*** 2017, PMID 28642008):** Randomized 547 pts with LS-SCLC to CHT with either BID RT (45 Gy/30 fx delivered BID over 3 weeks) or daily chemoRT (66 Gy/33 fx over 6.5 weeks), both with RT starting on day 1 of cycle 2 of EP CHT, followed by PCI if indicated. Primary endpoint: 2-yr OS. MFU 45 mos. Two-yr OS & MS were 56% and 30 mos for BID and 51% and 25 mos for daily tx (*p* = .14). Toxicities were comparable except for grade 4 neutropenia (increased from 38% in daily RT group to 49% in BID group, *p* = .05). In each arm, grade 3 esophagitis was 19%. Grade 3-4 pneumonitis was rare (~2% in each arm). **Conclusion: Similar results between arms support use of either regimen for LS-SCLC, but the superiority design of the trial suggests the standard arm (BID) remains standard as equivalence was not demonstrated.**

What is the optimal timing of chemoRT?

In an appropriately fit patient, chemoRT should be given concurrently and SER (start of any treatment until end of RT) should be <30 days per De Ruysscher's meta-analysis.[35] *There has historically been some controversy as to whether early versus delayed start is optimal. There are three trials (Murray, Jeremic, Takada) suggesting benefit to early RT, but three other trials (CALGB, Spiro, and Sun) suggesting no benefit. However, given findings of De Ruysscher meta-analysis (with particular attention on SER <30 days) as well as theoretical radiobiologic advantages to early* *treatment in SCLC (rapid cell turnover makes this disease prone to repopulation, which can thus be more vulnerable to accelerated treatment), most clinicians prefer cycle 1 or 2 start.*

Murray, NCIC (*JCO* 1993, PMID 8381164): PRT of 308 pts treated with concurrent CHT and randomized to early RT (cycle 2 at week 3) or delayed RT (cycle 6 at week 15). CHT was alternating CAV and EP for six cycles. RT dose was 40 Gy/15 fx at 2.67 Gy/fx. PCI in 25 Gy/10 fx was given to all pts w/o progressive disease after CHT. Results in Table 27.5. Toxicity was similar between arms. **Conclusion: Early thoracic RT with concurrent CHT is superior to delayed RT.** *Comment: Note that cycle 2 start was to avoid concurrent Adriamycin in CAV. Since then, a number of trials have compared CAV, CAV-EP, and EP alone, and found that response rate for EP alone is equivalent to CAV/EP and superior to CAV alone.*[36] *Thus, EP rather than combined EP-CAV is now standard in this setting and thus cycle 1 start, if feasible, may still be preferable to cycle 2.*

TABLE 27.5: Results of Murray NCIC Trial for Small-Cell Lung Cancer

Murray	CR	MS	2-yr OS	3-yr OS	5-yr OS	Brain Mets
Early RT	64%	21 mos	40%	30%	20%	18%
Delayed RT	56%	16 mos	34%	21.5%	11%	28%
p value	.14	.008			$p = .006$	.042

Jeremic, Yugoslavia (*JCO* 1997, PMID 9060525): PRT 107 pts were treated with RT 54 Gy/36 fx at 1.5 Gy BID (36/24 AP/PA, then off cord) with concurrent daily carboplatin/etoposide (30 mg/m² each) followed by four cycles of cisplatin (30 mg/m²)/etoposide (120 mg/m²). Group 1 started with concurrent carboplatin/etoposide + RT, then four cycles of EP. Group 2 started with two cycles EP, then RT with carbo/etop, then additional two cycles of EP. All responders received PCI to 25 Gy/10 fx. MS 34 versus 26 months, 5-yr OS 30% versus. 15% both in favor of group 1 ($p = .052$ on univariate analysis, $p = .027$ on MVA). MS 53 versus 15 mos for KPS 90 to 100 versus 50 to 80 ($p < .0001$). 96% versus 80% CR rates at 9 weeks. Grade 3-4 esophagitis 28% versus 24% (NS). **Conclusion: Accelerated BID RT to total dose of 54 Gy/36 fx has similar toxicities to Turrisi trial, with encouraging survival data.**

Takada, JCOG 9104 (*JCO* 2002, PMID 12118018): Compared concurrent chemoRT to sequential CHT then RT (specifically, cycle 1 chemoRT at 45 Gy BID versus same RT followed by CHT). MS 27 mos for cycle 1 start, 20 mos for sequential, $p = .097$. **Conclusion: EP and concurrent RT more effective than EP and sequential RT.**

Perry, CALGB 8083 (*JCO* 1998, PMID 9667265): Compared cycle 1 chemoRT versus cycle 4 chemoRT versus CHT alone. CHT was cyclophosphamide, etoposide, and vincristine, with doxorubicin replacing etoposide later in trial. RT was 50 Gy in 5 weeks (40 Gy to tumor and mediastinum + 10 Gy boost). All pts received PCI to 30 Gy. MS was approximately 13 to 14 mos for all three arms. However, via pairwise comparisons using log-rank test, authors showed that CHT alone was inferior to both RT-containing regimens. **Conclusion: With 10 years of follow-up, two arms that included thoracic RT**

TABLE 27.6: Long-Term Results of CALGB 8083 for Small-Cell Lung Cancer

CALGB 8083, 10-yr update	MS (mos)	Time to clinical failure (mos)
Arm I (Cycle 1 start)	13	11
Arm II (Cycle 4 start)	14.5	11.2
Arm III (CHT Alone)	13.6	8.7
Both MS and time to clinical failure were worse in arm III than I + II (SS) but could not demonstrate whether arm I or II was superior.		

remain superior to CHT alone. Addition of thoracic RT therapy to combination CHT improved both CR rates and survival, with increased but acceptable toxicity. *Comment: CHT regimen may have been inferior to EP.*

Spiro, UK London Lung Cancer Group (*JCO* 2006, PMID 16921033): PRT of 325 pts treated using NCIC regimen and randomization earlier again with both CAV and EP CHT. More pts in early arm were treated with RT than late arm, 92% versus 82% ($p = .01$). Fewer pts in early arm completed CHT than late arm, 69% versus 80% ($p = .003$). MS same, 13.7 versus 15.1 mo ($p = .23$). **Conclusion: Failed to replicate survival advantage noted in NCIC trial.** *Comment: Lower rate of CHT completion in early arm could have obscured detection of survival advantage when utilizing early thoracic RT.*

Sun, South Korea (*Ann Onc* 2013, PMID 23592701): Phase III trial comparing thoracic RT w/ first cycle versus third cycle of EP CHT; 220 pts. Outcomes were essentially same between two arms (CR, PFS, and OS) but neutropenic fever was worse in early arm (22% vs. 10%, $p = .002$). **Conclusion: Later RT start may be favorable.**

When combining the preceding trials, is there difference in early versus late administration of thoracic RT?

De Ruysscher, Netherlands Meta-analysis (*Ann Oncol* 2006, PMID 16344277): Meta-analysis of seven trials to determine whether timing of chest RT may influence survival of pts with LS-SCLC. When including all seven trials, 2- and 5-yr OS was not improved between early and late RT. Looking at only trials using concurrent platinum CHT w/ RT, 5-yr OS was significantly improved with early RT, OR 0.64 ($p = .02$). In studies with short RT (<30 days treatment time), 2-yr survival showed no difference, but 5-yr OS better (OR 0.56, SS).

De Ruysscher, RTT-SCLC Collaborative Group (*Ann Oncol* 2016, PMID 27436850): Individual patient level analysis of nine trials comprising 2,305 pts with MFU of 10 years. Authors rationalized this patient level update based on Spiro's combined RCT/meta-analysis, which showed that early delivery of thoracic RT may contribute to improved survival if pts received CHT regimen as prescribed.[37] When all trials were analyzed together, "earlier or shorter" versus "later or longer" thoracic RT did not affect OS. However, when limiting analysis to those who were compliant with planned CHT, benefit to those receiving "earlier or shorter" thoracic RT was observed when contrasted to those who received "later or longer" RT regimens (HR for survival 0.79, 95% CI: 0.69–0.91). That said, grade 3-5 toxicity was greater in "earlier or shorter" group: neutropenia increased from 59% to 69%, $p = .001$, and esophagitis increased from 8 to 14%, $p < .001$. Interestingly, reverse was shown in those unable to remain compliant with their planned CHT regimen (better OS with later/longer: HR 1.19, 95% CI: 1.05–1.34). Authors concluded that "earlier or shorter" delivery of thoracic RT in those who completed planned CHT significantly improves 5-yr OS at cost of increased toxicity.

Does package time for RT completion matter?

Yes, "start of any treatment until end of RT" (SER) <30 days is critical.

De Ruysscher (*JCO* 2006, PMID 16505424): Meta-analysis of four trials (Murray, Jeremic, Turrisi, Takada) to analyze influence of timing of chest RT and on local tumor control, survival and esophagitis. SER was most important predictor of outcome. 5-yr OS improved in shorter (<30 days) versus longer SER arms (RR 0.62, $p = .0003$). Each week extension of SER beyond that of study arm w/ shortest SER resulted in absolute 5-yr OS decrease of 1.83%. Shorter SER also associated with higher incidence of severe esophagitis (RR 0.55, $p < .0001$). SER did not correlate with local control rates.

What is the ideal field size? Should the pre- or post-CHT volume be targeted?

Based on subset randomization performed as part of SWOG 7924, it seems that post-CHT rather than pre-CHT volume leads to equivalent LC and OS.

Kies, SWOG 7924 *(JCO 1987, PMID 3031226)*: PRT of 473 LS-SCLC pts treated with induction CHT (VMV-VAC x 6). 153 pts (33%) who had CR to induction CHT were randomized to receive chest RT 48 Gy split course w/ PCI 30 Gy followed by CHT, versus continuing CHT w/ no chest RT. OS for CR pts did not differ according to whether chest RT was used due to distant relapses. However, patterns of tumor relapse were affected by chest RT, as 38 of 42 relapsing pts who did not receive RT had intrathoracic recurrences, in comparison to 20 of 36 radiated pts. 191 pts with PR/SD to induction CHT were treated with RT, randomized to "large-field" pre-CHT volume versus "small-field" post-CHT volume. There was no significant difference in relapse patterns or OS between large or small RT volumes. Myelosuppression was higher in pts treated with larger field, but there was no difference in radiation pneumonitis.

Should elective nodal volumes be included in the CTV?

In setting of recent imaging advances (both contrast enhanced CT and PET/CT), omission of ENI has led to low rates of isolated nodal failure (<5%) as evidenced by several studies. However, nearly all of trials in SCLC treated both gross and elective volumes; this is in contrast to NSCLC in which treating only PET-positive disease has been adopted as standard. Thus, it is still controversial whether or not only PET-positive disease is covered or if PET-positive disease PLUS ipsilateral hilum (as an elective volume) are both included, though a 2008 report helps provide some clarity.[38] Note that ENI has been omitted in recent prospective trials (both CONVERT and RTOG 0538).

Baas, Netherlands *(BJC 2006, PMID 16465191)*: Phase II study of 38 pts treated with carboplatin, etoposide, and paclitaxel x 4 cycles with concurrent RT 45 Gy/25 fractions, starting cycle #2 for LS-SCLC, treating only involved sites (primary and any involved nodes >1 cm) determined at simulation with IV contrast; PCI given to responders (30 Gy/10 fx). MS 19.5 months. 5-yr OS 27%. Grade 3 esophagitis 27%. Grade 3–4 heme toxicity 57%. In-field LR 16%.

Van Loon, Netherlands *(IJROBP 2010, PMID 19782478)*: Only prospective study to show value of PET for selective nodal irradiation (SNI) in LS-SCLC. 60 pts with LS-SCLC, RT dose 45 Gy/bid with EP. Only PET-avid primary and LN stations irradiated (SNI). PET altered nodal involvement in 30% of pts. Isolated nodal relapse occurred in only 3% (*N* = 2). Acute grade 3 esophagitis occurred in 12% (lower than on Turrisi trial). MS was 19 mos. **Conclusion: PET appears to help in selection of nodal stations for irradiation, which may reduce toxicity and keep regional failures low.**

Colaco, UK *(Lung Cancer 2012, PMID 22014897)*: Evaluated relapse patterns in pts whose CT-based treatment volumes included only primary tumor and involved nodes. All treatment was 3D conformal and PET was not routinely used. 38 pts were recruited and of 31 evaluable following treatment, 14 relapsed but there were no isolated nodal relapses. Authors concluded that omitting ENI based on CT imaging was not associated with high risk of isolated nodal recurrence.

Extensive stage small-cell lung cancer

Should consolidative chest RT be delivered to ES-SCLC pts with response to CHT?

One can consider chest RT in favorable pts who have demonstrated response to CHT.

Jeremic, Yugoslavia *(JCO 1999, PMID 10561263)*: PRT 210 pts w/ ES-SCLC treated w/ EP x 3. Pts w/ CR at distant level and either CR or PR at local level received either (Group 1) hyperfractionated RT to 54 Gy/36 fx over 18 days w/ concurrent carboplatin/etoposide followed by EP x 2 or (Group 2) EP x 4. All pts w/ CR at distant level received PCI (25 Gy/10 fx). RT fields included gross disease and ipsilateral hilum w/ 2 cm margin, mediastinum w/ 1 cm margin, and bilateral SCV. Pts w/ PR at distant level were treated nonrandomly with CHT and/or later HFX chemoRT, and pts w/ progressive disease received supportive care or oral etoposide. Among all pts, MS was 9 mo and 5-yr OS 3.4%. MS and 5-yr OS superior in Group 1: 17 versus 11 mo and 9.1% versus 3.7% (p = .041). LC nonsignificantly better in Group 1 (p = .062). No difference in DM. Acute Gr 3/4 toxicity higher in Group 2. **Conclusion: Addition of hyperfractionated RT for most favorable subset of pts leads to improved OS over CHT alone.**

TABLE 27.7: Results of Jeremic Trial for Consolidative Chest RT in ES-SCLC					
210 ES-SCLC pts treated w/ 3 cycles of EP, 109 pts with CR or PR, all received PCI and randomized to CHT alone vs. chemoRT		5-yr LRFS	5-yr DMFS	MS (mos)	Nausea and Vomiting
	ChemoRT (RT + carboplatin/etoposide CHT; 54 Gy/36 fx BID) + EP x2c	20%	27%	17	4%
	CHT alone (EP x4c)	8.1%	14%	11	20%
		p = .062	p = .35	p = .041	p = .0038

Slotman, Netherlands (*Lancet* 2015, PMID 25230595): Phase III RCT of 498 pts with WHO performance status 0-2 and ES-SCLC who responded to CHT, all of whom received PCI and were then randomized to either thoracic RT (30 Gy/10 fx) or observation. Primary endpoint was 1-yr OS; PFS was secondary endpoint. MFU 24 mos. OS at 1 yr was not significantly different between groups: 33% for thoracic RT arm versus 28% for control group (HR 0.84, p = .066). However, in secondary analysis, 2-yr OS was 13% versus 3% (p = .004). At 6 mos, PFS was 24% in thoracic RT group versus 7% in control group (p = .001). There was no significant difference in toxicity between two groups. **Conclusion: Thoracic RT + PCI should be considered for pts with ES-SCLC who respond to CHT.**

Gore, RTOG 0937 (*J Thorac Oncol* 2017, PMID 28648948): Randomized Phase II of pts with ES-SCLC with one to four extracranial metastases randomized to either PCI alone vs. PCI with consolidative RT given to the intrathoracic disease and extracranial metastases to 45 Gy/15 fx. 97 pts, MFU 9 mos. 1-yr OS was 60.1% (PCI) vs. 50.8% (PCI+consolidation, p = .21). 12-month progression was 79.6% (PCI) vs. 75% (PCI+consolidation), favoring consolidation (HR 0.53, p = .01). **Conclusion: OS analysis was underpowered due to high rate of survival. Consolidation may reduce progression but did not alter OS.**

Prophylactic cranial irradiation

Who should be treated with prophylactic cranial irradiation (PCI)?

Patients with CR or good PR after local chemoRT who have LS-SCLC as per Auperin meta-analysis should receive PCI. Some use findings of Slotman's 2007 study to justify PCI for any responders to CHT in ES-SCLC pts, but this remains controversial.

Auperin, French Meta-analysis (*NEJM* 1999, PMID 10441603): Meta-analysis of 987 pts w/ SCLC in CR from seven RCTs conducted between 1965 and 1995 comparing PCI to no PCI. Note that most pts on this meta-analysis were limited stage but ~15% were extensive stage. PCI was performed in varied doses and fractionations. An analysis of four dose groups was performed: 8 Gy/1 fx versus 24–25 Gy/8–12 fx versus 30 Gy/10 fx versus 36–40 Gy/18–20 fx. PCI improved 3-yr OS and reduced incidence of brain mets (see Table 27.8). Effect of PCI on OS did not differ significantly according to total dose. However, there was a trend toward lower risk of brain mets as RT dose increased. There was also trend toward greater effect of PCI on incidence of brain mets in pts randomized sooner (<6 mos) after CHT.

TABLE 27.8: Results of Auperin Meta-Analysis of PCI

	Incidence of Brain Mets	3-yr OS
PCI	33.3%	20.7%
No PCI	58.6%	15.3%
	$p < .001$	$p = .01$

Slotman, EORTC 08993-22993 (*NEJM* 2007, PMID 17699816): Phase III RCT of PCI in ES-SCLC, including pts aged 18 to 75, PS 0-2, response to CHT, no previous RT, no clinical suggestion of brain mets (imaging not required), N = 286. PCI ranged from 20 to 30 Gy with fractionation that was variable but consistent within an institution. Median interval between diagnosis and randomization was 4.2 mos. Note that primary endpoint was reduction in symptomatic brain metastases. There was no difference in extracranial disease progression between groups. There was no difference in cognitive and emotional function with PCI. **Conclusion: PCI reduces incidence of symptomatic brain metastases and prolongs DFS and OS.** *Comment: Brain imaging was not required prior to randomization.*

TABLE 27.9: Results of Slotman PCI for ES-SCLC

	Symptomatic Brain Mets at 1 yr	Median DFS (weeks)	MS (mos)	1-yr OS
No PCI	40.4%	12	5.4	13.3%
PCI	14.6%	14.7	6.7	27.1%
	$p < .001$	$p = .02$	$p = .03$	$p = .003$

Takahashi, Japanese (*Lancet Oncol* 2017, PMID 28343976): Phase III RCT of PCI in ES-SCLC including pts aged ≥20, PS 0-2, any response to platinum-based doublet CHT and no brain mets on MRI obtained within 4 weeks of PCI randomized to 25 Gy/10 fx versus no PCI. Post-PCI brain MRI was obtained at 3-month intervals up to 12 mos, at 18 mos and at 24 mos. Primary endpoint was OS. The trial was terminated early due to likely futility. **Conclusion: PCI does not improve OS in ES-SCLC in this prescreened population though does reduce the incidence of MRI-detected brain mets at all time points.** *Comment: Close MRI surveillance was performed and should be considered necessary to replicate results if PCI is omitted.*

TABLE 27.10: Results of Takahashi PCI for ES-SCLC

	MS (mos)	Incidence of brain mets at 12 mos	Overall grade 3-4 toxicity
PCI	11.6	32.9%	2.5%
No PCI	13.7	59.0%	4.0%
	$p = .094$	$p < .0001$	NS

What dose of PCI should be delivered?

25 Gy/10 fx is standard. This was investigated in the EORTC/RTOG 0212 prospective randomized trial[39] *composed of three treatment arms: 25 Gy/10 fx, 36 Gy/18 fx QD, and 36 Gy/24 fx BID. Incidence of brain mets at 2 yrs was approximately 25% in all arms with no statistical difference.*[40,41]

REFERENCES

1. Govindan R, Page N, Morgensztern D, et al. Changing epidemiology of small-cell lung cancer in the United States over the last 30 years: analysis of the surveillance, epidemiologic, and end results database. *J Clin Oncol.* 2006;24(28):4539–4544.
2. Siegel RL, Miller KD, Jemal A. Cancer statistics, 2016. *CA Cancer J Clin.* 2016;66(1):7–30.
3. Pesch B, Kendzia B, Gustavsson P, et al. Cigarette smoking and lung cancer: relative risk estimates for the major histological types from a pooled analysis of case-control studies. *Int J Cancer.* 2012;131(5):1210–1219.
4. Kreuzer M, Muller KM, Brachner A, et al. Histopathologic findings of lung carcinoma in German uranium miners. *Cancer.* 2000;89(12):2613–2621.
5. Travis WD, Brambilla E, Noguchi M, et al. International association for the study of lung cancer/American Thoracic Society/European Respiratory Society international multidisciplinary classification of lung adenocarcinoma. *J Thorac Oncol.* 2011;6(2):244–285.
6. NCCN Clinical Practice Guidelines in Oncology: Small-Cell Lung Cancer. 2016. https://www.nccn.org/professionals/physician_gls/pdf/sclc.pdf
7. Travis WD. Advances in neuroendocrine lung tumors. *Ann oncol.* 2010;21(Suppl 7):vii65–vii71.
8. Rivera MP, Mehta AC, Wahidi MM. Establishing the diagnosis of lung cancer: diagnosis and management of lung cancer, 3rd ed: American College of Chest Physicians evidence-based clinical practice guidelines. *Chest.* 2013;143(5, Suppl):e142S–e165S.
9. Nugent JL, Bunn PA Jr, Matthews MJ, et al. CNS metastases in small cell bronchogenic carcinoma: increasing frequency and changing pattern with lengthening survival. *Cancer.* 1979;44(5):1885–1893.
10. Seute T, Leffers P, ten Velde GP, Twijnstra A. Detection of brain metastases from small cell lung cancer: consequences of changing imaging techniques (CT versus MRI). *Cancer.* 2008;112(8):1827–1834.
11. Castillo JJ, Vincent M, Justice E. Diagnosis and management of hyponatremia in cancer patients. *Oncologist.* 2012;17(6):756–765.
12. Videtic GMM, Stitt LW, Dar AR, et al. Continued cigarette smoking by patients receiving concurrent chemoradiotherapy for limited-stage small-cell lung cancer is associated with decreased survival. *J Clin Oncol.* 2003;21(8):1544–1549.
13. Kalemkerian GP. Staging and imaging of small cell lung cancer. *Cancer Imaging.* 2012;11: 253–258.
14. Foster NR, Mandrekar SJ, Schild SE, et al. Prognostic factors differ by tumor stage for small cell lung cancer: a pooled analysis of North Central Cancer Treatment Group trials. *Cancer.* 2009;115(12):2721–2731.
15. Albain KS, Crowley JJ, LeBlanc M, Livingston RB. Determinants of improved outcome in small-cell lung cancer: an analysis of the 2,580-patient Southwest Oncology Group data base. *J Clin Oncol.* 1990;8(9):1563–1574.
16. Hermes A, Waschki B, Reck M. Hyponatremia as prognostic factor in small cell lung cancer: a retrospective single institution analysis. *Respir Med.* 2012;106(6):900–904.
17. Lassen UN, Osterlind K, Hirsch FR, et al. Early death during chemotherapy in patients with small-cell lung cancer: derivation of a prognostic index for toxic death and progression. *Br J Cancer.* 1999;79(3-4):515-519.
18. Fearon K, Strasser F, Anker SD, et al. Definition and classification of cancer cachexia: an international consensus. *Lancet Oncol.* 2011;12(5):489–495.
19. The Diagnosis and Treatment of Lung Cancer (Update). Cardiff (UK). National Collaborating Centre for Cancer. NICE Clinical Guidelines NC, Treatment of SCLC. http://www.ncbi.nlm.nih.gov/books/NBK99023
20. Kalemkerian GP, Gadgeel SM. Modern staging of small cell lung cancer. *JNCCN.* 2013;11(1): 99–104.
21. Fox W, Scadding JG. Medical Research Council comparative trial of surgery and radiotherapy for primary treatment of small-celled or oat-celled carcinoma of bronchus: ten-year follow-up. *Lancet.* 1973;2(7820):63–65.
22. Stahl JM, Corso CD, Verma V, et al. Trends in stereotactic body radiation therapy for stage I small cell lung cancer. *Lung Cancer.* 2017;103:11–16.

23. Roth BJ, Johnson DH, Einhorn LH, et al. Randomized study of cyclophosphamide, doxorubicin, and vincristine versus etoposide and cisplatin versus alternation of these two regimens in extensive small-cell lung cancer: a Phase III trial of the Southeastern Cancer Study Group. *J Clin Oncol.* 1992;10(2):282-291.

24. Sundstrom S, Bremnes RM, Kaasa S, et al. Cisplatin and etoposide regimen is superior to cyclophosphamide, epirubicin, and vincristine regimen in small-cell lung cancer: results from a randomized phase III trial with 5 years' follow-up. *J Clin Oncol.* 2002;20(24):4665-4672.

25. Noda K, Nishiwaki Y, Kawahara M, et al. Irinotecan plus cisplatin compared with etoposide plus cisplatin for extensive small-cell lung cancer. *N Engl J Med.* 2002;346(2):85-91.

26. Lara PN Jr, Natale R, Crowley J, et al. Phase III trial of irinotecan/cisplatin compared with etoposide/cisplatin in extensive-stage small-cell lung cancer: clinical and pharmacogenomic results from SWOG S0124. *J Clin Oncol.* 2009;27(15):2530-2535.

27. Rossi A, Di Maio M, Chiodini P, et al. Carboplatin- or cisplatin-based chemotherapy in first-line treatment of small-cell lung cancer: the COCIS meta-analysis of individual patient data. *J Clin Oncol.* 2012;30(14):1692-1698.

28. Verma V, Simone CB 2nd, Allen PK, et al. Multi-Institutional experience of stereotactic ablative radiation therapy for stage I small cell lung cancer. *Int J Radiat Oncol Biol Phys.* 2017;97(2):362-371.

29. Turrisi AT 3rd, Kim K, Blum R, et al. Twice-daily compared with once-daily thoracic radiotherapy in limited small-cell lung cancer treated concurrently with cisplatin and etoposide. *N Engl J Med.* 1999;340(4):265-271.

30. Murray N, Coy P, Pater JL, et al. Importance of timing for thoracic irradiation in the combined modality treatment of limited-stage small-cell lung cancer. The National Cancer Institute of Canada Clinical Trials Group. *J Clin Oncol.* 1993;11(2):336-344.

31. Movsas B, Moughan J, Komaki R, et al. Radiotherapy patterns of care study in lung carcinoma. *J Clin Oncol.* 2003;21(24):4553-4559.

32. Perry MC, Eaton WL, Propert KJ, et al. Chemotherapy with or without radiation therapy in limited small-cell carcinoma of the lung. *N Engl J Med.* 1987;316(15):912-918.

33. Bunn PA Jr, Lichter AS, Makuch RW, et al. Chemotherapy alone or chemotherapy with chest radiation therapy in limited stage small cell lung cancer: a prospective, randomized trial. *Ann Intern Med.* 1987;106(5):655-662.

34. Turrisi AT 3rd, Glover DJ, Mason BA. A preliminary report: concurrent twice-daily radiotherapy plus platinum-etoposide chemotherapy for limited small cell lung cancer. *Int J Radiat Oncol Biol Phys.* 1988;15(1):183-187.

35. De Ruysscher D, Pijls-Johannesma M, Vansteenkiste J, et al. Systematic review and meta-analysis of randomised, controlled trials of the timing of chest radiotherapy in patients with limited-stage, small-cell lung cancer. *Ann Oncol.* 2006;17(4):543-552.

36. Fukuoka M, Furuse K, Saijo N, et al. Randomized trial of cyclophosphamide, doxorubicin, and vincristine versus cisplatin and etoposide versus alternation of these regimens in small-cell lung cancer. *J Natl Cancer Inst.* 1991;83(12):855-861.

37. Spiro SG, James LE, Rudd RM, et al. Early compared with late radiotherapy in combined modality treatment for limited disease small-cell lung cancer: a London Lung Cancer Group multicenter randomized clinical trial and meta-analysis. *J Clin Oncol.* 2006;24(24):3823-3830.

38. Videtic GMM, Belderbos JS, Spring Kong FM, et al. Report from the International Atomic Energy Agency (IAEA) consultants' meeting on elective nodal irradiation in lung cancer: small-cell lung cancer (SCLC). *Int J Radiat Oncol Biol Phys.* 2008;72(2):327-334.

39. Le Pechoux C, Dunant A, Senan S, et al. Standard-dose versus higher-dose prophylactic cranial irradiation (PCI) in patients with limited-stage small-cell lung cancer in complete remission after chemotherapy and thoracic radiotherapy (PCI 99-01, EORTC 22003-08004, RTOG 0212, and IFCT 99-01): a randomised clinical trial. *Lancet Oncol.* 2009;10(5):467-474.

40. Le Pechoux C, Laplanche A, Faivre-Finn C, et al. Clinical neurological outcome and quality of life among patients with limited small-cell cancer treated with two different doses of prophylactic cranial irradiation in the intergroup phase III trial (PCI99-01, EORTC 22003-08004, RTOG 0212 and IFCT 99-01). *Ann Oncol.* 2011;22(5):1154-1163.

41. Wolfson AH, Bae K, Komaki R, et al. Primary analysis of a phase II randomized trial radiation therapy oncology group (RTOG) 0212: impact of different total doses and schedules of prophylactic cranial irradiation on chronic neurotoxicity and quality of life for patients with limited-disease small-cell lung cancer. *Int J Radiat Oncol Biol Phys.* 2011;81(1):77-84.

28: MESOTHELIOMA

Gregory M. M. Videtic and Bindu V. Manyam

QUICK HIT: Mesothelioma is a rare thoracic malignancy associated with progressive morbidity. Pts are rarely curable due to disease extent and comorbidity at diagnosis. Extrapleural pneumonectomy (EPP) or pleurectomy/decortication (P/D) is a surgical option for nonmetastatic, medically operable pts with epithelioid histology. CHT and RT are used mainly for palliation but when indicated, are considered in the perioperative setting with surgery.

TABLE 28.1: General Treatment Paradigm for Mesothelioma[1]	
Patient	Treatment Options
Clinical stage I–III Epithelial or biphasic histology Medically operable Resectable disease	• Induction CHT (cisplatin/pemetrexed), reassessment, P/D followed by observation • Induction CHT (cisplatin/pemetrexed), reassessment, EPP followed by hemithoracic RT (54 Gy) • EPP, sequential adjuvant CHT, hemithoracic RT (54 Gy) • P/D, CHT +/− IMRT consolidation
Clinical stage IV Sarcomatoid histology Medically inoperable Unresectable	• CHT and palliative RT

EPIDEMIOLOGY: U.S. incidence of mesothelioma is 3,000 cases per yr. Incidence peaked around 2000 and has been steadily declining secondary to OSHA limitations on acceptable asbestos exposure initiated in 1970s.[2]

RISK FACTORS: Exposure to asbestos is the most significant risk factor, with 90% of cases related to asbestos. Exposure can be occupational, most commonly (used as flame retardant in automobile brakes, shipbuilding, ceiling tiles, pool tiles), and more rarely, environmental. Also, occult transmission of asbestos fibers from workers to family members. Lifetime risk of an asbestos worker developing mesothelioma is as high as 10%. Dose–response relationship and latency period of 20 to 40 yrs exist between exposure and development of disease. Synergistic effect of asbestos and smoking known. Other risk factors include ionizing RT, carbon nanotubes, and potentially viral oncogenes and genetic susceptibility (BAP1 mutation).[2]

ANATOMY: Can arise from any mesothelial surface, including pleura (80%), and less commonly peritoneum, tunic vaginalis, or pericardium. Two areas of pleura particularly challenging to identify and adequately cover after EPP include ipsilateral diaphragmatic crura and lowest posterior point of diaphragm. Right crus extends to L3 and left crus extends to L2. Lowest point of pleural space can extend as low at L4. Distribution of pleural mesothelioma: 60% right-sided, 35% left-sided, 5% bilateral.[3]

PATHOLOGY: Three histologic variants: **epithelioid** (most common, 60% of cases), **sarcomatoid**, **biphasic** (combination of latter two), though several variations exist. Histology more prognostic than stage. Immunohistochemistry is crucial for diagnosis (mesothelin glycoprotein is 67% sensitive and 98% specific); osteopontin and gene expression assays may be helpful.[2]

SCREENING: There is no clearly advocated screening strategy for mesothelioma.

CLINICAL PRESENTATION: Majority of pts affected are aged 60 or higher and present 20 to 40 yrs after exposure to asbestos. Symptoms include weight loss, fatigue, chest pain, dyspnea, cough, hoarseness, and dysphagia. Physical exam findings are usually indicative of pleural effusion with unilateral dullness to percussion or decreased air exchange. Can present as incidental unilateral pleural effusion on CXR. Features on CXR suggestive of mesothelioma include unilateral pleural density or thickening, persistent pleural effusion, mediastinal shift, lung volume loss, asbestosis demonstrated as bibasilar interstitial fibrosis, and warrant further workup.

WORKUP: H&P with risk-factor assessment.

Labs: Assess operability with PFTs with DLCO, perfusion scanning (if FEV1 <80%), cardiac stress test.[4]

Imaging: CT chest with contrast necessary. PET/CT. MRI chest is optional, but may be helpful in determining resectability.

Pathology: Historically, thoracentesis used for histologic diagnosis, though only diagnostic in 26% of cases. In contrast, VATS biopsy diagnostic in 98% and provides evidence of stromal, fibroadipose or lung parenchymal invasion needed to differentiate between reactive hyperplasia, fibrous pleurisy, and malignancy. 10% risk of seeding biopsy tract, and tract should be excised at surgery. For pts who are potentially resectable, mediastinal staging with mediastinoscopy or EBUS.

PROGNOSTIC FACTORS: Stage and histology are most significant prognostic factors. Sarcomatoid and biphasic histologies have worse prognosis compared to epithelioid histology. Poor performance status, age >75, elevated LDH, and hematologic abnormalities (thrombocytosis, leukocytosis, anemia) are associated with worse prognosis.[4]

NATURAL HISTORY: Prognosis is poor, with OS 9 to 17 mos. Distant metastatic disease is less common, most common involves bone, liver, CNS. Most pts succumb to local progression of disease (painful) and respiratory failure, arrhythmia, heart failure, stroke.

STAGING

TABLE 28.2: AJCC 8th ed. (2017) Staging for Malignant Pleural Mesothelioma				
T/M	N	cN0	cN1	cN2
T1	• Ipsilateral parietal pleura with extension to visceral, mediastinal, or diaphragmatic pleura	IA		

T2	• Involving all ipsilateral pleural surfaces (parietal, mediastinal, diaphragmatic, and visceral) with at least of the following:
	  o Diaphragmatic muscle
	  o Underlying pulmonary parenchyma
		IB	II	

T3	• Involving all ipsilateral pleural surfaces with involvement of at least one of the following:
	  o Endothoracic fascia
	  o Mediastinal fat
	  o Solitary, resectable focus of tumor extending into chest wall soft tissue
	  o Nontransmural pericardium
			IIIA	

(continued)

TABLE 28.2: AJCC 8th ed. (2017) Staging for Malignant Pleural Mesothelioma (*continued*)				
T/M	N	cN0	cN1	cN2
T4	• Involving all ipsilateral pleural surfaces with involvement of at least one of the following: o Multifocal chest wall mass o Transdiaphragmatic extension to peritoneum o Direct extension to contralateral pleura o Direct extension to mediastinal organs o Direct extension into spine o Direct extension to inner surface of pericardium o Direct extension to myocardium	IIIB		
M1	• Distant metastasis	IV		

Significant changes from the AJCC 7th Edition: T1 and T1b in 7th edition were combined to become T1 in 8th edition. 7th edition N1 and N2 were combined into N1 in 8th edition. N3 in 7th edition was reassigned as N2 in 8th edition. Prognostic stage groups altered slightly.

cN1, ipsilateral bronchopulmonary, hilar, mediastinal (including internal mammary, peridiaphragmatic, pericardial fat pad, or intercostal) LNs; cN2, contralateral mediastinal or any supraclavicular LNs.

TREATMENT PARADIGM

Surgery: Radical surgery should be limited to carefully selected pts, as it is associated with significant morbidity and mortality (early series demonstrate 31% mortality with EPP). Surgical candidates are those pts who have resectable disease, limited to one hemithorax (clinical stage I-III), no metastatic disease, adequate cardiopulmonary function, and ECOG PS <2. Nearly all surgical series demonstrate survival benefit to surgery when limited to pure epithelial subtype alone. Pts with biphasic or sarcomatoid subtypes often have OS similar to or shorter than expected with nonoperative management.

Definitive surgical procedures include EPP or P/D. P/D provides opportunity to preserve lung parenchyma. Decision is based on surgeon's judgment on obtaining R0 resection. RRs suggest P/D may have less mortality and morbidity compared to EPP, with comparable OS. See Flores data in the following regarding outcomes for EPP versus P/D.

- EPP is an en bloc resection of parietal and visceral pleura, ipsilateral lung, pericardium, and diaphragm. If there is no involvement of pericardium or diaphragm, these structures can remain intact.
- Extended P/D is parietal and visceral pleurectomy, with removal of all gross tumor and resection of diaphragm and pericardium.
- P/D is parietal and visceral pleurectomy with removal of all gross tumor, without diaphragm and pericardial resection.

Pleurodesis is a surgical option used to palliate symptoms from pleural effusion, involves obliteration of pleural space through injection of sterile, asbestos-free talc to cause adhesion of visceral and parietal pleura. Complete drainage of pleural effusion by tube thoracostomy or video thoracoscopy usually precedes this procedure.

Chemotherapy: Roles exist for CHT in neoadjuvant, adjuvant, and palliative settings. Cisplatin and pemetrexed demonstrate prolonged OS in pts with unresectable disease. A phase II multicenter study by Krug used neoadjuvant pemetrexed and cisplatin for four cycles, followed by EPP in those pts who did not have disease progression, followed by adjuvant RT (54 Gy) and demonstrated an MS of 16.8 mos.[5] Those pts who were able to complete all therapy had MS of 29.1 mos. Alternative CHT regimens include cisplatin + gemcitabine and carboplatin + pemetrexed.

Radiation

Indications: RT has two main roles: adjuvant after EPP and palliative.

Dose: For EPP, dose for negative margins is 50 to 54 Gy and for positive margins boost of 54 to 60 Gy. See the following for data regarding benefit of RT therapy after EPP.

Toxicity: Fatigue, esophagitis, pneumonitis (caution with contralateral lung in postpneumonectomy pts).[6]

EVIDENCE-BASED Q&A

What is the benefit of EPP?

Local control is the main goal of EPP. There is high rate of mortality with EPP; however, with careful selection of pts, there may be survival benefit.

Treasure, MARS Study (*Lancet Oncol* 2011, PMID 21723781): PRT of 50 pts from 12 UK hospitals who received neoadjuvant CHT, randomized to EPP or no EPP, followed by RT. Of 24 pts randomized to EPP, 16 underwent EPP. 30-day mortality rate was 12.5%. HR for OS with EPP was 1.90 ($p = .082$). After adjustment for sex, histological subtype, stage, and age, HR for EPP was 2.75 ($p = .016$). **Conclusion: Despite study deficiencies EPP did worse in OS than no EPP suggesting importance of choosing EPP candidates very carefully.**

What are outcomes of EPP compared to P/D?

Data is conflicting, with some showing improved LC and OS with EPP, while others demonstrating improved outcomes with P/D. EPP shown to have higher perioperative morbidity and mortality.

Flores, MSKCC (*J Thorac Cardiovasc Surg* 2008, PMID 18329481): RR of 663 pts from three institutions treated between 1990 and 2006 with EPP or P/D. EPP had perioperative mortality rate of 7% versus P/D with perioperative mortality rate of 4%. Stage ($p < .001$), epithelioid histology ($p < .001$), EPP ($p < .001$), multimodality therapy ($p < .001$) were all significantly associated with improved survival. Multivariate analysis demonstrated hazard ratio of 1.4 for extrapleural pneumonectomy ($p < .001$) controlling for stage, histology, gender, and multimodality therapy.

Lang-Lazdunski, UK (*J Thorac Oncol* 2012, PMID 22425923): Nonrandomized prospective study of 22 pts who underwent neoadjuvant CHT, EPP, adjuvant RT and 54 pts who underwent neoadjuvant CHT, P/D, RT, and adjuvant CHT. 30-day mortality rate was 4.5% in EPP and 0% for P/D. Complications observed in 68% in EPP and 27.7% in P/D. Trimodality therapy completed by 68% in EPP and 100% in P/D. Survival was significantly better in P/D compared to EPP (2-yr OS 49% vs. 18.2%) and (5-yr OS 30.1% vs. 9%; $p = .004$). Epithelioid histology, P/D, and R0 resection all associated with improved survival on MVA.

Is trimodality therapy safe and effective? Which pts are best candidates?

Trimodality therapy is generally safe and effective in very carefully selected pts. Epithelioid histology, R0 resection, and N0 pts have been shown to have 5-yr OS as high as 50% with trimodality therapy.

Sugarbaker (*J Thorac Cardiovasc Surg* 1999, PMID 9869758): RR of 183 pts treated with EPP followed by adjuvant CHT and RT therapy. MFU 13 mos. Perioperative mortality rate 3.8% at 2 yrs with 50% morbidity. Survival was 37% at 1 yr and 15% at 5 years. MS was 19 mos. Three variables significantly associated with improved survival: (a). **Epithelial** type

(52% 2-yr OS, 21% 5-yr OS, 26-mo MS); (b) **negative resection margins** (44% 2-yr OS, 25% 5-yr OS, 23 MS); (c) EPP **negative lymph nodes** (42% 2-yr OS, 17% 5-yr OS). Pts with all three variables had 62% 2-yr OS, 46% 5-yr OS, MS 51 mos. **Conclusion: Trimodality therapy is feasible. Mediastinal lymph node evaluation is important in selecting optimal pts for trimodality therapy. Epithelioid type, R0 resection, and extrapleural node-negative pts have extended survival.**

Pagan (*J Thorac Cardiovasc Surg* **2006, PMID 17033611**): Prospective nonrandomized trial 32/44 pts who underwent EPP followed by carboplatin/paclitaxel and RT (50 Gy). 30-day mortality rate was 4.5% and overall complication rate was 50%. No major complications observed. MS was 20 mos and 5-yr OS 19%. Pts with epithelioid histology, R0 resection, and N0-1 had 5-yr OS 50%.

What is the benefit of postoperative RT therapy after EPP?

Local recurrence rates following EPP are reported as high as 80%. Addition of postoperative RT has been shown to decrease locoregional failure rates to 37%.

Rusch (*J Thorac Cardiovasc Surgery* **2001, PMID 11581615**): Phase II trial of 88 pts who underwent EPP or P/D followed by postoperative hemithoracic RT (54 Gy/30 fx) in 55 pts. RT was AP/PA with photons and electron boost to areas requiring shielding. Locoregional failure in 7/55 (12.7%), grade 4 pneumonitis in 9.1%. MS was 33.8 mos for stage I and II, 10 mos for stage III and IV tumors (*p* =.04).

Is there a role for postoperative RT after P/D?

There are series evaluating its use; however, this is not routinely recommended.

Gupta (*IJROBP* **2005, PMID 16054774**): RR of 123 pts who underwent P/D followed by RT (54 underwent intraoperative brachytherapy through LDR, HDR, or P32 solution to gross residual tumor), followed by hemithoracic RT (mean dose 42.5 Gy). MS 13.3 mos, 23% 2-yr OS, 5% 5-yr OS. Pts receiving brachytherapy had worse survival (11 vs. 18 mos). **1-yr LC was 42%, described as better than historical data for pts treated with P/D alone.**

Lee (*J Thorac Cardiovasc Surg* **2002, PMID 12447185**): RR of 26 pts with diffuse MPM received P/D with median 15 Gy IORT (24/26 pts) and/or median 41.4 Gy EBRT following surgery (24/26 pts), 12 received CHT; PFS 1 yr: 50%, most failed along resected pleura; pneumonitis in 4/24 (17%).

What is role and safety of IMRT after EPP?

With appropriate mean lung dose constraint for residual lung, IMRT can be safely employed post-EPP.

Allen (*IJROBP* **2006, PMID 16751058**): RR of 13 pts treated with hemithoracic IMRT (54 Gy/30 fx) after EPP and adjuvant CHT with cisplatin or cisplatin/pemetrexed. Fatal pneumonitis rate was 46%. Pts with fatal pneumonitis had V20 15.3% to 22.4%, V5 81% to 100%, and mean lung dose 13.3 Gy to 17 Gy.

Rice (*Ann Thorac Surg* **2007, PMID 17954086**): RR of 63 pts who underwent EPP followed by IMRT (45 Gy), CHT not routinely administered. Nonepithelioid histology represented 33% of pts, Stage III 72%, and ipsilateral nodal metastases in 54%. Perioperative mortality was 8%. MS was 14.2 mos for pts who received IMRT and 10.2 mos for pts who received 3DCRT. Node-negative pts with epithelioid histology had median survival 28 mos. Locoregional recurrence was 13% and only 5% had in-field recurrence. **Rate of fatal lung events was 9.5% and V20 predicted for pulmonary related death on MVA.**

What is role and safety of IMRT after P/D?

There are series evaluating its use; however, it remains investigational and likely best suited to centers with expertise.

Chance (*IJROPB* 2015, PMID 25442335): Matched pair analysis of 24 pts who underwent PD followed by adjuvant CHT and hemithoracic IMRT to dose of 45 Gy. Outcomes were compared to 24 pts who received EPP followed by IMRT, matched for age, nodal status, performance status, and CHT. MFU 12.2 mos. There was statistically significant decrease in FVC, FEV1, and DLCO between after P/D and after IMRT. MS was 28.4 versus 14.2 mos (*p* = .04) and median PFS was 16.4 versus 8.2 mos (*p* = .01) for PD/IMRT versus EPP/IMRT, respectively. There was no significant difference in grade 4–5 toxicity between two groups (0% vs. 12.5%; *p* = .23) for PD/IMRT versus EPP/IMRT.

Rimner, IMPRINT Trial (*JCO* 2016, PMID 27325859): Phase II study of 27 pts who received neoadjuvant platinum CHT and pemetrexed, P/D, followed by adjuvant hemithoracic IMRT (median dose 46.8 Gy). MFU 21.6 mos. Grade 2 pneumonitis was 22% and grade 3 pneumonitis was 7.4% and all resolved with steroids. Median PFS and OS were 12.4 mos and 23.7 mos, respectively. Two-yr OS was 59%.

Which CHT regimens are most effective?

Platinum doublet CHT has been shown to have superior outcomes compared to platinum alone in palliative setting. Good outcomes have been demonstrated with platinum doublet-based CHT in neoadjuvant setting as well. Addition of bevacizumab in palliative setting to platinum doublet suggested survival benefit.

Vogelzang, EMPHACIS Trial (*JCO* 2003, PMID 12860938): Single-blinded PRT of 456 pts not eligible for surgical resection, randomized to cisplatin only versus cisplatin and pemetrexed every 21 days. **MS was 12.1 versus 9.3 mos (*p* = .02) for cisplatin/pemetrexed versus cisplatin, respectively.** Median time to progression was significantly longer in cisplatin/pemetrexed arm (5.7 vs. 3.9 mos; *p* = .001) and response rates were significantly better with cisplatin/pemetrexed (41.3% vs. 16.7%; *p* < .0001). Folic acid and vitamin B12 were added after 117 pts, resulting in significant reduction in toxicities in cisplatin/pemetrexed arm.

Krug (*JCO* 2009, PMID 19364962): Phase II multicenter trial of 75 pts who received neoadjuvant cisplatin + pemetrexed, 50 received EPP, and 28 received adjuvant RT. Pts who had radiographic response to CHT had trend toward better OS (29.1 vs. 13.9 mos, *p* = .07). MS was 16.6 mos for whole cohort and median PFS was 13.1 mos.

Zelman (*Lancet* 2016, PMID 26719230): PRT of 448 pts with unresectable disease randomized to cisplatin/pemetrexed +/− bevacizumab in 21-day cycles for up to six cycles. **OS was significantly longer with addition of bevacizumab (18.8 vs. 16.1 mos; *p* = .0167).** There was more grade 3 hypertension and thrombotic events (23% vs. 0%) and (6% vs. 1%), with cisplatin/pemetrexed/bevacizumab compared to cisplatin/pemetrexed, respectively.

If biopsy tract is not surgically excised, can prophylactic RT reduce chance of tract recurrence?

Currently, the role of tract RT remains depending on the clinical setting and primary form of treatment.

Bydder (*Br J Cancer* 2004, PMID 15199394): PRT of 28 pts randomized to 10 Gy/1 fx with electrons following chest wall violation observation. **Tract metastasis was not significantly different (10% vs. 7%; *p* = .53) for RT and observation, respectively.** Freedom from tract metastasis survival was not significantly different as well (*p* = .82). Crude rates of tract metastases were 22% for Abrams needles, 9% for thoracic drains, and 4% for FNA, and these were not statistically significantly different (p = .23).

O'Rourke (*Radiother Oncol* 2007, PMID 17588698): PRT of 61 pts who underwent chest drain placement or pleural biopsy randomized to 21 Gy/3 fx after procedure versus observation. There were four drain site metastases in RT arm and three in observation arm. **Conclusion: There was no significant difference between rate of tract metastases associated with drain site (p = .75).**

Clive, SMART Trial (*Lancet Oncol* 2016, PMID 27345639): PRT of 203 pts from 22 UK hospitals who underwent large-bore pleural intervention were randomized to prophylactic RT (21 Gy/3 fx within 42 days of pleural intervention) versus deferred RT (21 Gy/3 fx upon procedure tract metastasis). Primary outcome was incidence of procedure tract metastasis within 7 cm of site of pleural intervention within 12 mos of randomization. **Conclusion: There was no significant difference in procedure tract metastasis between immediate and deferred RT (9% vs. 16%; p = .14).**

Is there benefit to dose-escalated RT in mesothelioma?

No evidence at this time to increase dose beyond 54 Gy in the adjuvant setting.

Allen (*IJROBP* 2007, PMID 17674974): RR of 39 pts treated with hemithoracic RT after EPP, with 24 treated to doses of 30 to 40 Gy and 15 treated with 54 Gy. Local failure was higher with lower doses of RT (50% vs. 27%), but was not statistically significant. There was no significant difference in OS.

Is RT useful for treating pain in mesothelioma?

Evidence supports palliative benefit of RT in MPM, with duration of sx control possibly function of dose.

McLeod (*J Thorac Oncol* 2015, PMID 25654216): Phase II, 40 pts, with assessments of pain and other symptoms at baseline, then received 20 Gy/5 fx to areas of pain. Primary end point measure was assessment of pain at the site of RT at 5 weeks. **Forty-seven percent of pts alive at week 5 had an improvement in their pain.**

de Graaf-Strukowska (*IJROBP* 1999, PMID 10078630): RR of 189 pts, higher local response rate for pts treated with 4 Gy per fx compared with less than 4 Gy per fx (50% vs. 39%). Duration of response was short, with pain recurring predominantly in the RT field after a median of 69 days (range 32–363).

REFERENCES

1. NCCN Clinical Practice Guidelines in Oncology: Malignant Pleural Mesothelioma. https://www.nccn.org/professionals/physician_gls/pdf/mpm.pdf. Published 2017.
2. Ai J, Stevenson JP. Current issues in malignant pleural mesothelioma evaluation and management. *Oncologist*. 2014;19(9):975–984.
3. Rosenzweig KE, Giraud P. Radiation therapy for malignant pleural mesothelioma. *Cancer Radiother*. 2017;21(1):73–76.
4. Patel SC, Dowell JE. Modern management of malignant pleural mesothelioma. *Lung Cancer (Auckl)*. 2016;7:63–72.
5. Krug LM, Pass HI, Rusch VW, et al. Multicenter phase II trial of neoadjuvant pemetrexed plus cisplatin followed by extrapleural pneumonectomy and radiation for malignant pleural mesothelioma. *J Clin Oncol*. 2009;27(18):3007–3013.
6. Allen AM, Czerminska M, Jänne PA, et al. Fatal pneumonitis associated with intensity-modulated radiation therapy for mesothelioma. *Int J Radiat Oncol Biol Phys*. 2006;65(3):640–645.

29: THYMOMA

Jonathan Sharrett and Gregory M. M. Videtic

QUICK HIT: Rare tumor of anterior mediastinum, for which surgery is primary management. Postoperative RT is indicated for stage III (locally advanced) disease, CHT is usually employed for potentially resectable tumors to facilitate surgery. Metastatic thymoma may have very long natural history, systemic therapy has limited benefits, "aggressive" local therapies (surgery, RT) may be appropriate as indicated by patient and tumor presentations.

TABLE 29.1: General Treatment Paradigm for Thymoma

Thymic neoplasm suspected and resection possible?	Yes, proceed to total thymectomy (biopsy may be omitted)	Stage I	No adjuvant RT
		Stage II, R0 Resection	No adjuvant RT (recently controversial)
		R1 resection or stage III–IVa	PORT 45–50 Gy (negative/close margins), 54 Gy (microscopic margins)
		R2 Resection	PORT±CHT (role of CHT in thymoma and thymic carcinoma controversial)
	No (locally advanced, solitary/ potentially resectable metastases)	Core needle biopsy followed by induction CHT	Individualized by disease burden/ pt status, including CHT +/– local therapy (surgery/RT) as indicated

EPIDEMIOLOGY: 1.5 cases per million person-years in the United States. Thymoma typically occurs in adults aged 40 to 60, slight male predominance. Comprises around 20% of all mediastinal tumors but half of all anterior mediastinal tumors. Incidence of thymic carcinoma is less than 1% of thymic tumors, is very aggressive, and carries worse survival with 5-yr OS in recent analyses around 60%.[1]

RISK FACTORS: No known etiologic factors. Up to 50% of pts with thymoma will present with myasthenia gravis (MG); it is less common for MG pts to acquire thymoma. Other less common disorders include other paraneoplastic syndromes (i.e., red cell aplasia, immune deficiency syndromes, and autoimmune disorders), and other malignancies (i.e., lymphomas, Kaposi sarcoma, GI/breast carcinoma).

ANATOMY: Thymus is an anterior mediastinal structure, with lymphatic drainage to lower cervical, internal mammary, and hilar nodes. Structurally, thymus consists of capsule, cortex, and medulla. Histologically, it includes epithelial cells, epithelioreticular cells (form Hassall's corpuscles), myoid cells, lymphocytes ("thymocytes"), and B-lymphocytes.

PATHOLOGY

TABLE 29.2: WHO Thymoma Grading

WHO Type[2,3]	Histology
A	Medullary thymoma

(continued)

TABLE 29.2: WHO Thymoma Grading (*continued*)	
AB	Mixed thymoma
B1	Predominantly cortical thymoma
B2	Cortical thymoma
B3	Well-differentiated thymic carcinoma
C	Thymic carcinoma

CLINICAL PRESENTATION: Often incidental finding on imaging. Local symptoms often based on mass effect and include chest pain, dyspnea, cough, phrenic nerve palsy, and potentially SVC syndrome. Paraneoplastic syndromes may be present with their associated side effects and myasthenia gravis is most common.

WORKUP: H&P.

Labs: Serum β-hCG and AFP (rule out germ cell tumor), CBC, CMP, serum level of anti-ACh antibodies to assess for MG.

Imaging: Chest CT with contrast, PET/CT (optional), PFTs.

Pathology: If thymoma suspected and considered resectable, biopsy may be omitted and resection performed. If unresectable/medically inoperable, obtain core needle biopsy to confirm diagnosis (open biopsy also possible; biopsy should not violate pleural space); multidisciplinary evaluation indicated.

PROGNOSTIC FACTORS: Masaoka stage, histology, degree of resection (R0, R1 vs. R2).[4]

NATURAL HISTORY: Indolent but locally aggressive with long natural history based on staging and malignant phenotypes/growth rate, even in setting of metastases.

STAGING: Koga Modification of Masaoka Staging System, surgically based. TNM staging system not commonly used and not officially adopted.

TABLE 29.3: Masaoka–Koga Staging System for Thymoma[5]	
Stage	**Definition**
I	Grossly and microscopically completely encapsulated tumor
IIa	Microscopic transcapsular invasion
IIb	Macroscopic invasion into surrounding fatty tissue or grossly adherent to but not breaking through mediastinal pleura or pericardium
III	Macroscopic invasion into neighboring organ (i.e., pericardium, great vessels or lung)
IVA	Pleural or pericardial involvement
IVB	Distant metastasis

TREATMENT PARADIGM

Surgery: Total thymectomy with negative margins is mainstay of therapy in resectable cases. This is typically performed with median sternotomy, albeit partial or total pneumonectomy or pericardiectomy may be required. Resection of both phrenic nerves should be avoided to prevent severe respiratory compromise. Signs and symptoms of MG should be controlled medically with anticholinesterase inhibitors prior to surgery.

Chemotherapy: Platinum-based CHT is indicated for thymic carcinoma, unresectable disease, medically inoperable with gross disease. CHT is often used for downstaging and postoperatively based on degree of resection. For diffuse metastases, consider CHT alone.

No randomized trials have identified superior regimen. Common regimens include cisplatin/adriamycin/cyclophosphamide, cisplatin/etoposide or carboplatin/paclitaxel (thymic carcinoma).

Radiation

Indications: Postoperative RT (PORT) should be offered for positive surgical margins, stage III disease and considered for any thymic carcinoma.

Dose: RT dosing is based on degree of resection with 45 to 54 Gy, 55 to 60 Gy, and 60 to 70 Gy given for R0, R1, and R2, respectively. Definitive RT indicated for medically inoperable disease, with the addition of CHT and its sequencing empiric.

Toxicity

Acute: Fatigue, cough, skin erythema. Late: Cardiac morbidity, hypothyroidism, second malignancy.

EVIDENCE-BASED Q&A

Resectable thymoma

What are outcomes for completely resected thymoma by stage and when should PORT be considered?

Surgery is the mainstay of therapy for operable pts with locoregional disease, with excellent LC and survival for R0 resections. The role of PORT has become controversial recently. Conventionally, stage III/IVA disease has been generally managed by surgery followed by the addition of PORT, independent of margins. Large RRs from Japan had however suggested no benefit to PORT if R0 resection in any stage. PORT remains always indicated for residual disease, if repeat resection not feasible. In 2008 Wright et al.[6] recommended PORT for stage II/III positive or close margin (<1 mm), gross fibrous adhesion to pleura or WHO high grade (B3), but otherwise no PORT for R0 resected thymoma. A recent publication in 2016 by Rimner et al. suggests an OS benefit with the use of PORT in completely resected stage II and III thymoma. At present, PORT for stage III would be generally recommended.

Kondo, Japan (*Ann Thorac Surg* 2003, PMID 12963221): RR of 1,320 pts with thymic epithelial tumors from 115 special thoracic surgery institutes across Japan. Pts with stage I thymoma received surgery alone and pts with stage II and III thymoma and thymic carcinoid underwent surgery + PORT. Pts with stage IV thymoma and thymic carcinoma were treated with RT or CHT. In stage III and IV thymoma, 5-yr survival rates of total resection, subtotal resection, and inoperable groups were 93%, 64%, and 36%, respectively. On other hand, in thymic carcinoma, 5-yr survival rates of total resection, subtotal resection, and inoperable groups were 67%, 30%, and 24%, respectively. PORT did not change LR rates in pts with totally resected stage II and III thymoma. Adjuvant therapy including RT or CHT did not improve prognosis in pts with totally resected III and IV thymoma and thymic carcinoma. **Conclusion: Total resection is the most important factor in treatment of thymic epithelial tumors. Adjuvant therapy may not improve outcomes for totally resected invasive thymoma and thymic carcinoma.**

TABLE 29.4: Results of Japanese Retrospective Study for Thymoma by Kondo et al.				
Masaoka Stage	I	II	III	IVA
Complete resection (%)	100	100	85	42
Recurrence (%)	1	4	28	34
5-yr OS (%)	100	98	89	71

Utsumi, Japan (*Cancer* 2009, PMID 19685527): RR of 324 pts from 1970 to 2005 who underwent complete resection of thymoma. PORT was performed for 134 pts. Survival rates and patterns of recurrence were determined according to Masaoka stage and WHO cell type. 10-year disease specific survival (DSS) with and without PORT was 92.8% and 94.4%, respectively ($p = .22$). Subset analyses after stratifying by Masaoka stage and WHO cell type: 10-year DSS for pts w/o PORT with Masaoka stage I and II, as well as WHO cell types A, AB, or B1, was 100%. For Masaoka stage III/IV and those with WHO cell types B2/B, PORT did not improve outcomes. **Conclusion: Suggests surgical resection alone is sufficient for thymoma pts with Masaoka stage I and II, and those with WHO cell types A, AB, and B1. Furthermore, optimal treatment strategy should be established for pts with Masaoka stage III/IV and WHO cell type B2/B3 thymoma.**

Forquer, Indiana SEER Analysis (*IJROP* 2010, PMID 19427738): SEER analysis to determine impact of PORT for thymoma (T) and thymic carcinoma (TC). Pts with surgically resected localized (Masaoka stage I) or regional (Masaoka stage II-III) thymoma analyzed for OS and CSS from 1973 to 2005. 901 T/TC pts were identified (275 localized; 626 regional). For all localized pts, PORT had no benefit and may adversely impact 5-year CSS rate (91% vs. 98%, $p = .03$). For pts with regional disease, 5-year OS rate was improved by adding PORT (76% vs. 66% for surgery alone, $p = .01$); however, 5-yr CSS rate was no better (91% vs. 86%, $p = .12$). No benefit was noted for PORT in regional disease after extirpative surgery (defined as radical or total thymectomy). On multivariate OS and CSS analysis, stage and age were independently correlated with survival. For multivariate CSS analysis, outcome of PORT is significantly better for regional disease than for localized disease (HR 0.167; $p = .001$). **Conclusion: PORT for T/TC had no advantage in pts with local disease, but possible OS benefit in pts with regional disease was found, especially after nonextirpative surgery.**

Rimner, ITMIG group (*J Thorac Oncol* 2016, PMID 27346413): Used large database of the International Thymic Malignancy Interest Group (ITMIG) to determine whether postoperative radiation therapy (PORT) is associated with an OS benefit in pts with completely resected Masaoka or Masaoka–Koga stage II and III thymoma. Of 1,263 pts meeting the selection criteria, 870 (69%) had stage II thymoma. 5- and 10-yr OS rates for pts having undergone an operation plus PORT were 95% and 86%, respectively, compared with 90% and 79% for pts receiving an operation alone ($p = .002$). This OS benefit remained significant when pts with stage II ($p = .02$) and stage III thymoma ($p = .0005$) were analyzed separately. **Conclusion: PORT improves OS in stage II/III resected thymoma.**

Is there role for PORT in Stage II thymoma specifically?

Until very recently, for R0 resected stage II thymoma, PORT was generally not indicated since it had not shown a decreased risk of LR or change survival. This has recently been brought into question by large RR suggesting survival benefit to PORT (see Rimner et al., above). Small RR suggests LR benefit specifically for pts with macroscopic pleural adherence.

Singhal, UPenn (*Ann Thorac Surg* 2003, PMID 14602300): RR of 167 pts comparing outcomes of stage I and II thymomas treated by resection alone with thymomas treated by resection plus radiation. All completely resected. No differences in OS or LR rates between stage II pts who did (20 pts) or did not (20 pts) receive PORT. **Conclusion: Margin-negative surgical resection alone is sufficient treatment for both stages I and II thymoma.**

Mangi, Harvard (*Ann Thorac Surg* 2002, PMID 12400741): RR of 49 pts with stage II thymoma +/− administration of PORT after resection. 14 pts had PORT, 35 did not receive PORT. Addition of PORT did not significantly alter local or distant recurrence rates. DSS at 10 yrs was 100% both with and without PORT ($p = .87$). **Conclusion: Stage II pts do not require adjuvant RT and can be observed after complete resection.**

Haniuda, Japan (*Ann Surg* 1996, PMID 8757387): RR from 1973 to 1992 of 80 pts with completely resected stage II thymoma. Recurrence of thymoma was observed in 13 of 80 (16.3%) pts. No recurrence was observed in 23 pts with noninvasive thymoma. In pts with invasive thymoma whose tumor was macroscopically adherent to pleura but not microscopically invasive, recurrence was observed in 4 of 11 pts (36.4%) when mediastinal PORT was not performed, but in 0/10 (0%) of pts who received PORT. However, in pts with microscopic pleural invasion, high recurrence rate was observed with mediastinal PORT (40%, 6/15 pts) or without mediastinal PORT (30%, 3/10 pts). PORT for pts with microscopic invasion to pericardium did not decrease recurrence rate. Analysis of mode of recurrence showed that PORT may have been effective in preventing LR, but it did not control pleural dissemination that was observed in 12 of 13 recurrent cases. **Conclusion: PORT is effective in pts with macroscopic adhesion to pleura but not microscopic invasion. PORT may not be sufficient for pts with microscopic pleural or pericardial invasion.**

When is post-op concurrent chemoRT recommended?

Empirically driven decision since there is very little data; extrapolation from other aerodigestive cancers suggest chemoRT for thymoma with gross residual disease (R2 resection), or any stage of resected thymic carcinoma.[7]

Unresectable/medically inoperable thymoma and thymic carcinoma

What are the management options for unresectable/inoperable thymic tumors?

In the unresectable setting, downstaging with neoadjuvant therapy may be attempted with induction CHT +/− RT. In those who are medically inoperable or remain unresectable, completion of definitive treatment using combined-modality therapy may be appropriate. Data for definitive RT is modest given this rare clinical scenario. Diffuse systemic metastatic disease is typically treated with CHT alone, with palliative RT considered for symptomatic progression.

Loehrer, SWOG/SECSG/ECOG (*JCO* 1997, PMID 9294472): Prospective single-arm study conducted from 1983 to 1995 involving 26 pts with limited-stage unresectable thymoma or thymic carcinoma. Pts received two to four cycles q3 weeks of cisplatin, doxorubicin, and cyclophosphamide (PAC) followed by RT with 54 Gy to primary tumor and regional lymph nodes for pts with stable, partial (PR), or complete response (CR) to CHT. 23 pts were evaluable. Toxicity was mild. There were 5 CR and 11 PR to CHT (overall response rate, 69.6%). Median time to treatment failure was 93.2 mos, and MS was 93 mos. 5-yr OS 52.5%. **Conclusion: PAC combination CHT produces response rates in management of pts with unresectable thymoma. Combined-modality therapy is feasible and associated with prolonged PFS. Benefit of combined-modality therapy over RT alone is suggested for pts with unresectable thymoma.**

Shin, MD Anderson (*Ann Intern Med* 1998, PMID 9669967): Prospective cohort study from 1990 to 1996 of 13 consecutively enrolled pts with newly diagnosed, histologically proven, unresectable malignant thymoma. Pts were treated with induction CHT consisting of 3 cycles of cyclophosphamide, doxorubicin, cisplatin, and prednisone along with surgical resection, PORT, and consolidation CHT with 3 more cycles of same regimen. 12 pts were evaluable. CR to CHT in 3 pts (25%), PR in 8 pts (67%), and 1 pt had minor response (8%). 11 pts underwent surgical resection with one refusing surgery. R0 resection in 9 (82%) and incompletely in 2 (18%) of 11 pts who had been receiving RT and consolidation CHT. All 12 pts alive at 7 yrs, with MFU of 43 mos, while 10/12 are disease-free (7-yr DFS 73%). **Conclusion: Aggressive multimodal treatment may be appropriate for locally advanced, unresectable malignant thymoma.**

REFERENCES

1. Ahmad U, Yao X, Detterbeck F, et al. Thymic carcinoma outcomes and prognosis: results of international analysis. *J Thorac Cardiovasc Surg*. 2015;149(1):95–100, 101.e1–101.e102.
2. Falkson CB, Bezjak A, Darling G, et al. Management of thymoma: systematic review and practice guideline. *J Thorac Oncol*. 2009;4(7):911–919.
3. Kondo K, Yoshizawa K, Tsuyuguchi M, et al. WHO histologic classification is prognostic indicator in thymoma. *Ann Thorac Surg*. 2004;77(4):1183–1188.
4. Safieddine N, Liu G, Cuningham K, et al. Prognostic factors for cure, recurrence and long-term survival after surgical resection of thymoma. *J Thorac Oncol*. 2014;9(7):1018–1022.
5. Masaoka A, Monden Y, Nakahara K, Tanioka T. Follow-up study of thymomas with special reference to their clinical stages. *Cancer*. 1981;48(11):2485–2492.
6. Wright CD. Management of thymomas. *Crit Rev Oncol Hematol*. 2008;65(2):109–120.
7. Clinical Practice Guidelines in Oncology: Thymomas and Thymic Carcinomas. 2017. https://www.nccn.org/professionals/physician_gls/pdf/thymic.pdf

VI: GASTROINTESTINAL

30: ESOPHAGEAL CANCER

Camille A. Berriochoa and Gregory M. M. Videtic

> **QUICK HIT:** Esophageal cancer historically was most commonly seen as squamous carcinomas arising from upper to middle esophagus, often associated with chronic alcohol and tobacco use. In the last decades, adenocarcinoma arising from the distal esophagus or gastroesophageal junction (GEJ) has escalated in incidence to become the most common esophageal malignancy, felt to be related to chronic reflux, obesity, and Barrett's esophagus. External beam RT is employed in definitive, neoadjuvant, adjuvant settings, since the appropriateness of, and sequencing of modalities in, tri-modality therapy (surgery, CHT, and RT) remains controversial. Brachytherapy may be beneficial for select pts as boost or for palliation.

TABLE 30.1: General Treatment Paradigm for Esophageal Cancer[1]	
Stage I	Tis/T1a (SCC or ACA): Endoscopic resection/ablation (preferred) vs. esophagectomy T1b (SCC): Endoscopic resection/ablation T1b (ACA): Esophagectomy
Stage II–IVA (T4a only)	1. Preoperative CRT (41.4–50.4 Gy with concurrent CHT) or 2. Definitive CRT (particularly for cervical esophagus), typically to a dose of 50.4 Gy but can consider 60–66 Gy for cervical location or 3. Postoperative CRT for pathologic stages IIA(T3N0)-IVA; any stage with R1/R2 resection Can consider esophagectomy for T2 low-risk lesions, <2 cm, well differentiated
Stage IVA (T4b)	Definitive CRT, 50.4 Gy; can consider CHT alone if invasion to trachea, great vessels, or heart
Stage IVB	Palliation with EBRT, brachytherapy, CHT, and/or best supportive care

EPIDEMIOLOGY: Approximately 17,000 new esophageal cancers diagnosed with nearly 16,000 deaths per year in the United States.[2] Incidence peaks in sixth and seventh decades. Globally, SCC accounts for 90% of cases with the majority of these cases arising in endemic regions of Eastern Europe and Asia. However, adenocarcinoma is more common in North America and Western European countries, comprising about 70% of cases.[3] Both histologic subtypes are more common in men but the relative increased incidence in males is more pronounced for adenocarcinoma.

RISK FACTORS: For squamous cell (mnemonic: ABCDEF)[3–5]: **A**chalasia, **B**ad diet (nutritional deficiency, high fat, low fruit/vegetables, drinking beverages at high temperatures causing thermal injury to mucosa), **C**austic stricture (lye ingestion), **C**igarette smoking, **D**ysplasia/**D**iverticuli, **E**sophageal webs (Plummer–Vinson syndrome includes iron-deficiency anemia, atrophic glossitis, webs), **E**thanol (alcohol), **F**amilial. For adenocarcinoma (mnemonic: BOG)[3–5]: **B**arrett's esophagus (squamocolumnar metaplasia; risk approximately 0.5%/year for nondysplastic lesions; ranges from 1% to 5% for dysplastic lesions),[6,7] **Obesity, GERD** (weekly symptoms increase risk by factor of 5, daily symptoms increase risk by factor of 7),[8] cigarette smoking (less so than squamous), also associated with hiatal hernia and EGFR polymorphisms. Rarely, hereditary predisposition syndromes may be implicated including tylosis, Bloom syndrome, Fanconi anemia for squamous cell, and familial Barrett's syndrome for adenocarcinoma.[1]

ANATOMY: Esophagus anatomic key features include: no true serosa, nonkeratinized squamous epithelium superiorly that transitions to glandular epithelium inferiorly, and extensive submucosal lymphatic plexus that often results in skip metastases. Approximately 25 cm long, begins at cricopharyngeus muscle at about 15 cm from incisors to GEJ, about 40 cm from incisors. Esophagus extends from vertebral levels C6-T10. GEJ tumors defined as within 5 cm from true GEJ (epithelial change) are frequently classified according to modified Siewert system, with class I tumors originating from 1 to 5 cm superior to true GEJ, class II tumors originating from 1 cm above to 2 cm below and class III tumors from 2 to 5 cm below GEJ.[9,10]

TABLE 30.2: Anatomic and Endoscopic Landmarks of the Esophagus		
Anatomic Site	**Description**	**Approximate Distance From Incisors**
Cervical	Upper esophageal sphincter (UES) to thoracic inlet (sternal notch)	15–20 cm
Upper thoracic	Sternal notch to azygos vein	20–25 cm
Middle thoracic	Azygos vein to inferior pulmonary vein	25–30 cm
Lower thoracic	Inferior pulmonary vein to esophagogastric junction (GEJ)	30–40 cm
Lower abdominal	GEJ to 5 cm below EGJ (see Chapter 31)	40–45 cm
GEJ/Cardia	GEJ to 5 cm below EGJ	40–45 cm

PATHOLOGY: As in the preceding, SCC accounts for 90% of cases globally but adenocarcinoma comprises 70% of cases in North America and Western Europe. Mixed adenosquamous and carcinomas, NOS are categorized as SCC for purposes of staging. Rare histologies included small cell carcinoma and sarcoma.

CLINICAL PRESENTATION[3]**:** Common symptoms include progressive dysphagia, weight loss, heartburn that does not respond to medical therapy, melena and/or symptoms of asymptomatic blood loss. Less commonly, pts may present with symptoms or laryngeal nerve paralysis such as hoarseness, cough, and pneumonia. Note that asymptomatic cases may be detected due to Barrett's esophagus screening. Given association with other aerodigestive malignancies, it is important to evaluate for symptoms related to H&N SCC.

WORKUP[1]**:** H&P with careful neck and abdominal exam.

Labs: CBC, CMP. Her2-neu testing for unresectable, recurrent, or metastatic adenocarcinoma (approximately 25% of esophageal cancers are Her2-neu positive).[11,12]

Imaging: Barium swallow, CT chest/abdomen/pelvis with oral and IV contrast; PET/CT for distant metastases (has poor sensitivity and specificity for nodal metastases: approximately 50% and 80% respectively).[13]

Pathology: Upper GI endoscopy with biopsy. EUS (more accurate than CT and PET-CT for local/nodal staging, can biopsy nodes if suspicious).[14] Upper- to midesophageal lesions at or above carina need bronchoscopy to rule out tracheoesophageal fistula.

PROGNOSTIC FACTORS: Age, KPS, stage, grade, weight loss, pretreatment and postinduction dysphagia.[15] RPA of esophageal pts showed only weight loss, specifically loss of ≥10% in preceding 6 months, as prognostic.[16]

NATURAL HISTORY: 5-year OS is approximately 40% if confined to primary site, 20% if spread to regional LNs, and 4% if distant metastases present.

STAGING

TABLE 30.3: AJCC 8th ed. (2017) Staging for Esophagus Cancer							
Tumor		**Node**		**Distant Metastasis**		**Grade**	
T1	a Invades lamina propria or muscularis mucosa	N0	• No regional LNs	M0	• No distant metastasis	G1	• Well differentiated
	b Invades submucosa						
T2	• Invades muscularis propria	N1	• 1–2 Regional LNs	M1	• Distant metastasis	G2	• Moderately differentiated
T3	• Invades adventitia	N2	• 3–6 Regional LNs			G3	• Poorly differentiated
T4	a Resectable[1]	N3	• ≥7 Regional LNs				
	b Unresectable[2]						

Notes: Resectable[1] = Invades pleura, pericardium, diaphragm, azygos vein, or peritoneum. Unresectable[2] = Invades aorta, vertebral body, airway. AJCC suggests ≥10 nodes removed for pT1 tumors, ≥20 for pT2 and ≥30 for pT3-4.

Stage Grouping (AJCC 8th)			
Note that the AJCC 8th Edition includes a pathologic TNM and postneoadjuvant pathologic TNM which are not displayed here.			
Squamous Cell Carcinoma		**Adenocarcinoma**	
Clinical Stage	**Clinical TNM**	**Clinical Stage**	**Clinical TNM**
0	Tis N0	0	Tis N0
I	T1 N0-1	I	T1 N0
II	T2 N0-1 T3 N0	IIA	T1 N1
		IIB	T2 N0
III	T3 N1 T1-3 N2	III	T2 N1 T3 N0-1 T4a N0-1
IVA	T4 N0-2 T any N3	IVA	T1-4a N2 T4b N0-2 T any N3
IVB	T any N any M1	IVB	T any N any M1

TREATMENT PARADIGM

Surgery: Surgery is a commonly utilized option for locoregionally confined disease and options are based on patient's medical condition, tumor location, and stage. Cervical tumors are typically treated nonoperatively because these lesions may also need laryngopharyngectomy with permanent stoma. For upper and middle thoracic tumors (>5 cm below cricopharyngeus), total esophagectomy with gastric pull-through is standard. Distal esophagogastrectomy is standard for lesions of GEJ and lower thoracic esophagus. Contraindications to surgery include distant metastases, T4b lesions (involvement of heart, great vessels, trachea, or other surrounding organs), bulky multistation adenopathy and medical comorbidity.

Three techniques are commonly employed in North America for total esophagectomy: Ivor Lewis, McKeown (tri-incisional), and transhiatal. Both Ivor Lewis esophagogastrectomy and McKeown esophagogastrectomy require right thoracotomy incisions, with the latter permitting access to more superiorly located tumors. Transhiatal esophagogastrectomy can be used for cervical, thoracic, and GEJ lesions and requires abdominal and left cervical incisions; thoracotomy is not performed (often resulting in shorter operative times). There is some evidence of lower postoperative morbidity with transhiatal approach[17]; however, several disadvantages associated with this technique include difficulty in resecting large, midesophageal and/or paratracheal tumors as well as lower lymph node retrieval. Postoperative mortality at high volume centers is typically less than 5%[18–20] but can be 10% or higher after neoadjuvant CRT.[21–23]

For most distal lesions, mediastinal and upper abdominal lymphadenectomy is performed. Minimum number of lymph nodes to optimize staging and survival is controversial, with recommendations varying widely from 6 to 23 LNs.[24–27] Retrospective evidence exists for improved survival with increased number of lymph nodes resected.[26]

Minimally invasive surgery is possible although data is evolving. Two randomized trials have reported reduction in postoperative complications with use of minimally invasive surgery (thoracoscopy with upper abdominal laparoscopy) as compared to open technique with thoracotomy.[28,29]

Chemotherapy: CHT is commonly utilized for T2–T4 or node-positive tumors in neoadjuvant, peri-operative, adjuvant or definitive settings.[30–35] In both preoperative and definitive settings, common regimens concurrent with RT include cisplatin + infusional 5-FU or carboplatin + paclitaxel. Infusional 5-FU is thought to be superior to bolus 5-FU based on data from gastric cancer.[1,36] Oral capecitabine can be substituted for infusional 5-FU.[1] Metastatic adenocarcinomas of GEJ should be tested for HER2-neu and trastuzumab can be considered if positive based on survival benefit demonstrated by TOGA trial.[37] Note that peri-operative ECF (epirubicin, cisplatin, and 5-FU) is common regimen for distal esophageal adenocarcinomas based on inclusion in gastric data.[31] Irinotecan, etoposide, and oxaliplatin are all also under investigation. Addition of cetuximab to standard cytotoxic therapy has shown no benefit.[38,39]

Radiation

Indications: Typically delivered with concurrent CHT in preoperative or definitive setting for T2–T4 or node-positive tumors.

Dose: With concurrent CHT, 50–50.4 Gy/25–28 fx is standard. Without CHT, 64 Gy/32 fx is standard (see Herskovic in the following). Randomized trials show benefit to concurrent CHT and no benefit to dose escalation beyond 50.4 Gy.[34,40] In preoperative setting, 41.4 Gy is appropriate dose based on the CROSS trial. Brachytherapy boost can be selectively employed though does not improve survival and may be associated with morbidity.[41,42]

Palliation: EBRT and brachytherapy can be used. Other options include dilation, laser therapy, endoscopic injection therapies, endoscopic mucosal resection, photodynamic therapy, stenting (preferable in those with malignant fistula). Safe to treat with palliative RT post-stenting.

Toxicity: Acute: esophagitis, fatigue, weight loss, subacute pneumonitis. Late: strictures, pulmonary fibrosis, pericarditis, coronary artery disease.

Procedure: See *Treatment Planning Handbook*, Chapter 6.[43]

Endoscopic therapy: Endoscopic management of early esophageal cancer may be performed using endoscopic mucosal resection (EMR) or endoscopic submucosal dissection (ESD). Both techniques allow resection of mucosa (and possibly a portion of the submucosa) containing early tumor without interruption of deeper layers. EMR can remove lesions less than 2 cm in size en bloc. Larger lesions may require resection in piecemeal fashion limiting assessment of margins of the lesion. ESD offers en bloc dissection of tumor regardless of its size. ESD is performed with specialized needle knives, which allow incision followed by careful dissection of lesion within submucosal layer. ESD is labor intensive and has increased risk of perforation. Esophageal stenosis remains a concern after extensive EMR or ESD.

Locally ablative modalities: Include thermal destruction by laser, multipolar electrocoagulation (MPEC), argon plasma coagulation (APC), or radiofrequency ablation; cryotherapy; and photodynamic therapy (PDT). PDT may eradicate high-grade dysplasia and Barrett's.

EVIDENCE-BASED Q&A

Unresectable/inoperable esophageal cancer

Is RT alone sufficient for esophageal cancer or should concurrent CHT be added?

RT alone is insufficient since OS is improved with the addition of the CHT to RT.

Herskovic, RTOG 8501 (*NEJM* 1992, PMID 1584260; Update Al-Sarraf *JCO* 1997, PMID 8996153; Update Cooper *JAMA* 1999, PMID 10235156): Phase III PRT of 129 pts with ACA (12%) or SCC (88%) cT1-3N0-1 randomized to RT alone (64 Gy/32 fx) versus CRT (concurrent cisplatin/5-FU + 50 Gy/25 fx). CHT was cisplatin 75 mg/m^2 and 5-FU 1,000 mg/m^2 on weeks 1, 5, 8, and 11. Initial RT field extended from SCV fossa to GEJ (except SCV was optional for distal-third tumors). For the CRT arm, extended field was taken to 30 Gy followed by 20 Gy boost to tumor +5 cm. For the RT-alone arm, extended field was taken to 50 Gy followed by 14 Gy boost to tumor +5 cm. Trial stopped early due to survival difference. 5-yr OS was 26% versus 0% favoring CRT. Persistent disease was the most common mode of failure: 26% in CRT arm and 37% in RT alone arm. Acute severe/life-threatening acute toxicity were 44%/20% with CRT, and 25%/3% with RT alone. No differences in late toxicity. **Conclusion: Concurrent when treating non-operatively, CHT is superior for T1-3N0-1 esophageal cancer.**

Does RT dose escalation improve survival in setting of CHT?

There is no evidence that dose escalation improves outcomes. Whether modern techniques may permit safer delivery of dose escalated treatment was evaluated in a 2016 NCDB analysis.[44] This analysis reviewed pts with stage I–III esophageal cancer who received RT between 2004 and 2012 to doses ≥50 Gy and found no benefit to dose escalation, consistent with the results of the Minsky trial.

Minsky, RTOG 94-05/INT 0123 (*JCO* 2002, PMID 11870157): Phase III PRT of 218 pts with T1-4N0-1 ACA (15%) or SCC (85%) treated with low dose (50.4 Gy) versus high-dose (64.8 Gy) RT with both arms receiving concurrent CHT (cisplatin + 5-FU). For the high dose arm, RT was 50.4 Gy/28 fx to tumor + 5 cm sup-inf (and 2 cm laterally), with 14.4 Gy boost to tumor + 2 cm. CHT was cisplatin 75 mg/m² and 5-FU 1000 mg/m² on weeks 1, 5, 9, and 13 in low dose arm, and weeks 1, 5, 11, and 15 in high dose arm. Closed early because no benefit seen in high dose arm. See Table 30.4. **Conclusion: No benefit to high dose RT with concurrent CHT, with higher incidence of treatment-related death in this trial. Note that 7 of 11 deaths in high dose arm occurred at ≤50.4 Gy.**

TABLE 30.4: RTOG 9405 Minsky, RT Dose Escalation for Esophageal Cancer				
	MS (mos)	2-yr OS	2-yr LR	Treatment-Related deaths
High dose CRT (64.8 Gy)	13.0	31%	56%	10% (7/11 deaths at ≤50.4 Gy)
Low dose CRT (50.4 Gy)	18.1	40%	52%	2%
p value	NS	NS	.71	

Comment: Some authors have commented that higher mortality observed in dose escalation arm may not be related to radiation dose given that majority of these deaths occurred before pts reached high dose portion of their treatment.

Should elective nodal stations be targeted when treating pts definitively?

There is no strong evidence to suggest that elective nodal stations should not be included. A single PRT examining elective versus involved nodal RT in esophageal SCC suggested equivalent outcomes and higher toxicity rates following elective nodal RT.[45]

Resectable/operable esophageal cancer

Is there benefit to trimodality therapy as compared to definitive CRT?

To date, there is no evidence to suggest that surgery improves overall survival, although PFS appears improved by reducing locoregional failure.

Stahl, "Stahl I" (*JCO* 2005, PMID 15800321): Phase III PRT of 172 pts with locally advanced SCC upper–midesophageal cancer, uT3-4N0-1M0, age ≤70, randomized to either (A) induction CHT, pre-op CRT (40 Gy/20 fx), then surgery, or (B) induction CHT, then definitive CRT (≥65 Gy) without surgery. Induction CHT was bolus 5-FU, LCV, etoposide and cisplatin q3 weeks for three cycles. Concurrent CHT was EP. In arm B, T4 and obstructing T3 tumors received 50 Gy/25 fx, with EBRT boost to 65 Gy with 15 Gy/10 fx BID over last week. For nonobstructing T3 tumors, pts received 60 Gy/30 fx, with HDR brachytherapy boost of 4 Gy x 2 fractions to 5 mm depth. MFU was 6 years. No difference in 2-yr OS (40% vs. 35%) or MS (16.4 vs. 14.9 mos). Surgery arm had better 2-yr PFS (64% vs. 41%, p = .003) due to improved LC, but also higher treatment-related mortality (13% vs. 4%, p = .03). Of arm A, only 66% proceeded to surgery, but complete resection was possible in 82% of those who did. Seventy percent of surgery pts had at least one severe complication; 11% post-op hospital mortality; 35% had pCR. Response to induction CHT was associated with improved survival. **Conclusion: Adding surgery to CRT improves LC but does not improve OS. Pts who respond to induction treatment may be treated definitively with CRT, while poor responders may benefit from surgery.**

Bedenne, French FFCD 9102 (*JCO* 2007, PMID 17401004): Phase III PRT of operable pts with T3N0-1M0 thoracic esophageal cancer comparing (A) neoadjuvant CRT followed by surgery versus (B) higher dose definitive CRT in those with response to up-front CRT. Pts received two cycles of 5-FU and cisplatin (days 1 to 5 and 22 to 26) and either conventional (46 Gy in 4.5 weeks) or split-course (15 Gy, days 1 to 5 and 22 to 26) concomitant RT (investigator choice). Subsequently, pts with response and no contraindication to either treatment were randomly assigned to surgery (arm A) or continuation of CRT (arm B; three additional cycles of 5-FU/cisplatin and either conventional [20 Gy] or split-course [15 Gy] RT). CRT was considered equivalent to surgery if difference in 2-year survival rate was less than 10%. Surgery arm: MS: 17.7 versus 19.3 mos in no surgery arm ($p = .44$). 2-yr LC: 66.4% in surgery arm compared with 57.0% in definitive CRT arm. Fewer stents were required in surgery arm (5% for surgical arm vs. 32% in CRT arm; $p < .001$). **Conclusion: LC is improved with surgery but no difference in OS.**

Does CHT with surgery improve OS compared to surgery alone?

Yes, multiple trials studied neoadjuvant and peri-operative regimens with most demonstrating OS benefit.[33,46] However, local response was often inadequate (pCR rates were typically <5%) and CRT may be superior. The MAGIC trial, investigating peri-operative ECF, continues to be a commonly utilized regimen for GEJ cancers (this was largely a gastric cancer trial of which approximately 20% were lower thoracic or GEJ adenocarcinomas).[31]

Does preoperative CRT improve OS compared to surgery alone?

Yes, although two early randomized trials showed no benefit to preoperative sequential CRT. [47,48] Several studies now demonstrate significant benefits to preoperative concurrent CRT, including CROSS which showed doubled OS with use of trimodality therapy.

Walsh, Ireland (NEJM 1996, PMID 8672151): Randomized 58 pts to preoperative CRT (cisplatin/5-FU with 40 Gy/15 fx) versus surgery alone, with results showing pCR rate of 25% in pre-op CRT arm and improved MS from 11 to 16 mos. ($p = .01$).[49]

Bosset, EORTC Trial (NEJM 1997, PMID 9219702): PRT, which randomized pts with stage I-II SCC to pre-op CRT (cisplatin and split course of 37 Gy in two 1-week courses of 18.5 Gy in five fractions separated by 2 weeks), versus surgery alone. Results showed pCR of 26% with CRT with improved 3-yr DFS in CRT arm (from 27% to 35%, $p = .003$) but no difference in MS (18.6 mos for both groups). Of note, this trial closed early due to higher rate of post-op mortality in CRT group (12% vs. 4%, $p = .012$).

Tepper, CALGB 9781 (JCO 2008, PMID 18309943): PRT of 56 pts (consisting of both ACA and SCC), again comparing pre-op CRT (cis/5-FU with 50.4 Gy in 28 fx) to surgery alone. Though study closed early due to poor accrual, it was able to demonstrate pCR rate of 40% and improvement in PFS from 1.0 to 3.5 years as well as improved MS (from 1.8 years to 4.5 years) with use of pre-op CRT ($p = .008$).[50]

Van Hagen, CROSS (NEJM 2012, PMID 22646630; Update Shapiro Lancet Oncol 2015, PMID 26254683): Phase III PRT of neoadjuvant CRT + surgery versus surgery alone. 366 potentially resectable pts randomized to carboplatin (AUC 2 mg/mm/min)/paclitaxel (50 mg/m^2) and concurrent RT (41.4 Gy/23 fx) followed by surgery (transthoracic or transhiatal approach) versus surgery alone. Surgery was performed within 4 to 6 weeks of completion of CRT. 75% ACA, 23% SCC, and 2% had large-cell undifferentiated carcinoma. Initial publication showed that MS improved from 24 mos to 49.4 mos with the addition of pre-op CRT ($p = .003$). Updated publication: MFU 84 mos. Complete resection (R0) rate was higher with CRT, 92% versus 69% ($p < .001$). pCR was achieved in 29% overall (49% in SCC subgroup) of those treated with CRT. MS was improved in CRT + surgery group versus surgery alone (see Table 30.5). 5-yr OS increased from 33% to 47% ($p = .003$). Estimated number needed to treat to prevent one additional death at 5 yrs was 7.1. **Conclusion: Preoperative CRT improved survival among pts with potentially curable esophageal or GEJ cancer.**

TABLE 30.5: CROSS Trial of Neoadjuvant CRT for Esophageal Cancer			
	Neoadjuvant CRT + Surgery	Surgery Alone	p value
MS, All	48.6 mos	24 mos	.003
MS, SCC	81.6 mos	21.1 mos	.008
MS, ACA	43.2 mos	27.1 mos	.038

Does neoadjuvant CRT improve OS as compared to neoadjuvant CHT?

Yes, the Stahl trial supports benefit to CRT as compared to CHT alone. Multiple meta-analyses also support this concept.

Stahl, "Stahl II" (*JCO* 2009, PMID 19139439): Phase III PRT of neoadjuvant CHT versus neoadjuvant CRT. 126 pts (goal 394, closed due to poor accrual), resectable T3-4NxM0 (staged by EUS, CT, and laparoscopy), randomized to (A) PLF x2.5 cycles (cisplatin/leucovorin/fluorouracil) versus (B) PLF x 2 cycles, then 3 weeks of combined CRT, 30 Gy/15 fx with cisplatin/etoposide. Both arms followed by tumor resection 3 to 4 weeks after induction. Complete (R0) resection in 70% versus 72%, CR 2% versus 15.6% ($p = .03$), 3-yr OS 28% versus 47% ($p = .07$). **Conclusion: Preoperative CRT has trend to improved OS compared with preoperative CHT alone.** *Comment: Trial closed early and is underpowered.*

Gebski, Australasian Group Meta-analysis (*Lancet Oncol* 2007, PMID 17329193): Study-level meta-analysis included 10 PRTs comparing neoadjuvant CRT versus surgery alone and 8 PRTs comparing neoadjuvant CHT versus surgery alone. HR for all-cause mortality with neoadjuvant CRT versus surgery alone was 0.81 (95% CI: 0.70–0.93; $p = .002$), corresponding to 13% absolute difference in survival at 2 yrs, HR for neoadjuvant CHT was 0.90 (0.81–1.00; $p = .05$), which indicates 2-yr absolute survival benefit of 7%. **Conclusion: CRT demonstrates larger effect size than neoadjuvant CHT alone.**

Pasquali, Network Meta-analysis (*Ann Surg* 2016, PMID 27429017): Study-level network (compares ≥3 treatment approaches) meta-analysis, which included 33 RCTs in which 6,072 pts were randomized to receive either surgery alone or neoadjuvant CHT, RT, or CRT followed by surgery OR surgery followed by adjuvant CHT, RT, and CRT. Neoadjuvant CRT demonstrated strongest effect on OS of all treatments. HR for OS of neoadjuvant CRT versus surgery alone was 0.77 ($p < .001$) whereas HR for OS of neoadjuvant CHT versus surgery alone was 0.89 ($p = .051$). **Conclusion: Neoadjuvant CRT appears the most effective strategy for resectable esophageal cancers.**

If patient gets surgery up front, should he/she receive adjuvant therapy?

Yes. The McDonald trial (INT 0116) evaluated role of adjuvant CRT in pts with GE junction or gastric cancer. Admittedly, only 20% of pts had GEJ cancer but this is nevertheless important study to consider when evaluating patient with stage IB-IV disease who underwent up-front esophagectomy as it demonstrated improvement in 3-yr OS (from 41% to 50%, $p = .005$) in those who received adjuvant CRT (bolus 5-FU and leucovorin with concurrent RT, 45 Gy/25 fx).[51] That said, as described previously, a recent meta-analysis reviewing outcomes for over 6,000 pts from 33 RCTs with resectable esophageal carcinoma found no significant advantage in OS in pts who received surgery + adjuvant therapy (HR 0.87, 95% CI: 0.67–1.14) whereas neoadjuvant therapies followed by surgery were associated with survival advantage (HR 0.83, 95% CI: 0.76–0.90).[30]

Is there benefit to IMRT for esophageal cancer?

3D-conformal RT via three or four fields is standard technique for esophageal cancer. Retrospective data suggests IMRT benefit with respect to cardiac toxicity but selection and follow-up bias remains the issue and further study is necessary. Guidelines for IMRT planning are available.[52]

Lin, MDACC (*IJROBP* 2012, PMID 22867894): Retrospective study of 676 pts treated at MDACC (413 3D-CRT, 263 IMRT) with stage IB-IVA esophageal cancer treated with CRT (46% also received surgery) between 1998 and 2008. Inverse probability-weighted adjusted Cox model was used to compare OS. OS was independently associated with stage, performance status, PET staging, induction CHT, and treatment modality (IMRT vs. 3D-CRT, HR 0.72, *p* < .001). Compared with IMRT, 3D-CRT pts had significantly greater risk of dying (72.6% vs. 52.9%, *p* < .0001) and of locoregional recurrence (*p* = .0038). No difference was seen in cancer-specific mortality (Gray's test, *p* = .86) or distant metastasis (*p* = .99) between two groups. Increased cumulative incidence of cardiac death was seen in 3D-CRT group (*p* = .049), as well as undocumented deaths (5-yr estimate: 11.7% in 3D-CRT vs. 5.4% in IMRT group, *p* = .0029). **Conclusion: IMRT can be considered in treatment of esophageal cancer.**

Esophageal brachytherapy

What is role for esophageal brachytherapy in modern era?

Classically, brachytherapy was developed as boost to external beam RT and for palliation of dysphagia related to esophageal cancer. ABS consensus guidelines have been established for brachytherapy.[42] *Brachytherapy is less utilized in modern era, likely due to availability of other advanced RT techniques, limited indications, and potential complications.*

Does brachytherapy boost improve outcomes when added to definitive CRT?

This was investigated in RTOG 9207, phase II study which showed high fistula rate that was lethal in 50% of pts and outcomes that were no better than prior trials looking at CRT alone. Note that CHT was given concurrently with brachytherapy in this trial, and this may have contributed to high toxicity rates.

Gaspar, RTOG 9207 (*Cancer* 2000, PMID 10699886): Phase I/II trial of 49 pts with cT1-2NX-1M0 with SCC (92%) or ACA (8%) <10 cm in length, ≥18 cm from incisors, ≥1 cm from GEJ and without bronchial invasion proven by bronchoscopy (for those <29 cm from incisors). Pts were treated with brachytherapy boost 2 weeks after concurrent CRT with cisplatin/5-FU + 50 Gy/25 fx as per RTOG 85-01. Brachytherapy dose for HDR was 15 Gy/3 fx (at weeks 8, 9, and 10) at first but then reduced to 10 Gy/2 fx, prescribed to 1-cm depth with uniform dwell times. If LDR was chosen, dose was 20 Gy x 1 at week 8. Note that CHT was delivered at weeks 8 and 11. 1-yr OS 49%, 3-yr OS 29%, MS 11 months. Local failure occurred in 63%. Grade 3 toxicity 59%, grade 4 toxicity 24%, mortality 10%, and 12% developed fistula at 0.5 to 6 mos from first day of brachytherapy, leading to death in 50% of these pts. HDR dose was decreased to 10 Gy/2 fx after toxicities noted, and no other fistulae were noted. LDR arm was dropped due to poor accrual (19 pts). **Conclusion: Brachytherapy boost is not recommended because it does not improve OS and is complicated by significant toxicity.**

Which is the most effective method of palliation: metal stent or brachytherapy?

Homs, Dutch SIREC (*Lancet* 2004, PMID 15500894): Phase III PRT, 209 pts with either metastatic disease or with medically inoperable esophageal or GEJ cancer. Randomized either to stent or to 12 Gy in 1 fx via brachytherapy (10-mm diameter applicator, prescribed to 1 cm from source axis, sucralfate x4 weeks, lifelong omeprazole). Excluded tumors >12 cm, fistula, tumor within 3 cm of upper esophageal sphincter, previous RT or stent. Primary endpoint was physician-reported dysphagia; patient-reported outcomes recorded as well. Stenting demonstrated more rapid relief, brachytherapy demonstrated more long-term relief. Late hemorrhage occurred more with stenting (33% vs. 22%, p = .02); QOL scores favored brachytherapy, medical costs were similar; fistula formation occurred in 3 pts in each group. **Conclusion: Brachytherapy has more durable dysphagia relief and fewer complications than stenting.**

REFERENCES

1. NCCN Clinical Practice Guidelines in Oncology: Esophageal Cancer. 2016. https://www.nccn.org/professionals/physician_gls/pdf/esophageal.pdf
2. SEER Cancer Statistics 2016. https://seer.cancer.gov/statfacts/html/esoph.html
3. Rustgi A, El-Serag HB. Esophageal carcinoma. *N Engl J Med.* 2015;372(15):1472–1473.
4. Lundell LR. Etiology and risk factors for esophageal carcinoma. *Dig Dis.* 2010;28(4–5):641–644.
5. American Cancer Society. https://www.cancer.org/cancer/esophagus-cancer/causes-risks-prevention/risk-factors.html
6. Hvid-Jensen F, Pedersen L, Drewes AM, et al. Incidence of adenocarcinoma among patients with Barrett's esophagus. *N Engl J Med.* 2011;365(15):1375–1383.
7. de Jonge PJ, van Blankenstein M, Looman CW, et al. Risk of malignant progression in patients with Barrett's oesophagus: a Dutch nationwide cohort study. *Gut.* 2010;59(8):1030–1036.
8. Rubenstein JH, Taylor JB. Meta-analysis: the association of oesophageal adenocarcinoma with symptoms of gastro-oesophageal reflux. *Aliment Pharmacol Ther.* 2010;32(10):1222–1227.
9. Siewert JR, Stein HJ. Classification of adenocarcinoma of the oesophagogastric junction. *Br J Surg.* 1998;85(11):1457–1459.
10. Rudiger Siewert J, Feith M, Werner M, Stein HJ. Adenocarcinoma of the esophagogastric junction: results of surgical therapy based on anatomical/topographic classification in 1,002 consecutive patients. *Ann Surg.* 2000;232(3):353–361.
11. Gowryshankar A, Nagaraja V, Eslick GD. HER2 status in Barrett's esophagus & esophageal cancer: a meta analysis. *J Gastrointest Oncol.* 2014;5(1):25–35.
12. Bartley AN, Washington MK, Ismaila N, Ajani JA. HER2 testing and clinical decision making in gastroesophageal adenocarcinoma: guideline summary from the college of American pathologists, American Society for Clinical Pathology, and American Society of Clinical Oncology. *J Oncol Pract.* 2017;13(1):53–57.
13. van Westreenen HL, Westerterp M, Bossuyt PM, et al. Systematic review of the staging performance of 18F-fluorodeoxyglucose positron emission tomography in esophageal cancer. *J Clin Oncol.* 2004;22(18):3805–3812.
14. Lightdale CJ, Kulkarni KG. Role of endoscopic ultrasonography in the staging and follow-up of esophageal cancer. *J Clin Oncol.* 2005;23(20):4483–4489.
15. McNamara MJ, Adelstein DJ, Allende DS, et al. Persistent dysphagia after induction chemotherapy in patients with esophageal adenocarcinoma predicts poor post-operative outcomes. *J Gastrointest Cancer.* 2016;48(2):181–189.
16. Thomas CR, Jr., Berkey BA, Minsky BD, et al. Recursive partitioning analysis of pretreatment variables of 416 patients with locoregional esophageal cancer treated with definitive concomitant chemoradiotherapy on Intergroup and Radiation Therapy Oncology Group trials. *Int J Radiat Oncol Biol Phys.* 2004;58(5):1405–1410.
17. Hulscher JB, van Sandick JW, de Boer AG, et al. Extended transthoracic resection compared with limited transhiatal resection for adenocarcinoma of the esophagus. *N Engl J Med.* 2002;347(21):1662–1669.
18. Karl RC, Schreiber R, Boulware D, et al. Factors affecting morbidity, mortality, and survival in patients undergoing Ivor Lewis esophagogastrectomy. *Ann Surg.* 2000;231(5):635–643.
19. Orringer MB, Marshall B, Chang AC, et al. Two thousand transhiatal esophagectomies: changing trends, lessons learned. *Ann Surg.* 2007;246(3):363–372; discussion 372–364.
20. Orringer MB, Marshall B, Iannettoni MD. Transhiatal esophagectomy: clinical experience and refinements. *Ann Surg.* 1999;230(3):392–400; discussion 400–393.

21. Bosset JF, Gignoux M, Triboulet JP, et al. Chemoradiotherapy followed by surgery compared with surgery alone in squamous-cell cancer of the esophagus. *N Engl J Med*. 1997;337(3):161–167.

22. Stahl M, Stuschke M, Lehmann N, et al. Chemoradiation with and without surgery in patients with locally advanced squamous cell carcinoma of the esophagus. *J Clin Oncol*. 2005;23(10):2310–2317.

23. Bedenne L, Michel P, Bouche O, et al. Chemoradiation followed by surgery compared with chemoradiation alone in squamous cancer of the esophagus: FFCD 9102. *J Clin Oncol*. 2007;25(10):1160–1168.

24. Bogoevski D, Onken F, Koenig A, et al. Is it time for a new TNM classification in esophageal carcinoma? *Ann Surg*. 2008;247(4):633–641.

25. Hu Y, Hu C, Zhang H, Ping Y, Chen LQ. How does the number of resected lymph nodes influence TNM staging and prognosis for esophageal carcinoma? *Ann Surg Oncol*. 2010;17(3):784–790.

26. Greenstein AJ, Litle VR, Swanson SJ, et al. Effect of the number of lymph nodes sampled on postoperative survival of lymph node-negative esophageal cancer. *Cancer*. 2008;112(6):1239–1246.

27. Peyre CG, Hagen JA, DeMeester SR, et al. The number of lymph nodes removed predicts survival in esophageal cancer: an international study on the impact of extent of surgical resection. *Ann Surg*. 2008;248(4):549–556.

28. Biere SS, van Berge Henegouwen MI, Maas KW, et al. Minimally invasive versus open oesophagectomy for patients with oesophageal cancer: a multicentre, open-label, randomised controlled trial. *Lancet*. 2012;379(9829):1887–1892.

29. Mariette C Meunier B, Pezet D, et al. Hybrid minimally invasive versus open oesophagectomy for patients with oesophageal cancer: a multicenter, open-label, randomized phase III controlled trial, the MIRO trial. *J Clin Oncol*. 2015;33(Suppl 3):5.

30. Pasquali S, Yim G, Vohra RS, et al. Survival after neoadjuvant and adjuvant treatments compared to surgery alone for resectable esophageal carcinoma: a network meta-analysis. *Ann Surg*. 2016; 265(3):481–491

31. Cunningham D, Allum WH, Stenning SP, et al. Perioperative chemotherapy versus surgery alone for resectable gastroesophageal cancer. *N Engl J Med*. 2006;355(1):11–20.

32. Allum WH, Stenning SP, Bancewicz J, et al. Long-term results of a randomized trial of surgery with or without preoperative chemotherapy in esophageal cancer. *J Clin Oncol*. 2009;27(30):5062–5067.

33. Boige V PJ, Saint-Aubert B. Final results of a randomized trial comparing preoperative fluorouracil/cisplatin to surgery alone in adenocarcinoma of the stomach and lower esophagus: FNLCC ACCORD 07 –FFCD 9703 trial. *J Clin Oncol*. 2007;25(18S):4510.

34. Herskovic A, Martz K, al-Sarraf M, et al. Combined chemotherapy and radiotherapy compared with radiotherapy alone in patients with cancer of the esophagus. *N Engl J Med*. 1992;326(24):1593–1598.

35. Stahl M, Walz MK, Stuschke M, et al. Phase III comparison of preoperative chemotherapy compared with chemoradiotherapy in patients with locally advanced adenocarcinoma of the esophagogastric junction. *J Clin Oncol*. 2009;27(6):851–856.

36. Wagner AD, Grothe W, Haerting J, et al. Chemotherapy in advanced gastric cancer: a systematic review and meta-analysis based on aggregate data. *J Clin Oncol*. 2006;24(18):2903–2909.

37. Bang YJ, Van Cutsem E, Feyereislova A, et al. Trastuzumab in combination with chemotherapy versus chemotherapy alone for treatment of HER2-positive advanced gastric or gastro-oesophageal junction cancer (ToGA): a phase 3, open-label, randomised controlled trial. *Lancet*. 2010;376(9742):687–697.

38. Crosby T, Hurt CN, Falk S, et al. Chemoradiotherapy with or without cetuximab in patients with oesophageal cancer (SCOPE1): a multicentre, phase 2/3 randomised trial. *Lancet Oncol*. 2013;14(7):627–637.

39. Suntharalingam M WK, Ilson D. The initial report of local control on RTOG 0436: a Phase 3 trial evaluating the addition of cetuximab to paclitaxel, cisplatin, and radiation for patients with esophageal cancer treated without surgery. *Oral Presentation*. ASTRO 2014 Annual Meeting. 2014.

40. Minsky BD, Pajak TF, Ginsberg RJ, et al. INT 0123 (Radiation Therapy Oncology Group 94-05) Phase III trial of combined-modality therapy for esophageal cancer: high-dose versus standard-dose radiation therapy. *J Clin Oncol*. 2002;20(5):1167–1174.

41. Gaspar LE, Winter K, Kocha WI, et al. A Phase I/II study of external beam radiation, brachytherapy, and concurrent chemotherapy for patients with localized carcinoma of the esophagus (Radiation Therapy Oncology Group Study 9207): final report. *Cancer*. 2000;88(5):988–995.

42. Gaspar LE, Nag S, Herskovic A, et al. American Brachytherapy Society (ABS) consensus guidelines for brachytherapy of esophageal cancer. Clinical Research Committee, American Brachytherapy Society, Philadelphia, PA. *Int J Radiat Oncol Biol Phys.* 1997;38(1):127–132.

43. Videtic GMM, Woody N, Vassil AD. *Handbook of Treatment Planning in Radiation Oncology.* 2nd ed. New York, NY: Demos Medical; 2015.

44. Brower JV, Chen S, Bassetti MF, et al. Radiation dose escalation in esophageal cancer revisited: a contemporary analysis of the National Cancer Data Base, 2004 to 2012. *Int J Radiat Oncol Biol Phys.* 2016;96(5):985–993.

45. Li T YA, Zhang X. Involved-field irradiation vs elective nodal irradiation for locally advanced thoracic esophageal squamous cell carcinoma: a comparative interim analysis of clinical outcomes and toxicities (NCT01551589, CSWOG 003). Plenary, ASTRO 2015 Annual Meeting. 2015.

46. Medical Research Council Oesophageal Cancer Working Group. Surgical resection with or without preoperative chemotherapy in oesophageal cancer: a randomised controlled trial. *Lancet.* 2002;359(9319):1727–1733.

47. Le Prise E, Etienne PL, Meunier B, et al. A randomized study of chemotherapy, radiation therapy, and surgery versus surgery for localized squamous cell carcinoma of the esophagus. *Cancer.* 1994;73(7):1779–1784.

48. Nygaard K, Hagen S, Hansen HS, et al. Pre-operative radiotherapy prolongs survival in operable esophageal carcinoma: a randomized, multicenter study of pre-operative radiotherapy and chemotherapy. The second Scandinavian trial in esophageal cancer. *World J Surg.* 1992;16(6):1104–1109; discussion 1110.

49. Walsh TN, Noonan N, Hollywood D, et al. A comparison of multimodal therapy and surgery for esophageal adenocarcinoma. *N Engl J Med.* 1996;335(7):462–467.

50. Tepper J, Krasna MJ, Niedzwiecki D, et al. Phase III trial of trimodality therapy with cisplatin, fluorouracil, radiotherapy, and surgery compared with surgery alone for esophageal cancer: CALGB 9781. *J Clin Oncol.* 2008;26(7):1086–1092.

51. Macdonald JS, Smalley SR, Benedetti J, et al. Chemoradiotherapy after surgery compared with surgery alone for adenocarcinoma of the stomach or gastroesophageal junction. *N Engl J Med.* 2001;345(10):725–730.

52. Wu AJ, Bosch WR, Chang DT, et al. Expert consensus contouring guidelines for intensity modulated radiation therapy in esophageal and gastroesophageal junction cancer. *Int J Radiat Oncol Biol Phys.* 2015;92(4):911–920.

31: GASTRIC CANCER

Bindu V. Manyam, Kevin L. Stephans, and Gregory M. M. Videtic

> **QUICK HIT:** Most gastric pts present with locoregionally advanced or metastatic disease. For cT2-4 or N+ locoregionally confined disease, most common approach in the United States is surgery followed by chemoRT but options include perioperative CHT. Surgery can be either partial or total gastrectomy depending on disease location and extent, with regional LND (D2 dissection recommended including ≥15 LNs).

TABLE 31.1: General Treatment Paradigm for Gastric Cancer	
Tis/T1a (≤3 cm, nonulcerated, well differentiated)	• Endoscopic mucosal resection or endoscopic submucosal dissection
T1a-bN0	• Gastrectomy and regional LND • No adjuvant therapy indicated
T2-4N0-3 or T1N+	• Gastrectomy and regional LND • Adjuvant CHT and RT indicated for T2-T4 or lymph node positive disease • Per INT 0116: 45 Gy/25 fx starting on day 29 of CHT (five cycles of bolus 5-FU/LCV)
T4N0-3	• Gastrectomy and regional lymph node dissection • Adjuvant CHT and RT • Bulk of disease may prompt consideration of neoadjuvant CHT alone (ECF) or neoadjuvant CHT (5-FU and LCV) with RT (45 Gy/25 fx) for downstaging, followed by gastrectomy and regional LND
M1	• Palliative CHT and/or RT

EPIDEMIOLOGY: Gastric cancer has estimated incidence of 26,370 cases and estimated 10,730 deaths in the United States in 2016. Gastric cancer is the 15th leading cause of cancer death in the United States and 4th leading cause of cancer death worldwide. It is most common in East Asia (China, Japan, Korea, and Taiwan), with lowest incidence in the United States and Canada. In the United States, most common location is within proximal stomach (gastroesophageal junction [GEJ] and cardia).[1]

RISK FACTORS: Increased salt intake, salt-preserved foods (salted fish, cured meat, and salted vegetables), nitrates, smoked and processed meats, fried food, low consumption of fruits and vegetables, and low vitamin A and C.[2-4] Obesity (BMI ≥25, OR 1.22).[5] Smoking[6] and pathogens such as Helicobacter pylori and Epstein–Barr virus.[7,8] Hereditary syndromes due to hereditary diffuse gastric cancer (HDGC), gastric adenocarcinoma, and proximal polyposis of stomach (GAPPS), and familial intestinal gastric cancer (FIGC) represent about 1% to 3% of cases.[9]

ANATOMY

Stomach: Starts at GEJ (40–45 cm from incisions) and ends at pylorus. There are three main parts: fundus/cardia, body, and antrum/pylorus. There are five layers of stomach (starting from luminal surface): mucosa, submucosa, muscularis (outer longitudinal, middle circular, inner oblique), subserosa, and serosa. Gastric submucosal plexus is rich and carcinoma can spread superficially along stomach to esophagus, which also has rich submucosal plexus. Access to subserosal channels allows distal tumor spread to duodenum via subserosal lymphatic plexus.

Vascular: Vascular supply is derived from **celiac axis**, which is composed of three branches (Table 31.2).

TABLE 31.2: Vascular Supply of Stomach		
Celiac axis	Branches	Supply
Left gastric	-	Lesser curvature/right portion of stomach
Common hepatic	Right gastric	Lesser curvature/inferior right stomach
	Right gastroepiploic	Greater curvature
Splenic	Left gastroepiploic	Upper portion of greater curvature
	Short gastrics	Fundus/proximal stomach

Lymphatics: Japanese Research Society for Gastric Cancer (JRSGC) proposed 16 regional lymph node stations for stomach in 1963. See Table 31.3. N1/2 lymph node stations are considered regional and N3/4 are considered distant.[10]

PATHOLOGY: Adenocarcinoma is the most common histology (90%–95%) and MALT lymphoma is the second most common. Rare histologies include leiomyosarcoma (2%), carcinoid (1%), adenoacanthoma (1%), and squamous cell carcinoma (1%).

Lauren histological classification: There are two distinct types of adenocarcinoma (intestinal and diffuse types). Intestinal type is more likely to be associated with environmental exposures (H. pylori, chronic gastritis, tobacco, diet), is more prevalent in high-incidence areas, and has better prognosis. Diffuse type (also known as "linitis plastic") tends to present as diffuse involvement of gastric mucosa, is characterized by organized clusters of signet ring (mucin-rich) cells, is more predominant in younger women, and is associated with poorer prognosis.[11]

Siewert classification of GEJ tumors (based on location): Class I: arises from metaplasia of distal esophagus and invades distally into stomach; Class II: arises from gastric cardia; Class III: arises from subcardia and invades proximally into esophagus.[12]

Bormann classification: Class I: polypoid/fungating; Class II: ulcerative with raised borders; Class III: ulceration with invasion into gastric wall; Class IV: diffuse infiltration (linitis plastic).[13]

GENETICS: Her2-positivity was seen in 22% of pts screened for ToGA trial.[14]

SCREENING: Observational studies suggest screening in high-incidence areas may reduce gastric cancer mortality; however, there is no randomized data to support this finding.[15,16] Population-based screening has been implemented in Japan, Korea, Venezuela, and Chile, though screening intervals and modalities vary, and randomized data has not established optimal program.[15,17,18] In Japan, universal screening is recommended for all individuals >50 years of age with upper endoscopy every 2 to 3 years or double-contrast barium study every year. Alternatively, in Korea, upper endoscopy is recommended every 2 years for those 40 to 75 years of age.[19] In the United States, screening can be considered for pts with atrophic gastritis, pernicious anemia, gastric adenomas, Barrett's esophagus, and familial gastric cancer syndromes.

CLINICAL PRESENTATION: Symptoms include weight loss, epigastric pain, nausea, vomiting, anorexia, dysphagia, early satiety, melena, weakness. Characteristic physical exam findings include palpable stomach, succussion splash, palpable lymphadenopathy: Virchow's node (left supraclavicular), Irish's node (left axillary node), Sister Mary Joseph node (periumbilical node), Blumer's shelf (rectal shelf), Krukenberg tumor (metastatic deposit to ovary).

WORKUP: H&P.

Labs: CBC, CMP.

Imaging: Includes CT chest, abdomen, pelvis with IV and oral contrast. Consider PET/CT in absence of M1 disease on CT scans.

Pathology: Esophagogastroduodenoscopy (EGD) with biopsies (six–eight biopsies should be obtained), and endoscopic ultrasound to assess for tumor invasion and lymph node staging. Diagnostic laparoscopy to assess peritoneal cavity prior to surgery is indicated for clinical stage T1b and higher.[20] Obtain Her2-Neu status if metastatic.

PROGNOSTIC FACTORS: Poor KPS, advanced T and N stage, subtotal resection or gross residual disease (R2>R1>R0), diffuse type histology are all poor prognostic features.[21] Retrospective multicenter study from Italy demonstrated that pts with 0, 1 to 3, 4 to 6, and >6 lymph nodes had 10-yr OS after surgery of 92%, 82%, 73%, and 27%, respectively.[21] Metabolic response (≥35% decrease in PET SUV max) after neoadjuvant CHT is associated with improved MS.[22]

NATURAL HISTORY: Majority of pts (90%) present with locally advanced or metastatic disease, with 80% presenting with nodal metastases, 40% peritoneal metastases, and 30% liver metastases, for which prognosis is poor. Patients with early-stage gastric cancer (≤T1bN0) have excellent outcomes: 5-yr OS of 100% with mucosal invasion and 80% to 90% with submucosal involvement.[23]

STAGING: Cancers with midpoint in lower thoracic esophagus, GEJ, or within proximal 5 cm of stomach *and* extending to GE junction or esophagus are staged as *esophageal neoplasms*. Cancers with midpoint in stomach >5 cm distal to GEJ or within 5 cm of GEJ, but *not* involving GEJ or esophagus are staged as gastric cancer. AJCC is based on number of nodes, whereas JRSGC is based on anatomic location. Positive peritoneal cytology is defined as pM1.

TABLE 31.3: AJCC 8th ed. (2017) Gastric Cancer Staging[24]						
T/M	N	cN0	cN1	cN2	cN3a	cN3b
T1	a Lamina propria or muscularis mucosae	I		IIA		
	b Submucosa	I		IIA		
T2	• Muscularis propria	I		IIA		
T3	• Subserosal connective tissue	IIB		III		
T4	a Visceral peritoneum	IIB		III		
	b Adjacent organs	IVA				
M1	• Distant metastasis	IVB				
cN1, 1-2 regional LNs; cN2, 3-6 regional LNs; cN3a, 7-15 regional LNs; cN3b, ≥16 regional LNs.						

TREATMENT PARADIGM

Surgery: Surgery is mainstay of therapy, which includes endoscopic resection (small subset of pts), partial or total gastrectomy. Endoscopic resection includes endoscopic mucosal resection and endoscopic submucosal dissection, both shown in retrospective data to have high rate of local control in appropriately selected pts.[25] Optimal selection criteria for endoscopic resection are evolving, with routine features being high likelihood of en bloc resection, intestinal type histology, tumor limited to mucosa, no LVSI, and tumor size <2 cm without ulceration.[26-28]

Survival is similar between partial and total gastrectomy in setting of satisfactory margins, with partial gastrectomy associated with improved nutritional status and quality of life, except in proximal lesions, in which partial gastrectomy was associated with higher rates of reflux and anastomotic stenosis compared to total gastrectomy.[29,30] Therefore, total gastrectomy is typically utilized for lesions in upper third of stomach and partial gastrectomy is utilized for lesions in lower two-thirds.[30] Total gastrectomy involves esophagojejunostomy with Roux-en-Y anastomosis to prevent reflux of bile and pancreatic fluid. Billroth I is end-to-end gastrojejunal anastomosis using gastric resection margin. Billroth II is end-to-side gastrojejunal anastomosis, with closure of duodenal stump and lesser curvature (gastric resection margin not used for anastomosis). Complications include anastomotic failure, bleeding, ileus, B-12 deficiency, dumping syndrome, and reflux.

Lymph node dissection (LND): Extent of LND is controversial, but it is recommended that at least 15 lymph nodes be resected for adequate staging. See Table 31.4 for data regarding extent of LND. Gastrectomy with D2 LND is standard of care in eastern Asia.[31]

JRSGC Nodal stations		
N1	1	Right Cardia
	2	Left Cardia
	3	Lesser Curvature
	4	Greater Curvature
	5	Suprapyloric
	6	Infrapyloric
N2	7	Left gastric artery
	8	Common hepatic artery
	9	Celiac axis
	10	Splenic hila
	11	Splenic artery
N3	12	Hepatoduodenal lig.
	13	Post. Pancreatic head
	14	Mesenteric root
N4	15	Transverse mesocolon
	16	Paraaortic

TABLE 31.4: Definition of Extent of Lymph Node Dissection for Gastric Cancer	
D0	No LND
D1	JRSGC N1 nodes
D2	D1 dissection + JRSGC N2 nodes with distal pancreatectomy and splenectomy
D3	D2 dissection + JRSGC N3 nodes
D4	D3 dissection + JRSGC N4 nodes

Chemotherapy: GASTRIC meta-analysis demonstrated OS benefit of about 6% with use of 5-FU based CHT in adjuvant setting compared to surgery alone.[32] Standard options in the United States are either peri-operative epirubicin, cisplatin, and 5-FU (ECF) as per MAGIC trial[33] or adjuvant CHT with bolus 5-FU and leucovorin (LCV) concurrent with RT as per INT 0116.[34] 5-FU is inhibitor of thymidylate synthase. LCV is derivative of tetrahydrofolate and enhances effect of 5-FU. ToGA trial demonstrated OS benefit to trastuzumab in addition to standard CHT (5-FU or capecitabine with cisplatin, 13.8 vs. 11.1 months; $p = .0046$) for locally advanced, recurrent, or metastatic and inoperable Her-2 Neu amplified cancers of GEJ and stomach.[14]

Radiation

Indications: Indications for adjuvant RT include T2-4, node-positive disease, or positive margins. Preoperative RT is option for borderline resectable or definitive RT for unresectable disease.

Dose: Dosing for adjuvant RT is 45 Gy/25 fx. Consider 5.4 to 5.9 Gy boost for positive margins or gross residual disease.[20] Tumor bed is covered and coverage of gastric remnant is dependent on risk and organs at risk. Lymph node coverage in adjuvant setting is dependent on anatomic site of primary (see the following). Can consider omission of nodal coverage in pts with T2-3N0 and >15 lymph nodes removed.[35-37]

Perigastric lymph nodes: Always covered, except for proximal T1-2aN0 pts with negative margins >5 cm and 10 to 15 LNs removed.

Celiac and suprapancreatic lymph nodes: Cover for T4, N+, or T3N0 with <15 LN resected.

Porta-hepatic LN: Cover all T4 or N+, except proximal lesions with only one to two involved LN and >15 LN resected.

Splenic LN: Cover for all T4 or N+, except distal lesions with only one to two involved LN and >15 LN resected.

Distal paraesophageal LN: Lesions with esophageal extension.

Toxicity: Acute: Fatigue, nausea, vomiting, diarrhea, gastritis/esophagitis. Late: Stricture, renal insufficiency, second malignancy.

Procedure: See *Treatment Planning Handbook*, Chapter 7.[38]

EVIDENCE-BASED Q&A

What is the optimal extent of LND?

It is recommended that at least 15 lymph nodes be dissected for satisfactory staging with NCCN recommending D2 dissection. However, extent of LND is controversial. There are four randomized clinical trials and meta-analysis demonstrating no survival advantage and higher postoperative morbidity and mortality with extensive LND.[39–42] *On the other hand, several nonrandomized clinical trials have suggested improvement in survival with more radical LND.*[29,43]

Bonenkamp, Dutch Gastric Cancer Group (*NEJM* 1999, PMID 10089184): Prospective randomized trial (PRT) of 711 pts with gastric cancer undergoing curative resection were randomized to D1 LND (N = 380) or D2 LND (N = 331). Patients who received D2 LND had significantly higher rates of postoperative complications compared to D1 LND (43% vs. 25%; *p* < .001) and postoperative deaths (10% vs. 4%; *p* = .004). 5-yr OS was similar between two groups (45% vs. 47%), for D1 and D2 LND, respectively. **Conclusion: D2 LND resulted in significantly higher toxicity and no survival benefit compared to D1 LND.**

Is there benefit to neoadjuvant CHT compared to surgery alone?

There are two PRTs (MAGIC/FFCD), which demonstrate significant survival benefit with use of neoadjuvant CHT compared to surgery alone, while EORTC 40954 demonstrated no survival benefit.[44] *Neoadjuvant CHT may be particularly beneficial in pts at high risk of developing distant metastases (T3/T4 tumors, high clinical nodal burden, diffuse histology).*

Cunningham, MAGIC (*NEJM* 2006, PMID 16822992): PRT of 503 pts with stage II-IV (M0) potentially resectable adenocarcinoma of stomach (74%), GEJ (11%), or lower third of esophagus (14%) randomized to either surgery alone or preoperative epirubicin 50 mg/m^2, cisplatin 60 mg/m^2, 5-FU 200 mg/m^2/day for three cycles, surgery, and postoperative ECF for three cycles. Extent of LND was at discretion of surgeon. MFU was 4 years. See Table 31.5. There was no significant difference in postoperative complications (45% vs. 46%) for perioperative CHT and surgery alone, respectively.

Ychou, French FFCD/FNCLCC Trial (*JCO* 2011, PMID 21444866): PRT of 224 pts with resectable adenocarcinoma of stomach, GEJ, lower third of esophagus randomized to either surgery alone or perioperative cisplatin 100 mg/m^2 on day 1 and 5-FU 800 mg/m^2, on days 1 to 5 for two to three cycles every 28 days, surgery, and same postoperative CHT for three or four cycles. See Table 31.5. On multivariable analysis (MVA), perioperative CHT (*p* = .01) and stomach tumor location (*p* < .01) were favorable prognostic factors. Perioperative CHT significantly improved R0 resection rate (84% vs. 73%; *p* = .04) and postoperative morbidity was similar between two groups.

TABLE 31.5: Neoadjuvant/Perioperative CHT Phase III Trials in Gastric Cancer						
Trial	N	CHT	R0 resection	Local recurrence	Distant Metastasis	OS
MAGIC Perioperative CHT Surgery	250 253	Epirubicin/ Cisplatin/5-FU	69% 66%	14% 21%	24% 37%	5-yr 36%* 23%*
FFCD/FNCLCC Perioperative CHT Surgery	113 111	Cisplatin/5-FU	87%* 74%*	24% 26%	42% 56%	5-yr 38%* 24%*
EORTC 40954 Neoadjuvant CHT Surgery	72 72	Cisplatin/5-FU/ LCV	82%* 67%*	-	-	2-yr 72.7% 69.9%
*Statistically significant.						

Xiong, China (*Cancer Invest* 2014, PMID 24800782): Meta-analysis that included the preceding three trials and nine other PRT (n = 1,820) comparing variety of neoadjuvant CHT regimens versus surgery alone for resectable gastric and GEJ cancer. **Conclusion: Neoadjuvant CHT was associated with significantly improved OS (OR 1.32, *p* = .01),**

3-yr PFS (OR 1.85, $p < .0001$), and R0 resection (OR 1.38, $p = .01$), with no significant increase in operative complications, perioperative morality, or grade 3 or 4 adverse effects.

Is there benefit to neoadjuvant CHT and RT?

The impact of RT, in addition to neoadjuvant CHT, is unclear but Stahl and RTOG 9904 suggest some benefit. TOPGEAR trial, which is currently accruing, will assess neoadjuvant ECF with RT + adjuvant ECF versus neoadjuvant and adjuvant ECF alone.

Stahl, Germany (*JCO* 2009, PMID 19139439): PRT of 354 pts with locally advanced adenocarcinoma of lower third of esophagus or gastric cardia undergoing surgery randomized to induction CHT for 15 weeks (cisplatin, 5-FU, LCV) followed by surgery or induction CHT for 13 weeks followed by concurrent CHT (cisplatin and etoposide) and RT (30 Gy/15 fx) followed by surgery. Neoadjuvant chemoRT demonstrated higher rate of pCR (15.6% vs. 2%) and N0 status (64.6% vs. 37.7%), compared to neoadjuvant CHT alone. Three-yr OS was (47.7% vs. 27.7%; $p = .07$) for neoadjuvant chemoRT and neoadjuvant CHT, respectively. **Conclusion: Neoadjuvant chemoRT had higher pCR and trend toward improved survival, though not statistically significant compared to neoadjuvant CHT alone.**

Ajani, RTOG 9904 (*JCO* 2006, PMID 16921048): Phase II trial of 49 pts with potentially resectable T2-3NxM0 gastric adenocarcinoma treated with induction CHT (cisplatin, 5-FU, LCV) for two cycles, followed by concurrent CHT (5-FU, paclitaxel) and RT (45 Gy/25 fx) and then surgery (D2 LND recommended). pCR was 26% and R0 resection was obtained in 77% of pts. One-yr OS was 82% for pts who had pCR and 69% for pts who had less than pCR. **Conclusion: Neoadjuvant chemoRT had 26% pCR rate, which may be associated with higher OS.**

Is there benefit to adjuvant CHT compared to surgery alone?

The role of adjuvant CHT is unclear for Western pts, as trials performed in European populations have not shown survival benefit (GOIRC/GOIM). Only one trial (ACTS-GC) has demonstrated OS benefit in Japanese population, while CLASSIC trial demonstrated DFS benefit in pts from South Korea, China, and Taiwan. Summary of these trials is provided in Table 31.6.

TABLE 31.6: Summary of Adjuvant CHT Trials in Gastric Cancer					
Trial	N	CHT	LRR	DM	OS
ACTS-GC Adjuvant CHT Surgery	 529 530	Tegafur/gimeracil/oteracil	 8% 13%	 26% 32%	5-yr 72%* 61%*
GOIM Adjuvant CHT Surgery	 112 113	Epirubicin/LCV/5-FU/etoposide	- 	- 	5-yr 41% 34%
GOIRC Adjuvant CHT Surgery	 130 128	Epirubicin/LCV/5-FU/cisplatin	- 	- 	5-yr 48% 49%
CLASSIC Adjuvant CHT Surgery	 520 515	Oxaliplatin/capecitabine	- 	- 	3-yr DFS 74%* 60%*
*Statistically significant.					

Sakuramoto, ACTS-GC (*NEJM* 2007, PMID 17978289): PRT of 1,059 pts with stage II-III gastric cancer who underwent surgical resection with D2 LND randomized to observation versus 1 year of oral S-1 (combination of tegafur, gimeracil, and oteracil). Median follow-up was 3 years. Ninety-five percent of pts had D2 LND and 5% had D3 LND. OS at 3 years was significantly higher with adjuvant CHT compared to observation (80.1% vs. 70.1%; p = .002). **Conclusion: Adjuvant CHT with oral S-1 had significant overall survival benefit in East Asian population of pts who underwent D2 LND.**

GASTRIC Group Meta-analysis (*JAMA* 2010, PMID 20442389): Meta-analysis of 17 PRTs comparing surgery alone versus surgery and adjuvant CHT in pts with resectable gastric cancer. Adjuvant CHT was associated with significant PFS benefit (HR 0.82; p < .001) and 5-year OS benefit (55.3% vs. 49.6%; p < .001). **Conclusion: Adjuvant CHT was shown to provide survival benefit compared to surgery alone.**

Is there benefit to adjuvant chemoRT compared to surgery alone?

In the United States, for pts undergoing surgery first, adjuvant chemoRT is preferred.

MacDonald, INT0116 (*NEJM* 2001, PMID 11547741; Update Smalley *JCO* 2012, PMID 22585691): PRT of 556 pts with stage IB-IV (M0) gastric cancer or GEJ adenocarcinoma with R0 resection randomized to surgery alone versus surgery followed by adjuvant chemoRT. CHT was bolus 5-FU 425 mg/m^2 and LCV 20 mg/m^2/day on days 1 to 5 for two cycles. RT was 45 Gy/25 fx and was started on day 1 of cycle 2 with 5-FU dose reduced to 400 mg/m^2 during RT and cycle 3 as 5-FU alone. After completion of RT, bolus 5-FU and LCV was given for two more cycles. Median follow-up was 5 years. See Table 31.7. D0 LND (54%), D1 LND (36%), and D2 LND (10%). 69% were T3-4 and 85% N+. With MFU >10 years, OS remained significantly improved with chemoRT (HR 1.32, p = .0046) and there was benefit in all subsets except diffuse histology.

TABLE 31.7: Results of INT0116 Adjuvant ChemoRT for Gastric Cancer						
	3-yr RFS	Median DFS	DM	LRR	MS	3-yr OS
Surgery	31%	19 months	18%	29%	27 months	41%
Surgery + Adjuvant chemoRT	48%	30 months	33%	19%	36 months	50%
***p* value**	<.001	<.001	NS		.006	.005

Is there benefit to adjuvant chemoRT compared to adjuvant CHT alone?

This is unclear. ARTIST trial demonstrated trend to DFS benefit in pts who had R0 resection with D2 LND. Subset analysis demonstrated DFS benefit in N+ or intestinal-type histology pts. ARTIST II trial is currently accruing to evaluate adjuvant CHT versus adjuvant chemoRT.

Lee, ARTIST Trial (*JCO* 2015, PMID 25559811): PRT of 458 pts with R0 resection and D2 LND randomized to adjuvant capecitabine and cisplatin (XP) for six cycles or capecitabine and cisplatin for two cycles followed by RT (45 Gy/25 fx) with capecitabine, followed by capecitabine and cisplatin for two cycles. OS was similar between two groups. Subgroup analysis demonstrated that addition of XRT to XP significantly improved 3-yr DFS for pts with node-positive disease (76% vs. 72%, p = .04) and intestinal histology (94% vs. 83%, p = .01). **Conclusion: Adjuvant chemoRT did not significantly improve DFS and OS compared to adjuvant CHT alone.** *Comment: There may be subset of pts with N+ and intestinal type histology who have DFS benefit from adjuvant chemoRT.*

Verheji, CRITICS (*ASCO* 2016, Abstract 4000): PRT of 788 pts from Netherlands, Denmark, and Sweden with stage IB-IV (M0) gastric cancer who received neoadjuvant CHT (epirubicin, capecitabine, and cisplatin or oxaliplatin: ECX or EOX) for three cycles and resection with D2 dissection, then randomized to three cycles of ECX/EOX or chemoRT (45 Gy/25 fx with weekly cisplatin and capecitabine). See Table 31.8. 87% of pts had ≥D1 LND and removal of median 20 lymph nodes. Only 47% of pts completed adjuvant CHT and 55% completed adjuvant chemoRT.

TABLE 31.8: Results of CRITICS Gastric Cancer Trial

	5-yr OS	≥Grade 3 GI toxicity
CHT + Surgery + Adjuvant CHT	41%	37%
CHT + Surgery + Adjuvant chemoRT	41%	42%
p value	.99	.14

REFERENCES

1. PDQ Adult Treatment Editorial Board. *PDQ Gastric Cancer Treatment.* Bethesda, MD: National Cancer Institute. Updated February 2, 2017. https://www.cancer.gov/types/stomach/hp/stomach-treatment-pdq
2. Kono S, Hirohata T. Nutrition and stomach cancer. *Cancer Causes Control.* 1996;7(1):41–55.
3. Gonzalez CA, Jakszyn P, Pera G, et al. Meat intake and risk of stomach and esophageal adenocarcinoma within the European Prospective Investigation Into Cancer and Nutrition (EPIC). *J Natl Cancer Inst.* 2006;98(5):345–354.
4. Zhu H, Yang X, Zhang C, et al. Red and processed meat intake is associated with higher gastric cancer risk: a meta-analysis of epidemiological observational studies. *PloS One.* 2013;8(8):e70955.
5. Yang P, Zhou Y, Chen B, et al. Overweight, obesity and gastric cancer risk: results from a meta-analysis of cohort studies. *Eur J Cancer.* 2009;45(16):2867–2873.
6. Ladeiras-Lopes R, Pereira AK, Nogueira A, et al. Smoking and gastric cancer: systematic review and meta-analysis of cohort studies. *Cancer Causes Control.* 2008;19(7):689–701.
7. Fox JG, Dangler CA, Taylor NS, King A, Koh TJ, Wang TC. High-salt diet induces gastric epithelial hyperplasia and parietal cell loss, and enhances Helicobacter pylori colonization in C57BL/6 mice. *Cancer Res.* 1999;59(19):4823–4828.
8. Boysen T, Mohammadi M, Melbye M, et al. EBV-associated gastric carcinoma in high- and low-incidence areas for nasopharyngeal carcinoma. *Br J Cancer.* 2009;101(3):530–533.
9. Oliveira C, Pinheiro H, Figueiredo J, et al. Familial gastric cancer: genetic susceptibility, pathology, and implications for management. *Lancet Oncol.* 2015;16(2):e60–e70.
10. Moron FE, Szklaruk J. Learning the nodal stations in the abdomen. *Br J Radiol.* 2007;80(958):841–848.
11. Correa P. Human gastric carcinogenesis: a multistep and multifactorial process—first American Cancer Society Award Lecture on Cancer Epidemiology and Prevention. *Cancer Res.* 1992;52(24):6735–6740.
12. Siewert JR, Holscher AH, Becker K, Gossner W. [Cardia cancer: attempt at a therapeutically relevant classification]. *Der Chirurg; Zeitschrift fur alle Gebiete der operativen Medizen.* 1987;58(1):25–32.
13. Hu B, El Hajj N, Sittler S, et al. Gastric cancer: classification, histology and application of molecular pathology. *J Gastrointest Oncol.* 2012;3(3):251–261.
14. Bang YJ, Van Cutsem E, Feyereislova A, et al. Trastuzumab in combination with chemotherapy versus chemotherapy alone for treatment of HER2-positive advanced gastric or gastro-oesophageal junction cancer (ToGA): a phase 3, open-label, randomised controlled trial. *Lancet.* 2010;376(9742):687–697.
15. Mizoue T, Yoshimura T, Tokui N, et al. Prospective study of screening for stomach cancer in Japan. *Int J Cancer.* 2003;106(1):103–107.
16. Kunisaki C, Ishino J, Nakajima S, et al. Outcomes of mass screening for gastric carcinoma. *Ann Surg Oncol.* 2006;13(2):221–228.
17. Llorens P. Gastric cancer mass survey in Chile. *Semin Surg Oncol.* 1991;7(6):339–343.
18. Pisani P, Oliver WE, Parkin DM, et al. Case-control study of gastric cancer screening in Venezuela. *Br J Cancer.* 1994;69(6):1102–1105.
19. Choi IJ. Endoscopic gastric cancer screening and surveillance in high-risk groups. *Clin Endosc.* 2014;47(6):497–503.
20. National Comprehensive Cancer Network. Gastric Cancer (Version 3.2017). https://www.nccn.org/professionals/physician_gls/pdf/gastric_blocks.pdf

21. Roviello F, Rossi S, Marrelli D, et al. Number of lymph node metastases and its prognostic significance in early gastric cancer: a multicenter Italian study. *J Surg Oncol*. 2006;94(4):275–280; discussion 274.

22. Lordick F, Ott K, Krause BJ, et al. PET to assess early metabolic response and to guide treatment of adenocarcinoma of the oesophagogastric junction: the MUNICON Phase II trial. *Lancet Oncol*. 2007;8(9):797–805.

23. Okada K, Fujisaki J, Yoshida T, et al. Long-term outcomes of endoscopic submucosal dissection for undifferentiated-type early gastric cancer. *Endoscopy*. 2012;44(2):122–127.

24. Amin MB, Edge S, Greene F, et al, (Eds.). *AJCC Cancer Staging Manual*. 8th ed. New York, NY: Springer Publishing; 2017.

25. Takekoshi T, Baba Y, Ota H, et al. Endoscopic resection of early gastric carcinoma: results of a retrospective analysis of 308 cases. *Endoscopy*. 1994;26(4):352–358.

26. Soetikno R, Kaltenbach T, Yeh R, Gotoda T. Endoscopic mucosal resection for early cancers of the upper gastrointestinal tract. *J Clin Oncol*. 2005;23(20):4490–4498.

27. Min YW, Min BH, Lee JH, Kim JJ. Endoscopic treatment for early gastric cancer. *World J Gastroenterol*. 2014;20(16):4566–4573.

28. Gotoda T. Endoscopic resection of early gastric cancer: the Japanese perspective. *Curr Opin Gastroenterol*. 2006;22(5):561–569.

29. Bozzetti F, Marubini E, Bonfanti G, et al. Subtotal versus total gastrectomy for gastric cancer: five-year survival rates in a multicenter randomized Italian trial. Italian Gastrointestinal Tumor Study Group. *Ann Surg*. 1999;230(2):170–178.

30. Pu YW, Gong W, Wu YY, et al. Proximal gastrectomy versus total gastrectomy for proximal gastric carcinoma. A meta-analysis on postoperative complications, 5-year survival, and recurrence rate. *Saudi Med J*. 2013;34(12):1223–1228.

31. Degiuli M, De Manzoni G, Di Leo A, et al. Gastric cancer: current status of lymph node dissection. *World J Gastroenterol*. 2016;22(10):2875–2893.

32. Group G, Paoletti X, Oba K, et al. Benefit of adjuvant chemotherapy for resectable gastric cancer: a meta-analysis. *JAMA*. 2010;303(17):1729–1737.

33. Cunningham D, Allum WH, Stenning SP, et al. Perioperative chemotherapy versus surgery alone for resectable gastroesophageal cancer. *N Engl J Med*. 2006;355(1):11–20.

34. Macdonald JS, Smalley SR, Benedetti J, et al. Chemoradiotherapy after surgery compared with surgery alone for adenocarcinoma of the stomach or gastroesophageal junction. *N Engl J Med*. 2001;345(10):725–730.

35. Tepper JE, Gunderson LL. Radiation treatment parameters in the adjuvant postoperative therapy of gastric cancer. *Semin Radiat Oncol*. 2002;12(2):187–195.

36. Smalley SR, Gunderson L, Tepper J, et al. Gastric surgical adjuvant radiotherapy consensus report: rationale and treatment implementation. *Int J Radiat Oncol Biol Phys*. 2002;52(2):283–293.

37. Wo JY, Yoon SS, Guimaraes AR, et al. Gastric lymph node contouring atlas: a tool to aid in clinical target volume definition in 3-dimensional treatment planning for gastric cancer. *Pract Radiat Oncol*. 2013;3(1):e11–e19.

38. Videtic GMM, Woody N, Vassil AD. *Handbook of Treatment Planning in Radiation Oncology*. 2nd ed. New York, NY: Demos Medical; 2015.

39. Bonenkamp JJ, Hermans J, Sasako M, et al. Extended lymph-node dissection for gastric cancer. *N Engl J Med*. 1999;340(12):908–914.

40. Cuschieri A, Weeden S, Fielding J, et al. Patient survival after D1 and D2 resections for gastric cancer: long-term results of the MRC randomized surgical trial. Surgical Co-operative Group. *Br J Cancer*. 1999;79(9–10):1522–1530.

41. Sasako M, Sano T, Yamamoto S, et al. D2 lymphadenectomy alone or with para-aortic nodal dissection for gastric cancer. *N Engl J Med*. 2008;359(5):453–462.

42. Seevaratnam R, Bocicariu A, Cardoso R, et al. A meta-analysis of D1 versus D2 lymph node dissection. *Gastric Cancer*. 2012;15(Suppl 1):S60–S69.

43. Schwarz RE, Smith DD. Clinical impact of lymphadenectomy extent in resectable gastric cancer of advanced stage. *Ann Surg Oncol*. 2007;14(2):317–328.

44. Schuhmacher C, Gretschel S, Lordick F, et al. Neoadjuvant chemotherapy compared with surgery alone for locally advanced cancer of the stomach and cardia: European Organisation for Research and Treatment of Cancer randomized trial 40954. *J Clin Oncol*. 2010;28(35):5210–5218.

32: **HEPATOCELLULAR CARCINOMA**

Neil McIver Woody and Kevin L. Stephans

QUICK HIT: Hepatocellular carcinoma (HCC) is associated with liver disease, particularly hepatitis B and C. Screening of pts with chronic HBV infection and those with cirrhosis for select other causes may result in early detection and better outcomes. Diagnosis may be either pathologic or based on AFP and imaging characteristics. Pts are staged according to Barcelona Clinic Liver Cancer staging system and early tumors are treated with surgical resection or liver transplantation if within Milan criteria. Pts with multiple tumors, larger tumors, or reduced functional status may be treated with focal therapies including radiofrequency ablation (RFA), transarterial chemoembolization (TACE), radioembolization (Y90), or RT (proton or SBRT). Pts with advanced disease may be candidates for sorafenib, which has been shown to improve OS in advanced disease.

EPIDEMIOLOGY: HCC is the second leading cause of cancer death worldwide in men and sixth leading cause of cancer death in women. In the United States, incidence of HCC is six cases per 100,000.[1] HCC is more common in areas with high rates of hepatitis B and C infection. Incidence has been increasing in the United States due to prevalence of hepatitis C infection.

RISK FACTORS: HCC is most strongly associated with liver inflammation and cirrhosis, and primarily related to hepatitis B and C viral infection, which are present in ~80% of cases. Treatment of viral infection has been shown to reduce future cancer risk in HBV by 50% to 60%, while data are still emerging after treatment of HCV. Other risk factors include male gender (RR 2–3), diabetes (RR 2), smoking, hereditary hemochromatosis, alcohol use, chemical exposure, obesity, and exposure to environmental toxins including aflatoxin and microcystin.

ANATOMY: The liver is the largest solid organ in body, surrounded by peritoneal membrane (Glisson's capsule) and can be divided based on vasculature into eight segments. On the left numbering begins with caudate lobe (segment 1), followed by lateral (segments 2 and 3), and medial portion (segment IV). On the right numbering starts with anterior inferior segment (5) and moves in clockwise direction; posterior inferior, posterior superior, and anterior superior segments are numbered 6, 7, and 8 respectively. There are no anatomic borders between segments, and thus no barriers to intrahepatic spread of disease. Liver supplied by dual blood supply portal vein (75%) and hepatic artery.

PATHOLOGY: HCC can be diagnosed based on biopsy or combination of AFP and radiographic criteria alone (see the workup section). HCC can be conventional type, which is graded from I to IV based on presence of trabecular organization and nuclear appearance. Molecular markers including HepPar1, albumin, fibrinogen, a1-antitrypsin, and AFP and GPC-3 can help to confirm diagnosis. Approximately 1% of HCC are fibrolamellar type, which presents more commonly in young adults, and have more indolent growth pattern and more favorable prognosis.

SCREENING: The American Association of Liver Diseases (AASLD) has developed screening guidelines (updated 2010) for pts with chronic hepatitis B infection and/or cirrhosis.[2,3]

Recommendation is for surveillance with ultrasound every 6 mos for: all cirrhotic HBV carriers; noncirrhotic HBV carriers of Asian descent age >40 for males and >50 for females; all HBV carriers with family history of HCC or Africans age >20. In addition cirrhotic pts with HCV infection, alcoholic cirrhosis, hemochromatosis, and primary biliary cirrhosis should be screened. Finally all pts on transplant waiting list should be screened to ensure they do not develop HCC while awaiting transplant. For pts found to have lesion on ultrasound 3-month follow-up is recommended for lesions <1 cm while pts with larger lesions should receive four-phase CT or MRI to evaluate. A randomized trial[4] of 18,816 pts in China using AFP and ultrasound showed low compliance rate of 58.2% but achieved 37% reduction in HCC mortality (no equivalent U.S.-based study). NCCN guidelines recommend screening with AFP and ultrasound every 6 to 12 mos.[5]

CLINICAL PRESENTATION: HCC most commonly presents as asymptomatic disease except for symptoms related to pt's chronic liver disease. Pts may have mild to moderate abdominal pain, weight loss, early satiety, diarrhea, fever, and fatigue. It is important to be alert for signs and symptoms of decompensated cirrhosis including ascites, encephalopathy, jaundice, and variceal bleeding. Pts with HCC may present with paraneoplastic syndromes including erythrocytosis, hypercalcemia, hypoglycemia, and watery diarrhea. Paraneoplastic symptoms save for erythrocytosis are associated with worsened prognosis. HCC can be associated with cutaneous features including dermatomyositis, pemphigus foliaceus, sign of Leser–Trelat, pityriasis rotunda, porphyria cutanea tarda although these are not specific to HCC.

WORKUP: Detailed H&P including evaluation of prior liver disease and treatment history.

Labs: HBV and HCV serology and AFP. Evaluate liver function with complete metabolic panel for (bilirubin, albumin, liver transaminases), PT/INR for coagulation, renal function (BUN, creatinine) and blood counts (CBC).

Imaging: 4-phase CT or MRI to evaluate lesion, and biopsy as indicated. Phases must include hepatic arterial phase, portal venous phase, and delayed phase and may include precontrast phase as well. For cirrhotic (or other high-risk pts), multiple criteria have been suggested by AASLD, OPTN, EASL, and LI-RADS for lesions ≥1 cm (lesions <1 cm are indeterminate).[6–9] Features include arterial hyperenhancement, pseudocapsule, venous washout, and growth. Criteria do not apply to pts without risk factors for HCC. Note that lesions with vascular invasion may have different features. Complete systemic staging with CT of chest, abdomen, and pelvis. Bone scan if symptoms are present. PET/CT not recommended.

Pathology: Biopsy not necessary in most cases (if previous diagnostic criteria are met). Biopsy may be associated with small risk of tract seeding and in cases where indeterminate lesion is resectable, it may be preferable to resect for simultaneous diagnosis and cure.

PROGNOSTIC FACTORS: Tumor stage, functional status, Child–Pugh score (Table 32.1), and presence of metastatic disease are all prognostic of survival, which in some cases is more determined by cirrhosis than tumor.

TABLE 32.1: Child–Pugh Functional Status for Chronic Liver Disease			
Measure	1 point	2 points	3 points
Total bilirubin mg/dL	<2	2-3	>3
Serum albumin g/dL	>3.5	2.8–3.5	<2.8

(continued)

TABLE 32.1: Child–Pugh Functional Status for Chronic Liver Disease (*continued*)

Measure	1 point	2 points	3 points
Prothrombin time (s)	<4.0	4.0–6.0	>6.0
or			
INR	<1.7	1.7–2.3	>2.3
Ascites	None	Moderate	Severe
Encephalopathy	None	Grade I–II or suppressed with medication	Grade III or IV or refractory

Child–Pugh Scoring

Points	Class	2-yr OS
5–6	A	85%
7–9	B	57%
10–15	C	35%

STAGING: Although AJCC TNM staging system exists for HCC, most pts are typically staged according to Barcelona Clinic Liver Cancer Staging System (BCLC).[10] This staging system includes liver and pt functional status as well as tumor characteristics and is accompanied by recommended treatment strategy.

TABLE 32.2: Barcelona Clinic Liver Cancer Staging System (BCLC) for HCC

	Stage Characteristics	Suggested Treatment
Very early stage (0)	ECOG PS 0, Child–Pugh A, single lesion <2 cm	Resection
Early stage (A)	ECOG PS 0, Child–Pugh A-B, 1–3 <3 cm	Liver transplantation, radiofrequency ablation
Intermediate stage (B)	ECOG PS 0, Child–Pugh A-B, multiple nodules not meeting stage A	Transarterial chemoembolization (TACE)
Advanced stage (C)	ECOG PS 02, Child–Pugh A-B, portal invasion, nodal or distant metastasis	Sorafenib
Terminal stage (D)	ECOG PS >2 or Child–Pugh C	Supportive care

TABLE 32.3: AJCC 8th ed. Staging System for HCC

T/M		N	cN0	cN1
T1	a Solitary tumor ≤2 cm		IA	
	b Solitary tumor >2 cm without vascular invasion		IB	
T2	• Solitary tumor >2 cm with vascular invasion • Multiple tumors <5 cm		II	IVA
T3	• Multiple tumors, at least one >5 cm		IIIA	
T4	• Involvement of major branch of portal or hepatic vein • Direct invasion of adjacent organs (other than gall bladder) • Perforation of visceral peritoneum		IIIB	
M1	• Distant metastasis		IVB	

cN1, regional LNs.

TREATMENT PARADIGM: As per BCLC staging system, treatment is based on tumor, pt, and liver function. Surgical resection or transplantation is preferred as curative option for early-stage pts while nonsurgical options including radiofrequency ablation (RFA), Y_{90} embolization, TACE, and RT may be used for definitive treatment or as bridge to liver transplantation.[11–14] Systemic therapy is reserved for advanced disease.

Prevention: Vaccination of infants reduces rates of development of HBV infection and reduces incidence of development of HCC. Studies of universal vaccination in Taiwan beginning in 1984 revealed 50% decline in pediatric cases of HCC.[15] Similarly treatment of HBV and HCV should be undertaken in affected pts and precautions should be taken to avoid transmission.[5]

Surgery: For early-stage pts surgical resection is mainstay of cure. For very small early lesions partial hepatectomy can provide good rate of cure.[16] However, many pts are not candidates for partial hepatectomy based on tumor features or liver function. In such cases orthotopic liver transplantation may provide alternative. For pts without cirrhosis, partial hepatectomy has equivalent cure rates to liver transplantation.[17] Since liver transplant is also used for noncancer indications pts are carefully selected to receive liver on basis of Milan criteria defined as single tumor ≤5 cm or ≤3 tumors ≤3 cm, with no extrahepatic spread or macrovascular involvement. Following Milan criteria resulted in 5-yr OS of approximately 70%, and recurrence rate is less than 15%.[18] UCSF has validated expanded criteria for HCC: single lesion ≤6.5 cm in diameter or two lesions ≤4.5 cm with total tumor diameter ≤8 cm and demonstrated low rates of recurrence when expanded criteria were met.[19] Pts listed for transplantation are stratified based on risk of death MELD (model for end-stage liver disease) scoring system.[20] MELD score is equation based on creatinine, bilirubin, and INR and serves similar purpose to older Child–Pugh score. In addition, pts with HCC can be listed based on exception points reflecting risk that their tumor could progress and make them ineligible for transplantation. Number of points granted has changed over time to try to balance access to organs for cancer and noncancer transplant candidates. For example, United Network for Organ Sharing (UNOS) uses criteria of single HCC between 2 and 5 cm, or 2 to 3 lesions, none >3 cm and assigns MELD score of 22.

CHT: CHT is difficult to administer in pts with HCC who often have associated poor liver function. Multiple agents have been studied with small benefits at cost of significant toxicity. Randomized SHARP trial was completed comparing sorafenib to placebo in pts with advanced disease (not candidate for other surgical or locoregional therapies).[21] Sorafenib demonstrated significant improvement in MS from 7.9 to 10.7 mos. The radiographic response rate to sorafenib was 2% and pts on sorafenib had higher incidence of adverse events relative to placebo 80% versus 52%. Dosage of sorafenib is 400 mg BID.

RT

Indications: Traditionally, RT has played minor role in treatment of pts with HCC due to intrinsic sensitivity of liver itself. However, improved techniques including SBRT and proton therapy suggest that RT is feasible LC modality to treat HCC and in some situations may be preferable to other ablative techniques. Although comparative data are evolving, RT may be preferred to interventional techniques for those with vascular invasion, tumor thrombosis, inaccessible lesions or those with vascular shunting (see question on portal vein thrombosis in the following). RT to Child–Pugh C pts is not recommended and caution is necessary for Child–Pugh B.

Dose: Dose varies by technique. Three- and five-fraction regimens have been described up to 54–60 Gy/3 fx or 50 Gy/5 fx with dose reduction based on dose limits to normal liver.

Toxicity: Radiation-induced liver disease (RILD) is the most feared complication, occurring 1 to 2 mos after RT (range 0.5–8 mos). Two types: classic (fatigue, pain, hepatomegaly, anicteric ascites, elevated alkaline phosphatase but not AST/ALT) and nonclassic (jaundice, elevated ALT/AST). No effective treatment for RILD exists.[22]

Procedure: See *Treatment Planning Handbook*, Chapter 7.[11–13]

Radiofrequency Ablation (RFA): RFA is percutaneous or laparoscopic technique, which involves thermal ablation of lesion. One or more probes may be used to achieve optimal ablation. Larger lesions and difficult locations such as hepatic dome, caudate lobe, central biliary tree, proximal to major blood vessels, subcapsular location, abutting gall bladder, small bowel, kidney, and stomach can be problematic. Advantages include single-day treatment and high control rates particularly for small tumors.[23,24]

Embolization: Transarterial chemoembolization (TACE): Combines arterial embolization of tumor vasculature with infusion of chemotherapeutic agents, thereby increasing transit time of chemotherapeutic agent, and thus increasing apoptosis and necrosis. TACE is generally considered for pts with encapsulated lesions without vascular invasion or extrahepatic spread and preserved liver function. There is limited data for safety and efficacy of TACE in setting of portal vein thrombus. Previously pts can receive TACE or bland embolization but a randomized controlled trial of 112 pts comparing TACE to bland embolization and conservative treatment showed OS advantage to TACE over conservative treatment (HR 0.47 $p = .025$) and 2-yr OS was 63% with TACE, 50% with bland embolization, and 27% for control.[25] There is controversy regarding survival benefit of TACE as other randomized studies of TACE have not shown survival benefit over conservative management.[26] TACE can be given using either CHT mixed with lipiodol or on drug-eluting beads (DEB). Studies have not shown significant difference between conventional and DEB TACE. Chemotherapeutic agents employed included cisplatin, doxorubicin, and mitomycin C. 80% of pts undergoing TACE will develop post embolization syndrome which includes RUQ pain, nausea, ileus, fatigue, fever, and transaminitis lasting typically 3 to 4 days. As many as 15% of pts may develop irreversible hepatotoxicity.

Radioembolization: Yttrium-90 microspheres: Y-90 is pure β-emitter, with average energy ~1 MeV. Microspheres are delivered via hepatic artery as HCC receives significantly more blood flow from arterial system than portal system. Prior to radioembolization pts undergo pretreatment ^{99}mTc macro-aggregated albumin scan, which facilitates prediction of distribution of radioactive beads. If lung exposure ≥30 Gy is anticipated or if lung shunt fraction exceeds 20% or if significant GI tract dose is observed then catheter needs to be repositioned. If liver target cannot be isolated without significant shunting then procedure is contraindicated. Encephalopathy, Child–Pugh C status or biliary obstruction are other contraindications. Longitudinal cohort study of Y_{90} of 291 pts receiving 526 treatments revealed overall time to progression of 7.9 mos. Child-Pugh A pts had median survival of 17.2 mos compared to 7.7 mos for B pts, and Child-Pugh B pts with portal vein thrombus had median survival of 5.6 mos.[27] Y-90 may be particularly useful in setting of portal vein thrombus and prospective study of 30 pts was completed revealing MS of 13 mos. However, 13% developed grade II hepatobiliary toxicity and 17% required hospitalization.[28] Alternatively, iodine 131-labeled Lipiodol has also been employed for radioembolization.

EVIDENCE-BASED Q&A

What are key studies defining current role of SBRT for HCC?

Bujold, Princess Margaret Phase I & II (*JCO* 2013, PMID 23547075): Combined analysis of prospective phase I and phase II studies of liver SBRT in Canada. 102 pts with HCC unsuitable for TACE, RFA and surgery were enrolled and treated to doses of 24 to 54 Gy in 6 fx. 52% of pts had received prior liver directed therapy and 55% had tumor vascular thrombus. 1-yr LC was 87% and 30% of pts experienced grade III toxicity and 7 pts experienced possible grade V toxicity. MOS was 17 mos. OS was significantly worse in pts with tumor vascular thrombosis 42% versus 27%.

Sanuki, Japan (*Acta Oncol* 2014, PMID 23962244): RR from Japan of 185 pts with 277 HCC tumors not candidates for surgery or percutaneous ablative therapy treated with SBRT 35 (Child–Pugh B) or 40 Gy (Child–Pugh A) in 5 fx. MFU 24 mos. 3-yr LC and OS were 91% and 70% respectively. 13% of pts had grade III toxicity and 10.3% of pts experienced worsening of Child–Pugh score by two points.

Yoon, Korea (*PLoS One* 2013, PMID 24255719): Registry study of 93 pts treated with SBRT for HCC <6 cm not candidates for surgery or other percutaneous therapies, Child–Pugh or B, >2 cm from tumor or organs at risk. Dose was 30 to 60 Gy in 3 to 4 days. Pts with vascular invasion or extrahepatic metastases were excluded. MFU was 25.6 mos and 3-yr LC and OS were 92.1% and 53.8% respectively; 6.5% of pts experienced hepatic toxicity and one pt developed septic shock from fiducial placement. **Conclusion: SBRT is associated with high rate of LC and good OS. Toxicity rates are not trivial particularly in higher risk pts.**

Is SBRT safe in Child–Pugh B and C pts?

Select Child–Pugh B pts may be candidates.

Culleton, Princess Margaret (*Radiother Oncol* 2014, PMID 24906626): RR of 29 pts with Child–Pugh B (n = 28) and C (n = 1) pts treated to 30 Gy/6 fx. MS was 7.9 mos and for 16 pts with post-treatment liver function testing available, 63% of pts experienced decline in Child–Pugh index of two or more points at 3 mos. **Conclusion: SBRT is feasible in selected Child–Pugh B pts but data is lacking for Child–Pugh C pts.**

What are data for use of SBRT as bridge to liver transplantation?

Outcomes following transplantation in most series have been excellent.

O'Connor, Baylor University (*Liver Transpl* 2012, PMID 22467602): RR from Baylor of 10 pts with 11 tumors treated with 33 to 54 Gy/3 fx SBRT as bridge to transplant. Median tumor size was 3.4 cm and all pts proceeded to transplant after median transplant wait time of 163 days. MFU was 62 mos and all pts were alive and disease-free. Explant pathology revealed pCR to SBRT in 3 of 11 treated tumors.

Facciuto, Mount Sinai, (*J Surg Oncol* 2012, PMID 21960321): RR of 27 pts with 39 lesions listed for liver transplant treated with SBRT. Pts received 24 to 36 Gy in 2 to 5 fx with most pts receiving 28 Gy/4 fx. 17 pts (63%) proceeded to transplantation and 37% of tumors exhibited complete or partial response.

Andolino, Indiana University (*IJROBP* 2011, PMID 21645977): RR of 60 pts treated with SBRT for HCC confined to liver treated to 40 to 44 Gy in 3 to 5 fx. MFU was 27 mos. 2-yr LC and OS were 90% and 67% respectively. 23 pts (38.3%) proceeded on to transplantation. **Conclusion: SBRT is feasible as bridge to transplantation.**

What prospective evidence is available for conventional RT for HCC?

Mornex, French Phase II (*IJROBP* 2006, PMID 17145534): Prospective phase II trial of 66 Gy/33 fx for Child–Pugh A/B HCC one nodule <5 cm, or two nodules ≤3 cm not suitable for resection. 27 pts were enrolled and 25 were assessable. 92% of pts experienced treatment response including 80% complete response. 2 of 11 pts with Child–Pugh B disease had grade IV toxicity compared to 3 of 16 Child–Pugh pts developing grade

III toxicity. **Conclusion: Focal high-dose conventional RT is associated with excellent control rate for HCC.**

Can conventional RT or SBRT be combined with TACE to improve outcomes?

It appears safe and effective to give SBRT either combined with TACE or as salvage treatment.

Jacob, UAB (*HPB [Oxford]* 2015, PMID 25186290): RR of pts with HCC >3 cm treated with TACE (n = 124) versus TACE + SBRT 45 Gy/3 fx over 7 days (n = 37). LR was significantly lower in pts receiving TACE + SBRT 10.8% versus 25.8% p = .04. When censored for liver transplant TACE + SBRT pts exhibited higher overall survival than TACE alone pts.

Seong Korea Series (*IJROBP* 2003, PMID 12527045): RR of 158 pts with unresectable HCC treated with local RT combined with TACE. Mean RT dose of 48.2 in 1.8 Gy fx. Response rate was 67.1% with OS of 30.5% and 9% at 2 and 5 yrs, respectively from time of diagnosis.

Honda, Japan (*Hepatogastroenterology* 2014, PMID 24895789): RR of 28 HCC pts meeting Milan criteria treated with TACE followed by SBRT. 1-yr LC and OS were 96.3% and 92.6% respectively. No severe toxicities were noted.

Honda, Japan (*J Gastroenterol Hepatol* 2013, PMID 23216217): Case-control study of 30 pts treated with TACE followed by SBRT compared with 38 pts treated with TACE alone. No grade III events observed with combination of TACE and SBRT and DFS was improved from 4.2 mos to 15.7 mos with addition of SBRT to TACE. **Conclusion: It is feasible to give both conventional RT and SBRT after TACE.**

Can conventional RT or SBRT improve outcomes in setting of portal vein tumor and can it be safely combined with other treatments?

Zhang, China (*IJROBP* 2005, PMID 15667964): RR of 158 pts HCC with tumor thrombus including portal vein or IVC thrombus including pts receiving no therapy, TACE, resection, or RT 30 to 60 Gy. Use of RT was associated with improved survival with median survival for EBRT with or without additional therapies, TACE, resection, and conservative treatment of 8 vs. 5, 4, and 1 mos, respectively.

Kang, Beijing (*Mol Clin Oncol* 2014, PMID 24649306): Prospective study of 101 pts with HCC and portal vein tumor thrombus randomized to SBRT followed by TACE, TACE followed by SBRT and SBRT alone. SBRT was given in 6 fractions to total dose ranging from 21 to 60 Gy with median dose of 40.2 Gy. 1-yr local control trended toward improvement in SBRT followed by TACE 55.9% versus 48.6% with TACE followed by SBRT and 43.3% for SBRT alone. CR of tumor thrombus to SBRT was achieved in 17.8% of pts and partial response achieved in 52.5%. TACE followed by SBRT was associated with slightly higher rate of increase in Child–Pugh score of 40.5% compared to 32% and 30% in other arms. **Conclusion: Conventional RT and SBRT improve outcomes in HCC in portal vein thrombus and can be safely combined with TACE. It may be most advantageous to sequence SBRT followed by TACE to preserve liver function.**

What data is available to compare efficacy of ablative treatments for HCC?

Data comparing efficacy of numerous therapies are limited.

Lin, Taiwan (*Gut* 2005, PMID 16009687): PRT of 187 pts with HCC <3 cm randomized to RFA, ethanol ablation, or acetic acid embolization. RFA was associated with significantly higher 3-yr OS of 74% compared to ethanol and acetic acid 51% and 53% respectively. RFA was associated with 4.8% major complication rate compared to 0% in the other arms.

Wahl, Michigan (*JCO* 2016, PMID 26628466): RR of 224 pts treated with RFA (161 pts 250 tumors) or SBRT (63 pts, 83 tumors). Pts treated with SBRT had lower Child–Pugh scores and higher pretreatment AFP and more prior treatments. 1-yr freedom from local progression (FFLP) was increased with SBRT 97.4% versus 83.6%. Increasing size was associated with reduced control for RFA but not for SBRT. For tumors >2 cm, SBRT has significantly higher FFLP HR 3.35 p = 0.025. No differences in 1- or 2-yr OS.

Bush, Loma Linda (*IJROBP* 2016, PMID 27084661): PRT of 69 pts with new diagnosis of HCC meeting either Milan or San Francisco criteria for transplantation randomized to TACE versus proton therapy 70.2 Gy/15 fx. Median tumor size was 3.2 cm and median AFP was 23. At MFU of 28 mos, 2-yr LC was higher in proton group 88% versus 45% (p = .06) and 2-yr OS was not significantly different. Total hospitalization days within 30 days of treatment was significantly higher with TACE 166 versus 24 days (p < .001) and proton therapy was associated with higher CR rate among pts proceeding on to transplant 25% versus 10% (p = .38). **Conclusion: RFA is superior to ethanol ablation. SBRT may be preferable to RFA in HCC lesions >2 cm and proton therapy may have better efficacy and lower toxicity than TACE as bridge to transplantation.**

Salem, Northwestern (*Gastroenterology* 2016, PMID 27575820): Randomized phase II study of 45 pts with BCLC stages or B randomized to TACE versus Y-90. Excluded Child–Pugh C patients or vascular invasion. Median time to progression was 6.8 mos with TACE versus not reached (>26 mos) in Y-90 group (p = .007). 13 of 15 pts receiving Y-90 went on to transplant compared to 7 of 10 of TACE patients with no differences in OS.

Is there advantage to proton therapy for HCC?

Given dosimetric characteristics of protons, there may be an advantage to spare normal liver but the clinical benefits of this remain to be defined.

Hong, Proton Phase II (*JCO* 2016, PMID 26668346): Prospective Phase II study of 58.0 to 67.5 GyE/15 fx proton therapy for unresectable HCC or cholangiocarcinoma. Tumors within 2 cm of porta hepatis received 58 GyE while more peripheral tumors received 67.5 GyE. 49 HCC pts enrolled but five did not receive protocol therapy and were excluded. 2-yr OS was 63.2% for HCC pts and only two pts experienced LF.

Fukumitsu, Japan (*IJROBP* 2009, PMID 19304408): Prospective study from Japan of 51 pts with HCC >2 cm from porta hepatis treated to 66 GyE/10 fx. 3-yr OS of 49.2% and 3-yr LC of 94.5%. Only three pts developed grade II toxicity.

Bush, Loma Linda (*Gastroenterology* 2004, PMID 15508084): Phase II study of proton therapy for HCC pts Child–Pugh 63 GyE/15 fx. 34 pts completed treatment. MFU 20 mos, median tumor size 5.7 cm. 2-yr LC and OS were 75% and 55%, respectively.

Hata, Japan (*Cancer* 2005, PMID 15981284): RR of 12 pts with portal vein thrombus treated with proton therapy 50–72 GyE/10–22 fx. At MFU of 2.3 yrs, PFS was 67% and two pts remained disease-free long term at 4.3 and 6.4 yrs post-RT. **Conclusion: Proton therapy is associated with excellent LC of HCC and is feasible in setting of portal vein thrombus.**

REFERENCES

1. Liu M, Cheng S, Huang A. Chapter 60: Cancer of the liver and hepatobiliary tract. In: Halperin E, Wazer D, Perez C, Brady L, eds. *Perez and Brady's Principles and Practice of Radiation Oncology*. 6th ed. Philadelphia, PA: Lippincott Williams & Wilkins; 2013:1203–1215.

2. Bruix J, Sherman M, Practice Guidelines Committee, American Association for the Study of Liver Diseases. Management of hepatocellular carcinoma. *Hepatology*. 2005;42(5):1208–1236. doi:10.1002/hep.20933

3. Bruix J, Sherman M, American Association for the Study of Liver Diseases. Management of hepatocellular carcinoma: an update. *Hepatology*. 2011;53(3):1020–1022. doi:10.1002/hep.24199

4. Zhang BH, Yang BH, Tang ZY. Randomized controlled trial of screening for hepatocellular carcinoma. *J Cancer Res Clin Oncol*. 2004;130(7):417–422. doi:10.1007/s00432-004-0552-0

5. NCCN Panel Members. NCCN Guidelines version 1. 2016. Hepatobiliary Cancers. https://www.nccn.org/professionals/physician_gls/pdf/hepatobiliary.pdf

6. Bruix J, Sherman M, American Association for the Study of Liver Diseases. Management of hepatocellular carcinoma: an update. *Hepatology*. 2011;53(3):1020–1022. doi:10.1002/hep.24199

7. European Association for the Study of the Liver, European Organisation for Research and Treatment of Cancer. EASL-EORTC clinical practice guidelines: management of hepatocellular carcinoma. *J Hepatol*. 2012;56(4):908–943. doi:10.1016/j.jhep.2011.12.001

8. Pomfret EA, Washburn K, Wald C, et al. Report of a national conference on liver allocation in patients with hepatocellular carcinoma in the United States. *Liver Transpl*. 2010;16(3):262–278. doi:10.1002/lt.21999

9. American College of Radiology. Liver Imaging Reporting and Data System (LI-RADS). 2017. https://www.acr.org/Quality-Safety/Resources/LIRADS

10. Forner A, Reig ME, de Lope CR, Bruix J. Current strategy for staging and treatment: the BCLC update and future prospects. *Semin Liver Dis*. 2010;30(1):61–74. doi:10.1055/s-0030-1247133

11. Graziadei IW, Sandmueller H, Waldenberger P, et al. Chemoembolization followed by liver transplantation for hepatocellular carcinoma impedes tumor progression while on the waiting list and leads to excellent outcome. *Liver Transpl*. 2003;9(6):557–563. doi:10.1053/jlts.2003.50106

12. Kulik LM, Atassi B, van Holsbeeck L, et al. Yttrium-90 microspheres (TheraSphere) treatment of unresectable hepatocellular carcinoma: downstaging to resection, RFA and bridge to transplantation. *J Surg Oncol*. 2006;94(7):572–586. doi:10.1002/jso.20609

13. O'Connor JK, Trotter J, Davis GL, et al. Long-term outcomes of stereotactic body radiation therapy in the treatment of hepatocellular cancer as a bridge to transplantation. *Liver Transpl*. 2012;18(8):949–954. doi:10.1002/lt.23439

14. Llovet JM, Fuster J, Bruix J. Intention-to-treat analysis of surgical treatment for early hepatocellular carcinoma: resection versus transplantation. *Hepatology*. 1999;30(6):1434–1440.

15. Chang MH, Chen CJ, Lai MS, et al. Universal hepatitis B vaccination in Taiwan and the incidence of hepatocellular carcinoma in children. Taiwan Childhood Hepatoma Study Group. *N Engl J Med*. 1997;336(26):1855–1859. doi:10.1056/NEJM199706263362602

16. Poon RT, Fan ST, Lo CM, et al. Long-term survival and pattern of recurrence after resection of small hepatocellular carcinoma in patients with preserved liver function: implications for a strategy of salvage transplantation. *Ann Surg*. 2002;235(3):373–382.

17. Iwatsuki S, Starzl TE, Sheahan DG, et al. Hepatic resection versus transplantation for hepatocellular carcinoma. *Ann Surg*. 1991;214(3):221–228; discussion 228–229.

18. Mazzaferro V, Regalia E, Doci R, et al. Liver transplantation for the treatment of small hepatocellular carcinomas in patients with cirrhosis. *N Engl J Med*. 1996;334(11):693–699. doi:10.1056/NEJM199603143341104

19. Yao FY, Xiao L, Bass NM, et al. Liver transplantation for hepatocellular carcinoma: validation of the UCSF-expanded criteria based on preoperative imaging. *Am J Transplant*. 2007;7(11):2587–2596.

20. Wiesner R, Edwards E, Freeman R, et al. Model for end-stage liver disease (MELD) and allocation of donor livers. *Gastroenterology*. 2003;124(1):91–96. doi:10.1053/gast.2003.50016

21. Llovet JM, Ricci S, Mazzaferro V, et al. Sorafenib in advanced hepatocellular carcinoma. *N Engl J Med*. 2008;359(4):378–390. doi:10.1056/NEJMoa0708857

22. Benson R, Madan R, Kilambi R, Chander S. Radiation induced liver disease: a clinical update. *J Egypt Natl Canc Inst*. 2016;28(1):7–11. doi:10.1016/j.jnci.2015.08.001

23. Tateishi R, Shiina S, Teratani T, et al. Percutaneous radiofrequency ablation for hepatocellular carcinoma: an analysis of 1000 cases. *Cancer*. 2005;103(6):1201–1209. doi:10.1002/cncr.20892

24. Tanabe KK, Curley SA, Dodd GD, et al. Radiofrequency ablation: the experts weigh in. *Cancer*. 2004;100(3):641–650. doi:10.1002/cncr.11919

25. Llovet JM, Real MI, Montana X, et al. Arterial embolisation or chemoembolisation versus symptomatic treatment in patients with unresectable hepatocellular carcinoma: a randomised controlled trial. *Lancet*. 2002;359(9319):1734–1739.

26. Groupe d'Etude et de Traitement du Carcinome Hépatocellulaire. A comparison of lipiodol chemoembolization and conservative treatment for unresectable hepatocellular carcinoma. *N Engl J Med*. 1995;332(19):1256–1261. doi:10.1056/NEJM199505113321903

27. Salem R, Lewandowski RJ, Mulcahy MF, et al. Radioembolization for hepatocellular carcinoma using Yttrium-90 microspheres: a comprehensive report of long-term outcomes. *Gastroenterology*. 2010;138(1):52–64. doi:10.1053/j.gastro.2009.09.006

28. Kokabi N, Camacho JC, Xing M, et al. Open-label prospective study of the safety and efficacy of glass-based yttrium 90 radioembolization for infiltrative hepatocellular carcinoma with portal vein thrombosis. *Cancer*. 2015;121(13):2164–2174. doi:10.1002/cncr.29275

33: PANCREATIC ADENOCARCINOMA

Charles Marc Leyrer and Mohamed E. Abazeed

QUICK HIT: Pancreatic cancer has a poor prognosis, because it is prone to wide dissemination, often presents in a locale that precludes surgical removal and is relatively resistant to CHT and RT. MS can range from 3 to 24 months depending on the stage of disease and the performance status of the patient. Only 15% of pts have resectable disease at presentation. Twenty percent present with borderline resectable disease; however, only ~60% of these patients will undergo surgery to a clear margin.

TABLE 33.1: General Treatment Paradigm for Pancreatic Cancer			
Setting	**Initial Option**	**Additional Treatment(s)**	
Resectable disease	Surgery	CHT alone[1] - 5-FU - Gemcitabine +/− capecitabine - 5-FU-based multiagent regimen (e.g., FOLFIRINOX)	
		CHT followed by chemoRT to 45–54 Gy with concurrent 5-FU or gemcitabine	
	Neoadjuvant CHT	Surgery	Adjuvant CHT or chemoRT
Borderline resectable	Neoadjuvant CHT followed by chemoRT (45–54 Gy), reassessment, then surgery		
Locally advanced/ unresectable	Initial CHT	ChemoRT or SBRT (*maturing data favors the latter*)	
	SBRT (if symptomatic)	CHT	
	CHT Alone		
Metastatic	Treated with single or multiagent systemic therapy +/− palliative surgery/biliary stent/RT		

EPIDEMIOLOGY: Estimated 53,670 new cases in 2017 in the United States, with 43,090 deaths; fourth leading cause of cancer mortality in the United States.[2] Higher incidence in males versus females (1.3:1); higher incidence in African Americans versus Caucasians, and more common in developed nations.[3-6] Rare under 40 years of age with median age of 60 at diagnosis.[7] Peak incidence sixth to seventh decade, which makes aggressive treatment challenging.

RISK FACTORS: Chronic pancreatitis (RR 16–69), cigarette smoking (RR 1–3), high BMI (RR 1–2), chronic diabetes (RR 1–3), heavy alcohol consumption (RR 2–4), red meat (RR 1–1.5), and exposure to hydrocarbon compounds/pesticides/heavy metals.[8-10] There is emerging evidence for increased risk in those previously infected with H. pylori, HBV, and HCV.[8,11] Hereditary conditions include familial predisposition, hereditary pancreatitis (*PRSS1/SPINK1*, RR 50–67), Peutz–Jeghers (*STK11/LKB1*, RR 132), familial atypical multiple mole melanoma (FAMMM syndrome, *CDKN2A/TP16*, RR 48), mutations in *BRCA1/ BRCA2* (RR 2–7), Lynch syndrome (*MLH1/MSH2/MSH6/PMS2*), or ataxia telangiectasia.[8,12–17] Five to ten percent of cases have inherited component although if one first-degree relative, RR 1.5 to 13; if two relatives RR 18; if three relatives RR 57.[18–21] Other risk factors include non-O blood type (RR 1–2), partial gastrectomy/cholecystectomy/appendectomy, and coffee/tea.[8,22–24]

ANATOMY: Pancreas: retroperitoneal and located anterior to L1/L2. It is divided into head (including uncinate process), neck, body, and tail. Head lies in duodenal flexure, to right of SMV, with tail extending toward spleen. Peritoneal involvement is more common with body and tail tumors. Venous drainage is via portal system. Tumor invasion posteriorly can lead to lung/pleural metastasis via vena cava drainage. Pancreatic duct and accessory duct combine with common bile duct and enter duodenum via sphincter of Oddi at ampulla of Vater. Pancreas is directly adjacent to or in close proximity to stomach, duodenum, jejunum, kidneys, spleen, and several blood vessels (celiac axis, superior mesenteric artery, splenic artery, and associated veins as well as portal vein), and common bile duct. Celiac axis at T11/T12, SMA at L1.

Lymphatics/patterns of spread: Regional drainage is to peripancreatic, celiac, superior mesenteric, porta hepatic, and para-aortic lymph nodes. Frequently metastasizes to liver via portal venous network. Tumors of head and neck drain along common bile duct, common hepatic artery, portal vein, posterior/anterior pancreaticoduodenal arcades, SMV, and right lateral wall of SMA. Tumors of body and tail drain along common hepatic artery, celiac axis, splenic artery, and splenic hilum.

PATHOLOGY: Greater than 80% are ductal adenocarcinoma.[25] Approximately 60% arise from head, 15% in body or tail, and 20% diffusely involve pancreas.[25] Periampullary tumors can originate from head of pancreas, distal common bile duct, ampulla of Vater, or adjacent duodenum. Acinar cell tumors associated with fat necrosis, elevated lipase, rash, eosinophilia, polyarthralgia, and poor prognosis. Others include mucinous cystadenoma and adenosquamous carcinoma.[26] Other histologies include signet ring, medullary, adenosquamous, serous, and mixed acinar/ductal/neuroendocrine carcinoma. Approximately 5% of all pancreatic tumors are indolent endocrine tumors with long natural history and circulating polypeptides.[27]

GENETICS: Can be defined by *KRAS* and *p53* oncogene mutation >90%.[25,28] Overexpression of matrix metalloproteinases (MMP) or EGFR in 60% to 70%. *TP53* mutation in 60%. *SMAD4* tumor suppressor mutated/deleted in ~30% of pancreatic cancers; poor prognostic marker linked to higher predisposition for metastatic disease and shortened survival.[25,28]

SCREENING: International Cancer of Pancreas Screening (CAPS) consortium recommends screening with EUS and/or MRI/MRCP for high-risk individuals (not CT) defined as pts with Peutz–Jeghers; hereditary pancreatitis; first-degree relative with pancreatic cancer and three or more first/second/third degree relatives with pancreatic cancer; carriers of *BRCA1/2, p16, and HNPCC* mutations with one or more first-degree relative with pancreatic cancer.[29,30] No consensus exists on age to initiate or terminate screening/surveillance, how to manage detected lesions, and interval of screening required. Higher detection rate when screened with EUS over MRI or CT imaging.[31]

CLINICAL PRESENTATION: *Pain* (40%–60%) particularly in upper abdomen radiating to the back, which is intermittent and can be exacerbated by eating and/or alleviated specific positions such as leaning forward, lying on left side or in fetal position; *weight loss* (80%–85%); fatigue (85%); nausea (~25%); diarrhea/steatorrhea; *jaundice* (~55%), often with acholic stools and/or dark urine; hepatomegaly.[32–34] Classically, painless jaundice in resectable pts as associated with origination in pancreatic head with more favorable prognosis than those with obstructive jaundice. Pts may develop diabetes in 2 to 3 years prior to presentation. *Eponyms:* Enlarged nontender gallbladder (Courvoisier's sign), migratory thrombophlebitis (Trousseau's sign), left SCV lymph node (Virchow's node), left axillary node (Irish's node), periumbilical node (Sister Mary Joseph node), rectal shelf (Blumer's shelf), periumbilical ecchymosis (Cullen's sign), or flank ecchymosis (Grey Turner sign).

WORKUP: H&P, CBC, metabolic panel (including LFTs), CA 19-9 (may be undetectable in Lewis antigen-negative patients), pancreatic protocol CT (arterial and venous phases), or MRI (abdomen and pelvis). Systemic staging with CT (PET/CT controversial, detected unsuspected CT-occult DM in 33% of patients).[35] Biopsy via EUS, ERCP, or CT-guided. Biopsy is not necessarily required before surgery in pt with resectable disease. However, biopsy is necessary before administration of neoadjuvant therapy, in pts with locally advanced unresectable disease or metastatic disease (biopsy of metastatic site may be preferable), or enrollment in clinical trial. EUS provides optimal T/N staging, and is favored method of biopsy because of better diagnostic yield, safety, and potentially lower risk of peritoneal seeding.[31,36,37] ERCP (with brushing/biopsy) may be useful for symptomatic obstructive jaundice requiring stent placement. MRCP useful when looking for occult primary (benefits are no contrast and no increased risk of post-ERCP pancreatitis).[38] Staging laparoscopy may be considered to assess for peritoneal disease; however, this varies by institution as by quality of pre-op imaging.[39-41]

PROGNOSTIC FACTORS: Age, stage, grade, KPS, histology, location (head lesions are more favorable and present earlier), visceral artery involvement, extent of resection, response to neoadjuvant therapy, perineural invasion, lymph node status/ratio, and both pre- and postoperative serum CA 19-9 levels.[42-46]

NATURAL HISTORY: Local recurrence 35%, distant metastases 34%, both 27% in ESPAC-1 (see Neoptolemos later).

STAGING

TABLE 33.2: AJCC 8th ed. (2017) Staging for Exocrine Pancreatic Cancer		cN0	cN1	cN2
T1	a ≤0.5 cm	IA	IIB	III
	b >0.5 & <1 cm	IA		
	c 1–2 cm			
T2	• 2.1–4 cm	IB		
T3	• >4 cm	IIA		
T4	• Involvement[1]			
M1	• Distant metastasis	IV		

*Changes to AJCC 7th Edition include T1a-c subclassification and addition of N2 category (previously N0-1 only).

Notes: Involvement[1] = celiac axis, SMA, and/or common hepatic artery.

cN1, 1-3 LNs; cN2, ≥4 LNs.

TREATMENT PARADIGM

Surgery: Surgery is currently the only potentially curative option for pancreatic cancer. 20% present with apparently resectable disease. Approximately 20% of pts thought to have resectable disease do *not* have resectable disease at time of surgery (e.g., peritoneal involvement, etc.). Approximately 50% of pts present with disseminated disease (commonly liver, peritoneum, and lungs). Remainder have borderline resectable disease (i.e., tumor is neither clearly resectable nor clearly unresectable) or locally advanced unresectable disease. Ultimately, ~15% pts with newly diagnosed pancreatic cancer have up-front resectable disease. Whipple procedure (pancreaticoduodenectomy) is standard therapeutic operation, and involves en bloc resection of pancreatic head/body, distal stomach, duodenum, proximal jejunum, gallbladder, and distal common bile duct. Four PRTs have shown no difference in survival between variations on pancreaticoduodenectomy including pylorus-preserving, subtotal stomach-preserving, and minimally invasive techniques.[47–50] In addition, more extensive surgery, including extended lymphadenectomy and arterial en bloc resection, does not improve outcomes.[50,51] Operative mortality at high-volume centers is <5%.[52] After Whipple, remnant organs are attached to jejunum (pancreaticojejunostomy, gastrojejunostomy, and choledochojejunostomy) with vagotomy. Most common site of positive margin is retroperitoneal margin. Tail lesions can be considered for distal pancreatectomy depending on disease involvement. For highly selected pts with body/tail lesions with celiac artery involvement, Appleby procedure may be option (includes splenectomy, distal pancreatectomy and celiac artery resection, relies on collateral circulation for hepatic perfusion). Postoperative complications include anastomotic leaks, which can lead to peritonitis, abscess, autodigestion, hemorrhage, and delayed gastric emptying.

TABLE 33.3: NCCN Criteria for Resectability[53]	
Clearly resectable	1. No arterial tumor contact of celiac axis, SMA, and common hepatic artery 2. No radiographic evidence of SMV or portal vein contact or ≤180° contact without vein contour irregularity

Borderline resectable	1. Involvement of SMV/portal vein of >180° OR ≤180° with contour irregularity of vein
	2. SMV/Portal impingement (distortion/narrowing/occlusion/thrombosis), which can be resected/reconstructed
	3. Head/uncinate process tumor:
	  a. Involvement of common hepatic artery without celiac axis or hepatic bifurcation involved.
	  b. Abutment of SMA of ≤180°
	  c. Contact with anatomic arterial variant (e.g., replaced or accessory artery)
	4. Body/Tail tumors: Involvement of ≤180° of celiac axis or >180° without aorta involvement and uninvolved gastroduodenal artery
	5. Limited involvement of IVC

Unresectable	1. Distant metastases, including lymph nodes beyond field of resection 2. Contact with first jejunal SMA branch for head/uncinate process lesions OR contact with CA and aortic involvement for body/tail lesions. 3. Involvement with >180 degrees of celiac axis 4. Unreconstructable SMV/portal vein occlusion due to tumor involvement or occlusion (even bland thrombus) 5. Aortic invasion or encasement 6. Contact with proximal draining jejunal branch into SMV for head/uncinate process tumors.

Chemotherapy: Used in adjuvant and neoadjuvant settings as well as in context of locally advanced unresectable disease or metastatic disease. Historically, 5-FU has been the most common agent used although gemcitabine is increasingly favored (see the following discussion) as both have been associated with improved overall survival. Multidrug regimens such as FOLFIRINOX have also shown promise, with phase III data in metastatic setting demonstrating improved survival relative to single-agent gemcitabine.[54] Gemcitabine-based combination therapies (e.g., gem/nab-paclitaxel) have also shown survival advantage.[55,56] In Japanese population, the oral fluoropyrimidine S-1 versus gemcitabine after resection has shown higher survival with reduced toxicity; however, this has not been replicated in the United States.[57]

Radiation

Indications: RT can be delivered in postoperative, neoadjuvant, definitive, or palliative settings. Preoperative RT is used commonly for borderline resectable pts in attempt to optimize downstaging and provide local control in event resection does not occur. Adjuvant RT is controversial (see the following trials) but may improve outcomes. Definitive RT for unresectable/locally advanced cases may improve survival (see the following trials), reduce LF, and reduce pain. For locally advanced tumors, many prefer initial CHT followed by chemoRT or SBRT in setting of local progression or stable disease to avoid overtreatment of those who may ultimately succumb to metastatic disease (see ASCO Guidelines).[58]

Dose: Definitive, adjuvant and neoadjuvant typically given to 50.4 Gy/25 fx.

Toxicity: Acute: Fatigue, dermatitis, N/V, diarrhea, appetite loss, weight loss, stomach ulcers *Late*: Fatigue, skin discoloration, liver/renal dysfunction, bowel obstruction, stomach/bowel ulcers, dry/hyperpigmented skin.

Procedure: See *Treatment Planning Handbook*, Chapter 7[59] or RTOG Contouring Guidelines.[60]

Palliation: Palliative RT can improve pain control in up to 65% of patients.[61,62] Whipple procedure can offer palliation for duodenal obstruction and jaundice. Other surgeries include hepaticojejunostomy ± gastrojejunostomy. Endoscopic stent placement (frequently plastic for resectable disease and expandable metal stent for unresectable disease) is preferred method (compared to percutaneous stents). Celiac plexus and intrapleural nerve blocks can provide effective and long-lasting pain for some patients. However, relief can be transient in those who respond and other pts derive minimal pain relief after procedure.[63–65]

EVIDENCE-BASED Q&A

Resectable pancreatic cancer

Is surgery necessary in management of pancreatic cancer?

Surgery, if possible, carries a significant survival benefit. Retroperitoneal lymphadenectomy is not necessary as it provides no OS advantage; and pylorus preservation carries higher risk of positive margins (21% vs. 5%) as per Riall et al.[51]

Doi, Japan (*Surg Today* 2008, PMID 18958561): Japanese multi-institution RCT. *Eligibility*: Age 20–75, PS 0-2 with resectable pancreatic ACA (no involvement of SMA/common hepatic artery, no para-aortic LN+). *Randomization*: Surgery (pancreaticoduodenectomy or distal pancreatectomy + regional LN dissection) versus chemoRT (continuous infusion 5-FU at 200 mg/m^2/day with 50.4 Gy/28 fx, 4-field technique, Tumor + 1–3 cm margin covering regional LN). Closed early due to survival benefit (42/150 enrolled). All survival results favored surgical resection. MS 12.1 vs. 8.9 months, 3-yr OS 20% versus 0% ($p <$ .03); 5-yr OS 10% versus 0% (NS). LC not reported. **Conclusion: Surgery significantly improves OS in resectable pancreatic cancer.**

Riall, Johns Hopkins (*Ann Surg* 2002, PMID 12192322; Update Riall, *J Gastrointest Surg* 2005, PMID 16332474): RCT of pancreaticoduodenectomy with pylorus preservation versus distal gastrectomy with retroperitoneal LN dissection for periampullary adenocarcinoma. 299 pts (57% pancreatic, 22% ampullary, 17% distal bile duct, 3% duodenal). MFU 5.3 years. 5-yr OS 13% versus 29% (standard vs. radical; $p =$ .13). Margin positivity rate: 21% vs. 5% (standard vs. radical; $p =$ .002). **Conclusion: No evidence of survival benefit with distal gastrectomy and retroperitoneal lymphadenectomy when compared to pylorus-preserving pancreaticoduodenectomy. Similar mortality with increased morbidity and operative time with radical pancreaticoduodenectomy.**

Is there benefit to adjuvant chemoRT compared to surgery alone?

The benefit to adjuvant chemoRT compared to surgery alone is controversial given results of the following two trials.

Kalser, GITSG 91-73 (*Arch Surg* **1985, PMID 4015380; Confirmation Arm,** *Cancer* **1987, PMID 3567862):** PRT of 43 pts. *Eligibility:* Negative margins following resection without peritoneal mets. Pts w/ periampullary, islet cell and cystadenocarcinoma were excluded. *Randomization:* Post-op chemoRT versus observation. Treatment was split-course 40 Gy w/ 2-wk break + 5-FU 500 mg/m^2 d1-3 w/ each 20 Gy course, then weekly 5-FU for 2 years or until recurrence. RT covered pancreas, pancreatic bed and regional LNs. Subtotal Whipple in 68%, total Whipple in 32%. 25% did not start adjuvant treatment for >10 weeks post-op. ChemoRT increased MS (20 vs. 11 mos) and 2-yr OS (42% vs. 15%). **Conclusion: combined use of chemoRT as adjuvant therapy after curative resection is effective and is preferred to no adjuvant therapy.** *Comment: Terminated early after 8 years due to poor accrual and early benefit to chemoRT presented in 1985. Also, additional 30 pts were accrued to receive adjuvant chemoRT after closure presented in 1987 to demonstrate replication of results ("confirmation arm").*

TABLE 33.4: Results of GITSG 91-73 Adjuvant Pancreas Trial

GITSG	MS (Mos)	2-yr OS	5-yr OS
Surgery alone	11	15%	5%
Adjuvant chemoRT	20	42%	15%
Confirmation arm	18	46%	17%

Klinkenbijl, EORTC 40891 (*Ann Surg* **1999, PMID 10615932; Reanalysis Garofalo,** *Ann Surg* **2006 PMID 16858208; Update Smeenk,** *Ann Surg* **2007, PMID 17968163):** PRT of 218 pts with T1-2N0-1a pancreatic head ACA (n = 114) or T1-3N0-1a periampullary ACA (n=104) s/p resection. N1a was defined as LNs within resection specimen. Positive margins were included. *Randomization:* Adjuvant concurrent chemoRT (40 Gy split course, with 5-FU 25 mg/kg on d1-5 and 29-34) versus no adjuvant therapy. CHT was similar to GITSG 9173 with NO maintenance CHT. Adjuvant treatment arm had more pancreatic head tumors than observation arm, and fewer periampullary tumors. Overall, no difference in survival, but study was underpowered. Trend of benefit to adjuvant chemoRT for pancreatic head tumors (excluding periampullary). Garofalo et al. showed SS advantage in 2-yr OS with adjuvant chemoRT for pts with pancreatic head cancer (37% vs. 23%; p = .049), though this was with one-sided test. **Conclusion: Routine use of post-op chemoRT not recommended; 12-yr update confirmed no benefit.** *Comment: Study limitations included: pts with positive margins, no maintenance CHT, split-course RT, low RT dose, no RT QA, and inclusion of periampullary and N1a pts. 20% of pts randomized to CRT did not receive it.*

TABLE 33.5: Results of EORTC 40891 Adjuvant ChemoRT for Pancreas Cancer

EORTC 40891 (12-Year Update)	MS (Yrs)	5-yr OS	10-yr OS	Median PFS (Yrs)	5-yr PFS	10-yr PFS	MS Pancreatic Head (Yrs)
Surgery alone	1.6	22%	18%	1.2	20%	17%	1
Adjuvant chemoRT	1.8	25%	17%	1.5	21%	16%	1.3
p value	NS	NS	NS	NS	NS	NS	NS

Is there benefit to postoperative chemoRT compared to postoperative CHT?

Controversial. On basis of ESPAC-1 trial, postoperative CHT is beneficial, whereas postoperative chemoRT is not beneficial and possibly detrimental.[66,67] However, both EORTC 40891 and

ESPAC-1 had several flaws and thus results do not preclude chemoRT as acceptable choice in adjuvant setting based on GITSG 91-73. This is currently ongoing Phase III trial question in RTOG 0848.

Neoptolemos, ESPAC-1 (*Lancet* 2001 PMID 11716884; Update Neoptolemos *NEJM* 2004, PMID 15028824): PRT of 541 pts with grossly resected pancreatic ductal carcinoma randomized to 2x2 factorial design to surgery followed by observation versus CHT alone versus chemoRT versus chemoRT + consolidative CHT. Altered to boost accrual with randomization into one of main treatment comparisons (chemoRT vs. no chemoRT or CHT vs. no CHT). CHT was 5-FU 425 mg/m^2 d1-5 + LCV 20 mg/m^2 q28d x 6 cycles. ChemoRT regimen was 40 Gy split course (20 Gy/10 fx + bolus 5-FU 500 mg/m^2 followed by 2-week break followed by 20 Gy/10 fx + bolus 5-FU 500 mg/m^2). 285 pts randomized to 2x2 design: 68 to +/– chemoRT and 188 to +/– CHT. MFU 47 months. 81% with R0 resection, 19% had positive margins. Median time from resection to treatment was 46 days in CHT arm and 61 days in chemoRT arm. Prognostic factors were higher grade, LN+, tumor >2 cm. QOL parameters were equivalent between groups. When adjusted for prognostic factors, there was no benefit for adjuvant chemoRT (MS 16.1 vs. 15.5 for chemoRT, HR 1.18, CI: 0.90–1.55, *p* = .24). There was survival benefit for adjuvant CHT (MS 14 vs. 19.7 for CHT, HR 0.66, *p* = .0005). **Conclusion: CHT alone improved survival compared to observation. Adjuvant 5-FU based chemoRT did not improve survival, and may have had deleterious effect.** *Comment: Study limitations included: no central QA, selection bias (physician allowed to select which randomization), background treatment allowed by clinician choice (CHT or chemoRT), nearly 1/3 of observation arm and 1/3 of CHT arm received RT. RT dose was inconsistent—designed at 40 Gy, but choice of up to 60 Gy allowed.*

TABLE 33.6: Results of ESPAC 1 for Pancreas Cancer

ESPAC 1: 2x2 Subset Only (2004)	MS (mos)	TTF (mos)	5-yr OS
ChemoRT	15.9	10.7	10%
No chemoRT	17.9	15.2	20%
p value (+/– chemoRT)	.05	.04	
CHT	20.1	15.3	21%
No CHT	15.5	10.5	8%
p value (+/– CHT)	.009	.02	

Stocken, Pancreatic Cancer Meta-Analysis Group (*Br J Cancer* 2005, PMID 15812554): Systematic review and meta-analysis of 5 RT (GITSG, Norway, EORTC, Japan, ESPAC-1) of adjuvant CHT and chemoRT for 1,136 patients. CHT showed reduction in risk of death by 25% (HR 0.75, CI: 0.64–0.90, *p* = .001) and improved MS at 19 months versus 13.5 months without CHT. No significant difference in risk of death with chemoRT (HR 1.09, CI: 0.89–1.32, *p* = .43). Subgroup analysis showed chemoRT more effective with positive margins and CHT alone less effective. **Conclusion: CHT is effective adjuvant therapy while chemoRT is not unless pt has margin-positive disease.**

TABLE 33.7: Results of Stocken Meta-Analysis

Stocken Meta-Analysis	MS (mos)	2-yr OS	5-yr OS
CHT alone	19.0	38%	19%
Observation (hemo)	13.5	28%	12%
ChemoRT	15.8	30%	12%
Observation (chemoRT)	15.2	34%	17%

Morganti, Multi-Institution Retrospective Pool (*IJROBP* 2014, PMID 25220717): Multicenter RR of 955 consecutive pts who underwent R0-1 resection for invasive carcinoma (T1-4, N0-1, M0) of pancreas. MFU 21.0 mo. 623 received RT, 575 received chemoRT, and 462 received adjuvant CHT. 5-yr OS was 41.2% in pts treated with CRT versus 25.7% without. Benefit of CRT remained significant on multivariate analysis (HR=0.72, CI: 0.6–0.87, p = .001). R1 resection, LN+, higher pT stage, and tumor diameter >20 mm were negatively associated w/ survival on MVA. CRT and treatment at centers with >10 pancreatic resections/yr were associated with improved survival (HR=1.14, CI: 1.05–1.23] p = .002). **Conclusion: Although retrospective, OS appeared improved in pts who received chemoRT.**

Is postoperative CHT with gemcitabine beneficial over surgery alone?

Yes, like ESPAC-1 (which used 5-FU), German CONKO-001 showed benefit for adjuvant CHT.

Oettle, CONKO-001 (*JAMA* 2007 PMID 17227978, Update Oettle, *JAMA* 2013, PMID 24104372): PRT of 354 pts. *Eligibility:* T1-4N0-1M0 s/p R0-1 resection. Pts with postoperative CA 19-9 or CEA >2.5x upper limit of normal were excluded. *Randomization:* Observation or six cycles of gemcitabine (4-week cycles, 1000 mg/m² on days 1, 8, 15). Intention-to-treat analysis, but also included prespecified "qualified" survival analysis based on pts who had received at least one complete cycle of gemcitabine in adjuvant group and no adjuvant cytotoxic or RT therapy in control group. MFU 136 months. 83% received R0 resection. Median DFS improved in adjuvant treatment group (HR 0.55, p < .001) along with improved OS and MS (HR 0.76, p = .01) based on 2013 *JAMA* publication. **Conclusion: Gemcitabine improves DFS and OS in resected pancreatic cancer.**

TABLE 33.8: Results of CONKO-001 German Adjuvant CHT Trial			
CONKO-001 2013 update	Median DFS	5-yr OS	10-yr OS
Surgery alone	6.7 m	10.4%	7.7%
Adjuvant gemcitabine	13.4 m	20.7%	12.2%
p value	<.001	.01	.01

What is optimal adjuvant CHT regimen?

Gemcitabine, 5-FU/leucovorin, and combination gemcitabine/capecitabine are all recommended as per NCCN.[53]

Neoptolemos, ESPAC-3 (JAMA 2010, PMID 20823433): PRT of 1088 pts with resected pancreatic ACA randomized to 5-FU 425 mg/m² IV bolus with LCV 20 mg/m² IV bolus on d1-5 of 28d cycle x6 cycles versus gemcitabine 1000 mg/m² IV infusion over 30 min weekly for 3 out of every 4 weeks (1 cycle) x6 cycles. MFU 34.2 months. No significant difference in QOL scores. **Conclusion: Gemcitabine did not show benefit over 5-FU/ LCV in survival or PFS but had less toxicity.** *Comment: 5-FU regimen was more intense than Burris (see in the following).*

TABLE 33.9: Results of ESPAC-3 Adjuvant CHT for Pancreas Cancer				
ESPAC-3	Median PFS (mos)	MS (mos)	2-yr OS	Treatment-related Serious Adverse Events
Adjuvant 5-FU/LCV	14.1	23.0	48.1 %	14%
Adjuvant gemcitabine	14.3	23.6	49.1 %	7.5%
p value	.53	.39	NS	<.001

Neoptolemos, ESPAC-4 (Lancet 2017, PMID 28129987): Phase III PRT of 730 pts *Eligibility:* Age >18 s/p R0-1 resection of pancreatic ACA. *Randomization:* Six cycles of gemcitabine (1000 mg/m² once weekly on week 1-3 q4 weeks) OR gemcitabine (same regimen) with capecitabine (1,660 mg/m² D1-21 q28 days). Primary Endpoint was OS. MFU 43.2 months. MS significantly higher for gemcitabine+capecitabine versus gemcitabine alone (HR 0.82, $p = .032$). Treatment type, positive margins, higher grade, LN+, higher postoperative CA 19-9, and larger tumor size significant for worse OS on MVA. No significant difference in QOL (HR 0.10, CI: 0.29–0.09, $p = .3$). Significantly higher grade 3-4 neutropenia, diarrhea, and hand/foot/mouth syndrome with gemcitabine and capecitabine. **Conclusion: Adjuvant gemcitabine+capecitabine recommended as new SOC for adjuvant therapy in resected pancreatic ACA.**

TABLE 33.10: Results of ESPAC-4 CHT for Pancreas Cancer

ESPAC-4	MS (mos)	5-yr OS	LR	5-yr PFS
Gemcitabine	25.5	16.3%	66%	11.9%
Gemcitabine + capecitabine	28	28.8%	65%	18.6%
p value	.032		.715	

What is optimal adjuvant chemoRT regimen?

Regine, RTOG 97-04 (*JAMA* 2008, PMID 18319412; Update Regine *Ann Surg Oncol* 2011, PMID 21499862): PRT of 451 pts *Eligibility:* GTR of T1-4N0-1M0 pancreatic ACA (excluded ampullary cancers) with KPS >60. *Randomization:* PVI 5-FU (250 mg/m²/d) x 3 wks → chemoRT → PVI 5-FU 4 wks on/2 wks off for 2 months OR weekly gemcitabine (weekly 1000 mg/m² 30-minute infusion) x 3 → chemoRT → gemcitabine 3 wks on/1 wk off for 2 months. ChemoRT was to 50.4 Gy/28 fx (cone-down after 45 Gy) w/ concurrent PVI 5-FU 250 mg/m²/d. Primary endpoints of OS in all pts and/or in pts with pancreatic head tumors. Toxicity was secondary endpoint. MFU 1.48 years overall and 6.98 for alive pts. 67% were N1, 75% were T3-4 (more in gemcitabine arm), 34% had positive margins (25% had unknown margin status), 86% were pancreatic head tumors. Overall, there was no difference in OS or DFS. After adjustment for protocol-specified stratification variables of nodal status, tumor diameter and margin status on MVA, no benefit of gemcitabine vs. 5-FU with MS of 20.5 versus 17.1 months and 5-year OS of 22% versus 18% respectively (HR 0.84, $p = .12$). **Conclusion: No difference in survival of pts with gemcitabine or 5-FU given before/after chemoRT. Gemcitabine was associated with greater heme toxicity.** *Comment: Second analysis of RTOG 97-04 demonstrated effect between RT QA and protocol compliance on survival.[68] Furthermore, significantly worse survival reported in pts with postresection CA19-9 >90 U/mL (HR 3.1, p < .0001).[69]*

TABLE 33.11: Results of RTOG 97-04 chemoRT for Pancreas Cancer

RTOG 97-04 (All Pts)	LR	MS	3-yr OS	Grade 4 Heme Toxicity
5-FU arm	28%	16.9 m	22 %	1%
Gemcitabine arm	23%	20.5 m	31 %	14%
p value	NS	.09		<.001

Borderline resectable

What is rationale for neoadjuvant chemoRT?

Neoadjuvant chemoRT may help downstage patients, reduce nodal burden, reduce rate of positive margins, and improve resectability of borderline patients. Treatment regimens include 5-FU/RT and gemcitabine/RT. Recently, attention is being paid to neoadjuvant regimens incorporating more aggressive CHT with or without RT, such as FOLFIRINOX, modified FOLFIRINOX, and gemcitabine/docetaxel/capecitabine or gemcitabine/capecitabine + RT.[70–72]

Strobel, Heidelberg Germany (*Surgery* 2012, PMID 22770956): From prospective database, 257 pts identified who received neoadjuvant chemoRT (77.4%) or CHT (22.6%) for locally advanced unresectable pancreatic cancer. All pts underwent resection (46.7%) or underwent exploration only (53.3%). There were 6 (5%) ypT0 neoplasms, 36 (30.0%) R0, 61 (50.8%) R1, and 16 (13.3%) R2 resections. Median postoperative survival was greater after resection than exploration alone (12.7 months vs. 8.8 months; $p < 0.0001$). Median postoperative survival was 24.6 months after R0, 11.9 months after R1, and 8.9 months after R2 resection. 3-yr OS after R0 resection was 24%. **Conclusion: R0/R1 resections can be achieved in up to 40% of pts with unresectable pancreatic cancer with similar survival rates for initially resectable patients.**

Laurence, Australian Meta-Analysis (*J Gastrointest Surg* 2011, PMID 21913045): Systematic review and meta-analysis of 19 studies to evaluate benefits and complications associated with neoadjuvant chemoRT for both resectable and initially unresectable pancreatic cancer. Pts with unresectable pancreatic cancer showed similar survival outcomes to pts with resectable disease. Only 40% were ultimately resected after neoadjuvant therapy. Neoadjuvant chemoRT was associated with reduced margin+ rate. There was increase in risk of perioperative death, but no significant increase in pancreatic fistula formation or total complications. **Conclusion: Available data for OS of given studies was poor and unable to draw definitive conclusion. However, neoadjuvant therapy may reduce risk of positive margins while increasing risk of peri-operative complications/ death.**

Gillen, Munich Meta-Analysis (*PLoS Med* 2010, PMID 20422030): Systematic review and meta-analysis of prospective and retrospective studies evaluating neoadjuvant chemoRT, RT, or CHT followed by restaging and surgical exploration/resection. 111 studies (4,934 pts) were divided according to whether they were assessing initially resectable tumors or tumors considered unresectable/borderline. MS was 23.3 months after resection for with resectable disease and 20.5 months for initially unresectable patients. Initially resectable tumors had CR rate of 3.6% and PR rate of 30.6% while initially unresectable tumors showed CR rate of 4.8% and PR rate of 30.2%. **Conclusion: Neoadjuvant therapy with reassessment should be considered for pts thought unresectable as one-third of pts ultimately underwent surgery with survival similar to those initially thought resectable.**

Locally advanced/unresectable pancreatic cancer

Does CHT improve symptoms for advanced pancreatic cancer?

Burris (*JCO* 1997, PMID 9196156): Multi-institution PRT of 126 pts. *Eligibility:* Symptomatic locally advanced (unresectable) or metastatic disease randomized to gemcitabine 1000 mg/m^2 weekly x7 followed by 1 week of rest, then weekly x3 every 4 weeks OR 5-FU (600 mg/m^2) once weekly. Evaluated "clinical benefit response," which was composite measurement of pain (analgesic consumption and pain intensity), KPS, and weight. Clinical benefit required sustained (defined as ≥4 weeks) improvement in ≥1 parameter without decrease in others. Median time to clinical benefit response was 7 weeks for gemcitabine and 3 weeks for 5-FU patients, mean duration was 18 weeks versus 13 weeks respectively. Gemcitabine demonstrated more treatment-related side effects. **Conclusion: Gemcitabine increased clinical benefit of response in advanced, symptomatic pt population while also improving OS. Treatment was well tolerated.**

TABLE 33.12: Results of Burris Trial Pancreas Cancer			
	Clinical Benefit Response	MS (mos)	1-yr OS
5-FU	4.8%	4.41	2%
Gemcitabine	23.8%	5.65	18%
p value	.0022	.0025	

What is rationale for definitive chemoRT in locally advanced unresectable pancreatic cancer?

As with resectable pancreatic adenocarcinoma, use of RT therapy as part of standard management of locally advanced or unresectable pancreatic cancer is controversial because of conflicting results of randomized studies. In general, biliary stent (if jaundice) can be performed first followed by induction CHT with restaging followed by chemoRT or continued CHT alone (see ASCO guidelines).[58] Following trials (see Table 33.13) support use of chemoRT, whereas later trials (Chauffert, Krishnan, and Hammel) do not support chemoRT.

TABLE 33.13: Trials Supporting Use of ChemoRT for Locally Advanced/Unresectable Pancreatic Cancer				
Trial	Year	Arms	Results	Notes
Mayo Clinic[73]	1969	RT alone ChemoRT (35–40 Gy±5-FU)	MS 10.4 (chemoRT) vs. 6.3 mo (RT alone)	
GITSG 9273[74]	1981	RT alone (60 Gy) ChemoRT (40 Gy) ChemoRT (60 Gy)	1-yr OS 40% vs. 10%	RT given with 2-week break every 20 Gy, CHT 5-FU concurrent and maintenance
GITSG 9283[75]	1988	CHT alone ChemoRT	1-yr OS 41% vs. 19%	CHT alone: SMF (streptozocin, MMC, and 5-FU) ChemoRT was 54 Gy+ 5-FU concurrent
ECOG E4201[76]	2008	CHT alone (gemcitabine) ChemoRT (gemcitabine + 50.4 Gy/28 fx)	MS 9.2 vs. 11.1 in favor of gem/RT (p = .017)	Closed early due to poor accrual

Chauffert, French FFCD-SFRO (*Ann Oncol* 2008, PMID 18467316): PRT of 119 pts with locally advanced pancreatic cancer and WHO PS-0. *Randomization:* induction chemoRT (60 Gy/30 fx with PVI 5-FU, 300 mg/m², d1-5 x6 weeks and cisplatin 20 mg/m², d1-5 during weeks 1 and 5) or induction gemcitabine alone (1,000 mg/m² weekly x7 weeks). Maintenance gemcitabine (1000 mg/m² weekly, 3/4 weeks) was given in both arms until disease progression or toxicity. Stopped early due to worse chemoRT survival. MS was lower with chemoRT (8.6 vs. 13 months, p = .03), while toxicity was higher (grade 3-4 toxicity 36% vs. 22% during induction and 32% vs. 18% during maintenance). **Conclusion: Induction chemoRT as described earlier showed increased toxicity and decreased effectiveness than gemcitabine alone.** *Comment: ChemoRT regimen in this trial was nonstandard and toxic.*

Krishnan, MD Anderson (*Cancer* 2007, PMID 17538975): RR of 323 pts with locally advanced pancreatic cancer. 247 underwent chemoRT (concurrent 5-FU or Gemcitabine),

76 had induction gemcitabine with RT (~85% received 30 Gy/10 fx) with concurrent 5-FU (41%), gemcitabine (39%), or capecitabine (20%). MFU was 5 months. Induction chemoRT improved MS (12 months vs. 8 months; $p < .001$] and local progression (6 months vs. 9 months; $p = .003$]. **Conclusion: Optimal pt selection is by determining chemoRT based on progression after induction CHT may be ideal treatment strategy and merits prospective randomized evaluation.**

Hammel, LAP07 (*JAMA* 2016, PMID 27139057): PRT of 442 pts. Two randomizations: first to either gemcitabine (1,000 mg/m² weekly x3 weeks) or gemcitabine with erlotinib (100 mg/d for 4 months). Those with no progression after 4 months were randomized again to further CHT +/− RT (54 Gy and capecitabine 1600 mg/m²/d). Pts receiving erlotinib received maintenance erlotinib after completion. MFU 36.7 mos. 269 pts had no progression after 4 months. MS was 16.5 with CHT and 15.2 months with CHT+RT ($p = .83$). MS was 13.6 mos in those undergoing gemcitabine and 11.9 mos for gemcitabine+erlotinib ($p = .09$). Reduced LR was noted with chemoRT (32% versus 46%, $p = .03$) with no increased grade 3-4 toxicity except nausea. **Conclusion: No significant difference in OS with chemoRT versus CHT OR with addition of gemcitabine in conjunction with erlotinib used as maintenance CHT.** *Comment: After formal RT QA, only 32% of pts in chemoRT arm were treated per protocol, while 50% had minor deviations and 18% had major deviations.*

Is SRS/SBRT for pancreatic cancer safe and effective?

SBRT offers attractive solution to safely decrease local failure without delaying CHT. NCCN now allows for SBRT in select patients.

Chang, Stanford (*Cancer* 2009, PMID 19117351): RR of 77 pts with unresectable pancreatic cancer (58% locally advanced; 14% medically inoperable; 8% locally recurrent; 19% metastatic) treated with 25 Gy in single fraction with CyberKnife®. 21% also received between 45 and 54 Gy of fractionated EBRT. Various gemcitabine-based regimens in 96% of patients, remaining 4% did not receive CHT until they had distant failure. Isolated local failure at 6 and 12 months was 5%. PFS at 6 and 12 months was 26% and 9%, respectively. OS at 6 and 12 months was 56% and 21%. Grade ≥2 acute toxicity was 5%. Grade ≥3 late toxicity was 9%. **Conclusion: 25 Gy in one fraction provides effective local control with concerns about late toxicity, with the most common toxicity being ulceration. In fact, a subsequent dose-volume analysis of duodenal toxicity in a cohort of 73 previously unirradiated patients treated with 25 Gy in one fraction showed that the 12-month risk of duodenal toxicity was 29%.**[77]

Pollom, Stanford Update (*IJROBP* 2014, PMID 25585785): RR of 167 pts treated with SBRT with either single fx (45.5%) or 5 fx (54.5%) regimens. MFU 7.9 mo. No difference in recurrence by fractionation scheme with 6/12 month rates of LR 5.3%/9.5% for single fraction while 3.4%/11.7% for multi-fx, respectively. No difference in survival by fractionation scheme with 6/12 month rates of survival 67%/30.8% for single fraction while 75.7%/34.9% for multi-fx respectively. Significantly less grade ≥2 toxicity with 5 fx regimen. In single-fx group, 6/12 month rates of GI toxicity grade ≥3 were 8.1%/12.3% respectively while both were 5.6% in multi-fx group without significant difference. **Conclusion: Multifraction SBRT reduces GI toxicity without reducing local control.**

Mahadevan, Harvard (*IJROBP* 2011, PMID 21658854): RR of 47 pts who received gemcitabine (1,000 mg/m²/wk x3 wks then 1 wk off) until intolerance, at least six cycles or progression. Pts without metastases after two cycles received SBRT (normal tissue tolerance-based dose of 24–36 Gy in three fractions) between third and fourth cycles without interrupting CHT. MFU for survivors was 21 months. Of initial 47 pts, 17% found to have metastatic disease after two cycles of gemcitabine. MS for all pts who received SBRT was 20 months, with median PFS 15 months. LC was 85%. 54% of pts (21/39) developed metastases. Late grade 3 toxicities such as GI bleeding and obstruction in 9% (3/39). **Conclusion: Pts can be appropriately selected for local failure by identifying those with early metastatic disease. Local therapy can be accomplished safely with SBRT without disrupting CHT.**

Moningi, Johns Hopkins (*Ann Surg Oncol* 2015, PMID 25564157): RR of 88 pts with pancreatic adenocarcinoma receiving SBRT from 2010-2014. Goal was evaluation of OS and local PFS. 74 pts were locally advanced and 14 were borderline resectable. MFU was 14.5 months for locally advanced disease and 10.3 months for borderline resectable. Most pts received pre-SBRT CHT 25 to 33 Gy/5 fx. MS was 18.4 months and median PFS was 9.8 months. Only three pts had ≥grade 3 toxicity and five pts had late ≥grade 2 GI toxicity. 19 pts underwent resection, of whom 15 (79%) had locally advanced disease and 16 (84%) had margin-negative surgery. **Conclusion: SBRT after CHT for either locally advanced or borderline resectable pancreatic cancer results in low acute and late toxicity. Majority of pts completed resection without significant radiographic response.**

Are there any data for IORT/IOERT in pancreatic cancer?

Current data is limited. Sindelar et al. showed surgery with 60 Gy EBRT split course versus 25 Gy IOERT w/ 18 to 22 MeV electrons followed by 50 Gy EBRT at 1.5 to 1.75 Gy/fx was not significantly different in survival.[78] Both groups had MS of 12 months (NS), DFS (20 vs. 12 months) but not significant, and significant difference in LC (80% versus 0%) both favoring IOERT. Willett et al. at reviewed 150 pts with unresectable nonmetastatic disease treated with IOERT and EBRT/5-FU.[79] IORT started at 15 Gy; however, increased to 20 Gy due to local failures with 1-year OS of 54%, 2-year OS 15%, and 3-year OS 7% with smaller tumors having significantly better OS. Late complications noted in 15% with few long-term survivors (8/150) beyond 3 to 4 years.

REFERENCES

1. Twombly R. Adjuvant chemoradiation for pancreatic cancer: few good data, much debate. *J Natl Cancer Inst.* 2008;100(23):1670–1671.
2. Siegel RL, Miller KD, Jemal A. Cancer statistics, 2017. *CA Cancer J Clin.* 2017;67(1):7–30.
3. Boyle P, Hsieh CC, Maisonneuve P, et al. Epidemiology of pancreas cancer (1988). *Int J Pancreatol.* 1989;5(4):327–346.
4. Hariharan D, Saied A, Kocher HM. Analysis of mortality rates for pancreatic cancer across the world. *HPB (Oxford).* 2008;10(1):58–62.
5. Yao JC, Eisner MP, Leary C, et al. Population-based study of islet cell carcinoma. *Ann Surg Oncol.* 2007;14(12):3492–3500.
6. Ma J, Siegel R, Jemal A. Pancreatic cancer death rates by race among US men and women, 1970–2009. *J Natl Cancer Inst.* 2013;105(22):1694–1700.
7. Yao JC, Hassan M, Phan A, et al. One hundred years after "carcinoid": epidemiology of and prognostic factors for neuroendocrine tumors in 35,825 cases in the United States. *J Clin Oncol.* 2008;26(18):3063–3072.
8. Barone E, Corrado A, Gemignani F, Landi S. Environmental risk factors for pancreatic cancer: an update. *Arch Toxicol.* 2016;90(11):2617–2642.
9. Fuchs CS, Colditz GA, Stampfer MJ, et al. A prospective study of cigarette smoking and the risk of pancreatic cancer. *Arch Intern Med.* 1996;156(19):2255–2260.
10. Michaud DS, Giovannucci E, Willett WC, et al. Physical activity, obesity, height, and the risk of pancreatic cancer. *JAMA.* 2001;286(8):921–929.
11. Hassan MM, Li D, El-Deeb AS, et al. Association between hepatitis B virus and pancreatic cancer. *J Clin Oncol.* 2008;26(28):4557–4562.
12. Giardiello FM, Brensinger JD, Tersmette AC, et al. Very high risk of cancer in familial Peutz-Jeghers syndrome. *Gastroenterology.* 2000;119(6):1447–1453.
13. van Lier MG, Wagner A, Mathus-Vliegen EM, et al. High cancer risk in Peutz-Jeghers syndrome: a systematic review and surveillance recommendations. *Am J Gastroenterol.* 2010;105(6):1258–1264.

14. Lim W, Olschwang S, Keller JJ, et al. Relative frequency and morphology of cancers in STK11 mutation carriers. *Gastroenterology*. 2004;126(7):1788–1794.

15. de Snoo FA, Bishop DT, Bergman W, et al. Increased risk of cancer other than melanoma in CDKN2A founder mutation (p16-Leiden)-positive melanoma families. *Clin Cancer Res*. 2008;14(21):7151–7157.

16. Roberts NJ, Jiao Y, Yu J, et al. ATM mutations in patients with hereditary pancreatic cancer. *Cancer Discov*. 2012;2(1):41–46.

17. Iqbal J, Ragone A, Lubinski J, et al. The incidence of pancreatic cancer in BRCA1 and BRCA2 mutation carriers. *Br J Cancer*. 2012;107(12):2005–2009.

18. Olson SH, Kurtz RC. Epidemiology of pancreatic cancer and the role of family history. *J Surg Oncol*. 2013;107(1):1–7.

19. Klein AP. Genetic susceptibility to pancreatic cancer. *Mol Carcinog*. 2012;51(1):14–24.

20. Klein AP, Hruban RH, Brune KA, et al. Familial pancreatic cancer. *Cancer J*. 2001;7(4):266–273.

21. Solomon S, Das S, Brand R, Whitcomb DC. Inherited pancreatic cancer syndromes. *Cancer J*. 2012;18(6):485–491.

22. Amundadottir L, Kraft P, Stolzenberg-Solomon RZ, et al. Genome-wide association study identifies variants in the ABO locus associated with susceptibility to pancreatic cancer. *Nat Genet*. 2009;41(9):986–990.

23. Wolpin BM, Chan AT, Hartge P, et al. ABO blood group and the risk of pancreatic cancer. *J Natl Cancer Inst*. 2009;101(6):424–431.

24. Genkinger JM, Li R, Spiegelman D, et al. Coffee, tea, and sugar-sweetened carbonated soft drink intake and pancreatic cancer risk: a pooled analysis of 14 cohort studies. *Cancer Epidemiol Biomarkers Prev*. 2012;21(2):305–318.

25. Esposito I, Konukiewitz B, Schlitter AM, Kloppel G. Pathology of pancreatic ductal adenocarcinoma: facts, challenges and future developments. *World J Gastroenterol*. 2014;20(38):13833–13841.

26. La Rosa S, Sessa F, Capella C. Acinar Cell carcinoma of the pancreas: overview of clinicopathologic features and insights into the molecular pathology. *Front Med (Lausanne)*. 2015;2:41.

27. Klimstra DS. Nonductal neoplasms of the pancreas. *Mod Pathol*. 2007;20(Suppl 1):S94–S112.

28. Winter JM, Maitra A, Yeo CJ. Genetics and pathology of pancreatic cancer. *HPB (Oxford)*. 2006;8(5):324–336.

29. Canto MI, Goggins M, Hruban RH, et al. Screening for early pancreatic neoplasia in high-risk individuals: a prospective controlled study. *Clin Gastroenterol Hepatol*. 2006;4(6):766–781; quiz 665.

30. Canto MI, Harinck F, Hruban RH, et al. International Cancer of the Pancreas Screening (CAPS) Consortium summit on the management of patients with increased risk for familial pancreatic cancer. *Gut*. 2013;62(3):339–347.

31. Canto MI, Hruban RH, Fishman EK, et al. Frequent detection of pancreatic lesions in asymptomatic high-risk individuals. *Gastroenterology*. 2012;142(4):796–804; quiz e714–e795.

32. Porta M, Fabregat X, Malats N, et al. Exocrine pancreatic cancer: symptoms at presentation and their relation to tumour site and stage. *Clin Transl Oncol*. 2005;7(5):189–197.

33. Kalser MH, Barkin J, MacIntyre JM. Pancreatic cancer: assessment of prognosis by clinical presentation. *Cancer*. 1985;56(2):397–402.

34. Bakkevold KE, Arnesjo B, Kambestad B. Carcinoma of the pancreas and papilla of Vater: presenting symptoms, signs, and diagnosis related to stage and tumour site: a prospective multicentre trial in 472 patients. Norwegian Pancreatic Cancer Trial. *Scand J Gastroenterol*. 1992;27(4):317–325.

35. Chang JS, Choi SH, Lee Y, et al. Clinical usefulness of (1)(8)F-fluorodeoxyglucose-positron emission tomography in patients with locally advanced pancreatic cancer planned to undergo concurrent chemoradiation therapy. *Int J Radiat Oncol Biol Phys*. 2014;90(1):126–133.

36. Poley JW, Kluijt I, Gouma DJ, et al. The yield of first-time endoscopic ultrasonography in screening individuals at a high risk of developing pancreatic cancer. *Am J Gastroenterol*. 2009;104(9):2175–2181.

37. Langer P, Kann PH, Fendrich V, et al. Five years of prospective screening of high-risk individuals from families with familial pancreatic cancer. *Gut*. 2009;58(10):1410–1418.

38. Hennedige TP, Neo WT, Venkatesh SK. Imaging of malignancies of the biliary tract: an update. *Cancer Imaging*. 2014;14:14.

39. Ahmed SI, Bochkarev V, Oleynikov D, Sasson AR. Patients with pancreatic adenocarcinoma benefit from staging laparoscopy. *J Laparoendosc Adv Surg Tech A*. 2006;16(5):458–463.

40. Allen VB, Gurusamy KS, Takwoingi Y, et al. Diagnostic accuracy of laparoscopy following computed tomography (CT) scanning for assessing the resectability with curative intent in pancreatic and periampullary cancer. *Cochrane Database Syst Rev.* 2013;(11):CD009323.

41. Warshaw AL, Gu ZY, Wittenberg J, Waltman AC. Preoperative staging and assessment of resectability of pancreatic cancer. *Arch Surg.* 1990;125(2):230–233.

42. Gillen S, Schuster T, Meyer Zum Buschenfelde C, et al. Preoperative/neoadjuvant therapy in pancreatic cancer: a systematic review and meta-analysis of response and resection percentages. *PLoS Med.* 2010;7(4):e1000267.

43. Andren-Sandberg A. Prognostic factors in pancreatic cancer. *N Am J Med Sci.* 2012;4(1):9–12.

44. Bilici A. Prognostic factors related with survival in patients with pancreatic adenocarcinoma. *World J Gastroenterol.* 2014;20(31):10802–10812.

45. Tas F, Sen F, Keskin S, et al. Prognostic factors in metastatic pancreatic cancer: older patients are associated with reduced overall survival. *Mol Clin Oncol.* 2013;1(4):788–792.

46. Eloubeidi MA, Desmond RA, Wilcox CM, et al. Prognostic factors for survival in pancreatic cancer: a population-based study. *Am J Surg.* 2006;192(3):322–329.

47. Tran KT, Smeenk HG, van Eijck CH, et al. Pylorus preserving pancreaticoduodenectomy versus standard Whipple procedure: a prospective, randomized, multicenter analysis of 170 patients with pancreatic and periampullary tumors. *Ann Surg.* 2004;240(5):738–745.

48. Lin PW, Shan YS, Lin YJ, Hung CJ. Pancreaticoduodenectomy for pancreatic head cancer: PPPD versus Whipple procedure. *Hepatogastroenterology.* 2005;52(65):1601–1604.

49. Seiler CA, Wagner M, Bachmann T, et al. Randomized clinical trial of pylorus-preserving duodenopancreatectomy versus classical Whipple resection-long term results. *Br J Surg.* 2005;92(5):547–556.

50. Yeo CJ, Cameron JL, Lillemoe KD, et al. Pancreaticoduodenectomy with or without distal gastrectomy and extended retroperitoneal lymphadenectomy for periampullary adenocarcinoma, part 2: randomized controlled trial evaluating survival, morbidity, and mortality. *Ann Surg.* 2002;236(3):355–366; discussion 366–358.

51. Riall TS, Cameron JL, Lillemoe KD, et al. Pancreaticoduodenectomy with or without distal gastrectomy and extended retroperitoneal lymphadenectomy for periampullary adenocarcinoma—Part 3: update on 5-year survival. *J Gastrointest Surg.* 2005;9(9):1191–1204; discussion 1204–1196.

52. Langer B. Role of volume outcome data in assuring quality in HPB surgery. *HPB (Oxford).* 2007;9(5):330–334.

53. NCCN Clinical Practice Guidelines in Oncology: Pancreatic Adenocarcinoma. 2017. https://www.nccn.org

54. Conroy T, Desseigne F, Ychou M, et al. FOLFIRINOX versus gemcitabine for metastatic pancreatic cancer. *N Engl J Med.* 2011;364(19):1817–1825.

55. Goldstein D, El-Maraghi RH, Hammel P, et al. nab-Paclitaxel plus gemcitabine for metastatic pancreatic cancer: long-term survival from a phase III trial. *J Natl Cancer Inst.* 2015;107(2). doi:10.1093/jnci/dju413

56. Moore MJ, Goldstein D, Hamm J, et al. Erlotinib plus gemcitabine compared with gemcitabine alone in patients with advanced pancreatic cancer: a phase III trial of the National Cancer Institute of Canada Clinical Trials Group. *J Clin Oncol.* 2007;25(15):1960–1966.

57. Maeda A, Boku N, Fukutomi A, et al. Randomized phase III trial of adjuvant chemotherapy with gemcitabine versus S-1 in patients with resected pancreatic cancer: Japan Adjuvant Study Group of Pancreatic Cancer (JASPAC-01). *Jpn J Clin Oncol.* 2008;38(3):227–229.

58. Balaban EP, Mangu PB, Khorana AA, et al. Locally advanced, unresectable pancreatic cancer: American Society of Clinical Oncology clinical practice guideline. *J Clin Oncol.* 2016;34(22):2654–2668.

59. Videtic GMM, Woody N, Vassil AD. *Handbook of Treatment Planning in Radiation Oncology.* 2nd ed. New York, NY: Demos Medical; 2015.

60. Goodman KA, Regine WF, Dawson LA, et al. Radiation Therapy Oncology Group consensus panel guidelines for the delineation of the clinical target volume in the postoperative treatment of pancreatic head cancer. *Int J Radiat Oncol Biol Phys.* 2012;83(3):901–908.

61. Morganti AG, Trodella L, Valentini V, et al. Pain relief with short-term irradiation in locally advanced carcinoma of the pancreas. *J Palliat Care.* 2003;19(4):258–262.

62. Ceha HM, van Tienhoven G, Gouma DJ, et al. Feasibility and efficacy of high dose conformal radiotherapy for patients with locally advanced pancreatic carcinoma. *Cancer.* 2000;89(11):2222–2229.

63. Arcidiacono PG, Calori G, Carrara S, McNicol ED, Testoni PA. Celiac plexus block for pancreatic cancer pain in adults. *Cochrane Database Syst Rev.* 2011;(3):CD007519.

64. Wong GY, Schroeder DR, Carns PE, et al. Effect of neurolytic celiac plexus block on pain relief, quality of life, and survival in patients with unresectable pancreatic cancer: a randomized controlled trial. *JAMA.* 2004;291(9):1092–1099.

65. Eisenberg E, Carr DB, Chalmers TC. Neurolytic celiac plexus block for treatment of cancer pain: a meta-analysis. *Anesth Analg.* 1995;80(2):290–295.

66. Neoptolemos JP, Dunn JA, Stocken DD, et al. Adjuvant chemoradiotherapy and chemotherapy in resectable pancreatic cancer: a randomised controlled trial. *Lancet.* 2001;358(9293):1576–1585.

67. Neoptolemos JP, Stocken DD, Friess H, et al. A randomized trial of chemoradiotherapy and chemotherapy after resection of pancreatic cancer. *N Engl J Med.* 2004;350(12):1200–1210.

68. Abrams RA, Winter KA, Regine WF, et al. Failure to adhere to protocol specified radiation therapy guidelines was associated with decreased survival in RTOG 9704: a Phase III trial of adjuvant chemotherapy and chemoradiotherapy for patients with resected adenocarcinoma of the pancreas. *Int J Radiat Oncol Biol Phys.* 2012;82(2):809–816.

69. Berger AC, Winter K, Hoffman JP, et al. Five year results of US intergroup/RTOG 9704 with postoperative CA 19-9 ≤90 U/mL and comparison to the CONKO-001 trial. *Int J Radiat Oncol Biol Phys.* 2012;84(3):e291–e297.

70. Paniccia A, Edil BH, Schulick RD, et al. Neoadjuvant FOLFIRINOX application in borderline resectable pancreatic adenocarcinoma: a retrospective cohort study. *Medicine (Baltimore).* 2014;93(27):e198.

71. Blazer M, Wu C, Goldberg RM, et al. Neoadjuvant modified (m) FOLFIRINOX for locally advanced unresectable (LAPC) and borderline resectable (BRPC) adenocarcinoma of the pancreas. *Ann Surg Oncol.* 2015;22(4):1153–1159.

72. Sherman WH, Chu K, Chabot J, et al. Neoadjuvant gemcitabine, docetaxel, and capecitabine followed by gemcitabine and capecitabine/radiation therapy and surgery in locally advanced, unresectable pancreatic adenocarcinoma. *Cancer.* 2015;121(5):673–680.

73. Moertel CG, Childs DS Jr, Reitemeier RJ, et al. Combined 5-fluorouracil and supervoltage radiation therapy of locally unresectable gastrointestinal cancer. *Lancet.* 1969;2(7626):865–867.

74. Moertel CG, Frytak S, Hahn RG, et al. Therapy of locally unresectable pancreatic carcinoma: a randomized comparison of high dose (6000 rads) radiation alone, moderate dose radiation (4000 rads + 5-fluorouracil), and high dose radiation + 5-fluorouracil: The Gastrointestinal Tumor Study Group. *Cancer.* 1981;48(8):1705–1710.

75. Treatment of locally unresectable carcinoma of the pancreas: comparison of combined-modality therapy (chemotherapy plus radiotherapy) to chemotherapy alone. Gastrointestinal Tumor Study Group. *J Natl Cancer Inst.* 1988;80(10):751–755.

76. Loehrer PJ Sr, Feng Y, Cardenes H, et al. Gemcitabine alone versus gemcitabine plus radiotherapy in patients with locally advanced pancreatic cancer: an Eastern Cooperative Oncology Group trial. *J Clin Oncol.* 2011;29(31):4105–4112.

77. Murphy JD, Christman-Skieller C, Kim J, et al. A dosimetric model of duodenal toxicity after stereotactic body radiotherapy for pancreatic cancer. *Int J Radiat Oncol Biol Phys.* 2010;78(5):1420–1426.

78. WF S, TJ K. Randomized trial of intraoperative radiotherapy in resected carcinoma of the pancreas. *Int J Radiat Oncol Biol Phys.* 1986;12(1):148.

79. Willett CG, Del Castillo CF, Shih HA, et al. Long-term results of intraoperative electron beam irradiation (IOERT) for patients with unresectable pancreatic cancer. *Ann Surg.* 2005;241(2):295–299.

34: RECTAL CANCER

Ehsan H. Balagamwala and Sudha R. Amarnath

QUICK HIT: Colorectal cancer (CRC) is the third most common cancer in the United States. Pts with FAP or HNPCC are at increased risk for developing CRC at younger age. Surgical resection is standard and involves total mesorectal excision (TME) accomplished by either low anterior resection (LAR, sphincter sparing) or abdominoperineal resection (APR, not sphincter sparing). Neoadjuvant RT is standard for high-risk pts, typically defined as either node-positive or cT3-4 and reduces LRR. Typical RT dose is 50.4 Gy/28 fx with concurrent continuous infusion 5-FU or capecitabine followed by surgery ~7–8 weeks later, although 25 Gy/5 fx RT alone with surgery 7 to 10 days later is also an accepted standard.

TABLE 34.1: General Treatment Paradigm for Rectal Cancer	
	Treatment Options
Stage I	cT1N0: consider transanal local excision alone followed by observation for low-risk lesions (pT1 lesion <3 cm, <30% circumference, within 8 cm of anal verge, grade 1-2, margin >3 mm, no LVSI).[1] If pT1 with high-risk features (+margins, LVSI, poorly differentiated tumors) or pT2, proceed with APR/LAR with TME followed by adjuvant therapy as indicated. cT2N0: APR/LAR as indicated with TME. No adjuvant treatment if pT1-2N0. If pT3N0 or pT1-3N1-2, adjuvant chemoRT +/− adjuvant CHT.
Stage II/III	Preoperative chemoRT/RT, then LAR/APR with TME, then adjuvant CHT (controversial). *Short-course RT not recommended for T4 or multiple clinical LNs. If obstructed may need diverting colostomy prior to induction therapy.*
Stage IVA (resectable metastasis)	Individualize therapy based on multidisciplinary discussion and presentation. General options include: Combination CHT followed by RT (short or long course), then staged or synchronous resection (primary with metastasis) and adjuvant CHT *or* ChemoRT followed by staged or synchronous resection (primary and metastasis) and adjuvant CHT
Isolated pelvic or anastomotic recurrence	Resectable: preoperative chemoRT → resection +/− IORT Unresectable: CHT +/− RT If prior pelvic RT, consider BID re-irradiation.

EPIDEMIOLOGY: Colorectal cancer (CRC) is the third leading cause of cancer in the United States, second most common cause of cancer-related deaths in males, and third most common in females. In 2017, estimated incidence of CRC is 135,430 of which 95,520 are rectal cancers. Incidence of CRC is higher in men and in African Americans compared to women and Caucasians. Incidence is declining in both genders but has risen sharply in young patients.[2] In the United States, average lifetime risk of developing CRC is 5%.[3]

RISK FACTORS: Age, male sex, IBD (especially UC[4]), high fat, low fiber, alcohol use, tobacco, family history, genetic syndromes (Table 34.2), diabetes, red meat, cholecystectomy. Protective factors: NSAIDs, fiber, vitamin B6.

TABLE 34.2: Familial Colorectal Cancer Syndromes	
FAP	Autosomal dominant germline mutation in adenomatous polyposis coli (APC) gene located on chromosome 5. CRC occurs at younger age than general population and usually does not arise from adenoma. Variants include Gardener's (sarcomas, osteomas, desmoid tumors) and Turcot's (GBM, medulloblastoma).
HNPCC (Lynch)	Due to microsatellite instability as result of mutations in mismatch repair genes, most commonly hMLH1, hMSH2, hMSH6, or PMS2. Synchronous and metachronous tumors are possible. Pts with HNPCC also have increased risk of endometrial, ovarian, stomach, small bowel, hepatobiliary system, brain, renal pelvis, and ureteral cancers.

ANATOMY: Rectal cancer defined as lesion straddling or inferior to peritoneal reflection (landmark is middle transverse fold at ~11 cm from anal verge) OR lesion within 12 cm of verge. If lesion completely above this level, treated as colon cancer (note: trials have used anywhere up to 16 cm from verge). Layers of rectum: mucosa, muscularis mucosa, submucosa, muscularis propria, serosa, fat. Rectum is ~12–15 cm in length, beginning proximally at rectosigmoid junction (~S3) and extending to anorectal ring, just proximal to dentate line. Proximal third is peritonealized anteriorly and laterally, supplied by superior rectal artery (from IMA). Middle third is peritonealized anteriorly, and is supplied by middle rectal artery from internal iliac. Lower rectum is not peritonealized, and is supplied by inferior rectal artery from internal pudendal artery. Anorectal ring is composed of internal and external sphincters and levator ani muscles. Mesorectum is not true mesentery but rather loose connective tissue that is thicker posteriorly. It contains terminal branches of IMA and needs to be removed for adequate surgery (see TME later). Anorectal ring: (a) represents internal anal sphincter muscle and is necessary for anal continence, (b) represents inferior limit for functional sphincter preservation surgery, and (c) defines lymphatic watershed for rectal cancer spread. Tumors arising above anorectal ring tend to metastasize along distribution of middle rectal vessels to internal iliac lymph nodes as compared to tumors that may extend into anal canal, which may spread to superficial inguinal nodes via nodes along inferior rectal and external iliac pathways. *Nodal drainage*: Superior half of rectum drains along superior rectal artery to pararectal, presacral, sigmoidal, and inferior mesenteric nodes. Inferior half of rectum drains along middle rectal artery to internal iliac nodes. Tumors extending to anal canal (below dentate line) may drain to superficial inguinal nodes. Tumors that invade anteriorly (into pelvic organs) can drain to external iliac nodes. Pattern of metastasis: Liver is the most common site of metastatic disease in both colon and rectal cancer, but rectal cancer has increased propensity for lung as compared to colon cancer. Upper rectal tumors spread along superior rectal vein to portal system and into liver. Middle and inferior rectal tumors spread along middle and inferior rectal veins, into internal iliac lymph nodes, into systemic circulation and into lung.

PATHOLOGY: More than 90% of rectal cancers are adenocarcinomas. Approximately 15% to 20% of adenocarcinomas have colloid (extracellular mucin); however, there is no prognostic significance. However, tumors with signet ring (intracellular mucin) compose 1% to 2% of adenocarcinomas and have worse prognosis. Other histologies: small cell, carcinoid, leiomyosarcoma, lymphoma.

SCREENING[5,6]**:** For average-risk pts, NCCN suggests colonoscopy at 50 years of age and every 10 years if negative. If polyps identified, repeat colonoscopy every 3 or 5 years depending on risk of polyp. Other options include stool-based testing, imaging with CT colonoscopy, or combination of flexible sigmoidoscopy with stool guaiac. Stool-based tests include stool guaiac, fecal immunochemical (FIT), or fecal DNA; if positive, proceed to colonoscopy. In high-risk pts, start screening at 40 years of age or 10 years before first diagnosis in affected first-degree relative, then repeat colonoscopy every 5 years. If IBD, annual colonoscopy starting 8 to 10 yrs after symptom onset. If FAP, elective colectomy or proctocolectomy after onset of polyposis. If HNPCC, colonoscopy every 1 to 2 yrs starting at 20 to 25 years of age.

CLINICAL PRESENTATION: Hematochezia is the most common presenting symptom in rectal and lower sigmoid cancers. Abdominal pain is more common in colon cancer. Other symptoms: constipation, diarrhea, reduced stool caliber and in locally advanced disease, tenesmus, rectal urgency, inadequate emptying, urinary symptoms, buttock and perineal pain.

WORKUP: H&P, including DRE (size, location, mobility, sphincter function) and pelvic exam in women.

Labs: CBC, LFTs, CEA (adverse impact on survival independent of stage).

Procedures: Colonoscopy w/ biopsies.

Imaging: CT chest, abdomen, pelvis. MRI pelvis with contrast standard clinical staging. Rectal ultrasound can be utilized if MRI not available. PET/CT is not routine, but is utilized in many practices.

PROGNOSTIC FACTORS: Stage (both T and N classifications), circumferential resection margin (CRM), and LVI are most important factors. Performance status, AJCC stage, grading (G3 worse), surgery, administration of CHT and hemoglobin levels before (<12 vs. ≥12 g/dL) and during RT all predicted for improved survival.[7] Preoperative CEA >5 ng/mL has been associated with inferior RFS and OS. Gunderson et al. performed pooled analysis of 3,791 pts enrolled on five clinical trials treated with surgery and adjuvant therapy consisting of CHT and/or RT. Both T and N stage were independent factors for survival.[8] Four risk groups were identified: low (T1-2N0), intermediate (T1-2N1/T3N0), moderately high (T1-2N2, T3N1 or T4N0), and high risk. Moderately high and high risk were felt to warrant trimodality treatment; intermediate was felt to be borderline.

STAGING

TABLE 34.3: AJCC 8th ed. (2017) Staging for Rectal cancer		cN0	cN1a	cN1b	cN1c	cN2a	cN2b
T/M	**N**						
T1	• Invades submucosa	I	IIIA				
T2	• Invades muscularis mucosa	I					
T3	• Invades into pericolorectal soft tissue	IIA	IIIB				
T4	a Invades into visceral peritoneum[1]	IIB					
	b Invades or adherent to adjacent organs/ structures	IIC	IIIC				
M1a	• Distant metastasis to 1 organ without peritoneal metastasis	IVA					
M1b	• Distant metastasis to ≥2 organs without peritoneal metastasis	IVB					
M1c	• Metastasis to peritoneal surface with or without other organ or site	IVC					

No major changes from AJCC 7th edition; M1c category was added.

Notes: Peritoneum[1] = Includes gross perforation of bowel through tumor and continuous invasion of tumor through areas of inflammation to surface of visceral peritoneum.

cN1a, 1 regional LN; cN1b, 2-3 regional LNs; cN1c, no positive regional LNs, but subserosal, mesenteric, non-peritoneal peri-colic or peri-rectal tumor deposits; cN2a, 4-6 regional LNs; cN2b, ≥7 regional LNs.

TREATMENT PARADIGM

Surgery: Surgery is mainstay of treatment. T1 tumors can be initially managed with transanal excision. All other tumors should undergo transabdominal resection (LAR or APR) with sharp TME with at least 12 lymph nodes resected for staging.

Local Excision (Transanal Excision or Transanal Endoscopic Microsurgery): Possible for T1 tumors that are <3 cm in greatest diameter, no more than 30% of rectal circumference, within 8 cm of dentate line or below middle rectal valve, low-grade histology and no LVSI.[1]

Low Anterior Resection (LAR): Sphincter-sparing surgery with coloanal anastomosis (or alternatively colonic J-pouch or coloplasty). Distal margins of 2 cm or even less is now adequate and crucial margin is circumferential resection margin (CRM).

Abdominoperineal Resection (APR): Historically for tumor <5 cm from anal verge where sphincter sparing was not thought possible. Rectosigmoid is oversewn via abdominal incision and pulled out with anal canal via perineal incision. Requires permanent colostomy, with more morbidity. NSABP R-04 did not show worse QOL at 1 year between APR compared to sphincter-sparing surgery but profiles of QOL were different.[9]

Total Mesorectal Excision: STANDARD OF CARE regardless of APR or LAR. Involves sharp en bloc removal of mesorectum including associated vascular and lymphatic structures, fatty tissue, and mesorectal fascia as "package" through sharp dissection, designed to spare autonomic nerves. TME improves LC and autonomic nerve damage (impotence, retrograde ejaculation, and urinary incontinence) compared with standard blunt dissection of conventional surgery, but with higher rate of anastomotic leaks.

Chemotherapy: Utilization of CHT leads to improved LC and OS as well as decreased risk for developing DM.[10]

Indications: in pre/post-op setting for T3/T4, N1/N2 disease, positive margins or at high risk for local recurrence (high-grade positive or close margin).

Concurrent CHT:

1. PVI 5-FU: With concurrent RT improves LC, DFS and OS (as per the following Mayo Clinic/NCCTG study); protracted venous infusion (PVI) 5-FU with concurrent RT, when compared to bolus 5-FU, had lower rate of recurrence and DM, with improvement in 4-yr OS from 60% to 70%.[11] PVI 5-FU dose is 225 mg/m^2 c throughout RT (7 days/week).
2. Capecitabine: Several trials suggest noninferiority relative to PVI 5-FU. German phase III trial (included pre- and post-op chemoRT) showed significant reduction in DM and trend toward OS and DFS benefit.[12] NSABP R-04 trial confirmed equivalency and showed equivalence of capecitabine to PVI 5-FU.[13] Capecitabine is associated with more hand foot syndrome, fatigue, proctitis, and less leukopenia compared to 5-FU. Concurrent dose is 825 mg/m^2 BID 5 days per week. Without RT, dose is 1,000 to 1,250 mg/m^2 BID days 1 to 14, q3 weekly cycle.
3. Oxaliplatin: Not recommended as no benefit was observed on multiple trials despite increased toxicity.[13–16]
4. Irinotecan and bevacizumab: Multiple phase 2 trials showing good tolerability in combination with capecitabine as part of long-course chemoRT; however, use remains investigational.[17–19]

Adjuvant CHT: Role for adjuvant CHT is presently controversial but often performed given German rectal trial (see Sauer et al). Common regimens included FOLFOX, CAPEOX, 5-FU or 5-FU+LCV. Adore trial showed improved 3-yr DFS (72% vs. 63%) with adjuvant FOLFOX.[20] Similarly CAO/ARO/AIO-04 trial comparing preoperative chemoRT with

5-FU +/− oxaliplatin followed by surgery and adjuvant 5-FU LCV +/− oxaliplatin showed improved DFS with oxaliplatin.[21] In contrast, recent patient level meta-analysis shows no benefit to adjuvant CHT over no adjuvant CHT in pts who underwent concurrent pre-op chemoRT followed by surgery.[22,23]

Radiation: RT improves LC, reduces deaths from rectal cancer as well as possible improvement in OS.[24]

Preoperative RT: Indications include cT3-4 or cN1-2. Two options include short course (25 Gy/5 fx with surgery within 1 week and adjuvant CHT if node-positive) or long course (50.4 Gy/28 fx with concurrent CHT followed by surgery 7–8 weeks later). After short-course RT, postoperative complications increase after 5 days and substantially increase after 10 days (between surgery and RT). Although waiting 4 to 5 weeks after short course leads to improved downstaging (44% vs. 13%), there is no improvement in sphincter-sparing surgery.[25]

Post-operative RT: Indications include pT3-4, pN1-2 (stage II-III), positive margin, poor differentiation.[26] Consider boost to 55 to 60 Gy for gross residual disease. Consider colostomy prior to XRT in select pts including pts with severe obstruction. Relative contraindications for RT: active IBD, connective tissue disorder.

Procedure: See *Treatment Planning Handbook*, Chapter 7.[27]

Other Modalities: Other options for small T1 tumors include thermal electrocoagulation or endocavitary RT, HDR brachytherapy.

EVIDENCE-BASED Q&A

Long-course RT

Why is addition of chemoRT to surgery standard for rectal cancer?

GITSG 7175 (*NEJM* 1985, PMID 2859523; Update Thomas, *Radiother Oncol* 1988, PMID 3064191): PRT of 227 pts with Dukes B2 and C rectal (T3-4 or N+) ACA, R0 resection, no mets, distal edge of tumor <12 cm from verge. Randomized to either (a) surgery alone, (b) post-op CHT (bolus IV 5-FU/M-CCNU), (c) post-op RT 40 or 48 Gy standard fraction, or (d) post-op chemoRT: 40 or 44 Gy standard fraction + 5-FU 500 mg/m^2 followed by adjuvant 5-FU/M-CCNU as in CHT alone arm. Trial ended early due to significant benefit to chemoRT. Overall, CHT reduced DM (20% vs. 30%) and RT decreased LR (16% vs. 25%). **Conclusion: Adjuvant chemoRT improves LR and OS in rectal cancer.**

TABLE 34.4: Results of GITSG 7175 Rectal Cancer		
	7-yr LR	7-yr OS
Surgery	24%	36%
Surgery + RT	27%	46%
Surgery + CHT	20%	46%
Surgery + chemoRT + adjuvant CHT	11%	56%

Fisher, NSABP R-01 (*JNCI* 1988, PMID 3276900): PRT of 555 pts with Dukes B (AJCC T3N0) and C (node-positive) rectal cancer after curative resection randomized to (a) surgery alone, (b) post-op CHT with Me-CCNU, vincristine, and 5-FU (MOF), or (c) post-op RT alone (46–47 Gy). CHT improved 5-yr OS (53% vs. 43%, $p = .05$) and 5-yr DFS (42% vs. 30%, $p = .006$) while RT improved 5-yr LR (16% vs. 25%, $p = .06$) but did not improve OS. **Conclusion: adjuvant CHT improves OS while RT reduces LR.**

Krook, NCCTG 794751 (*NEJM* 1991, PMID 1997835): PRT of 204 pts with T3-4 or N+, within 12 cm of anal verge randomized to (a) post-op RT 45 Gy/25 fx + 5.4 Gy boost to tumor bed and adjacent LN or (b) post-op chemoRT with 5-FU bolus + semustine x1 month, then bolus 5-FU 500 mg/m^2 concurrent with RT, then 2 mos consolidative 5-FU/semustine. ChemoRT improved OS, DFS, LR and rate of DM compared to RT alone. **Conclusion: Adjuvant chemoRT is preferred to RT alone.**

What is the value of adding RT to CHT in adjuvant setting?

Wolmark, NSABP R-02 (*JNCI* 2000, PMID 106990969): PRT of 694 pts with resected Dukes B (AJCC T3N0) and C (node-positive) rectal cancer randomized to receive either (a) postoperative adjuvant CHT alone (n = 348) or (b) CHT with postoperative RT (n = 346). All female pts (n = 287) received 5-FU plus LV CHT; male pts received either MOF (n = 207) or 5-FU plus LV (n = 200). RT significantly improved LC in chemoRT arm. **Conclusion: Addition of RT to CHT improves LC but not OS.**

TABLE 34.5: Results of NSABP R-02 Rectal Trial

NSABP R-02	5-yr OS	5-yr DFS	5-yr LR
Post-op CHT	60%	54%	13%
Post-op chemoRT	62%	56%	8%
p value	.38	.90	.02

What is the benefit of pre-op chemoRT over postoperative chemoRT?

Sauer, German Rectal Study (*NEJM* 2004, PMID 15496622, Update *JCO* 2012, PMID 22529255): PRT of 823 pts ≤75 years of age with cT3-4 or cN+ rectal ACA with inferior margin ≤16 cm from anal verge, randomized to (a) preoperative chemoRT 50.4 Gy/28 fx and concurrent continuous infusion 5-FU followed by TME in 6 weeks, (b) Postop chemoRT 50.4 Gy/28 fx with 5.4 Gy boost to tumor bed 4 weeks following surgery. All pts had TME, and adjuvant CHT started 4 weeks after surgery or after completion of post-op chemoRT composed of four cycles of FU 500 mg/m^2 intravenous bolus. Primary endpoint was OS. Compliance higher in pre-op arm 90% versus ~50% in post-op arm. Overall, sphincter-preserving surgery was not more common in pre-op group, although pre-op therapy improved likelihood of sphincter-preservation surgery in those initially felt to require APR (39% vs. 19% *p* = .004). ChemoRT improved acute and late toxicity (14% vs. 25% late toxicity), and 10-yr LR with RT. Pre-op therapy improved likelihood of sphincter-sparing operation via downstaging. pCR was 8%, nodal involvement decreased (40% vs. 25%). No improvement in DR, OS, or DFS. 18% of pts in postoperative arm were overstaged by clinical staging. **Conclusion: Preoperative chemoRT improves LC, tumor downstaging, reduces late effects, and is preferred to postoperative chemoRT.**

TABLE 34.6: Long-term Results of German Rectal Study

	10-yr LR	10-yr DM	10-yr OS	10-yr DFS	Acute Grade 3-4	Late Grade 3-4
Pre-op chemoRT	7%	29.8%	59.6%	68.1%	27%	14%
Post-op chemoRT	10%	29.6%	59.9%	67.8%	40%	24%
p value	.048	.9	.85	.65	.001	.01

Roh, NSABP R-03 (*JCO* 2009, PMID 19770376): PRT of 267 pts (900 planned) with cT3-4 or N+ rectal ACA, lesion <15 cm from verge, M0 randomized to (a) pre-op 5-FU 500 mg/m^2 and leucovorin 500 mg/m^2 x6 weeks followed by chemoRT 50.4 Gy/28 fx with concurrent 5-FU+LV or (b) Postop chemoRT (same as pre-op) with primary endpoints DFS and OS. Trial was underpowered with improved DFS with pre-op chemoRT 64.7% versus 53.4% $p = .01$ but no difference in OS. Trial had 15% pCR rate. **Conclusion: Although underpowered, supports pre-op chemoRT as preferred approach.**

Does concurrent CHT improve outcomes over long-course RT alone?

Gérard, FFCD 9203/France (*JCO* 2006, PMID 17008704): PRT of T3-4NxM0 rectal ACA, accessible to DRE randomized to (a) Pre-op RT 45 Gy/25 fx or (b) pre-op chemoRT with bolus 5-FU + LCV on weeks 1 and 5. 50% of pts in both arms received adjuvant 5-FU CHT and primary endpoint was OS. ChemoRT reduced LF (8.1% vs. 16.5%, $p < .05$) and pCR (11.4% vs. 3.6%, $p < 0.05$) at cost of increased grade 3-4 toxicity (15% vs. 3%, $p < .05$) with chemoRT. No change in sphincter preservation.

Bosset, EORTC 22921 (*NEJM* 2006, PMID 16971718, Update *JCO* 2007, PMID 17906203): PRT of 1,011 pts (≤80 y/o) with T3 or resectable T4 rectal ACA within 15 cm of anal verge, randomized to (a) pre-op RT, (b) pre-op chemo, (c) pre-op RT and post-op CHT, or (4) pre-op chemoRT and post-op CHT. RT was 45 Gy/25 fx to posterior pelvis and 5-FU was given 350 mg/m^2/day. TME not routine. Primary endpoint OS. 5-yr incidence of LR was 17.1%, 8.7%, 9.6%, and 7.6% per arms of study, respectively. There was no effect on OS. **Conclusion: Preoperative chemoRT is superior to long-course RT alone with respect to LC.**

Does increased interval of time between pre-op chemoRT and surgery impact pCR rates?

Lefevre, GRECCAR-6 (*JCO* 2016, PMID 27432930): PRT of 265 pts from 24 centers. cT3/4 or cN+ pts in mid or lower rectum were eligible. ChemoRT included 45 to 50 Gy with 5-FU or capecitabine. Randomization was chemoRT, then randomized to surgery at either 7 or 11 weeks. Primary endpoint was pCR rate. 82% of tumors were cT3. Surgery not performed in 3.4% of pts due to development of metastatic disease or other reasons. Overall, 47 pts (18.6%) achieved pCR. pCR rates were not different between 7 and 11 weeks (15% vs. 17.4%, $p = .598$). However, morbidity was significantly increased in 11-week group (44.5% vs. 32%, $p = .04$) and quality of TME was also worse (complete mesorectum 78.7% vs. 90%, $p = .02$). **Conclusion: Waiting 11 weeks after chemoRT did not increase rate of pCR. Longer waiting period may be associated with higher morbidity and more difficult surgical resection.**

Since pCR is associated with improved outcomes, can additional CHT after pre-op long-course chemoRT increase pCR rates?

Garcia-Aguilar (*Lancet Oncol* 2015, PMID 26187751): Phase 2, nonrandomized study with four consecutive groups: group 1 underwent chemoRT followed by surgery 6 to 8 weeks later; groups 2 to 4 received two, four, or six cycles of mFOLFOX6, respectively, after long-course chemoRT followed by surgery. Primary endpoint pCR (intention to treat). 292 pts registered, 259 analyzable. pCR rates: 18% (group 1), 25% (group 2), 30% (group 3), 38% (group 4), $p = .0036$. Study group was independently associated with pCR ($p = .011$). Grades 3 and 4 toxicities were increased with total neoadjuvant therapy: group 2 (3%), group 3 (18%), group 4 (28%). **Conclusion: mFOLFOX6 prior to surgery is being evaluated for nonoperative management of rectal cancer.**

In pts who achieve cCR after pre-op therapy, can surgery be omitted?

This is active area of investigation on protocol but is not standard off protocol.

Habr-Gama, Brazil (*Ann Surg* 2004, PMID 15383798): RR of 265 pts with distal rectal adenocarcinoma (cT2-4, 24% node-positive) treated with 50.4 Gy/28 fx and 5-FU/LCV. 71 pts (26.8%) developed cCR and additional 8.3% were pT0 on resection. All were followed. Pts with cCR had 100% 5-yr OS and in pT0 group 5-yr OS was 88%.

Habr-Gama, Brazil (*Semin Radiat Oncol* 2011, PMID 21645869): Review and RR of 173 pts from 1991 to 2009 treated with neoadjuvant chemoRT 50.4 to 54 Gy with concurrent 5-FU; 63% cT3/T4, 21% cTxN1-2. MFU of 65 mos. 67 pts (39%) developed cCR. Of these 67 pts, 13% underwent rectal biopsy and 87% were managed without surgical procedures. Recurrences were observed in 15 pts (21%): 8 pts developed local only recurrence and seven developed DM. Median time to recurrence was 38 mos. Of 8 pts who recurred locally, seven were successfully salvaged. 5-yr OS was 96% and 5-yr DFS was 72%. **Conclusion: Early retrospective data suggests it may be feasible to reserve surgery for salvage after cCR to chemoRT.**

Renehan, OnCoRe (*Lancet Oncol* 2016, PMID 26705854): Propensity matched cohort study from UK evaluating "watch and wait" strategy in pts who achieve clinical CR after preoperative chemoRT. 259 pts were included of which 228 underwent surgery and 31 (12%) had complete CR and underwent watch and wait. Additional 98 pts with clinical CR were included via national registry for total of 129 pts managed by watch and wait. MFU 33 mos. Of 129 pts, 44 (34%) had LR and 36 of 41 pts were salvaged. In matched analysis, there was no difference in non-regrowth DFS between watch and wait and immediate post-chemoRT surgery (88% and 78%, $p = .04$). No difference in 3-yr OS (96% vs. 87%, $p = .02$). Improved 3-yr colostomy-free survival in watch and wait cohort (74% vs. 47%). **Conclusion: Watch and wait can be considered in many pts without detriment in 3-yr OS.**

Can RT be omitted in pts with cT3N0 rectal cancer?

This cohort is considered "borderline" and may not benefit from RT in all cases. However, given concerns with accuracy of preoperative staging and nonequivalence of postoperative RT, many recommend pre-op RT for cT3N0 pts.[28]

Guillem, MSKCC (*JCO* 2008, PMID 18202411): RR review of 188 pts with cT3N0 rectal cancer who underwent preoperative chemoRT followed by resection. Despite pCR rate of 20% in pts, 22% of pts had pathologically involved mesorectal lymph nodes.

Is tumor response after pre-op chemoRT predictive of outcomes?

Patel, Mercury Study (*JCO* 2011, PMID 21876084): Prospective cohort study of 111 pts treated with pre-op long-course RT alone or long-course chemoRT who underwent pre-operative MRI 4 to 6 weeks following pre-op treatment. All pts had to have at least 5 mm of initial tumor extension beyond muscularis propria. Results: Tumor regression on MRI was significantly predictive of OS (HR 4.4) and DFS (HR 3.3). If CRM was involved based on post-treatment MRI, there was significantly increased risk of LR (28% vs. 12%, $p < .05$). 5-yr OS for pts with involved pCRM was 30% versus 63% ($p = .001$), DFS was 34% versus 63% ($p < .001$) and LR was 26.4% versus 6.5% ($p < .001$). **Conclusion: Tumor regression as documented by MRI predicts DFS and OS and MRI predicted CRM involvement is associated with increased risk of LR.**

Fokas, German Rectal Trial Posthoc Analysis (*JCO* 2014, PMID 24752056): See details on German Rectal trial previously. Authors evaluated pathologic response based on viable tumor versus fibrosis—Tumor Regression Grading (TRG): Grade 0, no regression; Grade 1, minor regression (dominant tumor mass with obvious fibrosis in ≤25% of tumor mass); Grade 2, moderate regression (dominant tumor mass with obvious fibrosis in 26% to 50% of tumor mass); Grade 3, good regression (dominant fibrosis outgrowing tumor mass [i.e., >50% tumor regression]); and Grade 4, total regression (no viable tumor cells; fibrotic mass only). MFU 132 mos. Multivariate analysis showed that ypN+ and TRG were only independent prognosticators for DM and DFS. ypN+ and LVSI were predictive of LR. Cienfuegos et al. also showed that in pts with PNI/LVSI, TRG had no impact on OS. However, in pts without PNI/LVSI, TRG was predictive for OS and DFS.[29] Finally, pathologic response correlated with DFS, LR, and DM.

TABLE 34.7: German Rectal Trial Secondary Analysis on Tumor Regression Grade

10-yr results	DM	DFS
TRG 4	10.5%	89.5%
TRG 2/3	29.3%	73.6%
TRG 0/1	39.6%	63%
p value	.005	.008

Short-course RT

Is short course of preoperative RT effective compared to surgery alone?

Folkesson, Swedish Rectal Cancer Trial (*NEJM* 1997, PMID 9091798; Update *JCO* 2005, PMID 16110023): PRT of 1,168 pts with resectable rectal carcinoma, age <80, planned abdominal surgery, and no mets randomized to (a) 25 Gy/5 fx followed by surgery within 1 week or (b) surgery alone. Primary endpoints were LR and postoperative mortality. See Table 34.8 for results. **Conclusion: Pre-op RT is associated with significantly improved LC and OS compared to surgery alone.** *Comment: Unclear how many T1 included, non-TME surgery, increase risk of late small bowel obstruction in RT group.*

TABLE 34.8: Results of Short-Course Swedish Rectal Trial

	13-yr LR	13-yr OS	13-yr CSS
Pre-op 25 Gy/5 fx	9%	38%	72%
Surgery alone	26%	30%	62%
p value	<.001	.004	<.001

If TME is performed, is short-course RT still beneficial?

Kapiteijn, Dutch CKVO 9504 (*NEJM* 2001, PMID 11547717; Updates *Ann Surg* 2007 PMID 17968156, *Lancet Oncol* 2011 PMID 21596621): PRT of 1,861 pts with clinically resectable adenocarcinoma of rectum, no mets, inferior tumor margin <15 cm from anal verge randomized to (a) 25 Gy/5 fx followed by TME or (b) TME alone. Primary endpoint was LR. 10-yr LR was reduced from 11% to 5% (p < .0001) with no change in OS or DM. Of note, there was statistically significant OS benefit in stage III pts who had negative circumferential margins (50% vs. 40%, p = .03). **Conclusion: Preoperative RT with 25 Gy/5 fx significantly improves LC, even with good surgery (TME), but does not improve OS.**

Is pre-op short course better than post-op chemoRT?

Sebag-Montefiore, MRC CR 07 (*Lancet* 2009, PMID 19269519): PRT of 1,350 pts with resectable rectal ACA, (distal tumor <15 cm from verge), no mets randomized to (a) 25 Gy/5 fx followed by surgery or (b) surgery followed by post-op chemoRT (45 Gy/25 fx with concurrent 5-FU) for those with positive circumferential margin. Primary endpoint was LR. Most node-positive pts received adjuvant CHT. Pre-op short course was associated with improved LR (4.4% vs. 10.6%, $p < .0001$) and DFS (77.5% vs. 71.5%, $p = .013$) but not OS (70.3% vs. 67.9%, $p = .40$). **Conclusion: Pre-op short course is superior to selected post-op chemoRT.**

How does pre-op long-course chemoRT compare to short-course pre-op RT?

Bujko, Polish Study (*Br J Surg* 2006, PMID 16983741): PRT of 312 pts with cT3-4 with no evidence of sphincter involvement randomized to (a) 25 Gy/5 fx followed by TME within 7 days or (b) 50.4 Gy/28 fx with concurrent bolus 5-FU+LV followed by TME 4 to 6 weeks later. Primary endpoint was sphincter preservation. No difference in sphincter preservation, LR, OS, or DFS (Table 34.9). **Conclusion: Long-course chemoRT did not increase OS, LC, or late toxicity compared to short-course RT.** *Comment: Limitations to this study include clinical staging (no US or MRI), no standard post-op chemotherapy, not all TME, and no RT QA.*

TABLE 34.9: Polish Rectal Cancer Short-Course Trial

	4-yr LR	4-yr DFS	5-yr OS	Grade 3-4 Early Toxicity	Grade 3-4 Late Toxicity	Positive CRM
Pre-op chemoRT	15.5%	55.6%	66%	18%	7%	4.4%
Pre-op short-course RT	10.6%	58.4%	67%	3%	10%	12.9%
p value	.2	NS	NS	<.001	.36	.017

Ngan, TROG Intergroup Trial (*JCO* 2012, PMID 23008301): PRT of 326 pts with cT3N0-2M0 rectal ACA, within 12 cm of verge (US or MRI staged) randomized to (1) 25 Gy/5 fx (given in 1 week), surgery in 3 to 7 days, six cycles 5-FU with folinic acid or (2) 50.4 Gy/28 fx + CONTINUOUS INFUSION 5-FU (225 mg/m^2), surgery in 4 to 6 weeks, four cycles of 5-FU with folinic acid. Primary endpoint was LR. MFU 5.9 yrs. No differences in LR, DR, OS or late grade 3-4 toxicity (Table 34.10). For distally located tumors, LR was 12.5% in arm 2 versus 3% in arm 1, p = NS. **Conclusion: Short-course pre-op RT is equivalent to pre-op chemoRT without increased late toxicity. Unclear if short course is equivalent to long course for distally located tumors.**

TABLE 34.10: Results of TROG Short Versus Long-Course Rectal Trial

TROG 01.04	3-yr LR	5-yr DR	5-yr OS	Late Grade 3-4 Toxicity
Long course	4.4%	30%	70%	8.2%
Short course	7.5%	27%	74%	5.8%
p value	.24	.92	.62	NS

How long after short-course RT should surgery be performed?

Pach, Polish (*Langenbecks Arch Surg* 2012, PMID 22170083): Polish study of 154 pts randomized to early surgery (7–10 days) versus delayed (4–5 weeks) after short-course RT. Significantly higher rate of downstaging was achieved, (44% vs. 13%), for those who underwent delayed surgery. No differences were seen in sphincter sparing procedures, LC or OS. **Conclusion: In limited size prospective trial, delayed surgery after short-course RT is feasible and associated with higher rate of downstaging.**

Erlandsson, Stockholm III Trial (*Lancet Oncol* 2017, PMID 28190762): PRT (noninferiority) of 840 pts with resectable rectal adenocarcinoma without evidence of metastasis. Pts were randomized to (1) short-course RT (25 Gy/5 fx), then surgery (within 1 week), (2) short-course RT then surgery (4–8 weeks after RT), or (3) long-course RT only (50

Gy/25 fx) then surgery (4–8 weeks after RT). LR was 2.2%, 2.8%, 5.5% per arms of study, respectively (*p* = NS). Postoperative complications were similar between three arms of study. However, when evaluating only short-course pts, risk of postoperative complications was lower in arm (2) compared to arm (1) (41% versus 53%, *p* = .001). **Conclusion: Oncologic outcomes were similar between immediate surgery and delayed surgery after short-course RT. Similarly, long-course RT is similar to both short-course regimens. Postoperative complications were lower in pts who underwent delayed surgery after short-course RT.** *Comment: No CHT in long-course arm, protocol amendment allowed centers to enroll only on short-course arm, use of neoadjuvant CHT not reported, very few pts (<20%) received adjuvant CHT. Due to these deficiencies, it is difficult to interpret the results of this trial.*

Is IMRT for rectal cancer safe and effective?

Hong, RTOG 0822 (*IJROBP*** 2015, PMID 26163334):** Phase II study of cT3-4, N0-2 low to mid rectal cancer treated with IMRT 45 Gy/25 fx followed by 3D-chemoRT boost of 5.4 Gy/3 fx with concurrent capecitabine and oxaliplatin. Primary endpoint was improvement in grade II GI toxicity seen on RTOG 0247. 79 pts enrolled, 68 analyzable, 51% of pts developed grade II or higher GI toxicity, which was not significantly improved relative to historical controls. 15% of pts developed pCR and 4-yr LRF was 7.4%. **Conclusion: IMRT is feasible but did not demonstrate significant toxicity improvement relative to historical controls.**

Arbea, Spain (*IJROBP*** 2012, PMID 22079731):** Phase II study of T3/T4 and or N+ rectal cancer treated with preoperative IMRT 47.5 Gy/19 fx with concurrent capecitabine and oxaliplatin. 100 pts enrolled. pCr in 13% of pts and downstaging in 78%. **Conclusion: Preoperative IMRT with concurrent capecitabine and oxaliplatin is feasible.**

Recurrent rectal cancer

What are outcomes with reirradiation of recurrent rectal cancer?

Valentini, STORM (*IJROBP*** 2006, PMID 16414206):** Phase II nonrandomized trial of pelvic recurrences of rectal cancer in pts with previous RT <55 Gy and KPS ≥60. Pre-op RT: PTV2 (GTV + 4 cm) 30 Gy/25 fx at 1.2 Gy/fx BID followed by boost to PTV1 (GTV+2 cm) to 10.8 Gy/9 fx at 1.2 Gy/fx BID with concurrent PVI 5-FU. Pts who were resectable underwent surgery 6 to 8 weeks later. 59 pts enrolled. Median time to reirRT was 27 mos (min. 9 mos). Majority of pts (86.4%) completed therapy; 8.5% of pts developed pCR. Grade 3 GI toxicity was 5.1%. Overall response rate was 44.1%.

Guren, Norway (*Radiother Oncol*** 2014, PMID 25613395):** Systematic review of reirRT identified seven prospective and retrospective studies. Median initial dose was 50.4 Gy. Most studies used 1.2 Gy BID or 1.8 Gy daily fractionation with concurrent 5-FU. Median total dose was 30–40 Gy to GTV + 2–4 cm margin. Among pts who could be resected, MS was 39 to 60 mos and 12 to 16 mos for unresectable pts. Good symptomatic relief in 82% to 100%. Acute diarrhea reported in 9% to 20% of pts; however, late toxicity was insufficiently reported.

Mohiuddin, Kentucky (*Cancer*** 2002, PMID 12209702):** RR 103 pts previously treated w/ median dose 50.4 Gy. ReirRT dose was 30 Gy (1.2 Gy/fx BID) or 30.6 Gy (1.8 Gy/fx QD) with 6 to 20 Gy boost (median total dose 34.8 Gy). 34 pts were able to undergo resection, six had sphincter preservation. 5-yr OS was 19%. Palliation of bleeding achieved in 100%.

Ng, Peter MacCallum, Australia (*J Med Imaging Radiat Oncol*** 2013, PMID 23870353):** RR of 56 pts treated with reirRT to 39.6 Gy/22 fx at 1.8 Gy/fx QD (80% received concurrent PVI 5-FU). Overall, 91% completed tx. MS was 39 mos for resected and 15 mos for unresected pts; 12.5% developed grade 3 acute toxicity. **Conclusion: ReirRT is safe and feasible in rectal cancer and provides excellent palliation. Survival is higher in pts going on to radical resection.**

In pts with isolated liver metastasis, is cure still possible?

Choti, Johns Hopkins (*Ann Surg* 2002, PMID 12035031): RR of 226 pts from 1984 to 1999 treated with liver resection for colorectal metastases. MFU 46 mos. 5-yr OS was 40% overall (31% in early years and 58% in later years). 10-yr OS was 26%. **Conclusion: Cure and long-term survival after liver resection, particularly anatomical resection is possible in colorectal cancer.**

REFERENCES

1. NCCN Rectal Cancer Guidelines. 2017. https://www.nccn.org/professionals/physician_gls/pdf/rectal.pdf
2. Siegel RL, Fedewa SA, Anderson WF, et al. Colorectal cancer incidence patterns in United States, 1974–2013. *J Natl Cancer Inst.* 2017;109(8). doi:10.1093/jnci/djw322
3. Siegel RL, Miller KD, Jemal A. Cancer Statistics, 2017. *CA Cancer J Clin.* 2017;67(1):7–30. doi:10.3322/caac.21387
4. Ekbom A, Helmick C, Zack M, Adami HO. Ulcerative colitis and colorectal cancer. *N Engl J Med.* 1990;323(18):1228–1233. doi:10.1056/NEJM199011013231802
5. NCCN Colorectal Screening Guidelines. 2017. https://www.nccn.org/professionals/physician_gls/pdf/colorectal_screening.pdf
6. NCCN Genetic/Familial High-Risk Assessment: Colorectal. 2017. https://www.nccn.org/professionals/physician_gls/pdf/genetics_colon.pdf
7. Rades D, Kuhn H, Schultze J, et al. Prognostic factors affecting locally recurrent rectal cancer and clinical significance of hemoglobin. *Int J Radiat Oncol Biol Phys.* 2008;70(4):1087–1093. doi:10.1016/j.ijrobp.2007.07.2364
8. Gunderson LL, Sargent DJ, Tepper JE, et al. Impact of T and N stage and treatment on survival and relapse in adjuvant rectal cancer: pooled analysis. *J Clin Oncol Off J Am Soc Clin Oncol.* 2004;22(10):1785–1796. doi:10.1200/JCO.2004.08.173
9. Russell MM, Ganz PA, Lopa S, et al. Comparative effectiveness of sphincter-sparing surgery versus abdominoperineal resection in rectal cancer: patient-reported outcomes in National Surgical Adjuvant Breast and Bowel Project randomized trial R-04. *Ann Surg.* 2015;261(1):144–148. doi:10.1097/SLA.0000000000000594
10. Buyse M, Zeleniuch-Jacquotte A, Chalmers TC. Adjuvant therapy of colorectal cancer: why we still don't know. *JAMA.* 1988;259(24):3571–3578.
11. O'Connell MJ, Martenson JA, Wieand HS, et al. Improving adjuvant therapy for rectal cancer by combining protracted-infusion fluorouracil with RT therapy after curative surgery. *N Engl J Med.* 1994;331(8):502–507. doi:10.1056/NEJM199408253310803
12. Hofheinz R-D, Wenz F, Post S, et al. ChemoRT with capecitabine versus fluorouracil for locally advanced rectal cancer: randomised, multicentre, non-inferiority, phase 3 trial. *Lancet Oncol.* 2012;13(6):579–588. doi:10.1016/S1470-2045(12)70116-X
13. Allegra CJ, Yothers G, O'Connell MJ, et al. Neoadjuvant 5-FU or capecitabine plus RT with or without oxaliplatin in rectal cancer patients: phase III randomized clinical trial. *J Natl Cancer Inst.* 2015;107(11). doi:10.1093/jnci/djv248
14. Aschele C, Cionini L, Lonardi S, et al. Primary tumor response to preoperative chemoRT with or without oxaliplatin in locally advanced rectal cancer: pathologic results of STAR-01 randomized phase III trial. *J Clin Oncol Off J Am Soc Clin Oncol.* 2011;29(20):2773–2780. doi:10.1200/JCO.2010.34.4911
15. Gérard J-P, Azria D, Gourgou-Bourgade S, et al. Comparison of two neoadjuvant chemoRT regimens for locally advanced rectal cancer: results of phase III trial ACCORD 12/0405-Prodige 2. *J Clin Oncol Off J Am Soc Clin Oncol.* 2010;28(10):1638–1644. doi:10.1200/JCO.2009.25.8376

16. Hong TS, Moughan J, Garofalo MC, et al. NRG oncology RT Therapy Oncology Group 0822: phase 2 study of preoperative ChemoRT therapy using intensity modulated RT therapy in combination with capecitabine and oxaliplatin for patients with locally advanced rectal cancer. *Int J Radiat Oncol Biol Phys.* 2015;93(1):29–36. doi:10.1016/j.ijrobp.2015.05.005

17. Cai G, Zhu J, Palmer JD, et al. CAPIRI-IMRT: Phase II study of concurrent capecitabine and irinotecan with intensity-modulated RT therapy for treatment of recurrent rectal cancer. *Radiat Oncol Lond Engl.* 2015;10:57. doi:10.1186/s13014-015-0360-5

18. García M, Martinez-Villacampa M, Santos C, et al. Phase II study of preoperative bevacizumab, capecitabine and RT for resectable locally-advanced rectal cancer. *BMC Cancer.* 2015;15:59. doi:10.1186/s12885-015-1052-0

19. Salazar R, Capdevila J, Laquente B, et al. Randomized phase II study of capecitabine-based chemoRT with or without bevacizumab in resectable locally advanced rectal cancer: clinical and biological features. *BMC Cancer.* 2015;15:60. doi:10.1186/s12885-015-1053-z

20. Hong YS, Nam B-H, Kim K-P, et al. Oxaliplatin, fluorouracil, and leucovorin versus fluorouracil and leucovorin as adjuvant CHT for locally advanced rectal cancer after preoperative chemoRT (ADORE): open-label, multicentre, phase 2, randomised controlled trial. *Lancet Oncol.* 2014;15(11):1245–1253. doi:10.1016/S1470-2045(14)70377-8

21. Rodel C, Liersch T, Fietkau R, et al. Preoperative chemoRT and postoperative CHT with 5-fluorouracil and oxaliplatin versus 5-fluorouracil alone in locally advanced rectal cancer: results of German CAO/ARO/AIO-04 randomized phase III trial. *J Clin Oncol.* 2014;32:5s(Suppl; abstr 3500). http://meetinglibrary.asco.org/content/133115-144

22. Breugom AJ, Swets M, Bosset J-F, et al. Adjuvant CHT after preoperative (chemo)RT and surgery for patients with rectal cancer: systematic review and meta-analysis of individual patient data. *Lancet Oncol.* 2015;16(2):200–207. doi:10.1016/S1470-2045(14)71199-4

23. Colorectal Cancer Collaborative Group. Adjuvant RT for rectal cancer: systematic overview of 8,507 patients from 22 randomised trials. *Lancet Lond Engl.* 2001;358(9290):1291–1304. doi:10.1016/S0140-6736(01)06409-1

24. Cammà C, Giunta M, Fiorica F, et al. Preoperative RT for resectable rectal cancer: meta-analysis. *JAMA.* 2000;284(8):1008–1015.

25. Pach R, Kulig J, Richter P, Gach T, et al. Randomized clinical trial on preoperative RT 25 Gy in rectal cancer–treatment results at 5-year follow-up. *Langenbecks Arch Surg.* 2012;397(5):801–807. doi:10.1007/s00423-011-0890-8

26. Song C, Song S, Kim J-S, et al. Impact of postoperative chemoRT versus CHT alone on recurrence and survival in patients with stage II and III upper rectal cancer: propensity score-matched analysis. *PloS One.* 2015;10(4):e0123657. doi:10.1371/journal.pone.0123657

27. Videtic GMM, Woody N, Vassil AD, eds. *Handbook of Treatment Planning in RT Oncology.* 2nd ed. New York, NY: Demos Medical; 2015.

28. Wo JY, Mamon HJ, Ryan DP, Hong TS. T3N0 rectal cancer: RT for all? *Semin Radiat Oncol.* 2011;21(3):212–219. doi:10.1016/j.semradonc.2011.02.007

29. Cienfuegos JA, Rotellar F, Baixauli J, et al. Impact of perineural and lymphovascular invasion on oncological outcomes in rectal cancer treated with neoadjuvant chemoRT and surgery. *Ann Surg Oncol.* 2015;22(3):916–923. doi:10.1245/s10434-014-4051-5

35: ANAL CANCER

Aditya Juloori and Sudha R. Amarnath

> **QUICK HIT:** Squamous carcinoma of the anal canal is a relatively rare but often curable cancer. Standard of care is concurrent chemoRT with 5-fluorouracil (5-FU) and mitomycin C (MMC). Select T1N0 pts with well-differentiated anal margin cancers may be treated with WLE with 1-cm margins. Acute treatment-related toxicities are often severe but treatment breaks should be avoided as prolonged treatment time has been associated with increased failure rates. IMRT has been shown to reduce hematologic, GI, and skin toxicities but expertise is required with this approach.

TABLE 35.1: General Treatment Paradigm for Anal Cancer

Stage	Treatment Recommendations*
T1N0 (anal margin, well differentiated)	WLE ± chemoRT if inadequate margins
T1–T2N0 (anal canal)	50.4 Gy/28 fx to primary, 42 Gy/28 fx to LN
T3/T4N0	54 Gy/30 fx to primary, 45 Gy/30 fx to LN
Node-positive	54 Gy/30 fx to primary **Nodes:** ≤3 cm: 50.4 Gy/28 fx >3 cm: 54 Gy/30 fx
*IMRT doses per RTOG 0529[1].	

EPIDEMIOLOGY: Approximately 8,000 new diagnoses of anal cancer with 1,000 anal cancer–related deaths in the United States in 2016. Lifetime risk 1 in 500.[2] Comprises 2.5% of GI malignancies[3] (rectal cancer is 10x as common). Incidence in men and women has increased over last 30 years. Average age at diagnosis is in early 60s.[2] Incidence of anal cancer is twice as high in females as it is in males.[2] Incidence has not decreased in era of HAART.[4]

RISK FACTORS: HPV (most commonly HPV-16, but also 18, 31, 33, and 45).[2] High-risk HPV DNA has been detected in up to 84% of specimens in large-scale anal cancer studies.[5] Other risk factors include HIV infection, history of cervical, vulvar, or vaginal cancer (HPV-related), immunosuppression after organ transplant, smoking, history of receptive anal intercourse.

ANATOMY: *Anal canal* is 4-cm long and extends proximally from *anal verge* (palpable junction between non-hair-bearing and hair-bearing squamous epithelium) to *dentate line* (line between simple columnar epithelium proximally to stratified squamous epithelium distally). *Anal margin* is skin within 5 cm of anal verge. Canal is surrounded by internal and external anal sphincters.

Histology: Three zones: *Cutaneous zone* is anal margin. *Transition zone* is in canal and ends at dentate line, contains squamous epithelium without hair. *True mucosa* starts at dentate line and contains columns of Morgagni and holds transitional epithelium for about 2 cm before true mucosa of rectum begins.

Lymphatics: For tumors that arise below dentate line, drainage pattern is to inguinal and femoral nodes that arise from external iliacs. Above dentate line, nodal drainage pattern is similar to that of rectal cancer: perirectal and internal iliacs.

PATHOLOGY: 75% to 80% are squamous cell carcinoma. Other, more rare anal cancers include adenocarcinoma (treated like rectal cancer), melanoma, neuroendocrine, carcinoid, Kaposi's, leiomyosarcoma, and lymphoma. Perianal skin tumors (SCC, BCC, melanoma, Bowen's, Paget's) should be treated as skin cancer.

CLINICAL PRESENTATION: 45% of pts present with rectal bleeding, 30% will experience either pain or sensation of rectal mass.[6] Pts with more proximally located tumors can also present with alteration in bowel movements. At presentation roughly 50% of pts will present with localized disease, 30% will present with regional LN involvement, 10% will present with distant metastases (most commonly liver and lung).[7] Risk of nodal involvement is higher in pts with sphincter involvement or poorly differentiated tumors.

WORKUP: H&P (with careful attention to inguinal node exam and digital rectal exam to determine extent of tumor and sphincter function). GYN exam/cervical screening for females.

Labs: CBC, BMP, LFTs, CEA, HIV if there are risk factors (and CD4 if HIV+). Anoscopy with biopsy of primary, excisional biopsy or FNA of suspicious inguinal LNs and HPV status. Sigmoidoscopy/colonoscopy often performed as well.

Imaging: CT chest, abdomen, and pelvis, MRI of pelvis with contrast, PET/CT.

PROGNOSTIC FACTORS: Male sex, positive nodes, and tumor size >5 cm were independently prognostic for worse OS on analysis of RTOG 98-11.

STAGING

TABLE 35.2: AJCC 8th ed. (2017) Staging for Anal Cancer		cN0	cN1a	cN1b	cN1c
T/M					
T1	• ≤2 cm	I			
T2	• 2.1–5 cm	IIA		IIIA	
T3	• >5 cm	IIB			
T4	• Invasion into adjacent organs[1]	IIIB		IIIC	
M1	• Distant metastasis		IV		

Significant changes from 7th Edition include: revised N-staging (previous N1: perirectal, N2: unilateral internal iliac and/or inguinal, N3: perirectal and inguinal or bilateral internal iliac or bilateral inguinal), revised group staging (new IIA/B delineation, new IIIC).

Notes: Organs[1] = Invasion of vagina, urethra, bladder. Invasion of rectal wall, perirectal skin, subcutaneous tissue, or sphincter muscle are not always T4.

cN1a, metastasis in inguinal, mesorectal, or internal iliac nodes; cN1b, metastasis in external iliac nodes; cN1c, metastasis in external iliac node as well as any of inguinal, mesorectal, or internal iliac node involvement.

TREATMENT PARADIGM

Surgery: Before 1970s, anal cancer was treated with abdominal perineal resection (APR) and permanent colostomy with historical 5-yr OS rates of 60% for T1/2 disease, 40% for T3 disease and 20% for LN+ disease. In 1970s, the Nigro regimen was established after high CR rates to neoadjuvant chemoRT were noted. Concurrent chemoRT is now standard but has never prospectively compared with surgery. Local excision is treatment option as per

NCCN for those with T1N0 well-differentiated tumors of anal margin.[8] Pts with adequate margins (>1 cm) can be observed. Those resected with positive margins require re-excision, adjuvant RT, or chemoRT.

Chemotherapy: Definitive chemoRT as established by Nigro regimen is indicated for T2+ or any N+ disease. Standard of care is two cycles of 5-FU/MMC concurrent with radiation; 5-FU dose is 1,000 mg/m^2 days 1 to 4 and 29 to 32 (start of week 5). MMC given concurrently with 5-FU, two cycles on d1 and 29, 10 mg/m^2 IV bolus. Major limiting toxicity of MMC is neutropenia.

Radiation

Indications: RT is indicated in all cases except T1N0 tumors of anal margin treated with WLE, although RT alone may be appropriate for T1N0 (controversial). For others (cT2-4 or N+), organ-preservation therapy is standard with concurrent chemoRT.

Dose: No prospective data exists to guide RT dosing strategies. One common standard is as defined by RTOG 0529 (see Table 35.1 for dosing). IMRT is considered appropriate option for anal cancer in modern era.

Toxicity: Acute: Skin desquamation, fatigue, nausea, vomiting, diarrhea, urethritis, cystitis, pain, neutropenia.

Late: Cystitis, proctitis, sexual dysfunction (females), infertility, sacral insufficiency fracture, second malignancy, bowel stricture, fistula, hyperpigmentation, bowel incontinence.

EVIDENCE-BASED Q&A

What is the basis for nonsurgical management of anal cancer?

Historically, primary treatment was APR. Use of preoperative chemoRT in Wayne State study demonstrated excellent rates of CR and thus established that chemoRT alone was adequate. There has not been direct phase III comparison with surgery though definitive chemoRT compares favorably in retrospective reviews with benefit of allowing for sphincter preservation. T1 pts were not included in original Nigro studies.

Leichman, Wayne State "Nigro Regimen" (*Am J Med* 1985, PMID 3918441): RR of 45 pts (T2 or greater) treated with continuous infusion 5-FU (1000 mg mg/m^2) for 96 hours x two cycles days 1 to 4 and 29 to 32 as well as one cycle bolus MMC (15 mg/m^2) on day 1. RT was 30 Gy/15 fx over 3 weeks in AP/PA technique to pelvis and inguinal nodes. Post-treatment biopsy was taken 4 to 6 weeks after completion of chemoRT. Originally APR was required for all pts but in first six pts, five had PCR. Thus, in remainder of study, APR was required only for those with positive post-treatment biopsy. 84% of pts had negative biopsy after chemoRT, and there were no recurrences observed in this population with rate of 89% OS at 50 mos. Overall, 5-yr OS was 67% and 5-year CFS was 59%. **Conclusion: Definitive treatment with chemoRT alone is effective treatment for anal cancer.**

Is concurrent chemoRT superior to RT alone?

Two major randomized trials have been performed to answer this question. Both trials included more locally advanced pts and demonstrated that addition of CHT to RT improves pCR rates, LC, CSF, and DSS, though there was no noted improvement in OS. Addition of CHT did not significantly increase late toxicity. Update of ACT I shows that benefit provided by adjuvant chemoRT persists at 13 years.

UK ACT I (*Lancet* 1996, PMID 8874455; **Update Northover,** *Br J Cancer* 2010, PMID 20354531): PRT of 577 pts with stage II-IV anal SCC randomized to treatment with RT alone versus chemoRT. RT regimen was either 45 Gy/20 fx or 45 Gy/25 fx depending on institutional preference. In chemoRT arm, regimen was two cycles of continuous infusion 5-FU (1,000 mg/m^2 days 1–4 or 750 mg/m^2 days 1–5) during first and last week of RT. One cycle of bolus MMC was given on day 1 (12 mg/m^2). Clinical response was assessed at 6 weeks and those with response received additional 15 Gy boost with EBRT or 25 Gy boost with Ir-192 brachytherapy. Those without response had salvage surgery. Primary endpoint was LF. See Table 35.3. Addition of concurrent CHT to RT significantly improved LC and CSS. Acute toxicity was worse with CHT but there was no observed increase in late toxicity in pts treated with concurrent CHT. 13-year update demonstrated that for every 100 pts treated with chemoRT, there were 25 fewer locoregional relapses and 12.5 fewer anal cancer deaths with no difference in late toxicity. Though there was initial increase in nonanal cancer related deaths in first 5 years in pts treated with chemoRT, this was not seen in long-term FU. **Conclusion: CHT in addition to RT improves LC and CSS without increasing late toxicity.**

TABLE 35.3: Initial Results of ACT I Concurrent ChemoRT for Anal Cancer

	3-yr LF	3-yr OS	3-yr CSS	Acute Morbidity	Late Morbidity
RT	61%	58%	61%	39%	38%
RT + 5-FU/MMC	39%	65%	72%	48%	42%
p value	<.0001	.25	.02	.03	.39

Bartelink, EORTC 22861 (*JCO* 1997, PMID 9164216): PRT of 103 pts with T3/T4 or N+ disease randomized to RT versus chemoRT. RT was 45 Gy/25 fx with assessment at 6 weeks followed by 20 Gy boost for PR and 15 Gy boost for CR. APR was used if there was no response. CHT regimen was continuous infusion 5-FU 750 mg/m^2 on days 1 to 5 and days 29 to 33 and single dose of MMC 15 mg/m^2 on day 1. See Table 35.4. Addition of concurrent CHT improves LC, CFS, and CR rates but not OS. No significant difference in severe toxicities. **Conclusion: ChemoRT improves oncologic outcomes over use of definitive RT alone.**

TABLE 35.4: Results of EORTC ChemoRT for Anal Cancer

	5-yr CR	5-yr LC	5-yr CFS	5-yr OS
RT (n = 52)	54%	50%	40%	56%
RT + 5-FU/MMC (n = 51)	80%	68%	72%	56%
p value	.02	.02	.002	.17

Is concurrent 5-FU alone sufficient in comparison to 5-FU/MMC?

Multiple studies have shown that addition of MMC to 5-FU based chemoRT improves outcomes of LC, CFS, and OS despite greater toxicity. Most notable is RTOG 87-04 as follows but Princess Margaret study also confirmed importance of adding MMC.[9]

Flam, ECOG 1289/RTOG 8704 (*JCO* 1996, PMID 8823332): PRT of 291 pts with anal cancer of any T/N-stage treated with definitive chemoRT and randomized to either concurrent 5-FU and MMC or 5-FU alone. Regimen was 5-FU 1,000 mg/m^2 continuous infusion days 1 to 4 and 28 to 33, MMC 10 mg/m^2 IV bolus days 1 and 28. RT was 45 Gy/25 fx to pelvis with 5.4 Gy boost if palpable disease present at end of initial RT course. Biopsy was performed 4 to 6 weeks after chemoRT. If biopsy positive, further 9 Gy was given with concurrent 5-FU and cisplatin. Pts with residual tumor underwent APR. With use of concurrent MMC, at 4 years, rates of colostomy was lower (9% vs. 22%, *p* = .002), CFS was higher (71% vs. 59%, *p* = .014), and DFS was higher (73% vs. 51%, *p* = .003). No significant difference was observed in terms of OS. Grade 4 and 5 toxicity was higher in MMC arm (23% vs. 7%, $p \leq .001$). Of 24 pts who underwent salvage chemoRT after initial course of chemoRT, 50% were cured. **Conclusion: Though it is associated with greater toxicity, use of MMC improves DFS and colostomy-free survival. Salvage chemoRT may be reasonable for pts with residual disease as opposed to salvage APR.**

Can MMC be replaced with cisplatin?

RTOG 98-11 showed that replacing MMC with cisplatin and addition of induction CHT signifi- cantly decreased hematologic toxicities but also increased colostomy rates and reduced disease-free survival and overall survival. However, ACT II trial established that replacement of MMC with cisplatin does not affect rate of complete response. Because of ACT II showing that CHT regimens are equal in terms of response rate, some have suggested results of 98-11 show that induction CHT may be detrimental.

Ajani, RTOG 9811 (*JAMA* 2008, PMID 18430910; Update Gunderson *JCO* 2012, PMID 23150707): PRT of 649 pts with T2-T4, N0-N3 disease randomized to (a) RT + concurrent 5-FU/MMC or (b) RT + induction/concurrent 5-FU/cisplatin. RT was 45 Gy/25 fx with 2 Gy/fx boost to primary tumor and involved nodes to between 55 and 59 Gy for those with T3-T4, N+ or T2 pts with residual disease after 45 Gy. Elective nodal sites were treated to 30.6–36 Gy/17-20 fx. CHT in standard arm was 5-FU 1,000 mg/m^2 continuous infusion days 1 to 4 and 29 to 32 and MMC 10 mg/m^2 IV bolus days 1 and 29. In experimental arm, two cycles of induction 5-FU were given and RT started on day 57 with third cycle of 5-FU and was continued through end of fourth cycle. Cisplatin was also given in four bolus administrations: 75 mg/m^2 IV days 1, 29, 57, and 85, with two cycles prior to start of RT. See Table 35.5. OS and DFS were superior in standard arm. **Conclusion: Use of concur- rent 5-FU/MMC without induction CHT should remain standard of care.**

TABLE 35.5: Results of RTOG 98-11					
	5-yr OS	5-yr CFS	5-yr DFS	Grade 3-4 Heme Toxicity	Grade 3-4 Nonheme Toxicity
RT+ concurrent 5-FU/ MMC	78.3%	71.9%	67.8%	61%	74%
RT+ induction/ concurrent 5-FU/ cisplatin	70.7%	65%	57.8%	42%	74%
p value	.026	.05	.006	.0013	NS

James, UK ACT II (*Lancet Oncol* 2013, PMID 23578724): PRT of 940 T1-T4 pts rand- omized in 2 x 2 fashion to either concurrent 5-FU/cisplatin or concurrent 5-FU/MMC followed by second randomization to 5-FU x two cycles after completion of chemoRT (maintenance) or observation. RT dose was 50.4 Gy/28 fx. MFU 5.1 years. CR was ~90% with either concurrent CHT regimen. 3-yr PFS was 74% with maintenance CHT versus 73% with observation (p = NS). **Conclusion: MMC/5-FU+RT remains standard. There was no benefit to addition of maintenance CHT after completion of standard therapy.**

Are there any advantages to dose escalation?

RTOG 9208[10] demonstrated that there is no role for dose escalation, though study was limited by use of treatment break. Pts were treated to 59.4 Gy with concurrent 5-FU/MMC with mandatory 2-week break (then amended to be continuous without break). Higher dose in this study was associ- ated with increased colostomy rate and no significant difference in OS or LC compared to historical standards (RTOG 8704). These findings are supported by more recent ACCORD 03 trial, which also showed no improvement in oncologic outcomes with high dose boost (see the following).

Should we add induction CHT or high dose boost?

The results of ACCORD 03 are in line with findings of RTOG 9811—there is no benefit to induction CHT. One retrospective study has suggested there may be benefit in colostomy-free survival with use of induction CHT in T4 pts, though this has not been validated prospectively.[11] There is no role for high dose boost at this time.

Peiffert, ACCORD 03 (JCO 2012, PMID 22529257): PRT of 307 pts with anal SCC (tumor either ≥4 cm or N+) randomized in 2x2 fashion: ±induction CHT and either standard or high dose boost in addition to concurrent chemoRT (45 Gy/25 fx with concurrent 5-FU/cisplatin). Standard boost was 15 Gy. High dose boost was 20 Gy for CR or greater than 80% reduction and was 25 Gy for PR (less than 80% reduction). See Table 35.6. At MFU 50 mos, there was no statistically significant difference between four arms. Colostomy-free survival (CFS) was main endpoint with no advantage of induction CHT ($p = .37$) or high dose ($p = .067$) RT boost. **Conclusion: No benefit to induction CHT or high dose boost. Authors concluded that there should be further evaluation of dose intensification given that high dose boost had trend to improved CFS.**

TABLE 35.6: Results of ACCORD 03 for Anal Cancer			
Arm	5-Yr CFS	5-Yr LC	5-Yr DSS
Induction+chemoRT+ standard boost	69.6%	72.0%	76.6%
Induction+chemoRT+high dose boost	82.4%	87.9%	88.8%
chemoRT+standard boost	77.1%	83.7%	80.6%
chemoRT+high dose boost	72.7%	78.0%	75.9%

Is there benefit to IMRT?

RTOG 0529[1] was phase II trial evaluating use of IMRT for anal cancer. It demonstrated significant reduction in hematologic, GI, and skin toxicity compared to historic 3D-CRT standards. NCCN consensus is that IMRT is preferred over 3D conformal RT; however, IMRT requires expertise in its application. 81% of pts on study required replanning on central review. RTOG 0529 is appropriate guideline for use of IMRT in anal cancer.

What salvage options are available for recurrence after definitive chemoRT?

APR is used for salvage in setting of failure after definitive chemoRT. Salvage surgery results vary widely in literature due to small patient populations and selection bias. One study from Washington University of 22 pts undergoing salvage APR demonstrated only 65% of operations achieved negative margins and ultimately 50% of cohort recurred after salvage APR at median of 9 months.[12]

What is recommendation for T1N0 pts?

This patient subset was not included in original Nigro studies; these pts were also not included in RTOG 9811, ACT I, ACT II, or EORTC 22861. NCCN recommends local excision with adequate margins (defined as 1 cm) for anal margin cancers and chemoRT for anal canal lesions. Options for inadequate margins include re-excision (preferred) or local radiation with or without concurrent CHT. Retrospective series have suggested good outcomes with definitive RT for this patient subset.

REFERENCES

1. Kachnic LA, Winter K, Myerson RJ, et al. RTOG 0529: phase 2 evaluation of dose-painted inten-
    sity modulated radiation therapy in combination with 5-fluorouracil and mitomycin-C for reduc-
    tion of acute morbidity in carcinoma of anal canal. *Int J Radiat Oncol Biol Phys.* 2013;86(1):27–33.
2. American Cancer Society-Anal Cancer. What is anal cancer? 2016. http://old.cancer.org/
    cancer/analcancer/detailedguide/anal-cancer-what-is-anal-cancer
3. Siegel RL, Miller KD, Jemal A. Cancer statistics, 2016. *CA Cancer J Clin.* 2016;66(1):7–30.
4. Crum-Cianflone NF, Hullsiek KH, Marconi VC, et al. Anal cancers among HIV-infected persons:
    HAART is not slowing rising incidence. *AIDS (London, England).* 2010;24(4):535–543.
5. Frisch M, Glimelius B, van den Brule AJ, et al. Sexually transmitted infection as cause of anal
    cancer. *N Engl J Med.* 1997;337(19):1350–1358.
6. Ryan DP, Compton CC, Mayer RJ. Carcinoma of anal canal. *N Engl J Med.* 2000;342(11):792–800.
7. Altekruse SF, Kosary CL, Krapcho M, et al, eds. *SEER Cancer Statistics Review, 1975–2007, National
    Cancer Institute.* Bethesda, MD. (Based on November 2009 SEER data submission, posted to the
    SEER website, 2010). http://seer.cancer.gov/csr/1975_2007
8. NCCN Clinical Practice Guidelines in Oncology: Anal Carcinoma. 2017. https://www.nccn.org
9. Cummings BJ, Keane TJ, O'Sullivan B, et al. Epidermoid anal cancer: treatment by radiation
    alone or by radiation and 5-fluorouracil with and without mitomycin C. *Int J Radiat Oncol Biol
    Phys.* 1991;21(5):1115–1125.
10. Konski A, Garcia M Jr, John M, et al. Evaluation of planned treatment breaks during radiation
    therapy for anal cancer: update of RTOG 92-08. *Int J Radiat Oncol Biol Phys.* 2008;72(1):114–118.
11. Moureau-Zabotto L, Viret F, Giovaninni M, et al. Is neoadjuvant chemotherapy prior to
    radio-chemotherapy beneficial in T4 anal carcinoma? *J Surg Oncol.* 2011;104(1):66–71.
12. Stewart D, Yan Y, Kodner IJ, et al. Salvage surgery after failed chemoradiation for anal canal can-
    cer: should paradigm be changed for high-risk tumors? *J Gastrointest Surg.* 2007;11(12):1744–1751.

VII: **GENITOURINARY**

36: LOW-RISK PROSTATE CANCER

Yvonne D. Pham and Rahul D. Tendulkar

QUICK HIT: Low-risk prostate cancer includes organ-confined disease typically detected by a screening PSA or on DRE (T1-T2a), with a PSA <10 ng/mL and Gleason score (GS) ≤6. Standard treatment options include active surveillance, prostatectomy, EBRT, or brachytherapy (see Table 36.1). Prostate cancer–specific survival is >95% for each. Therefore, treatment selection is guided by side effect profiles and patient preference. Most guidelines recommend treatment only if life expectancy is >10 years. Dose-escalated RT improves biochemical control compared to "conventional" doses. Concurrent ADT is not indicated in low-risk prostate cancer. PROST-QA and ProtecT trials include patient-reported outcomes and are helpful to inform patient decisions.

TABLE 36.1: General Overview of Treatment Options for Low-Risk Prostate Cancer

Treatment Option	General Overview/ Example	Pros	Cons	Patient Selection
Watchful waiting	No further testing, treatment only when symptoms develop	No risk of overtreatment, reduces cost	Progression may occur without notice	Pts with severe comorbidity and/or limited life span
Active surveillance	Regimented follow-up with PSA testing and repeat biopsies; consider genomic testing and MRI-guided biopsy	Avoids immediate side effects and cost of treatment	Patient anxiety; risk of disease progression; costs increase over time	Compliant pts with low-risk or favorable intermediate-risk disease motivated toward deferring treatment
Radical prostatectomy	Robotic or open, usually with pelvic lymph node dissection	Removes all tumor/ prostate, relieves obstructive symptoms; obtains pathologic staging; avoids radiation exposure	Operative risk; higher risk of ED and incontinence than nonoperative options	Younger, healthier pts motivated toward avoiding RT or with significant obstructive symptoms or with concern regarding urinary or bowel effects of RT

(continued)

TABLE 36.1: General Overview of Treatment Options for Low-Risk Prostate Cancer (*continued*)

Treatment Option	General Overview/ Example	Pros	Cons	Patient Selection
IMRT (standard fractionation)	74–80 Gy over 7–9 weeks	"Gold standard" RT regimen with long-term follow-up	Protracted course is inconvenient; potential late effects include cystitis, proctitis, ED, second malignancy	
IMRT (moderate hypofractionation)	60–70 Gy over 4–5.5 weeks	Reduces treatment time, large randomized trials supporting treatment, reduced cost over conventional IMRT	Treatment time still moderately protracted; potential late effects include cystitis, proctitis, ED, second malignancy	Pts motivated toward nonoperative intervention or specific concerns of erectile dysfunction or incontinence from RP
SBRT (extreme hypofractionation)	35–40 Gy/5 fx QOD	Significantly reduces overall treatment time; late effects appear favorable	Long-term follow-up data not available; potential late effects include cystitis, proctitis, ED, second malignancy	
Brachytherapy	LDR with I-125/P-103 or HDR with Ir-192	Single-day procedure (LDR); minimally invasive; long-term follow-up available	Pronounced acute LUTS; potential late effects include urinary retention, cystitis, ED, second malignancy	

EPIDEMIOLOGY: There were an estimated 180,890 new cases and 26,120 deaths predicted for 2016.[1] 14% lifetime risk for U.S. males. Prostate cancer is the most common noncutaneous malignancy in U.S. men and second most common cause of cancer death in men (behind lung cancer). Due to screening, the median age of diagnosis is 60 years of age. The incidence is highest in Scandinavia and lowest in Asia. In the United States, incidence is higher in African Americans compared to Caucasians (1.5–2:1).

RISK FACTORS: Increasing age, African American (earlier onset and often more aggressive even after adjustment for confounders), and family history are the strongest known factors.[2,3,4] Germline mutations in genes responsible for DNA repair: germline BRCA2 mutation may be associated with a higher GS and a worse prognosis.[5,6] Other general syndromes associated with increased risk of prostate cancer are Lynch syndrome, BRCA2, Fanconi's anemia, and HOXB13.[7-9]

ANATOMY: The prostate is composed of ⅔ glandular elements and ⅓ fibromuscular stroma. The glandular part is divided into three zones: peripheral zone (comprises 70% of prostate volume, with the majority of prostate cancer arising from this zone), central zone (comprises 25% of prostate volume, with 5% of prostate cancer arising from this zone), and the transition zone (comprises 5% of the prostate volume and is the site of benign prostatic hyperplasia). The neurovascular bundles are located posterolaterally. The fibromuscular stroma (or anterior zone) extends superiorly from the smooth muscle of the bladder neck and inferiorly to the urethra, prostate apex, and external sphincter. The seminal vesicles (SVs) are coaxial with the gland and adjacent to the posterolateral aspect of the prostate, joining the vas deferens to the ejaculatory duct and entering the prostatic urethra at the verumontanum. The position of the prostate and SVs varies w/ filling of the rectum and bladder. Typical prostate variability is as follows (standard deviation): A-P—2.4 mm, Inf-Sup—2.1 mm, and Med-Lat—0.4 mm; SV displacement: A-P—3.5 mm, Inf-Sup—2.1 mm, and Med-Lat—0.8 mm.[10] Lymphatic drainage of the prostate includes internal iliac, external iliac, obturator, and presacral lymph nodes, with occasional draining directly to the common iliac nodes. The lymphatics of the SVs typically drain to the external iliacs.

PATHOLOGY: 95% of prostate cancers are adenocarcinomas. Other histologies such as small cell (neuroendocrine) carcinoma, ductal adenocarcinoma, transitional cell carcinoma, sarcomatoid carcinoma, and sarcoma are associated with a worse prognosis.[11–14] The GS is based on the architectural structure of the malignant cells. Current recommendation for needle core biopsies is that the most prevalent and highest grade are summed together for the GS since any amount of high-grade tumor may indicate a more significant amount within the prostate. Tertiary grades are given only in radical prostatectomy specimens if there is a component (<5%) of higher grade tumor than the two predominant patterns.[15] Extracapsular extension (ECE) is seen in approximately 45% of pts w/ clinically localized disease and is within 2.5 mm in 96% of cases.[16] SV involvement increases with risk group: low risk ~1%, intermediate risk ~15%, and high risk ~30%, with a median 1.0-cm length of involvement and ~1% risk of SV involvement beyond 2.0 cm.[17] Recently a grouping system was developed by the International Society of Urological Pathology based on GS, which demonstrated an increased risk of biochemical recurrence with increasing group.[18]

TABLE 36.2: ISUP Consensus Grouping[18]		
Grade Group	**Gleason Score(s)**	**HR of Biochemical Recurrence**
1	≤6	Reference
2	3 + 4 = 7	1.9
3	4 + 3 = 7	5.4
4	8	8.0
5	9 or 10	11.7

SCREENING: The American Urological Association (AUA) recommends PSA screening every 1 or 2 years for men with life expectancy >10 years and 55 to 69 years of age. Screening decisions should be individualized for men between 40 and 54 years of age with higher risk features (African American race or family history).[19] Free PSA (ratio of free PSA/total PSA, with lower free PSA predicting higher risk of cancer) and PSA velocity (>0.75 ng/mL/year) can increase the positive predictive value of screening.[20] PSA velocity of >2 ng/mL in the year previous to diagnosis has been associated with increased risk of death due to prostate cancer.[21] The half-life of PSA is ~2.2 days. PSA levels can be increased by prostatitis, urinary retention, DRE, ejaculation, TRUS biopsy, TURP, and BPH. Medical treatment for BPH with 5α-reductase inhibitors such as finasteride decreases PSA by ~50% within 6 mos of use, and thus correct PSA by multiplying by 2 in the first 2 yrs and by

2.3x for longer term use.[22,23] National screening guidelines do not recommend DRE alone for screening (poor PPV of 4%–11%).[24] Combined DRE and PSA screening is left to the discretion of physicians and DRE is recommended in any patient with suspicious PSA.[19] DRE palpates only the posterior and lateral aspects of the prostate gland, which inherently limits its screening utility, but 85% of prostate cancers arise from these locations. DRE has a sensitivity of 53% and specificity of 86% in one study.[25] A multicenter screening study demonstrated that PSA detected significantly more prostate cancer than DRE (82% vs. 55%; $p = .001$).[26] Prostate cancer antigen 3 (PCA3) is an RNA biomarker overexpressed by malignant cells and can be found in urine after an "attentive" DRE with a "minimum of six pressed strokes on the prostate from lateral to medial"; this test may be a useful surrogate to repeat biopsies in the detection of cancer with a high negative predictive value (88%), but its use is not routine.[27]

CLINICAL PRESENTATION: Prostate cancer is usually asymptomatic, with the majority determined by PSA value or as an incidental finding on TURP. Suspicious DRE findings include areas of nodularity, asymmetry, or induration. Some pts with locally advanced disease may present with obstructive urinary symptoms (weak or interrupted stream), polyuria, and less frequently, dysuria and hematuria. Unexplained bony pain may suggest metastatic disease, but this is rare in patients with otherwise low-risk prostate cancer.

WORKUP: H&P, including DRE and assessment of baseline urinary, bowel, and sexual function. The AUA score (aka International Prostate Symptom Score or IPSS) can be used to assess urinary function (range 0–5 points for seven questions; total score 35 with higher score implying worse symptoms) based on incomplete emptying, frequency, intermittency, urgency, weak stream, straining, and nocturia. The Sexual Health Inventory in Men (SHIM) score is commonly used to assess baseline erectile function (range 0/1–5 points for five questions; total score 25 with higher score signifying better erections).

Labs: PSA, preoperative workup if surgery indicated.

Pathology: TRUS-guided random biopsy involving removal of 8 to 12 cores of tissue is the most common approach for diagnosis. A systematic review suggested that MRI targeted biopsy may detect clinically significant cancers with less core samples compared to conventional prostate biopsy techniques.[28]

Imaging: No role for routine staging scans in low-risk prostate cancer.

PROGNOSTIC FACTORS: Risk stratification of prostate cancer is based primarily upon clinical staging by DRE, pretreatment PSA, GS/grade group on biopsy, and the number of biopsy cores involved with cancer. Several risk classifications exist, including the NCCN, D'Amico, and American Joint Committee on Cancer (AJCC) risk categories (Tables 36.3 and 36.4). An unfavorable intermediate-risk category has been proposed by MSKCC: primary GS pattern 4, percentage of positive biopsy cores ≥50%, or multiple intermediate-risk factors (cT2b-c, PSA 10–20 ng/mL, or GS 7), which independently predicted for increased PCSM, DM, and inferior PSA RFS compared to favorable intermediate-risk disease.[29] Other prognostic factors also exist, including cancer volume (>4 cm³ demonstrated shorter time to PSA failure),[30] PNI on biopsy (associated with higher rate of positive margin, but has not been shown to be an independent predictor of PSA recurrence),[31] and the presence of disseminated cancer cells (>5 disseminated cancer cells per 7.5 mL associated with shorter OS in three randomized trials).[32] The UCSF-CAPRA nomogram includes age (≥50 years vs. <50 years), PSA, GS, clinical stage (T1/T2 vs. T3a), percentage of biopsy core involved (<34% vs. ≥34%) to predict likelihood of disease recurrence or progression.[33] Several tissue-based tests have been developed to determine prognosis, including Oncotype DX Genomic Prostate Score (Genomic Health, Redwood City, California),which is a 17-gene expression panel used in pts with very low, low, and "modified intermediate" risk cancer, which predicts for risk of recurrence, prostate cancer death, and aggressive features on pathology (Gleason ≥4 + 3 or pT3) after radical prostatectomy (RP).[34] This test as well as others can be used in pts with at least 10-yr life expectancy who might be candidates for active surveillance (AS) or definitive therapy.[35]

NATURAL HISTORY: The risk of death from early-stage, early-risk disease is <10% at 10 yrs. Many tumors follow an indolent course for the first 10 to 15 yrs after diagnosis, but beyond 15 yrs, the PCSM rate triples (15/1,000 person-yrs to 44/1,000 person years).[36] As per the Pound study of pts with biochemical failure after prostatectomy, metastases developed at a median of 8 years after biochemical failure and death occurred at a median of 5 years from the development of DM.[37]

STAGING

TABLE 36.3: AJCC 8th ed. (2017) Prostate Cancer Staging								
cT			**pT**		**N**		**M**	
T1	**a**	Incidental finding in ≤5% of tissue resected			**N0**	• No regional LNs	**M1a**	• Non regional LNs
	b	Incidental finding in >5% of tissue resected						
	c	Identified by needly biopsy (e.g., PSA), but not palpable						
T2	**a**	Palpable ≤½ of one lobe or less	**T2**	• Organ confined disease	**N1**	• Metastasis in regional LNs	**M1b**	• Metastasis to bone
	b	Palpable >½ of one lobe, but not both lobes						
	c	Palpable both lobes						
T3	**a**	EPE	**T3**	**a** EPE or microscopic bladder neck invasion			**M1c**	• Metastasis to other sites with or without bone disease
	b	SV invasion		**b** SV invasion				
T4	Invasion[1]		**T4**	• Invasion[1]				

AJCC 8th ed. 2017, Prognostic Stage Groups	
I	cT1a-c, cT2a or pT2 + PSA <10 ng/mL + Grade Group 1
IIA	cT1a-c or cT2a + PSA ≥10 and <20 ng/mL + Grade Group 1 cT2b-c + PSA <20 ng/mL + Grade Group 1
IIB	T1-T2, PSA <20 ng/mL, Grade Group 2
IIC	T1-T2, PSA<20 ng/mL, Grade Group 3 T1-T2, PSA<20 ng/mL, Grade Group 4
IIIA	T1-T2, PSA ≥20, Grade Groups 1–4
IIIB	T3-T4, Any PSA, Grade Groups 1–4

(continued)

AJCC 8th ed. 2017, Prognostic Stage Groups (*continued*)	
IIIC	Any T, Any PSA, Grade Group 5
IVA	Any T, N1, Any PSA, Any Grade Group
IVB	Any T, M1, Any PSA, Any Grade Group

Significant changes in the 8th Edition include removal of the pT2 subclassifications, incorporation of the grade grouping, updates to M1 subclassification, and updates to the definition of stage II & III.

Notes: Invasion[1] = Invasion into bladder, external sphincter, rectum, levator muscles, pelvic wall.

TABLE 36.4: Risk Stratifications for Prostate Cancer (Other Than AJCC Staging)			
NCCN Risk Classification[35]		**D'Amico Risk Categories**[38]	
Very low risk	T1 GS ≤6 PSA <10 ng/mL <3 positive biopsy cores <50% cancer in any core PSA density <0.15 ng/mL/gram		
Low risk	T1-T2a, and GS ≤6/grade group 1, and PSA <10 ng/mL	Low risk	T1-2a, and GS ≤6, and PSA <10 ng/mL
Intermediate risk	T2b-T2c, or GS 3 + 4 = 7/grade group 2, or GS 4 + 3 = 7/grade group 3, or PSA 10–20 ng/mL	Intermediate risk	T2b, or GS 7, or PSA 10–20 ng/mL
High risk	T3a, or GS 8/grade group 4, or GS 9–10/grade group 5, or PSA >20 ng/mL	High risk	≥T2c, or GS 8–10, or PSA >20 ng/mL
Very high risk	T3b-T4, or Primary Gleason pattern 5/grade group 5, or >4 cores with GS 8–10/grade group 4 or 5		

TREATMENT PARADIGM

Active Surveillance (AS) and Watchful Waiting (WW): AS involves regular monitoring of pts with PSA, DRE, and biopsy and evidence of progression will prompt conversion to potentially curative treatment. This is different from WW in which monitoring continues but treatment is typically initiated only when symptoms develop. Recommendations for AS criteria vary but can include most pts who have low-risk disease (GS ≤6) with a "reasonable" life expectancy,[39] while NCCN recommends it for very low-risk disease and life expectancy ≤20 yrs.[35] Genomic profiling may help identify pts appropriate for AS. WW recommendations also vary and can be considered for pts with low-risk cancer and limited life expectancy (<10 yrs).[35,39]

Prevention: The role of 5α-reductase inhibitors to prevent cancer progression in the setting of AS is debatable among consensus guidelines, but the REDEEM trial revealed lower 3-yr rates of prostate cancer progression with dutasteride compared to placebo (38% vs. 48%, $p = .009$).[40] Finasteride is currently not approved by the FDA for prevention of prostate cancer.

Surgery: Radical prostatectomy (RP) approaches include retropubic or laparoscopic/ robotic approach. Robotic surgery has been compared to open surgery in one single-institution RCT, which reported early outcomes at 6 and 12 weeks and demonstrated similar rates of positive surgical margins, postoperative complications, intraoperative adverse events, and similar patient-reported urinary and sexual function scores for both techniques.[41] A perineal approach omits lymphadenectomy and seminal vesicle removal and has been shown to be associated with higher rates of biochemical failure, +margins, capsular incisions, and rectal injury.[42] The positive margin rates for open, laparoscopic, and robotic techniques are estimated to be 23%, 15%, and 14%, respectively.[43] Perioperative complications are rare and include mortality (<1%), rectal injury (<1%), thromboembolism (1%–3%), myocardial infarction (1%–8%), wound infection (<1%), <1 L blood loss and pelvic pain. [44,45] Impotence and incontinence are most common. Bilateral nerve sparing procedure is associated with an estimated ~50% rate of impotence and unilateral nerve sparing is associated with impotence rate of ~75%. An estimated 32% of pts reported total urinary control, 40% with occasional leakage, and 7% frequent leakage, and 1%–2% reported no urinary control.[46] A standard lymph node dissection involves sampling of the obturator and external iliac lymph nodes alone.

Radiation

Indications: Definitive RT is an option for low-risk prostate cancer without contraindications such as prior pelvic RT or inflammatory bowel disease.

Dose: Dose escalation with conventional EBRT has been shown to improve biochemical outcomes in several randomized trials, but without an improvement in OS (see the following). Dose and fractionation vary widely in practice. Common conventionally fractionation regimens: 78 Gy/39 fx or 79.2 Gy/44 fx. Moderately hypofractionated options such as 70 Gy/28 fx or 60 Gy/20 fx have been tested in large prospective trials. For SBRT, 36.25 Gy in 5 fx delivered QOD is a commonly utilized regimen, although SBRT has not been tested against IMRT in a randomized trial. Brachytherapy is frequently used for low-risk prostate cancer with comparable outcomes to surgery and EBRT, but no randomized trial has compared these modalities head to head for assessment of clinical outcomes. Dose for LDR brachytherapy is 144 to 145 Gy for I-125 or 125 Gy for Pd-103. For low-risk and favorable intermediate-risk prostate cancer, there is no role for combining EBRT with brachytherapy boost or with ADT; monotherapy is sufficient. After RT, PSA surveillance should occur ~q6 months. Per the RTOG-ASTRO Phoenix Consensus, the definition of biochemical failure is a rise of 2 ng/ml above the post-treatment nadir PSA.[47] A PSA "bounce" phenomenon may occur in some pts, particularly after brachytherapy, and is not associated with worse outcomes.

Toxicity: Acute: Fatigue, dysuria, frequency, retention, rectal urgency, diarrhea. Late: Stricture, cystitis, proctitis, sexual dysfunction, second malignancy. QOL outcomes have been compared between these therapies and each modality is associated with distinct patterns of change in terms of urinary, bowel, and sexual function (see the ProtecT and PROST-QA trials).

Procedure: See *Treatment Planning Handbook,* Chapter 8.[48]

Other: Other treatments such as high frequency ultrasound (HIFU) and cryotherapy are emerging techniques but are not recommended as first-line options per NCCN guidelines.

EVIDENCE-BASED Q&A

Screening and prevention

What is the value of PSA screening? Why did the U.S. Preventive Services Task Force (USPSTF) previously recommend against PSA screening?

Despite stage migration toward early localized disease and a decrease in metastatic rates in the PSA era, the USPSTF recommended against routine PSA screening in 2012 (revised guidelines in progress at time of publication).[49] *There are three major screening trials, and the methodology suggests that the magnitude of screening may be likely larger than represented. The ERSPC and Swedish Trial show a PCSM benefit for PSA screening while PLCO did not. Notably, it is difficult to keep people in the "observation" arm from being screened, which is one of the criticisms of the PLCO trial.*

Schröder, European Randomized Study of Screening for Prostate Cancer (ERSPC) (*NEJM* 2009, PMID 19297566; Update *Lancet* 2014, PMID 25108889): 162,388 men (55–69 years of age) randomized to a PSA q4 years (on average) versus no screening. PSA ≥3 ng/mL was indication for biopsy in most centers; 1° endpoint was prostate cancer mortality (PCM). Incidence of prostate cancer was 9.55/1,000 person-years for screening versus 6.23/1,000 person-years for control group. 355 men in screening group and 545 men in control died from prostate Ca, yielding a PCM rate ratio of 0.79 at 13 years ($p = .001$), corresponding to a number needed to screen (NNS) of **781** and a NNT of **27** to prevent one death. No difference in all-cause mortality. **Conclusion: Reduction in PCM was observed in the cohort randomized to PSA screening.** *Comment: Did not report treatment type, assumed arms were balanced, and overall rate of screening in control group was not reported; there was variance amongst European centers for recruiting, use of DRE, TRUS, and screening intervals. There is increased survival and decreased progression but at a cost of overdetection and overtreatment.*

Hugosson, Swedish Trial (*Lancet Oncol* 2010, PMID 20598634): 20,000 men 50 to 64 years of age living in Göteborg, Sweden, randomly selected by computer to be screened by PSA every other year or not (no informed consent). PSA >3 ng/mL was indication for DRE and biopsies; 1° endpoint was PCM. 78% reached max follow-up of 14 years, 76% compliance with screening. Incidence and metastatic burden decreased by screening. Prostate cancer incidence of 12.7% in screening group versus 8.2% in control group (HR 1.64; 95% CI: 1.50%–1.80; $p < .0001$). Rate ratio for PCM was 0.56 (95% CI: 0.39%–0.82; $p = .002$) for screening versus control group. 46 screened men versus 87 controls were dx with metastatic disease ($p = .003$). NNS = 293, NNT = 12 to prevent one prostate cancer death. Risk of PC was only 2.6% if the first PSA was <1. **Conclusion: PSA screening is worth it and reduces risk of death by almost half.** *Comment: This is the most "pure" trial because of the randomization and lack of informed consent with good follow-up, and also had the lowest NNS.*

Andriole, Prostate, Lung, Colorectal, and Ovarian (PLCO) Cancer Screening Trial (*NEJM* 2009, PMID 19297565; Update *J Natl Cancer Inst* 2012, PMID 22228146; Update Shoag, *NEJM* 2016, PMID 27144870): 76,693 men between 55 and 74 years of age randomized to annual screening with PSA + DRE versus usual care. PSA of >4 ng/mL or abnormal DRE was indication for biopsy. 92% of participants followed to 10 years. Incidence of PCa was 108 versus 97 per 10,000 person-years for screening arm versus control arm, which is a 12% relative increase in incidence rates (RR 1.12) but there was no statistical difference in PCM in screening versus control arm, 3.7 versus 3.4 deaths per 10,000 person-years. **Conclusion: No evidence of PCM benefit from annual screening.** *Comment: 45% men had PSA in the 3 yrs preceding randomization, eliminating prostate cancer prior to randomization; 52% (85% at the update) of men in control arm underwent PSA testing. Because of the crossover contamination and prescreening PSA, many feel these data are insufficient to conclude PSA screening is not useful.*

Can prostate cancer be prevented with 5α-reductase inhibitors?

Yes, although 5-ARIs reduce primarily the risk of low-grade cancer.

Thompson, PCPT Trial (*NEJM* 2003, PMID 12824459; Update *NEJM* 2013, PMID 23944298): 18,880 men randomized to finasteride (5 mg/day) versus placebo. Cutoff level PSA ≤3 ng/mL; 10.5% in the finasteride versus 14.9% in the placebo were diagnosed with prostate cancer (RR 0.7, 95% CI: 0.65–0.76; $p < .001$). Finasteride group compared to placebo had a significant relative risk reduction of low-grade cancers (GS 2-6) (RR 0.57; 95% CI: 0.52–0.63; $p < .001$). The finasteride group compared to placebo had more high-grade cancers (GS 7-10; 3.5% vs. 3.0%, RR 1.17, $p = .05$) with no difference in survival between groups for this subset of pts. 15-yr OS rates did not differ for finasteride versus placebo (78% vs. 78.2%). **Conclusion: Finasteride decreases the risk of prostate cancer by about 1/3 and is "due entirely to a relative reduction of 43% in the risk of low-grade cancer."**

Andriole, REDUCE Trial (*NEJM* 2010, PMID 20357281): 6,729 men randomized to dutasteride 0.5 mg daily versus placebo. Included men with PSA of 2.5 to 10 ng/mL (ages 50–60) or 3.0–10 ng/ml (>60 y/o). During study period of 4 yrs, 19.9% in dutasteride versus 25.1% in placebo group had a diagnosis of prostate cancer, with relative risk reduction for prostate cancer of 22.8% and absolute risk reduction of 5.1% with dutasteride. Dutasteride group had less GS 5-6 cancers compared to placebo (13.2% vs. 18.1%, $p < .001$) and accounted for 70% of cancers. GS 7-10 tumors did not differ between groups. During years 3 and 4, there were more GS 8-10 tumors in dutasteride group versus placebo ($p = .003$). No difference in OS between groups. **Conclusion: Dutasteride reduced the risk of prostate cancer mainly due to reduction in GS 5-6 cancers.** *Comment: Increase in high GS tumors may be due to gland shrinkage and increased biopsy yield.*

Active surveillance

What are the long-term outcomes of men on active surveillance?

Klotz (*JCO* 2010, PMID 19917860; Update *JCO* 2015, PMID 25512465): Single-arm cohort of 993 pts followed under AS. Between 1995 and 1999, included all GS ≤6 and PSA ≤10 ng/mL. If >70 yrs of age, PSA ≤15 ng/mL or GS ≤ 3+4 (7). From 2000, restricted to GS ≤6 and PSA ≤10 ng/mL or pts with favorable intermediate-risk disease (PSA 10–20 ng/mL and/or GS 3+4) with significant comorbidities and life expectancy <10 years. Excellent 10- and 15-yr actuarial prostate cancer survival rates of 98.1% and 94.3%, respectively. Only 15 of 933 (1.5%) died of prostate cancer and 2.8% developed metastatic disease. The 10- and 15-yr OS rates were 80% and 62%, respectively. At 5, 10, and 15 years, 75.7%, 63.5%, and 55.0% of pts remained untreated and on AS. Pts were 9.2x more likely to die of causes other than prostate cancer. **Conclusion: AS for low-risk and select favorable intermediate-risk pts seems safe.**

Can a 5α-reductase inhibitor aid pts undergoing active surveillance?

Fleshner, REDEEM Trial (*Lancet* 2012, PMID 22277570): 302 men with Gleason 5-6, PSA ≤11 placed on AS randomized to dutasteride 0.5 mg daily versus placebo. Pts followed q3 months for 1 year, then q6 months with a PSA and DRE at each visit q18 months. All pts had a repeat bx at 18 months and 3 years or if concerning PSA/DRE. Progression defined as ≥4 cores involved, ≥50% of one core or Gleason pattern 4. At 3 years, prostate cancer progression decreased from 48% to 38% with dutasteride (HR 0.62, 95% CI: 0.43–0.89; $p = .009$). **Conclusion: Dutasteride may be beneficial for reducing progression in AS pts.**

Is early treatment better than active surveillance or watchful waiting?

Bill-Axelson, Scandinavian Prostate Cancer Group-4 (SPCG-4) (*NEJM* 2011, PMID 21542742; QOL *Lancet Onc* 2011, PMID 21821474; *NEJM* 2014, PMID 24597866): PRT of 695 pts with early prostate cancer randomized to RP versus WW. Progression for WW group defined as palpable ECE or symptoms of obstruction w/ voiding requiring intervention. T2 were 76%, T1c were 12% (not the current population in post-PSA era). Eligibility: age <75 years of age, T1-2, PSA <50 ng/mL, and life expectancy >10 yrs; 6.6%

were LN+ at RP. RP has higher rates of at least daily urinary leakage (41% vs. 11%) and reported ED (84% vs. 80%) but lower rates of urinary obstruction (29% vs. 40%). The rates of bowel dysfunction, anxiety, depression, well-being, and subjective QOL were similar. NNT to prevent one death at 18-yr FU was 8. **Conclusion: RP is associated with a statistically significant reduction in all endpoints.** *Comment: Due to stage migration, these results may not be readily applicable to low-risk population.*

TABLE 36.5: Results of SPCG-4 Prostatectomy Trial

	18-yr DSM	18-yr DM	18-yr OM
WW	28.7%	38.3%	68.9%
RP	17.7%	26.1%	56.1%
p value	.001	<.001	<.001

Wilt, PIVOT Trial (*NEJM* 2012, PMID 22808955; Update *NEJM* 2017, PMID 28700844): PRT of 731 men randomized to AS versus RP. Included T1-2, any grade, PSA <50, <75 years of age, life expectancy >10 yrs. 40% low-risk, 34% intermediate, 21% high-risk. AS group: definitive treatment offered for pts with a PSA doubling of <3 yrs, GS progression to 4+3 (or greater) or clinical progression. MFU 12.7 yrs (update). In RP arm, 7.4% died from prostate cancer or treatments versus 4.0% men in observation arm (p = .06, not SS). No difference in all-cause mortality for RP versus AS (61.3% versus 66.8%, p = .06) but RP reduced ACM in intermediate but not low-risk. **Conclusion: RP did not significantly reduce ACM or PCM as compared with AS.** *Comment: Effect size is reasonable (5.5% absolute risk reduction in all-cause mortality) and more power may have led to a significant p-value.*

Hamdy, UK ProtecT (*NEJM* 2016, PMID 27626136; QOL Donovan *NEJM* 2016, PMID 27626365): 1,643 pts 50 to 69 years of age with localized prostate cancer randomized to "active monitoring" (AM, PSA monitoring only), surgery (RP), or RT with ADT. Median age 62 years of age, median PSA 4.6 ng/mL (range 3–19.9), 77% had GS 6, 76% had T1c. AM group had PSA q3 months first year, q6-12 months thereafter; increase in 50% PSA in previous 12 months triggered a review to continue monitoring or pursue treatment. RT arm had ADT for 3 to 6 months before and concurrent with 3D-CRT to 74 Gy/37 fx. RP arm had post-op PSA q3 months for first year, then q6–12 months. Primary outcome: prostate cancer–specific survival (PCSS). MFU 10 yrs. AM, RP, and RT had 1.5, 0.9, and 0.7 prostate cancer specific deaths per 1,000 person-years, respectively, without any significant difference among groups (p = .48). More DM and disease progression in AM groups than RP or RT group. In AM arm (n = 545): 54.8% received a radical treatment at 10 years. RP arm (n = 391): 2% had PSA >0.2 ng/mL post-op, five had salvage RT, nine had adjuvant RT w/i a year after surgery due to pT3 or +margins; pT3 in 29%, 24% had +margins. RP NNT = 27 and RT NNT = 33 to avoid one pt having metastatic disease. 9 pts NNT with either RP or RT to avoid one pt having clinical progression. **Conclusion: Irrespective of treatment arm, PCM remained low at ~1%. Rate of disease progression and metastatic disease significantly lower for RP or RT compared to AM. ACM and PCSM were much lower in the ProtecT trial than SPCG-4 or PIVOT trials.**

TABLE 36.6: Results of ProtecT Randomized Trial

	5-yr PCSS	10-yr PCSS	Clinical Progression Per 1,000 Person-yrs	Metastatic Disease Per 1,000 Person-yrs	All-Cause Deaths Per 1,000 Person-yrs
Active monitoring	99.4%	98.8%	22.9	6.3	10.9
Surgery	100%	99%	8.9	2.4	10.1

(continued)

TABLE 36.6: Results of ProtecT Randomized Trial (*continued*)					
	5-yr PCSS	10-yr PCSS	Clinical progression per 1,000 person-yrs	Metastatic disease per 1,000 person-yrs	All-cause deaths per 1,000 person-yrs
Radiation	100%	99.6%	9.0	3.0	10.3
p value	.48	.48	<.001	.004	.87

External beam radiation therapy

With conventional EBRT, does dose escalation improve outcomes?

There have been at least five major randomized trials investigating "dose escalation" with each one showing a biochemical control benefit (but no difference in OS) for higher doses compared to "conventional" lower doses (~70 Gy at 1.8–2.0 Gy/fx), but also higher rates of rectal bleeding. The current standard dose is 78 to 80 Gy with conventional fractionation (see Table 36.7).

TABLE 36.7: Summary of Phase III Dose Escalation Trials for Prostate Cancer					
	Pollack, MDACC[50]	Zietman, MGH[51]	Al-Mamgani, Dutch[52]	Dearnaley, MRC[53]	Michalski, RTOG 0126 (ASCO 2015)
Doses	70 vs. 78 Gy	70.2 vs. 79.2 Gy	68 vs. 78 Gy	64 vs. 74 Gy	70.2 vs. 79.2 Gy
N	301	393	669	843	1,499
Technique	4-field box and 3D-CRT	4-field box and proton boost	3D	3D	3D or IMRT
MFU (yrs)	8.7	8.9	5.8	5.3	7
Biochemical Control	59% vs. 78%, *p* = .004	67.6% vs. 83.3% (*p* < .0001)	45% vs. 56% (*p* = .03)	60% vs. 71% (*p* = .0007)	55% vs. 70% (*p* < .0001)

Is moderate hypofractionation safe and effective?

There have been several randomized trials examining moderate hypofractionation (2.4–4 Gy/fx to 60–70 Gy) compared to conventional fractionation. The potential advantages include improved convenience for pts, lower cost, and potentially improved outcomes (due to hypothesized low α/β ratio). Follow-up is moderate, with MFU ranging from 5 to 8 years. This is a reasonable option but longer follow-up will be helpful to establish noninferiority for clinical effectiveness and toxicity profiles.

TABLE 36.8: Summary of Moderate Hypofractionation Trials in Prostate Cancer					
Author, Institution	MFU	Eligibility	Hypofx Arm	Conventional Arm	Outcome
Hoffman, MDACC (ASTRO 2016)	8.4 yrs	LR-IR	72 Gy at 2.4 Gy/fx	75.6 at 1.8 Gy/fx	8-yr bRFS 89.3% vs. 84.6%, 10-yr 89.3% vs. 76.3%, *p* = .034 favoring hypofx arm. No diff in OS or late GI or GU toxicity (but hypofx arm had nonsignificantly more rectal bleeding after treatment). Better control emerged after 5 yrs.
Pollack, Fox Chase[54]	5.7 yrs	IR-HR	70.2 Gy at 2.7 Gy/fx	76 Gy at 2 Gy/fx	5-yr bRFS: 76.7% vs. 78.6% (*p* = NS). No diff in late toxicity (except those with poor urinary function IPSS >12 had higher toxicity in hypofx arm).

(continued)

TABLE 36.8: Summary of Moderate Hypofractionation Trials in Prostate Cancer (*continued*)					
Author, Institution	MFU	Eligibility	Hypofx Arm	Conventional Arm	Outcome
Lee, RTOG 0415[55]	5.8 yrs	LR	70 Gy at 2.5 Gy/fx	73.8 at 1.8 Gy/fx	No SS difference in DFS (HR 0.85; CI: 0.64–1.14) or BF (HR 0.77; CI: 0.51–1.17). Hypofx arm noninferior to conventional arm. Hypofx arm more late grade 2 GI (18.3% vs. 11.4%, $p = .002$) and GU toxicity (26.2% vs. 20.5%, $p = .06$), but this was not clinically significant in patient-reported outcomes (ASTRO 2016).
Dearnaley, CHHiP[56]	5.2 yrs	All (most IR)	60 or 57 Gy at 3 Gy/fx	74 at 2 Gy/fx	5-yr bRFS: 88.3% (74 Gy) vs. 90.6% (60 Gy) vs. 85.9% (57 Gy). 60 Gy not inferior to 74 Gy but noninferiority could NOT be claimed for 57 Gy vs. 74 Gy. No diff in GI/GU toxicity between arms.
Incrocci, HYPRO/ Dutch[57]	5 yrs	IR-HR	64.6 Gy at 3.4 Gy/fx	78 Gy at 2 Gy/fx	Treatment failure: 20% hypofx vs. 22% conventional. 5-yr RFS: 80.5% in hypofx arm vs. 77.1% in conventional arm ($p = .36$). Grade ≥3 late GU toxicity was significantly greater for hypofx vs. conventional (19.0% vs. 12.9%; $p = .021$).
Arcangeli, Italian[58,59]	9 yrs	HR	62 Gy at 3.1 Gy/fx	80 at 2 Gy/fx	10-yr FFBF 72% hypofrac vs. 65% conventional ($p = .148$). No difference in late effects.
Catton, PROFIT[60]	6 yrs	IR	60 Gy at 3 Gy/fx	78 at 2 Gy/fx	5-yr BF in both arms was 15% (HR = 0.96; 90% CI: 0.77–1.2). Hypofx arm not inferior to conventional arm. No SS difference in late grade 3+ GI and GU toxicity.
HR, high risk; IR, intermediate risk; LR, low risk.					

Is extreme hypofractionation (>4–10 Gy/fx) delivered with SBRT safe and effective?

Biochemical control and toxicity outcomes with SBRT are comparable to historical outcomes of dose-escalated 3D/IMRT but longer follow-up is needed. Pts should be aware of the shorter follow-up and lack of randomized data with SBRT.

TABLE 36.9: Summary of Select SBRT Series for Prostate Cancer						
Study	N	Dose (Gy/Fx)	Fx	Total Dose	MFU (Years)	Biochemical Control
Meier et al. (2016)[61]	309	7.25–8	5	36.25 Gy to PTV and 40 Gy (SIB) to prostate	5.1	97.1%
Kotecha et al. (2016)[62]	24	7.25–10	5	36.25 Gy to PTV and 50 Gy (SIB) to prostate (sparing urethra, bladder, rectum)	2.1	95.8%

(continued)

TABLE 36.9: Summary of Select SBRT Series for Prostate Cancer (*continued*)						
Study	N	Dose (Gy/Fx)	Fx	Total Dose	MFU (Years)	Biochemical Control
Katz et al. (2016)[63]	515	7–7.25	5	35–36.25 Gy	7	8 yrs: Low risk: 93.6%, Intermediate risk: 84.3% High risk: 65%
Chen et al. (2013)[64]	100	7–7.25	5	35–36.25 Gy	2.3	99%
King et al. (2012)[65]	67	7.25	5	36.25 Gy	2.7	94%
Boike et al. (2011)[66]	45	9–10	5	45–50 Gy	2.5	100%
Freeman et al. (2011)[67]	41	7.25	5	35–36.25 Gy	5	93%
Madsen et al. (2007)[68]	40	6.7	5	33.5 Gy	3.4	90%

What data exist regarding late effects of SBRT?

Many studies have published low rates of late GI/GU toxicity in short follow-up, but longer follow-up is necessary to observe late effects. Katz et al.[69] found that 90% of toxicity events occurred within 3 years of treatment. The early experience from Stanford found that QOD treatment resulted in less toxicity than once daily SBRT, and so most have adopted a QOD schedule.[65]

TABLE 36.10: Summary of Toxicity Outcomes in Select Prostate SBRT Series				
Study	Dose	MFU (Years)	Late GI Toxicity	Late GU Toxicity
Meier et al. (2016)[61]	36.25 Gy (SIB to 40 Gy)/5 fx	5.1	2% G2	12% G2
Kotecha et al. (2016)[62]	36.25 Gy (SIB to 50 Gy)/5 fx	2.1	8% G2	8% G2
Katz et al. (2014)[69]	35–36.25 Gy/5 fx	6	4% G2	9% G2 2% G3
King et al. (2012)[65]	36.25 Gy/5 fx	2.7	16% G1-2	23% G1 5% G2 3% G3
Freeman et al. (2011)[67]	36.25 Gy/5 fx	5	15.5% G1-2	32% G1-2 2.5% G3

How does the side effect profile compare between RP, EBRT, and brachytherapy?

Generally, RP has worse incontinence and impotence, EBRT has worse bowel/rectal irritation, and brachytherapy has worse urinary irritation/obstruction. Placement of a rectal spacer can significantly reduce rectal dose and side effects from RT.[70]

Sanda, PROST-QA (*NEJM* 2008, PMID 18354103): First major prospective study (nonrandomized) to document patient- and partner-reported QOL outcomes. Prospective questionnaire of 1,201 pts and 625 spouses given pre- and post- (up to 24 months) definitive RP, brachytherapy, and EBRT for localized T1-T2 cancer. Pts who received EBRT had greatest number of baseline comorbidities followed by brachytherapy and RP. RP was associated with worse sexual and urinary incontinence scores despite higher baseline function. Nerve sparing surgical procedures had better recovery of sexual QOL. EBRT was associated with more irritative and obstructive side effects as well as bowel toxicity. Large prostates had greater urinary irritation with brachytherapy and greater relief w/ RP. The use of ADT decreased vitality scores. On MVA, the most important factors associated with overall patient satisfaction were sexual function, vitality, and urinary function, in descending order. Patient-related factors that diminished health-related QOL included obesity, large prostate size, elevated initial PSA, older age, and African American race.

Donovan, ProtecT Trial QOL (*NEJM* 2016, PMID 27626365): Same trial as noted previously (Hamdy et al). Patient-reported outcomes through questionnaires given before diagnosis, 6 and 12 mos, then annually and reported through 6 yrs. RP had greatest negative effect on sexual function (erections firm enough for intercourse at 6 mos: 52% AS, 22% RT, 12% surgery) and urinary incontinence. RT had a peak negative effect on sexual function at 6 mos but recovered and stabilized (note: all pts received short-term ADT). RT had little effect on urinary continence but urinary voiding and nocturia problems peaked at 6 mos, then recovered by 12 mos to be similar to other groups. RT had worse bowel function at 6 mos compared to other arms but then recovered (except for frequency of bloody stools, which remained ~5%) while other groups had stable bowel function. Sexual function gradually declined in AM group (erections firm enough for intercourse: 41% yr 3 and 30% at yr 6) as well as urinary function. No differences among groups for anxiety, depression, general health-related or cancer-related QOL.

REFERENCES

1. Siegel RL, Miller KD, Jemal A. Cancer statistics, 2016. *CA Cancer J Clin*. 2016;66(1):7–30.
2. Hoffman RM, Gilliland FD, Eley JW, et al. Racial and ethnic differences in advanced-stage prostate cancer: the Prostate Cancer Outcomes Study. *J Natl Cancer Inst*. 2001;93(5):388–395.
3. Hamilton RJ, Aronson WJ, Presti JC Jr, et al. Race, biochemical disease recurrence, and prostate-specific antigen doubling time after radical prostatectomy: results from the SEARCH database. *Cancer*. 2007;110(10):2202–2209.
4. Hemminki K, Ji J, Forsti A, et al. Concordance of survival in family members with prostate cancer. *J Clin Oncol*. 2008;26(10):1705–1709.
5. Agalliu I, Gern R, Leanza S, Burk RD. Associations of high-grade prostate cancer with BRCA1 and BRCA2 founder mutations. *Clin Cancer Res*. 2009;15(3):1112–1120.
6. Castro E, Goh C, Olmos D, et al. Germline BRCA mutations are associated with higher risk of nodal involvement, distant metastasis, and poor survival outcomes in prostate cancer. *J Clin Oncol*. 2013;31(14):1748–1757.
7. Raymond VM, Mukherjee B, Wang F, et al. Elevated risk of prostate cancer among men with Lynch syndrome. *J Clin Oncol*. 2013;31(14):1713–1718.
8. Tischkowitz M, Easton DF, Ball J, et al. Cancer incidence in relatives of British Fanconi Anaemia patients. *BMC Cancer*. 2008;8:257.
9. Ewing CM, Ray AM, Lange EM, et al. Germline mutations in HOXB13 and prostate-cancer risk. *N Engl J Med*. 2012;366(2):141–149.
10. Deurloo KE, Steenbakkers RJ, Zijp LJ, et al. Quantification of shape variation of prostate and seminal vesicles during external beam radiotherapy. *Int J Radiat Oncol Biol Phys*. 2005;61(1):228–238.
11. Tetu B, Ro JY, Ayala AG, et al. Small cell carcinoma of the prostate: Part I: a clinicopathologic study of 20 cases. *Cancer*. 1987;59(10):1803–1809.
12. Robinson B, Magi-Galluzzi C, Zhou M. Intraductal carcinoma of the prostate. *Arch Pathol Lab Med*. 2012;136(4):418–425.
13. Palou J, Wood D, Bochner BH, et al. ICUD-EAU International Consultation on Bladder Cancer 2012: urothelial carcinoma of the prostate. *Eur Urol*. 2013;63(1):81–87.
14. Markowski MC, Eisenberger MA, Zahurak M, et al. Sarcomatoid carcinoma of the prostate: retrospective review of a case series from the Johns Hopkins Hospital. *Urology*. 2015;86(3):539–543.
15. Gordetsky J, Epstein J. Grading of prostatic adenocarcinoma: current state and prognostic implications. *Diagn Pathol*. 2016;11:25.

16. Davis BJ, Pisansky TM, Wilson TM, et al. The radial distance of extraprostatic extension of prostate carcinoma: implications for prostate brachytherapy. *Cancer.* 1999;85(12):2630–2637.

17. Kestin L, Goldstein N, Vicini F, et al. Treatment of prostate cancer with radiotherapy: should the entire seminal vesicles be included in the clinical target volume? *Int J Radiat Oncol Biol Phys.* 2002;54(3):686–697.

18. Epstein JI, Egevad L, Amin MB, et al. The 2014 International Society of Urological Pathology (ISUP) consensus conference on Gleason Grading of Prostatic Carcinoma: definition of grading patterns and proposal for a new grading system. *Am J Surg Pathol.* 2016;40(2):244–252.

19. Gershman B, Van Houten HK, Herrin J, et al. Impact of prostate-specific antigen (PSA) screening trials and revised PSA screening guidelines on rates of prostate biopsy and postbiopsy complications. *Eur Urol.* 2016;71(1):55–65.

20. Catalona WJ, Partin AW, Slawin KM, et al. Use of the percentage of free prostate-specific antigen to enhance differentiation of prostate cancer from benign prostatic disease: a prospective multicenter clinical trial. *JAMA.* 1998;279(19):1542–1547.

21. D'Amico AV, Chen MH, Roehl KA, Catalona WJ. Preoperative PSA velocity and the risk of death from prostate cancer after radical prostatectomy. *N Engl J Med.* 2004;351(2):125–135.

22. Guess HA, Heyse JF, Gormley GJ. The effect of finasteride on prostate-specific antigen in men with benign prostatic hyperplasia. *Prostate.* 1993;22(1):31–37.

23. Thompson IM, Goodman PJ, Tangen CM, et al. The influence of finasteride on the development of prostate cancer. *N Engl J Med.* 2003;349(3):215–224.

24. Schroder FH, van der Maas P, Beemsterboer P, et al. Evaluation of the digital rectal examination as a screening test for prostate cancer. Rotterdam section of the European Randomized Study of Screening for Prostate Cancer. *J Natl Cancer Inst.* 1998;90(23):1817–1823.

25. Mistry K, Cable G. Meta-analysis of prostate-specific antigen and digital rectal examination as screening tests for prostate carcinoma. *J Am Board Fam Pract.* 2003;16(2):95–101.

26. Catalona WJ, Richie JP, Ahmann FR, et al. Comparison of digital rectal examination and serum prostate specific antigen in the early detection of prostate cancer: results of a multicenter clinical trial of 6,630 men. *J Urol.* 1994;151(5):1283–1290.

27. Wei JT, Feng Z, Partin AW, et al. Can urinary PCA3 supplement PSA in the early detection of prostate cancer? *J Clin Oncol.* 2014;32(36):4066–4072.

28. Moore CM, Robertson NL, Arsanious N, et al. Image-guided prostate biopsy using magnetic resonance imaging-derived targets: a systematic review. *Eur Urol.* 2013;63(1):125–140.

29. Zumsteg ZS, Spratt DE, Pei I, et al. A new risk classification system for therapeutic decision making with intermediate-risk prostate cancer patients undergoing dose-escalated external-beam radiation therapy. *Eur Urol.* 2013;64(6):895–902.

30. D'Amico AV, Whittington R, Malkowicz SB, et al. Calculated prostate cancer volume greater than 4.0 cm^3 identifies patients with localized prostate cancer who have a poor prognosis following radical prostatectomy or external-beam radiation therapy. *J Clin Oncol.* 1998;16(9):3094–3100.

31. D'Amico AV, Wu Y, Chen MH, et al. Perineural invasion as a predictor of biochemical outcome following radical prostatectomy for select men with clinically localized prostate cancer. *J Urol.* 2001;165(1):126–129.

32. Goldkorn A, Ely B, Quinn DI, et al. Circulating tumor cell counts are prognostic of overall survival in SWOG S0421: a phase III trial of docetaxel with or without atrasentan for metastatic castration-resistant prostate cancer. *J Clin Oncol.* 2014;32(11):1136–1142.

33. Punnen S, Freedland SJ, Presti JC Jr, et al. Multi-institutional validation of the CAPRA-S score to predict disease recurrence and mortality after radical prostatectomy. *Eur Urol.* 2014;65(6):1171–1177.

34. Cullen J, Rosner IL, Brand TC, et al. A biopsy-based 17-gene genomic prostate score predicts recurrence after radical prostatectomy and adverse surgical pathology in a racially diverse population of men with clinically low- and intermediate-risk prostate cancer. *Eur Urol.* 2015;68(1):123–131.

35. National Comprehensive Cancer Network. Prostate Cancer (Version 2) 2017. www.nccn.org/professionals/physician_gls/PDF/prostate.pdf

36. Johansson JE, Andren O, Andersson SO, et al. Natural history of early, localized prostate cancer. *JAMA.* 2004;291(22):2713–2719.

37. Pound CR, Partin AW, Eisenberger MA, et al. Natural history of progression after PSA elevation following radical prostatectomy. *JAMA*. 1999;281(17):1591–1597.

38. D'Amico AV, Whittington R, Malkowicz SB, et al. Biochemical outcome after radical prostatectomy, external beam radiation therapy, or interstitial radiation therapy for clinically localized prostate cancer. *JAMA*. 1998;280(11):969–974.

39. Chen RC, Rumble RB, Loblaw DA, et al. Active surveillance for the management of localized prostate cancer (cancer care ontario guideline): American Society of Clinical Oncology Clinical Practice Guideline Endorsement. *J Clin Oncol*. 2016;34(18):2182–2190.

40. Fleshner NE, Lucia MS, Egerdie B, et al. Dutasteride in localised prostate cancer management: the REDEEM randomised, double-blind, placebo-controlled trial. *Lancet*. 2012;379(9821):1103–1111.

41. Yaxley JW, Coughlin GD, Chambers SK, et al. Robot-assisted laparoscopic prostatectomy versus open radical retropubic prostatectomy: early outcomes from a randomised controlled phase 3 study. *Lancet*. 2016;388(10049):1057–1066.

42. Boccon-Gibod L, Ravery V, Vordos D, et al. Radical prostatectomy for prostate cancer: the perineal approach increases the risk of surgically induced positive margins and capsular incisions. *J Urol*. 1998;160(4):1383–1385.

43. Sooriakumaran P, Srivastava A, Shariat SF, et al. A multinational, multi-institutional study comparing positive surgical margin rates among 22,393 open, laparoscopic, and robot-assisted radical prostatectomy patients. *Eur Urol*. 2014;66(3):450–456.

44. Alibhai SM, Leach M, Tomlinson G, et al. 30-day mortality and major complications after radical prostatectomy: influence of age and comorbidity. *J Natl Cancer Inst*. 2005;97(20):1525–1532.

45. Van Hemelrijck M, Garmo H, Holmberg L, et al. Thromboembolic events following surgery for prostate cancer. *Eur Urol*. 2013;63(2):354–363.

46. Stanford JL, Feng Z, Hamilton AS, et al. Urinary and sexual function after radical prostatectomy for clinically localized prostate cancer: the Prostate Cancer Outcomes Study. *JAMA*. 2000;283(3):354–360.

47. Roach M, 3rd, Hanks G, Thames H, Jr., et al. Defining biochemical failure following radiotherapy with or without hormonal therapy in men with clinically localized prostate cancer: recommendations of the RTOG-ASTRO Phoenix Consensus Conference. *Int J Radiat Oncol Biol Phys*. 2006;65(4):965–974.

48. Videtic GMM, Woody N, Vassil AD. *Handbook of Treatment Planning in Radiation Oncology*. 2nd ed. New York, NY: Demos Medical; 2015.

49. U.S. Preventive Services Task Force. Prostate cancer: screening. 2012. https://www.uspreventiveservicestaskforce.org/Page/Document/UpdateSummaryFinal/prostate-cancer-screening

50. Kuban DA, Tucker SL, Dong L, et al. Long-term results of the M. D. Anderson randomized dose-escalation trial for prostate cancer. *Int J Radiat Oncol Biol Phys*. 2008;70(1):67–74.

51. Zietman AL, Bae K, Slater JD, et al. Randomized trial comparing conventional-dose with high-dose conformal radiation therapy in early-stage adenocarcinoma of the prostate: long-term results from Proton Radiation Oncology Group/American College of Radiology 95-09. *J Clin Oncol*. 2010;28(7):1106–1111.

52. Al-Mamgani A, van Putten WL, Heemsbergen WD, et al. Update of Dutch multicenter dose-escalation trial of radiotherapy for localized prostate cancer. *Int J Radiat Oncol Biol Phys*. 2008;72(4):980–988.

53. Dearnaley DP, Sydes MR, Graham JD, et al. Escalated-dose versus standard-dose conformal radiotherapy in prostate cancer: first results from the MRC RT01 randomised controlled trial. *Lancet Oncol*. 2007;8(6):475–487.

54. Pollack A, Walker G, Horwitz EM, et al. Randomized trial of hypofractionated external-beam radiotherapy for prostate cancer. *J Clin Oncol*. 2013;31(31):3860–3868.

55. Lee WR, Dignam JJ, Amin MB, et al. Randomized phase III noninferiority study comparing two radiotherapy fractionation schedules in patients with low-risk prostate cancer. *J Clin Oncol*. 2016;34(20):2325–2332.

56. Dearnaley D, Syndikus I, Mossop H, et al. Conventional versus hypofractionated high-dose intensity-modulated radiotherapy for prostate cancer: 5-year outcomes of the randomised, non-inferiority, phase 3 CHHiP trial. *Lancet Oncol*. 2016;17(8):1047–1060.

57. Incrocci L, Wortel RC, Alemayehu WG, et al. Hypofractionated versus conventionally fractionated radiotherapy for patients with localised prostate cancer (HYPRO): final efficacy results from a randomised, multicentre, open-label, phase 3 trial. *Lancet Oncol.* 2016;17(8):1061–1069.

58. Arcangeli S, Strigari L, Gomellini S, et al. Updated results and patterns of failure in a randomized hypofractionation trial for high-risk prostate cancer. *Int J Radiat Oncol Biol Phys.* 2012;84(5):1172–1178.

59. Arcangeli G, Saracino B, Arcangeli S, et al. Moderate hypofractionation in high-risk, organ-confined prostate cancer: final results of a phase III randomized trial. *J Clin Oncol.* 2017;35:1891–1897. doi:10.1200/JCO.2016.70.4189

60. Catton CN, Lukka H, Gu CS, et al. Randomized trial of a hypofractionated radiation regimen for the treatment of localized prostate cancer. *J Clin Oncol.* 2017;35(17):1884–1890. doi:10.1200/JCO.2016.71.7397

61. Meier R, Beckman A, Henning G, et al. Five-year outcomes from a multicenter trial of stereotactic body radiation therapy for low- and intermediate-risk prostate cancer. *Int J Radiat Oncol Biol Phys.* 2016;96(2, Suppl):S33–S34.

62. Kotecha R, Djemil T, Tendulkar RD, et al. Dose-escalated stereotactic body radiation therapy for patients with intermediate- and high-risk prostate cancer: initial dosimetry analysis and patient outcomes. *Int J Radiat Oncol Biol Phys.* 2016;95(3):960–964.

63. Katz A, Formenti SC, Kang J. Predicting biochemical disease-free survival after prostate stereotactic body radiotherapy: risk-stratification and patterns of failure. *Front Oncol.* 2016;6:168.

64. Chen LN, Suy S, Uhm S, et al. Stereotactic body radiation therapy (SBRT) for clinically localized prostate cancer: the Georgetown University experience. *Radiat oncol.* 2013;8:58.

65. King CR, Brooks JD, Gill H, Presti JC, Jr. Long-term outcomes from a prospective trial of stereotactic body radiotherapy for low-risk prostate cancer. *Int J Radiat Oncol Biol Phys.* 2012;82(2):877–882.

66. Boike TP, Lotan Y, Cho LC, et al. Phase I dose-escalation study of stereotactic body radiation therapy for low- and intermediate-risk prostate cancer. *J Clin Oncol.* 2011;29(15):2020–2026.

67. Freeman DE, King CR. Stereotactic body radiotherapy for low-risk prostate cancer: five-year outcomes. *Radiat Oncol.* 2011;6:3.

68. Madsen BL, Hsi RA, Pham HT, et al. Stereotactic hypofractionated accurate radiotherapy of the prostate (SHARP), 33.5 Gy in five fractions for localized disease: first clinical trial results. *Int J Radiat Oncol Biol Phys.* 2007;67(4):1099–1105.

69. Katz AJ, Kang J. Quality of life and toxicity after SBRT for organ-confined prostate cancer, a 7-year study. *Front Oncol.* 2014;4:301.

70. Hamstra DA, Mariados N, Sylvester J, et al. Continued benefit to rectal separation for prostate radiation therapy: final results of a phase III trial. *Int J Radiat Oncol Biol Phys.* 2017;97(5):976–985.

37: INTERMEDIATE- AND HIGH-RISK PROSTATE CANCER

Bindu V. Manyam and Rahul D. Tendulkar

QUICK HIT: Prostate cancer demonstrates highly heterogeneous clinical behavior. Most patients with intermediate-risk and nearly all with high-risk disease are thought to benefit from definitive therapy (as opposed to active surveillance). Treatment paradigms for definitive therapy are evolving and a clear standard of care is difficult to identify given the currently available data.

TABLE 37.1: General Treatment Paradigm for Intermediate- and High-Risk Prostate Cancer[1]	
Definitions (NCCN)	**Treatment Options**
Intermediate risk cT2b-c or GS 7 or PSA 10–20 ng/mL	• Active surveillance (if life expectancy <10 yrs) • EBRT ± short-term ADT (4–6 months) • Brachytherapy alone • RP: Consider adjuvant or salvage EBRT for adverse features (+ margins, seminal vesicle invasion, extracapsular extension, detectable postoperative PSA)
High Risk cT3a or GS 8–10 or PSA >20 ng/mL **Very High Risk** T3b-4 Primary GS 5 >4 cores with GS 8-10	• EBRT + long-term ADT (2–3 yrs) • EBRT + brachytherapy boost ± long-term ADT • RP (in select patients): Consider adjuvant or salvage EBRT for adverse features (+ margins, seminal vesicle invasion, extracapsular extension, detectable postoperative PSA). If lymph node positive, consider ADT ± pelvic EBRT • ADT alone in select patients who are not otherwise candidates for local therapy
Clinically node-positive	• RT + long-term ADT (2–3 yrs) • ADT alone

EPIDEMIOLOGY: Prostate cancer is the most common noncutaneous malignancy and second leading cause of cancer death in men. There is an estimated incidence of 180,890 cases, 15% of which represent high-risk disease.[2,3] It is estimated that the proportion of men diagnosed with intermediate- or high-risk prostate cancer increased by 6% between 2011 and 2013.[4]

RISK FACTORS: Increasing age is the strongest risk factor for prostate cancer. Prostate cancer is more common in African American men, in whom it presents at earlier age of onset, and many studies have demonstrated higher prostate-specific antigen (PSA) levels, higher Gleason score (GS), more advanced stage of disease at diagnosis, and significantly higher biochemical disease recurrence (HR 1.28, 95% CI: 1.07–1.54, $p = .006$), even when adjusting for socioeconomic, clinical, and pathologic confounders.[5,6] Family history, specifically having a father who survived less than 24 months from prostate cancer, has been associated with higher risk disease.[7] Germline mutations in genes responsible for DNA repair are more common in prostate cancer. Most commonly, germline BRCA2 mutation may be associated with a higher GS and a worse prognosis.[8,9] Other general syndromes associated with increased risk of prostate cancer are Lynch syndrome, Fanconi's anemia, and HOXB13.[10-12]

ANATOMY, PATHOLOGY, SCREENING, CLINICAL PRESENTATION: See Chapter 36. The risk of pelvic nodal involvement has been evaluated by both the Partin tables and the Roach formula (2/3*PSA+[Gleason-6]*10; tends to over-estimate in the modern era).[33,34]

WORKUP: H&P including DRE and assessment of baseline urinary, bowel, and sexual function.

Labs: PSA, preoperative workup as indicated.

Imaging: Bone scan is indicated for pts at high risk for metastases (indications per NCCN guidelines include any of the following: T1 and PSA ≥20; T2 and PSA ≥10; GS ≥8; T3/T4; symptomatic). As per NCCN, CT or MRI pelvis is indicated for pts with T3/T4 disease or pts with T1/T2 disease and "nomogram-indicated probability of lymph node involvement >10%." 18F sodium fluoride PET/CT has been shown to have higher sensitivity and specificity in the detection of skeletal metastatic disease, though its routine use is not recommended at this time and decisions to utilize it should be individualized. Other novel imaging modalities (e.g., PSMA PET) are under development.

NATURAL HISTORY: A study of the Connecticut Tumor Registry demonstrated the probability of dying from untreated prostate cancer within 15 yrs in a patient with GS 8–10 disease was 60% to 87%.[13] Among intermediate- and high-risk patients on the PIVOT trial, treatment with RP significantly decreased all-cause mortality by an absolute amount of 10.5% (HR 0.7, 95% CI: 0.54–0.92, $p = .01$). Prostate cancer mortality was also lower with radical prostatectomy compared to observation for patients with PSA >10 ng/mL (5.6% vs. 12.8%; $p = .02$).[14]

PROGNOSTIC FACTORS, STAGING: See Chapter 36 for prognostic factors, AJCC 8th Edition staging and risk classifications.

TREATMENT PARADIGM

Active surveillance: Observation is not a standard management option for intermediate- and high-risk prostate cancer, but may have a role in select patients with low-volume, favorable intermediate-risk (GS 3 + 4 = 7) prostate cancer and/or those with a limited life expectancy and multiple medical comorbidities.[15]

Surgery: Radical prostatectomy is an option for intermediate- and high-risk prostate cancer although some pts will require postoperative RT after surgery for a rising PSA. There have been no randomized trials comparing RP with EBRT for high-risk prostate cancer. See Chapter 36 for details regarding surgical options.

Androgen Deprivation Therapy (ADT): The decision to use ADT, timing, and sequencing is dependent on disease characteristics and patient factors. Generally, 2 to 3 yrs of ADT is recommended with high-risk disease treated with EBRT, and 4 to 6 months of ADT can be considered for intermediate-risk disease treated with EBRT. Most commonly used are GnRH agonists alone or with oral antiandrogens (combined androgen blockade). ADT alone is used for treatment of metastatic prostate cancer or for select patients who are not otherwise candidates for definitive local therapy. Side effects include impotence, decreased libido, fatigue, weight gain, hot flashes, cognitive changes, depression, osteoporosis, and potentially cardiovascular disease.

TABLE 37.2: Androgen Deprivation Therapy Medications		
Method	**Mechanism**	**Examples**
Surgical castration	Removes 90%–95% of circulating testosterone and results in prompt decline in testosterone.	Bilateral orchiectomy
Gonadotropin releasing hormone (GnRH) agonists	Induce initial stimulation of LH and subsequent testosterone release, followed by gradual decline. By days 20–28, testosterone levels are in castration range. Initial transient elevation in testosterone can exacerbate pain in patients with metastatic disease. An antiandrogen is commonly used concurrently for 1 month on initiation of LHRH agonist to avoid this flare reaction.	Leuprolide (7.5 mg/month), goserelin acetate (3.6 mg/month), buserelin, triptorelin
GnRH antagonists	Suppress testosterone while avoiding flare reaction.	Degarelix
Steroidal antiandrogens	Inhibition of testosterone and dihydrotestosterone (DHT) from binding to the androgen receptor in prostatic nuclei.	Megestrol acetate, cyproterone acetate
Nonsteroidal antiandrogens	Binds to androgen receptors and inhibit binding of testosterone and DHT in prostatic nuclei.	Bicalutamide (50 mg), flutamide *(hepatotoxicity)*, enzalutamide *(gynecomastia)*
Adrenal suppression	Suppresses synthesis of multiple adrenal steroids.	Ketoconazole *(most rapid drug for reducing testosterone)*
5α-reductase inhibitors	Suppresses the enzyme that catalyzes the conversion of testosterone to DHT.	Finasteride, dutasteride
CYP17A1 inhibitors	Inhibits the formation of DHEA and androstenedione, precursors of testosterone. Given with prednisone. Approved for the use in castrate-resistant metastatic prostate cancer with recent data also suggesting a benefit when given with ADT[16,17] when castrate sensitive.	Abiraterone

Radiation

Indications: Generally, EBRT is an appropriate option for all patients with intermediate- and high-risk prostate cancer. EBRT with brachytherapy boost can be considered in high-intermediate and high-risk patients. Select intermediate-risk patients may be candidates for short-term ADT (4–6 months) in combination with EBRT. High-risk patients are candidates for pelvic lymph node irradiation and the addition of neoadjuvant and adjuvant ADT for a total of 2 to 3 yrs.[18]

Dose: Several randomized trials have demonstrated 10% to 20% improvement in biochemical PFS with dose escalation (compared to conventional doses), ranging from 74 to 79.2 Gy to the prostate and seminal vesicles, but dose escalation has not improved survival (see Chapter 36 for details).[19–22] If brachytherapy boost is planned, EBRT dose is typically 45 Gy.[23]

Pathologic analysis of prostatectomy specimens by Kestin et al. demonstrated the median length of seminal vesicle invasion to be 1 cm, with 90% within 2 cm. SV invasion was found most commonly in patients with PSA ≥10 ng/mL, GS ≥ 7, or ≥cT2b. Therefore, the proximal 2 to 2.5 cm of the seminal vesicles are typically included within the CTV for intermediate and high-risk patients.[24] Sohayda et al. analyzed prostatectomy specimens and determined that extracapsular extension extended 4 mm in 90% of cases, which has implications for CTV margins (typically ≥5 mm).[25]

Toxicity: Common acute effects of EBRT include fatigue, dysuria, urinary frequency, rectal urgency. If treating pelvic nodes, diarrhea and cramping are common. Late effects are less common and include radiation cystitis, urethral stricture, radiation proctitis, bowel obstruction, fistula, and secondary malignancies.

Procedure: See *Treatment Planning Handbook*, Chapter 8.[26]

EVIDENCE-BASED Q&A

For locally advanced prostate cancer, is there a benefit to EBRT over ADT alone?

Two trials demonstrated an OS benefit to EBRT with ADT over ADT alone. One older trial (Fellows) did not demonstrate advantage to the addition of EBRT to ADT, although there were several limitations in this trial.

Widmark, SPCG-7/SFU0-3 (*Lancet* 2009, PMID 19091394): PRT of 875 pts from 47 centers with T1b-T2 and G2-G3 disease or T3, PSA <70 ng/mL, N0, M0 randomized to ADT (3 months total androgen blockage followed by continuous flutamide 250 mg) or ADT + EBRT (70 Gy) to prostate/SVs. MFU 7.6 yrs. **Conclusion: The addition of RT to ADT improved biochemical-progression–free survival (bPFS), cancer-specific survival (CSS), and overall survival (OS), but was associated with increased toxicity in pts with high-risk prostate cancer.**

TABLE 37.3: SPCG-7 Trial Results							
10 Yr Data	bPFS	CSS	OS	Erectile Dysfunction	Urethral Stricture	Urgency	Incontinence
ADT	25%	76%	61%	81%	0%	8%	3%
ADT + EBRT	74%	88%	70%	89%	2%	14%	7%
All results statistically significant.							

Warde, NCIC CTG PR.3/MRC UK PR 07 (*Lancet* 2011, PMID 22056152; update Mason *JCO* 2015, PMID 25691677): PRT of 1,205 pts with T3-4N0, or T1-2 and PSA >40 ng/mL, or PSA >20 ng/mL and GS >8 randomized to lifelong ADT (bilateral orchiectomy or GnRH agonist) or ADT + EBRT (64–69 Gy to prostate, SVs, and 45 Gy to pelvic nodes). MFU 8 yrs. The addition of EBRT to ADT improved OS at 7 yrs (74% vs. 66%; $p = .033$). Deaths from prostate cancer were significantly reduced by the addition of RT to ADT (HR 0.46, $p < .001$). **Conclusion: The addition of EBRT to lifelong ADT improves OS in pts with high-risk prostate cancer.**

Fellows, British MRC Study (*BJU* 1992, PMID 1422689): PRT of 277 pts with cT2-T4N0M0 prostate cancer randomized to EBRT alone (88), orchiectomy alone (90), or combination therapy (99). Results: Orchiectomy had significant reduction in time to metastases compared to EBRT, but the addition of EBRT to ADT did not significantly improve LC or OS. **Conclusion: EBRT provided no advantage of orchiectomy monotherapy for locally advanced prostate cancer.** *Comment: Study was underpowered to demonstrate a survival difference, EBRT was suboptimal, and survival in both arms was lower than expected.*

For intermediate-risk pts, is there a benefit to ADT with EBRT over EBRT alone?

RTOG 9408 demonstrated an improvement in all outcomes by the addition of 4 months ADT to 66.6 Gy EBRT. RTOG 0815 is investigating this question in the setting of modern, dose-escalated radiation.

Jones, RTOG 9408 (*NEJM* 2011, PMID 21751904): PRT of 1,979 pts with prostate cancer T1b-T2b and PSA ≤ 20 ng/mL randomized to EBRT (46.8 Gy to whole pelvis with 19.8 Gy boost to prostate—total 66.6 Gy) alone or with neoadjuvant and concurrent ADT (goserelin or leuprolide x 4 months starting 2 months before RT). 35% low risk, 54% intermediate risk, 11% high risk. MFU 9.1 yrs. **Conclusion: The use of short-term neoadjuvant and concurrent ADT with EBRT significantly decreased BF, DM, and PCSM and improved OS. Post hoc risk analysis demonstrated that significant benefit in outcomes was limited to intermediate-risk pts, but not low-risk pts.**

TABLE 37.4: RTOG 9408 Results				
10-Yr Data	BF	DM	PCSM	OS
EBRT	41%	8%	8%	57%
EBRT + ADT (4 months)	26%	6%	4%	62%
All results statistically significant.				

For high-risk or locally advanced prostate cancer, is there a benefit to ADT with EBRT over EBRT alone?

Multiple trials demonstrated a survival benefit to the addition of ADT to EBRT. These trials largely did not utilize dose-escalated EBRT, and all included pelvic nodal irradiation. The following trials used heterogeneous inclusion criteria and sequencing and duration of ADT.

Bolla, EORTC 22863 (*Lancet Oncol* 2010, PMID 20933466): PRT of 415 pts with T1-2N0 and grade 3 (17%) or T3-T4N0-1 (93%) randomized to EBRT (50 Gy/25 fx to whole pelvis with 20 Gy/10 fx cone down to prostate and seminal vesicles) + ADT (goserelin x 3 yrs on day 1 of EBRT + concurrent cyproterone acetate x 1 month) or EBRT alone. MFU 65.7 months. **Conclusion: Immediate androgen suppression with GnRH agonist for 3 yrs with EBRT improves bPFS, DFS, and OS in pts with high-risk or locally advanced prostate cancer.**

TABLE 37.5: EORTC 22863 Results			
10-Yr Data	bPFS	DFS	OS
EBRT	18%	23%	40%
EBRT + ADT (3 yrs)	38%	48%	58%
All results statistically significant.			

Roach, RTOG 8610 (*JCO* 2008, PMID 18172188): PRT of 456 pts with T2-T4N0-1 prostate cancer randomized to EBRT (44–46 Gy whole pelvis with boost to prostate of 20–25 Gy, for total 65–70 Gy) + neoadjuvant and concurrent ADT (goserelin x 4 months starting 2 months before EBRT + flutamide x 4 months). **Conclusion: The addition of 4 months of neoadjuvant and concurrent ADT improved DFS, PCSM but had no OS benefit, with no increase in cardiovascular mortality.** *Comment: Subset of GS 2-6 patients had improved OS, but those with GS 7-10 did not, suggesting that 4 months ADT may be insufficient in high-risk patients.*

TABLE 37.6: RTOG 8610 Results					
10-Yr Data	LF	DM	PCSM	OS	Cardiovascular Mortality
EBRT	42%	47%	3%	34%	9%
EBRT + ADT (4 months)	30%	35%	11%	43%	12.5%
All results statistically significant except OS.					p = .32

Pilepich, RTOG 8531 (*IJROBP* 2005, PMID 15817329): PRT of 945 pts with T3 or N1 prostate cancer randomized to EBRT (44–46 Gy to whole pelvis with boost to prostate of 20–25 Gy) + ADT (goserelin during last day of RT, then monthly indefinitely) or EBRT alone. MFU 7.6 yrs. 10-yr biochemical failure was not significantly different for GS ≤6 (57% vs. 51%; p = .26), but was significantly higher with EBRT alone for GS ≥7 (52% vs. 42%; p = .026). Cardiovascular mortality was not significantly different between the two groups (8% ADT vs. 11% no ADT). **Conclusion: The addition of ADT to EBRT improved outcomes particularly in pts with GS ≥7.**

TABLE 37.7: RTOG 8531 Results				
10-Yr Data	LF	DM	bNED	OS
EBRT	38%	39%	9%	39%
EBRT + ADT (lifelong)	23%	24%	31%	49%
All results statistically significant.				

D'Amico, Dana Farber 95-096 (*JAMA* 2004, PMID 15315996; update D'Amico *JAMA* 2008, PMID 18212313; update D'Amico *JAMA* 2015, PMID 26393854): PRT of 206 intermediate- to high-risk pts randomized to 70 Gy (without nodal RT) with or without 6 months of ADT. Updated at an MFU of 4.5, 7.6, and 16.6 yrs. First two reports suggested improved OS and CSS with ADT. Final results suggested no long-term difference overall, but men with no to minimal comorbidity benefited whereas in men with moderate to severe comorbidity, overall mortality was worse with ADT. **Conclusion: ADT benefits men with minimal comorbidity, caution in those with comorbidity (see the following meta-analyses).**

Does concurrent ADT continue to add a benefit to dose-escalated EBRT?

Early results suggest at least a biochemical and perhaps a distant metastasis benefit to adding ADT in the dose-escalation era.

Bolla, EORTC 22991 (*JCO* 2016, PMID 26976418): PRTs of 819 pts with intermediate- or high-risk prostate cancer (T1b-c and PSA >10 ng/mL or GS ≥7 or cT2aN0 and PSA ≤50 ng/mL) were randomized to concurrent and adjuvant ADT (GnRH agonist x 6 months) and EBRT (70, 74, or 78 Gy, per institution preference) or EBRT alone. By D'Amico, 75% intermediate risk and 25% high risk. RT was by 3D-CRT (83%) or IMRT (17%); 25% received 70 Gy, 50% 74 Gy, and 25% 78 Gy (IMRT was used in >50% of 78 Gy pts). The addition of ADT improved 5-yr bDFS (HR 0.52, p < .001) and 5-yr cDFS (HR 0.63, p = .001), with a similar effect across all three dose groups. **Conclusion: 6 months ADT improves bDFS and cDFS for dose-escalated RT.**

TABLE 37.8: EORTC 22991 Results				
5-Yr Data	bDFS	cDFS	DM	OS
EBRT	70%	81%	8%	88%
EBRT + ADT	83%	89%	4%	91%
p value	<.001	.001	.05	Not available

Nabid, Canadian (*GU ASCO* 2015, abstract 5): PRT of 600 pts with intermediate-risk prostate cancer randomized to short-term ADT (bicalutamide and goserelin for 6 months) with conventional dose EBRT (70 Gy, Arm 1) or dose-escalated EBRT (76 Gy, Arm 2) or dose-escalated EBRT alone (76 Gy, Arm 3). MFU 75.4 months. BFs for arms 1 to 3 were 12.5%, 8%, and 21.5%, with a statistically worse BF between arms 1 and 3 (p = .023) and arms 2 and 3 (p = .001). There was no significant difference in OS between the arms.

Conclusion: Combination short-term ADT+EBRT, even with lower RT doses, leads to superior biochemical control and DFS compared to dose-escalated EBRT alone in intermediate-risk prostate cancer.

What is the optimal duration of hormone therapy?

For pts with high-risk prostate cancer, an OS benefit has been demonstrated with long-term ADT in the dose-escalated EBRT era compared to shorter term regimens, with most recent data demonstrating a benefit to 2 to 3 yrs of ADT even in the dose escalation era (DART). For pts with intermediate-risk prostate cancer receiving ADT, short-term ADT (4–6 months) has been shown to be similar to longer term regimens.

Hanks, RTOG 9202 (*JCO* 2003, PMID 14581419; update Horwitz *JCO* 2008, PMID 18413638): PRT of 1,554 pts with cT2c-4 prostate cancer and PSA <150 ng/mL randomized to neoadjuvant and concurrent short-term ADT (goserelin and flutamide x 4 months) and EBRT (45 Gy to whole pelvis and boost to 65–70 Gy to prostate) or long-term ADT x 28 months and EBRT. **Conclusion: Long-term ADT provided DFS benefit for all pts, but not OS benefit. Long-term ADT had significant survival benefit for pts with GS 8-10 disease.**

TABLE 37.9: RTOG 9202 Results							
10-Yr Data	DFS	BF	LF	DM	DSS	OS (all GS)	OS (GS [8–10])
4-month ADT + EBRT	13%	68%	22%	26%	84%	52%	32%
28-month ADT + EBRT	22%	52%	12%	18%	89%	54%	45%
p value	.0001	<.0001	.0002	.0002	.0001	.25	.006

Bolla, EORTC 22961 (*NEJM* 2009, PMID 19516032): PRT of 970 pts with cT2c-4 or N1 and PSA <150 ng/mL prostate cancer randomized to short-term ADT (triptorelin x 6 months) and EBRT (50 Gy to whole pelvis with boost to prostate and seminal vesicles to 70 Gy) or long-term ADT (36 months) and EBRT. MFU 6.4 yrs. **Conclusion: Long-term ADT (3 yrs) demonstrated significant survival benefit compared to short-term ADT (6 months), with comparable quality of life and no difference in fatal cardiac events (4% vs. 3%).**

TABLE 37.10: EORTC 22961 Results				
5-Yr Data	bPFS	CSS	OS	Gynecomastia	Incontinence
6-month ADT + EBRT	59%	95%	81%	7%	10%
36-month ADT + EBRT	78%	97%	85%	18%	18%
All results statistically significant.					

Pisansky, RTOG 9910 (*JCO* 2015, PMID 25534388): PRT of 1,579 pts with intermediate-risk prostate cancer randomized to neoadjuvant ADT for 8 weeks versus 28 weeks prior to EBRT (70.2 Gy/39 fx) followed by 8 weeks of concurrent ADT (total 16 vs. 36 weeks). MFU 8.7 yrs. **Conclusion: Short-term and long-term ADT with EBRT yielded similar outcomes in pts with intermediate-risk prostate cancer.**

TABLE 37.11: RTOG 9910 Results			
10-Yr Data	Biochemical recurrence	CSS	OS
4-month ADT + EBRT	27%	95%	66%
9-month ADT + EBRT	27%	96%	67%
p value	.77	.45	.62

Denham, TROG 9601 (*Lancet Oncol* 2011, PMID 21440505): PRT of 802 pts with cT2b-4N0, stratified by stage (T2b/c vs. T/T4) and PSA (<20 and ≥20 ng/mL) randomized to neoadjuvant and concurrent ADT (goserelin and flutamide x 3 months) + EBRT (66 Gy to prostate and seminal vesicles) or neoadjuvant and concurrent ADT (6 months) + EBRT or EBRT alone. 85% were high risk. Compared to EBRT alone, 3 months of ADT decreased PSA progression (HR 0.72, $p = .003$) and improved event-free survival (HR 0.63, $p < .0001$). 6 months of ADT further reduced PSA progression (HR 0.57, $p < .0001$) and led to a greater improvement in event-free survival (HR 0.51, $p < .0001$), compared with EBRT alone. While 3-month ADT had no effect on distant progression, PCSM, or ACM, 6-month ADT decreased distant progression (HR 0.49, $p = .001$), PCSM (HR 0.49, $p = .0008$), and ACM (HR 0.63, $p = .0008$) significantly, compared to EBRT alone. **Conclusion: 6-month ADT had superior overall outcomes compared to 3-month ADT for pts with high-risk prostate cancer.**

Zapatero, DART 01/05 GICOR (*Lancet Oncol* 2015, PMID 25702876): PRTs of 355 pts with intermediate- (47%) and high-risk (53%) prostate cancer (cT1c-T3aN0M0 and PSA <100 ng/mL) randomized to neoadjuvant and concurrent short-term ADT (goserelin x 4 months) and dose-escalated EBRT (76–82 Gy) or long-term ADT (goserelin x 28 months) and EBRT. Pelvic RT optional. MFU 63 months. **Conclusion: Long-term ADT significantly improved outcomes, including OS, compared to short-term ADT, even with dose-escalated EBRT. The benefit was more evident in pts with high-risk prostate cancer ($p = .01$).**

TABLE 37.12: DART 01/05 GICOR Results			
5-Yr Data	Biochemical DFS	Metastasis-Free Survival	OS
Short-term ADT + EBRT	81%	83%	86%
Long-term ADT + EBRT	89%	94%	95%
p value	.019	.009	.009

Is there significant cardiovascular toxicity associated with ADT?

Multiple pooled analyses have been performed, with mixed results. Some demonstrated no significant difference in cardiovascular mortality with the use of ADT, while others demonstrated increased cardiovascular death and shorter time to fatal myocardial infarction, particularly in men over 65 years of age. Studies have consistently demonstrated that the duration of ADT does not seem to significantly influence cardiovascular risk.[27-29]

D'Amico, Meta-Analysis (*JCO* 2007, PMID 17557956): Pooled analysis of 1,372 pts from 3 PRT, who received 0, 3, or 6 months ADT. Men ≥65 yrs of age who received 6 months of ADT had shorter times to fatal myocardial infarction ($p = .017$). There was no difference between 3- and 6-month ADT and no difference in men <65 yrs of age. **Conclusion: The use of ADT appears to shorten the time to fatal myocardial infarction compared to EBRT alone.**

Nguyen, Meta-Analysis (*JAMA* 2011, PMID 22147380): Systematic review of 4,141 pts from eight randomized trials. Demonstrated that cardiovascular death was not significantly different between pts who received ADT and those who did not (11% vs. 11.2%, RR 0.93; $p = .41$). There was no excess cardiovascular death in long-term ADT (>3 yrs) versus short-term ADT (≤6 months). **Conclusion: In pts with intermediate- or high-risk prostate cancer, use of ADT was not associated with an increased risk of cardiovascular death; however, ADT did reduce PCSM and overall mortality.**

Is there a role for ADT prior to prostatectomy?

Klotz, Canada (*J Urol* 2003, PMID 12913699): PRT of 213 pts randomized to prostatectomy with neoadjuvant ADT (cyproterone x 3 months) or prostatectomy alone. MFU 6 yrs. The positive margin rate was reduced by 50% with addition of ADT; however, there was no difference in rates of BF (34% vs. 37%; *p* = .07). **Conclusion: The use of ADT has not been shown to significantly improve clinical outcomes and its use is not considered standard of care.**

Is there a benefit to pelvic nodal irradiation and which pts should be considered?

The data is conflicting regarding the benefit of pelvic nodal irradiation. RTOG 9413 has been a difficult trial to interpret, but demonstrates a PFS benefit to nodal irradiation in pts with ≥15% risk of lymph node metastasis. On the other hand, other trials have demonstrated limited benefit to pelvic nodal irradiation. However, because most of the preceding high-risk trials used whole pelvic fields, high-risk pts can be considered candidates for elective nodal irradiation. The question is currently being investigated in pts with unfavorable intermediate and favorable high-risk prostate cancer on RTOG 0924.

Roach, RTOG 9413 (*JCO* 2003, PMID 12743142; update Lawton *IJROBP* 2007, PMID 17531401; update Roach *ASTRO* 2013 Abstract 260): PRT of 1,275 pts with clinically localized prostate cancer with PSA ≤100 ng/mL with an estimated ≥15% risk of lymph node positive disease according to Roach formula. See Table 37.13 for treatment arms. Primary endpoint PFS. ADT was goserelin or leuprolide with flutamide for 2 months before EBRT and 2 months during EBRT in the neoadjuvant and concurrent arm. Adjuvant ADT was also 4 months. EBRT dose was 50.4 Gy to the whole pelvis with 4-field box and boost of 19.8 Gy to the prostate. Initial publication demonstrated PFS improvement with pelvic nodal RT (both arms) compared to prostate-only RT (both arms). In the second update (Lawton), this PFS difference was not found overall but a trend was demonstrated in the WPRT+Neoadj arm compared pairwise to the others (*p* = .065). **Conclusion: Neoadjuvant/concurrent ADT and whole pelvis EBRT improves PFS when compared to the other arms in pts with ≥15% risk of lymph node metastasis.** *Comment: This trial is controversial due to the 2x2 design and is being further investigated by RTOG 0924.*

TABLE 37.13: RTOG 9413 Results			
2013 Update	PFS	BF	OS
Neoadjuvant/concurrent ADT and whole pelvis EBRT	60%	30%	88%
Neoadjuvant/concurrent ADT and prostate only EBRT	44%	43%	83%
Adjuvant ADT and whole pelvis EBRT	49%	37%	81%
Adjuvant ADT and prostate only EBRT	50%	37%	82%
p value	.03	.01	NS*

Roach, RTOG 9413 subset (*IJROBP* 2006, PMID 17011443): Secondary analysis of RTOG 9413 to determine if pelvic field size had an effect on PFS. A "mini-pelvis" (MP) field was defined as ≥10 x 11 cm, but <11 x 11 cm. 7-yr PFS was 40%, 35%, and 27% for whole pelvis, MP, and prostate only fields, respectively (*p* = .02). Increasing field size correlated with late grade 3–4 GI toxicity, but not grade 3-4 GU toxicity. **Conclusion: RT field size significantly affected PFS and the results support comprehensive nodal treatment for pts with ≥15% risk of lymph node involvement.**

Pommier, GETUG-01 (*IJROBP* 2016, PMID 27788949): PRT of 446 pts with cT1b-3N0 prostate cancer randomized to whole pelvis EBRT (46 Gy with boost to prostate 66–70 Gy) or prostate only EBRT (66–70 Gy). Pts stratified into low risk (cT1-2, GS 6, and PSA <3x upper limit normal) versus high risk (cT3 or GS >6 or PSA >3x upper limit normal). High-risk pts received 6-month ADT. MFU 11.4 yrs. No difference in EFS or OS. A post hoc subgroup analysis demonstrated a significant benefit to whole pelvis RT in pts who did not receive ADT. **Conclusion: Pelvic nodal irradiation did not appear to improve EFS or OS.** *Comment: The trial has been criticized for using low doses (median 68 Gy) and inferior coverage with superior border at S1/S2.*

TABLE 37.14: GETUG-01 Results		
10-Yr Results	EFS	OS
Whole pelvis EBRT	52%	71%
Prostate only EBRT	54%	71%
p value	.485	.517

Is hypofractionation safe and effective for high-risk pts?

The following trials are hypofractionation trials enrolling intermediate- to high-risk men only. See Chapter 36 for additional details, including the CHHiP trial, which enrolled 12% high-risk pts.

Dearnaley, CHHiP UK (*Lancet Oncol* 2016, PMID 27339115): PRT three-arm noninfe-riority trial. Men randomized 1:1:1 to either 74 Gy/37 fx, 60 Gy/20 fx over 4 weeks or 57 Gy/19 fx over 3.8 weeks. Primary endpoint was biochemical or clinical failure. Enrolled 3,216 men, MFU 62 months. 73% were intermediate, 12% were high risk. 97% received ADT for a median of 24 months. 5-yr failure-free rates were 88.3% (74 Gy), 90.6% (60 Gy), and 85.9% (57 Gy). The 60 Gy but not the 57 Gy arm was noninferior to 74 Gy. Side effects were similar. **Conclusion: 60 Gy/20 fx recommended as the standard of care.**

Incrocci, HYPRO Netherlands (*Lancet Oncol* 2016, PMID 27339116): PRT (superiority design) of 804 intermediate- (26%) to high-risk (74%) prostate cancer randomized to either 64.6 Gy/19 fx given 3 per week versus 78 Gy/39 fx. ADT prescribed by center choice, 66% received ADT for a median of 32 months. Primary outcome: 5-yr RFS (any biochemical, locoregional, distant, or ADT). MFU 60 months. 5-yr RFS was 80.5% (hypo) versus 77.1% (conventional), *p* = .36. Physician-reported acute GU toxicity was not noninferior and acute GI toxicity was significantly increased by hypofractionation.[30] **Conclusion: This hypofractionation dose schedule was not superior and should not be standard.**

Catton, PROFIT Canada (*JCO* 2017, PMID 28296582): PRT of 1,206 pts with intermedi-ate-risk prostate cancer (cT1-2, GS 6, and PSA 10–20 ng/mL; T2b-c, GS 6, PSA <20 ng/mL; cT1-2, GS 7, and PSA <20 ng/mL) randomized to CF (78 Gy/39 fx) or HF (60 Gy/20 fx) to the prostate and base of the seminal vesicles without ADT. MFU 6 yrs. 5-yr BF was not inferior for hypofractionation (21% vs. 21%; *p* = .044). Acute grade 3 GI/GU toxicity was statistically similar between the two groups and numerically improved late grade >3 tox-icity with HF (3.5% vs. 5.4%). **Conclusion: HF was not inferior to CF, with no apparent increase in acute or late toxicity in pts with intermediate-risk prostate cancer.**

Arcangeli, Italy (*IJROBP* 2012, PMID 22537541; update *JCO* 2017, PMID 28355113): PRT of 168 pts with high-risk prostate cancer randomized conventional fractionation (CF; 80 Gy/40 fx in 8 weeks) or hypofractionation (HF; 62 Gy/20 fx in 5 weeks) with 9 months of ADT. MFU 9 years. No significant difference in the incidence or severity of late GI/GU toxicity. For CF versus HF, 10-yr FFBF (72% vs. 65%), OS (64% vs. 75%), PCSS (88% vs. 95%) were not significantly different. Hypofractionation was a prognostic factor for PCSS and FFBF on unplanned MVA. **Conclusion: HF appeared to have similar cancer-related and toxicity outcomes compared to CF, but the trial did not meet the primary endpoint of a reduction in late toxicity.**

Can brachytherapy boost improve outcomes in addition to EBRT?

Brachytherapy boost is associated with increased toxicity but may benefit higher risk pts.[31,32]

Morris, ASCENDE-RT (*IJROBP* 2016, PMID 28262473): PRT of 398 pts with intermediate- (31%) and high-risk (69%) prostate cancer treated with neoadjuvant and concurrent ADT for 8 months and EBRT (46 Gy/23 fx to the whole pelvis) and then randomized to conformal EBRT boost to prostate (32 Gy/16 fx) or I-125 LDR brachytherapy boost (prescribed to minimum peripheral dose of 115 Gy). The 9-yr RFS (defined as nadir + 2 ng/mL) was significantly higher for the brachytherapy boost arm compared to EBRT boost arm (83% vs. 62%; $p < .001$), but also had higher risk of GU toxicity. **Conclusion: LDR brachytherapy boost significantly increased biochemical control compared to EBRT boost in pts with intermediate- and high-risk prostate cancer, but also had higher risk of GU toxicity.**

Is LDR brachytherapy alone sufficient treatment for favorable intermediate-risk prostate cancer?

Prestige, RTOG 0232 (*ASTRO* 2016, abstract 7): PRT of 579 pts with favorable intermediate-risk prostate cancer, defined as: T1c-T2b; GS 2-6 with PSA 10–19 ng/mL or GS 7 with PSA <10 ng/mL) randomized to EBRT (45 Gy/25 fx to prostate and seminal vesicles; lymph nodes optional) followed by LDR brachytherapy with Pd-103 (100 Gy) or I-125 (110 Gy) or brachytherapy alone with Pd-103 (125 Gy) or I-125 (145 Gy). Freedom from progression was not improved at 5 yrs with the addition of EBRT. Grade ≥2 and grade ≥3 acute toxicity were similar, but grade ≥2 (53% vs. 37%; $p = .0001$) and grade ≥3 (12% vs. 7%; $p = .039$) late toxicity were higher in the EBRT + brachytherapy arm. **Conclusion: The addition of EBRT to brachytherapy did not significantly improve 5-yr freedom from progression, but did increase late toxicity in pts with favorable intermediate-risk prostate cancer.**

Is there a role for the use of chemotherapy in high-risk prostate cancer?

The OS benefit of the addition of chemotherapy to long-term ADT and dose-escalated EBRT in the modern era for pts with high-risk prostate cancer is unclear. PRTs currently have limited follow-up, but demonstrate significantly improved biochemical control, and NCCN guidelines currently report the use of chemotherapy as a category 1 recommendation for high-risk prostate cancer.[1] The decision to use chemotherapy should be individualized, based on patient and disease characteristics.

Rosenthal, RTOG 9902 (*IJROBP* 2015, PMID 26209502): PRT of 397 pts with high-risk prostate cancer (68% with GS 8-10 and 24% with cT3-4) randomized to EBRT + long-term ADT (GnRH agonist x 24 months) with adjuvant paclitaxel, estramustine, oral etoposide chemotherapy (CHT) versus EBRT + ADT alone. MFU 9.2 yrs. **Conclusion: The addition of CHT to standard of care EBRT + long-term ADT was not shown to improve outcomes in pts with high-risk prostate cancer.**

TABLE 37.15: RTOG 9902 Results					
10-yr Results	BF	LF	DM	DFS	OS
EBRT + ADT + CHT	54%	7%	14%	26%	63%
EBRT + ADT	58%	11%	16%	22%	65%
p value	.82	.09	.42	.61	.81

Sandler, RTOG 0521 (*ASCO GU* 2015): PRT of 612 pts with high-risk prostate cancer (GS 7-8 with PSA >20 ng/mL, and any T stage; GS 8, cT2, and any PSA; or GS 9-10, any T stage, any PSA) randomized to EBRT (75.6 Gy) + long-term ADT (24 months) followed by CHT (docetaxel x 6 cycles) or EBRT + long-term ADT alone. EBRT + ADT + CHT had significantly higher 4-yr OS (93% vs. 89%; $p = .04$) and 5-yr DFS (73% vs. 66%; $p = .05$), compared to EBRT + ADT alone. **Conclusion: Adjuvant CHT, in addition to EBRT and long-term ADT may provide a survival benefit in pts with high-risk prostate cancer.**

Fizazi, GETUG 12 (*Lancet Oncol* 2015, PMID 26028518): PRT of 207 pts with high-risk prostate cancer (cT3-T4 or GS ≥8; PSA >20 ng/mL; pN1) randomized to long-term ADT (GnRH agonist x 3 yrs) with CHT (docetaxel and estramustine x 4 cycles) or ADT alone. Local therapy with RP or EBRT was performed 3 months after systemic treatment. MFU 8.8 yrs. RFS at 8 yrs was significantly higher with the addition of CHT (62% vs. 50%; $p = .017$). **Conclusion: Docetaxel and estramustine CHT in combination with long-term ADT and local therapy (RP or EBRT) significantly improved RFS in pts with high-risk prostate cancer.**

Lymph node positive prostate cancer

What is the management of pts with clinically lymph node–positive disease?

Historically, node-positive disease was treated according to a similar treatment paradigm to distant metastases, with early trial questions evaluating immediate versus delayed ADT at the time of progression. Current practice patterns have shifted, as newer data, though only retrospective, suggests a benefit to EBRT in these pts (see Chapter 38 for further details in the adjuvant setting).

Lin, NCDB (*JNCI* 2015, PMID 25957435): RR of 3,450 pts with clinically node-positive prostate cancer without DM. ADT + EBRT was associated with a 50% decreased risk of 5-yr ACM (HR 0.50, 95% CI: 0.37–0.67; $p < .001$). **Conclusion: The combination of ADT+ EBRT may be associated with a significant survival benefit in men with clinically node-positive prostate cancer.**

Rusthoven, SEER (*IJROBP* 2014, PMID 24661660): SEER study of 796 clinically and 2,991 pathologically node-positive pts. In the clinical cohort, 43% were treated with EBRT and 57% without local therapy. 10-yr OS in the clinical cohort was 45% versus 29% ($p < .001$) and prostate cancer-specific survival was 67% versus 53% ($p < .001$) in favor of EBRT. Results similar in the pathologic cohort. **Conclusion: Retrospective data suggest that node-positive pts benefit from local therapy in addition to systemic therapy.**

REFERENCES

1. Network NCC. Clinical Practice Guidelines in Oncology Prostate Cancer. 2017. https://www.nccn.org/professionals/physician_gls/pdf/prostate_blocks.pdf
2. Cooperberg MR, Broering JM, Carroll PR. Time trends and local variation in primary treatment of localized prostate cancer. *J Clin Oncol*. 2010;28(7):1117–1123.
3. Institute NC. Surveillance, Epidemiology, and End Results Program Prostate Cancer. 2016. https://seer.cancer.gov/statfacts/html/prost.html
4. Drazer MW, Huo D, Eggener SE. National prostate cancer screening rates after the 2012 US preventive services task force recommendation discouraging prostate-specific antigen-based screening. *J Clin Oncol*. 2015;33(22):2416–2423.
5. Hoffman RM, Gilliland FD, Eley JW, et al. Racial and ethnic differences in advanced-stage prostate cancer: the Prostate Cancer Outcomes Study. *J Nat Cancer Inst*. 2001;93(5):388–395.
6. Hamilton RJ, Aronson WJ, Presti JC Jr, et al. Race, biochemical disease recurrence, and prostate-specific antigen doubling time after radical prostatectomy: results from the SEARCH database. *Cancer*. 2007;110(10):2202–2209.
7. Hemminki K, Ji J, Forsti A, et al. Concordance of survival in family members with prostate cancer. *J Clin Oncol*. 2008;26(10):1705–1709.

8. Agalliu I, Gern R, Leanza S, Burk RD. Associations of high-grade prostate cancer with BRCA1 and BRCA2 founder mutations. *Clin Cancer Res.* 2009;15(3):1112–1120.

9. Castro E, Goh C, Olmos D, et al. Germline BRCA mutations are associated with higher risk of nodal involvement, distant metastasis, and poor survival outcomes in prostate cancer. *J Clin Oncol.* 2013;31(14):1748–1757.

10. Raymond VM, Mukherjee B, Wang F, et al. Elevated risk of prostate cancer among men with Lynch syndrome. *J Clin Oncol.* 2013;31(14):1713–1718.

11. Tischkowitz M, Easton DF, Ball J, et al. Cancer incidence in relatives of British Fanconi Anaemia patients. *BMC cancer.* 2008;8:257–261.

12. Ewing CM, Ray AM, Lange EM, et al. Germline mutations in HOXB13 and prostate-cancer risk. *N Engl J Med.* 2012;366(2):141–149.

13. Albertsen PC, Hanley JA, Fine J. 20-year outcomes following conservative management of clinically localized prostate cancer. *JAMA.* 2005;293(17):2095–2101.

14. Wilt TJ, Brawer MK, Jones KM, et al. Radical prostatectomy versus observation for localized prostate cancer. *N Engl J Med.* 2012;367(3):203–213.

15. Chen RC, Rumble RB, Loblaw DA, et al. Active surveillance for the management of localized prostate cancer (Cancer Care Ontario Guideline): American Society of Clinical Oncology Clinical practice guideline endorsement. *J Clin Oncol.* 2016;34(18):2182–2190.

16. James ND, de Bono JS, Spears MR, et al. Abiraterone for prostate cancer not previously treated with hormone therapy. *NEJM.* 2017;377(4):338–351.

17. Fizazi K, Tran N, Fein L, et al. Abiraterone plus prednisone in metastatic, castration-sensitive prostate cancer. *NEJM.* 2017;377(4):352–360.

18. Zapatero A, Guerrero A, Maldonado X, et al. High-dose radiotherapy with short-term or long-term androgen deprivation in localised prostate cancer (DART01/05 GICOR): a randomised, controlled, phase 3 trial. *Lancet Oncol.* 2015;16(3):320–327.

19. Pollack A, Zagars GK, Starkschall G, et al. Prostate cancer radiation dose response: results of the M. D. Anderson phase III randomized trial. *Int J Radiat Oncol Biol Phys.* 2002;53(5):1097–1105.

20. Zietman AL, Bae K, Slater JD, et al. Randomized trial comparing conventional-dose with high-dose conformal radiation therapy in early-stage adenocarcinoma of the prostate: long-term results from Proton Radiation Oncology Group/American College of Radiology 95-09. *J Clin Oncol.* 2010;28(7):1106–1111.

21. Al-Mamgani A, van Putten WL, Heemsbergen WD, et al. Update of Dutch multicenter dose-escalation trial of radiotherapy for localized prostate cancer. *Int J Radiat Oncol Biol Phys.* 2008;72(4):980–988.

22. Dearnaley DP, Sydes MR, Graham JD, et al. Escalated-dose versus standard-dose conformal radiotherapy in prostate cancer: first results from the MRC RT01 randomised controlled trial. *Lancet Oncol.* 2007;8(6):475–487.

23. Orio PF 3rd, Nguyen PL, Buzurovic I, et al. The decreased use of brachytherapy boost for intermediate and high-risk prostate cancer despite evidence supporting its effectiveness. *Brachytherapy.* 2016;15(6):701–706.

24. Kestin L, Goldstein N, Vicini F, et al. Treatment of prostate cancer with radiotherapy: should the entire seminal vesicles be included in the clinical target volume? *Int J Radiat Oncol Biol Phys.* 2002;54(3):686–697.

25. Sohayda C, Kupelian PA, Levin HS, Klein EA. Extent of extracapsular extension in localized prostate cancer. *Urology.* 2000;55(3):382–386.

26. Videtic GMM. *Handbook of Treatment Planning in Radiation Oncology.* 2nd ed. New York, NY: Demos Medical; 2014.

27. Nguyen PL, Je Y, Schutz FA, et al. Association of androgen deprivation therapy with cardiovascular death in patients with prostate cancer: a meta-analysis of randomized trials. *JAMA.* 2011;306(21):2359–2366.

28. D'Amico AV, Denham JW, Crook J, et al. Influence of androgen suppression therapy for prostate cancer on the frequency and timing of fatal myocardial infarctions. *J Clin Oncol.* 2007;25(17):2420–2425.

29. Tsai HK, D'Amico AV, Sadetsky N, et al. Androgen deprivation therapy for localized prostate cancer and the risk of cardiovascular mortality. *J Natl Cancer Inst.* 2007;99(20):1516–1524.

30. Aluwini S, Pos F, Schimmel E, et al. Hypofractionated versus conventionally fractionated radiotherapy for patients with prostate cancer (HYPRO): acute toxicity results from a randomised non-inferiority phase 3 trial. *Lancet Oncol.* 2015;16(3):274–283.

31. Hoskin PJ, Rojas AM, Bownes PJ, et al. Randomised trial of external beam radiotherapy alone or combined with high-dose–rate brachytherapy boost for localised prostate cancer. *Radiother Oncol.* 2012;103(2):217–222.

32. Morton G, Loblaw A, Cheung P, et al. Is single fraction 15 Gy the preferred high-dose–rate brachytherapy boost dose for prostate cancer? *Radiother Oncol.* 2011;100(3):463–467.

33. Eifler JB, Feng Z, Lin BM, et al. An updated prostate cancer staging nomogram (Partin tables) based on cases from 2006 to 2011. *BJU Int.* 2013;111(1):22–29. https://www.ncbi.nlm.nih.gov/pubmed/22834909

34. Nguyen PL, Chen MH, Hoffman KE, et al. Predicting the risk of pelvic node involvement among men with prostate cancer in the contemporary era. *Int J Radiat Oncol Biol Phys.* 2009;74(1):104–109. https://www.ncbi.nlm.nih.gov/pubmed/19286330

38: POST-PROSTATECTOMY RADIATION THERAPY

Camille A. Berriochoa and Rahul D. Tendulkar

QUICK HIT: After radical prostatectomy (RP), approximately 25% to 30% will have PSA progression postoperatively (over 50% among men with pT3 disease or positive margins). Adjuvant RT versus observation with salvage treatment at the time of biochemical relapse remains controversial. Three randomized trials (SWOG 8794, German ARO 9602, and EORTC 22911) showed that immediate treatment (i.e., RT within 6 months) improves bRFS by about 20% to 25%. Of these, only the SWOG study detected an improvement in DMFS and OS. Several trials (RAVES, RADICALS, GETUG-17, and EORTC 22043-30031) are ongoing or recently closed. If observation is conducted, early salvage RT at low PSA levels is associated with improved bRFS and DM rates, and concurrent ADT led to improved outcomes in two trials (RTOG 9601 and GETUG 16). A common dose regimen for salvage RT is 70 Gy/35 fractions; the RTOG uses 64.8 to 70.2 Gy in 1.8 Gy fractions on protocols. More practitioners utilize salvage rather than adjuvant RT,[1] though some argue that in pts with multiple adverse pathologic features (+margins, high GS, SVI) or high risk by genomic profile testing, adjuvant RT should be employed.

TABLE 38.1: General Treatment Paradigm for Postoperative Prostate Cancer[2]		
Initial Treatment	Pathologic Findings	Subsequent Treatment Options
Radical prostatectomy	No adverse features or LN mets	Close monitoring*
	Adverse features (+margin, SVI, ECE) but no LN mets	Adjuvant EBRT
		Close monitoring*
	Positive for LN mets	ADT +/− EBRT
		Close monitoring*
	Detectable postoperative PSA and no evidence of distant metastases	Salvage EBRT +/−ADT
		Close monitoring* (if low grade with slow PSA doubling time and/or limited life expectancy)
*Close monitoring: PSA q6–12 mos + annual DRE.		

EPIDEMIOLOGY: Approximately 230,000 diagnoses of prostate cancer per year, with 30,000 deaths annually. Over 90% have localized disease and over half undergo RP. Following RP, PSA is highly sensitive and biochemical failure is not uncommon: for men with intermediate-risk prostate cancer, 5-yr bRFS ~80%, 10-yr bRFS ~65%. For high/very high risk disease, 5-yr bRFS ~70%, 10-year bRFS ~55%.[3] Laparoscopic/robotic surgery has become more common, with 85% undergoing this approach rather than open technique.[4] Overall, after RP, 25% to 30% have PSA progression post-op (>50% if pT3 or positive margins).

RISK FACTORS, ANATOMY, PATHOLOGY, SCREENING, CLINICAL PRESENTATION: See Chapter 36 for details.

GENETICS: Role of multigene assays to improve selection for adjuvant RT is evolving.

WORKUP: H&P to rule out distant metastatic disease. Palpation of nodule on DRE highly sensitive and specific for anastomotic recurrence.

Labs: PSA.

Imaging

Bone Scan (Tc-99m): Consider for high PSA, short PSADT, symptomatic, or after prior ADT. In a study of 414 bone scans, 14% were + for metastatic cancer, and only 4% of those with a PSA between 0 and 10 had a positive scan.[5]

CT Abdomen/Pelvis: Consider preoperatively for T3-4 disease or T1-2 disease with a >10% risk of nodal metastases per nomogram. Postoperatively, consider if PSA does not fall to undetectable levels.

Prostascint: In-111 capromab pendetide: monoclonal antibody to PSMA (prostate-specific membrane antigen). Sensitivity 27% to 76%, so utility is uncertain at this point.[6] Highly technique and interpretation dependent.

18F-NaF PET-CT: ^{18}F-sodium fluoride PET (not the usual ^{18}F-glucose PET). Fluoride uptake by bone. Compared to Tc-99m bone scan: superior pharmacokinetics with a shorter time from injection to imaging, higher bone uptake, faster blood clearance, lower radiation dose, and superior image quality.

11-Choline PET-CT: C-11 is preferentially taken up by high densities of cellular membranes, which arise in areas where cancer cells are rapidly multiplying. May be able to detect LR or DM in about half of pts.[7]

Note that for both F18 and C11 PET, false positive scans remain a significant concern and there is a steep learning curve associated with interpretation of these approaches. The Prostate Cancer Radiographic Assessments for Detection of Advanced Recurrence (RADAR) Working Group recommends using 18F-NaF PET/CT for skeletal assessment in biochemical recurrence as an initial scan with PSA >5 ng/mL or for doubling of PSA after a prior negative scan.[8]

MRI: Emerging data reporting on visualization of postsurgical failure[9,10] and may also help with treatment planning.[11] Note that for a prostate MRI, a 3T magnet is preferred for sufficient resolution.

Pathology: Generally no role for biopsy unless a suspicious finding is discovered on exam or imaging. Pathology from prostatectomy sample should be analyzed.

PROGNOSTIC FACTORS: As per the Stephenson and Tendulkar nomogram paper: surgical margins (positive margins are favorable for response to salvage RT), Gleason score, PSA level, PSA doubling time, PSA response (ratio of rate of climb to rate of fall before and after ADT, ratio <1 has >3X OS), interval from surgery to bF, lack of SV involvement.[12,13] Tertiary pattern of 4 or 5 in prostatectomy specimens should be categorized as having high-risk disease.

NATURAL HISTORY: Most common sites of local recurrence following RP: (a) vesicourethral anastomosis (approximately 2/3 of LR) (b) bladder neck (c) retrotrigone.[14] Survival following bF is highly variable ranging from 4 to 15+ yrs in various series.[15] Historically, median time to radiographic mets after post-prostatectomy bF is 8 yrs and median time to death after developing macrometastatic disease another 5 yrs.[16]

STAGING: See Chapter 36 for AJCC 8th Edition staging and risk classifications.[17]

TREATMENT PARADIGM

Surgery: RP remains the most common procedure performed for clinically localized prostate cancer.[12] Retropubic, laparoscopic ± robot and perineal approaches can be used. The perineal approach is distinguished by a lack of lymph node dissection (outcomes not compromised w/ early risk), omission of SV removal (associated with higher biochemical failure rate), and higher rates of rectal injury or fecal incontinence.[18] Positive margins arise in approximately 20% to 25% of cases and are most often located along the posterolateral aspect of the prostate, in part due to the proximity of the nerves in that area.[19]

Definition of biochemical failure after RP: AUA definition is detectable or rising PSA value after surgery ≥0.2 ng/mL with a second confirmatory level ≥0.2 ng/mL.[20] Note that the ASTRO and Phoenix definitions refer to post-RT biochemical recurrence. Risk of PSA progression after RP: if low-risk disease: bF <10%; if positive margins or T3 disease: bF ~50%; if LN +, bF ~80%.[12,21]

Acute adverse events: 0.5 to 1 L blood loss, pelvic pain, 0% to 2% mortality, impotence, incontinence, rectal injury (<1%), thromboembolic events (1%–3%), MI (1%–8%), wound infection (<1%), slight shortening of penile length.[22,23]

Late adverse events: The Prostate Cancer Outcomes Study (PCOS) quantified patient-reported outcomes following prostatectomy. At 18+ mos following surgery, 60% of men were impotent and 8% were incontinent. Among men who were potent before surgery, the proportion reporting impotence at 18+ mos depended on whether bilateral NS (56% impotent) versus unilateral NS (58% impotent) versus non-NS (66% impotent) RP was performed. Regarding urinary control, 32% of men had total control, 40% had occasional leakage, 7% had frequent leakage, and 1% to 2% were incontinent.[24] The PCOS results were updated in 2013 and found that pts undergoing RP were more likely to have urinary incontinence (5-yr OR: 5.10) and ED (5-yr OR: 1.96) than those undergoing RT, though no significant differences were noticed at 15 yrs.[25] PROST-QA was the first trial to report patient and partner QOL and is further detailed in Chapter 36.[26] The UK ProtecT trial provided the first randomized trial (RP vs. EBRT vs. active monitoring) for early-stage prostate cancer and found that RP had the greatest negative effect on sexual function and urinary incontinence.[27]

Chemotherapy: No current role for adjuvant cytotoxic chemotherapy in the early salvage setting. The STAMPEDE trial found an overall survival benefit to the use of docetaxel administered at the time of first-line ADT in metastatic hormone-sensitive prostate cancer patients, although it is unclear if this applies to nonmetastatic recurrent pts (HR 0.95, 95% CI: 0.62–1.47).

Androgen deprivation: Consider ADT concurrent with salvage RT for pts with a pre-salvage PSA between 0.2 and 4 ng/mL. See Chapter 37 for details on ADT dosing and administration.

Radiation

Indications

Adjuvant therapy: Treatment in absence of detectable disease, generally within 6 months after surgery (although defined as within 4 months on the ongoing RAVES trial). Typically starts ~3–4 mos after surgery so that incontinence or other post-op complications are allowed time for recovery. Rationale: Prevent recurrence in those at high risk when disease burden is minimal. Classic indications: +margins, ECE (pT3a), SVI (pT3b).

Salvage therapy: Treatment in presence of detectable disease (elevated PSA or palpable nodule). Rationale: RT may eradicate locally recurrent/residual prostate cancer. Clinical indications: palpable local recurrence, persistently elevated post-op PSA, rising PSA.

Pelvic lymph nodes: Pelvic nodal RT indicated in the pN+ pts (see the following for discussion). For pN0 pts, elective nodal irradiation is an evolving paradigm. RTOG 0534 is investigating this question and enrolled pT2-3N0/X pts regardless of surgical margins.

Dose: Typically ranges from 64 to 70.2 at 1.8 to 2 Gy/fx. Doses above 66 Gy are associated with improved outcomes.

Procedure: See *Treatment Planning Handbook*, Chapter 8.

EVIDENCE-BASED Q&A

Is there a benefit to salvage RT versus observation after biochemical failure?

Trock, Hopkins (*JAMA* 2008, PMID 18560003): RR of 635 men s/p RP 1982-2004 with bF and/or local recurrence; 397 were observed, 160 received salvage RT alone, and 78 received salvage RT + ADT. Prostate CSS defined from time of recurrence until death from disease. MFU 6 yrs after recurrence (9 yrs after RP). Salvage RT associated with threefold increase in CSS versus observation (HR 0.34, $p < .001$). Benefit was observed primarily in men w/ PSADT ≤6 mo and salvage RT <2 yrs after bF. No additional benefit to ADT.

Does immediate post-prostatectomy RT improve outcomes for pts with high-risk features?

Rates of bF after prostatectomy are 70% to 75% in those with pT3 disease, +margins and high Gleason score.[28,29] Therefore, three major trials evaluated the role of immediate ("adjuvant") RT to the prostate bed versus observation. In all three, immediate RT improved bRFS by about 20% to 30%, but only the SWOG study detected an improvement in DMFS and OS. Two meta-analyses (Ontario and Cochrane) were also performed, with conflicting results. In the current ultrasensitive PSA era, some argue that the low risk of toxicity may warrant prompt adjuvant treatment in these populations. However, none of these trials specified the timing or type of salvage treatment provided to pts who failed observation. This was instead left to the treating physician and ultimately a wide range of treatments were given, including no salvage therapy for some pts.

Swanson, SWOG 8794 (*JCO* 2007, PMID 17105795; Update *J Urology* 2009, PMID 19167731): PRT of 425 pts w/ pT3N0 and/or +margins randomized to immediate RT (60–64 Gy) versus observation. No concurrent ADT. PSA q 3 mo for 1 yr, q6 mo for 2 yrs, then annually. Primary endpoint: metastasis-free survival. Secondary endpoint: bRFS (bF defined as PSA ≥0.4 ng/mL). MFU 12.7 yrs. 33% of observation pts eventually received RT, 50% of observation pts eventually required ADT. All endpoints improved with adjuvant RT: bF (decreased from 64% to 34%, $p < .005$), median met free survival (14.7 yrs vs. 12.9 yrs, HR 0.71, $p = .016$, NNT=12 to prevent one death at 12.6 yrs), and OS (median 15.2 yrs vs. 13.3 yrs, HR 0.72, $p = .023$, NNT = 9.1 to prevent one death at 12.6 yrs). QOL was worse w/ RT at 6 mo and 2 yrs but equivalent by 5 yrs. Benefit to RT seen in all three risk groups. **Conclusion: Immediate RT improved OS, DM, and BF for pts with pT3 or**

margin-positive prostate cancer. *Comment: approximately 30% had a detectable PSA >0.2 ng/mL prior to "adjuvant" RT, so not truly an adjuvant trial.*

Bolla, EORTC 22911 (*Lancet*** 2005, PMID 16099293; Update** *Lancet* **2012, PMID 23084481):** PRT of 1,005 pts treated with immediate RT to 60 Gy versus "wait and see" (W&S) after RP, pT3N0, and/or +margins. RT started within 16 weeks after RP. RT was 4-field to a dose of 50 Gy/25 fx + 10 Gy boost to the prostate bed. bF defined as increase of 0.2 ng/mL over the nadir on three separate occasions 2 weeks apart. MFU 10.6 yrs and 7 PSAs per pt. In the W&S group, 56% pts received salvage RT and 23% received ADT. Primary endpoint: bRFS. *Comment: Like the SWOG study, ~30% of pts had a detectable PSA >0.2 ng/mL prior to "adjuvant" RT.*

TABLE 38.2: EORTC Adjuvant RT for Prostate Cancer Results							
	10-yr bRFS	5-yr Clinical PFS	10-yr LRF	Grade 3 Acute Toxicity	10-yr Toxicity	10-yr OS	10-yr DM
Adjuvant RT	62%	70%	7%	5.3%	70.8%	77%	10.1%
Wait and see	39%	65%	16%	2.5%	59.7%	80%	11%
p **value**	<.0001	.054	<.0001	.052	.001	NS	NS

Wiegel, German ARO 96-02 (*JCO*** 2009, PMID 19433689; Update** *Eur Urol* **2014, PMID 24680359):** PRT of 385 pts w/ pT3N0 prostate cancer (any margin status) randomized to adjuvant RT versus W&S. Primary endpoint: bRFS. RT (60 Gy/30 fx) with 3DCRT to prostatic bed + SVs, 1 cm PTV margins, starting 8 to 12 wks after surgery. 70 of 78 pts who did not reach "undetectable PSA" received 66.6 Gy RT and were excluded from study. bF defined as undetectable to detectable and another increase at 3 months. 19% of pts randomized to RT did not receive it. 3% of observation pts elected to receive RT. Neither DMFS nor OS was significantly improved by adjuvant RT. Only one grade 3 bladder toxicity, and five total grade 2 urinary and/or rectal toxicities reported. **Conclusion: Adjuvant RT reduced the risk of biochemical progression with a hazard ratio of 0.51 in pT3 PCa and is safe.** *Comment: ARO used the most modern RT technique, used the most sensitive PSA assay, required an undetectable PSA prior to randomization, and included only pT3 pts.*

TABLE 38.3: Results of German ARO 9602 Adjuvant Radiotherapy for Prostate Cancer			
	5-yr bRFS (PSA undetectable)	≥Gr 1 toxicity	10-yr bRFS
Adjuvant RT	72%	22%	56%
Observation	54%	4%	35%
p value	.0015	<.001	<.0001

When combining the three immediate RT trials, is there a clear benefit to RT?

Morgan, Ontario Meta-analysis (*Radiother Oncol*** 2008, PMID 18501455):** Study-level meta-analysis of three PRTs that comprised 1,743 pts with pT3 and/or +margins. No benefit for OS; significant benefit to immediate RT for bRFS (HR 0.47, $p < .00001$). EORTC 22991 was the only trial to report on toxicity, finding no significant difference in grade 3+ GI or GU toxicity at 5 yrs (both <5%) but an increase in any grade of toxicity (54%–64%, $p = .005$) with the use of adjuvant RT. **Conclusion: No OS benefit to immediate post-op RT over active surveillance, but significant improvement in bRFS without severe late toxicity.**

Daly, Cochrane Review (*Cochrane Database Syst Rev*** 2011, PMID 22161411):** Study-level analysis with longer follow-up than Ontario. Concluded that adjuvant RT does indeed improve DMFS as well as OS. However, this was found only at 10 yrs of follow-up. 5-yr follow-up was not significant for these results. Investigators found an NNT of 10.

Is early salvage RT superior to adjuvant RT?

Early salvage therapy may reduce the number of pts needlessly irradiated but may also compromise outcomes if the disease progresses. This is the subject of several ongoing trials (RAVES, RADICALS, GETUG-17, EORTC 22043-30031). If salvage RT is initiated early, the strategies are likely similar. Retrospective data from VCU suggests that as long as the pt's pretreatment PSA was <1 ng/mL, outcomes were similar between adjuvant and salvage therapy (N = 157).[30] UCLA data (King) shows that with every 0.1 ng/mL increase, the likelihood of cure decreases by ~3%, suggesting that earlier intervention may lead to better outcomes.[31] Other retrospective data shown later also suggests improved outcomes with earlier initiation of salvage RT.

Stish, Mayo Clinic (*JCO* 2016, PMID 27480153): Single-institution RR of 1,106 pts s/p RP who received salvage RT between 1987 and 2013. Pts with a post-op PSA ≥0.1 ng/mL were excluded. MFU 9 yrs. On MVA, pathologic tumor stage, GS, and presalvage PSA were associated with bF, DM, and PCM. The use of ADT was associated with bRFS; RT dose >68 Gy was also associated with bRFS. **Conclusion: Early salvage RT significantly reduced the risk of bF, DM, and PCM even when calculating outcomes from date of RP.**

TABLE 38.4: Mayo Clinic Outcomes of Early Salvage RT (Stish et al.)

	10-yr outcomes		*p* value
	PSA ≤0.5 ng/mL	PSA >0.5 ng/mL	
bF	60%	68%	<.001
DM	13%	25%	<.001
PCM	6%	13%	.02
OS	83%	73%	.14

Is there a nomogram that can be used to delineate which pts may be good candidates for salvage RT?

The Stephenson nomogram has been utilized to predict outcomes after salvage RT. This nomogram was updated by Tendulkar to help elucidate the efficacy of salvage therapy in the ultrasensitive PSA era.

Stephenson, Multi-Institution Nomogram (*JCO* 2007, PMID 17513807): Multi-institution RR of 1,540 pts examining predictors of 6-yr bRFS after salvage RT. All pts were treated at a PSA ≥0.2 ng/mL. Six-yr bRFS was 32% overall. 48% of pts w/RT at PSA ≤0.50 ng/mL were disease-free at 6 yrs, including 41% w PSADT ≤10 m or Gleason grade 8-10. Significant variables were surgical margins, PSA before RT, Gleason score, PSADT, ADT before or during RT (all *p* < .001), and LN mets (*p* = .019).

Tendulkar, Multi-Institution Nomogram (*JCO* 2016, PMID 27528718): Multi-institution RR of 2,460 LN- pts s/p RP with a detectable post-RP PSA treated with salvage RT w/ or w/o ADT with this study including pts whose post-op PSA was <0.2 ng/mL. Both bRFS and DM rates improved when salvage RT delivered at lower PSA levels, even before meeting AUA criteria for bF.

TABLE 38.5: Tendulkar Nomogram Results

PSA at salvage RT	0.01–0.20 ng/mL	0.21–0.5 ng/mL	0.51–1.0 ng/mL	1.01–2 ng/mL	>2.0 ng/mL	*p* value
5-yr bRFS	71%	63%	54%	43%	37%	<.001
10-yr DM	9%	15%	19%	20%	37%	<.001

Can genomic analyses help risk-stratify pts?

Den, 22-Gene Classifier (*JCO* 2015, PMID 25667284): 22 prespecified biomarkers combined into one genomic classifier (GC) score. With a low GC score (<0.4), no difference in adjuvant versus salvage RT. With a high GC score (≥0.4), the incidence of metastases was decreased (6% vs. 23%) in those treated with adjuvant RT versus salvage RT. **Conclusion: GC may identify ideal candidates for adjuvant RT.** *Comment: May require prospective validation.*

What is the benefit of adding ADT to salvage RT?

Two randomized trials comparing salvage RT +/− ADT have both shown a bRFS benefit to the addition of ADT, and RTOG 96-01 found an OS benefit of 5% at 12 yrs. Of note, RTOG 96-01 utilized 2 yrs of bicalutamide, whereas the GETUG trial used 6 months of goserelin. Some clinicians have used the GETUG trial to justify limiting ADT to 6 months, although the optimal duration and method of ADT in the postoperative setting is unknown.

Shipley, RTOG 9601 (*NEJM* 2017, PMID 28146658): PRT of 761 pts with biochemical failure (post-op PSA 0.2–4.0 ng/mL) and either pT2 w/ +margins or pT3, N0, who then received salvage RT (64.8 Gy/36 fx) randomized to 24 mos of 150 mg daily bicalutamide versus placebo. Median PSA at entry 0.6 ng/mL. MFU 12.6 yrs. **Conclusion: The addition of ADT to salvage RT improved bF, DM, PCM, and OS with tolerable side effects.** *Comment: Relatively high PSA at entry, low RT dose by modern standards.*

TABLE 38.6: RTOG 9601 Clinical Outcomes							
	12-yr bF	12-yr DM	12-yr PCM	12-yr OS	Late grade 3/4 bladder toxicity	Late grade 3/4 bowel toxicity	Gynecomastia
RT + placebo	68%	23%	13%	71%	6.7%	1.6%	11%
RT + bicalutamide	44%	14%	6%	76%	7%	2.7%	70%
p value	<.001	<.001	<.001	.04	NS	NS	<.001

Carrie, GETUG-AFU 16 (*Lancet Oncol* 2016, PMID 27160475): PRT of 743 men s/p RP with initially undetectable and subsequently rising post-op PSA between 0.2 and 2.0 ng/mL, randomized to RT alone versus RT + 6 mos of goserelin (10.8 mg day 1 and 3 mos later). RT was 66 Gy in 33 fx via 3DCRT or IMRT. MFU 63 mos. RT+ADT arm had improved 5-yr bRFS (from 62% without ADT to 80% with ADT, *p* < .0001). No difference in the rates of GU toxicity or sexual disorders between the two arms (all ≤8%).

Is there a hypofractionated regimen that can be considered when delivering salvage radiotherapy?

A University of Wisconsin study (Kruser et al.) evaluated 108 pts treated with salvage RT to 65 Gy/26 fractions of 2.5 Gy/fx. The 4-yr bRFS was 67% and authors concluded that "hypofractionation may provide a convenient, resource-efficient, and well-tolerated salvage approach."[32] Additionally, the German PRIAMOS trial utilized 54 Gy/18 fx to the prostate bed; toxicity outcomes were favorable, although at early follow-up.[33] Gladwish et al. (Toronto) published their phase I/II toxicity results using 51 Gy/17 fx.[34] These two trials each included 40 or fewer pts and oncologic outcomes are pending.

When should salvage ADT be initiated in the post-RP or post-EBRT setting?

Duchesne, TOAD (*Lancet Oncol* 2016, PMID 27155740): PRT from Australia, NZ, and Canada. Randomized 293 men with either PSA relapse (N = 261) or de novo incurable disease (N = 32) to immediate ADT (within 8 weeks of randomization) or delayed ADT (recommended to start ADT ≥2 yrs after randomization unless clinically indicated). Included men who received either RP, EBRT, or salvage RT following RP. For post-EBRT pts, investigators initially used the ASTRO definition but then transitioned to the Phoenix definition later in the study. Pts post-RP required a PSA ≥0.2 ng/mL. Excluded pts with overt metastases, those who received ≥12 mos of ADT as part of up-front tx or any pt whose time from completing up-front ADT was ≤12 mos. MFU 5 yrs. The 5-yr OS improved from 86% with delayed ADT to 91% with immediate ADT ($p = .047$). After Cox regression, the unadjusted HR for OS for immediate versus delayed ADT was 0.55, $p = .05$. Median time to starting ADT in the delayed arm was 18 mos, shorter than the prespecified 2-yr time frame because of clinical progression in 58%. **Conclusion: Immediate ADT improves OS compared with delayed initiation.** *Comment: The survival curves did not begin to separate until 5 yrs. Note that the curves were significant when all pts were included (both post-op and incurable pts) but not when limited to the post-op group alone.*

How should we treat pts who have lymph node–positive disease following prostatectomy?

There are no randomized radiation trials evaluating post-operative radiotherapy for LN+ prostate cancer. Classic studies are the Messing trial and the Briganti matched pair analysis.

Messing (*NEJM* 1999, PMID 10588962; Update Messing *Lancet Oncol* 2006, PMID 16750497): Multi-institution PRT of 98 men with pT1b-T2 prostate cancer s/p RP found to have LN+ disease randomized to immediate versus delayed ADT. Arm 1: Immediate ADT, either 3.6 mg goserelin monthly or bilateral orchiectomy (at pt discretion). Arm 2: ADT delayed until disease progression. MFU 11.9 yrs. Immediate ADT improved OS (HR 1.84, $p = .04$), PCSS (HR 4.09, $p = .0004$), and PFS (3.42 $p < .0001$). 79% of those in arm 2 entered an active treatment by 5 yrs. **Conclusion: Immediate post-operative ADT improves OS for LN+ prostate cancer.** *Comment: Study conducted in the pre-PSA era and PSA was not used to guide decision making (e.g., only clinically palpable nodules were considered local failures); average pretreatment PSA in the delayed ADT arm was 14 ng/mL at time of initiating ADT; Gleason score information was not available from 14 of 36 institutions; an imbalance may exist that accounts for differences in survival.*

Briganti (*Eur Urol* 2011, PMID 21354694): Retrospective matched pair analysis for pT2-4, LN+ prostate cancer comparing ADT + RT versus ADT alone. 703 pts matched for age, T stage, Gleason, margin status, number of nodes, follow-up time. MFU 100 months. 10-yr OS 55% versus 74% ($p < .001$) and 10-yr CSS 70% versus 86% ($p = .004$) in favor of ADT+RT. **Conclusion: Adding RT to ADT may improve CSS and OS for LN+ disease.** *Comment: Retrospective; lack of standardized RT dose and length of ADT; PSA data at time of RT not available.*

Is there a way by which to risk-stratify pts who are found to have LN+ disease following prostatectomy?

Abdollah et al. examined the role of adjuvant RT in treating pts with pN1 prostate cancer in their 2014 publication.[35] They evaluated over 1,100 pts with pN1 prostate cancer who had undergone RP and PLND between 1988 and 2010 treated with ADT with or without RT. Investigators found four variables that could be used to stratify pts according to PCM risk including number of involved LNs, pathologic GS, tumor stage, and margin status. Combined ADT and RT was associated with greatest benefit in pts with either (a) ≤2 +LNs, GS 7-10, pT3b/pT4 disease, or +margins (HR 0.30, $p = .002$) or (b) 3 to 4 +LNs (HR 0.21, $p = .02$). These results were confirmed when OS was examined as an endpoint.

Are there any significant differences between open and robotic prostatectomy?

In a series of over 20,000 men who underwent prostatectomy between 2000 and 2011, the overall rates of positive surgical margins were approximately 18% overall with no SS difference. Lower volume centers were shown to have increased risk of positive margin, reflecting the importance of the experience of the center and the surgeon.[36] Two large observational studies suggested that a minimally invasive approach reduced length of stay and decreased complications. The Trinh series from Henry Ford found that pts undergoing robotic surgery were less likely to receive a blood transfusion (OR 0.34), less likely to experience an intra-op (OR 0.47) or post-op (OR 0.86) complication, and less likely to require a prolonged length of stay (defined as >2 days, OR 0.28).[37] A SEER study found that robotic prostatectomy was associated with increased rate of GU complications (4.7% vs. 2.1%), incontinence (15.9% vs. 12.2% per 100 person-yrs), and erectile dysfunction (27% vs. 19% per 100 person-yrs).[38] However, single-institution series from academic centers suggest that both approaches result in similar lengths of stay without differences in post discharge recovery.[39] A Medicare claims study showed that ~30% have incontinence following surgery, and ~90% have sexual dysfunction regardless of the type of surgery performed. In the United States, up to 85% of prostatectomies are now being performed robotically.[4] A randomized trial out of Australia comparing robotic to open prostatectomy reported on 6- and 12-week results and found urinary and sexual functions were similar between groups.[40] Caveats of this study include the relatively small number of pts (n = 326) and short follow-up time.

REFERENCES

1. Kalbasi A, Swisher-McClure S, Mitra N, et al. Low rates of adjuvant radiation in patients with nonmetastatic prostate cancer with high-risk pathologic features. *Cancer*. 2014;120:3089–3096.
2. Prostate Cancer, NCCN Clinical Practice Guidelines in Oncology. 2016. https://www.nccn.org/professionals/physician_gls/pdf/prostate.pdf
3. Boorjian SA, Karnes RJ, Rangel LJ, et al. Mayo Clinic validation of the D'amico risk group classification for predicting survival following radical prostatectomy. *J Urol*. 2008;179:1354–1360; discussion 1360–1361.
4. Barry MJ, Gallagher PM, Skinner JS, et al. Adverse effects of robotic-assisted laparoscopic versus open retropubic radical prostatectomy among a nationwide random sample of Medicare-age men. *J Clin Oncol*. 2012;30:513–518.
5. Dotan ZA, Bianco FJ Jr., Rabbani F, et al. Pattern of prostate-specific antigen (PSA) failure dictates the probability of a positive bone scan in patients with an increasing PSA after radical prostatectomy. *J Clin Oncol*. 2005;23:1962–1968.
6. Beresford MJ, Gillatt D, Benson RJ, et al. A systematic review of the role of imaging before salvage radiotherapy for post-prostatectomy biochemical recurrence. *Clin Oncol (R Coll Radiol)*. 2010;22:46–55.
7. Brush JP. Positron emission tomography in urological malignancy. *Curr Opin Urol*. 2001;11:175–179.
8. Crawford ED, Stone NN, Yu EY, et al. Challenges and recommendations for early identification of metastatic disease in prostate cancer. *Urology*. 2014;83:664–669.
9. Sella T, Schwartz LH, Swindle PW, et al. Suspected local recurrence after radical prostatectomy: endorectal coil MR imaging. *Radiology*. 2004;231:379–385.
10. Silverman JM, Krebs TL. MR imaging evaluation with a transrectal surface coil of local recurrence of prostatic cancer in men who have undergone radical prostatectomy. *AJR Am J Roentgenol*. 1997;168:379–385.
11. Miralbell R, Vees H, Lozano J, et al. Endorectal MRI assessment of local relapse after surgery for prostate cancer: a model to define treatment field guidelines for adjuvant radiotherapy in patients at high risk for local failure. *Int J Radiat Oncol Biol Phys*. 2007;67:356–361.
12. Tendulkar R, Stephans K. Contemporary external beam radiotherapy. In Klein EA, Jones JS, eds. *Management of Prostate Cancer*. 3rd ed. New York, NY: Humana Press; 2012:243–261.

13. Stephenson AJ, Scardino PT, Kattan MW, et al. Predicting the outcome of salvage radiation therapy for recurrent prostate cancer after radical prostatectomy. *J Clin Oncol.* 2007;25:2035–2041.

14. Connolly JA, Shinohara K, Presti JC, Jr., et al. Local recurrence after radical prostatectomy: characteristics in size, location, and relationship to prostate-specific antigen and surgical margins. *Urology.* 1996;47:225–231.

15. Freedland SJ, Humphreys EB, Mangold LA, et al. Risk of prostate cancer-specific mortality following biochemical recurrence after radical prostatectomy. *JAMA.* 2005;294:433–439.

16. Pound CR, Partin AW, Eisenberger MA, et al. Natural history of progression after PSA elevation following radical prostatectomy. *JAMA.* 1999;281:1591–1597.

17. Edge SB, Byrd DR, Compton CC, et al., eds. *AJCC Cancer Staging Manual.* 7th ed. New York, NY: Springer Publishing; 2010.

18. Lance RS, Freidrichs PA, Kane C, et al. A comparison of radical retropubic with perineal prostatectomy for localized prostate cancer within the Uniformed Services Urology Research Group. *BJU Int.* 2001;87:61–65.

19. Iczkowski KA, Lucia MS. Frequency of positive surgical margin at prostatectomy and its effect on patient outcome. *Prostate Cancer.* 2011;2011:1–12.

20. Cookson MS, Aus G, Burnett AL, et al. Variation in the definition of biochemical recurrence in patients treated for localized prostate cancer: the American Urological Association Prostate Guidelines for Localized Prostate Cancer Update Panel report and recommendations for a standard in the reporting of surgical outcomes. *J Urol.* 2007;177:540–545.

21. Soloway M, Roach M, 3rd. Prostate cancer progression after therapy of primary curative intent: a review of data from prostate-specific antigen era. *Cancer.* 2005;104:2310–2322.

22. Martis G, Diana M, Ombres M, et al. Retropubic versus perineal radical prostatectomy in early prostate cancer: eight-year experience. *J Surg Oncol.* 2007;95:513–518.

23. Alibhai SM, Leach M, Tomlinson G, et al. 30-day mortality and major complications after radical prostatectomy: influence of age and comorbidity. *J Natl Cancer Inst.* 2005;97:1525–1532.

24. Stanford JL, Feng Z, Hamilton AS, et al. Urinary and sexual function after radical prostatectomy for clinically localized prostate cancer: the Prostate Cancer Outcomes Study. *JAMA.* 2000;283:354–360.

25. Resnick MJ, Koyama T, Fan KH, et al. Long-term functional outcomes after treatment for localized prostate cancer. *N Engl J Med.* 368:436–445.

26. Sanda MG, Dunn RL, Michalski J, et al. Quality of life and satisfaction with outcome among prostate-cancer survivors. *N Engl J Med.* 2008;358:1250–1261.

27. Donovan JL, Hamdy FC, Lane JA, et al. Patient-reported outcomes after monitoring, surgery, or radiotherapy for prostate cancer. *N Engl J Med.* 2016;375(15):1425–1437.

28. Han M, Partin AW, Zahurak M, et al. Biochemical (prostate specific antigen) recurrence probability following radical prostatectomy for clinically localized prostate cancer. *J Urol.* 2003;169:517–523.

29. Nguyen CT, Reuther AM, Stephenson AJ, et al. The specific definition of high risk prostate cancer has minimal impact on biochemical relapse-free survival. *J Urol.* 2009;181:75–80.

30. Hagan M, Zlotecki R, Medina C, et al. Comparison of adjuvant versus salvage radiotherapy policies for postprostatectomy radiotherapy. *Int J Radiat Oncol Biol Phys.* 2004;59:329–340.

31. King CR. The timing of salvage radiotherapy after radical prostatectomy: a systematic review. *Int J Radiat Oncol Biol Phys.* 2012;84:104–111.

32. Kruser TJ, Jarrard DF, Graf AK, et al. Early hypofractionated salvage radiotherapy for postprostatectomy biochemical recurrence. *Cancer.* 117:2629–2636.

33. Katayama S, Striecker T, Kessel K, et al. Hypofractionated IMRT of the prostate bed after radical prostatectomy: acute toxicity in the PRIAMOS-1 trial. *Int J Radiat Oncol Biol Phys.* 2014;90:926–933.

34. Gladwish A, Loblaw A, Cheung P, et al. Accelerated hypofractioned postoperative radiotherapy for prostate cancer: a prospective phase I/II study. *Clin Oncol (R Coll Radiol).* 2015;27:145–152.

35. Abdollah F, Karnes RJ, Suardi N, et al. Impact of adjuvant radiotherapy on survival of patients with node-positive prostate cancer. *J Clin Oncol.* 2014;32:3939–3947.

36. Sooriakumaran P, Srivastava A, Shariat SF, et al. A multinational, multi-institutional study comparing positive surgical margin rates among 22,393 open, laparoscopic, and robot-assisted radical prostatectomy patients. *Eur Urol.* 2014;66:450–456.

37. Trinh QD, Sammon J, Sun M, et al. Perioperative outcomes of robot-assisted radical prostatectomy compared with open radical prostatectomy: results from the nationwide inpatient sample. *Eur Urol*. 2014;61:679–685.
38. Chamie K, Williams SB, Hu JC. Population-based assessment of determining treatments for prostate cancer. *JAMA Oncol*. 2015;1:60–167.
39. Wood DP, Schulte R, Dunn RL, et al. Short-term health outcome differences between robotic and conventional radical prostatectomy. *Urology*. 2007;70:945–949.
40. Yaxley JW, Coughlin GD, Chambers SK, et al. Robot-assisted laparoscopic prostatectomy versus open radical retropubic prostatectomy: early outcomes from a randomised controlled phase 3 study. *Lancet*. 2016;388:1057–1066.

39: BLADDER CANCER

Michael A. Weller, Camille A. Berriochoa, and Rahul D. Tendulkar

QUICK HIT: Bladder cancer is the second most common GU malignancy, and >90% are urothelial carcinomas. About 70% have superficial disease and are managed with TURBT +/- intravesical therapy. Pts with muscle-invasive bladder cancer (MIBC) are most often managed with radical cystectomy and perioperative CHT. Selective bladder preservation (SBP) may be utilized in certain pts. Up to 80% achieve a CR to induction chemoRT, and 70% to 80% will remain free of local recurrence and retain their native bladder.

TABLE 39.1: General Treatment Paradigm for Bladder Cancer	
	Treatment Options
Superficial tumors (Ta, Tis, T1)	TURBT followed by surveillance OR intravesical therapy (BCG vs. mitomycin) OR cystectomy (for high risk)
T2-T4a (cystectomy candidates)	Radical cystectomy +/- neoadjuvant cisplatin-based CHT OR SBP: maximal TURBT, then chemoRT 40–45 Gy, then cystoscopy, then if CR* boost to 65 Gy, then surveillance
T2-T4 (inoperable)	ChemoRT (preferred, if CHT candidate) OR RT alone (if not CHT candidate)
Metastatic	CHT (e.g., cisplatin/gemcitabine) + palliative RT as needed

*CR = T0/Tis/Ta; if ≥ T1 on cystoscopy after induction chemoRT, salvage cystectomy.

Candidates for selective bladder preservation: Unifocal tumor <5 cm after complete TURBT, cT2-T3 (and selected T4a), cN0, adequate bladder function, compliant with surveillance protocol, no hydronephrosis, no associated CIS, no IBD, no prior RT.

EPIDEMIOLOGY: In 2016, ~77,000 new cases (80% male), ~16,000 deaths.[1] Median age 70 years.[2] Highest rates in North America/western Europe.[3] Incidence in white males roughly double that of African American or latino populations.

RISK FACTORS: Majority of cases are related to environmental exposures. Smoking is the most important with RR of 2 to 5 compared with nonsmokers and is associated with about 50% of cases. Others include chemical exposures (industrial aromatic amines, polycyclic aromatic hydrocarbons, hair dyes, chlorinated water, arsenic), drugs (phenacetin-containing analgesics, cyclophosphamide), schistosomiasis (associated with squamous cell carcinoma), chronic inflammation (chronic UTIs, cystitis, stones), radiation exposure.[3]

ANATOMY: The bladder can be divided into the body (above the ureteral orifices), the trigone (area between the ureteral and urethral orifices), and bladder neck. Layers from internal to external: urothelium (epithelial lining made up of transitional cells bounded by a thin basement membrane), lamina propria (thick layer of fibroelastic connective tissue), and detrusor muscle (smooth muscle arranges in inner longitudinal, middle circular, and outer longitudinal layers). The bladder is anchored to anterior abdominal wall by the urachus. It is bounded superiorly by peritoneum, and anteriorly/inferiorly/laterally by perivesical fat. Primary lymph nodes include external iliac, internal iliac, obturator, perivesical, and presacral nodes. The common iliacs are a secondary drainage site.[4]

PATHOLOGY: Urothelial carcinoma (>90% of cases in the United States), squamous cell carcinoma (~3%), adenocarcinoma (~2%), small cell carcinoma (~1%), all others <1% (sarcomas, lymphomas, melanoma, mets). In schistosoma haematobium endemic areas, squamous cell carcinomas comprise the majority of cases. Urachal tumors are commonly adenocarcinomas, and have better outcomes than nonurachal adenocarcinoma.

CLINICAL PRESENTATION: Gross or microscopic hematuria most common presenting symptoms. If gross hematuria, risk of a bladder tumor is 10% to 20%. Less commonly, pts may note obstructive/irritative bladder symptoms or pain.

WORKUP: H&P

Labs: Urine cytology. Cytology has poor sensitivity (34%) but high specificity (>98%).[5] CBC, CMP, alk phos.

Procedures: Cystoscopy. If a suspicious lesion is noted in the bladder, proceed to TURBT. TURBT is diagnostic and often therapeutic for T1 disease. Random or targeted biopsies of sites adjacent to tumor are performed to assess for field defect/CIS, as well as biopsy of the prostate. Biopsy specimen should include muscle to assess for invasion.

Imaging: If cystoscopic appearance of the tumor is solid, high grade, or MIBC, consider CT or MRI of abdomen and pelvis prior to TURBT. The entire urinary tract should be imaged (e.g., CT urogram with and without contrast including delayed images or MRI urogram). Obtain chest imaging if muscle invasive. Bone scan if alk phos elevated or bone pain. No role for PET/CT.

PROGNOSTIC FACTORS

Stage, grade, multicentricity, size, recurrence, presence of CIS, LVI, growth pattern (micropapillary and nested variants are worse).

STAGING

TABLE 39.2: AJCC 8th ed. (2017) Staging for Urinary Bladder Cancer						
T/M		**N**	**cN0**	**cN1**	**cN2**	**cN3**
T1	• Invades lamina propria (subepithelial connective tissue)	I				
T2	a Invades muscularis propria (inner half)	II				
	b Invades muscularis propria (outer half)			IIIA	IIIB	
T3	a Invades perivesical tissue (microscopic)					
	b Invades perivesical tissue (macroscopic)					
T4	a Invades prostatic stroma, seminal vesicles, uterus, vagina					
	b Invades pelvic wall or abdominal wall			IVA		
M1a	Non-regional LNs					
M1b	Distant metastasis			IVB		
Updates from the AJCC 7th Edition include subdivision of M1, stage III and stage IV. cN1, single pelvic node (true pelvis, perivesicular, obturator, internal iliac, external iliac, or sacral); cN2, multiple LNs in the true pelvis; cN3, common iliac LNs.						

TREATMENT PARADIGM

Surgery

TURBT: First step in diagnosis, therapeutic for Ta/Tis/T1 non-muscle-invasive disease. Observation can be considered after TURBT in select pts with Ta or low-grade T1 disease without risk factors. Adjuvant intravesical therapy recommended for Tis, high-grade Ta or T1, positive cytology, recurrent disease, or multifocality. TURBT for maximal debulking is the initial therapy in SBP for MIBC.

Cystectomy: Radical cystectomy with urinary diversion is a standard of care for multiply recurrent superficial tumors, high-grade T1 tumors with CIS, and MIBC, as well as variant histologies. The technique includes en bloc resection of bladder, peritoneal covering, urachus, perivesical fat, lower ureters, bilateral pelvic LNs, proximal urethra (men), entire urethra (all women, and men with CIS/multicentric tumors/involvement of bladder neck or prostatic urethra), prostate, seminal vesicles, pelvic vas deferens (men), uterus, fallopian tubes, ovaries, cervix, vaginal cuff (women). Per NCCN, bilateral pelvic lymphadenectomy should be performed and include at a minimum the obturator, external iliac, internal iliac, and common iliac lymph nodes.[6] SWOG 8710 demonstrated improved survival when at least 10 LNs were removed[7]. A 2016 ASCO guideline stated that the standard treatment for cT2-T4a bladder cancer is neoadjuvant cisplatin-based combination CHT followed by radical cystectomy, reserving chemoRT as an alternative in appropriately selected pts and in pts for whom cystectomy is not an option.[8]

Urinary diversions: Diversion may be either noncontinent or continent. Historically, noncontinent diversions were standard (e.g., ileal conduit). Advances in technique resulted in continent diversion for most pts in the modern era. Broadly, these techniques are categorized as continent cutaneous diversions (e.g., Kock, Indiana, Miami pouches) that require self-catheterization or (more commonly) orthotopic neobladders that connect directly to the native urethra using the external sphincter for continence.

Intravesical therapy: Allows for high concentrations of agents to be delivered locally in an effort to eradicate viable tumor and prevent recurrences. Bacillus Calmette-Guerin (BCG) is a live attenuated mycobacterium bovis that functions as immunotherapy, and is considered the adjuvant treatment of choice for high-grade Ta, Tis, or T1 tumors after TURBT. BCG is initiated 3 to 4 weeks after resection, and given weekly for 6 weeks. Meta-analyses have shown BCG to be superior to mitomycin C in Tis[9] as well as Ta and T1 disease.[10] Common toxicities of BCG include urinary frequency (71%), cystitis (67%), fever (25%), and hematuria (23%).[10] Note that the frequency and dysuria associated with BCG treatment can be severe and that many pts do not complete the full 6-week course due to acute toxicity.

Chemotherapy: Can be used perioperatively before or after cystectomy, concurrent with RT as part of bladder preservation therapy, or in the metastatic setting. Evidence is stronger for neoadjuvant CHT rather than for adjuvant—a meta-analysis demonstrated a 5% survival benefit with neoadjuvant platinum-based CHT compared to surgery alone.[11]

Perioperative: Cisplatin-based regimens including dose-dense methotrexate, vinblastine, doxorubicin, and cisplatin (DD-MVAC), gemcitabine/cisplatin, and methotrexate, cisplatin, and vinblastine (MCV). The different regimens have not been directly compared in randomized trials.

Concurrent with RT: Typically a cisplatin doublet. NCCN considers options to be: cisplatin 15 mg/m^2 days 1–3, 8–10, 15–17 and paclitaxel 50 mg/m^2 on days 1, 8, and 15; cisplatin 15 mg/m^2 days 1–3, 8–10, 15–17 and 5-FU 400 mg/m^2 days 1–3, 8–10, and 15–17; or 5-FU 500 mg/m^2 days 1–5 and 16–20 and mitomycin C 12 mg/m^2 day 1.

Metastatic: Category 1 evidence exists for gemcitabine/cisplatin or DD-MVAC.

Radiation

Indications: RT may be given for organ preservation as an alternative to cystectomy (SBP), as definitive management in pts who are not candidates for and/or refuse cystectomy, or for palliation. The role for adjuvant RT after cystectomy is evolving but may be considered for select cases of pT3-4, positive margins, or ECE (54–60 Gy to positive margin with tumor bed and pelvic nodes to 45–50.4 Gy, see adjuvant guidelines[12]).

Selective bladder preservation: Candidates include those with a unifocal tumor <5 cm after complete TURBT, cT2-T3 (and selected T4a), cN0, adequate bladder function, compliant with surveillance protocol, no hydronephrosis, no associated CIS, no IBD, and no prior pelvic RT.

Schema: Maximal TURBT → chemoRT 40 to 45 Gy → cystoscopy → if CR (T0/Tis/Ta) boost to ~64 Gy → surveillance. If ≥T1 on cystoscopy after induction chemoRT, proceed to salvage cystectomy.

Dose: Multiple regimens have been used, typically treating the pelvis to 40–45 Gy followed by a boost to ~64 Gy at 1.8–2.0 Gy/fraction. If treating definitively with chemoRT (e.g., not a cystectomy candidate) no break for cystoscopy is required. An alternative fractionation is 55 Gy/20 fx as per BC2001.[13] Elective nodal irradiation was typically utilized in RTOG trials, but not in BC2001 (see the following). For clinical node-positive disease, consider boosting the involved node up to 64 Gy if safely achievable.

Toxicity: Acute: fatigue, nausea, diarrhea, urinary urgency, frequency. Late: cystitis, fibrosis, proctitis, enteritis.

Procedure: See *Treatment Planning Handbook,* Chapter 8.[14]

EVIDENCE-BASED Q&A

What is the rationale for SBP?

Strategies to preserve the native bladder and avoid the potential complications of radical cystectomy and urinary diversion are appealing, particularly for those who are elderly or with significant comorbidities. A series of phase II trials were conducted by the RTOG in the 1980s and 1990s.[15–21] Pooled analysis of these trials demonstrated low rates of toxicity with survival outcomes similar to historical cystectomy series for clinically staged pts.[22] There have been no randomized trials comparing SBP with radical cystectomy. Of note, clinical understaging is very common; therefore, caution must be taken when comparing retrospective series of SBP versus cystectomy.

Mak, RTOG pooled analysis (*JCO* 2014, PMID 25366678): Pooled analysis of five RTOG prospective phase II trials. 468 pts, clinical T2 (61%), T3 (35%), T4 (4%). MFU 4.3 years among all pts, 7.8 years among survivors. Following chemoRT, CR was observed in 69% of pts. 5-yr OS associated with T stage: 62% for T2 versus 49% for T3-4 ($p = .002$). **Conclusion: Long-term DSS is comparable to cystectomy series and can be considered as an alternative to surgery.**

TABLE 39.3: RTOG Pooled Analysis of Selective Bladder Trials					
	OS	DSS	Muscle-invasive LF	Non-muscle-invasive LF	DM
5 years	57%	71%	13%	31%	31%
10 years	36%	65%	14%	36%	35%

Are the rates of toxicity after selective bladder preservation prohibitive?

Although survival rates are comparable to cystectomy, there is concern regarding late effects. RTOG pooled analysis suggests high-grade toxicity is uncommon.

Efstathiou, RTOG pooled analysis (*JCO* 2009, PMID 19636019): 285 pts from four RTOG trials. MFU of 5.4 years. The late grade ≥3 toxicity rates were 5.7% GU and 1.9% GI. No late grade 4 events, and no pts required a cystectomy due to treatment-related toxicity. **Conclusion: Late effects do not appear prohibitive after SBP.**

Is there a benefit to neoadjuvant CHT prior to SBP?

Neoadjuvant CHT improves survival when delivered prior to radical cystectomy.[11] RTOG 8903 tested this concept in the SBP setting, but both this trial and other retrospective series[23] showed no benefit to neoadjuvant CHT prior to definitive chemoRT.

Shipley, RTOG 8903 (*JCO* 1998, PMID 9817278): PRT to assess the addition of neoadjuvant CHT to SBP. 123 pts with cT2-4a MIBC received TURBT and then were randomized to +/− 2 cycles of neoadjuvant MCV (methotrexate, cisplatin, vinblastine). All pts were treated to a dose of 39.6 Gy at 1.8 Gy/fx to pelvic field with cisplatin, then underwent cystoscopy at 4 weeks. If <CR, pts proceeded to cystectomy. If CR, pts received a 25.2 Gy tumor boost with cisplatin. MFU 5 years. No difference in CR rate (61% vs. 55%), 5-yr OS (48% vs. 49%), DM (33% vs. 39%), or survival with intact bladder (36% vs. 40%). **Conclusion: Neoadjuvant CHT prior to SBP increased toxicity without improving outcomes.**

Does the addition of CHT to RT improve outcomes with definitive (nonoperative) management?

Local recurrence rates with RT alone are high, and early data suggested a benefit to concurrent CHT.[24] This led to the UK Bladder Cancer 2001 (BC2001) trial.

James, BC2001 (*NEJM* 2012, PMID 22512481): PRT of 360 pts with T2-T4a bladder cancer (adenocarcinoma, TCC, and SCC included). Allowed but did not require neoadjuvant CHT. Randomized to RT alone versus RT and concurrent CHT with 5-FU 500 mg/m² days 1–5 and 16–20 and mitomycin C 12 mg/m² on day 1. RT either 55 Gy/20 fx or 64 Gy/32 fx, and the pelvic nodes were not electively targeted. Of note, mid-treatment cystoscopy was not performed on this protocol; as a result, all patients were treated definitively. Primary endpoint was LRFS. **Conclusion: The addition of 5-FU/mitomycin C to RT improves LRFS over RT alone, with a trend toward improved OS (but not powered for OS).**

TABLE 39.4: UK BC2001 Trial of Definitive RT for Bladder Cancer					
BC2001	2-yr LRFS	Invasive LR	Non-invasive LR	2-yr Cystectomy	5-yr OS
RT	54%	19%	17%	17%	35%
ChemoRT	67%	11%	14%	11%	48%
p value	.03	.01		.07	.16

Do target volumes need to include the entire bladder? Is there a benefit to elective nodal irradiation?

Given the difficulties with tumor localization as well as the propensity for multifocality of bladder cancer, standard RT techniques included the entire bladder in the target volume, even in localized disease. However, sparing the uninvolved bladder could potentially reduce toxicity, leading to interest in partial bladder-sparing techniques, which was assessed by the BC2001 trial. Most

RTOG trials incorporate elective nodal irradiation using a "mini-pelvis" field, with the superior border at S2-S3 to allow sparing of bowel in the potential future event of a urinary diversion. BC2001 did not intentionally target elective nodes, but did include the low pelvis/obturator nodes given the field design of whole bladder + 1.5 cm margin. Only 10 of 76 locoregional recurrences were in the pelvic nodes.

Huddart, BC2001 (*IJROBP* 2013, PMID 23958147): 219 pts (subset of BC2001) randomized to standard whole bladder RT (PTV included outer bladder wall plus extravesical extent of tumor + 1.5 cm) versus reduced high-dose volume RT (2 PTVs defined: PTV1 was the same as the control group and was treated to 80% of the prescribed dose, and PTV2 was defined as GTV + 1.5 cm). Pts were simulated with bladder empty. No difference in 2-yr LRFS (61% vs. 64%), grade 3–4 acute toxicity (23% vs. 23%), 2-yr grade 3–4 late toxicity (2.4% vs. 5.4%), or reduction in bladder capacity (76 mL difference in reduction favoring the reduced volume group was not statistically significant). **Conclusion: No differences in 2-year LRFS or late toxicity with reduced high-dose volume RT.**

Is there a benefit to hyperfractionation?

Evidence for hyperfractionation is mixed, as two older PRTs showed improved outcomes with hyperfractionation over standard fractionation, while a more recent PRT demonstrated no benefit and increased toxicity.[25] None of these trials included concurrent CHT, and thus the role of hyperfractionation is unclear in this setting. However, hyperfractionated chemoRT was one of the arms in the completed RTOG 0712 phase II randomized trial and may be considered in select pts.

Is there a benefit to adjuvant RT after cystectomy?

Adjuvant RT after cystectomy is rarely utilized. However, certain patient populations are known to have high rates of local failure (~30% for T3-4, ~70% for positive margins[7]). A randomized trial published in 1992 demonstrated a LC and DFS benefit in pts with T3-T4 disease; however, 80% of the pts on this study had squamous cell carcinoma.[26] A patterns-of-failure analysis showed that in pts with negative margins and >pT3 disease, 76% of all LF sites would have been covered within a small CTV covering only the iliac/obturator nodes, which would limit dose to bowel and neobladder. In pts with positive margins, failure in the cystectomy bed and presacral nodes increases substantially, necessitating larger CTV and the subsequent increase in potential toxicity,[27] leading to consensus contouring guidelines.[12] If treating adjuvantly, a typical regimen would consist of 45–50.4 to the cystectomy bed and a possible boost to positive margin/ECE to 54–60 Gy.[6]

Is there a role for RT in select cases of T1 non-muscle-invasive disease?

TURBT followed by intravesical therapy is the standard of care for most pts with high-grade superficial cancers. However, many will still recur locally after this approach. For recurrent disease, standard therapy is cystectomy. RT may offer a bladder-sparing option for some pts with high-grade T1 or recurrent T1 cancers after BCG. The evidence supporting this approach is mixed, and RTOG 0926 is addressing this question.

REFERENCES

1. Siegel RL, Miller KD, Jemal A. Cancer statistics, 2016. *CA Cancer J Clin.* 2016;66(1):7–30.
2. Scosyrev E, Noyes K, Feng C, Messing E. Sex and racial differences in bladder cancer presentation and mortality in the US. *Cancer.* 2009;115(1):68–74.
3. Pelucchi C, Bosetti C, Negri E, et al. Mechanisms of disease: the epidemiology of bladder cancer. *Nat Clin Pract Urol.* 2006;3(6):327–340.
4. Edge SB, American Joint Committee on Cancer. *AJCC Cancer Staging Manual.* 7th ed. New York, NY: Springer Publishing; 2010.

5. Lotan Y, Roehrborn CG. Sensitivity and specificity of commonly available bladder tumor markers versus cytology: results of a comprehensive literature review and meta-analyses. *Urology*. 2003;61(1):109–118; discussion 118.

6. National Comprehensive Cancer Network. Bladder cancer. Clinical practice guidelines in oncology. *J Natl Compr Canc Netw*. 2017;1:2017.

7. Herr HW, Faulkner JR, Grossman HB, et al. Surgical factors influence bladder cancer outcomes: a cooperative group report. *J Clin Oncol*. 2004;22(14):2781–2789.

8. Milowsky MI, Rumble RB, Booth CM, et al. Guideline on muscle-invasive and metastatic bladder cancer (European Association of Urology Guideline): American Society of Clinical Oncology Clinical Practice Guideline Endorsement. *J Clin Oncol*. 2016;34(16):1945–1952.

9. Sylvester RJ, van der Meijden AP, Witjes JA, Kurth K. Bacillus calmette-guerin versus chemotherapy for the intravesical treatment of patients with carcinoma in situ of the bladder: a meta-analysis of the published results of randomized clinical trials. *J Urol*. 2005;174(1):86–91; discussion 91–82.

10. Shelley MD, Court JB, Kynaston H, et al. Intravesical bacillus calmette-guerin in Ta and T1 bladder cancer. *Cochrane Database Syst Rev*. 2000(4):CD001986.

11. Collaboration ABCM-a. Neoadjuvant chemotherapy in invasive bladder cancer: a systematic review and meta-analysis. *Lancet*. 2003;361(9373):1927–1934.

12. Baumann BC, Bosch WR, Bahl A, et al. Development and validation of consensus contouring guidelines for adjuvant radiation therapy for bladder cancer after radical cystectomy. *Int J Radiat Oncol Biol Phys*. 2016;96(1):78–86.

13. James ND, Hussain SA, Hall E, et al. Radiotherapy with or without chemotherapy in muscle-invasive bladder cancer. *N Engl J Med*. 2012;366(16):1477–1488.

14. Videtic GMM, Woody N, Vassil AD. *Handbook of Treatment Planning in Radiation Oncology*. 2nd ed. New York, NY: Demos Medical; 2015.

15. Shipley WU, Prout GR, Einstein AB, et al. Treatment of invasive bladder cancer by cisplatin and radiation in patients unsuited for surgery. *JAMA*. 1987;258(7):931–935.

16. Kaufman DS, Shipley WU, Griffin PP, et al. Selective bladder preservation by combination treatment of invasive bladder cancer. *N Engl J Med*. 1993;329(19):1377–1382.

17. Tester W, Porter A, Asbell S, et al. Combined modality program with possible organ preservation for invasive bladder carcinoma: results of RTOG protocol 85-12. *Int J Radiat Oncol Biol Phys*. 1993;25(5):783–790.

18. Tester W, Caplan R, Heaney J, et al. Neoadjuvant combined modality program with selective organ preservation for invasive bladder cancer: results of Radiation Therapy Oncology Group phase II trial 8802. *J Clin Oncol*. 1996;14(1):119–126.

19. Kaufman DS, Winter KA, Shipley WU, et al. The initial results in muscle-invading bladder cancer of RTOG 95-06: phase I/II trial of transurethral surgery plus radiation therapy with concurrent cisplatin and 5-fluorouracil followed by selective bladder preservation or cystectomy depending on the initial response. *Oncologist*. 2000;5(6):471–476.

20. Hagan MP, Winter KA, Kaufman DS, et al. RTOG 97-06: initial report of a phase I–II trial of selective bladder conservation using TURBT, twice-daily accelerated irradiation sensitized with cisplatin, and adjuvant MCV combination chemotherapy. *Int J Radiat Oncol Biol Phys*. 2003;57(3):665–672.

21. Kaufman DS, Winter KA, Shipley WU, et al. Phase I–II RTOG study (99-06) of patients with muscle-invasive bladder cancer undergoing transurethral surgery, paclitaxel, cisplatin, and twice-daily radiotherapy followed by selective bladder preservation or radical cystectomy and adjuvant chemotherapy. *Urology*. 2009;73(4):833–837.

22. Stein JP, Lieskovsky G, Cote R, et al. Radical cystectomy in the treatment of invasive bladder cancer: long-term results in 1,054 patients. *J Clin Oncol*. 2001;19(3):666–675.

23. Shipley WU, Kaufman DS, Zehr E, et al. Selective bladder preservation by combined modality protocol treatment: long-term outcomes of 190 patients with invasive bladder cancer. *Urology*. 2002;60(1):62–67; discussion 67–68.

24. Coppin CM, Gospodarowicz MK, James K, et al. Improved local control of invasive bladder cancer by concurrent cisplatin and preoperative or definitive radiation. The National Cancer Institute of Canada Clinical Trials Group. *J Clin Oncol*. 1996;14(11):2901–2907.

25. Horwich A, Dearnaley D, Huddart R, et al. A randomised trial of accelerated radiotherapy for localised invasive bladder cancer. *Radiother Oncol*. 2005;75(1):34–43.
26. Zaghloul MS, Awwad HK, Akoush HH, et al. Postoperative radiotherapy of carcinoma in bilharzial bladder: improved disease free survival through improving local control. *Int J Radiat Oncol Biol Phys*. 1992;23(3):511–517.
27. Baumann BC, Guzzo TJ, He J, et al. Bladder cancer patterns of pelvic failure: implications for adjuvant radiation therapy. *Int J Radiat Oncol Biol Phys*. 2013;85(2):363–369.

40: TESTICULAR CANCER

Ehsan H. Balagamwala and Rahul D. Tendulkar

QUICK HIT: Of testicular tumors, approximately 40% are seminomatous and 60% are nonseminomatous germ cell tumors (NSGCT). 85% of seminomas present as clinical stage I disease. Initial management is inguinal orchiectomy with high ligation of the spermatic cord (not trans-scrotal biopsy). Treatment paradigm for seminomatous testicular cancer is summarized in Table 40.1. For NSGCT, adjuvant therapy after inguinal orchiectomy is nsRPLND, CHT, or surveillance depending on stage.

TABLE 40.1: General Treatment Paradigm for Testicular Seminoma

Seminoma	Initial Treatment	Adjuvant Treatment Options
Stage I	Radical inguinal orchiectomy with high ligation of spermatic cord	Active surveillance: 15%–20% relapse Carboplatin (AUC 7 x1-2c): <5% relapse (TE19 trial) RT (para-aortic strip, 20 Gy/10 fx): <5% relapse (TE10/TE18 trials)
Stage II		Stage IIA: Modified dogleg RT, 20 Gy/10 fx with boost to 30 Gy Stage IIB: CHT preferred. Modified dogleg RT, 20 Gy/10 fx with boost to 36 Gy Stage IIC: EP x4 OR BEP x3 (RT/surgery for salvage)
Stage III		EP x4 OR BEP x3 (RT/surgery for salvage)

EPIDEMIOLOGY: Annually ~8,700 cases with ~380 deaths.[1] Most common solid tumor in men 15 to 34 years of age, and accounts for 1% of all male cancers. Up to 5% are bilateral (synchronous or metachronous). 10-year survival >95%. Two broad categories are recognized: seminomas, which present at 30 to 40 years of age, and NSGCTs, which present at 20 to 30 years of age. Worldwide incidence has more than doubled in the past four decades. Lymphoma is the most common testicular tumor in men over 60.[1,2]

RISK FACTORS: Abdominal cryptorchid testes have 1/20 (5%) risk of cancer and must be resected. Inguinal cryptorchid testes have 1/80 risk of cancer and should undergo orchiopexy before puberty. 20% of GCTs in patients with history of cryptorchidism occur in the contralateral, normally descended testicle. Intratubular germ cell neoplasia of unclassified type (ITGCNU) have 50% risk of progression to invasive malignancy at 5 years.[3] Other risk factors include hypospadias, androgen insensitivity syndrome, gonadal dysgenesis, previous contralateral testicular cancer,[4] extragonadal GCT, family history, white race, HIV.

ANATOMY: Layers (from external to internal): skin, dartos fascia, external spermatic fascia, cremasteric fascia, internal spermatic fascia, parietal layer of tunica vaginalis, visceral layer of tunica vaginalis, and tunica albuginea. Seminiferous tubules merge to form the rete testis. Testicular arteries arise directly from abdominal aorta. Right testicular vein joins IVC inferior to right renal vein; left testicular vein joins left renal vein. Lymphatic drainage is from rete testes via spermatic cord along testicular veins to retroperitoneal/

para-aortic LNs at vertebral levels T11-L4, then via cisterna chyli and thoracic duct to posterior mediastinum, left SCV, and axilla. Inguinal nodes are not involved in testicular cancer unless the scrotum is surgically disrupted (usually by trans-scrotal biopsy, hernia repair, vasectomy, etc.).

PATHOLOGY[5]: Majority (95%) of testicular cancers are GCTs: seminomas (40%), NSGCTs (60%). Minority (5%) are non-GCTs: Leydig cell, Sertoli cell, rhabdomyosarcoma, lymphoma. Seminomas include classic (85%), anaplastic (10%), or spermatocytic (5%), which are all treated the same. Anaplastic has high mitotic activity, but does not have a worse outcome. Spermatocytic type occurs in older men (age >50) and has a favorable prognosis. Pure seminomas with syncytiotrophoblastic cells (still considered pure) may have elevated β-HCG in 10% to 15%. NSGCTs include embryonal, teratoma, choriocarcinoma, yolk sac (endodermal sinus tumors), and mixed tumors. CIS precedes invasive GCTs by 3 to 5 years and is found adjacent to invasive tumor in nearly 100% (except spermatocytic seminoma and infant tumors). AFP never elevated in pure seminoma but β-HCG may be elevated in 10% to 15% of seminomas with syncytiotrophoblastic cells. AFP can also be elevated in hepatocellular carcinoma and liver disease. β-HCG is very high with choriocarcinoma, can also be elevated with high luteinizing hormone, GI, GU, lung and breast cancers. LDH is nonspecific and can be elevated in about half of germ cell tumors.

TABLE 40.2: Characteristics of Testicular Histologies

GCT Histology	Age	Characteristics	% with AFP Elevation	% with β-hCG Elevation
Seminoma (40%)	30–40	Radiosensitive; 80% local at presentation; lymphatic spread; relapse occurs later	0%	9%
NSGCTs (60%)	20–30	Radioresistant; 70% distant at presentation; often hematogenous spread; relapse occurs earlier	50%	60%
• **Embryonal**	25–35	Most common pure NSGCT; more aggressive, >60% DM (lung, liver) at presentation	70%	60%
• **Teratoma**	25–35	Second most common NSGCT; multiple germ layers; mature vs. immature; >75% NSGCTs have teratoma component	38%	25%
• **Choriocarcinoma**	20–30	Rare; very high hCG (gynecomastia), AFP always normal; most aggressive; spreads hematogenously; may hemorrhage	0%	100%
• **Yolk sac**	<10	Most common pediatric GCT, 80% <2 y/o; in adults, presents in mediastinum and is chemoresistant; Schiller–Duval bodies	75%	25%

CLINICAL PRESENTATION: Classically painless testicular mass. Minority will have a dull ache (acute pain in 10%), swelling, heavy sensation in lower abdomen or perianal area, or fullness of scrotum. Infertility seen in 50%. Gynecomastia secondary to estrogenic effect of hCG in 5%. Distant metastasis causes presenting symptoms in 10%.

DIFFERENTIAL DIAGNOSIS: Testicular cancer, testicular torsion, epididymitis, hydrocele, varicocele, hernia, hematoma, or spermatocele.

WORKUP: H&P with bimanual exam of scrotal contents. A firm or fixed mass is cancer until proven otherwise. Palpate abdomen for nodal disease or visceral involvement, SCV nodes and examine chest for gynecomastia. Bilateral scrotal color Doppler ultrasound demonstrates a hypoechoic mass; seminomas are well defined without cystic areas while NSGCTs are inhomogeneous with calcifications, cystic areas, and indistinct margins. Ultrasound insufficient for staging; surgery required for staging (accuracy 44% of seminomas and 8% in NSGCTs).[6]

Labs: CBC, CMP, serum tumor markers (AFP, β-hCG, LDH).

Imaging: CXR, CT abdomen/pelvis (add CT chest if suspicious). PET is of limited utility for workup; may be more useful for seminoma than NSGCTs and alters staging in 10%.[7] Brain imaging if symptomatic, significant lung metastases, or with high β-hCG. Offer semen analysis/sperm banking prior to treatment.

Other: Trans-scrotal biopsy or orchiectomy is absolutely contraindicated because of risk of tumor seeding into the scrotal sac, lymphatic disruption, or metastatic spread of tumor into the inguinal lymph nodes. Retroperitoneal LN dissection (RPLND) for select patients with NSGCT. Repeat the serum tumor markers (AFP, β-hCG, and LDH) since S stage in the AJCC system is based on postorchiectomy values. The half-life of β-HCG is 24 to 36 hours and of AFP is 5 to 7 days.[8]

PROGNOSTIC FACTORS

Seminoma: stage, nonpulmonary visceral mets (NPVM).

NSGCT: LVI, NPVM, S3, mediastinal primary, embryonal predominant.[9]

NATURAL HISTORY: Risk for relapse after orchiectomy approximately 12.2% for stage I seminoma with size <3 cm and 20.3% with size ≥3 cm. However, for patients who did not relapse in the first 2 years, their risk for relapse in the next 5 years was 3.9% and 5.6%, respectively.[10] 90% of nodal relapses on surveillance occur in the para-aortic lymph nodes ("landing zone") and 10% also have positive pelvic LN.[11] Nodal crossover may occur from right to left (~15%), but rarely from left to right. Late distant relapses are possible.

STAGING

TABLE 40.3: AJCC 8th ed. (2017) Staging for Testicular Cancer						
pT		**cN**		**pN**		**M**
Tis	• Carcinoma in situ	N1	• Regional LNs ≤2 cm	N1	• Regional LN ≤2 cm • ≤5 LNs positive	M1a	• Non-retroperitoneal LNs • Pulmonary metastasis
T1	a Limited to testis/epididymis[1], no LVSI, <3 cm	N2	• Regional LN >2 cm and ≤5 cm	N2	• Regional LN >2 cm and ≤5 cm • >5 regional LNs, ≤5 cm and no ECE	M1b	• Non-pulmonary visceral metastasis
	b Limited to testis/epididymis, no LVSI, ≥3 cm						
T2	• Limited to testis with LVSI • Involves[2]	N3	• Regional LNs >5 cm	N3	• Regional LN >5 cm		

(continued)

TABLE 40.3: AJCC 8th ed. (2017) Staging for Testicular Cancer (*continued*)			
pT	**cN**	**pN**	**M**
T3 • Invasion of spermatic cord		**S Staging (Serum Tumor Markers)**	
T4 • Invasion of scrotum			**AFP (ng/mL)**	**LDH**	**Beta-hCG (mIU/mL)**
		S0	WNL	WNL	WNL
		S1	<1,000 or	<5,000 or	<1.5 x normal
		S2	1,000–10,000 or	5,000–50,000 or	1.5–10 x normal
		S3	>10,000 or	>50,000 or	> 10 x normal

Stage Grouping				
IA	T1	N0	M0	S0
IB	T2-4	N0	M0	S0
IS	any T	N0	M0	S1-3
IIA	any T	N1	M0	S0-1
IIB	any T	N2	M0	S0-1
IIC	any T	N3	M0	S0-1
IIIA	any T	any N	M1a	S0-1
IIIB	any T	N1-3	M0	S2
	any T	any N	M1a	S2
IIIC	any T	N1-3	M0	S3
	any T	any N	M1a	S3
	any T	any N	M1b	any S

*Major changes from the 7th edition include: subclassifcation of T1a/b, epididymal invasion is now T2 (was T1), hilar invasion is T2, discontinuous involvement of the spermatic cord (metastasis) is considered M1.

Notes: Epididymis[1] = can include rete testis invasion. Involves[2] = involves hilar soft tissue, epididymis, penetrating visceral mesothelial layer covering the external surface of tunica albuginea.

SEMINOMA TREATMENT PARADIGM: Mixed seminomas/NSGCT are treated based on the NSGCT component. Pure seminomas are treated as follows.

Active surveillance: Recommended option for stage I seminoma. Must be compliant with follow-up. NCCN recommends H&P every 3 to 6 months for year 1, every 6 to 12 months for years 2 to 3, then annually. A CT abdomen/pelvis is recommended at 3, 6, and 12 months in the first year, then every 6 to 12 months for years 2 to 3, then every 12 to 24 months for years 4 to 5.[12]

Surgery: The standard surgery is a radical inguinal orchiectomy with high ligation of the spermatic cord. RPLND is indicated for select NSGCT but not in seminoma.

Chemotherapy: Adjuvant CHT is based on pathologic stage. Single-agent carboplatin (AUC 7) x 1–2 cycles is an option for stage I patients. BEP (bleomycin, etoposide, cisplatin) x 3 cycles or EP (etoposide, cisplatin) x 4 cycles are options for stage II–III patients.

Radiotherapy: For stage I patients, a para-aortic strip may be treated to 20 Gy/10 fx. For stage IIA patients, a modified dogleg field can be delivered to 20 Gy/10 fx with a boost to 30 Gy. For stage IIB patients, a modified dogleg field to 20 Gy/10 fx followed by boost to 36 Gy to the gross disease is appropriate.[5] Most recommend coverage of the left renal hilum (see TE10 in the following). Contraindications include horseshoe kidney, inflammatory bowel disease, and genetic syndromes with an increased risk of further malignancies or prior radiation. Side effects include nausea, vomiting, diarrhea, fatigue, second malignancy. Offer sperm banking prior to treatment if fertility is desired.

Procedure: See *Treatment Planning Handbook,* Chapter 8 for details.

EVIDENCE-BASED Q&A

Stage I seminoma

What data supports active surveillance as an option for patients with stage I seminoma?

The risk of relapse and death from a stage I seminoma is small. Although no prospective trials support this approach directly, a systematic literature review (14 studies with 2,060 men) showed that relapse occurred in 17% (9% relapsed >2 years) and mortality from seminoma was 0.3% due to effective salvage therapies.[13] Another study demonstrated that the risk of relapse can be as low as 6% if tumor size <4 cm and no rete testis invasion.[14] A Danish retrospective cohort study of 1,954 men showed that the median time to relapse was 13.7 months with 73.4% of patients developing relapse during the first 2 years, 22.2% between years 3 and 5, and 4.3% after year 5. The 15-year DSS and OS were 99.3% and 91.6%, respectively.[15] Therefore, it is reasonable to recommend surveillance for a compliant patient with a stage I seminoma. Despite the push toward increasing surveillance in these patients, approximately 40% of patients continue to receive adjuvant therapy.[16,17]

Is a full dogleg field necessary for stage I patients treated with adjuvant RT, or will a PA strip suffice?

For stage I patients, pelvic relapse is rare. MRC TE10 showed that para-aortic strip is the standard RT field and dogleg fields should be reserved for patients with prior inguinal or scrotal surgery due to aberrant lymphatic drainage.

Fossa, MRC TE10 (*JCO* 1999, PMID 10561173): Noninferiority PRT of 478 pts with stage I (T1-T3) seminoma randomized to dogleg (DL: para-aortic strip plus ipsilateral iliac lymph node) versus para-aortic strip (PAS; T11-L5) fields. All treated to 30 Gy/15 fx. MFU 4.5 years. No difference in 3-year RFS or OS. Each group had nine relapses, although the PAS group had four pelvic relapses compared to none in the DL group. PAS had less acute toxicity (N/V, diarrhea, leukopenia) and higher sperm counts than DL fields (11% vs. 35% had azoospermia). One patient in the para-aortic arm died of seminoma. **Conclusion: PAS irradiation is considered standard treatment for stage I (T1-T3), with DL fields reserved for patients with prior inguinal or scrotal surgery.**

TABLE 40.4: Results of MRC TE10				
MRC TE10	3-yr RFS	3-yr OS	# Pelvic Relapses	Azoospermia
PAS	96.0%	99.3%	4 (2%)	11%
DL	96.6%	100%	0 (0%)	35%
p value	NS	NS	–	<.001

What is the optimal RT dose for patients with stage I seminoma?

Based on MRC TE18, the standard dose for stage I seminoma is 20 Gy in 10 fx.

Jones, MRC TE18 (*JCO* 2005, PMID 15718317): PRT of 625 pts with stage I seminoma (pT1-3N0) randomized to 20 Gy/10 fx versus 30 Gy/15 fx, all to para-aortic strip (T11-L5). Designed to assess noninferiority, and powered to exclude a 4% difference in 2-year relapse rates. MFU 61 m. No difference in OS or RFS; 30 Gy arm had 10 relapses, compared to 11 relapses in the 20 Gy arm (*p* = NS); 20 Gy arm had less acute side effects (moderate–severe fatigue and inability to conduct normal work) at 4 weeks, but differences returned to baseline by 12 weeks. Six new primary cancers diagnosed, all in the 30 Gy arm. **Conclusion: 20 Gy/10 fx as effective as 30 Gy/15 fx, with less acute SE.**

TABLE 40.5: Results of MRC TE18			
MRC TE18	2-yr RFS	Moderate–Severe Lethargy	Inability to Work at 4 wks
20 Gy	97.0%	5%	28%
30 Gy	97.7%	20%	46%
p value	NS	<.001	<.001

What is the role for CHT in patients with stage I seminoma?

Based on MRC TE19, carboplatin is noninferior to RT, and has reduced side effects.

Oliver, MRC TE19 (*Lancet* 2005, PMID 16039331; Oliver *JCO* 2011, PMID 21282539): PRT of 1,477 pts with stage I seminoma randomized to adjuvant carboplatin (1 cycle, AUC 7) versus adjuvant RT (20 Gy/10 fx [36%] or 30 Gy/15 fx [54%] or an intermediate dose [10%]; dogleg [13%] or para-aortic strip [87%]) after orchiectomy. Powered to exclude absolute differences in 2-year relapse rates of >3%. MFU 6.5 years. Carboplatin had more para-aortic node-only relapses, but fewer pelvic, mediastinal, or SCV relapses compared to RT. Carboplatin arm had fewer second GCTs (carboplatin n = 2, RT n = 15, HR 0.22, *p* = .03) and significantly less acute dyspepsia (8% vs. 17%), moderate–severe lethargy (7% vs. 24%), and inability to do normal work (19% vs. 38%), but more thrombocytopenia (12% vs. 2%). Only one seminoma death, which was in the RT arm. Those getting more of the prescribed CHT (>99% AUC 7) had improved RFS (96.1% vs. 92.6%) than those who received less CHT. **Conclusion: Adjuvant carboplatin is not inferior to RT for stage I seminoma, and has fewer acute SE.**

TABLE 40.6: Results of MRC TE19				
MRC TE19	2-yr RFS	3-yr RFS	5-yr RFS (not SS)	New GCT
RT	96.7%	95.9%	96%	15 (1.7%)
Carboplatin	97.7%	94.8%	94.7%	2 (0.3%)

Oliver, *ASCO* 2005:[18] Pooled analysis of phase II reports of two cycles versus one cycle of adjuvant carboplatin for stage I seminoma. 521 patients received two courses of carboplatin with 2.9% relapse, 0 second GCT, 0 GCT deaths, and 1.3% non-GCT deaths (NS). 316 patients received one course with 4.4% relapse (8.6% in those receiving 400 mg/m² and 2.5% in those receiving AUC 7), 1% second GCT, no GCT, or non-GCT deaths. **Conclusion: Results suggest a dose–response relationship and future studies should be conducted.**

What are the outcomes in patients with stage I seminoma who experience a relapse?

Choo, Toronto (*IJROBP* 2005, PMID 15708251): Prospective, single-arm observational study in 88 pts with stage I seminoma. MFU 12.1 years. 15-year RFS rate was 80%. 17 pts relapsed, 88% of which were below the diaphragm. Salvage therapy: 14 treated with RT

(25 Gy–35 Gy), 3 treated with CHT (3–4 cycles of BEP). All 17 ultimately were salvaged successfully. **Conclusion: Surveillance with the reservation of RT or CHT for salvage is a safe alternative to up-front adjuvant therapy for stage I testicular seminoma.**

Mead, UK TE pooled analysis (*JNCI* 2011, PMID 21212385): Pooled analysis of the TE10, TE18, TE19 trials. A total of 3,049 pts included in these three noninferiority studies. MFU 6.4 to 12 years in the three trials; 99.8% CSS overall. 98 relapses, but only 4 (0.2%) relapsed after 3 years. Four died of metastatic failure. Among pts treated with dogleg who relapsed, 11/16 (65%) failed in the mediastinum or neck. Among pts treated with a para-aortic strip who relapsed, 20/54 (37%) failed in the pelvis and 14/54 (26%) failed in the mediastinum or neck. Among pts treated with carboplatin who relapsed, 18/27 (67%) failed in the retroperitoneum. **Conclusion: Patterns of relapse depend on adjuvant treatment received.**

Stage II seminoma

Why may RT be preferred over CHT in patients with stage IIA/B seminoma?

Krege, German Testicular Cancer Study Group (*Ann Oncol* 2006, PMID 16254023): Phase II trial of single-agent carboplatin (AUC 7) q4 weeks x 3 cycles in stage IIA (n = 51) or x 4 cycles in stage IIB (n = 57). CR was achieved in 81% of pts, 16% with PR, and 2% had no change. 13% who initially achieved a CT relapsed and required salvage therapy. Overall failure rate was 18%. OS 99% and DSS 100%. **Conclusion: CHT used was not effective in eradicating RP metastasis in stage IIA/B seminoma.**

Toxicity and secondary malignancy risk

What is the risk for developing secondary malignancy after adjuvant therapy for testicular cancer?

After adjuvant therapy (CHT or RT), patients with testicular cancer are at a higher risk for developing secondary malignancy. Given the increased risk of mortality from secondary malignancies, it is important to appropriately select patients for adjuvant therapy.

Travis, NIH (*JNCI* 2005, PMID 16174857): Population-based registries of >40,000 testicular cancer survivors used to calculate relative and absolute risks of second solid cancers. Among 10-year survivors diagnosed at 35 years of age, the relative risk of a second solid tumor was 1.9, and remained statistically significantly elevated for 35 years. Cancers of the lung, colon, bladder, pancreas, and stomach accounted for ~60% of the excess malignancies. There was also an increased risk of pleural (malignant mesothelioma) and esophagus cancers. Overall relative risk of second solid malignancy for patients treated with RT alone was 2, CHT alone 1.9, and both 2.9. For patients diagnosed with seminoma or NSGCT at 35 years of age, cumulative risk of solid cancer in the next 40 years was 36% or 31%, respectively (the corresponding risk of solid cancer in the general population was 23%). Note that the authors estimate about 16% of the evaluated patients received chest RT. **Conclusion: Testicular cancer survivors treated with RT and/or CHT are at increased risk of solid tumors for at least 35 years.**

Kier, Danish Nationwide Cohort (*JAMA Oncology* 2016, PMID 27711914): Danish nationwide cohort of 5,190 pts (2,804 seminoma, 2,386 nonseminoma) treated with adjuvant therapy. Pts underwent surveillance, retroperitoneal RT, BEP (bleomycin, etoposide, cisplatin) CHT, or MTOL (more than one line) of CHT. MFU 14.4 years. The 20-year cumulative incidence of second malignancy (death used as a competing risk) was 7.8% for surveillance, 7.6% for BEP (HR 1.7), 13.5% for RT (HR 1.8), 9.2% for MTOL (HR 3.7), and 7.0% for controls. Excess mortality due to second malignancy was found with BEP (HR 1.6), RT

(HR 2.1), and MTOL (HR 5.8). **Conclusion: Excess mortality due to second malignancy from adjuvant therapy suggests that approaches to define the best candidates for adjuvant therapy are needed.**

REFERENCES

1. Siegel RL, Miller KD, Jemal A. Cancer statistics, 2016. *CA Cancer J Clin.* 2016;66(1):7–30. doi:10.3322/caac.21332
2. Yacoub JH, Oto A, Allen BC, et al. ACR Appropriateness criteria staging of testicular malignancy. *J Am Coll Radiol.* 2016;13(10):1203–1209. doi:10.1016/j.jacr.2016.06.026
3. Von der Maase H, Rørth M, Walbom-Jørgensen S, et al. Carcinoma in situ of contralateral testis in patients with testicular germ cell cancer: study of 27 cases in 500 patients. *Br Med J Clin Res Ed.* 1986;293(6559):1398–1401.
4. Fosså SD, Chen J, Schonfeld SJ, et al. Risk of contralateral testicular cancer: a population-based study of 29,515 U.S. men. *J Natl Cancer Inst.* 2005;97(14):1056–1066. doi:10.1093/jnci/dji185
5. Wilder RB, Buyyounouski MK, Efstathiou JA, Beard CJ. Radiotherapy treatment planning for testicular seminoma. *Int J Radiat Oncol Biol Phys.* 2012;83(4):e445–e452. doi:10.1016/j.ijrobp.2012.01.044
6. Marth D, Scheidegger J, Studer UE. Ultrasonography of testicular tumors. *Urol Int.* 1990;45(4):237–240.
7. Ng SP, Duchesne G, Tai KH, et al. Can positron emission tomography (PET) complement conventional staging of early-stage testicular seminoma? *Int J Radiat Oncol.* 2016;96(2, Suppl):E253. doi:10.1016/j.ijrobp.2016.06.1258
8. *AJCC Cancer Staging Manual.* New York, NY: Springer Science+Business Media; 2016.
9. International Germ Cell Consensus Classification: a prognostic factor-based staging system for metastatic germ cell cancers. International Germ Cell Cancer Collaborative Group. *J Clin Oncol.* 1997;15(2):594–603.
10. Nayan M, Jewett MAS, Hosni A, et al. Conditional risk of relapse in surveillance for clinical stage I testicular cancer. *Eur Urol.* 2017;71(1):120–127. doi:10.1016/j.eururo.2016.07.013
11. Von der Maase H, Specht L, Jacobsen GK, et al. Surveillance following orchidectomy for stage I seminoma of the testis. *Eur J Cancer Oxf Engl 1990.* 1993;29A(14):1931–1934.
12. NCCN Guidelines: Testicular Cancer Version 2.2017. https://www.nccn.org/professionals/physician_gls/pdf/testicular.pdf
13. Groll RJ, Warde P, Jewett MAS. A comprehensive systematic review of testicular germ cell tumor surveillance. *Crit Rev Oncol Hematol.* 2007;64(3):182–197. doi:10.1016/j.critrevonc.2007.04.014
14. Albers P, Albrecht W, Algaba F, et al. Guidelines on testicular cancer: 2015 Update. *Eur Urol.* 2015;68(6):1054–1068. doi:10.1016/j.eururo.2015.07.044
15. Mortensen MS, Lauritsen J, Gundgaard MG, et al. A nationwide cohort study of stage I seminoma patients followed on a surveillance program. *Eur Urol.* 2014;66(6):1172–1178. doi:10.1016/j.eururo.2014.07.001
16. Matulewicz RS, Oberlin DT, Sheinfeld J, Meeks JJ. The evolving management of patients with clinical stage I seminoma. *Urology.* 2016;98:113–119. doi:10.1016/j.urology.2016.07.037
17. Wymer KM, Pearce SM, Harris KT, et al. Adherence to National Comprehensive Cancer Network Guidelines for Testicular Cancer. *J Urol.* 2016;197(3 Pt 1):684–689. doi:10.1016/j.juro.2016.09.073
18. Oliver T, Dieckmann K-P, Steiner H, Skoneczna I. Pooled analysis of phase 2 reports of 2 v 1 course of carboplatin as adjuvant for stage 1 seminoma. *ASCO Meet Abstr.* 2005;23(16, Suppl):4572.

41: PENILE CANCER

Rupesh Kotecha, Omar Y. Mian, and Rahul D. Tendulkar

> **QUICK HIT:** Penile cancer is a rare disease. The primary nodal drainage is to inguinal LNs—about 50% of clinically enlarged LNs are pathologically involved (the rest are reactive). Surgical management can include a partial or total penectomy, with inguinal and/or pelvic node dissection depending on clinical risk factors and staging outcomes. Organ preservation can be performed for select early-stage pts with either EBRT or brachytherapy (ideally for T1-T2 tumors <4 cm and <1 cm of corpora invasion). Locally advanced pts should be considered for neoadjuvant CHT (TIP x 4 cycles) +/– RT followed by surgery or definitive chemoRT.

TABLE 41.1: General Treatment Paradigm for Penile Cancer	
Stage	**Treatment Options**
Tis or Ta	Topical therapy, WLE, laser therapy, glansectomy, Mohs surgery
T1	Grade 1–2: WLE, glansectomy, Mohs, laser therapy, RT Grade 3: WLE, partial penectomy, total penectomy, RT, chemoRT
T2-T4	Partial penectomy, total penectomy, RT, chemoRT, neoadjuvant CHT (TIP), and surgery

EPIDEMIOLOGY: Rare cancer in the United States, accounting for ~0.1% of all solid tumors with ~2,100 new cases and 360 deaths in 2017.[1] More common in the less developed world. Mean age 60. A significant proportion of men have delayed treatment due to incorrect diagnosis or perceptions of social stigma.

RISK FACTORS: Epidemiologic factors: single, never married, lack of circumcision. Medical factors: HPV exposure, genital warts, UTI, penile injury, urethral stricture, phimosis (circumferential fibrosis of the prepuce causing inability to retract the foreskin over the glans), HIV, tobacco exposure, psoralen, and UVA photochemotherapy. 30% to 50% are HPV+ (most commonly 16 and 18) w/ some suggestion of a more favorable prognosis.

ANATOMY: Generally divided into the root, shaft, and glans. Penis is anchored to the public ramus. Two corporal bodies share a perforated midline septum terminating at the glans. The urethra is surrounded by the corpus spongiosum. Two layers of fascia cover the corpora: the superficial fascia is continuous with the dartos fascia of the scrotum and the deep fascia (Buck's) surrounds the erectile bodies (acts as barrier to corporal invasion). Blood supply is from the common penile artery from the internal pudendal artery, which is a branch of the internal iliac. LN drainage occurs bilaterally and sequentially, from the superficial inguinal to the deep femoral LNs, then into the pelvis. Regional LNs include superficial inguinal, deep inguinal, and iliac LNs. The sentinel LNs (Cloquet) are located anteromedial to the superficial epigastric and saphenous vessels.

PATHOLOGY: 95% are squamous cell carcinoma. Other rarer subtypes include melanoma, TCC, BCC, Kaposi sarcoma, lymphoma, extramammary Paget's disease, or metastasis from other sites. Penile squamous cell carcinomas can be subclassified by microscopic histologic features: usual type SCC (most common), papillary, warty, basaloid, verrucous, and sarcomatoid subgroups. Low-grade (1–2) carcinomas comprise 80% of cases. Poorly differentiated (grade 3), basaloid and sarcomatoid subgroups have poorer prognosis. Verrucous and low-grade tumors are more commonly local diseases and rarely metastasize.

CLINICAL PRESENTATION: Often presents with a penile mass or skin abnormality, occurring typically on the glans, in the coronal sulcus, or prepuce (involvement of the shaft is rare, <10%). Presenting symptoms include rash, ulceration, bleeding, or with a secondary infection. May be mistaken for premalignant lesions such as bowenoid papulosis (papules on the penile shaft), Bowen's disease (plaque on follicle-bearing epithelium of penile shaft), erythroplasia of Queyrat (red lesion on mucocutaneous epithelium of the glans or prepuce), lichen sclerosis, condylomas, Buschke–Lowenstein (giant condyloma), and Kaposi sarcoma. Bowenoid papulosis, Bowen's disease, and erythroplasia of Queyrat are associated with HPV+ and are considered in situ lesions (Cis). Locoregionally advanced cases progress in an orderly fashion to inguinal LNs, followed by spread to pelvic or RP LNs. Only 50% of clinically apparent inguinal lymphadenopathy is due to metastatic nodal disease (other 50% are reactive adenopathy, often from infection); <10% have DM at presentation.

WORKUP: H&P with careful examination of penile lesion and inguinal LNs. If infection is suspected, consider a 4- to 6-week course of antibiotics.

Pathology: Punch or incisional biopsy of the penile lesion can usually be performed, reserving excisional biopsy if the initial biopsy is not diagnostic. Cystourethroscopy should be performed to examine lower urinary tract.

Imaging: CT abdomen/pelvis and CXR are standard. MRI and ultrasound may clarify depth of invasion. MRI should be performed if corporal involvement is suspected. Bone scan if advanced disease is suspected. PET/CT should be considered in high-risk pts, particularly those with LN+ by FNA or node dissection.

Labs: CBC, CMP, alkaline phosphatase.

PROGNOSTIC FACTORS: LN+ (correlates with T stage and grade, p53+, LVSI, PNI, tumor emboli in venous/lymphatic channel), ENE. There is some evidence that HPV may have better prognosis (but not reproducible across series).

STAGING

TABLE 41.2: AJCC 8th ed. (2017) Staging for Penile Cancer[2]		N	cN0	cN1	cN2	cN3
T/M						
T1[1]	a No LVSI, PNI, or Grade 3/sarcomatoid		I			
	b LVSI, PNI or Grade 3/sarcomatoid		IIA	IIIA	IIIB	
T2	• Invades corpus spongiosum with or without urethral invasion		IIA	IIIA	IIIB	
T3	• Invades corpus cavernosum with or without urethral invasion		IIB			
T4	• Invades adjacent structures (scrotum, prostate, pubic bone)		IV			
M1	• Distant metastasis					

(continued)

TABLE 41.2: AJCC 8th ed. (2017) Staging for Penile Cancer[2] (*continued*)
Major changes from the AJCC 7th Ed. include T1 cancers being staged by site (glans, foreskin, shaft), T2 cancers being defined by corpus spongiosum invasion and T3 cancers being defined by corpus cavernosum invasion.
Notes: T1[1] = Glans: invades lamina propria; Foreskin: invades dermis, lamina propria or dartos fascia; Shaft: invades connective tissue between epidermis and corpora.
cN1, palpable, mobile unilateral inguinal LN; cN2, palpable, mobile, ≥2 unilateral inguinal or bilateral inguinal LN; cN3, palpable, fixed inguinal nodal mass or pelvic lymphadenopathy.

TREATMENT PARADIGM: The European Association of Urology published guidelines, which are summarized as follows.[3]

Surgery: In general, men with low-risk operable tumors (Tia, Ta, T1a) should undergo organ-preserving treatment (Table 41.3). High-risk pts with T1 G3 or T2-T4 tumors should undergo penile amputation with either a total penectomy or partial penectomy (removal of the glans +/− underlying corpora cavernosa), depending on extent of disease and location of tumor. For T1 G3 without involvement of the glans or underlying corporal tissues, can consider excision of the penile shaft skin alone. Distal T2-3 tumors can be treated with limited excision if a negative margin can be attained (need to leave >2 cm for standing void). In a large review, most pts are able to undergo partial penectomy (total penectomy accounted for 23%).[4] LR is <10% in most series. The most common side effect is meatal stenosis (4%–9%). Psychological trauma is also common and some pts have attempted or committed suicide after penectomy. Men should be counseled about penile reconstruction options. For pts who refuse surgery, interstitial brachytherapy can be considered. Those with unresectable primary tumor or bulky lymphadenopathy should receive neoadjuvant CHT +/− RT prior to consideration of surgery.

TABLE 41.3: Summary of Management Options for Early-Stage Penile Cancer		
Candidates	**Treatment**	**Notes**
Tis, Ta, or T1a	Limited excision	Goal is to preserve penile length and sexual function
Tis	Topical therapy	5-FU cream and imiquimod cream for 4–6 weeks
Tis	Laser ablation	CO2, argon, Nd:YAG and potassium titanyl phosphate laser ablation; high rate of preserving sexual activity and satisfaction
Tis	Total glans resurfacing	Removal of epithelial and subepithelial layers of glans down to corpus spongiosum, followed by skin graft
Tis or T1	Mohs surgery	Layer-by-layer excision to maximize organ preservation
Tis or T1	RT	Brachytherapy or EBRT

LN assessment: In addition to assessment of the primary tumor, evaluation of LNs should be performed, noting high rates of false positives and negatives on clinical exam (Tables 41.4 and 41.5).[5] Factors such as T stage, grade, and LVSI predict for LN involvement and risk categories have been identified to guide management of the inguinal LNs. If no palpable or radiographic adenopathy, consider dynamic SLNB (high sensitivity, but requires expertise in technique).[6] A superficial inguinal node dissection or modified inguinal node dissection may be performed by clinicians without experience in dynamic SLNB, but have higher complication rates than SLNB. For pts with palpable inguinal adenopathy or enlarged LNs on imaging (CT, MRI, or US), perform FNA first. If FNA is positive, then perform a complete (superficial and deep) ipsilateral inguinal node dissection. All pts with pLN+ should also undergo a contralateral superficial inguinal node dissection and cross-sectional imaging for staging. After inguinal node dissection, if only a single LN is positive without ENE, no pelvic node dissection is needed. If multiple LN+ or ENE is present, then a pelvic node dissection is indicated. For N2 disease, consider neoadjuvant chemo (TIP x 4 cycles) +/– RT followed by surgery.

TABLE 41.4: Summary of Inguinal Node Evaluation in Clinically LN- pts

Risk Category	Primary Tumor Factors (all cN0)	Management of cN0 Inguinal LNs
Low risk	pT1is, Ta, or T1 G1, and no LVSI	Surveillance (consider SLNB, or superficial or modified inguinal node dissection for noncompliant pts)
Intermediate risk	pT1a G2 and no LVSI	SLNB (alternatively, superficial or modified inguinal node dissection; surveillance in well-informed and compliant pts) • If LN– → surveillance • If 1 LN+, no ENE → complete inguinal node dissection • If 2 LN+ or ENE → complete inguinal and pelvic node dissection
High risk	pT1b or higher (G3 or LVSI)	SLNB or superficial or modified inguinal node dissection • If LN– →surveillance • If 1 LN+, no ENE → complete inguinal node dissection • If 2 LN+ or ENE → complete inguinal and pelvic node dissection

TABLE 41.5: Summary of Inguinal Node Evaluation in Clinically LN+ Pts After Initial FNA of Suspicious LN(s)

Clinical scenario (all cN+)	Management of cN+ inguinal LNs
Single enlarged LN <4 cm, low-risk primary tumor (pTis, pTa, pT1 G1)	If FNA– → excisional biopsy of enlarged LN If FNA+ → complete inguinal node dissection • If 1 LN+, no ENE → surveillance • If 2 LN+ or ENE → pelvic node dissection
Single enlarged LN <4 cm, high-risk primary tumor (pT1 or higher with G3 or LVSI)	If FNA– → superficial or modified inguinal node dissection If FNA+ → complete inguinal node dissection • If 1 LN+, no ENE → surveillance • If 2 LN+ or ENE → pelvic node dissection
Multiple or bilateral enlarged LNs	If FNA– → superficial inguinal node dissection with intra-op frozen evaluation If FNA+ → complete inguinal (and pelvic node dissection if 2 LN+ or ENE) OR neoadjuvant CHT (TIPx4) followed by surgery

Chemotherapy: CHT options are summarized in Table 41.6. TIP resulted in a response in 39/60 men in a phase II study of men with advanced penile cancer with 10 pts ypN0.[7] The 5-yr OS for those who responded to neoadjuvant CHT was 50% versus 8% for those who progressed during CHT. TPF has relatively poor response rates and tolerance. Adjuvant CHT recommendations are largely extrapolated from the neoadjuvant and metastatic setting, but may be applied to men with high-risk features.

TABLE 41.6: CHT Options for Penile Cancer

Type	Indications	CHT Options
Neoadjuvant	- Unresectable primary tumor - Bulky inguinal LN+ - Bilateral inguinal LN+	• TIP (paclitaxel [175 mg/m2 d1], ifosfamide [1,200 mg/m2 d1-3], cisplatin [25 mg/m2 d1-3]) q3-4 weeks x 4 • TPF (docetaxel, cisplatin and fluorouracil)

(continued)

TABLE 41.6: CHT Options for Penile Cancer (*continued*)

Type	Indications	CHT options
Adjuvant	- Pelvic LN+ - ENE - Bilateral inguinal LN+ - >3 LN+	• TIP
Metastatic	KPS ≥80	• TIP • Cisplatin (100 mg/m² d1) + 5-FU (1000 mg/m²/day d1-5) q3–4 weeks • Cisplatin (80 mg/m² on day 1) + irinotecan (60 mg/m² d1/8/15) on a 28-day cycle • Consider panitumumab, cetuximab alone, or in combo w/ chemo

Radiation: Used in the definitive setting for organ preservation (either RT alone or concurrent chemoRT, extrapolating from cervical cancer and anal cancer), neoadjuvant setting if locally advanced unresectable disease, or for symptom palliation in those with metastatic disease. First step in management is circumcision, which allows for full exposure and can prevent radiation balanitis and phimosis. Definitive RT for organ preservation of early-stage lesions can consist of either EBRT (LC 44%–65%, penile preservation 58%–86%) or brachytherapy (LC 70%–86%, penile preservation 74%–88%). Brachytherapy alone can be considered for lower risk (T1-T2) lesions <4 cm with corpora invasion <1 cm. For more advanced lesions, either EBRT alone or combined EBRT and CHT or brachytherapy boost may be considered.

TABLE 41.7: General Principles of RT for Penile Cancer

Group	RT Treatment Options
Early stage (T1-T2, N0) <4 cm	Definitive brachytherapy alone or EBRT or chemoRT to primary site +/– LNs
Early stage (T1-T2, N0) >4 cm	Definitive chemoRT (primary site + LNs)
Locally advanced (T3-4 or N+)	Definitive chemoRT (primary site + LNs)
Resected w/positive margins	Adjuvant EBRT to primary site and surgical scar +/– LNs if inadequate LND
Resected LN+	Adjuvant chemoRT to primary site and regional LNs, including pelvic LNs (extrapolating from vulvar cancer trials)

EBRT: For details, see *Treatment Planning Handbook*, Chapter 8.[8] Setup may be prone or supine with immobilizing bolus to position the penis (wax mold, Perspex block, plastic cylinder, water bath, etc.). Setup frog-leg if planning on inguinal node treatment via AP/PA technique (wide AP fields with electron supplementation). The entire length of the penis should be covered, with LNs included if clinically involved or at risk.

Dose: Historically doses of 50 to 55 Gy were used,[9,10] but in the modern era 45 to 50 Gy is given to the entire penile shaft followed by a boost to 65 to 70 Gy to treat gross disease. A hypofractionated schedule of 52.5 Gy/16 fx may be considered.[11] When electively treating LNs, uninvolved nodes should receive 45 to 50 Gy and gross/unresected groin nodes should be boosted to 65 to 70 Gy.

Brachytherapy: ABS-GEC-ESTRO guidelines by Crook et al. are summarized here.[12] Brachytherapy is ideally restricted to lesions <4 cm with <1 cm invasion of the corpora cavernosa (typically T1-T2 lesions and select T3 cases). Larger size associated with higher LR and increased risk of late effects. Superficial molds may be created to contain sources or interstitial implant. Pt placed under general anesthesia or penile block with systemic sedation. Foley catheter is placed to aid in urethral identification. Templates placed on either side of the penis for stabilization. Up to six needles inserted perpendicular to penis, 1 cm apart and in planes. Target volume includes tumor plus 1.5- to 2-cm margin for small lesions; include glans and shaft for larger lesions. Needles are loaded after edema has subsided. LDR dose is 60 to 65 Gy, limiting urethra to 50 Gy over 6 to 7 days. Dose rates with pulse dose rate technique (PDR) are typically ~50–60 cGy/hr. If using HDR brachy, no consensus standard dosing exists. A common HDR dose is 54 Gy in BID fx of 3 Gy each delivered over 9 days and 38.4 Gy in BID fx of 3.2 Gy/fx over 6 days is well tolerated. Interfraction interval should be ≥6 hours. To reduce risk of penile necrosis, limit V125 <40% and V150 <20%. To decrease risk of urethral strictures, limit urethra V115 <10% and V90 <95%. Minimize confluent areas of 125%.

Toxicity: Dermatitis, dysuria, skin telangiectasia, urethral stricture (10%–40%), urethral fistula, impotence, penile fibrosis, penile necrosis (3%–15%, higher with interstitial technique), bowel obstruction.

EVIDENCE-BASED Q&A

What are the general historical outcomes of penile cancer? Does surgery or RT provide better outcomes?

Surgery and RT are both appropriate modalities. Some retrospective series suggest better LC with surgical resection; however, psychosexual morbidity with penectomy is high.

Sarin (*IJROBP* 1997, PMID: 9240637): RR of 101 pts with stage I–IV disease treated with EBRT (59), brachytherapy (13), or penectomy (29). MFU 5.2 yrs. In 36 failures, 23 received partial penectomy, 3 had penectomy, 2 had RT, and 6 received CHT. 5-yr and 10-yr OS were 57% and 39%. 5-yr and 10-yr CSS were 66% and 57%. 5-yr and 10-yr LC were 60% and 55%. No difference between surgery and RT in LC after salvage. Among EBRT pts, five had moderate stricture, two had severe stricture, and two had penectomy (one for necrosis and one for urethral damage.). In surgical pts, there were two suicide attempts after penectomy.

Ozsahin (*IJROBP* 2006, PMID: 16949770): RR of 60 men w/ SCC s/p either surgery (n = 27) or RT (n = 29); 70% cN0. 22 pts received post-op RT for either + margins or LNs. 29 pts received RT for organ preservation and four pts refused RT. Median EBRT dose 52 Gy (26–74.5 Gy) with brachytherapy boost given in 7 (15–25 Gy). 1 pt treated with brachytherapy alone. 19 of 29 pts received nodal RT (36–66 Gy). LF was 13% in surgery group and 56% in organ sparing. Clinically + LNs controlled in 9/11 pts w/ lymphadenectomy and 5/7 pts with RT alone. 73% of LF salvaged with surgery. 5-yr OS 43%, 10-yr OS 25%.

What are the expected outcomes with limited excision?

Limited excision has been used more recently for pts with early-stage disease with a low risk for LR (Tis, Ta, or T1a). Recent long-term data show low rates of LR. Importantly, the historic standard was for a 2-cm margin, but in the current era, negative margin excision with a goal of 5 mm is appropriate.

Philippou (*J Urol* 2012, PMID: 22818137): UK study of 179 pts with invasive penile cancer treated from 2002 to 2010 w/ organ-preserving surgery: circumcision (involving skin shaft), WLE w/ primary closure, removal of the glans, or removal of the glans and distal corpora. Median distance to resection margin was 5 mm. MFU 43 months. After excision, LR in 9%, regional recurrence in 11%, and DM in 5%. 5-yr DSS 55%. For pts with isolated LR, 5-yr DSS was 92% versus 38% for those with a regional recurrence. 5-yr LRFS 86%. On MVA, tumor grade, stage, and LVSI were independent predictors of LR. Distance to margin was not a significant predictor of recurrence. **Conclusion: Penile-conserving surgery is safe and excision with 5-mm margin is still associated with low risk of LR. LR has no impact on OS.**

Is RT alone an adequate modality for early-stage lesions?

RT alone is an option for organ preservation. Nodal disease has poor prognosis. Close follow-up is required as relapses are frequent.

McLean (IJROBP 1993, PMID: 8454480): RR of 26 pts w/ invasive SCC stage I–II and 11 pts with CIS from 1970 to 1985. RT dose ranged from 35 to 60 Gy. Nodal dose ranged from 38 to 51 Gy. Median age 61 w/ MFU 9.7 yrs. 5-yr OS 62% and was 79% for LN- versus 12% for LN+. 21 of 26 pts had initial CR but 11/21 responders recurred (three in penis alone, two penis + LNs, 4 in LNs alone, two DM). 7 pts developed meatal stenosis/ phimosis, seven pts had other late effects (severe telangiectasia, fibrosis, urethral stenosis, ulceration) and eight pts later underwent penectomy (six for recurrence, two for RT complications).

What is the efficacy of brachytherapy for early-stage penile cancer?

Brachytherapy is effective with high rates of LC for early-stage tumors.

Crook (World J Urol 2009, PMID: 18636264): RR of 67 pts w/ MFU 4 yrs. 5-yr OS 59%, 10-yr CSS 84%; 5-yr and 10-yr penile preservation rates were 88% and 67%. Soft tissue necrosis in 12% and urethral stenosis in 9%. 6 of 11 pts with regional recurrence salvaged by LND+/− EBRT.

de Crevoisier (IJROBP 2009, PMID: 19395183): RR of 144 pts w/ SCC of glans treated with brachytherapy to median dose of 65 Gy. 10-yr penile recurrence 20%, inguinal node recurrence 11%, inguinal node met 6%. 10-yr CSS 92%. 10-yr probability of avoiding penile surgery was 72%. Stenosis in 23% and pain/necrosis in 22%,

Are there data to support adjuvant RT in pts with LN+ penile cancer?

Given the rarity of penile cancer, data on the benefit of adjuvant RT in pts with LN+ disease are often extrapolated from vulvar cancer trials, which showed a benefit in LC and OS to pelvic RT. One series from the Netherlands provides support when compared to older series and also highlights shortcomings of RT in pts with ENE and pelvic LN+ disease.

Graafland (J Urol 2010, PMID: 20723934): RR of 156 pts with LN+ penile cancer s/p therapeutic regional lymphadenectomy. Post-op RT (50 Gy/25 fx) was given if >1 pLN+ per institution paradigm and was performed in 45% of pts. MFU 57.8 months. 5-yr CSS was 61%. Men with ENE had decreased 5-yr CSS (42% vs. 80%). On MVA, ENE and pelvic LN+ disease were associated with decreased CSS. **Conclusion: Despite RT, ENE and pelvic LN+ disease are associated with inferior survival. Note that these numbers are higher than other series of men not receiving adjuvant RT.**

REFERENCES

1. Siegel RL, Miller KD, Jemal A. Cancer statistics, 2017. *CA Cancer J Clin.* 2017;67(1):7–30.
2. *AJCC Cancer Staging Manual, Eighth Edition.* 8th ed. New York, NY: Springer Publishing; 2017.
3. Hakenberg OW, Comperat EM, Minhas S, et al. EAU guidelines on penile cancer: 2014 update. *Eur Urol.* 2015;67(1):142–150.
4. Solsona E, Bahl A, Brandes SB, et al. New developments in the treatment of localized penile cancer. *Urology.* 2010;76(2 Suppl 1):S36–S42.

5. Heyns CF, Fleshner N, Sangar V, et al. Management of the lymph nodes in penile cancer. *Urology.* 2010;76(2 Suppl 1):S43–S57.
6. Graafland NM, Lam W, Leijte JA, et al. Prognostic factors for occult inguinal lymph node involvement in penile carcinoma and assessment of the high-risk EAU subgroup: a two-institution analysis of 342 clinically node-negative patients. *Eur Urol.* 2010;58(5):742–747.
7. Dickstein RJ, Munsell MF, Pagliaro LC, Pettaway CA. Prognostic factors influencing survival from regionally advanced squamous cell carcinoma of the penis after preoperative chemotherapy. *BJU Int.* 2016;117(1):118–125.
8. Videtic GMM, Woody N, Vassil AD. *Handbook of Treatment Planning in Radiation Oncology.* 2nd ed. New York, NY: Demos Medical; 2015.
9. Neave F, Neal AJ, Hoskin PJ, Hope-Stone HF. Carcinoma of the penis: a retrospective review of treatment with iridium mould and external beam irradiation. *Clin Oncol (R Coll Radiol).* 1993;5(4):207–210.
10. Munro NP, Thomas PJ, Deutsch GP, Hodson NJ. Penile cancer: a case for guidelines. *Ann R Coll Surg Engl.* 2001;83(3):180–185.
11. Azrif M, Logue JP, Swindell R, et al. External-beam radiotherapy in T1-2 N0 penile carcinoma. *Clin Oncol (R Coll Radiol).* 2006;18(4):320–325.
12. Crook JM, Haie-Meder C, Demanes DJ, et al. American Brachytherapy Society–Groupe Europeen de Curietherapie–European Society of Therapeutic Radiation Oncology (ABS-GEC-ESTRO) consensus statement for penile brachytherapy. *Brachytherapy.* 2013;12(3):191–198.

42: URETHRAL CANCER

Rupesh Kotecha and Rahul D. Tendulkar

QUICK HIT: Rare tumor that often presents with locally advanced disease, particularly proximal tumors, which have a worse prognosis. Squamous cell carcinomas are most common followed by urothelial carcinomas. Management involves surgery for early-stage disease (with organ preservation if possible) and combined modality therapy for advanced stage. Unfortunately, no prospective randomized trials guide management.

EPIDEMIOLOGY: Very rare tumor (<1% of GU malignancies). In a SEER registry from 1973 to 2002, there were 1,075 urethral carcinomas in men and 540 in women.[1] Annual incidence is ~500 cases. Up to 1/2 die of their disease.[2]

RISK FACTORS: Chronic inflammation: prior history of STD, urethritis, urethral strictures (potentially secondary to trauma), urethral diverticuli, urinary stasis, infection. HPV infection, or prior urothelial cancer.

ANATOMY

Men: male urethra extends from bladder neck proximally to urethral meatus distally (~20–21 cm in length), and is divided into the prostatic urethra (10% of cancer cases; composed of transitional epithelium), bulbomembranous (60%; transitional epithelium), and penile (30%; pseudostratified columnar epithelium) portions, with squamous epithelium at the meatus.

Women: female urethra is shorter than males (3–4 cm) and is divided into the posterior segment (proximal 1/3, transitional cells) and anterior segment (distal 2/3, squamous epithelium).

PATHOLOGY: In general, the majority of urethral cancers are squamous cell carcinomas, followed by urothelial carcinomas. Adenocarcinomas are rare and typically result from periurethral glandular tissue (Skene's glands). Mixed tumors are also seen.

CLINICAL PRESENTATION: May present with symptoms of a urethral stricture (urinary retention, difficulty voiding, dysuria), hematuria, urethral discharge, pain, swelling, priapism, irritative urinary symptoms, or dyspareunia. Often presents late because symptoms can be attributed to benign causes (e.g., UTI or strictures). Cancers can extend locally into the penis, spread to pelvic LNs (primary drainage for the proximal urethra) or to inguinal LNs (primary drainage for the distal urethra), which can present with palpable nodal metastasis. Clinically suspicious LNs are usually involved by urethral cancer metastases (in contrast to penile cancer where only ~50% of cN+ are pN+). DM present in only 10% at diagnosis (lung, liver, bone).

WORKUP: H&P with full GU exam (also GYN exam for women). EUA (palpation of the genitalia, urethra, rectum, perineum) and cystourethroscopy to evaluate extent of disease. Consider retrograde urethrogram.

Labs: CBC, CMP, urine cytology (more sensitive for urothelial carcinomas in pendulous urethra).[3]

Imaging: CT or MRI of the primary site and pelvis. Chest CT +/− bone scan. PET is not standard.

Biopsy: Transurethral biopsy.

PROGNOSTIC FACTORS: Poor prognosis associated with advanced age, tumor location (proximal worse than distal), tumor size (>2 cm vs. <2 cm), higher clinical nodal stage, higher histologic grade, presence of metastatic disease.[4-7]

STAGING

TABLE 42.1A: AJCC 8th ed. (2017) Staging for Male Penile Urethra and Female Urethra		N	cN0	cN1	cN2
T/M					
T1	• Invades subepithelial connective tissue	I			
T2	• Invades corpus spongiosum or periurethral muscle	II	III	IV	
T3	• Invades corpus cavernosum or anterior vagina				
T4	• Invades adjacent organs				
M1	• Distant metastasis				

Notes: Regional LNs include inguinal (superficial or deep), perivesical, obturator, internal, and external iliac cN1, single regional LN; cN2, multiple regional LNs.

TABLE 42.1B: AJCC 8th ed. (2017) Staging for Prostatic Urethra	
Tis	Carcinoma in situ involving prostatic urethra or periurethral or prostatic ducts without stromal invasion
T1	Invades subepithelial connective tissue
T2	Invades prostatic stroma surrounding ducts by direct extension from urothelial surface or prostatic ducts
T3	Invades periprostatic fat
T4	Invades other adjacent organs (e.g., bladder wall, rectal wall)

TREATMENT PARADIGM: Without prospective trials to guide management, only retrospective series are available. Treatment based on gender, location, extent of disease, and histology.

General principles

Localized disease: Surgical management, with transurethral resection for small lesions or segmental resection for larger lesions (partial or total urethrectomy). Consider RT for organ preservation.

Locally advanced disease: Neoadjuvant CHT +/− RT followed by surgery.

Metastatic disease: CHT +/− palliative local therapy.

TABLE 42.2: General Treatment Paradigm	
Men (Ta, Tis, T1 low grade)	Transurethral (endoscopic) resection or fulguration; distal urethrectomy for distal lesions
Men (T1 high grade)	Segmental resection with primary anastomosis

(continued)

TABLE 42.2: General Treatment Paradigm (*continued*)	
Men (T2)	Subtotal urethrectomy and perineal urethrostomy
Women (Ta, T1, and T2)	Local excision vs. definitive RT
T3/T4 or LN+	Neoadjuvant CHT +/– RT followed by surgery (likely exenteration), or definitive chemoRT (reserving surgery for salvage). Inguinal LN dissection for pts with LN+ disease

Surgery: In both men and women, inguinal LN dissection is controversial but is generally recommended in pts with clinically or radiographically positive LNs. No data on sentinel LN biopsy, although performed at some centers.

Men: For small Tis-T1 tumors, endoscopic resection is appropriate. Distal tumors can undergo distal urethrectomy. For larger tumors or if unable to obtain a negative margin resection endoscopically, perform a segmental resection with anastomosis. Subtotal urethrectomy and perineal urethrostomy for T2 cancers (spongiosum but not cavernosa involvement). T3-T4 tumors often require total penectomy, cystoprostatectomy, and anterior exenteration with perineal reconstruction.

Women: T1 tumors can be treated with endoscopic resection (must maintain urethral sphincter to preserve continence). More advanced tumors are treated by total urethrectomy with bladder neck closure and urinary diversion. Extensive locoregional disease may require pelvic exenteration and vaginectomy.

Chemotherapy: Neoadjuvant CHT indicated for locally advanced disease +/– RT prior to surgery based on histology. Squamous cell carcinomas often treated with 5-FU + cisplatin or 5-FU + MMC. Urothelial carcinomas typically receive cisplatin-based regimens such as gemcitabine + cisplatin or ddMVAC (dose-dense methotrexate, vinblastine, doxorubicin, and cisplatin).

Radiation: Prior to RT, perform circumcision in men to prevent balanitis and phimosis.

Adjuvant: Consider post-op RT for pts with locally advanced (pT3-4) primary disease depending on surgery extent or positive margins.

Neoadjuvant: Consider pre-op RT or chemoRT to reduce tumor burden and extent of surgery required.

Definitive: Consider organ preservation for distal tumors in men and proximal tumors in women. T1-T2 tumors can potentially be treated with RT alone, but for more advanced disease consider sequential or concurrent chemoRT.

Palliative: Indicated for symptomatic locally advanced disease not amenable to curative therapy.

Dose: EBRT dose is 45 to 50.4 Gy to primary site and inguinal, external and internal iliac LNs. Brachytherapy may be considered for lesions <2–3 cm with negative LNs or prior to EBRT for pts with larger tumors or LN+ disease. Brachytherapy dose is generally ~20–25 Gy after EBRT.

Toxicities: Acute: Radiation dermatitis, local pain, fibrosis, radiation cystitis, urethritis. Late: Chronic penile edema, fistula, and urethral stricture (consider biopsy to rule out recurrent disease).

Procedure: See *Treatment Planning Handbook*, Chapter 8.[8]

EVIDENCE-BASED Q&A

Can an organ-preservation approach be used for pts with early-stage urethral cancer?

Select series show promising outcomes with definitive RT (brachytherapy +/– EBRT) as an alternative to surgery.

Sharma, All India Institute (*J Contemp Brachytherapy* 2016, PMID 26985196): RR of ten female pts with periurethral cancer (five recurrent and five primary cancers) treated with HDR brachytherapy (2–3 plane free-hand implant with plastic catheters to tumor + 5-mm margin) +/– EBRT (primary site, inguinal LNs, external iliac LNs, internal iliac LNs). Brachytherapy alone 42 Gy/14 fx over 7 days BID for pts with lesions <3 cm in size, and brachytherapy boost 18–21 Gy/6–7 fx BID after EBRT (50.4 Gy up-front or 36 Gy for recurrent cases after prior RT) for pts with lesions >3 cm. Brachytherapy was performed prior to EBRT since tumors are well-delineated and easier to implant; no desquamation from EBRT to delay treatment and higher dose able to be delivered over a short period. MFU 25 mos. 6 pts were disease-free and four pts had recurrence (two in inguinal LNs, one LR, and one both). All five pts treated with brachytherapy developed moist desquamation. Grade II toxicity 30%. **Conclusion: Small sample size but brachytherapy provides good LRC with acceptable toxicity. Regional nodal RT recommended for pts with tumors >2 cm given the higher than expected nodal failure rate.**

Can an organ-preservation approach be used for pts with locally advanced urethral cancer?

Select series show promising outcomes with definitive chemoRT for pts who refuse surgery or are not surgical candidates (as an alternative to surgery). However, those who do not respond to therapy have dismal outcomes (despite salvage surgery).

Kent, Lahey Clinic (*J Urol* 2015, PMID 25088950): RR of 26 male pts treated with two cycles of 5-FU 1,000 mg/m^2 + MMC 10 mg/m^2 with concurrent EBRT 45–55 Gy/25 fx to genitals, perineum, inguinal and external iliac LN. All but one pt had squamous histology; 88% had at least T3 or LN+ disease; 79% had CR and 21% had no response to treatment (all of these pts died of their disease, regardless of salvage surgery). Of the CR pts, 42% ultimately had disease recurrence at a median of 12.5 mos. 5-yr DSS 68%, DFS 43%, and OS 52%. **Conclusion: ChemoRT may allow for organ preservation in select pts.**

Are there any data supporting the use of neoadjuvant CHT or chemoRT in pts with locally advanced urethral cancer?

For significant locally advanced disease, neoadjuvant therapy can decrease the burden of disease and reduce the extent of surgery needed.

Gakis, Multi-Institutional (*Ann Oncol* 2015, PMID 25969370): Multicenter RR of 124 pts (86 men, 38 women) with urethral cancer treated at 10 centers from 1993 to 2012. 31% received neoadjuvant CHT, 15% neoadjuvant chemoRT + adjuvant CHT, and 54% received adjuvant CHT. Neoadjuvant therapy was more likely to be used in pts with LN+ disease and reduced extent of surgery (avoiding cystectomy). RR to neoadjuvant CHT was 25% and to neoadjuvant chemoRT was 33%. 3-yr OS was 100% for those who received neoadjuvant CHT or neoadjuvant chemoRT, but was only 50% after surgery and 20% after surgery + adjuvant CHT. Neoadjuvant treatment was associated with improved 3-yr RFS and OS. **Conclusion: Neoadjuvant CHT or chemoRT for pts with T3 or LN+ disease associated with improved outcomes compared to up-front surgery or surgery + CHT.**

REFERENCES

1. Swartz MA, Porter MP, Lin DW, Weiss NS. Incidence of primary urethral carcinoma in the United States. *Urology*. 2006;68(6):1164–1168.
2. Visser O, Adolfsson J, Rossi S, et al. Incidence and survival of rare urogenital cancers in Europe. *Eur J Cancer*. 2012;48(4):456–464.
3. Touijer AK, Dalbagni G. Role of voided urine cytology in diagnosing primary urethral carcinoma. *Urology*. 2004;63(1):33–35.
4. Gakis G, Morgan TM, Efstathiou JA, et al. Prognostic factors and outcomes in primary urethral cancer: results from the international collaboration on primary urethral carcinoma. *World J Urol*. 2016;34(1):97–103.
5. Rabbani F. Prognostic factors in male urethral cancer. *Cancer*. 2011;117(11):2426–2434.
6. Champ CE, Hegarty SE, Shen X, et al. Prognostic factors and outcomes after definitive treatment of female urethral cancer: a population-based analysis. *Urology*. 2012;80(2):374–381.
7. Dalbagni G, Zhang ZF, Lacombe L, Herr HW. Female urethral carcinoma: an analysis of treatment outcome and a plea for a standardized management strategy. *Br J Urol*. 1998;82(6):835–841.
8. Videtic GMM, Woody N, Vassil AD. *Handbook of Treatment Planning in Radiation Oncology*. 2nd ed. New York, NY: Demos Medical; 2015.

VIII: **GYNECOLOGIC**

43: CERVICAL CANCER

Monica E. Shukla and Sheen Cherian

QUICK HIT: The vast majority of cervical cancer cases are HPV-mediated. Incidence and mortality significantly declined with introduction of screening with Pap smears. Three FDA approved vaccines are available that prevent development cervical cancer. Treatment at early stages is often surgical, while radiation therapy (RT) +/- chemotherapy (CHT) is employed in later stages. When treating definitively, external beam RT (EBRT) is followed by an intra-cavitary brachytherapy boost. Post-operative RT +/- chemotherapy is occasionally indicated for adverse pathologic features.

TABLE 43.1: Cervical Cancer General Treatment Paradigm[1]

Early Stage	
IA1 (Non-fertility sparing)	Extrafascial hysterectomy (Class I) or brachytherapy alone
IA1 (Fertility sparing)	w/o LVSI: CKC w/ 3-mm negative margins w/ LVSI: CKC w/ 3-mm negative margins + PLND (+/- PALNS) OR Radical trachelectomy + PLND (+/- PALNS)
IA2 (Non-fertility sparing)	Modified radical hysterectomy (Class II) + PLND (+/- PALNS) OR Pelvic EBRT + brachytherapy
IA2 (Fertility sparing)	CKC w/ 3-mm negative margins + PLND (+/- PALNS) OR Radical trachelectomy + PLND (+/- PALNS)
IB1 or IIA1 (Non-fertility sparing)	Radical hysterectomy (Class III) + PLND (+/- PALNS) OR Definitive EBRT + brachytherapy +/- concurrent CHT
Small (<2 cm) IB1 only (Fertility sparing)	Radical trachelectomy + PLND (+/- PALNS)
Locally Advanced	
IB2, IIA2-IVA	Definitive EBRT + brachytherapy + concurrent CHT

EPIDEMIOLOGY: In the United States, there were estimated 12,900 new cases of and 4,100 deaths due to invasive cervical cancer in 2016.[2] Disease burden in less developed countries is much higher (~85% of new cases). With screening, precancerous lesions are diagnosed far more often than invasive lesions. Incidence and death rate have decreased steadily over decades due to screening, which detects earlier lesions. Median age is 49. There is higher incidence among Hispanic and African American women.

RISK FACTORS: HPV infection is associated with >90% of cervical cancer cases. HPV 16/18 confer highest risk of carcinogenesis and account for 65% to 70% of cases (other cancer-causing strains are 31, 33, 45, 52, 58).[3] Other risk factors include: smoking, immunocompromised status (transplant, AIDS), history of STDs, young age at first intercourse, multiple sexual partners, multiparity, low SES, diethylstilbestrol (DES) exposure in utero (associated with clear cell adenocarcinoma of cervix/vagina).

ANATOMY: Cervix: Lower part of uterus that is cylindrical in shape. Endocervical canal, lined by columnar epithelium, runs through it and connects uterine cavity to vagina. Distal part of cervix projects into vagina (called ectocervix) and is lined by squamous epithelium. Squamocolumnar junction is located at external os and is most common site for carcinogenesis. Broad and cardinal ligaments attach uterus and cervix, respectively, to pelvic sidewall. Uterosacral ligament attaches low uterus to sacrum. Lymphatic drainage of cervix is through these ligaments to following lymphatic beds: presacral, obturator, internal iliac, external iliac, common iliac, and para-aortic LNs. Most common sites of distant spread are lungs, supraclavicular LNs (via thoracic duct), bones, and liver.

PATHOLOGY: Squamous cell carcinoma (70%–75%); adenocarcinoma (20%–25%); adenosquamous (5%). Higher incidence of adenocarcinoma histologies in younger patients. Adenocarcinoma often presents with larger tumors ("barrel cervix") with higher risk of local failure. Incidence is increasing and Pap screening is less sensitive for this histology. HPV testing may increase sensitivity. Less common histologies: clear cell adenocarcinoma, small cell, neuroendocrine, sarcoma (rhabdomyosarcoma in adolescents), melanoma, adenoid cystic carcinoma.

SCREENING: Current ACOG recommendation for cervical cancer screening (2016)[4]: **Ages 21–29:** Pap test alone q3 years, HPV testing is not recommended. **Ages 30–65:** Pap test with HPV test (cotesting) every 5 years (preferred) or Pap test alone every 3 years; **≥65 years:** No further screening if no history of moderate/severe dysplasia and three negative Paps in row or two negative cotests in row within 10 years, most recent within 5 years. Having HPV vaccination does not alter screening recommendations.

CLINICAL PRESENTATION: Asymptomatic and detected on screening, abnormal vaginal discharge, postcoital bleeding, dyspareunia, pelvic pain.

WORKUP: H&P with attention to GYN history with careful abdomen/pelvic exam with attention to inferior extension into vagina, lateral extension into parametria, posterior extension into uterosacral ligament or rectum, examine supraclavicular and inguinal LNs. Smoking cessation counseling; consider HIV testing.

Labs: CBC/CMP, pregnancy test.

Pathology: Colposcopy with cervical biopsy, cold-knife conization (CKC) if cervical biopsy is inadequate to determine DOI or if part of lesion is not well visualized on colposcopy or as definitive procedure in select early cases desiring fertility preservation. EUA with cystoscopy/rectosigmoidoscopy (for advanced disease or if bladder or rectal extension is suspected), ureteral stent placement if necessary.

Imaging: PET/CT (nodal staging),[5] pelvic MRI (to delineate local disease extent and guide decisions on fertility vs. non-fertility sparing approaches). As per FIGO only following studies are allowed to influence staging: colposcopy, CKC, cystoscopy, rectosigmoidoscopy, CXR, intravenous pyelogram (IVP).

PROGNOSTIC FACTORS: Stage, age, tumor size (≥4 cm worse), lymph node involvement, LVSI, persistent uptake on post-treatment PET/CT,[6] prolonged on treatment time (>56 days), low hemoglobin (<10 g/dL).

STAGING

TABLE 43.2: AJCC 8th ed. (2017) Staging for Cervical cancer		
AJCC		**FIGO**
T1	**IA Confined to cervix, microscopic lesion** **1a1** ≤ 3 mm DOI, ≤7 mm in horizontal spread **1a2** 3-5 mm DOI, ≤7 mm in horizontal spread	**I**
	IB Confined to cervix, clinically visible **1b1** ≤4 cm **1b2** >4 cm	
T2	**II Extension beyond uterus, but not to side wall or lower 1/3 vagina** **2a1** ≤ 4 cm, clinically visible **2a2** >4 cm **2b** Parametrial invasion	**II**
T3	**a** Involves lower 1/3 vagina, no extension to pelvic side wall **b** Extends to pelvic side wall and/or causes hydronephrosis or non-functioning kidney	**III**
T4	• Invasion of bladder, rectum, and/or extends beyond true pelvis	**IVA**
N0	• No regional LNs	
N0 (i+)	• Isolated tumor cells <0.2 mm	
N1	• Regional LNs (including para-aortic)	
M0	• No distant metastasis	
M1	• Distant metastasis	**IVB**
Significant changes from 7th Edition include: para-aortic nodes no longer staged as M1, N1 removed from FIGO IIIB.		

TREATMENT PARADIGM

Observation: Please refer to current ACOG guidelines on management for ASCUS, LSIL, HSIL, ASC-H, AGC.

Prevention: ACS, CDC, and ACOG recommend routine vaccination of 11- to 12-year-old boys and girls with 9-valent HPV vaccine (covers: 6, 11, 16, 18, 31, 33, 45, 52, 58), with "catch-up" vaccination through age 26. HPV 6 and 11 cause ~90% cases of anogenital warts.

Surgery: Reserved mainly for IA1-IB1 and IIA. BSO is optional, but spared when fertility preservation is desired. Goal of up-front surgery is to select patients at low risk of needing adjuvant radiation since bi-modality therapy increases morbidity.

Cold Cone Biopsy (CKC): Removal of cone-shaped piece of tissue containing ectocervix and endocervical canal en bloc with scalpel to avoid electrosurgical artifact. This facilitates accurate margin status assessment.

Radical trachelectomy: Fertility-sparing surgery that removes cervix, upper vagina, and parametria, while leaving uterine body in place. Cerclage or "purse-string stitch" is made at distal end of uterine body.

Class I aka "simple" or "extrafascial" hysterectomy: Removal of uterus and cervix, parametria left intact.

Class II aka "modified-radical" hysterectomy: Removes uterus, cervix, 1 to 2 cm vagina, and WLE of parametria.

Class III aka "radical" hysterectomy: Removal of uterus, cervix, ¼ to 1/3 of vagina, parametria divided at pelvic sidewall or sacral origin.

Adjuvant hysterectomy: Not generally performed, no additional benefit seen in DFS and OS.[7] Caveat: Persistent metabolic activity following up-front RT or chemoRT, and otherwise nonmetastatic, surgery is often performed as salvage in the hope of improving outcomes.

Chemotherapy

Definitive: Concurrent CHT with RT for locally advanced disease improves DFS and OS survival over RT alone (see the following). Weekly cisplatin 40 mg/m² has become standard of care. Common alternative is cisplatin/5-FU. Other concurrent regimens: weekly cisplatin + gemcitabine (increased pCR rate, PFS, and OS compared to cisplatin alone at the cost of very high acute toxicity)[8] and weekly cisplatin + bevacizumab (evaluated in RTOG 0417, proved to be tolerable with encouraging results, OS of 81%).[9]

Adjuvant: Concurrent CHT with postoperative RT improves OS in patients with positive margins, parametrial involvement, and positive lymph nodes (see the following). Adjuvant CHT following definitive chemoRT is active area of study (OUTBACK Trial— GOG 274/RTOG 1174/ANZGOG0902, which is phase III trial of definitive cisplatin with RT randomized to +/- adjuvant carboplatin/paclitaxel x 4).

Metastatic: Doublet CHT shows better outcomes than single-agent therapy.[10] GOG 240 showed significant improvement in PFS (2 months) and OS (3.7 months) with addition of bevacizumab to cisplatin/paclitaxel or topotecan/paclitaxel.[11]

Radiation

Definitive EBRT

Indications: EBRT is indicated in all cases stage ≥IA2 treated nonoperatively. Ensure coverage of uterus, cervix, parametria, uterosacral ligament, lymph nodes at risk determined by imaging and/or surgical nodal staging. Give sufficient vaginal margin (2–3 cm below inferior most extent of gross disease). For LN negative cases, cover external and internal iliac, obturator, and presacral LNs (superior border L4-5, some routinely cover common iliac LNs). For pelvic LN+, add common iliac coverage. For high pelvic LN+, extended field RT to renal vessels or higher is indicated. Add inguinal coverage for distal 1/3 vaginal extension.

Dose: 45 Gy/25 fx. Consider conformal boost to 50 to 54 Gy for parametrial involvement or grossly involved LNs. For bulky lymph nodes theoretically requiring ≥65–66 Gy to control, consider excision followed by microscopic dose RT. Central primary tumor is boosted to 80 Gy (small volume) or 85 to 90 Gy (large volume) with brachytherapy (see the following). Use of IMRT for intact cervix is controversial and evolving. If considering IMRT in definitive setting, it is important to have thorough imaging workup to understand full extent of disease, contouring must be complete and accurate, and one must account for pelvic organ motion due to bowel/bladder filling.[12]

Postoperative EBRT

Indications: Recommended following hysterectomy for those at higher risk for recurrence. Post-op RT alone recommended for any two of three Sedlis risk factors (simplified): LVSI, middle or deep 1/3 stromal invasion and tumor size ≥4 cm. Rotman update showed RT improved outcomes in adenocarcinoma or adenosquamous histology as well (see the following). Add concurrent CHT for 3 Ps: positive LNs, positive surgical margins, and parametrial involvement (see Peters later). Consider vaginal brachytherapy boost for close or positive vaginal margin or deep 1/3 stromal invasion.

Dose: 45–50.4 Gy/25–28 fx. IMRT reduces small bowel and iliac crest (bone marrow) dose, especially when treating extended field to cover PA LNs and/or when boosting grossly involved nodes.[13] IMRT is more commonly used in postoperative setting.[14] See RTOG 0418 and accompanying atlas for details.

Brachytherapy: Can be used as monotherapy for select early-stage cases (IA1), but more commonly following pelvic EBRT to boost gross residual primary to curative intent dose. Vaginal cuff brachytherapy considered postoperatively following EBRT as vaginal apex boost in cases of close or positive vaginal margin. Most commonly used with definitive EBRT. EBRT + brachytherapy improves OS over EBRT alone even in setting of concurrent CHT.[15] Proper applicator placement and dosing are critical to achieving optimal outcomes.[16] Repeat clinical exam and imaging prior to first insertion allows selection of applicator. Generally, intracavitary therapy is employed, but interstitial technique may be necessary in certain circumstances (e.g., narrow anatomy not accommodating intracavity applicator, wide lateral extent of disease, distal vaginal involvement, inaccessible cervical os). Hybrid devices exist that combine intracavitary and interstitial components. Anesthesia is often needed for patient comfort and to achieve high-quality insertion. ABS 2012 guidelines recommend 3D imaging for volume delineation and planning.[17] MRI-based planning is preferred; better coverage of tumor, while potentially limiting dose to bladder, sigmoid, and rectum as compared to conventional planning.[18] GEC-ESTRO guidelines[19] define high-risk CTV (HR-CTV) and intermediate-risk CTV (IR-CTV) for 3D planning.

Dose: Intended dose should cover ≥90% of HR-CTV (D_{90}). ABS recommends EQD2 of ≥80 Gy (~5.5 Gy x 5 fx) for <4 cm of residual disease and EQD2 of 85 to 90 Gy (~6 Gy x 5 fx) for nonresponders or ≥4 cm residual disease.[20] IR-CTV should receive ≥60 Gy. It is still required to report dose to point A.

Toxicity: Acute: Fatigue, diarrhea, rectal urgency, bloating/cramping, bladder/urethral irritation, skin erythema, and possible desquamation if inguinal LNs or distal vagina/vulva covered in fields. Late: Rectal bleeding, bowel obstruction, hematuria, fistula (GI or urinary), vaginal ulceration/necrosis (5%–10% within 1 yr, generally heals within 6 months with local care), vaginal stenosis (use dilators), infertility (~2 Gy), ovarian failure (5–10 Gy), osteopenia leading to hip and sacral insufficiency fractures.

Procedure: See *Treatment Planning Handbook*, Chapter 9.[21]

EVIDENCE-BASED Q&A

Surgical management

What factors portend higher risk of pelvic LN involvement or unfavorable outcome?

Delgado, GOG 49 (*Gynecol Oncol* 1989, PMID 2599466; Delgado *Gynecol Oncol* 1990, PMID 2227547):

Prospective registry of stage I cervical cancer patients with ≥3-mm invasion treated with radical hysterectomy with pelvic and para-aortic nodal dissection. 645 SCC patients with negative para-aortic LNs were included in this report. Factors associated with positive lymph nodes included: DOI, parametrial invasion, tumor grade and gross versus occult tumors. 3-yr disease-free interval (DFI) for positive nodes was 74% and for negative nodes was 86%. Factors associated with worse 3-yr DFI were: DOI (deep 1/3 < middle 1/3 < superficial 1/3 invasion), tumor size (occult vs. <3 cm vs. ≥3 cm), parametrial invasion, and LVSI. Led to development of GOG 92 (Sedlis) trial (see the following).

What are postoperative indications for adjuvant RT after hysterectomy?

The Sedlis trial defined these risk factors. Although inclusion criteria are challenging to remember, "any two of three risk factors" is good way of simplifying it and will often be correct. Risk factors: LVSI, middle or deep 1/3 stromal invasion, and tumor size ≥4 cm.

Sedlis, GOG 92 (*Gynecol Oncol* 1999, PMID 10329031; Update Rotman *IJROBP* 2006, PMID 16427212): Phase III PRT of 277 patients with FIGO IB cervical cancer randomized to radical hysterectomy + pelvic LND +/− adjuvant RT. Postoperatively, patients had negative nodes and (a) +LVSI and deep 1/3 stromal invasion; (b) +LVSI, middle 1/3 stromal invasion, and tumor ≥2 cm; (c) +LVSI, superficial 1/3, and tumor ≥5 cm; OR (d) no LVSI, deep or middle 1/3, and tumor ≥4 cm. Whole-pelvis RT given 4 to 6 weeks postoperatively to 46–50.4 Gy/23–28 fx. RT decreased local recurrence (28%–15%, p = .019) and improved RFS (79%–88%, p = .008). At longer term follow-up, LR benefit persisted and post-op RT also decreased risk of recurrence for adenocarcinoma/adenosquamous histologies (44% to 9%).

What factors postoperatively are indications for adjuvant chemoRT rather than RT alone?

The Peters criteria include any one of three factors ("three Ps"): positive margins, parametrial involvement, and positive nodes and serve as indications for adjuvant chemoRT.

Peters, GOG 109 (*JCO* 2000, PMID 10764420; Monk *Gynecol Oncol* 2005, PMID 15721417): Phase III PRT of 243 patients with FIGO IA2-IIA cervical cancer with positive margins, positive pelvic nodes or microscopic parametrial involvement randomized to adjuvant RT 49.3 Gy/29 fx with or without concurrent cisplatin 70 mg/m^2 and 5-FU 1,000 mg/m^2/day over 96 hr. Four cycles of CHT were given, first two concurrent with RT. 95% were FIGO IB. **Conclusions: CHT improved OS (71%–81%, p = .007) and PFS (63%–80%, p = .003). Subsequent retrospective analysis by Monk questioned CHT benefit for smaller (≤2 cm) tumors and for patients with only one LN+.**

Should FIGO IB-IIA patients be managed with surgery or RT?

Stage IA patients can easily be managed with extrafascial hysterectomy and stage IIB-IVA are typically better candidates for chemoRT given extent of disease. However, management of stage IB-IIA tumors is challenging and patient-specific. Main advantages of surgery over RT are preserved sexual and ovarian function and elimination of secondary malignancy risk.

Landoni, Italian Trial (*Lancet* 1997, PMID 9284774): Phase III PRT of 343 patients with FIGO stage IB or IIA cervical cancer randomized to radical hysterectomy or definitive RT. 69% of IBs were ≤4 cm. EBRT was 40 to 53 Gy followed by Cs-137 LDR implant to 70 to 90 Gy to point A. When lymphangiography showed common iliac or PA LNs+, 45 Gy was given to these beds; involved LNs boosted another 5 to 10 Gy. In surgical arm, adjuvant RT recommended for >pT2a disease, <3 mm of "safe" cervical stroma, tumor cut-through or positive nodes. Adjuvant RT was 50.4 Gy to WP (+/− 45 Gy to PA LNs based on pathologic involvement). Median FU was 87 months. Identical 5-yr OS and DFS in both groups, 83% and 74%, respectively. Recurrence rates were 25% in surgery group and 26% in RT group. Severe toxicity was seen in 28% of surgery group and 12% of RT group (p = .0004). Adenocarcinoma had inferior outcomes with RT as compared to surgery (DFS 66% vs. 47%, p = .05; OS 70% vs. 59%, p = .02). **Conclusion: Both surgery and RT are options for stage IB-IIA cervical cancer. Although RT may be better tolerated, surgery may improve outcomes for adenocarcinoma. Toxicity with combined treatment is worse than RT alone.**

Does adjuvant hysterectomy following RT improve overall survival?

Keys, GOG 71 (*Gynecol Oncol* 2003, PMID 12798694): Phase III PRT of 256 patients with FIGO IB "suboptimal or bulky" (current IB2) cervical cancer randomized to RT +/– adjuvant simple extrafascial hysterectomy. Whole-pelvis RT was 40 Gy for RT arm and 45 Gy for hysterectomy arm; both were followed by intracavitary boost to 40 Gy (RT only arm) or 30 Gy (hysterectomy arm) to point A. Extrafascial hysterectomy was performed 2 to 6 weeks later. No difference in OS (58% vs. 56%) or PFS (62% vs. 53%, $p = .09$). 10% grade 3 to 4 toxicity in both arms. Interaction was demonstrated with tumor sizes of 4, 5 and 6 cm possibly benefitting from surgery. **Conclusion: Adjuvant hysterectomy did not improve survival.**

Definitive management

Is there benefit for concurrent CHT in addition to RT compared to RT (EFRT) alone?

Yes. Based on mounting evidence, NCI issued clinical alert in 1999 recommending concurrent cisplatin be administered with RT for invasive cervical cancer. In addition to the following classic trials, there have been several randomized trials and meta-analyses demonstrating DFS and OS benefit for concurrent chemoRT over RT alone in invasive cervical cancer.[22,23]

Morris, RTOG 9001 (*NEJM* 1999, PMID 10202164; Update Eifel *JCO* 2004, PMID 14990643): Phase III PRT of 389 cervical cancer patients, stage IIB-IV or stage IB/IIA with tumor size ≥5 cm or biopsy-proven pelvic nodal metastasis randomized to EFRT or whole-pelvis RT with concurrent cisplatin 75 mg/m² and 5-FU 4,000 mg/m² over 96 hr for three cycles given every 3 weeks. Patients in CHT arm were treated from L4/5 interspace down to midpubis or 4 cm below distal edge of tumor. Patients in EFRT arm received RT to L1/2 interspace. Both arms received 45 Gy/25 fx. Updated results with MFU of 6.6 yrs showed 8-year OS improved from 41% to 67% with CHT. Late toxicity was similar. 5-yr LR and DM were also improved. **Conclusions: Concurrent cisplatin/5-FU improved OS without significant increase in late effects.**

Keys, GOG 123 (*NEJM* 1999, PMID 10202166): Phase III PRT of 369 women with bulky IB cervical cancer (current IB2) w/o radiographic lymphadenopathy treated with RT (45 Gy + LDR boost) +/– concurrent CHT (weekly cisplatin 40 mg/m² for up to six cycles) followed by extrafascial hysterectomy. PFS and OS were improved in CHT group (PFS HR 0.51, OS HR 0.54, both $p < .01$). **Conclusion: Concurrent cisplatin improves OS.**

To whom should concurrent CHT be added?

NCCN recommends addition of concurrent platinum-based CHT for "bulky" tumors (stage IB2, IIA2, and higher). For stage IB1 and IIA1, CHT is optional. For IA1 with LVSI or IA2 tumors, surgery is good option, but if treated nonoperatively, CHT can be omitted.[1]

What is standard concurrent CHT regimen?

Multiple single- and multiagent regimens have been studied but currently single-agent cisplatin, given weekly, is most common. Cisplatin/5-FU is common alternative.

Rose, GOG 120 (*NEJM* 1999, PMID 10202165; Update Rose *JCO* 2007, PMID 17502627): Three-arm PRT of 526 women with stage IIB-IVA cervical carcinoma without para-aortic involvement randomized to either concurrent cisplatin (40 mg/m² weekly for 6 weeks), concurrent hydroxyurea or combination cisplatin, 5-FU, and hydroxyurea. EBRT delivered to dose of 40.8 Gy/24 fx (or 51 Gy/30 fx for stages IIB, IIIB-IVA) followed by brachytherapy boost. Superior border of pelvic field was L4/5 interspace. MFU was 35 months. Hydroxyurea alone arm demonstrated worse PFS and OS, but cisplatin and multiagent arms were similar. Acute toxicity was worse in three-drug arm. **Conclusion: Cisplatin-based chemoRT improves PFS and OS. No increased late toxicity seen at long-term follow-up.**

What is impact of overall treatment time (OTT) on outcomes of patients treated definitively?

OTT for EBRT + brachytherapy should be ≤56 days.[24] Other OTT limits have been identified: ≤49 days[25]; ≤63 days.[26] Brachytherapy should begin no more than 1 to 7 days post-EBRT if downsizing of bulky disease is required. Alternatively, for favorable anatomy or small primary tumor, practitioners can interdigitate brachytherapy during last couple weeks of EBRT. It is generally recommended to avoid CHT and EBRT administration on brachytherapy days.

Is there benefit to IMRT in postoperative setting?

An early report of phase III data confirms benefit, safety, and efficacy of IMRT for gynecologic malignancies after hysterectomy.

Klopp, RTOG 1203/TIME-C (ASTRO 2016, Abstract #5): Phase III PRT of patient-reported toxicity and QOL during post-op pelvic IMRT versus conventional 4-field RT (included patients with cervical and endometrial cancer). Cisplatin was given based on disease characteristics. 5 weeks from start of RT, conventional arm experienced more high-level adverse events by PRO-CTCAE for diarrhea/fecal incontinence and greater decline in FACT-Cx score.

Chopra, TATA Memorial, India (ASTRO 2015, Abstract #8): Phase III PRT of 3DCRT versus IG-IMRT in pts undergoing adjuvant (chemo)RT. Primary aim: reduce grade ≥2 late bowel toxicity. 120 pts enrolled, MFU 20 months. Late grade ≥2 bowel toxicity was 25% versus 11.4% ($p = .13$) and late grade ≥3 bowel toxicity was 17.6% versus 3.2% ($p = .02$). **Conclusion: No difference in late grade ≥2 bowel effects, but late grade ≥3 was improved with use of IG-IMRT.**

What are differences between high-dose rate (HDR) and low-dose rate (LDR) brachytherapy?

LDR is generally administered over 1 to 2 fx, each over 1 to 3 days during which patient stays on strict bed rest with applicator and sources held in place. Despite best efforts, it is difficult to keep patients comfortable and immobilized for prolonged period of time. Change in applicator position can lead to changes in dose distribution. RT exposure to health care personnel is also major issue. Main theoretical advantage to LDR over HDR is much lower dose rate, which allows for enhanced sublethal damage repair. Concerns over years about HDR leading to increased toxicity have not consistently been borne out in studies.[27] HDR, used by 85% of surveyed U.S. institutions,[28] requires more frequent insertions, but treatment time is short (~10 min). Remote afterloading by and large eliminates exposure risk to health care personnel. Several different dwell positions and times allow for shaping of dose to treat target and avoid OARs. PDR (pulsed dose-rate) used in some institutions combines advantages of LDR and HDR. LDR: Dose rate 0.6 to 0.8 Gy/hr, generally with Cs-137 source, T½ = 30 years, β-decay, energy 662 keV. HDR: Dose rate >12 Gy/hr with Ir-192 source, T½ = 74 days, γ-decay with ~380 keV.

What is difference between brachytherapy dose prescriptions to HR-CTV versus point A?

Before CT/MRI were readily available, applicator placement was confirmed via AP and lateral films. Dose prescription was to 2D point (2 cm superior and 2 cm lateral to os, in plane of tandem), roughly corresponding to medial aspect of broad ligament (where uterine artery and ureter cross). Dose was estimated to point B (5 cm lateral to midline at level of point A), which represented pelvic sidewall/obturator LNs. Based on ICRU 38 report, max doses to bladder and rectum were recorded at following points: Bladder: posterior surface of Foley balloon on lateral film; Rectum: 0.5 cm posterior to vaginal wall at intersection of tandem and ovoids/ring. CT/MRI studies have shown that adequate dose to point does not always indicate good coverage of HR-CTV[29] and ICRU bladder and rectal points do not always accurately estimate max doses to these OARs[30,31]. In volumetric planning era, targets (HR-CTV, IR-CTV) and OARs (bladder, rectum, sigmoid, small bowel) can be accurately contoured in 3D and dose to these structures evaluated spatially and quantitatively using DVHs. Dose distribution during planning can be modified to adequately cover target while avoiding OARs. This is now the preferred method of planning/reporting.

REFERENCES

1. National Comprehensive Cancer Network. Cervical cancer (Version I.2017). https://www.nccn.org

2. National Cancer Institute: Surveillance, Epidemiology and End Results Program. Cancer Stat Facts: Cervix Uteri Cancer. https://seer.cancer.gov/statfacts/html/cervix.html

3. Cancer NCI-C. Causes and Prevention–HPV and Cancer. https://www.cancer.gov/about-cancer/causes-prevention/risk/infectious-agents/hpv-fact-sheet

4. Gynecologists TACoOa. Cervical Cancer Screening. http://www.acog.org/Patients/FAQs/Cervical-Cancer-Screening

5. Tsai CS, Lai CH, Chang TC, et al. Prospective randomized trial to study impact of pretreatment FDG-PET for cervical cancer patients with MRI-detected positive pelvic but negative para-aortic lymphadenopathy. *Int J Radiat Oncol Biol Phys.* 2010;76(2):477–484.

6. Schwarz JK, Siegel BA, Dehdashti F, Grigsby PW. Metabolic response on post-therapy FDG-PET predicts patterns of failure after RTy for cervical cancer. *Int J Radiat Oncol Biol Phys.* 2012;83(1):185–190.

7. Keys HM, Bundy BN, Stehman FB, et al. Radiation therapy with and without extrafascial hysterectomy for bulky stage IB cervical carcinoma: randomized trial of Gynecologic Oncology Group. *Gynecol Oncol.* 2003;89(3):343–353.

8. Duenas-Gonzalez A, Cetina-Perez L, Lopez-Graniel C, et al. Pathologic response and toxicity assessment of chemoRTy with cisplatin versus cisplatin plus gemcitabine in cervical cancer: randomized phase II study. *Int J Radiat Oncol Biol Phys.* 2005;61(3):817–823.

9. Schefter T, Winter K, Kwon JS, et al. RTOG 0417: efficacy of bevacizumab in combination with definitive radiation therapy and cisplatin CHT in untreated patients with locally advanced cervical carcinoma. *Int J Radiat Oncol Biol Phys.* 2014;88(1):101–105.

10. Long HJ, 3rd, Bundy BN, Grendys EC, Jr., et al. Randomized phase III trial of cisplatin with or without topotecan in carcinoma of uterine cervix: Gynecologic Oncology Group Study. *J Clin Oncol.* 2005;23(21):4626–4633.

11. Tewari KS, Sill MW, Long HJ, 3rd, et al. Improved survival with bevacizumab in advanced cervical cancer. *N Engl J Med.* 2014;370(8):734–743.

12. Lim K, Small W, Jr., Portelance L, et al. Consensus guidelines for delineation of clinical target volume for intensity-modulated pelvic RTy for definitive treatment of cervix cancer. *Int J Radiat Oncol Biol Phys.* 2011;79(2):348–355.

13. Vargo JA, Kim H, Choi S, et al. Extended field intensity modulated radiation therapy with concomitant boost for lymph node-positive cervical cancer: analysis of regional control and recurrence patterns in positron emission tomography/computed tomography era. *Int J Radiat Oncol Biol Phys.* 2014;90(5):1091–1098.

14. Klopp AH, Moughan J, Portelance L, et al. Hematologic toxicity in RTOG 0418: phase 2 study of postoperative IMRT for gynecologic cancer. *Int J Radiat Oncol Biol Phys.* 2013;86(1):83–90.

15. Gill BS, Lin JF, Krivak TC, et al. National Cancer Data Base analysis of radiation therapy consolidation modality for cervical cancer: impact of new technological advancements. *Int J Radiat Oncol Biol Phys.* 2014;90(5):1083–1090.

16. Viswanathan AN, Moughan J, Small W, Jr., et al. Quality of cervical cancer brachytherapy implantation and impact on local recurrence and disease-free survival in radiation therapy oncology group prospective trials 0116 and 0128. *Int J Gynecol Cancer.* 2012;22(1):123–131.

17. Viswanathan AN, Thomadsen B, American Brachytherapy Society Cervical Cancer Recommendations C, American Brachytherapy S. American Brachytherapy Society consensus guidelines for locally advanced carcinoma of cervix. Part I: general principles. *Brachytherapy.* 2012;11(1):33–46.

18. Zwahlen D, Jezioranski J, Chan P, et al. Magnetic resonance imaging-guided intracavitary brachytherapy for cancer of cervix. *Int J Radiat Oncol Biol Phys.* 2009;74(4):1157–1164.

19. Potter R, Haie-Meder C, Van Limbergen E, et al. Recommendations from gynaecological (GYN) GEC ESTRO working group (II): concepts and terms in 3D image-based treatment planning in cervix cancer brachytherapy-3D dose volume parameters and aspects of 3D image-based anatomy, radiation physics, radiobiology. *Radiother Oncol.* 2006;78(1):67–77.

20. Viswanathan AN, Beriwal S, De Los Santos JF, et al. American Brachytherapy Society consensus guidelines for locally advanced carcinoma of cervix. Part II: high-dose–rate brachytherapy. *Brachytherapy.* 2012;11(1):47–52.

21. Videtic GMM, Woody N, Vassil AD. *Handbook of Treatment Planning in Radiation Oncology.* 2nd ed. New York, NY: Demos Medical; 2015.

22. Green JA, Kirwan JM, Tierney JF, et al. Survival and recurrence after concomitant CHT and RTy for cancer of uterine cervix: systematic review and meta-analysis. *Lancet.* 2001;358(9284):781–786.

23. ChemoRTy for Cervical Cancer Meta-Analysis C. Reducing uncertainties about effects of chemoRTy for cervical cancer: systematic review and meta-analysis of individual patient data from 18 randomized trials. *J Clin Oncol.* 2008;26(35):5802–5812.

24. Song S, Rudra S, Hasselle MD, et al. Effect of treatment time in locally advanced cervical cancer in era of concurrent chemoRTy. *Cancer.* 2013;119(2):325–331.

25. Perez CA, Grigsby PW, Castro-Vita H, Lockett MA. Carcinoma of uterine cervix: I. impact of prolongation of overall treatment time and timing of brachytherapy on outcome of radiation therapy. *Int J Radiat Oncol Biol Phys.* 1995;32(5):1275–1288.

26. Chen SW, Liang JA, Yang SN, et al. adverse effect of treatment prolongation in cervical cancer by high-dose-rate intracavitary brachytherapy. *Radiother Oncol.* 2003;67(1):69–76.

27. Liu R, Wang X, Tian JH, et al. High dose rate versus low dose rate intracavity brachytherapy for locally advanced uterine cervix cancer. *Cochrane Database Syst Rev.* 2014(10):CD007563.

28. Viswanathan AN, Erickson BA. Three-dimensional imaging in gynecologic brachytherapy: survey of American Brachytherapy Society. *Int J Radiat Oncol Biol Phys.* 2010;76(1):104–109.

29. Potter R, Kirisits C, Fidarova EF, et al. Present status and future of high-precision image-guided adaptive brachytherapy for cervix carcinoma. *Acta Oncologica.* 2008;47(7):1325–1336.

30. Pelloski CE, Palmer M, Chronowski GM, et al. Comparison between CT-based volumetric calculations and ICRU reference-point estimates of radiation doses delivered to bladder and rectum during intracavitary RTy for cervical cancer. *Int J Radiat Oncol Biol Phys.* 2005;62(1):131–137.

31. Hashim N, Jamalludin Z, Ung NM, et al. CT based 3-dimensional treatment planning of intracavitary brachytherapy for cancer of cervix: comparison between dose-volume histograms and ICRU point doses to rectum and bladder. *Asian Pac J Cancer Prev.* 2014;15(13):5259–5264.

44: ENDOMETRIAL CANCER

Shireen Parsai, Jonathan Sharrett, and Sudha R. Amarnath

> **QUICK HIT:** Endometrial cancer is the most common gynecologic malignancy in the United States. Medically operable pts should undergo TAH/BSO (or radical hysterectomy if cervical stromal involvement) with peritoneal cytology. Need for pelvic and para-aortic lymphadenectomy for staging is controversial and could be considered for risk factors such as large, deeply invasive, or high-grade tumors. Postoperative management is dictated by pathologic features. Pts are grouped into low-, intermediate-, or high-risk groups, which were defined by GOG 33, GOG 99, and PORTEC studies. Management paradigm for locally advanced endometrial cancer is evolving but generally consists of surgery followed by combination chemoRT.

TABLE 44.1: General Treatment Paradigm for Endometrial Cancer (see ASCO/ASTRO guidelines for details)[1,2]

Stage	Adjuvant Treatment Options (After TAH/BSO)
Stage IA, grade I–II	Observation*
Stage IA, grade III or stage IB, grade I–II	Favor vaginal cuff brachytherapy**
Stage IB, grade III	Favor pelvic RT
Stage II	Pelvic RT + VBT boost ± CHT
Stage III–IV	ChemoRT vs. CHT +/– tumor-directed RT
Medically inoperable	Tumor-directed EBRT to uterus, cervix, upper vagina, pelvic LN, other involved areas (45–50.4 Gy) + intracavitary boost ± CHT

*Can consider vaginal cuff brachytherapy if higher risk features (age >60, LVSI).
**Can consider pelvic RT if other high-risk factors are present (age >60, LVSI) and surgical staging was inadequate.

EPIDEMIOLOGY: Endometrial cancer is the most common gynecologic malignancy in the United States (note: cervical cancer is the second most common gynecologic malignancy), with >60,000 new cases and >10,000 deaths per year (second most common cause of gynecologic cancer deaths).[3] Lifetime risk of endometrial cancer is 2.8%.[4] Worldwide, endometrial cancer represents the second most common gynecologic cancer after cervical cancer.[5] Median age at diagnosis is 62 years of age with 7% of cases occurring in pts <45 years of age.[4]

RISK FACTORS: Main risk factor is excess of endogenous/exogenous estrogen without opposing progestin: (a) *physiologic*: obesity, nulliparity, early menarche, and late menopause;[6-8] (b) *pathologic*: diabetes mellitus, polycystic ovarian syndrome[6,8]; (c) *exposure*: unopposed estrogen therapy, tamoxifen[9]; (d) *protective*: combined OCPs, progestin, exercise[6,10]; (e) *family_history/genetics*: Lynch II, subset of hereditary nonpolyposis colorectal cancer (aka HNPCC) has been associated with increased risk of endometrial cancer. HNPCC is autosomal dominant mutation in DNA mismatch repair genes (MMR). HNPCC increases lifetime risk of endometrial cancer to 27% to 71% as compared to 3% lifetime risk in general population.[11,12] In pts diagnosed with endometrial cancer <50 years of age, consider screening for HNPCC.[13] Screening for endometrial cancer recommended as follows for this patient population. Prophylactic TAH/BSO can be considered for carriers.[14]

ANATOMY: Uterine corpus is defined as upper 2/3 of uterus above internal cervical os (composed of fundus and body). Cervix and lower uterine segment comprise lower 1/3 of uterus. Oviducts (aka fallopian tubes) and round ligaments enter uterus at upper outer corners (cornu). Fundus and body of uterus are separated by line connecting tubo-uterine orifices. Uterine wall is composed of endometrium, myometrium, and serosa from innermost to outermost layers. There are three major ligaments that support the uterus including the broad ligament, uterosacral ligament, and transverse (aka Mackendrodt's or Cardinal) ligament.

Lymphatics: Regional lymphatics include bilateral parametrial, obturator, internal iliac (aka hypogastric), external iliac, common iliac, para-aortic (PA), presacral, and sacral.[3,15,16] Fundal lesions can drain directly to para-aortic lymph nodes whereas cervical lesions drain laterally to parametrium, obturator, and pelvic nodes.

PATHOLOGY: Two distinct pathogenic types have been described:

- **Type I** (~80%): Favorable course, presents at early stage. Grade 1-2. Endometrioid histology. Estrogen-responsive (and therefore main risk factors are related to excess of estrogen without opposing progestin as described previously). Diploid. Type I malignancies are thought to have multistep process leading to carcinogenesis: simple endometrial hyperplasia progresses to complex atypical hyperplasia, which becomes precursor lesion, and subsequently develops into endometrial intraepithelial neoplasia (EIN), which ultimately becomes endometrial carcinoma.[17]
- **Type II** (10%–20%): Aggressive course. Grade 3. Nonendometrioid histologies including serous, clear cell. Independent of estrogen or endometrial hyperplasia and develops from atrophic endometrium. Aneuploid. *TP53* is mutated early (81% of cases) and may account for different rates of progression in these two subtypes.[6,18,19]

In addition to appropriate staging, grade of tumor must also be reported. Grading system reports degree of glandular differentiation (which is described as percentage of nonsquamous or nonmorular solid growth pattern) and corresponds to aggressiveness of tumor. **Grade 1, 2, and 3 tumors have ≤5%, 6% to 50%, and >50% nonsquamous or nonmorular solid growth patterns respectively**. In addition, papillary serous and clear cell histologies are considered grade 3. Note: nuclear atypia out of proportion to architectural grade raises grade by 1 for grade 1 and 2 tumors.[3,19] More recently, "MELF" pattern (microcystic, elongated, and fragmented) has been described as correlating with more advanced pathologic features and may necessitate nodal staging, although its impact on survival outcomes is unclear.[20,21]

GENETICS: Many genetic mutations have been identified, most commonly in PIK3CA pathway and more specifically *PTEN* mutations, which are thought to be early event in carcinogenesis. *TP53* mutations are only seen in grade 3 endometrioid carcinomas (may represent late step in carcinogenesis though pathway not completely elucidated as of yet). 30% to 40% of cases have loss of DNA mismatch repair mechanisms resulting from loss of MLH1 promoter hypermethylation both among sporadic cases and hereditary Lynch syndrome.[6,19,22,23]

SCREENING: Cancer Genetics Consortium recommends screening for patient diagnosed with HNPCC with annual endometrial sampling and TVUS beginning at 30 to 35 years of age.[24]

CLINICAL PRESENTATION: The most common presenting symptom is vaginal bleeding (~90%). Other symptoms include abdominal/pelvic pain, abdominal distension, urinary/rectal bleeding, and constipation may be symptoms of advanced disease.[6,13,16]

WORKUP

H&P: Careful inspection of external genitalia, vagina, and cervix, rectal exam, and bimanual pelvic exam. Attention for enlargement of uterus, or tumor extension to cervix, vagina, or parametrium.

Labs: CBC; optional: LFTs and CA-125 for high-risk subtypes.[13]

Imaging: Goal is to guide surgical approach based on risk of recurrence as estimated per myometrial/cervical invasion and LN metastases. Endometrial stripe should be assessed with TVUS. If endometrial stripe is abnormally thickened, it should be further evaluated with a biopsy. Chest imaging with CXR. MRI is preferred imaging modality for preoperative local staging. However, it is *not* particularly helpful in detecting LN or peritoneal involvement and is performed only for suspicion of locally advanced disease or in medically inoperable setting. PET/CT remains best imaging modality for detecting LN metastases but is not routinely performed. May consider CT chest/abdomen/pelvis for high-grade tumors.[3,6,13]

Procedures: Gold standard is biopsy under hysteroscopy. Endometrial biopsy for histological information as preoperative evaluation. If endometrial biopsy nondiagnostic and concern for malignancy persists, fractional D&C should be performed.[6,13]

PROGNOSTIC FACTORS: Poor prognostic factors include age, grade, tumor size, LVSI, depth of invasion, grade, clear cell/papillary serous histology, lymph node involvement, and tumor involvement of lower uterine segment.[25,26]

NATURAL HISTORY: May arise from background of hyperplasia. Simple hyperplasia is associated with approximately 1% risk of malignancy, complex hyperplasia approximately 3%, simple atypia approximately 10% and complex atypia 30% to 40%. In general, complexity refers to glandular structure whereas atypia refers to cellular morphology. At diagnosis, disease is found localized/organ-confined (67%), spread to regional LN and organs (21%), and metastatic to distant sites (8%).[6] Most common metastatic sites include vagina and lung.[19] Clear cell tumors have been associated with metastases to abdominal or pelvic peritoneal surfaces or omentum.[3] The most common site of locoregional recurrence is vagina.[27]

STAGING: AJCC TNM staging system is both clinical and pathologic whereas FIGO staging system uses surgical and pathological data. Clinical staging system is assigned before CHT or RT if those are initial modalities of therapy.[3]

TABLE 44.2: AJCC 8th ed. (2017) Staging for Corpus Uteri Carcinoma and Carcinosarcoma		
AJCC		FIGO
T1	a Tumor limited to endometrium or invades <50% of myometrium	IA
	b Tumor invades ≥50% of myometrial invasion	IB
T2	• Invades cervical stroma, but does not extend beyond uterus	II
T3	a Invades serosa and/or adnexa via direct extension or metastasis*	IIIA
	b Invades vagina via direct extension or metastasis or parametrial involvement*	IIIB
N0 (i+)	• Isolated tumor cells ≤0.2 mm	
N1mi	• Positive pelvic LNs (0.2–2.0 mm)	IIIC1
N1a	• Positive pelvic LNs (>2.0 mm)	

(continued)

AJCC		FIGO
TABLE 44.2: AJCC 8th ed. (2017) Staging for Corpus Uteri Carcinoma and Carcinosarcoma		
N2mi	• Positive para-aortic LNs (with or without pelvic LNs) (0.2–2.0 mm)	IIIC2
N2a	• Positive para-aortic LNs (with or without pelvic LNs) (>2.0 mm)	
T4	• Invasion of bladder and/or bowel mucosa (bullous edema not sufficient)	IVA
M1	• Distant metastasis	IVB

Notable changes from the 7th Edition include a new definition for uterine sarcoma, endometrial intraepithelial carcinoma now considered T1, removal of Tis and new definition of N1mi/N2mi.

*Positive cytology should be reported, but it does not change stage.

FIGO 1988 system differed from the 2009 system as follows: IA: tumor limited to endometrium; IB: Invades <50% of myometrium; IC: Invades ≥50% of myometrial invasion; IIA: Endocervical glandular involvement only; IIB: Cervical stromal invasion.

TREATMENT PARADIGM

Surgery: TAH/BSO (aka simple or type I hysterectomy) is standard of care for early disease. Laparoscopic approaches are becoming increasingly utilized. Radical hysterectomy is done for cases of gross cervical invasion. Surgical staging requires evaluation of peritoneal surfaces. Omental and peritoneal biopsies are performed for high-risk disease.[6] Pelvic and PA lymphadenectomy is controversial (see the following ASTEC trial) and if performed, most appropriate technique remains unknown ranging from sentinel lymph node mapping to complete pelvic and PA lymphadenectomy. To avoid overtreatment, surgeon should consider pts at low risk for LN metastases including: (a) <50% myometrial invasion; (b) tumor size <2 cm; (c) well or moderately differentiated histology.[28,29] As per FIGO, any suspicious LNs should be removed and complete pelvic lymphadenectomy with resection of enlarged PA nodes should be performed for high-risk pts.[19]

Complications: Lymphedema (8%–50% risk depending on number of LNs removed, adjuvant CHT/RT, preoperative NSAID use).[30] Management of type II endometrial cancers include TAH/BSO, pelvic and PA lymphadenectomy, omentectomy, and peritoneal biopsies.[6]

Chemotherapy: Adjuvant CHT is *not* considered standard of care for pts w/ low or intermediate-risk disease. High-risk pts should be encouraged to participate in ongoing clinical trials. If utilized, carboplatin/paclitaxel is most common adjuvant regimen. Concurrently, weekly cisplatin is commonly delivered during RT (see the following trials).

Radiation

Indications: RT is used as adjuvant therapy after TAH/BSO or as primary therapy for pts who are not candidates for surgery. Indications for vaginal cuff brachytherapy include high-intermediate risk disease, generally defined as grade 1–2 tumors with ≥50% myometrial invasion or grade 3 tumors with <50% invasion (see the following trials and ABS guidelines[1,31]) or as boost following pelvic EBRT (not generally warranted except when risk factors such as cervical stromal invasion or positive margin). Pelvic EBRT is given to early-stage pts at high risk (grade 3 tumors with ≥50% invasion).

Dose: For vaginal cuff brachytherapy, PORTEC 2 (see the following) used 21 Gy/3 fx prescribed to 0.5-cm depth given weekly, but other regimens are also common (see ABS guidelines). As boost after EBRT, 45 to 50 Gy is given via EBRT in adjuvant setting with IMRT commonly utilized in postoperative setting.[13] For medically inoperable pts, see ABS consensus statement for guidelines.[32]

Toxicity: Acute: Fatigue, diarrhea, nausea, myelosuppression, dysuria, urinary frequency. Late: Vaginal stenosis, vaginal dryness, rarely RT cystitis, proctitis, sacral insufficiency fractures, bowel obstruction, fistula.

Procedure: See *Treatment Planning Handbook*, Chapter 9.[33]

EVIDENCE-BASED Q&A

Early-stage endometrial cancer

How are women with endometrial cancer categorized?

Endometrial cancers are historically classified into low-, intermediate-, and high-risk groups. Aalders trial (see the following) was one of first to demonstrate differences by risk group. GOG 33 (see the following) was a surgical study demonstrated that noninvasive (old stage IA) tumors were "low" risk, invasive cancers (old stage IB, IC, and occult stage IIA-B) were "intermediate" risk and any stage III–IV or invasive clear cell/papillary were "high" risk. GOG 33 further subdivided "intermediate" risk into low- and high-intermediate risk (see GOG 99 later). GOG 99 and PORTEC clarified benefit of adjuvant therapy in each of these subsets.

What pathologic findings correlate with risk of nodal involvement?

Early studies from GOG suggest that depth of invasion and grade highly correlate with nodal involvement.

Creasman, GOG 33 Staging (*Cancer* 1987, PMID 3652025): Prospective observational study of 681 women treated with TAH/BSO, pelvic, and para-aortic dissection with peritoneal cytology from 1977 to 1983. On MVA, grade, depth of invasion, and intraperitoneal disease were predictive of LN metastasis. See Table 44.3.

TABLE 44.3: Results of GOG 33 for Endometrial Cancer						
Depth of Invasion	% Para-Aortic and Pelvic LN Involvement					
	Grade 1		Grade 2		Grade 3	
	PA	Pelvic	PA	Pelvic	PA	Pelvic
Endometrium Only	0%	0%	3%	3%	0%	0%
Superficial Myometrial Invasion	1%	3%	4%	5%	4%	9%
Middle Myometrial Invasion	5%	0%	0%	9%	0%	4%
Deep Myometrial Invasion	6%	11%	14%	19%	23%	34%

Note: Risk of PA LN involvement is ⅔ risk of pelvic LN involvement, 30%–55% of +pelvic LNs have +PA LNs.

Morrow, GOG 33 (*Gynecol Oncol* 1991, PMID 1989916): Same study as the preceding but correlated surgical pathology findings and recurrence patterns prospectively. 895 pts with FIGO stage I and II (occult) of endometrioid type. (a) Isolated positive PA LNs in setting of negative pelvic LNs is uncommon (2.2%). (b) Only 5.4% (n = 48) had positive PA LNs. Of these, 47 had ≥1 of: grossly positive pelvic LNs, grossly positive adnexal mets, or deep myometrial penetration (accounted for 98% of cases with positive PA LNs and could be used to select pts for nodal staging) (c). **Conclusion: Among pts without metastases, lymphovascular space invasion, depth of invasion, and grade correlate with recurrence-free interval.** (d) LRF rate (32.4% vs. 48.4%) appears to favor adjuvant RT for pts with >⅓ myometrial invasion and Gr 2-3 tumor.

Katsoulakis, SEER (*Int J Gynaecol Obstet* 2014, PMID 25194213): SEER analysis from 1998 to 2003 ("contemporary era") including 4,052 pts. Pelvic nodal metastases identified as per Table 44.4.

TABLE 44.4: SEER Patterns of Nodal Spread					
	Grade 1		Grade 2		Grade 3	
	Pelvic	Para-aortic	Pelvic	Para-aortic	Pelvic	Para-aortic
IA	1%	0%	2%	0%	1%	1%
IB	2%	0%	3%	1%	3%	2%
IC	3%	3%	8%	5%	12%	8%
IIA	7%	3%	10%	4%	10%	5%
IIB	8%	4%	13%	8%	19%	12%

Is pelvic nodal dissection necessary in early-stage disease?

Without suspicious intraoperative lymph nodes, elective pelvic and para-aortic nodal dissection likely does not change oncologic outcomes but may help to guide treatment in few who are upgraded pathologically. Two trials did not show difference in DFS or OS.

Kitchener, ASTEC Trial (*Lancet* 2009, PMID 19070889). PRT of 1,408 women underwent TAH/BSO then randomized to +/− lymphadenectomy; 80% stage I/IIA; 40% had EBRT in both arms. MFU 37 mos. OS was similar in both arms (HR 1.04; $p = .83$). RFS was slightly better in "no lymphadenectomy" arm (HR 1.25; $p = .14$). **Conclusion: No significant OS or RFS benefit for lymphadenectomy in early stage endometrial cancer.**

Bendetti, Italian Trial (*JNCI* 2008, PMID 19033573): PRT of 514 women with clinical stage I randomized to *TAH/BSO* +/− lymphadenectomy. Excluded if grade I <50% invasion; ~80% Stage I/IIA. MFU 49 mo. 13% versus 3% of pts were found to have nodal involvement ($p < .001$). No improvement with LND in 5-yr DFS (82 vs. 81%) or 5-yr OS (90 vs. 86%). **Conclusion: LND improves staging but did not change DFS or OS.**

Which pts benefit from adjuvant RT after TAH/BSO?

Early-stage pts w/ adverse path features are at risk for extrauterine disease and recurrence. High-risk features vary but overall included: deep myometrial invasion, tumor grade, cervical involvement, older age, LVSI, tumor size (from GOG33 earlier).

Keys, GOG-99 (*Gynecol Oncol* 2004, PMID 14984936): PRT of 392 pts with "intermediate-risk" endometrial cancer evaluating TAH/BSO with pelvic and para-aortic nodal sampling, cytology randomized to no adjuvant therapy or WPRT. Eligibility: old FIGO IB-occult stage II (2009 FIGO stages IA, IB, and occult II) disease. Inclusion criteria were revised during trial to include only high-intermediate risk (HIR) subgroup (based on GOG 33): (a) age >70 yrs with one risk factor (grade 2 or 3, LVSI, outer one-third myometrial invasion), (b) age >50 yrs with two risk factors, and (c) any age with three risk factors. All others were LIR. RT 50.4 Gy/28 fx. Primary endpoint was cumulative incidence of recurrence (CIR) and study not powered for OS. MFU 69 mos. 59% of pts had stage IA disease and 82% of pts had Gr 1 or 2 disease. Greatest benefit in LR was in high-intermediate risk pts from 26% vs. 6% versus low-intermediate risk pts from 6% vs. 2%. Of three pelvic and vaginal recurrences in RT arm, two actually refused RT. RT had worse hematologic, GI, GU, and cutaneous toxicities. **Conclusion: Adjuvant RT in early-stage intermediate-risk endometrial cancer decreases risk of recurrence in HIR pts.** *Comment: Grade 2 was grouped with grade 3 even though grade 2 tends to behave more similarly to grade 1.*

TABLE 44.5: Results of GOG-99

GOG-99	2-yr Any Recurrence (All pts)	2-yr Any Recurrence for HIR Pts	4-yr OS
Surgery	12%	26%	86%
Surgery + RT	3%	6%	92%
p value	.007	.007	.557

Scholten, PORTEC 1 (*IJROBP* 2005, PMID 15927414; Update Creutzberg *IJROBP* 2011, PMID 21640520): PRT of 714 pts w/ stage I endometrial ca evaluating TAH/BSO + cytology ± pelvic RT (no IVRT or PLND). Eligibility: <½ MI and G2-3 OR ≥½ MI and G1-2 (stage IB/IC at time) endometrial ca. 99 pts w/ stage IC, G3 disease not randomized, but received post-op RT. RT 46 Gy/23 fx in two to four fields within 8 wks postop. MFU 97 mos. On MVA, RT and age <60 were favorable prognostic factors for LRR. Pts w/ ≥2 of 3 risk factors (age ≥60 y/o, >50% myometrial invasion, and Gr 3) had highest benefit from RT. In pts w/ isolated vaginal relapse, CR was obtained in 31/35 pts (89%), and 24 pts (77%) were still in CR after further f/u. 3-yr OS after vaginal relapse was 73%. On MVA of 15-year data (with 13.3 yr median follow-up), *grade 3, age >60, and invasion were prognostic for both LRR and endometrial cancer death.* Note: ~75% of LRs were in vaginal vault. On central pathology review, there was significant shift from G2 to G1. **Conclusion: Post-op RT in stage IB, G1-2 or stage IA, G2-3 endometrial ca reduces LRR with no impact on OS.** Post-op RT is *not* indicated in pts w/ stage IA, G2 disease, or for pts <60 years of age w/ stage IB, G1-2 or stage IA, G2-3 disease. OS after relapse is significantly better in pt group w/o prior RT. Treatment for vaginal relapse is effective. Pts w/ stage IB, G3 disease have high risk of early DM and endometrial ca-related death. Adjuvant WPRT should be avoided for pts at low or intermediate risk of recurrence.

TABLE 44.6: Results of PORTEC 1

15-yr Data	LRR	OS	DM	(-) Physical Function	Urinary/Bowel Symptoms	Second Malignancy
NAT	16%	60%	7%	61.60%	23.6%/14.1%	13%
WPRT	6%	52%	9%	50.50%	28.1%/19.5%	19%
p value	<.0001	.14	.26	.004	<.001	.12

Is there benefit to adding pelvic RT to vaginal brachytherapy?

Aalders, Norway (*Obstet Gynecol* 1980, PMID 6999399): PRT of 540 pts with stage I endometrial cancer evaluating TAH/BSO (without LND/sampling or peritoneal cytology) followed by VBT, then randomized to no further treatment or pelvic EBRT (4000 rads [sic] to pelvic LNs with midline block at 2000 rads [sic]). Overall, pelvic RT arm had decreased 9-yr LR (6.9%–1.9%) but more DM (5.4% vs. 9.9%). There was no difference overall in 5-yr OS. On subset analysis, pelvic RT improved 9-yr OS for pts with G3 and >50% MI or LVSI (72%–82%). **Conclusion: Only pts with Gr 3 tumors and >50% MI or LVSI may benefit from pelvic RT. All other stage I pts should get intravaginal BRT alone.**

TABLE 44.7: Results of Aalders (Norway) Trial of Pelvic RT for Endometrial Cancer

	5-yr OS	9-yr OS	LRR	DM	Deaths from DM
No pelvic RT	91%	90%	6.9%	5.4%	4.6%
Pelvic RT	89%	87%	1.9%	9.9%	9.5%
p value	NS	NS	<.01	NS	.10 > p > .05

Blake, MRC ASTEC-NCIC EN.5 Pooled Results (*Lancet* 2009, PMID 19070891): PRT study of 905 pts with *high-risk* endometrial cancer treated with TAH/BSO +/– adjuvant EBRT. Lymphadenectomy was optional (29% of pts underwent lymphadenectomy, of which 4% were found to have positive LN) and intracavitary was optional but had to be stated up front whether institution would deliver it and it had to be offered to both arms if given (used in 51% vs. 52%). High-risk disease: Gr 3, Stage IB, endocervical glandular involvement, serous papillary, or clear cell type. + PA nodes excluded. RT was 40–46 Gy/20–25 fx. Median age 65. EBRT had higher acute (60% vs. 26%) and late (7% vs. 3%) toxicity. 5-yr OS 84%, DSS 89%, RFS 78%. No diff between arms. Isolated vaginal/pelvic relapse (3.2% vs. 6.1% favoring EBRT, p = .038). **Conclusion: EBRT should not be routinely recommended for intermediate- or high-risk pts and although EBRT reduces local recurrence, it is not without toxicity.**

Kong (*J Natl Cancer Inst* 2012, PMID 22962693): Meta-analysis of seven RCTs comparing EBRT versus no EBRT (includes VBT) and one trial comparing VBT to no additional treatment. EBRT significantly reduced LRR (HR 0.36, p < .001) but did not improve OS (HR 0.99, p = .95), CSS, or DM. EBRT associated with increased severe acute and late toxicity. **Conclusion: EBRT reduces LRR but no impact on survival and is associated with significant morbidity and reduction in QOL.**

Sorbe, Swedish Intermediate Risk (*IJROBP* 2012, PMID 21676554): PRT of 527 pts randomized to TAH/BSO+VBT+/– WPRT. *Eligibility*: Stage I endometrioid histology with one RF (G3, IB, or DNA aneuploidy) RF 46 Gy + VBT or VBT alone (3 Gy x 6, 5.9 Gy x 3, or 20 G x 1 to 5 mm) 15 pelvic recurrences in VBT alone arm, one in WPRT+VBT (LR 5% vs. 1.5% at 5 years). 5-yr OS was 89% and 90% (p = .548). Deep MI was prognostic but not grade or DNA ploidy. WPRT had low toxicity (<2%) but difference favored VBT alone. **Conclusion: Even with LR benefit for WPRT+VBT, combined RT should be reserved for high-risk cases with two or more high-risk factors given toxicity and no OS benefit. VBT alone should be adjuvant treatment option for purely medium-risk cases.**

Does vaginal cuff brachytherapy reduce recurrence in low-risk women?

Sorbe, Swedish Low Risk (*Int J Gyn Cancer* 2009, PMID 19574776). PRT of 645 pts to TAH/BSO +/– VBT (HDR or LDR). *Eligibility*: FIGO 1988 Stage IA/B and G1-2. RT with Perspex applicators or ovoids Rx to 3–8 Gy with 3–6 fx 5 mm from surface. Vaginal recurrence 1.2% with VBT and 3.1% without (p = .114). Few side effects with G1-2. Toxicity at 2.8% with VBT and 0.6% without. **Conclusion: VBT is associated with nonsignificant reduction in recurrence. Observation is appropriate for this subgroup.** *Comment: Possible that certain other subgroups of low- or medium-risk pts (only stage IB, G-2, or tumors w/ LVSI, or pts w/ higher age) may benefit from vaginal brachytherapy.*

How should one select between adjuvant vaginal cuff brachytherapy and adjuvant EBRT?

Appropriate patient selection is key. Most recurrences in GOG 99 and PORTEC were in vaginal vault. Caveat: 28% were noncentral (sidewall). Also, GOG 99 pts were surgically staged. In PORTEC-2, however, after central pathology review, many of pts on study were found to be lower risk.

Nout, PORTEC-2 (*Lancet* 2010, PMID 20206777): PRT of 427 HIR pts s/p TAH/BSO (no PLND) w/ EBRT (46 Gy /23) versus VBT (21 Gy/3 fx HDR or 30 Gy LDR). *Eligibility*: Age ≥60 and IB G1-2 or IA G3; or endocervical glandular involvement grades 1-3, any age, but >½ *myometrial invasion w/ G3 excluded*. MFU 45 mo. QOL better in VBT (social function, diarrhea, fecal incontinence, and limit of ADLs). Central path review: Tumor G2 showed poor reproducibility and on re-review, many pts considered grade 1 (see Table 44.8). On MVA, high-risk profile and LVSI were only RFs for OS and RFS. **Conclusion: No**

difference in VR, OS, and DFS for VBT versus EBRT. In view of QOL benefit, VBT should be treatment for HIR endometrial cancer. Late Gr 3 GI tox was 2% versus none.

5-yr Results	VR	LRR	Pelvic Only Recurrence	DFS	OS	Gr 1-2 GI Toxicity	Path Distribution	G-1	G-2	G-3
TABLE 44.8: Results of PORTEC-2 for Endometrial Cancer										
EBRT	1.6%	2.1%	1.5%	82.7%	84.8%	53.8%	Original	48%	45%	7%
VBT	1.8%	5.1%	0.5%	78.1%	79.6%	12.6%	Review	79%	9%	12%
p value	.74	.17	.30	.74	.57	NS after 24 mos				

McMeekin, GOG 0249 (*SGO* 2014, Late-Breaking Abstract 1): PRT of TAH/BSO, then randomizing women with FIGO stage I endometrioid meeting HIR criteria as per GOG 99, all stage II, or stage I/II serous/clear cell carcinoma. After surgery randomized to whole-pelvis EBRT (45–50.4 Gy/25–28 fx) versus vaginal cuff brachytherapy followed by carboplatin/paclitaxel for three cycles given q3 weeks. Optional cuff boost in EBRT arm for stage II pts or papillary/clear cell histology. MFU 24 months. No difference in 2-yr RFS (EBRT 82% vs. 84% VBT/CHT) or OS (EBRT 93% vs. 92% VBT/CHT). No differences were seen for all subgroup recurrences (vaginal [5 vs. 3], pelvic [2 vs. 19], PA [2 vs. 3], distant [32 vs. 24]). Increased toxicities with VBT/CHT (nausea, heme, and neuropathy) versus EBRT (diarrhea). No clear subset benefiting from either regimen. **Conclusion: CHT/VCB is not superior to pelvic RT, is associated with more acute toxicity (long-term outcomes and QOL pending), and does not prevent pelvic recurrence.**

How strong of a risk factor is LVSI?

LVSI has consistently been shown to be strong risk factor for local and distant recurrence.

Bosse, Pooled PORTEC 1 & 2 (*Eur J Cancer* 2015, PMID 26049688): Pooled analysis from PORTEC-1 and PORTEC-2 showed that substantial LVSI (diffuse or multifocal LVSI as opposed to focal or no LVSI) was strongest independent prognostic factor for pelvic regional recurrence (HR 6.2), DM (HR 3.6) and OS (HR 2.0). 5-year risk of pelvic failure was 1.7%, 2.5%, and 15.3% for no, focal, and substantial LVSI, respectively. In pts with substantial LVSI, 5-yr pelvic recurrence was 4.3% after EBRT compared to 27.1% with brachytherapy alone and 30.7% after no additional treatment.

Does postoperative IMRT reduce treatment-related toxicity while maintaining control rates?

IMRT may decrease risk of bowel, bladder, rectal toxicity.

Klopp, RTOG 1203/TIME-C (*ASTRO* 2016, Abstract #5): PRT of patient-reported toxicity and QOL of during post-op pelvic IMRT versus conventional four-field RT (included pts with cervical and endometrial cancer). Cisplatin was given based on disease characteristics. 5 weeks from start of RT, conventional arm experienced more high-level adverse events by PRO-CTCAE for diarrhea/fecal incontinence and greater decline in FACT-Cx score. These differences decreased at later time points. **Conclusion: IMRT improves acute effects and QOL.**

Klopp, RTOG 0418 (*IJROBP* 2013, PMID 23582248): Phase II trial of 83 pts who underwent postoperative pelvic IMRT versus conventional four-field RT (included pts with cervical and endometrial cancer). Pts with endometrial cancer received IMRT alone, pts with cervical cancer received IMRT + weekly cisplatin. RT: IMRT to 50.4 Gy/28 fx to pelvic lymphatics and vagina. **Conclusion: In pts who received weekly cisplatin, V40 of bone**

marrow >37% was associated with grade 2 or higher hematologic toxicity compared to V40 of bone marrow <37% (75% vs. 40% respectively).

Viswanathan, RTOG 0921 (*Cancer* 2015, PMID 25847373): Phase II study of post-op IMRT w/ concurrent CDDP/bevacizumab followed by carboplatin/paclitaxel in 34 high-risk endometrial carcinoma. Eligible pts include: Gr 3/papillary serous/clear cell carcinoma w/ stage IC or IIA; Gr 2/3 w/ stage IIB; or stages III–IVA, any grade. Objectives were AEs, OS, pelvic failure, regional failure, distant failure, and DFS. Total of 30 evaluable pts; 23.3% grade ≥3 treatment-related nonhematologic toxicity within 90 days, with additional 20% within year from treatment. 2-yr OS was 96.7% and DFS was 79.1%. No in-field failures and no FIGO stage I to IIIA had recurrence after MFU of 26 months. **Conclusion: IMRT and bevacizumab is safe and effective.**

Advanced endometrial cancer

What is definition of advanced endometrial cancer?

The clearest definition of advanced endometrial cancer is any stage III–IVA although multiple trials also included high-risk early-stage pts typically defined by GOG 99 and PORTEC 1 as stage IB, grade 3, stage II, or those with aggressive histologies (papillary serous or clear cell).

Is adjuvant CHT alone superior to adjuvant RT alone for locally advanced disease?

Randall, GOG 122 (*JCO* 2006, PMID 16330675): PRT of 422 pts (396 assessable) with stage III–IV endometrial carcinoma receiving whole-abdominal RT (WART) versus doxorubicin–cisplatin (AP) CHT. *Eligibility*: Tumor invading beyond uterus s/p TAH/BSO, surgical staging w/ <2 cm residual tumor (P-A LNs allowed). RT 30 Gy/20 fx AP/PA +15 Gy boost to pelvic +/− PA LNs. AP was given every 3 weeks × seven cycles followed by one additional cycle of cisplatin (P). Median age was 63. MFU 74 mos. 50% had endometrioid histology. Most (>75%) were IIIC-IVA/B. 84% of pts completed RT, only 63% completed CHT. AP had more Gr 3-4 hematologic (88% vs. 14%), gastrointestinal, cardiac, and neurologic toxicity. However, AP improved 5-yr PFS (50% vs. 38%; *p* < .01) and OS (55% vs. 42%; *p* < .01), and reduced crude percentage of initial extra-abdominal failures (10% vs. 19%) compared to WART. There were pelvic failures in 13% of pts on WART arm and 18% of pts on AP arm, and abdominal recurrences occurred in 16% and 14%, respectively. **Conclusion: Surgical stage III or IV treated w/ AP had improved OS and PFS, but also more toxicity.** *Comment: Results were questioned because, although this was randomized trial, post hoc stage adjustment without reporting PRT endpoint (unadjusted) weakens results. Additionally, for pts with unresected lesions up to 2 cm who received RT, dose delivered would be considered inadequate, which limits findings.*

Maggi, Italy (*Br J Ca* 2006, PMID 16868539): PRT of 345 pts w/ high-risk endometrial carcinoma comparing adjuvant CHT versus RT. All pts underwent TAH/BSO and selective pelvic and PA LN sampling. *Eligibility*: FIGO stage IC G3, II G3 w/ >50% myometrial invasion, and III (224 pts) limited to pelvis. Pts randomized to RT received EBRT to 45–50 Gy to pelvis; LN+ disease also received lumbo-aortic RT to 45 Gy. Randomized to CHT received cyclophosphamide 600 mg/m², doxorubicin 45 mg/m², and cisplatin 50 mg/m² q28d x five cycles. MFU 95.5 mos. For RT and CHT, 7-yr OS was 62% for both arms, and 7-yr PFS was 56% versus 60% (ns), respectively. While nonsignificant, cumulative incidence curves of local and distant relapse favor RT for LRC and CHT for DM. **Conclusion: No difference of improvement in PFS and OS between two protocols with acceptable toxicity for both. Randomized trials of pelvic RT combined with adjuvant cytotoxic therapy compared with RT alone are eagerly awaited.**

Susumu, JGOG 2033 (*Gynecol Oncol* **2008, PMID 17996926):** Multicenter phase III PRT of adjuvant pelvic RT versus cisplatin-based CHT in pts with intermediate- and high-risk endometrioid adenocarcinoma w/ >50% MI. 385 eligible pts (193 RT vs. 192 CHT) were randomized to adjuvant pelvic RT of at least 40 Gy versus cyclophospha-mide–doxorubicin–cisplatin (CAP). *Eligibility:* >50% MI, including pts with stages IC–IIIC (only 11.9% IIIC) disease s/p TAH/BSO and surgical staging. RT 45 to 50 Gy AP/PA. CHT was given for ≥three cycles. 5-year PFS in pelvic RT and CAP groups was 83.5% and 81.8% (NS), while 5-year OS was 85.3% and 86.7% (NS). Unplanned subset analysis of high-risk subgroup consisting of (a) stage IC in >70 years of age or G3 endo-metrioid adenocarcinoma or (b) stage II or IIIA (positive cytology), showed higher PFS rate (83.8% vs. 66.2%, $p = .024$) and OS rate (89.7% vs. 73.6%, $p = .006$) for CAP CHT. **Conclusion: Adjuvant CHT may be useful as alternative to RT for HIR endometrial cancer.** *Comment: Study was not stratified for subset analysis, neither was it planned, limiting utility of this observation. Only 11.9% Stage IIIC. Randomization was not stratified by stage of disease.*

Johnson (*Gynecol Oncol* **2010, PMID 21975736):** Meta-analysis of five PRTs with over 2,000+ women comparing adjuvant CHT with any other adjuvant treatment or no other treatment. Four of these trials compared platinum-based CHT versus RT. Addition of Pt-based CHT is associated with 5% ARR for first recurrence outside pelvis and 4% ARR for relative risk of death regardless of addition of RT. **Conclusion: Postoperative plati-num CHT associated with small benefit of PFS and OS irrespective of RT.** *Comment: Analysis of pelvic rate recurrences is underpowered, with no direct comparison against RT, so cannot determine if more effective based on this. Could be alternative to RT for select pts and has added value when used with RT.*

Galaal (*Cochrane Database Syst Rev* **2014, PMID 24832785):** Pooled planned meta-anal-ysis of four RCTs involving 1,269 women treated with adjuvant CHT compared with RT or chemoRT in those with FIGO stage III and IV endometrial carcinoma. *Eligibility:* JGOG 2033, Italian trial by Maggi et al. and GOG 122 were all included. Only two of these trials (Maggi et al., GOG 122) provided survival data; thus only these two trials were combined leaving 620 evaluable pts. Of note, the fourth trial was GOG 184 PRT, which was CHT question following adjuvant RT comparing cisplatin/doxorubicin/paclitaxel versus cisplatin/doxorubicin. OS and PFS favored adjuvant CHT over RT (OS: HR 0.75, 95% CI: 0.57–0.99, and PFS: HR 0.74, 95% CI: 0.59–0.92). Sensitivity analysis for adjusted/unadjusted OS data and subgroup analysis showed results did not differ within stage III or between stage III and IV. Adverse effects were higher with CHT than RT, and no difference in treatment-related deaths. **Conclusion: Report increased survival time around 25% with adjuvant CHT versus RT in stage III/IV endometrial carcinoma. CHT versus chemoRT should be further explored with one large trial ongoing (see the following).**

Is it safe and effective to give RT along with CHT?

Multiple studies have demonstrated safety of various forms of CHT along with RT and compared to previous results, these regimens may be more effective.

Greven, RTOG 9708 (2-yr: *IJROBP* **2004, PMID 15093913; 4-yr:** *Gynecol Oncol* **2006, PMID 16545437):** Phase II study of 44 eligible pts w/ high-risk endometrial carcinoma evaluating safety and toxicity of CHT when combined w/ pelvic RT. All pts underwent TAH/BSO. *Eligibility:* Stage IB G2-3, II, or III disease. Pelvis RT consisted of 45 Gy/25 fx. CHT with cisplatin dose of 50 mg/m² was given on d 1 and 28. After pelvic RT, intra-cavitary RT was delivered with single dose LDR 20 Gy or three high-dose–rate applications totaling 18 Gy to vaginal surface. After RT, four additional courses of cis-platin 50 mg/m² and paclitaxel 175 mg/m² at 28-day intervals. Protocol completion rate was 98%. At median of 4.3-yr follow-up, maximum tolerated late toxicity was grade 1 in 16%, grade 2 in 41%, grade 3 in 16%, and grade 4 in 5%. Additionally, at 4 years pelvic, regional and distant recurrence rates were 2%, 2%, and 19%, respectively. 4-yr OS and DFS were 85% and 81%, respectively. 4-yr OS and DFS for stage III pts were 77% and 72%, respectively. No recurrences for remaining stages. **Conclusion: LRC is excellent following combined modality treatment in all pts, suggesting additive effects of CHT and RT.**

Homesley, GOG 184 (*Gynecol Oncol* 2009, PMID 19108877): PRT of 552 pts with stage III/IV (changed to exclude abdominal disease other than para-aortics) s/p hysterectomy/BSO. LN sampling was not required and pelvic/EFRT (50.4 Gy to pelvis, 43.5 Gy to para-aortics when + PA or inadequate LND) randomized to cisplatin+ doxorubicin (CD) +/− paclitaxel (P). RFS at 3 yrs: 62% for CD versus 64% for CDP. However, in subgroup analysis CDP was associated with 50% reduction in risk of recurrence or death among pts with gross residual disease (95% CI: 0.26–0.92). **Conclusion: Addition of paclitaxel to cisplatin and doxorubicin following surgery and RT was not associated with significant improvement in RFS but was associated with increased toxicity.** *Comment: Difficult to compare to GOG 122, as stage IV pts became ineligible early in GOG 184.*

Is combined chemoRT superior to either modality alone?

The preceding trials seemed to support that RT reduces locoregional failure whereas CHT reduces distant metastases. Therefore, combined chemoRT may be superior regimen, although this has not been demonstrated clearly and details on sequencing are in flux.

de Boer, PORTEC 3 (*ASCO* 2017, Abstract 5502): PRT of 686 women with high-risk endometrial cancer (FIGO stage IB, grade 3 and/or LVSI, stage II–III or serous/clear cell histology) underwent hysterectomy and randomized to either adjuvant RT or chemoRT. RT was 48.6 Gy/27, CHT was concurrent cisplatin 50 mg/m2 weeks 1 and 4 followed by adjuvant carboplatin AUC5/paclitaxel 175 mg/m2 q3 weeks for four cycles. MFU 60.2 mos. 5-yr OS 83.9% vs. 76.7% for RT vs. chemoRT (HR 0.79, 95% CI 0.57-1.12, p = .183). 5-yr FFS was 71.8% vs. 75.5% for RT vs. chemoRT, respectively. Subset analysis showed stage III pts had the greatest benefit to chemoRT. **Conclusion: ChemoRT did not improve FFS or OS but may improve FFS for stage III pts.**

Matei, GOG 255 (*ASCO* 2017, Abstract 5505): PRT of 813 women with stage III–IVA uterine cancer or stage I–II serous/clear cell (with positive cytology) randomized after optimal debulking (<2 cm residual) to either chemoRT followed by carboplatin/paclitaxel for four cycles vs. carboplatin/paclitaxel alone for six cycles. MFU 47 mos. RFS (primary endpoint) no different (HR 0.9). ChemoRT reduced vaginal (3% vs. 7%) and pelvic/paraaortic (10% vs. 21%) but distant failure more common in chemoRT arm (28% vs. 21%). Overall grade 3 toxicity less in the chemoRT arm (58% vs. 63%). **Conclusion: ChemoRT did not improve RFS in optimally debulked stage III–IVA endometrial cancer.**

Hogberg, EORTC 55991 (*ASCO* 2007, Abstract 5503): Phase III study of 382 pts s/p TAH/BSO (most w/o lymphadenectomy) + pelvic RT +/− CHT. *Eligibility*: Stage I, occult stage II, IIIA (only positive peritoneal fluid cytology) or IIIC (pelvic LN only), or any stage clear cell carcinoma, serous papillary carcinoma, or undifferentiated (anaplastic) carcinoma. Most had two or more of following: Grade 3, >50% MI, or DNA nondiploidy. RT dose was 44 Gy + optional brachytherapy boost. CHT was originally AP, then allowed carboplatin/paclitaxel, TAP or TEP. Terminated early because of slow accrual. MFU 4.3 yrs. 50% were stage IC, 50% were G3, and 92% completed EBRT. Brachytherapy given to ~40% in both arms. 27% of pts did not receive full CHT schedule. 5-yr PFS was 72% versus 79% (p = .03, ss) and OS 76% versus 83% (p = .10, ns), favoring adjuvant CHT. For endometrioid histology, PFS 73% versus 83% (p = .03) and OS 75% versus 86% (p = .08). **Conclusion: RT+CHT better than RT alone for high-risk pts, albeit no difference in OS.**

Kuoppala (*Gyn Oncol* 2008, PMID 18534669): PRT of 156 pts s/p TAH/BSO (P LND in 80%) and randomized to split-course pelvic RT (28 Gy/14 fx with 3-wk break) versus interdigitated chemoRT (28 Gy → CHT → 28 Gy → CHT, where CHT used was cisplatin/epirubicin/cyclophosphamide). *Eligibility:* Pts with (a) FIGO stage IA-B grade 3 or stage IC-IIIA grade 1-3. There was no difference in 5-yr DFS, LR, DM, or OS. **Conclusion: Adjuvant CHT failed to improve OS or lower LR rate in pts operated on and radiated for high-risk endometrial carcinoma. CHT was associated with low rate of acute toxicity but appeared to increase risk of bowel complications.**

Hogberg, Pooled results of MaNGO ILIADE-III and EORTC 55991 (*Eur J Cancer* 2010, PMID 20619634): Data from two PRTs of sequential adjuvant CHT and RT. Arm 1—adjuvant RT and arm 2—adjuvant CHT and RT. Pts with serous, clear cell, or anaplastic carcinomas were eligible regardless of risk factors; however, serous/clear cell carcinoma was excluded in ILIADE-III. RT was 45 Gy/25 fx. VBR was allowed if cervical stromal involvement. CHT was doxorubicin 60 mg/m^2 and cisplatin 50 mg/m^2 q3 weeks x three cycles. 5-yr PFS was 69% versus 78% and 5-yr OS was 75% versus 82% (p = .07) for arms 1 and 2, respectively. CSS was SS for chemoRT. Subset analysis showed no benefit to CHT for serous/clear cell carcinoma. **Conclusion: Addition of adjuvant CHT improves PFS with trend to OS improvement.** *Comment: Subset analyses was not planned and not powered to address question of endometrioid vs. serous/clear cell histology.*

What is ideal sequencing of CHT with RT?

Optimal sequencing of CHT is unclear but Geller and Secord demonstrated benefit of "sandwich" regimen (CHT->RT->CHT); however, these were small and retrospective evaluations, with imbalances in histologic subtypes between treatment groups requiring complex modeling.

Geller (*Gynecol Oncol* 2011, PMID 21239048): Phase II trial of carboplatin and docetaxel followed by RT and then consolidation CHT given in "sandwich" method for stages III, IV, and recurrent endometrial cancer (two pts). 42 pts with surgically staged III–IV (excluding IIIA from cytology alone) or biopsy-proven recurrent disease were eligible. 3 cycles of docetaxel and carboplatin followed by IFRT (45 Gy) ± brachytherapy and three additional cycles of docetaxel and carboplatin. 7 pts expired with median follow-up of 28 months. KM estimates of OS at 1, 3, and 5 years was 95%, 90%, and 71%, respectively. KM estimates of PFS at 1, 3, and 5 years were 87%, 71%, and 64%, respectively. **Conclusion: "Sandwiching" RT between CHT for advanced or recurrent endometrial cancer should be further investigated in PRTs.**

Secord (*Gynecol Oncol* 2007, PMID 17688923): RR of 356 pts from 1975 to 2006 at Duke/UNC with surgical stage III/IV with TAH/BSO +/− pelvic/PA LND followed with CHT +/− RT. Subset of 51 pts treated with "sandwich regimen" CHT->RT->CHT had highest 3-yr OS (91%) and PFS (69%) compared to nine pts treated with CHT>RT (47% and 19%) or 15 pts treated with RT>CHT (65% and 60%), respectively. **Conclusion: Promising results warrant further investigation on sequencing of therapy.** *Comment: Retrospective study, small number of pts, histology imbalance, and complex modeling of study are significant limitations.*

Secord (*Gynecol Oncol* 2009, PMID 19560193): Multicenter RR of 109 pts with surgical stage III and IV endometrial cancer treated from 1993 to 2007 who received postoperative adjuvant therapies. Subset of 44 pts (41%) received CHT followed by RT and then CHT aka "sandwich" therapy. 17% received RT followed by CHT, and 42% CHT followed by RT. **Conclusion: There was SS better 3-yr PFS (69% vs. 52% vs. 47%, p = .025) and 3-yr OS (88% vs. 57% vs. 54%) for sandwich approach (CHT>RT>CHT) versus CHT>RT**

or **RT>CHT, respectively.** *Comment: Small patient numbers, and needs further investigation prospectively.*

Carcinosarcoma

What is carcinosarcoma and how does its management differ from other endometrial carcinomas?

Carcinosarcoma is a high-grade carcinoma mixed with mesenchymal elements. Historically named "malignant mixed Müllerian tumor," it was considered one of the uterine sarcomas (see uterine sarcoma studies) but now is often treated similar to a high-grade carcinoma. General management is similar to other high-grade endometrial cancers: thorough workup followed by surgery, including omentectomy, peritoneal washings, pelvic and para-aortic nodal dissection.

These are rare tumors, and often present at advanced stages, so evidence for adjuvant treatment is primarily retrospective. Carcinosarcomas were included in the EORTC 55874 study (see Uterine Sarcoma chapter for details), which demonstrated an LC benefit to adjuvant pelvic RT (47% vs. 24%) compared to observation. Similarly, the French SARCGYN (see Uterine Sarcoma chapter) also included carcinosarcoma and demonstrated a DFS improvement to chemoRT over pelvic RT alone. Others prefer multiagent CHT alone based on GOG 150 in the following. However, multiple retrospective series including NCDB, SEER, and other large experiences have demonstrated a benefit to either pelvic RT or cuff brachytherapy in addition to CHT, so the optimal adjuvant treatment remains unclear.[34-40]

Wolfson, GOG 150 (*Gynecol Oncol* 2007, PMID 17822748): PRT of stage I–IV uterine carcinosarcoma, <1 cm residual disease randomized to either WART or cisplatin/ifosfamide/mesna (CIM) x three cycles. WART delivered AP/PA to 30 Gy/30 fx given BID, then due to slow accrual, changed to 30 Gy/20 fx QD. After WART, whole pelvis boost to 20 Gy/20 fx BID but then changed to 19.8 Gy/11 fx QD boost (total 49.8 Gy). 232 pts, 44% stage I/II, 57% stage III/IV. MFU 5 years. After adjustment for age and stage, recurrence rate was 21% lower for CIM than WART and the death rate was 29% lower for CIM than for WART (relative hazard 0.712, $p = .085$). **Conclusion: Results favor multiagent CHT for carcinosarcoma.** *Comment: Trial used older obsolete RT techniques and does not answer the question in the modern era about combined CHT and pelvic RT.*

REFERENCES

1. Klopp A, Smith BD, Alektiar K, et al. The role of postoperative radiation therapy for endometrial cancer: executive summary of an American Society for Radiation Oncology evidence-based guideline. *Pract Radiat Oncol.* 2014;4(3):137–144.
2. Meyer LA, Bohlke K, Powell MA, et al. Postoperative radiation therapy for endometrial cancer: American Society of Clinical Oncology Clinical Practice Guideline Endorsement of the American Society for Radiation Oncology Evidence-Based Guideline. *J Clin Oncol.* 2015;33(26):2908–2913.
3. Siegel RL, Miller KD, Jemal A. Cancer statistics, 2016. *CA Cancer J Clin.* 2016;66(1):7–30.
4. Cancer stat facts: endometrial cancer. http://seer.cancer.gov/statfacts/html/corp.html
5. Torre LA, Siegel RL, Ward EM, Jemal A. Global cancer incidence and mortality rates and trends: an update. *Cancer Epidemiol Biomarkers Prev.* 2016;25(1):16–27.
6. Morice P, Leary A, Creutzberg C, et al. Endometrial cancer. *Lancet.* 2016;387(10023):1094–1108.
7. Renehan AG, Tyson M, Egger M, et al. Body-mass index and incidence of cancer: a systematic review and meta-analysis of prospective observational studies. *Lancet.* 2008;371(9612):569–578.
8. Hernandez AV, Pasupuleti V, Benites-Zapata VA, et al. Insulin resistance and endometrial cancer risk: a systematic review and meta-analysis. *Eur J Cancer.* 2015;51(18):2747–2758.
9. Shapiro S, Kelly JP, Rosenberg L, et al. Risk of localized and widespread endometrial cancer in relation to recent and discontinued use of conjugated estrogens. *N Engl J Med.* 1985;313(16):969–972.

10. Beavis AL, Smith AJ, Fader AN. Lifestyle changes and the risk of developing endometrial and ovarian cancers: opportunities for prevention and management. *Int J Women's Health.* 2016;8:151–167.

11. Barrow E, Robinson L, Alduaij W, et al. Cumulative lifetime incidence of extracolonic cancers in Lynch syndrome: a report of 121 families with proven mutations. *Clin Genet.* 2009;75(2):141–149.

12. Koornstra JJ, Mourits MJ, Sijmons RH, et al. Management of extracolonic tumours in patients with Lynch syndrome. *Lancet Oncol.* 2009;10(4):400–408.

13. NCCN Clinical practice guidelines in oncology. https://www.nccn.org/professionals/physician_gls/pdf/uterine.pdf

14. Schmeler KM, Lynch HT, Chen LM, et al. Prophylactic surgery to reduce the risk of gynecologic cancers in the Lynch syndrome. *N Engl J Med.* 2006;354(3):261–269.

15. AJCC on Cancer. 662–667. www.cancerstaging.org

16. Halperin EC, Wazer DE, Perez CA, Brady LW. *Perez and Brady's Principles and Practice of Radiation Oncology.* 6th ed. Philadelphia, PA: Lippincott Williams & Wilkins; 2013.

17. Owings RA, Quick CM. Endometrial intraepithelial neoplasia. *Arch Pathol Lab Med.* 2014;138(4):484–491.

18. Kuhn E, Wu RC, Guan B, et al. Identification of molecular pathway aberrations in uterine serous carcinoma by genome-wide analyses. *J Natl Cancer Inst.* 2012;104(19):1503–1513.

19. Amant F, Mirza MR, Koskas M, Creutzberg CL. Cancer of the corpus uteri. *Int J Gynaecol Obstet.* 2015;131(Suppl 2):S96–S104.

20. Kihara A, Yoshida H, Watanabe R, et al. Clinicopathologic association and prognostic value of microcystic, elongated, and fragmented (MELF) pattern in endometrial endometrioid carcinoma. *Am J Surg Pathol.* 2017.

21. Sanci M, Gungorduk K, Gulseren V, et al. MELF pattern for predicting lymph node involvement and survival in grade I–II endometrioid-type endometrium cancer. *Int J Gynecol Pathol.* 2017;1–5.

22. Mutter GL, Lin MC, Fitzgerald JT, et al. Altered PTEN expression as a diagnostic marker for the earliest endometrial precancers. *J Natl Cancer Inst.* 2000;92(11):924–930.

23. Kandoth C, Schultz N, Cherniack AD, et al. Integrated genomic characterization of endometrial carcinoma. *Nature.* 2013;497(7447):67–73.

24. Lindor NM, Petersen GM, Hadley DW, et al. Recommendations for the care of individuals with an inherited predisposition to Lynch syndrome: a systematic review. *JAMA.* 2006;296(12):1507–1517.

25. Benedetti Panici P, Basile S, Salerno MG, et al. Secondary analyses from a randomized clinical trial: age as the key prognostic factor in endometrial carcinoma. *Am J Obstet Gynecol.* 2014;210(4):363.e361–363.e310.

26. Doll KM, Tseng J, Denslow SA, et al. High-grade endometrial cancer: revisiting the impact of tumor size and location on outcomes. *Gynecol Oncol.* 2014;132(1):44–49.

27. Creutzberg CL, van Putten WL, Koper PC, et al. Surgery and postoperative radiotherapy versus surgery alone for patients with stage-1 endometrial carcinoma: multicentre randomised trial. PORTEC Study Group. Post Operative Radiation Therapy in Endometrial Carcinoma. *Lancet.* 2000;355(9213):1404–1411.

28. Milam MR, Java J, Walker JL, et al. Nodal metastasis risk in endometrioid endometrial cancer. *Obstet Gynecol.* 2012;119(2 Pt 1):286–292.

29. Neubauer NL, Lurain JR. The role of lymphadenectomy in surgical staging of endometrial cancer. *Int J Surg Oncol.* 2011;2011:1–7.

30. Beesley VL, Rowlands IJ, Hayes SC, et al. Incidence, risk factors and estimates of a woman's risk of developing secondary lower limb lymphedema and lymphedema-specific supportive care needs in women treated for endometrial cancer. *Gynecol Oncol.* 2015;136(1):87–93.

31. Small W, Jr., Beriwal S, Demanes DJ, et al. American Brachytherapy Society consensus guidelines for adjuvant vaginal cuff brachytherapy after hysterectomy. *Brachytherapy.* 2012;11(1):58–67.

32. Schwarz JK, Beriwal S, Esthappan J, et al. Consensus statement for brachytherapy for the treatment of medically inoperable endometrial cancer. *Brachytherapy.* 2015;14(5):587–599.

33. Videtic GMM, Woody N, Vassil AD. *Handbook of Treatment Planning in Radiation Oncology.* 2nd ed. New York, NY: Demos Medical; 2015.

34. Seagle BL, Kanis M, Kocherginsky M, et al. Stage I uterine carcinosarcoma: matched cohort analyses for lymphadenectomy, chemotherapy, and brachytherapy. *Gynecol Oncol.* 2017;145(1):71–77.

35. Odei B, Boothe D, Suneja G, et al. Chemoradiation versus chemotherapy in uterine carcinosarcoma: patterns of care and impact on overall survival. *Am J Clin Oncol*. 2017;1–8

36. Cha J, Kim YS, Park W, et al. Clinical significance of radiotherapy in patients with primary uterine carcinosarcoma: a multicenter retrospective study (KROG 13-08). *J Gynecol Oncol*. 2016;27(6):1–12.

37. Zwahlen DR, Schick U, Bolukbasi Y, et al. Outcome and predictive factors in uterine carcinosarcoma using postoperative radiotherapy: a rare cancer network study. *Rare Tumors*. 2016;8:42–48.

38. Manzerova J, Sison CP, Gupta D, et al. Adjuvant radiation therapy in uterine carcinosarcoma: a population-based analysis of patient demographic and clinical characteristics, patterns of care and outcomes. *Gynecol Oncol*. 2016;141(2):225–230.

39. Sozen H, Çiftçi R, Vatansever D, et al. Combination of adjuvant chemotherapy and radiotherapy is associated with improved survival at early stage type II endometrial cancer and carcinosarcoma. *Aust N Z J Obstet Gynaecol*. 2016;56(2):199–206.

40. Guttmann DM, Li H, Sevak P, et al. The impact of adjuvant therapy on survival and recurrence patterns in women with early-stage uterine carcinosarcoma: a multi-institutional study. *Int J Gynecol Cancer*. 2016;26(1):141–148.

45: VULVAR CANCER

Matthew C. Ward and Sudha R. Amarnath

> **QUICK HIT:** Vulvar cancers are rare, most commonly squamous cancer and occur in older women with history of either HPV or lichen sclerosis. Primary therapy is surgical with risk-adapted adjuvant RT as indicated. IMRT use postoperatively is becoming more routine but is technically challenging. Prospective data guiding use of concurrent CHT is lacking except in neoadjuvant setting.

TABLE 45.1: General Treatment Paradigm for Vulvar Cancer[1]		
Stage	**Initial Treatment**	**Subsequent Therapy**
VIN	Local excision, skinning vulvectomy, imiquimod, topical 5-FU, laser ablation	N/A
Stage IA	Wide local excision	Excision alone is appropriate if final pathology demonstrates ≤1 mm of invasion, negative margins, and no additional risk factors.
Stage IB–II	Radical local resection or modified radical vulvectomy with inguinal sentinel lymph node biopsy (can be unilateral SLNB for well-lateralized primary >2 cm from midline)	*RT to vulva*: margins <8 mm (also consider for LVSI, depth of invasion >5 mm, tumor size, diffuse or spray histology). *RT to inguinal and pelvic nodes*: ≥2 positive nodes, ECE. Treatment reasonable for 1 positive node, particularly if <12 nodes were dissection without SLNB. Concurrent CHT can be considered based on risk factors (no clear indications described).
Stage III/ IVA	Neoadjuvant chemoRT with concurrent weekly cisplatin	Biopsy for pathologic confirmation of complete response, consider groin dissection as well for confirmation. Organ-sparing surgery if complete response was not obtained and possible.

EPIDEMIOLOGY: Rare cancer, estimated 5,950 cases and 1,110 deaths in 2016.[2,3] Fourth most common gynecologic malignancy. White women at slightly higher risk than Black or Hispanic women.[4] Peak incidence is in the seventh decade of life.

RISK FACTORS: Generally the two major etiologies are HPV infection and vulvar dystrophy.[4] Risk factors relating to HPV: younger age at first intercourse, number of sexual partners, genital warts. Vulvar intraepithelial neoplasm (VIN) is related to HPV. Most common high-risk HPV subtypes are HPV 16, 18, and 33. Vaginal dystrophies, such as lichen sclerosis, are chronic inflammatory lesions and associated with vulvar cancer in older patients. Risk of malignant transformation of lichen sclerosis is approximately 5%.[4] Risk of malignant transformation of VIN III is 80%.[5]

ANATOMY: Vulva consists of mons pubis, clitoris, labia majora, and labia minora. Fourchette is merging of labia minora posteriorly. Vulva is bounded posteriorly by perineal body. Innervation is provided by pudendal nerve (S2-4). Bartholin glands are in posterior labia majora; Skene's are peri-urethral. Lymphatic drainage is to superficial inguinal nodes but can travel directly to deep inguinal nodes. In addition to inguinal nodes, clitoral lesions can drain directly to pelvic nodes (obturator, internal, or external).[4] Cloquet's/Rosenmüller's node is superior-most deep inguinal node classically associated with additional pelvic metastases.[6] As per AJCC, pelvic nodes are distant (FIGO stage IVB), a finding supported by poor outcome on GOG 37 (Homesley in the following) but questioned in modern era.[7]

PATHOLOGY: Approximately 90% are squamous cell carcinoma, 5% to 10% melanoma, and remaining are rare types such as adenocarcinomas arising from Bartholin gland. Basaloid carcinoma is associated with HPV; keratinizing associated with vulvar dystrophy. Verrucous carcinoma is squamous variant that is warty in appearance and rarely metastasizes. Of squamous carcinomas, two patterns of growth have been identified by NCCN as risk factor after surgery: spray or diffuse. Spray pattern is associated with "fingers" of tumor extending deeper than main tumor and into dermis. Diffuse pattern is connected tumor of >1 mm in dimension and is often deeply invasive with stromal desmoplasia.[4] Extramammary Paget's disease of vulva may be associated with invasive carcinoma in approximately 80%.[8] Risk of groin lymph nodes is related to tumor thickness with risk being 2.6% if ≤1 mm, 8.9%, 18.6%, 30.9%, 33.3% for 2 to 5 mm respectively and 47.9% if >5 mm (this is tumor thickness as measured in GOG 36 but not identical to depth of stromal invasion).[9] For unilateral lesions, risk of contralateral groin involvement was 8% on GOG 36. Inguinal nodal ratio of >20% is associated with 53% risk of contralateral nodal metastases.[10]

CLINICAL PRESENTATION: Erythematous, ulcerated lesion, may be associated with bleeding, pruritus, or pain. Groin nodes may be palpable and/or ulcerated. Dark discoloration should raise concern for melanoma. Synchronous cervical cancer may be present in approximately 20%. Lung is the most common site of distant metastases.

WORKUP: H&P with pelvic and rectal exam.

Labs: CBC, LFTs.

Pathology: Biopsy with HPV testing. Consider EUA with proctoscopy or sigmoidoscopy if concerning.

Imaging: CXR is sufficient unless symptoms of metastatic disease. MRI pelvis with and without contrast if helpful for surgical or RT planning (locally advanced lesions). Accuracy of contrasted MRI for tumor stage and lymph node metastases are both approximately 85%.[11] Consider PET/CT for clinically advanced or to evaluate for node-positive lesions.[1]

DIFFERENTIAL: Epidermal inclusion cyst, lentigo, benign Bartholin gland disorders, acrochordons, seborrheic keratoses, hidradenomas, lichen scleroses, condyloma acuminata.

PROGNOSTIC FACTORS: Most important factor for nonmetastatic pts is lymph node involvement. Margin status, depth of invasion, extracapsular extension, tumor grade, LVSI, tumor size, perineural invasion.

STAGING

TABLE 45.2: AJCC 8th ed. (2017) and FIGO 2009[12] staging for vulvar cancer		
AJCC		FIGO
T1	a Confined to vulva/perineum, ≤2 cm in size, stromal invasion ≤1 mm	IA
	b Confined to vulva/perineum, >2 cm in size, stromal invasion >1 mm	IB

(continued)

TABLE 45.2: AJCC 8th ed. (2017) and FIGO 2009[12] staging for vulvar cancer (*continued*)		
AJCC		**FIGO**
T2	• Adjacent spread to distal 1/3 of urethra and/or distal 1/3 vagina or anus	II
T3	• Extension to proximal 2/3 urethra and/or proximal 2/3 vagina, bladder/rectal mucosa or fixation to pelvic bones	IVA
N0 (i+)	• Isolated tumor cells <0.2 mm	
N1	a 1–2 LNs, <5 mm	IIIA
	b 1 LN, ≥5 mm	
N2	a ≥3 LNs, all <5 mm	IIIB
	b ≥2 LNs, all ≥5 mm	
	c Any LN with ECE	IIIC
N3	• Fixed or ulcerated LNs	IVA
M1	• Distant metastasis	IVB

*No major changes were implemented in the AJCC 8th Edition in comparison to the 7th. Vulvar melanoma is staged separately.

TREATMENT PARADIGM

Surgery: Surgical excision prior to RT is standard for vulvar cancer and is determined by size and location of the lesion. For small, T1 lesions, wide local excision is appropriate. For T2 or higher lesions, modified radical vulvectomy (also called "radical local excision"; spares noninvolved parts of vulva whereas radical vulvectomy takes entire vulva). For select well-localized lesions hemivulvectomy is appropriate. For large T3 lesions in which degree of resection necessary would not be tolerated, definitive nonoperative management is appropriate. For primary, gross tumor should be excised to deep fascia and periosteum with at least 1-cm clinical margin and 8-mm pathologic margin (see Heaps later).[13] For close or positive margins, re-excision should be considered. For clinically node-negative pts with depth of invasion ≤1 mm (FIGO stage IA), nodal dissection is likely unnecessary. For clinically node-negative stage IB-II patients, sentinel lymph node biopsy is usually appropriate. If both Tc-99m and blue dye is used, sensitivity is 91% with negative predictive value of 96%.[14] Unilateral nodal staging with sentinel biopsy can be performed for well-lateralized lesions (>2 cm from midline, not invading central structures). If sentinel node is positive, NCCN recommendations allow for either radiation, chemoRT or completion dissection followed by risk-adapted RT (see the following for indications). For clinically node-positive patients, at least sentinel node biopsy is recommended as even MRI is inaccurate in approximately 15% (in pre-MRI era, false negative rate of clinical exam was 23.9% on GOG 36).[9,11] If biopsy is positive and nodes are not fixed or ulcerated, inguinal node dissection is recommended (classically includes both superficial and deep inguinal nodes). If there are fixed nodal metastases, definitive RT is recommended and surgical management is variable based on surgeon preference. Historically, radical vulvectomy with bilateral groin dissection was common but associated with high wound complication rates (50%). Today, for those requiring full groin dissection, primary tumor is often managed independently from groin dissection with two to three incisions thus improving recovery. Tumor recurrence between primary and groin incision is possible but rare.

Chemotherapy: No prospective data exist to confirm benefit of concurrent CHT with RT for vulvar cancer. NCDB data suggests survival benefit for node-positive pts in the adjuvant setting.[15] Although patterns of practice vary, most common regimen is concurrent weekly cisplatin (typically 40 mg/m²).[16] For locally advanced patients, neoadjuvant chemoRT is an option and has been prospectively evaluated with various regimens including cisplatin/5-FU or 5-FU/mitomycin C.[16] NCCN allows for adjuvant chemoRT for stage T1b-2 pts with microscopic positive nodes. NCCN recommends neoadjuvant chemoRT for T2 pts with larger tumors >4 cm or T3 pts requiring visceral organs to be resected.[1]

Radiation

Indications: Data most clearly supports adjuvant RT for ≥2 positive nodes (GOG 37 in the following) or close (<8 mm) or positive margins.[17] Data is less clear for those with a single positive node, but RT may be beneficial when ≤12 nodes were removed on groin dissection (may not apply in sentinel era).[18] NCCN risk factors for primary tumor treatment include LVSI, margins <8 mm, tumor size, depth of invasion (cutoff unclear, some use >5 mm), diffuse or spray histology. Treatment to groin nodes indicated for ≥2 positive nodes, ECE, or clinically node-positive groin.

Dose (as per NCCN and Gaffney consensus guidelines[1,19]): For postoperative treatment with negative margins, recommended vulvar dose is 45 to 50.4 Gy but higher doses may be necessary for LVSI or positive margins. Optimal positive margin dose may be 54 to 59.9 Gy as per NCDB.[20] To gross disease (i.e., locally advanced case), recommended dose is 60 to >70 Gy (consider site, size, response, CHT, and toxicity when deciding dose). To uninvolved lymph nodes, 45 to 50 Gy is recommended. For gross unresectable nodal disease, 60 to 70 Gy is recommended based on size and safety.[1] For neoadjuvant RT with concurrent CHT dose is classically 45 Gy to regional nodes with cone-down boost to total of 57.6 Gy/32 fx (as per GOG 205 in the following), although open trial GOG 279 trial boosts to 64 Gy/34 fx to gross tumor (60 Gy to high-risk groin and 45 Gy to low-risk nodes). For ECE, consider 54 to 64 Gy. Acute side effects include wound breakdown, skin moist desquamation, cystitis, proctitis. Late effects include pelvic insufficiency fracture, vaginal and skin fibrosis, lymphedema, RT proctitis, cystitis, bowel obstruction.

Procedure: See *Treatment Planning Handbook*, Chapter 9.[21]

Other modalities: Laser ablation, topical 5-FU, or imiquimod (immune response modulator) are options for VIN.

EVIDENCE-BASED Q&A

Adjuvant therapy

Which resected pts benefit from adjuvant RT to vulva?

Classically, strongest data is for pts with close (<8 mm) or positive margin.[22] LVSI, tumor size, depth of invasion, and diffuse or spray histology are also recommended factors to consider per NCCN.[1] Note that node-negative pts with risk factors are often treated to vulva alone rather than comprehensively.

Heaps, UCLA (*Gynecol Oncol* 1990, PMID 2227541): Retrospective review of 135 pts with squamous cell carcinoma of vulva treated surgically between 1957 and 1985. 91 had margin ≥8 mm and 0 had local recurrence. 44 had margin <8 mm and 21 recurred locally. Other factors included LVSI, depth of invasion (>9.1 mm), and spray histologic pattern were also associated with higher local recurrence. **Conclusion: Final margin of <8 mm is associated with 50% chance of recurrence.**

Faul, Pittsburgh (*IJROBP* 1997, PMID 9226327): Retrospective review of 62 pts with vulvar carcinoma and margin <8 mm; 31 treated with RT, 31 observed. Local recurrence 58% versus 16% in favor of RT. RT improved local recurrence for both close and positive margin cases ($p < .01$ for both). **Conclusion: Adjuvant RT is indicated for this high-risk cohort.**

For pts with positive inguinal nodes, should pelvic nodes be managed surgically or with RT ?

Homesley, GOG 37 (*Obstet Gynecol* 1986, PMID 3785783; Kunos *Obstet Gyencol* 2009, PMID 19701032): Phase III PRT from 1977 to 1984 with squamous cell carcinoma of vulva and one or more pathologically positive inguinal nodes (51% clinically node-positive) demonstrated on radical vulvectomy and bilateral groin dissection (GOG 36 was overarching study looking at inguinal metastases,[9] if positive, pt was eligible for GOG 37). Pts randomized intraoperatively to either pelvic node dissection or RT to 45–50 Gy to groins and pelvis in 5 to 6.5 weeks. Groin dose prescribed to 2- to 3-cm depth. Fields were from L5/S1 to top of obturator foramen. Primary vulvar site was omitted. Trial closed early at 114 pts due to significant survival difference. 28% of pts in surgery arm had positive pelvic nodes (14% for N0-1 pts and 45% for N2-3 patients). Initial report demonstrated improvement in 2-yr OS from 54% to 68% ($p = .03$) with RT . Benefit to RT was particularly significant for those with ≥2 positive nodes. In 6-yr update, OS difference not evident for all pts but difference remained for fixed ulcerated groin nodes or ≥2 inguinal nodes. Isolated vulvar recurrence occurred in 9% in RT arm (vulva not targeted) versus 7% in surgery arm. 2-yr OS for those with positive pelvic node was 23% (10/15 died), and hence pelvic nodes are staged as FIGO IVB (this has been questioned in modern era[7]). Late effects were similar. **Conclusion: RT improves OS for pts with ≥2 positive groin nodes. Pelvic nodal dissection is not routinely indicated.**

TABLE 45.3: Results of GOG 37 for Vulvar Cancer				
	2-yr OS	6-yr OS	MS (N2/3)	2-yr Groin Relapse
RT	68%	51%	40 mos	5%
Pelvic LND	54%	41%	12 mos	24%
p value	.03	.18	.01	.02

Which resected pts benefit from adjuvant RT to groin and pelvic nodes?

Homesley/GOG 37 provides strongest data and supports comprehensive nodal irRT to groin and pelvic nodes for those with ≥2 positive nodes. NCCN recommends RT for any positive node, including sentinel lymph node, especially if node is >2 mm[1] as supported by SEER data in the following.

Parthasarathy, Stanford SEER Analysis (*Gynecol Oncol* 2006, PMID 16889821): SEER data from 1988 to 2001 identified vulvar squamous cell carcinomas with one positive node. 208 pts included. 92% treated with radical vulvectomy with either unilateral or bilateral inguinal dissection. Median of 13 nodes removed. 102 underwent adjuvant RT, 106 did not. 5-yr DSS was 77% vs. 61% ($p = .02$) in favor of RT. RT particularly beneficial in those with ≤12 nodes removed (DSS 77% vs. 55%, $p = .035$) but those with >12 nodes removed difference did not reach significance (77% RT vs. 67% no RT, $p = .23$). **Conclusion: Adjuvant RT may improve DSS for pts with single positive node, particularly when ≤12 nodes were resected.**

Is RT alone sufficient to treat groins or is groin dissection necessary?

Stehman, GOG 88 (*IJROBP* 1992, PMID 1526880): Phase III PRT of 52 pts with squamous cell carcinoma and clinically negative/nonsuspicious nodes treated with radical vulvectomy and randomized to either groin dissection or RT . T1-3 tumors were included but T1 tumors required LVSI or >5 mm of invasion to be eligible. RT was 50 Gy to depth of 3 cm with photons allowed but electrons recommended. Only inguinal nodes were treated; pelvic nodes and primary site were omitted. Pts in surgery arm with positive nodes received postoperative RT to groin and hemipelvis (based on GOG 37 in the preceding). Trial stopped early due to excessive recurrences in RT arm. 71% of tumors were 2.1 to 4.0 cm. 5 of 25 pts on groin dissection arm had positive nodes. PFS and OS were both inferior in RT arm. Lymphedema (28% vs. 0%) and acute grade 3-4 toxicity (22 vs. 10) were both worse in groin dissection arm. **Conclusion: Radiation, as delivered in this study, is inferior to groin dissection.** *Comment: Review of 50 cases by Koh et al. demonstrated median femoral vessel depth of 6.1 cm (range 2.0–18.5 cm).23 RT arm of GOG 88 may have undertreated pts as dose was prescribed to 3 cm.*

TABLE 45.4: Results of GOG 88 Vulvar Cancer		
	2-yr OS	2-yr PFS
Radical vulvectomy + groin RT	60%	65%
Radical vulvectomy + LND (with PORT if LN+)	85%	90%
p value	.035	.033

Which resected pts benefit from adjuvant chemoRT?

Benefits are unclear given absence of prospective data. If done, weekly cisplatin is recommended concurrent CHT regimen.[19]

Gill, Pittsburgh NCDB Analysis (*Gynecol Oncol* 2015, PMID 25868965): NCDB analysis from 1998 to 2011 of pts with squamous cell carcinoma who underwent surgery with positive inguinal nodes. CHT used in 26% (41% in yr 2006). CHT more common with greater number of nodes, stage IVA disease, and positive margins. CHT was associated with improved OS on propensity-adjusted modeling. **Conclusion: Adjuvant chemoRT may benefit node-positive patients.**

For whom is sentinel lymph node biopsy sufficient?

As per NCCN guidelines, SLNB is alternative standard of care to groin dissection for pts with negative physical exam, negative imaging, unifocal vulvar tumor <4 cm in diameter and no previous vulvar surgery that may have altered lymph drainage. If only unilateral SLNB is performed and is positive, contralateral side should be considered for RT based on NCCN guidelines.[1]

Levenback, GOG 173 (*JCO* 2012, PMID 22753905): Single-arm trial of 452 women with squamous cell carcinoma of vulva with ≥1 mm of invasion, tumor size of 2 to 6 cm and clinically negative groin. Pts underwent SLNB followed by inguinal dissection; 418 of 452 (92%) identified sentinel node. Incidence of nodal metastasis was 32%. False negative rate was 8.3%. Sensitivity 91.7%, false negative predictive value (1-negative predictive value) was 3.7% in all-comers and 2.0% in tumors <4 cm. **Conclusion: SLNB is reasonable alternative to inguinal dissection.**

Van der Zee, GROINSS-V (*JCO* 2008, PMID 18281661): Single-arm trial of 403 pts treated from 2000 to 2006 with unifocal vulvar squamous carcinoma staged T1-2 with tumor size of <4 cm and depth of invasion >1 mm with clinically negative lymph nodes. Pts underwent radical excision with SLNB. If SLNB was negative, groin dissection was omitted. Postoperative RT to 50 Gy recommended if ≥2 nodes were positive or for ECE. 623 groins underwent SLNB. Rate of groin recurrence if SLNB was negative was 2.3% with 3-yr OS of 97%. **Conclusion: Negative SLNB is associated with low rate of groin recurrence and should be standard.**

Neoadjuvant/definitive therapy for advanced disease

Is neoadjuvant therapy feasible option for pts whose disease would require radical surgery?

Multiple prospective trials and retrospective data[24] have demonstrated safety and feasibility of this approach for both unresectable vulvar primary tumors and unresectable adenopathy.

Moore, GOG 101 Unresectable Primary Cohort (*IJROBP* 1998, PMID 9747823): Multipart phase II study of 73 pts with stage III–IV squamous vulvar carcinoma (T3-4 regardless of nodal status) requiring more than radical vulvectomy. This part required unresectable primary tumor, Montana report that follows required unresectable inguinal nodes. Pts (both parts) were treated with split-course of RT via AP/PA fields to 47.6 Gy to primary and inguinal/pelvic nodes for N2-3 patients; 23.8 Gy was given during each course via 1.7 Gy BID for first 4 days during CHT and QD thereafter for total of 12 treatment days per course. Courses separated by 1.5 to 2.5 weeks. During each course, bolus cisplatin 50 mg/m² and 4-day infusion of 5-FU 100 mg/m² were given. Following induction therapy, surgery was performed 4 to 8 weeks later. Boost of 20 Gy was given for residual unresectable disease or 10–15 Gy to microscopically positive margins. Complete clinical response observed in 46.5%, 53.5% had gross residual cancer. Only two pts (2.8%) had residual unresectable disease and in three pts surgery required sacrificing bowel/bladder continence. **Conclusion: Preoperative chemoRT is feasible and may reduce rates of pelvic exenteration.**

Montana, GOG 101 Unresectable Lymph Node Cohort (*IJROBP* 2000, PMID 11072157): Second part of phase II study including 46 pts who underwent same treatment regimen as per Moore earlier except with fields including inguinal and pelvic nodes. Disease was resectable in 38/40 pts and pCR rate was 40.5%. Control of lymphatic disease achieved in 36/37 pts (97%). **Conclusion: Preoperative chemoRT is feasible and high rates of control were achieved.**

Moore, GOG 205 (*Gynecol Oncol* 2012, PMID 22079361): Single-arm phase II trial of locally advanced primary tumors treated with chemoRT using 57.6 Gy/32 fx with weekly cisplatin 40 mg/m² followed by surgery. 58 evaluable pts, 69% completed treatment. 37 (64%) had complete clinical response and 29 (78% of 64%) had complete pathologic response. Of note, pathologic response rate overall was 50% in GOG 205 and 31% in GOG 101. **Conclusion: Cisplatin and RT induction yielded high response rates with acceptable toxicity.**

REFERENCES

1. NCCN Clinical Practice Guidelines in Oncology: Vulvar Cancer; 2017. https://www.nccn.org/professionals/physician_gls/pdf/vulvar.pdf
2. Cancer Facts & Figures 2016; 2016. http://www.cancer.org/research/cancerfactsstatistics/cancerfactsfigures2016.
3. Siegel RL, Miller KD, Jemal A. Cancer statistics, 2016. *Cancer J Clin.* 2016;66(1):7–30.
4. Chino JP, Havrilesky LJ, Montana GS. Carcinoma of the vulva. In: Halperin EC, Wazer DE, Perez CA, Brady LW, eds. *Principles and Practice of Radiation Oncology.* 6th ed. Philadelphia, PA: Lippincott Williams & Wilkins; 2013:1502–1516.
5. Alkatout I, Schubert M, Garbrecht N, et al. Vulvar cancer: epidemiology, clinical presentation, and management options. *Int J Women's Health.* 2015;7:305–313.
6. Chu CK, Zager JS, Marzban SS, et al. Routine biopsy of Cloquet's node is of limited value in sentinel node positive melanoma patients. *J Surg Oncol.* 2010;102(4):315–320.
7. Thaker NG, Klopp AH, Jhingran A, et al. Survival outcomes for patients with stage IVB vulvar cancer with grossly positive pelvic lymph nodes: time to reconsider the FIGO staging system? *Gynecol Oncol.* 2015;136(2):269–273.

8. van der Linden M, Meeuwis KA, Bulten J, et al. Paget disease of the vulva. *Crit Rev Oncol Hematol*. 2016;101:60–74.

9. Homesley HD, Bundy BN, Sedlis A, et al. Prognostic factors for groin node metastasis in squamous cell carcinoma of the vulva (a Gynecologic Oncology Group study). *Gynecol Oncol*. 1993;49(3):279–283.

10. Kunos C, Simpkins F, Gibbons H, et al. Radiation therapy compared with pelvic node resection for node-positive vulvar cancer: a randomized controlled trial. *Obstet Gynecol*. 2009;114(3):537–546.

11. Kataoka MY, Sala E, Baldwin P, et al. The accuracy of magnetic resonance imaging in staging of vulvar cancer: a retrospective multi-centre study. *Gynecol Oncol*. 2010;117(1):82–87.

12. Pecorelli S. Revised FIGO staging for carcinoma of the vulva, cervix, and endometrium. *Int J Gynaecol Obstet*. 2009;105(2):103–104.

13. Heaps JM, Fu YS, Montz FJ, et al. Surgical-pathologic variables predictive of local recurrence in squamous cell carcinoma of the vulva. *Gynecol Oncol*. 1990;38(3):309–314.

14. Meads C, Sutton AJ, Rosenthal AN, et al. Sentinel lymph node biopsy in vulval cancer: systematic review and meta-analysis. *Br J Cancer*. 2014;110(12):2837–2846.

15. Gill BS, Bernard ME, Lin JF, et al. Impact of adjuvant chemotherapy with radiation for node-positive vulvar cancer: A National Cancer Data Base (NCDB) analysis. *Gynecol Oncol*. 2015;137(3):365–372.

16. Reade CJ, Eiriksson LR, Mackay H. Systemic therapy in squamous cell carcinoma of the vulva: current status and future directions. *Gynecol Oncol*. 2014;132(3):780–789.

17. Faul CM, Mirmow D, Huang Q, et al. Adjuvant radiation for vulvar carcinoma: improved local control. *Int J Radiat Oncol Biol Phys*. 1997;38(2):381–389.

18. Parthasarathy A, Cheung MK, Osann K, et al. The benefit of adjuvant radiation therapy in single-node-positive squamous cell vulvar carcinoma. *Gynecol Oncol*. 2006;103(3):1095–1099.

19. Gaffney DK, King B, Viswanathan AN, et al. Consensus recommendations for radiation therapy contouring and treatment of vulvar carcinoma. *Int J Radiat Oncol Biol Phys*. 2016;95(4):1191–1200.

20. Chapman BV, Gill BS, Viswanathan AN, et al. Adjuvant radiation therapy for margin-positive vulvar squamous cell carcinoma: defining the ideal dose-response using the National Cancer Data Base. *Int J Radiat Oncol Biol Phys*. 2017;97(1):107–117.

21. Kotecha R, Cherian S. Gynecologic radiotherapy. In: Videtic GMM, Woody NM, eds. *Handbook of Treatment Planning*. 2nd ed. New York, NY: Demos Medical; 2015.

22. Ignatov T, Eggemann H, Burger E, et al. Adjuvant radiotherapy for vulvar cancer with close or positive surgical margins. *J Cancer Res Clin Oncol*. 2016;142(2):489–495.

23. Koh WJ, Chiu M, Stelzer KJ, et al. Femoral vessel depth and the implications for groin node radiation. *Int J Radiat Oncol Biol Phys*. 1993;27(4):969–974.

24. Beriwal S, Coon D, Heron DE, et al. Preoperative intensity-modulated radiotherapy and chemotherapy for locally advanced vulvar carcinoma. *Gynecol Oncol*. 2008;109(2):291–295.

46: VAGINAL CANCER

Camille A. Berriochoa and Sudha R. Amarnath

QUICK HIT: Vaginal cancer is a rare malignancy that arises as a primary in the vagina without involvement of the cervix or vulva. The majority (>80%) are squamous cell carcinomas, arise in posterior aspect of upper third of vagina (60%–80%),[1,2] and are not amenable to organ-sparing surgical resection due to close proximity of urethra, bladder, and rectum. Thus treatment typically consists of definitive RT with or without CHT. Brachytherapy boost is often recommended and choice of intracavitary cylinder versus interstitial is based on depth of invasion (≤0.5 cm for cylinder vs. >0.5 cm for interstitial).

TABLE 46.1: General Treatment Paradigm for Vaginal Cancer[3,4]

STAGE	TREATMENT
VAIN 1–2	Often addressed with close surveillance as ~ 80% of lesions will spontaneously regress.[5]
CIS (VAIN 3)	Surgery (local excision, partial or complete vaginectomy), topical 5-FU, or RT. RT usually delivered via intracavitary brachytherapy of 60 Gy* to entire vagina + boost to involved vaginal mucosa to 70 Gy.*
STAGE I	Surgery or RT. For lesions in superior 1/3 of vagina, radical hysterectomy, pelvic lymphadenectomy, and partial vaginectomy may be performed. If located in inferior 2/3, total vaginectomy (or vulvovaginectomy) with inguinal node dissection and reconstruction (e.g., split thickness skin graft) may be required. If surgery is not feasible, treat with RT. If lesion is ≤0.5-cm depth, use intracavitary brachytherapy alone to achieve vaginal surface dose of 60–65 Gy* (HDR 21–25 Gy, 5–7 Gy/week), with additional 20–30 Gy* (HDR = 14–18 Gy) prescribed to tumor + 2-cm margin using shielded vaginal cylinder. If lesion >0.5 cm depth, treat whole pelvis to 45 Gy with EBRT, then interstitial brachytherapy to provide a boost dose of 25–35 Gy* prescribed 0.5 cm beyond implant.
STAGE II (subvaginal infiltration only ≤0.5 cm depth)	Treat whole pelvis to 45 Gy, then boost with intracavitary implant of 25–35 Gy.*
STAGE II–IVA	(Paravaginal/parametrial involvement): Treat whole pelvis to 45 Gy, then boost with interstitial implant 25–35 Gy* to achieve total dose of 75–80 Gy.* Surgical option is total exenteration with bilateral inguinal LAD with caveat that this is highly morbid surgery. For tumors involving lower third of the vagina, inguinal nodes should be treated 45–50.4 Gy. Boost clinically positive nodes additional 20–25 Gy. May need to consider bolus to adequately cover inguinal nodes.

*Note that these doses are referring to brachytherapy equivalents of 2 Gy EBRT per fraction assuming α/β of 10. When using LDR, available data suggests that achieving total dose of 70–85 Gy in 2 Gy EBRT equivalents should be utilized with preferred dose rate of 35–70 cGy/hour.[3] HDR approach is more variable; largest series reviewed 86 pts whose most common HDR regimen was 7 Gy x five fractions.[6] Additional details regarding brachytherapy dose can be found in the following.

EPIDEMIOLOGY: Vaginal cancer is rare and accounts for less than 3% of all gynecologic cancers with about 4,000 cases in the United States annually.[7] The most common histology is squamous cell carcinoma (≥80% of cases) followed by adenocarcinoma (~10% of cases), with several other uncommon histologies including melanoma, small cell, lymphoid, and carcinoid comprising remaining subtypes.[8] Median age of diagnosis for SCC of vagina is 65.

ANATOMY: The vagina is a fibromuscular tube lined with mucous membrane and extends from uterus to vestibule. Urethra and bladder are located directly anterior to the vagina. Posteriorly, superoposterior vaginal wall is separated from rectum by fold of peritoneum called "rectouterine pouch" (pouch of Douglas). Extending caudally, the vagina runs adjacent to the rectum with the perineal body separating the two at their inferior-most location. Pelvic fascia, ureters, and levator ani run lateral to vagina. Posterior wall (~9 cm) is longer than anterior wall (~7 cm) because the vagina joins uterus at angle of approximately 90 degrees. The cervix projects into the vaginal lumen thus creating anterior, posterior, and lateral fornices. Layers of vagina are as follows: *inner mucosa* (nonkeratinizing, stratified squamous epithelium, no glands) → *lamina propria* (connective tissue) → *muscularis* (inner circular and outer longitudinal layers) → *adventitia* (thin, outer connective tissue). The vagina has two embryologic origins: upper third derives from uterine canal and lower two-thirds from urogenital sinus (implications for lymphatic drainage). Upper third drains in patterns similar to cervix (parametrial, obturator, and pelvic nodes). Lower third drains to inguinal nodes and then to external iliacs. Lesions in middle third can go either direction. Distant metastases can be seen in para-aortic LNs, lungs, liver, and bone.

PATHOLOGY[9]

TABLE 46.2: Summary of Pathologic Types of Vaginal Cancer		
Prevalence	Vaginal Cancer Subtype	Notes
Rare	*CIS* aka *VAIN3* (vaginal intraepithelial neoplasia 3)	Most are multifocal and can involve all vaginal surfaces.
75%–95%	*Squamous cell carcinoma*	Most are nonkeratinizing and moderately differentiated.
5%–10%	*Adenocarcinoma* (non-clear-cell)	May be associated with another primary (ovarian, endometrial, renal, etc.). Otherwise, non-clear-cell adenocarcinoma of vagina has very poor prognosis.[10]
	Adenocarcinoma (clear cell)	Related to *in utero* DES exposure; 1/1,000 risk if exposed. Younger age. Preceded by vaginal adenosis in up to 95% of cases.
<5%	*Melanoma*	Projects into lumen, tends to involve the vaginal surface rather than invade into wall. Melanin differentiates this from sarcoma. Race: White more common than Black. OS <20%
RARE	*Sarcoma botryoides* (Embryonal rhabdomyosarcoma)	MOST COMMON vaginal neoplasm in infants and children. Characteristic "grape-like" exophytic mass. Aggressive. Treat with surgery, multiagent chemo, and XRT (OS = 90%)
RARE	*Verrucous carcinoma* (variant of SCC), *serous papillary* ACA, *small cell*, *spindle cell epithelioma*, other *sarcoma*, and *lymphoma*.	Verrucous CA presents as large, warty, fungating mass. Locally aggressive but rarely metastasizes and thus has overall favorable prognosis.

RISK FACTORS: Risk factors are similar to cervical cancer: current smoking, multiple lifetime sexual partners, and early age at first intercourse.[11,12] The latter two correlate with exposure to HPV, and multiple studies have shown that HPV DNA can be found in at least 75% of vaginal intraepithelial neoplasia (VAIN)/invasive vaginal cancers, and specifically HPV 16 and 18 subtypes.[13,14] Additionally, previous gynecologic malignancy, DES exposure in utero (clear cell adenocarcinoma), and alcohol consumption have all been associated with vaginal cancer, with some controversy regarding exposure to prior pelvic XRT.[11,15,16]

CLINICAL PRESENTATION: Vaginal bleeding, often postcoital, is the most common presenting symptom (~50%–60% of patients), though as many as 20% of pts may be asymptomatic.[1] Additional symptoms include vaginal discharge and dysuria. Frank vaginal and/or pelvic pain is often a late presenting symptom, suggestive of invasion to surrounding tissues.[1,2] If vaginal cancer is diagnosed <5 years after previous gynecologic malignancy, then new diagnosis should be categorized as recurrence. Differential diagnosis includes cervical cancer, vulvar cancer, and metastases from ovarian, renal cell, or other primaries.

WORKUP: H&P including thorough abdominopelvic exam. Note that speculum exam can easily miss anterior and posterior lesions; to avoid this, rotate speculum upon exiting vault. Pelvic should include bimanual exam, rectovaginal exam, EUA with vaginal AND cervical biopsies and colposcopy (with acetic acid application first, lesions are white; can confirm with Schiller's test—Lugol's solution stains normal mucosal cells but not malignant cells). Perform cystoscopy and proctosigmoidoscopy for more advanced lesions.

Labs: CBC, CMP (with particular attention to creatinine and LFTs).

Imaging: CT chest/abdomen/pelvis, CXR. Recommend MRI and PET for more advanced presentations. MRI has excellent sensitivity (95%) and specificity (90%).[17] Recall that FIGO staging permits only physical exam and the following five studies: CXR, IV pyelogram, cystoscopy, proctosigmoidoscopy, and barium enema.

PROGNOSTIC FACTORS

TABLE 46.3: Prognostic Factors for Vaginal Cancer	
Better	HPV (+), SCC, involving <1/3 length of vagina (*5-yr DFS 61% vs. 25%*),[18] location in upper 1/3 of vagina, >75 Gy total dose (*2-yr PFS 76% vs. 40%*).[19] Smaller size (<4–5 cm[10,20,21]). Prior hysterectomy also appears to be protective perhaps due to anatomy of tumor spread.[10,17,22]
Worse	Advanced clinical stage, larger size (≥4–5 cm as earlier), presence of symptoms, LN involvement, ACA, nonepithelial tumors, posterior wall, overexpression of *HER-2/ neu* in SCC, mutated p53, longer treatment time, NOT being associated with DES exposure,[19] HIV[23]

STAGING

TABLE 46.4: AJCC 8th ed. (2017) & FIGO Staging for Vaginal Cancer[8,20,24-26]				
AJCC			FIGO	Risk of LNs
T1	a	Confined to vagina, ≤2 cm	I	6%–14%
	b	Confined to vagina, >2 cm		
T2	a	Invades paravaginal tissues, but not pelvic wall, ≤2 cm*	II	23%–32%
	b	Invades paravaginal tissues, but not pelvic wall, >2 cm*		

(*continued*)

TABLE 46.4: AJCC 8th ed. (2017) Staging for Vaginal Cancer[8,20,24-26] (*continued*)			
AJCC		**FIGO**	**Risk of LNs**
T3	• Extends to pelvic side wall • Involves lower 1/3 of vagina • Hydronephrosis or non-functioning kidney *	III	78%
N1	• Pelvic or inguinal LNs		
T4	• Invasion into bladder, rectum, and/or extends beyond true pelvis**	IVA	83%
M1	• Distant metastasis	IVB	

AJCC Group Staging	
IA	T1aN0M0
IB	T1bN0M0
IIA	T2aN0M0
IIB	T2bN0M0
III	T3N0M0, T1-3N1M0
IVA	T4N0-1M0
IVB	M1

Major changes from the 7th Edition include addition of the T1a/b and T2a/b delineations.

*Pelvic wall is muscle, fascia, neurovascular structures, or skeletal portions of bony pelvis.

**Bullous edema is not sufficient to classify tumor as T4.

TREATMENT PARADIGM[3,4,9]

Surgery: Wide local excision may be possible for VAIN 3/CIS. For superior lesions, hysterectomy with partial vaginectomy may be feasible. For distal 1/3 lesions, excision with reconstruction may be possible but often exenteration (either total or anterior including vagina and bladder only but sparing rectum) may be necessary. Multiple surgical series have demonstrated pathologic nodal involvement of approximately 10% for stage I lesions and 30% for stage II lesions.[24,25] Thus, pelvic LN dissection is often performed, and inguinofemoral nodes are also dissected if lesion is in distal vagina. Because of the extent of surgery often required in these cases, organ-sparing treatment with RT may improve quality of life.

Chemotherapy: Concurrent weekly cisplatin 40 mg/m² can be considered with other series using various multiagent combinations such as cisplatin/5-FU. This is extrapolating from cervical data (see retrospective data in the following section).

Radiation

Indications: RT delivered definitively typically for stage II–IVA lesions.

Dose: RT is given via EBRT to whole pelvis to dose of 45 Gy/25 fx (50.4 Gy/28 fx also common). In postoperative setting or when treating inguinal lymph nodes, IMRT may be superior to four-field box. HDR brachytherapy is then given as boost, which may be intracavitary or interstitial depending on depth of invasion. One common dosing strategy for interstitial brachytherapy is 25 Gy/5 fx; see ABS guidelines for details.[3] If brachytherapy boost is not feasible, boost with EBRT to approximately 64–70 Gy to primary and 55–66 Gy to involved lymphadenopathy.

Toxicity: Acute: vaginal irritation, pain, dysuria, proctitis. Chronic: vaginal stenosis, proctitis, fistulae, bleeding, bowel obstruction, incontinence, hemorrhagic cystitis, urethral stricture, sexual dysfunction. Risk factors include location, stage, and smoking.[19] Late RT toxicity is approximately 5% for bowel and bladder (each) with "vaginal morbidity" of 64%.[27]

Procedure: See *Treatment Planning Handbook*, Chapter 9.[28]

EVIDENCE-BASED Q&A

What evidence supports current treatment approaches and outcomes?

Most data for vaginal cancer treatment is retrospective; the two most commonly cited series are in the following.

Frank, MDACC (*IJROBP* 2005, PMID 15850914). RR of 193 pts with SCC of vagina, no prior gynecologic cancers. FIGO I (26%), II (50%), III (20%), and IVA (4%), treated from 1970 to 2000. 119 (62%) pts had EBRT + brachytherapy (median = 85 Gy surface, 81 Gy to depth), 63 (32%) had EBRT alone (median = 66 Gy), 11 (6%) had brachytherapy alone (median = 65 Gy). 18 pts had gross excision. EBRT alone more likely for advanced lesions, bulky, or comorbid disease. 22% of advanced stage received CHT. In more recent years, EBRT was used in addition to brachytherapy even for stage I disease (see Table 46.5). Three of 9 pts w/ stage I treated with brachytherapy alone failed in regional lymph nodes. Four pts were treated with neoadjuvant CHT; all died of progressive disease. To the contrary, four of nine treated with concurrent CHT were NED. **Conclusion: Size (DSS 82% vs. 60% for <4 or >4 cm lesions, *p* = .027) was significant. Stage predictive of survival and toxicity. Predominant pattern of relapse was locoregional (I–II = 68%, III–IVA = 83%). Concurrent chemoRT reasonable for advanced disease.**

TABLE 46.5: Summary of MDACC Series on Vaginal Cancer				
FIGO Stage	**5-yr DSS**	**5-yr Vaginal Control**	**5-yr Pelvic Control**	**Severe Toxicity**
I	85%	91%	86%	4%
II	78%		84%	9%
III		83%		
IVA	58%		71%	21% (ss)

Tran, Stanford (*Gynecol Oncol* 2007, PMID 17363046): RR of 78 pts with SCC of vagina treated with RT between 1959 and 2005. Median age 65 years. FIGO I (42%); II (29%); III (17%); and IVA/B (11%). 62% treated with EBRT and brachytherapy, 22% EBRT alone, 13% with brachytherapy alone. Intracavitary RT (46%) delivered to mean dose of 41 Gy; interstitial RT (31%) delivered to mean dose of 33 Gy. 62% treated with EBRT and brachytherapy to whole vagina. On MVA, stage, Hgb (<12.5 mg/dL), and prior hysterectomy were prognostic for DSS (*p* < .02). These three factors and tumor size (<4 cm) were all prognostic for LRC (*p* = .01). 26 pts failed: 13/26 local, 9/26 regional, 10/26 distant; 16/26 (62%) failed in pelvis only. MS after local failure 14 months. Of 35 pts with lower third vaginal involvement, 22 (63%) received elective inguinofemoral RT with no treatment failures in this group. Of 13 pts with lower third vaginal involvement who did *not* receive elective inguinofemoral RT, one pt failed. Toxicity: 14% grade 3/4 complication; tumor size (≥4 cm) and tumor dose (70 Gy) were independently predictive (*p* < .05). **Conclusion: RT effective treatment for stage I/II disease. Advanced disease requires improved treatment. Most failures are local and most cancer-related deaths due to local failure not distant metastases. Hgb level at time of treatment appears to be clinically significant.** *Comment: Authors suggested that studies evaluating correction of anemia may be warranted; however, extrapolating from cervical cancer literature, transfusion may not be associated with improved prognosis for anemic patients.[29]*

TABLE 46.6: Stanford Vaginal Cancer Series			
FIGO Stage	**5-yr LRC**	**5-yr DMFS**	**5-yr DSS**
I	83%	100%	92%
II	76%	95%	68%
III	62%	65%	44%
IVA	30%	18%	13%

Should concurrent CHT be utilized?

No prospective trials are available. Nevertheless, many argue that similarities between vaginal cancer and cervical cancer in terms of epidemiology, risk factors, histology, and anatomy warrant extrapolation from multiple randomized trials in cervical cancer showing improved PFS and OS with addition of concurrent CHT. In the absence of randomized data, the following retrospective reviews provide some support for use of concurrent CHT.

Rajagopalan, UPMC (*Gynecol Oncol* 2014, PMID 25281493): NCDB analysis of almost 14,000 pts reviewing treatment approach and outcomes in vaginal cancer pts treated between 1998 and 2011. 60% of pts w/ vaginal cancer received RT. Of these, 48% received concurrent CHT, with increasing use from 1998 to 2011. Median survival was longer with use of concurrent chemo, improved from 41 → 56 months ($p < .0005$). On MVA, the following factors were independently prognostic for improved OS: younger age, higher facility volume, squamous histology, concurrent chemo, use of brachytherapy, and lower stage.

Miyamoto, Harvard (*PLoS One* 2013, PMID 23762284): Single-institution RR of 71 primary vaginal cancer pts treated with definitive RT (n = 51) or CRT (n = 20). MFU 3 yrs. 3-yr OS improved from 56% with RT alone to 79% with CRT, $p = .037$. 3-yr DFS also improved with chemo, from 43% w/ RT alone to 73% w/ CRT, $p = .011$. On MVA, use of concurrent CHT remained significant predictor of DFS (HR 0.31, $p = .04$). **Conclusion: Concurrent CHT leads to improved outcomes in vaginal cancer pts.**

Samant, Ottawa (*IJROBP* 2007, PMID 17512130): Single-institution RR of all primary vaginal cancer pts (n = 12) treated with curative intent using concurrent cisplatin based CRT. Median F/U 4 yrs. 10 of 12 pts had SCC, 2 of 12 pts had adenocarcinoma. Stage distribution: 6/12 stage II, 4/12 stage III, 2/12 stage IVA. All pts received pelvic EBRT to median dose of 45 Gy/25 fx followed by either interstitial brachytherapy (10/12 pts) or intracavitary brachytherapy (2/12 pts) to dose of 30 Gy. 5-yr LRC was 92% and 5-yr OS was 66%. Late toxicity necessitating surgery occurred in 2/12 pts. **Conclusion: Definitive CRT for management of vaginal cancer leads to excellent LC and acceptable toxicity.**

REFERENCES

1. Gallup DG, Talledo OE, Shah KJ, Hayes C. Invasive squamous cell carcinoma of the vagina: a 14-year study. *Obstet Gynecol*. 1987;69(5):782–785.
2. Rubin SC, Young J, Mikuta JJ. Squamous carcinoma of the vagina: treatment, complications, and long-term follow-up. *Gynecol Oncol*. 1985;20(3):346–353.
3. Beriwal S, Demanes DJ, Erickson B, et al. American Brachytherapy Society consensus guidelines for interstitial brachytherapy for vaginal cancer. *Brachytherapy*. 2012;11(1):68–75.
4. Lee LJ, Jhingran A, Kidd E, et al. ACR Appropriateness Criteria management of vaginal cancer. *Oncology*. 2013;27(11):1166–1173.
5. Aho M, Vesterinen E, Meyer B, et al. Natural history of vaginal intraepithelial neoplasia. *Cancer*. 1991;68(1):195–197.

6. Mock U, Kucera H, Fellner C, et al. High-dose–rate (HDR) brachytherapy with or without external beam radiotherapy in the treatment of primary vaginal carcinoma: long-term results and side effects. *Int J Radiat Oncol Biol Phys.* 2003;56(4):950–957.

7. Siegel RL, Miller KD, Jemal A. Cancer statistics, 2015. *Cancer J Clin.* 2015;65(1):5–29.

8. Creasman WT, Phillips JL, Menck HR. The National Cancer Data Base report on cancer of the vagina. *Cancer.* 1998;83(5):1033–1040.

9. Perez CA, Brady LW, Halperin EC, Wazer DE. *Principles and Practice of Radiation Oncology.* 6th ed. Wulters Kluwer, Lippincott Williams & Williams; 2013.

10. Chyle V, Zagars GK, Wheeler JA, et al. Definitive radiotherapy for carcinoma of the vagina: outcome and prognostic factors. *Int J Radiat Oncol Biol Phys.* 1996;35(5):891–905.

11. Madsen BS, Jensen HL, van den Brule AJ, et al. Risk factors for invasive squamous cell carcinoma of the vulva and vagina: population-based case-control study in Denmark. *Int J Cancer.* 2008;122(12):2827–2834.

12. Daling JR, Madeleine MM, Schwartz SM, et al. A population-based study of squamous cell vaginal cancer: HPV and cofactors. *Gynecol Oncol.* 2002;84(2):263–270.

13. Alemany L, Saunier M, Tinoco L, et al. Large contribution of human papillomavirus in vaginal neoplastic lesions: a worldwide study in 597 samples. *Eur J Cancer.* 2014;50(16):2846–2854.

14. Sinno AK, Saraiya M, Thompson TD, et al. Human papillomavirus genotype prevalence in invasive vaginal cancer from a registry-based population. *Obstet Gynecol.* 2014;123(4):817–821.

15. Lee JY, Perez CA, Ettinger N, Fineberg BB. The risk of second primaries subsequent to irradiation for cervix cancer. *Int J Radiat Oncol Biol Phys.* 1982;8(2):207–211.

16. Boice JD, Jr., Engholm G, Kleinerman RA, et al. Radiation dose and second cancer risk in patients treated for cancer of the cervix. *Radiat Res.* 1988;116(1):3–55.

17. Chang YC, Hricak H, Thurnher S, Lacey CG. Vagina: evaluation with MR imaging. Part II. Neoplasms. *Radiology.* 1988;169(1):175–179.

18. Stock RG, Chen AS, Seski J. A 30-year experience in the management of primary carcinoma of the vagina: analysis of prognostic factors and treatment modalities. *Gynecol Oncol.* 1995;56(1):45–52.

19. Frank SJ, Jhingran A, Levenback C, Eifel PJ. Definitive radiation therapy for squamous cell carcinoma of the vagina. *Int J Radiat Oncol Biol Phys.* 2005;62(1):138–147.

20. Shah CA, Goff BA, Lowe K, et al. Factors affecting risk of mortality in women with vaginal cancer. *Obstet Gynecol.* 2009;113(5):1038–1045.

21. Rajagopalan MS, Xu KM, Lin JF, et al. Adoption and impact of concurrent chemoradiation therapy for vaginal cancer: a National Cancer Data Base (NCDB) study. *Gynecol Oncol.* 2014;135(3):495–502.

22. Tran PT, Su Z, Lee P, et al. Prognostic factors for outcomes and complications for primary squamous cell carcinoma of the vagina treated with radiation. *Gynecol Oncol.* 2007;105(3):641–649.

23. Merino MJ. Vaginal cancer: the role of infectious and environmental factors. *Am J Obstet Gynecol.* 1991;165(4 Pt 2):1255–1262.

24. Al-Kurdi M, Monaghan JM. Thirty-two years' experience in management of primary tumours of the vagina. *Br J Obstet Gynaecol.* 1981;88(11):1145–1150.

25. Davis KP, Stanhope CR, Garton GR, et al. Invasive vaginal carcinoma: analysis of early-stage disease. *Gynecol Oncol.* 1991;42(2):131–136.

26. Cancer AJCo. *AJCC Cancer Staging Manual.* 8th ed. New York, NY: Springer Publishing; 2017.

27. Lian J, Dundas G, Carlone M, et al. Twenty-year review of radiotherapy for vaginal cancer: an institutional experience. *Gynecol Oncol.* 2008;111(2):298–306.

28. Videtic GMM, Woody N, Vassil AD. *Handbook of Treatment Planning in Radiation Oncology.* 2nd ed. New York, NY: Demos Medical; 2015.

29. Bishop AJ, Allen PK, Klopp AH, et al. Relationship between low hemoglobin levels and outcomes after treatment with radiation or chemoradiation in patients with cervical cancer: has the impact of anemia been overstated? *Int J Radiat Oncol Biol Phys.* 2015;91(1):196–205.

47: UTERINE SARCOMA

Michael A. Weller and Sudha R. Amarnath

> **QUICK HIT:** Uterine sarcomas are rare tumors, comprising ~3% of all uterine malignancies. They are stromal neoplasms arising from the myometrium and connective tissue elements (in contrast to endometrial carcinomas, which are epithelial), and generally behave more aggressively. They are broadly divided into nonepithelial tumors, including endometrial stromal sarcomas (ESS), leiomyosarcomas (LMS), and undifferentiated endometrial sarcomas (UES); and mixed epithelial–nonepithelial tumors, which include adenosarcomas. Of note, carcinosarcomas are no longer considered sarcomas and are treated similar to carcinoma paradigm (see Chapter 44). In general, patients with resectable disease should undergo total hysterectomy and BSO followed by adjuvant therapy depending on risk factors.

TABLE 47.1: General Adjuvant Treatment Guidelines for Uterine Sarcoma Following Hysterectomy

	LMS/UES	ESS/Adenosarcoma
Stage I	Observation (CHT under investigation)	Observation vs. endocrine therapy
Stage II	Observation (CHT under investigation)	Endocrine therapy +/– RT
Stage III–IVA	CHT +/– RT	Endocrine therapy +/– RT
Stage IVB	CHT +/– palliative RT	Endocrine therapy +/– palliative RT

EPIDEMIOLOGY: Rare tumors: 0.3/100,000 person years (estimates typically include carcinosarcomas).[1,2] Approximately 9% of uterine cases[3]; 1,600 cases estimated in 2015. Median age at diagnosis 60 years of age (younger in LMS/ESS, carcinosarcomas tend to be older).

RISK FACTORS: Increasing age, race (2x more likely in African Americans),[4] tamoxifen (black box warning), pelvic RT. Genetic syndromes: hereditary leiomyomatosis and renal cell carcinoma (HLRCC) syndrome.

ANATOMY: See Chapter 44.

PATHOLOGY: Both the WHO and ACP have published classifications.[5,6] Uterine carcinosarcoma (previously mixed Müllerian tumor) is classified as a carcinoma.

Nonepithelial (Mesenchymal)

- Endometrial stromal tumors
  - Endometrial stromal nodule—benign, cured with surgery alone
  - Endometrial stromal sarcomas (ESS)—low grade, tend to be ER/PR positive, mild atypia rare mitotic figures, "finger-like" projections
  - Undifferentiated endometrial sarcomas (UES)—high grade, marked atypia, high mitotic activity, invasive
- Leiomyosarcomas (LMS)—All are high grade. NOT believed to arise from leiomyomas. Abundant mitoses, prominent cellular atypia, and areas of coagulative necrosis. May express ER/PR. Two variants: epithelioid, myxoid.

Mixed epithelial–mesenchymal

- Adenosarcomas—Benign epithelial component is mixed with a malignant stromal element. A variant with "sarcomatous overgrowth" appears to have a worse prognosis.

CLINICAL PRESENTATION: Most commonly presents with abnormal uterine bleeding, pelvic pain, and a uterine mass. Many are discovered incidentally.

WORKUP: H&P with pelvic exam including bimanual exam and Pap smear.

Imaging: CT chest, abdomen, pelvis with contrast. MRI considered to assess resectability. PET/CT not routine but can be considered as per NCCN.[7]

Pathology: Histologic diagnosis by endometrial biopsy (carcinosarcomas arise from endometrial lining, so more likely diagnosed with biopsy). LMS or ESS more often diagnosed after hysterectomy.

PROGNOSTIC FACTORS: Age, race, stage, grade, surgical resection, LVSI

STAGING

TABLE 47.2: AJCC 8th ed. (2017) & FIGO Staging for Uterine Sarcoma[8]			
AJCC	Leiomyosarcoma & Endometrial Stromal Sarcoma	Adenosarcoma	FIGO
T1	a ≤5 cm in greatest dimension	Limited to endometrium/endocervix	IA
	b >5 cm in greatest dimension	Limited to <1/2 myometrium	IB
	c Not applicable	Limited to >1/2 myometrium	IC
T2	a Involves adnexae	Involves adnexae	IIA
	b Involves other pelvic tissue	Involves other pelvic tissue	IIB
T3	a Tumor infiltrates abdominal tissues (1 site)	Tumor infiltrates abdominal tissues (1 site)	IIIA
	b Tumor infiltrates abdominal tissues (>1 site)	Tumor infiltrates abdominal tissues (> 1 site)	IIIB
N1	• Regional LNs	• Regional LNs	IIIC
T4	• Invades bladder or rectum	• Invades bladder or rectum	IVA
M1	• Distant metastasis	• Distant metastasis	IVB
The AJCC 8th Edition added the uterine sarcoma system (was not present in 7th edition).			

TREATMENT PARADIGM

Surgery: In general, hysterectomy and BSO recommended in resectable patients. Omission of BSO may be reasonable in premenopausal women with LMS, as one RR demonstrated no difference in DFS with this approach.[9] However, caution if tumor is ER/PR positive. Morcellation is NOT recommended, and worse outcomes in women inadvertently undergoing morcellation for benign reasons resulted in an FDA safety alert in 2014.[10,11]

Lymph node dissection: All women with enlarged nodes or extrauterine disease should receive LND. If LMS confined to the uterus, lymph nodes are rare (<5% in stage I–II), and LND is probably unnecessary.[12] In ESS, rates of LN+ are variable in the literature. A SEER analysis suggested the risk is related to grade (~8% for low grade, 12% for high grade).[13] The presence of LN was prognostic; however, performing LND did not impact DFS or OS.

Chemotherapy: No role currently in ESS. In localized LMS, GOG 277 is investigating observation versus adjuvant CHT (four cycles gemcitabine plus docetaxel, followed by four cycles of doxorubicin). In advanced LMS or EUS, multiagent chemotherapy is typically recommended: regimens include docetaxel/gemcitabine (preferred for LMS), doxorubicin/ifosfamide, doxorubicin/dacarbazine, gemcitabine/dacarbazine, gemcitabine/vinorelbine. Clinical trials are strongly recommended for these pts.

Anti-Hormonal therapy: For low-grade ESS or ER/PR+ LMS. Options include medroxyprogesterone acetate, megestrol acetate, aromatase inhibitors, GnRH analogues.

Radiation

Indications: RT is generally not indicated. In LMS, the only randomized data showed no improvement in LR or survival.[14] In advanced ESS, retrospective evidence has inconsistently demonstrated a small benefit in local control, but no survival benefit with the addition of RT.[15]

Dose: If RT is to be employed, "tumor-directed RT" typically entails treatment of the pelvis +/- para-aortic nodes to 45–50 Gy with or without brachytherapy boost.

EVIDENCE-BASED Q&A

Should RT be offered as adjuvant treatment for patients with uterine sarcoma?

Evidence supporting the use of RT in uterine sarcomas is sparse and generally limited to retrospective reviews. These generally show small benefits in LC and no difference in survival. The only randomized data comes from EORTC 55874.

Sampath, UC Davis (*IJROBP* 2010 PMID 19700247): RR of 3,650 pts with uterine sarcoma identified from the National Oncology Database (NODB, proprietary dataset). Pts with sarcoma, myomatous neoplasm, and complex/mixed neoplasm identified. Of those included 51% were carcinosarcomas, 25% LMS, 15% ESS, 4% AS, 5% other. 30% were stage I, 37% unknown stage; 7%, 12%, and 13% were stages II–IV respectively. Adjuvant RT improved local control in the entire cohort as well as in all subgroups. No difference in survival (5-yr OS was 37%). On MVA age, stage, grade, histology, and nodal status significantly influenced OS. **Conclusion: RT may improve LRFFS for pts with uterine sarcoma.**

TABLE 47.3: Results of Sampath Study: RT for Uterine Sarcoma			
Group	5-yr LRFFS (%)		Log-rank *p* value
	No RT	RT	
Carcinosarcoma	80	90	<.001
LMS	84	98	<.01
ESS	93	97	<.05
Overall	85	93	<.01

Reed, EORTC 55874 (*European Journal of Cancer* 2008, PMID 18378136): Phase III PRT of 224 pts w/ stage I–II uterine sarcoma (99 LMS, 92 CS, 30 ESS, 3 other) s/p TAH BSO randomized to adjuvant pelvic RT (50.4 Gy/28 fx over 5 weeks) versus observation. Required 13 years to accrue. In all patients, the addition of RT decreased the rate of local recurrence (40% vs. 24%) with no impact on DFS or OS. On subgroup analysis, the improvement in local failure was driven by CS (47% vs. 24%) and there was no benefit in local recurrence in patients with LMS (24% vs. 20%). **Conclusion: The addition of adjuvant RT improves local control in patients with stage I–II carcinosarcoma, but not LMS. RT does not impact survival.**

Is chemoradiation more effective than RT alone?

Pautier, SARCGYN French Study (*Ann Oncol* 2013, PMID 23139262): Phase III PRT of 81 patients. Stage I–III CS (19), LMS (53), UDES (9) randomized to adjuvant polychemo-therapy (four cycles of doxorubicin 50 mg/m² day 1, ifosfamide 3 g/m²/day days 1–2, cisplatin 75 mg/m² day 3) followed by pelvic RT (45 Gy/25 fx) versus RT alone. Primary endpoint DFS. 50 pts also received brachytherapy. Stopped early due to poor accrual (planned 256 pts). The addition of CHT improved 3-yr DFS (55% vs. 41%, $p = .048$). Similarly, OS improved but not statistically (81% vs. 69%, $p = .41$). Two toxic deaths, 76% grade 3–4 thrombocytopenia in chemo arm. **Conclusion: Adjuvant chemoRT improves DFS for uterine sarcoma.** *Comment: Approximately ¼ were carcinosarcoma.*

REFERENCES

1. Nordal RR, Thoresen SO. Uterine sarcomas in Norway 1956–1992: incidence, survival and mortality. *Eur J Cancer*. 1997;33(6):907–911.
2. Toro JR, Travis LB, Wu HJ, et al. Incidence patterns of soft tissue sarcomas, regardless of primary site, in the surveillance, epidemiology and end results program, 1978-2001: an analysis of 26,758 cases. *Int J Cancer*. 2006;119(12):2922–2930.
3. Ueda SM, Kapp DS, Cheung MK, et al. Trends in demographic and clinical characteristics in women diagnosed with corpus cancer and their potential impact on the increasing number of deaths. *Am J Obstet Gynecol*. 2008;198(2):218.e211–e216.
4. Brooks SE, Zhan M, Cote T, Baquet CR. Surveillance, epidemiology, and end results analysis of 2,677 cases of uterine sarcoma 1989–1999. *Gynecol Oncol*. 2004;93(1):204–208.
5. Kurman RJ, International Agency for Research on Cancer., World Health Organization. *WHO Classification of Tumours of Female Reproductive Organs*. 4th ed. Lyon: International Agency for Research on Cancer; 2014.
6. Otis CN, Ocampo AC, Nucci MR, McCluggage WG. Protocol for the Examination of Specimens From Patients With Sarcoma of the Uterus. 3.1.0.0; 2016. http://www.cap.org/ShowProperty?nodePath=/UCMCon/Contribution%20Folders/WebContent/pdf/cp-uter-ine-sarcoma-15protocol-3100.pdf
7. NCCN Clinical Practice Guidelines in Oncology: Uterine Neoplasms; 2017. https://www.nccn.org
8. Cancer AJCo. *AJCC Cancer Staging Manual*. 8th ed: New York, NY: Springer Publishing; 2017.
9. Kapp DS, Shin JY, Chan JK. Prognostic factors and survival in 1,396 patients with uterine leiomyosarcomas: emphasis on impact of lymphadenectomy and oophorectomy. *Cancer*. 2008;112(4):820–830.
10. Einstein MH, Barakat RR, Chi DS, et al. Management of uterine malignancy found incidentally after supracervical hysterectomy or uterine morcellation for presumed benign disease. *Int J Gynecol Cancer*. 2008;18(5):1065–1070.
11. Oduyebo T, Rauh-Hain AJ, Meserve EE, et al. The value of re-exploration in patients with inadvertently morcellated uterine sarcoma. *Gynecol Oncol*. 2014;132(2):360–365.
12. Major FJ, Blessing JA, Silverberg SG, et al. Prognostic factors in early-stage uterine sarcoma: a Gynecologic Oncology Group study. *Cancer*. 1993;71(4 Suppl):1702–1709.
13. Chan JK, Kawar NM, Shin JY, et al. Endometrial stromal sarcoma: a population-based analysis. *Br J Cancer*. 2008;99(8):1210–1215.
14. Reed NS, Mangioni C, Malmström H, et al. Phase III randomised study to evaluate the role of adjuvant pelvic radiotherapy in the treatment of uterine sarcomas stages I and II: a European Organisation for Research and Treatment of Cancer Gynaecological Cancer Group Study (protocol 55874). *Eur J Cancer*. 2008;44(6):808–818.
15. Sampath S, Schultheiss TE, Ryu JK, Wong JY. The role of adjuvant radiation in uterine sarcomas. *Int J Radiat Oncol Biol Phys*. 2010;76(3):728–734.

IX: **HEMATOLOGIC**

48: ADULT HODGKIN'S LYMPHOMA

Senthilkumar Gandhidasan, Matthew C. Ward, and Chirag Shah

> **QUICK HIT:** Hodgkin's lymphoma accounts for 10% of lymphomas in the United States and is broadly grouped into classical and nodular lymphocyte predominant types. Risk stratification of classical Hodgkin's determines treatment and broadly includes early-stage favorable, early-stage unfavorable, and advanced (stage III–IV) disease. Each major study group (EORTC, German HSG, UK RAPID, Stanford) defines risk stratification differently. Most recent trials use PET response as judged by Deauville criteria to guide treatment. For early-stage favorable disease, despite multiple large trials, CHT alone is not noninferior to combined chemoRT (in terms of PFS). However, many favor CHT alone due to favorable salvage rates with autologous SCT and equivalent OS. Late effects with RT are of particular concern due to the disease's excellent prognosis. Although most trials delivered involved-field RT (IFRT), involved-site RT (ISRT) is well-accepted internationally and may reduce toxicity. Nodular lymphocyte predominant pts are treated similar to low-grade non-Hodgkin's lymphoma. Treatment paradigms are different in children (age <21, see Pediatric Hodgkin's Lymphoma chapter for details).

TABLE 48.1: General Treatment Paradigm for Adult Hodgkin's Lymphoma

	Stage/Status	Example Treatment Options (see trials for specifics)[1]	Recent Trials Defining Paradigm
Classic HL	Stage IA/IIA Favorable	Combined chemoRT: ABVD x2-4c and ISRT to 20–30 Gy or CHT Alone: ABVD x3-4c (if PET-negative after 2–3 cycles, i.e., Deauville 1–2) or Stanford V x 8 weeks + ISRT to 30 Gy	German HSG HD10, UK RAPID, EORTC H10F, Stanford G4
	Stage I/II Unfavorable	Combined chemoRT: ABVD x4c and ISRT 30 Gy or ABVD x 6c or Stanford V x 12 weeks + ISRT 30–36 Gy	German HSG HD11, HD14, EORTC H10U
	Stage III–IV	ABVD x6c (consider ISRT to initially bulky or select PET+ sites) or Escalated BEACOPP x 6c	RATHL, German HSG HD15, ECOG 2496
NLPHL Stage IA/IIA Stage IA/IIA bulky or IB/IIB Stage III–IV		ISRT alone to 30 Gy (consider +6 Gy boost for bulky disease) CHT + rituximab + ISRT CHT + rituximab ± ISRT OR local RT for palliation only	

Epidemiology: Relatively uncommon; 0.6% of new cancer diagnoses, estimated 8,260 cases and 1,070 deaths in 2017.[2] Accounts for 10% of all lymphomas diagnosed in the

United States. Slight male predominance, rare under age 10. Bimodal age distribution with peaks around 25 and 60 to 70 years of age.

RISK FACTORS: There is association between Hodgkin's lymphoma and EBV. EBV DNA has been isolated within Reed–Sternberg cell and pts with history of infectious mononucleosis are at higher risk of developing Hodgkin's lymphoma. EBV tied most closely with mixed cellularity subtype and pediatric HD in developing countries.

ANATOMY: Primarily nodal disease with predictable spread. Extranodal spread is rare. 80% of pts present with cervical nodes and >50% with mediastinal nodes. Most common site of extranodal disease is spleen. 13 individual lymphatic regions identified in 1965 now define Ann Arbor staging and include: Waldeyer's ring, cervical/SCV/occipital/pre-auricular, infraclavicular, axillary/pectoral, mediastinal, hilar, para-aortic, spleen, mesenteric, iliac, inguinal/femoral, popliteal, and epitrochlear/brachial. Right and left hilar and cervical regions are counted as separate regions. Waldeyer's ring and spleen are considered lymphatic but extranodal regions for staging purposes. EORTC and German groups count differently than classic Ann Arbor system: EORTC includes axilla and infraclavicular as one site. German HSG includes cervical and infraclavicular regions as one site. Both EORTC and German HSG consider mediastinum and hilar areas as one site. These definitions have implications in risk stratification (see the following).

PATHOLOGY: Classic diagnostic cells are Reed–Sternberg cells though these account for only 1% to 2% of tumor volume with rest being infiltration of lymphocytes, eosinophils, and plasma cells. RS cell classically binucleate with two prominent nucleoli, well-demarcated nuclear membrane, and eosinophilic cytoplasm with perinuclear halo. Likely origin is precursor B-cell. Monoclonal EBV DNA has been identified in RS cells in classical HL. Several subtypes of HL have slightly different pathologic and cytologic markers.

TABLE 48.2: Histologic Characteristics of Hodgkin's Disease

	Histology	Frequency	Clinicopathologic Features	Markers
CLASSICAL	Nodular Sclerosis (NS)	≥70%	Less favorable than lymphocyte rich. Broad bands of birefringent collagen surrounding nodules of lymphocytes, eosinophils, plasma cells, and tissue histiocytes, intermixed w/ atypical mononuclear cells and Reed–Sternberg cells. No gender predilection. Median age approximately 26. Mediastinum often involved. One-third have B symptoms.	CD15+, CD30+ Occasional CD20+
	Mixed Cellularity (MC)	~20%	Less favorable than nodular sclerosis. Diffuse effacement of LNs by lymphocytes, eosinophils, plasma cells and relatively abundant atypical mononuclear and Reed–Sternberg cells. Males and older pts more common. Often have abdominal involvement or advanced dz. One-third with B symptoms.	
	Lymphocyte Rich (LR)	5%	Best prognosis. Occasional Reed–Sternberg cell but mostly diffusely effaced with normal appearing lymphocytes. Male more common. Median age 30. Frequently stage I–II, <10% have B symptoms. Uncommon mediastinal/ abdominal involvement.	

(continued)

	Histology	Frequency	Clinicopathologic Features	Markers
CLASSICAL	**Lymphocyte Depleted (LD)**	<5%	Worst prognosis. Paucity of normal-appearing cells and abundance of abnormal mononuclear cells, Reed–Sternberg cells and variants. Difficult to differentiate from anaplastic large cell lymphoma. Males and older pts more common. Usually advanced disease. Two-thirds with B symptoms.	CD15+, CD30+ Occasional CD20+
	Nodular Lymphocyte Predominant (NLP)	5%	Likely distinct entity from other HD with natural history similar to low-grade NHL. Lacks Reed–Sternberg cells. Significant rate of transformation (to diffuse large B-cell lymphoma) and frequent late relapse. Some response to rituximab. EBV negative.	CD19+, **CD20+**, CD45+, **CD15-**, **CD30-**

TABLE 48.2: Histologic Characteristics of Hodgkin's Disease (*continued*)

CLINICAL PRESENTATION: Painless adenopathy most common. B symptoms: drenching night sweats, fever >38.0°C, weight loss >10% in 6 months (B symptoms present at diagnosis in 1/3 patients; combination of weight loss and fever carries poor prognosis). Generalized pruritus/alcohol-induced pain in infiltrated tissues. Disease foci contiguous in 90% of pts (including connection of supraclavicular nodes to upper celiac/splenic nodes via thoracic duct). Visceral involvement is most frequently splenic and there is correlation between burden of splenic disease and likelihood of hematogenous spread. Marrow and liver involvement occurs almost exclusively in setting of splenic disease. HL is not more common in HIV+ but can have a more aggressive course.

WORKUP: H&P with attention to LN regions, B symptoms, chest and abdominal (spleen/liver) exam.

Labs: Pregnancy test, HIV, CBC, ESR, albumin, BMP, LFT, LDH, PFTs including DLCO.

Imaging: CXR, PET/CT (≥90% sensitivity, changes treatment in 14%–25%), echocardiogram/MUGA (if doxorubicin CHT considered).

Pathology: Excisional biopsy recommended versus core needle biopsy (may be adequate if diagnostic of HL). FNA is inadequate. Bone marrow biopsy if PET is positive or cytopenias exist (overall frequency of bone marrow involvement 5% or less).[1]

PROGNOSTIC FACTORS: Several prognostic factors including stage, age, erythrocyte sedimentation rate (ESR), number of nodal sites involved, extranodal involvement, and lymph node bulk have been identified. In addition to Ann Arbor stage, these factors have defined risk stratification into early-stage favorable and early-stage unfavorable, which define treatment. For early-stage classic Hodgkin's disease (stage I–II), unfavorable factors vary by consensus statement and include:

- NCCN: ESR >50 or B symptoms, mediastinal mass-intrathoracic diameter >0.33, >3 nodal sites, >10 cm
- GHSG: ESR >50 with no B symptoms or >30 with B symptoms, mediastinal mass-intrathoracic diameter >0.33, >2 nodal sites, any extranodal lesion
- EORTC: ESR >50 with no B symptoms or >30 with B symptoms, mass width at T5-6 >0.35, >3 nodal sites, ≥50 years of age.

International Prognostic Score (IPS): Since outcomes are excellent in early-stage disease, a prognostic scoring system was developed for advanced Hodgkin's lymphoma composed of seven factors: albumin <4 g/dL, Hgb <10.5 g/dL, male gender, age ≥45, Ann Arbor stage IV, leukocytes ≥15,000, and lymphocytes <600/mm^3 or <8% of white count. Initial publication stratified PFS from 84% to 42% going from 0 to 7 points.[3] Scoring system was reanalyzed in 2012 and remained valid with PFS ranging between 88% and 69%.[4]

TABLE 48.3: Ann Arbor (Lugano Update) Staging System for Lymphoma** [5]		
I	One node or group of adjacent nodes **OR** single extranodal lesions without nodal involvement (IE)	**A:** No systemic symptoms
II	≥2 nodal groups on same side of diaphragm OR stage I or II by nodal extent with limited contiguous extranodal involvement	**B:** Unexplained weight loss >10% in 6 mos before diagnosis. Unexplained fever with temperatures above 38° C. Drenching night sweats.
III	Nodes on both sides of diaphragm; nodes above diaphragm with spleen involvement	**E*:** Extralymphatic involvement.
IV	Additional noncontiguous extralymphatic involvement	**X*:** Bulky disease (≥10 cm or >1/3 of thoracic diameter)
*Note that 2014 Lugano update suggests "X" and "A/B" modifiers are necessary only for Hodgkin's lymphoma and "E" unnecessary for stage III–IV disease.[5]		
**Number of involved regions may be designated with subscript (i.e., II3).		

TREATMENT PARADIGM

Surgery: There is typically no role for surgery in treatment of adult Hodgkin's lymphoma. In children with NLPHL, resection followed by observation with CHT at progression has been investigated.[6]

Chemotherapy: Several CHT regimens have been used over history of Hodgkin's lymphoma. Historical regimen MOPP (mustard, vincristine, procarbazine, prednisone) resulted in sterility (80% of men, age-linked in women) and secondary acute nonlymphocytic leukemia. Modern regimens are associated with less sterility and secondary malignancy risk and include:

ABVD: (Adriamycin, bleomycin, vinblastine, dacarbazine). Toxicities include nausea, vomiting, hair loss, and marrow suppression. Long-term toxicities include cardiac and pulmonary toxicity. German HD13 study examined if bleomycin, dacarbazine, or both could be omitted (ABV, AVD, and AV arms) in early-stage HL. All alternative regimens were associated with inferior outcomes relative to ABVD.[7] Each cycle is generally one month with two infusions per cycle.

Stanford V: (nitrogen mustard, doxorubicin, vinblastine, vincristine, bleomycin, etoposide, prednisone) is quicker treatment (8–12 weeks vs. 16–24 weeks for four to six cycles of ABVD) and includes lower cumulative doses of doxorubicin and bleomycin. Designed as combined modality therapy with RT, which should not be omitted. Studies suggest similar outcomes as ABVD assuming RT is delivered.[8–10]

BEACOPP: (bleomycin, etoposide, doxorubicin, cyclophosphamide, vincristine, procarbazine, prednisone). Intensified treatment studied in setting of poor response or for unfavorable pts. BEACOPP is associated with higher response rates but also higher incidence of marrow suppression and alopecia.[11]

Number of Cycles: Number of cycles delivered on trials varies by study group. Generally, risk group should be selected and treatment should proceed as per trials evaluating response and outcomes in that risk group. Overall, in PET era, Table 48.1 outlines common approaches and recent trials that defined each approach.

Response Evaluation: Favorable (rapid/early) response to CHT has become an important predictor of outcome and is increasingly being used to determine treatment paradigm.[12-15] For example, PET response after Stanford V regimen (including RT) identified FFP rates of 96% for PET- pts versus 33% for PET+ pts.[16] Deauville score (named after conference in Deauville, France) is standardized method of PET response, which consists of five levels. Level 1 includes no uptake above background; level 2 is uptake less than or equal to mediastinal blood pool; level 3 is uptake above mediastinal blood pool but less than or equal to liver uptake; level 4 is uptake moderately above liver; and level 5 is uptake markedly greater than liver or new lesions.[17,18] Typically, trials consider early response of Deauville 1 to 2 to be favorable (CR), Deauville 3 to 4 to initiate adaptive treatment (PR), and Deauville 5 to define refractory disease. Of note, Deauville 3 is considered a favorable response in some trials.

Radiation: RT, once the only curative treatment for Hodgkin's lymphoma, continues to play an important role in the combined treatment of Hodgkin's lymphoma together with CHT. Thus far no randomized trial has identified population of early-stage Hodgkin's lymphoma where omission of RT did not result in significantly higher recurrence rate. NCDB study of utilization of RT in stage I/II HL between 1998 and 2011 revealed that RT use had declined from 55% to 44% and receipt of RT was associated with significant improvement in 5-yr OS (94.5% vs. 88.9%).[19]

Indications: RT is used in combined modality treatment of early-stage pts and select advanced-stage pts. For early-stage pts, RT use is defined by CHT used and paradigm set by accompanying clinical trial. RT is delivered after CHT to pre-CHT sites. Historically, large RT fields such as mantle, inverted-Y, or total nodal RT (mantle + inverted Y) were used alone to doses >40 Gy. Most recent trials used involved-field RT (IFRT), but now involved-site RT (ISRT) is well accepted. ILROG guidelines are available to guide ISRT or involved node RT (INRT, less common in the United States).[20] Studies have shown that appropriate use of these techniques results in equivalent outcomes.[21] For advanced (stage III–IV) disease, although controversial, RT can be considered for initially bulky or select sites, which remain PET-positive after CHT.[1] If given, initiate RT within 3 to 6 weeks of completion of CHT.

Dose: RT dose should follow paradigm of clinical trial that applies to pt based on PET response and number of CHT cycles given. Typically, for early-stage favorable disease following CHT, 20–30 Gy/10–15 fx is sufficient after PET CR. For early-stage unfavorable disease, 30 Gy is recommended and for bulky disease, 30–36 Gy/15–20 fx. For advanced disease residual on PET/CT or for consolidation of initially bulky disease, consider 30–36 GY/15–20 fx.

Toxicity: Acute: Fatigue, RT dermatitis, esophagitis, odynophagia, cough, xerostomia, nausea, mucositis. Late: Site age dependent but may include: hypothyroidism, pneumonitis, cardiac disease, xerostomia, infertility. Second malignancy is of significant concern and may include leukemia (CHT related), breast cancer, lung cancer. Historic data shows cause of death in Hodgkin's lymphoma at 25 years is most commonly Hodgkin's (24% cumulative incidence), followed by second malignancy (13.5%) and cardiovascular disease (6.9%).[22] Note that late effects data is generally based on obsolete RT techniques and doses—late effects data in combined modality/ISRT era are evolving.

Procedure: See *Treatment Planning Handbook,* Chapter 10.[23]

EVIDENCE-BASED Q&A

Early-stage favorable Hodgkin's lymphoma

What trials define current standard of care in early-stage favorable Hodgkin's lymphoma?

Through great effort and international collaboration, Hodgkin's clinicians have answered many questions that have transitioned treatment from the 1950s standard of large-field RT alone, to modern PET-adapted combined-modality therapy. These questions have included dose reduction of RT alone, demonstrating efficacy of combined-modality therapy and field-size reduction from extended-field RT to IFRT.[24–31]

Although these trials are of great interest, it is more recent trials that define the current "standard" of care and these have focused mainly on the omission of IFRT from CHT alone. Most physicians prefer to pick an approach as defined by the following trials to guide treatment. Omission of RT from ABVD remains controversial, but because of excellent OS results relating to effective salvage with autologous SCT, many argue that RT for all is overtreatment and may increase late effects, though this has not been validated with modern RT techniques, volumes, and doses.

Engert, German HD10 (*NEJM* 2010, PMID 20818855; Update Sasse *JCO* 2017, PMID 28418763): 1,370 pts with early-stage favorable (as defined by German criteria); 2x2 design randomized to ABVD x 4c versus ABVD x 2c as well as IFRT 20 Gy versus 30 Gy. Primary endpoint FFTF. PET was not used to assess response. MFU at update was 98 mos. There were no significant differences in initial or follow-up between either randomization. Noninferiority was confirmed for both (10-yr PFS of ABVD x 4 c + 30 Gy vs. ABVD x 2 c + 20 Gy was 87.4% vs. 87.2%). **Conclusion: ABVD for two cycles and IFRT to 20 Gy is standard as per German paradigm.**

Raemaekers, EORTC H10 (JCO 2014, PMID 24637998; Update André JCO 2017, PMID 28291393): PRT of PET-adapted therapy including both favorable (H10F stratum) and unfavorable (H10U stratum) early-stage Hodgkin's pts as defined by EORTC criteria earlier. Trial evaluated both ability to omit INRT in those with rapid PET response and utility of escalating to BEACOPP in pts not responding on early PET. In H10F, pts randomized to PET-adapted tx versus standard treatment, then received ABVD x 2c followed by PET. In standard arm, pts received one additional cycle of ABVD with INRT to 30 Gy (6 Gy boost allowed for residual disease). In experimental PET-adapted arm, pts received two additional cycles of ABVD (total four) if PET was negative (Deauville 1–2). If positive, pts received escalated BEACOPP x 2 cycles and INRT to 30 Gy (6 Gy boost allowed for residual). See the following for H10U description/results. Primary endpoint PFS, designed as noninferiority, powered to detect 5-yr PFS decrease from 95% (H10F) to 85%. Randomization to PET-adapted therapy was stopped early as noninferiority was unlikely. In final report, 1,950 pts were recruited. In final report, 18.5% of PET scans were positive. Noninferiority of ABVD alone could not be established (H10F 5-yr PFS 99% vs. 87.1%, HR 15.8, 95% CI: 3.8–66.1, noninferiority margin was 3.2). Escalation to BEACOPP improved 5-yr PFS from 77.4% (ABVD+INRT) to 90.6% (BEACOPP+INRT, $p = .002$). **Conclusion: Even in pts with excellent PET response, omission of INRT is associated with increased risk of progression (but no difference in OS).**

Radford, UK RAPID (*NEJM* 2015, PMID 25901426): Noninferiority trial of pts with classic Hodgkin's lymphoma stage IA-IIA (baseline PET not performed) without bulk (≥33% thoracic diameter at T5-6). Pts received three cycles of ABVD, then underwent PET and if negative (Deauville 1-2) randomized to either 30 Gy IFRT or no further treatment. If positive, received total of four cycles of ABVD and 30 Gy IFRT. Primary endpoint PFS, noninferiority margin originally 10% decrease, then modified to 7%. Overall, 32% were unfavorable as per German criteria and 31% had ≥3 nodal sites. MFU 60 mos. 3-yr PFS 94.6% in RT group and 90.8% in no additional therapy group, difference -3.8% (95% CI: -8.8%–1.3%). **Conclusion: ABVD alone is not noninferior to ABVD+IFRT although prognosis is excellent regardless.**

What is Stanford V and how does it differ from other regimens?

Stanford V CHT is standard option consisting of abbreviated CHT with reduced anthracycline and bleomycin doses compared to ABVD. It was designed as a combined modality regimen and omission of RT is not recommended.

Advani, Stanford G4 (*Ann Oncol* 2013, PMID 23136225): Single-arm prospective trial of Stanford V CHT for nonbulky early-stage Hodgkin's lymphoma. CHT included mechlorethamine, doxorubicin, vinblastine, vincristine, bleomycin, and etoposide. In this trial, regimen was abbreviated to 8 weeks from 12 weeks (12 weeks remain standard option for early-stage unfavorable). 1 to 3 weeks after CHT, 30–30.6 Gy/17–20 fx of modified IFRT was delivered. 87 pts enrolled, MFU 10 years. FFP, DSS, and OS were 94%, 99%, and 94%, respectively. **Conclusion: Stanford V is well-tolerated with excellent results and is comparable to other standard options.**

Early-stage unfavorable Hodgkin's lymphoma

The following trials are the most recent to define "standard" of care in early-stage unfavorable Hodgkin's lymphoma. Note that many trials define subsets of early-stage pts with other high-risk features such as bulk, B symptoms, or extranodal disease as advanced rather than early-stage unfavorable, so it is important to identify inclusion criteria for each paradigm when deciding treatment.

What trials define current standard of care in early stage unfavorable Hodgkin's lymphoma?

Eich, German HD11 (*JCO* 2010, PMID 20713848; Update Sasse *JCO* 2017, PMID 28418763): Precursor trial to the following HD14. PRT of pts with early-stage unfavorable (by German criteria) Hodgkin's lymphoma randomized in 2x2 fashion to either ABVD x 4c or BEACOPP x 4c as well as either 20 Gy IFRT or 30 Gy IFRT. 1,395 pts included, FFTF primary endpoint, updated MFU 106 mos. BEACOPP+20 Gy was initially more effective than ABVD+20 Gy, but not confirmed on long-term follow-up. No difference in FFTF between BEACOPP+30 Gy and ABVD+30 Gy. Similarly, after BEACOPP, 20 Gy was noninferior to 30 Gy but after ABVD 20 Gy was not noninferior to 30 Gy (10-yr PFS difference -8.3%, 95% CI: -15.2 to -1.3%). **Conclusion: ABVD x4c + 30 Gy is standard for early-stage unfavorable Hodgkin's lymphoma.**

von Tresckow, German HD14 (*JCO* 2012, PMID 22271480): Follow-up to the preceding trial. Prospective superiority trial of pts <60 years of age with early-stage unfavorable (by German criteria) randomized to either ABVD x 4c or BEACOPP x 2c followed by ABVD x 2c ("2+2" regimen). No PET. Both arms received 30 Gy IFRT following CHT. Primary endpoint FFTF. 1,528 pts, MFU 43 mos. FFTF improved with "2+2" regimen (FFTF HR 0.44, $p < .001$). 5-yr difference in PFS 6.2% (95.4% down to 89.1%, $p < .001$). No difference in OS. **Conclusion: In pts <60 years of age, escalated "2+2" + 30 Gy is standard German HSG treatment for early-stage unfavorable pts.**

Raemaekers, EORTC H10 (*JCO* 2014, PMID 24637998; Update André *JCO* 2017, PMID 28291393): Pts with unfavorable early-stage disease underwent total of four cycles of ABVD+INRT on standard arm and either six cycles of ABVD for PET-negative pts (Deauville 1-2) or two cycles of ABVD, two cycles of BEACOPP, and INRT if PET-positive.

H10U stratum powered to detect PFS decrease from 90% to 80%. Similar to favorable group, if PET was negative, 5-yr PFS was not noninferior in ABVD alone group (ABVD+INRT 92.1% vs. ABVD alone 89.6%, HR 1.45, 95% CI: 0.8–2.5, noninferiority margin was 2.1). As above, if PET was positive, escalation to BEACOPP improved 5-yr PFS from 77.4% (ABVD+INRT) to 90.6% (BEACOPP+INRT, p = .002). **Conclusion: In both early-stage favorable and unfavorable Hodgkin's lymphoma, omission of INRT is associated with increased risk of recurrence even after excellent PET response (but no difference in OS).**

Advanced-stage Hodgkin's lymphoma

What trials define current standard of care in advanced Hodgkin's lymphoma?

The following trials are commonly cited to define treatment. Note that some unfavorable stage I–II pts were included in these trials. Consolidation RT to PET-positive disease and sometimes to pretreatment bulky disease is commonly delivered.

Engert, German HD15 (*Lancet* 2012, PMID 22480758): Prospective randomized noninferiority trial of pts with advanced stage Hodgkin's lymphoma with goal of reducing intensity of treatment. "Advanced" defined as stage III–IV or stage IIB with either extranodal lesions or mediastinal mass >33% maximum thoracic diameter. Pts randomized into three arms: BEACOPP x 8c, BEACOPP x 6c, or BEACOPP-14 (given over 14 instead of 21 days) x 8c. Pts with residual mass of ≥2.5 cm or positive PET received 30 Gy. 2,126 pts included, MFU 48 mos. 5-yr FFTF was 84.4% for standard BEACOPP x 8c, 89.3% for BEACOPP x 6c, and 85.4% for BEACOPP-14. Mortality was higher in intensified standard arm of BEACOPP x 8c. 11% received RT. **Conclusions: Treatment with BEACOPP x 6c followed by PET-guided RT should be standard for advanced Hodgkin's. PET post-CHT can guide need for additional RT.**

Johnson, UK RATHL (*NEJM* 2016, PMID 27332902): Prospective randomized noninferiority study of pts with advanced classic Hodgkin's. "Advanced" defined as stage IIB-IV or IIA with ≥3 involved sites or bulky disease (>33% of transthoracic diameter or in other sites >10 cm). Goal was to omit bleomycin in pts with good PET response. All pts received ABVD x two cycles, then PET/CT. If Deauville 1 to 3, pts randomized to ABVD or AVD (no bleomycin), both for four additional cycles (total of six). Pts with Deauville 4 to 5 received BEACOPP. Noninferiority margin was 5% in 3-yr PFS. 1,214 pts enrolled, MFU 41 mos; 83.7% of interim PET scans were negative (Deauville 1–3). 3-yr PFS (primary endpoint) was 85.7% (ABVD) versus 84.4% (AVD), absolute difference 1.6 (95% CI: -3.2%–5.3%). 32 pts received consolidation RT (2.6% ABVD vs. 4.3% AVD). Rate of pulmonary events were less in AVD group (3% vs. 1%, p < .05). **Conclusion: AVD is not noninferior but results remain excellent and bleomycin omission may be reasonable (as accepted by NCCN 2017[1]).**

Gordon, ECOG E2496 (*JCO* 2013, PMID 23182987): PRT to assess superiority of Stanford V over ABVD. Pts with classical Hodgkin's stage III–IV or stage I–II with either bulky adenopathy (mass >33% maximum intrathoracic diameter on PA chest x-ray). Pts randomized to either ABVD x 6–8 versus Stanford V for 12 weeks. Primary endpoint FFS. RT administered to all pts with bulky mediastinal adenopathy. Mediastinum, bilateral hila, and supraclavicular areas were treated to 36 Gy. For Stanford V pts, any pretreatment site >5 cm and macroscopic splenic disease were also treated to 36 Gy. 794 pts randomized, MFU 6.4 years. No difference in 5-yr FFS for ABVD versus Stanford V: 74% versus 71% (p = .32). Subset analysis demonstrated improved FFS in pts with IPS of 3 to 7. Toxicity overall was no different. **Conclusion: ABVD, with consolidation RT to sites of pretreatment bulky disease, remains standard of care for advanced and locally extensive Hodgkin's lymphoma for pts treated in North America.**

What evidence specifically addresses the role of consolidative RT in the modern era?

Multiple trials have investigated this question directly. Older meta-analysis and trials in MOPP era suggested no benefit.[32-34] *More recent trials in ABVD/BEACOPP era have suggested improvement.*[35,36] *Overall it seems that consolidative RT to sites not responding on PET/CT, or RT to initially bulky sites may be of value, although this is controversial and institution-dependent.*

Borchmann, German HD12 (*JCO* 2011, PMID 21990399): 2x2 PRT of advanced Hodgkin's defined as either stage III–IV or stage IIB with bulk (≥33% of maximal thoracic diameter) or extranodal lesions. Pts randomized 2x2 to either escalated BEACOPP x 8c versus escalated BEACOPP x 4 c followed by reduced BEACOPP x 4 c ("2+2") and to either consolidation RT versus no further therapy. RT was 30 Gy to initially bulky sites or sites with residual tumor ≥1.5 cm. PET not used to assess response. 1,670 pts, MFU 78 mos; 66% to 72% of pts in RT arm received RT compared to 11% in no RT arms. RT improved 5-yr FFTF (difference -3.4, 95% CI: -6.6% to -0.2%) and PFS (95% CI: -6.6% to -0.2%). **Conclusion: BEACOPP x 8 cycles remained standard, and results support use of consolidation RT.** *Comment: This trial was performed in pre-PET era, which may influence treatment selection process.*

Relapsed/refractory Hodgkin's lymphoma

Is there value to adjuvant brentuximab after autologous SCT?

Moskowitz, AETHERA (*Lancet* 2015, PMID 25796459): PRT of 329 pts with unfavorable risk relapsed or primary progressive Hodgkin's lymphoma treated with autologous SCT, then randomized to adjuvant brentuximab vedotin (anti-CD30 antibody bound to antitubulin) or placebo. Median PFS improved from 24.1 to 42.9 mos with brentuximab; 17% versus 16% of pts had died in brentuximab versus placebo groups, respectively. **Conclusion: Adjuvant brentuximab after autologous SCT improves PFS but not OS.**

Is there role for adjuvant RT in refractory pts undergoing autologous SCT?

This is controversial and is without significant modern data. Some authors recommend consolidation RT prior to SCT to induce response if CR is not obtained on PET or consolidation RT after SCT for bulky disease but this is informed by small retrospective series.[37,38]

Is there role for PD-1 inhibition in relapsed/refractory disease?

Ansell (*NEJM* 2015, PMID 25482239): 23 pts with refractory HL enrolled; 78% previous SCT and 78% previously treated with brentuximab. Pts were treated with nivolumab (anti-PD1) at 3 mg/kg every 2 weeks. Objective response rate was 87%. CR rate was 17%. **Conclusion: Nivolumab is effective in heavily pretreated pts with refractory Hodgkin's lymphoma.**

REFERENCES

1. NCCN Clinical Practice Guidelines in Oncology: Hodgkin Lymphoma. I.2017. https://www .nccn.org; Published 2017.
2. Siegel RL, Miller KD, Jemal A. Cancer statistics, 2017. *Cancer J Clin.* 2017;67(1):7–30.
3. Hasenclever D, Diehl V, Armitage JO, et al. Prognostic score for advanced Hodgkin's disease. *N Engl J Med.* 1998;339(21):1506–1514.
4. Moccia AA, Donaldson J, Chhanabhai M, et al. International prognostic score in advanced-stage Hodgkin's lymphoma: altered utility in modern era. *J Clin Oncol.* 2012;30(27): 3383–3388.

5. Cheson BD, Fisher RI, Barrington SF, et al. Recommendations for initial evaluation, staging, and response assessment of Hodgkin and non-Hodgkin lymphoma: Lugano classification. *J Clin Oncol*. 2014;32(27):3059–3068.

6. Mauz-Körholz C, Gorde-Grosjean S, Hasenclever D, et al. Resection alone in 58 children with limited stage, lymphocyte-predominant Hodgkin lymphoma-experience from European network group on pediatric Hodgkin lymphoma. *Cancer*. 2007;110(1):179–185.

7. Behringer K, Goergen H, Hitz F, et al. Omission of dacarbazine or bleomycin, or both, from ABVD regimen in treatment of early-stage favourable Hodgkin's lymphoma (GHSG HD13): open-label, randomised, non-inferiority trial. *Lancet*. 2015;385(9976):1418–1427.

8. Gobbi PG, Levis A, Chisesi T, et al. ABVD versus modified Stanford V versus MOPPEBVCAD with optional and limited RTin intermediate- and advanced-stage Hodgkin's lymphoma: final results of multicenter randomized trial by Intergruppo Italiano Linfomi. *J Clin Oncol*. 2005;23(36):9198–9207.

9. Hoskin PJ, Lowry L, Horwich A, et al. Randomized comparison of Stanford V regimen and ABVD in treatment of advanced Hodgkin's lymphoma: United Kingdom National Cancer Research Institute Lymphoma Group Study ISRCTN 64141244. *J Clin Oncol*. 2009;27(32):5390–5396.

10. Chisesi T, Bellei M, Luminari S, et al. Long-term follow-up analysis of HD9601 trial comparing ABVD versus Stanford V versus MOPP/EBV/CAD in pts with newly diagnosed advanced-stage Hodgkin's lymphoma: study from Intergruppo Italiano Linfomi. *J Clin Oncol*. 2011;29(32):4227–4233.

11. Federico M, Luminari S, Iannitto E, et al. ABVD compared with BEACOPP compared with CEC for initial treatment of pts with advanced Hodgkin's lymphoma: results from HD2000 Gruppo Italiano per lo Studio dei Linfomi Trial. *J Clin Oncol*. 2009;27(5):805–811.

12. Zittoun R, Audebert A, Hoerni B, et al. Extended versus involved fields irRTcombined with MOPP CHTin early clinical stages of Hodgkin's disease. *J Clin Oncol*. 1985;3(2):207–214.

13. Raemaekers J, Burgers M, Henry-Amar M, et al. Pts with stage III/IV Hodgkin's disease in partial remission after MOPP/ABV CHT have excellent prognosis after additional involved-field radiotherapy: interim results from ongoing EORTC-LCG and GPMC phase III trial. *Ann Oncol*. 1997;8(suppl 1):S111–S114.

14. Noordijk E, Carde P, Mandard A-M, et al. Preliminary results of EORTC-GPMC controlled clinical trial H7 in early-stage Hodgkin's disease. *Ann Oncol*. 1994;5(suppl 2):S107–S112.

15. Somers R, Carde P, Henry-Amar M, et al. Randomized study in stage IIIB and IV Hodgkin's disease comparing eight courses of MOPP versus alteration of MOPP with ABVD: European Organization for Research and Treatment of Cancer Lymphoma Cooperative Group and Groupe Pierre-et-Marie-Curie controlled clinical trial. *J Clin Oncol*. 1994;12(2):279–287.

16. Advani R, Maeda L, Lavori P, et al. Impact of positive positron emission tomography on prediction of freedom from progression after Stanford V CHTin Hodgkin's disease. *J Clin Oncol*. 2007;25(25):3902–3907.

17. Gallamini A, Fiore F, Sorasio R, Meignan M. Interim positron emission tomography scan in Hodgkin lymphoma: definitions, interpretation rules, and clinical validation. *Leuk Lymphoma*. 2009;50(11):1761–1764.

18. Meignan M, Gallamini A, Meignan M, et al. Report on first international workshop on interim-PET scan in lymphoma. *Leuk Lymphoma*. 2009;50(8):1257–1260.

19. Parikh RR, Grossbard ML, Harrison LB, Yahalom J. Early-stage classic Hodgkin lymphoma: utilization of RT therapy and its impact on overall survival. *Int J Radiat Oncol Biol Phys*. 2015;93(3):684–693.

20. Specht L, Yahalom J, Illidge T, et al. Modern RT therapy for Hodgkin lymphoma: field and dose guidelines from International Lymphoma RTOncology Group (ILROG). *Int J Radiat Oncol Biol Phys*. 2014;89(4):854–862.

21. Campbell BA, Voss N, Pickles T, et al. Involved-nodal RT therapy as component of combination therapy for limited-stage Hodgkin's lymphoma: question of field size. *J Clin Oncol*. 2008;26(32):5170–5174.

22. Aleman BM, van den Belt-Dusebout AW, Klokman WJ, et al. Long-term cause-specific mortality of pts treated for Hodgkin's disease. *J Clin Oncol*. 2003;21(18):3431–3439.

23. Videtic GMM, Woody N, Vassil AD. *Handbook of Treatment Planning in RT Oncology*. 2nd ed. New York, NY: Demos Medical; 2015.

24. Dühmke E, Franklin J, Pfreundschuh M, et al. Low-dose RT is sufficient for noninvolved extended-field treatment in favorable early-stage Hodgkin's disease: long-term results of randomized trial of RT alone. *J Clin Oncol.* 2001;19(11):2905–2914.

25. Sasse S, Bröckelmann PJ, Goergen H, et al. Long-term follow-up of contemporary treatment in early-stage Hodgkin lymphoma: updated analyses of German Hodgkin Study Group HD7, HD8, HD10, and HD11 Trials. *J Clin Oncol.* 2017;35(18):1999–2007.

26. Noordijk EM, Carde P, Dupouy N, et al. Combined-modality therapy for clinical stage I or II Hodgkin's lymphoma: long-term results of European Organisation for Research and Treatment of Cancer H7 randomized controlled trials. *J Clin Oncol.* 2006;24(19):3128–3135.

27. Fermé C, Eghbali H, Meerwaldt JH, et al. CHT plus involved-field RT in early-stage Hodgkin's disease. *N Engl J Med.* 2007;357(19):1916–1927.

28. Zittoun R, Audebert A, Hoerni B, et al. Extended versus involved fields irRT combined with MOPP CHT in early clinical stages of Hodgkin's disease. *J Clin Oncol.* 1985;3(2):207–214.

29. Hoskin PJ, Smith P, Maughan TS, et al. Long-term results of randomised trial of involved field RT vs extended field RT in stage I and II Hodgkin lymphoma. *Clin Oncol (R Coll Radiol).* 2005;17(1):47–53.

30. Engert A, Schiller P, Josting A, et al. Involved-field RT is equally effective and less toxic compared with extended-field RTafter four cycles of CHT in pts with early-stage unfavorable Hodgkin's lymphoma: results of HD8 trial of German Hodgkin's Lymphoma Study Group. *J Clin Oncol.* 2003;21(19):3601–3608.

31. Arakelyan N, Jais JP, Delwail V, et al. Reduced versus full doses of irRTafter 3 cycles of combined doxorubicin, bleomycin, vinblastine, and dacarbazine in early stage Hodgkin lymphomas: results of randomized trial. *Cancer.* 2010;116(17):4054–4062.

32. Loeffler M, Brosteanu O, Hasenclever D, et al. Meta-analysis of CHTversus combined modality treatment trials in Hodgkin's disease. International Database on Hodgkin's Disease Overview Study Group. *J Clin Oncol.* 1998;16(3):818–829.

33. Aleman BM, Raemaekers JM, Tomišič R, et al. Involved-field RT for pts in partial remission after CHT for advanced Hodgkin's lymphoma. *Int J Radiat Oncol Biol Phys.* 2007;67(1):19–30.

34. Aleman BM, Raemaekers JM, Tirelli U, et al. Involved-field RT for advanced Hodgkin's lymphoma. *N Engl J Med.* 2003;348(24):2396–2406.

35. Laskar S, Gupta T, Vimal S, et al. Consolidation RT after complete remission in Hodgkin's disease following six cycles of doxorubicin, bleomycin, vinblastine, and dacarbazine chemotherapy: is there need? *J Clin Oncol.* 2004;22(1):62–68.

36. Borchmann P, Haverkamp H, Diehl V, et al. Eight cycles of escalated-dose BEACOPP compared with four cycles of escalated-dose BEACOPP followed by four cycles of baseline-dose BEACOPP with or without RT in pts with advanced-stage Hodgkin's lymphoma: final analysis of HD12 trial of German Hodgkin Study Group. *J Clin Oncol.* 2011;29(32):4234–4242.

37. Poen JC, Hoppe RT, Horning SJ. High-dose therapy and autologous bone marrow transplantation for relapsed/refractory Hodgkin's disease: impact of involved field RT on patterns of failure and survival. *Int J Radiat Oncol Biol Phys.* 1996;36(1):3–12.

38. Mundt AJ, Sibley G, Williams S, et al. Patterns of failure following high-dose CHTand autologous bone marrow transplantation with involved field RT for relapsed/refractory Hodgkin's disease. *Int J Radiat Oncol Biol Phys.* 1995;33(2):261–270.

49: AGGRESSIVE NON-HODGKIN'S LYMPHOMA

Matthew C. Ward and Chirag Shah

QUICK HIT: Non-Hodgkin's lymphoma (NHL) is a heterogeneous disease. Aggressive NHL is a loosely defined group of B- and T-cell histologies with survival measured in months for those untreated. T-cell histologies are aggressive but uncommon. Multiagent CHT is indicated in almost all cases of aggressive NHL. Diffuse large B-cell lymphoma (DLBCL) is the most common of the aggressive NHL and the subject of the majority of clinical data. Limited-stage DLBCL is typically treated with R-CHOP for either three cycles followed by ISRT to 30–36 Gy or R-CHOP for six cycles. After six to eight cycles, the role for consolidative RT is controversial in the setting of a CR. Advanced-stage DLBCL can be treated with R-CHOP for six to eight cycles with consideration of consolidation RT. When selecting for consolidative RT, risk factors such as bulk (≥7.5 cm), skeletal involvement, inability to tolerate full CHT, residual disease after CHT on PET/CT, and perhaps genetic factors can be considered, although no clear standard exists.

TABLE 49.1: General Overview of Treatment Paradigm for DLBCL

Limited (Stage I–II)	R-CHOP x 3 cycles followed by: 30–36 Gy for CR 40–50 Gy for PR or R-CHOP x 6–8 cycles
Advanced (Stage III–IV)	R-CHOP x 6–8 cycles ± ISRT 30–36 Gy
Relapsed/Refractory	High dose CHT + autologous SCT +/− RT pre- or post-transplant

EPIDEMIOLOGY: Overall there are 72,240 cases of NHL expected in the United States in 2017, and 20,140 deaths with an incidence of approximately 1 in 50.[1] NHL is the seventh most common noncutaneous cancer and ninth most common cause of death. Slightly more common in males (lifetime risk 1.26:1). Approximately 50% to 60% of NHLs are classified as aggressive. Most common NHL: DLBCL (29%), follicular (26%), SLL/CLL (7%), MZL/MALT (9%), mantle cell (8%), MZL/nodal (3%), primary mediastinal DLBCL (2%) among others.[2,3] Aggressive NHL is more common in low-middle–income countries.

RISK FACTORS: NHL is a heterogeneous disease with a multitude of risk factors. Risk factors for any NHL[4]: older age, race, family history,[5] geographic region,[3] *viral infection* (EBV [NK-T-cell, Burkitt], HTLV-1, HHV8 [Kaposi sarcoma and various lymphomas in HIV+], hepatitis C [DLBCL and splenic MZL]), *bacterial infection* (H. pylori [gastric MALT], Chlamydia psittaci [orbital MALT], Borrelia burgdorferi [tick bite, mantle cell],[6] Campylobacter jejuni [intestinal MALT]), *autoimmune disease* (rheumatoid arthritis, Sjögren's syndrome, Lupus), *immune suppression* (HIV, organ transplant), *medication* (immunosuppressants, alkylating agents), *chemicals* (hair dye, pesticides), previous CLL/hairy cell leukemia (Richter's transformation into DLBCL in 5%–10%).

ANATOMY: 13 individual nodal groups identified in 1965 now define staging and include: Waldeyer's ring, cervical/SCV/occipital/pre-auricular, infraclavicular, axillary/pectoral, mediastinal, hilar, para-aortic, spleen, mesenteric, iliac, inguinal/femoral, popliteal, and epitrochlear/brachial. Waldeyer's ring and the spleen are considered lymphatic but extranodal regions for staging purposes.

PATHOLOGY: NHL includes cancers originating from cells which normally differentiate into T or B lymphocytes, whether originating from the bone marrow or peripheral nodal tissues. 85% to 90% of NHLs derive from B-cell origins.[4] In contrast, leukemias derive from cells that differentiate into erythrocytes, monocytes, or granulocytes. Originally, it was thought that leukemias arose from the bone marrow and lymphoma arises from a mass lesion. Today, cell lineage, morphology, genetics, and immunotyping classify leukemia and lymphomas. Over 60 types of NHL are identified in the WHO 2016 classification, which does not attempt to differentiate into aggressive/indolent due to variable clinical behavior.[7] Many treat grade 3 follicular lymphoma similar to DLBCL.

GENETICS: See Table 49.2.

TABLE 49.2: Common Translocations, Immunotype, and Clinical Pearls for Select "Aggressive" NHLs

Histology		Classic Genetics and Implications	Classic Immunotype	Pearls
B-Cell	Diffuse Large B-Cell Lymphoma (DLBCL)	t(14:18), BCL-2, BLC-6, ALK, many others	CD19+, CD20+, CD45+	Most common NHL. WHO 2016 subtypes: EBV+, germinal center, activated, primary cutaneous, ALK+, HHV8+, "double hit" (MYC and BCL2 or BCL6). Grey zone lymphoma is intermediate between DLBCL and Hodgkin's.
	Primary Mediastinal (Thymic) DLBCL	No classic translocations	CD19+, CD20+, CD5-	Anterior mediastinal (thymic) mass most common in young women. Treatment different than DLBCL.
	Mantle Cell	t(11:14), cyclin D1	CD19+, CD20+, CD5+	Older age and advanced stage more common. Radiosensitive.
	Burkitt	t(8:14) → C-MYC [transcription factor]	CD19+, CD20+, CD5-, CD10+	Classic "starry sky" appearance. Most common NHL in children, endemic type in Africa (jaw, EBV+). Also nonendemic (abdomen, visceral organs) and immune-deficient types
	Follicular, Grade 3B	Grade 3B genetically distinct from grades 1-3A	CD19+, CD20+	High-grade FL (especially grade 3B) is often treated as per DLBCL paradigm (grade 1-3A managed per low-grade NHL paradigm)
T-Cell	Peripheral T-Cell, NOS (PTCL)	t(7:14), t(11:14) or t(14:14)	Variable T-cell (±CD2, 3, 4, 5, 7)	Most common peripheral T-cell, older adults
	Anaplastic Large Cell	t(2:5) → ALK	CD30+, EMA+	More common in kids, good prognosis with ALK+. T-cell neoplasm.
	Angioimmunoblastic	No classic translocations	CD4+	Older adults
	Extranodal NK-T-Cell, Nasal Type	LOH 6q	CD2+, CD56+	More common in Asian males. EBV+ (EBV encoded RNA [EBER] by FISH)

(continued)

TABLE 49.2: Common Translocations, Immunotype, and Clinical Pearls for Select "Aggressive" NHLs (*continued*)			
Histology	Classic Genetics and Implications	Classic Immunotype	Pearls
Either Lymphoblastic Lymphoma/ Leukemia	t(1;19), t(9:22)	TdT+	Nodal presentation of ALL and treated similarly. Can be T- or B-cell presentation

CLINICAL PRESENTATION: Most commonly presents with a painless enlarging LN. B symptoms (fever >38°C, drenching night sweats, weight loss >10% in 6 mos) or numerous other symptoms may be present (fatigue, anemia, pain, cord compression, SVC syndrome, etc.) depending on location and degree of involvement.

WORKUP: H&P with attention to constitutional symptoms (B symptoms), enlarged LNs, or hepatosplenomegaly.

Labs: CBC, CMP, β2 microglobulin, LDH, uric acid, hepatitis B testing (reactivation with rituximab), pregnancy test. Lumbar puncture with flow cytometry if symptomatic, testicular, double hit, HIV-associated, or epidural lymphoma (see CNS prognostic model for risk factors).[8]

Imaging: PET/CT is standard in almost all lymphoma histologies except certain low-grade histologies (extranodal MZL and SLL).[9-11] Uptake (SUV >10) in indolent lymphoma suggests transformation.[12,13] CT with contrast should also be obtained. Echocardiogram or MUGA if CHT dictates. EBV viral load for extranodal NK/T-cell, nasal type.

Biopsy: At least a core needle biopsy but preferably excisional biopsy should be performed for adequate pathologic evaluation including morphology, nodal architecture, genetic and immunoprofiling. FNA is insufficient. A negative PET is usually sufficient at ruling out bone marrow involvement of DLBCL.[14,15] Bone marrow biopsy remains standard for most other NHL (~20% risk of BM involvement for aggressive NHL vs. 50%–80% of indolent NHLs).

PROGNOSTIC FACTORS: Age, bulk (classically defined as ≥10 cm or >1/3 thoracic diameter, but more recently defined as ≥7.5 cm). Germinal center subtype more favorable than nongerminal center as defined by tissue microarray (combination of CD10, BCL6, and MUM1).[16] Multiple prognostic models exist for pts with aggressive NHL treated with CHT. See Tables 49.3 and 49.4. The IPI[17] is classic (mnemonic "LEAPS": LDH, extranodal sites, age, performance status, and stage). NCCN-IPI is most recent (improved discrimination of low and high risk). Mantle cell may be best classified using the MIPI.[18] The Deauville (5-point) score is used to interpret PET scans and is prognostic, particularly at the end of treatment. This consists of five levels. Level 1 includes no update above background; level 2 is uptake less than or equal to mediastinal blood pool; level 3 is uptake above mediastinal blood pool but less than or equal to liver uptake; level 4 is uptake moderately above liver; and level 5 is uptake markedly greater than liver or new lesions.[19]

NATURAL HISTORY: Aggressive lymphoma, loosely defined, includes cancers with survival measured in months if untreated, as compared to indolent lymphoma, with survival measured in years. Compared to Hodgkin's disease, the pattern of spread is less predictable and can skip nodal levels/sites.

TABLE 49.3: Classic IPI Prognostic System (1993[17]) and NCCN-IPI (2014[20]) for Aggressive NHL

	IPI		Age-Adjusted IPI		NCCN-IPI	
	Factor	Score	Factor	Score	Factor	Score
Age	>60	1	N/A	1	>40 to ≤60 >60 to <75 ≥75	1 2 3
LDH	High	1	High	1	>1xULN but ≤3xULN >3xULN	1 2
Extranodal Sites	≥2	1	N/A	1	Bone marrow, CNS, liver/GI tract, lung	1
Performance Status (ECOG)	≥2	1	≥2	1	≥2	1
Stage (Ann Arbor)	III–IV	1	III–IV	1	I–II vs. III–IV	1

ULN, Upper limit normal.

TABLE 49.4: Aggressive NHL Outcome by IPI Score (see Table 49.3 for risk factors)

Risk Group	Original IPI (Prerituximab)[17]			Age-Adjusted IPI[17]				IPI in Rituximab Era[21]			NCCN-IPI[20]		
	Score	5-yr OS	5-yr RFS	Score	5-yr OS (≤60 y/o)	5-yr OS (>60 y/o)	5-yr RFS	Score	3-yr OS	3-yr PFS	Score	5-yr OS	5-yr PFS
Low	0–1	73%	70%	0	83%	56%	86%	0–1	91%	87%	0–1	96%	91%
Low-intermediate	2	51%	50%	1	69%	44%	66%	2	81%	75%	2–3	82%	74%
High-intermediate	3	43%	49%	2	46%	37%	53%	3	65%	59%	4–5	64%	51%
High	4–5	26%	40%	3	32%	21%	58%	4–5	59%	56%	≥6	33%	30%

STAGING

TABLE 49.5: Ann Arbor (Lugano) Staging System for Lymphoma**

I	One node or a group of adjacent nodes OR single extranodal lesions without nodal involvement (IE)	**A:** No systemic symptoms
II	≥2 nodal groups on the same side of the diaphragm OR stage I or II by nodal extent with limited contiguous extranodal involvement	**B:** Unexplained weight loss >10% in 6 mos before diagnosis. Unexplained fever with temperatures above 38°C. Drenching night sweats.
III	Nodes on both sides of the diaphragm; nodes above the diaphragm with spleen involvement	**E*:** Extranodal involvement.
IV	Additional noncontiguous extralymphatic involvement	**X*:** Bulky disease (Hodgkin's: >10 cm or mediastinal mass >1/3 the maximum thoracic diameter at T5-6 on PA CXR).

*Note that 2014 Lugano update suggests "X" and "A/B" modifiers are no longer necessary for NHL, and "E" unnecessary for stage III–IV disease.[22]
**Number of involved regions may be designated with a subscript (i.e., II_3).

TREATMENT PARADIGM

Observation: Unlike indolent lymphomas, there is generally no role for observation of aggressive lymphomas. Notable exceptions may be mantle cell with a low tumor burden.[23]

Surgery: Generally the role for surgery is limited to excisional biopsy.

Chemotherapy: CHT is the backbone of treatment for NHL. See Table 49.6 for regimens. Rituximab is an anti-CD20 antibody consistently demonstrated in the early 2000s to improve 5-yr OS for DLBCL by approximately 10% with minimal increase in toxicity.[24-26] R-CHOP: rituximab, cyclophosphamide, doxorubicin, vincristine, and prednisone, often given q21 days for six cycles. R-EPOCH consists of the same agents as R-CHOP but with etoposide and overall, across subtypes of DLBCL, did not demonstrate a benefit compared to R-CHOP in the CALGB/Alliance 50303 trial (although it is still an option in other subtypes, e.g., primary mediastinal DLBCL or double-hit DLBCL). Consolidation with autologous SCT is not routinely recommended for DLBCL but can be considered for "double hit" type.[27] CNS prophylaxis can be delivered to high-risk pts via either systemic MTX, intrathecal MTX or cytarabine.[8,9]

TABLE 49.6: Example Regimens for Aggressive NHL		
Diagnosis	Common/Example CHT Regimens	Notes
DLBCL, Germinal Center Type	R-CHOPx6 ± RT	Good outcomes with standard R-CHOP
	R-CHOPx3 + RT	
DLBCL, Activated B-Cell Type	R-CHOPx6-8 ± RT	Studies suggest inferior outcomes with standard R-CHOP, some intensify CHT
	R-ACVBP + MTX/ Leukovorin[28]	
	R-CHOP + Lenalidomide[29]	
DLBCL, "Double Hit"	R-EPOCH	Outcomes with standard R-CHOP are inferior, consider CNS prophylaxis or autologous SCT
	RHyper-CVAD	
DLBCL, Transformed Follicular	R-CHOP x6 ± RT	Diagnosis: biopsy regions of PET SUV >10[13]
Follicular, Grade 3b	R-CHOP ± RT	As per DLBCL paradigm
Primary Mediastinal DLBCL	R-EPOCH x6 ± RT[30]	
	R-CHOP x6 + RT	
Mantle Cell	R-CHOP + Autologous SCT[31]	
	R-Hyper-CVAD/Cytarabine/ MTX[32]	
	R-CHOP + RT	Select stage I–II pts
	R-CHOP	Not curative
	Bendamustine + Rituximab	
	Many others	
Burkitt's	CODOX-M[33]	
	CALGB Regimen[34]	
	R-EPOCH[35]	

(*continued*)

TABLE 49.6: Example Regimens for Aggressive NHL (*continued*)		
Diagnosis	Common/Example CHT Regimens	Notes
Extranodal NK-T-Cell, Nasal Type	HyperCVAD[36]	
	SMILE + RT[37]	
	DeVIC + Concurrent RT[38]	
	GELOX + Sandwhich RT[39]	

Radiation

Indications: The role for RT in aggressive NHL is either for consolidation or palliation. For select patients unable to receive CHT or in early-stage mantle cell lymphoma, definitive RT may be appropriate. RT decisions should be based off the CHT regimen chosen and response to induction therapy. Historic technique was IFRT, modern technique is now ISRT (when treated after CHT). ILROG guidelines delineate the technique for involved-site RT.[40]

Dose

TABLE 49.7: NCCN RT Dose Guidelines for Aggressive Non-Hodgkin's Lymphoma[9,10]		
Mantle Cell, stage I–II	RT alone	30–36 Gy
DLBCL*	Consolidation after CR	30–36 Gy
	Consolidation after PR	40–50 Gy
	Primary treatment (nonchemo candidate)	40–55 Gy
	Combined with SCT	20–36 Gy
	Scrotal RT after CHT	25–30 Gy
Peripheral T-Cell Lymphoma	Consolidation	30–40 Gy
Extranodal NK-T-Cell, Nasal Type	Concurrent with DeVIC	50 Gy
	Sequential after SMILE	45–50.4 Gy
	After GELOX	56 Gy
	RT alone	≥50 Gy
*Note that grade 3B follicular lymphoma is often managed according to DLBCL paradigm.		

Toxicity: Acute: Fatigue, skin erythema, other sequelae are site-dependent. Late: Site-dependent but include second malignancy, xerostomia, fibrosis, cardiotoxicity, and so on.

Procedure: See *Treatment Planning Handbook*, Chapter 10.[41]

EVIDENCE-BASED Q&A

Historically, what data exists regarding the role of RT in DLBCL?

Three cooperative groups (SWOG, ECOG, French GELA) investigated the role of consolidative IFRT after CHT with variable results in the pre-rituximab era. RT was effective at reducing in-field relapses but that RT only improved OS in the initial results of one trial (SWOG), though these studies used higher doses and older RT techniques. Overall, it appears that less-intense CHT with RT is comparable to intensive CHT alone. Toxicity is significant with intense CHT; therefore combined-modality treatment may be ideal for some pts.

Miller, SWOG 8736 (*NEJM* 1998, PMID 9647875, Update Stephens *JCO* 2016, PMID 27382104): PRT of 401 pts with localized intermediate or high-grade NHL stage I, IE (including bulky), nonbulky stage II or IIE disease. Bulk defined as ≥10 cm or >1/3 maximal chest diameter. Pts were randomized to CHOP x 8 cycles given q21 days vs. CHOP x 3 cycles followed by IFRT to 40–55 Gy. IFRT targeted any involved location pre-CHT. MFU 4.4 years. See Table 49.8. Long-term follow-up of a subset of original population (MFU 17.7 years) suggested continuous treatment failure despite RT in patients receiving limited CHT. **Conclusion: Combined-modality treatment is superior to CHOP alone and less toxic, although with long-term follow-up this did not persist.**

TABLE 49.8: Results of SWOG 8736 NHL

SWOG 8736	5-yr PFS	5-yr OS	Life-Threatening Toxicity
CHOP x 8	64%	72%	40%
CHOP x 3 + RT	77%	82%	30%
p value	.03	.02	.06

Horning, ECOG 1484 (*JCO* 2004, PMID 15210738): PRT of 352 pts with early-stage diffuse aggressive lymphoma. Stage I with mediastinal or retroperitoneal involvement, bulky disease >10 cm, stage IE, II, or IIE included. Treatment was CHOP x 8 cycles, then restaging by CT. PR received 40 Gy IFRT. Pts with CR randomized to observation versus 30 Gy IFRT. MFU 12 years; 61% had CR; 31% of PR pts had CR after IFRT. See Table 49.9. **Conclusion: IFRT improved DFS but not OS.** *Comment: Powered for 20% OS difference.*

TABLE 49.9: Results of ECOG 1484 NHL

ECOG 1484	6-yr DFS	6-yr OS
CHOP x 8 → PR → RT	63%	69%
CHOP x 8 → CR → Obs	53%	67%
CHOP x 8 → CR → RT	69%	79%
p value	.05	.23

Reyes, GELA LNH 93-1 (*NEJM* 2005, PMID 15788496): PRT of 647 pts <61 years of age with localized stage I–IIE aggressive lymphoma and no IPI risk factors. Pts randomized to CHOP x 3 cycles + IFRT versus ACVBP alone (doxorubicin, cyclophosphamide, vindesine, bleomycin, prednisone) with MTX, etoposide, ifosfamide, and cytarabine consolidation. IFRT was 40 Gy/22 fx. MFU 7.7 years. See Table 49.10. Grade 3-4 toxicity worse in the ACVBP arm (12% vs. 1%). Initial site relapse more common in ACVBP arm (41% vs. 23%) but out-of-field relapse more common in CHOP arm (72% vs. 38%). **Conclusion: In young pts, intensive CHT alone is superior to CHOP+IFRT. ACVBP is not a standard regimen in the United States.**

TABLE 49.10: Results of GELA LNH 93-1 NHL

GELA LNH 93-1	CR	5-yr EFS	5-yr OS
CHOP x 3 + IFRT	92%	74%	81%
ACVBP	93%	82%	90%
p value	NS	<.001	.001

Bonnet, GELA LNH 93-4 (*JCO* 2007, PMID 17228021): PRT of 576 pts >60 years of age with localized stage I–IIE aggressive NHL and no IPI risk factors. Pts randomized to CHOP x 4 cycles ± IFRT to 40 Gy. MFU 7 years. CR (89% vs. 91%), 5-yr EFS (61% vs. 64%),

5-yr OS (72% vs. 68%, p = .5) were no different with the addition of RT. **Conclusion: For older pts with favorable risk factors, CHOP alone appears adequate.**

What was the impact of rituximab on outcomes with chemotherapy alone?

The preceding historic trials were performed in the pre-rituximab era. The introduction of rituximab in the early 2000s markedly improved outcomes above CHOP alone, with approximately a 10% improvement in OS at 5 years.[24–26,42] Therefore, many argue consolidation with RT is unnecessary, though there is no level I evidence to support this conclusion at this time.

How many cycles of R-CHOP are necessary for DLBCL?

Trials performed either six or eight cycles for DLBCL given every 21 days. The RICOVER-60 trial directly addressed this question.

Pfreundschuh, RICOVER-60 (*Lancet Oncol* 2008, PMID 18226581): PRT of 1,222 pts, 61 to 80 years of age with aggressive B-cell lymphoma; 2x2 randomization: CHOP versus R-CHOP and six versus eight cycles (both q14 days, rather than conventional q21 days). IFRT to 36 Gy was recommended to sites initially ≥7.5 cm (bulky) or extranodal sites regardless of response. R-CHOP improved DFS and OS, but no difference between six versus eight cycles. **Conclusion: Six cycles of R-CHOP is the preferred regimen for elderly pts.**

Is consolidative RT necessary for early-stage DLBCL in the rituximab era?

This is a controversial question and use of RT has been declining.[43] There may be some pts who benefit, but no high-quality data exists to guide decisions. Retrospective and nonrandomized data below supports the role of RT. This includes at least four large databases (NCDB, SEER, NCCN) and multiple retrospective reviews.[43–50] Of note, the German UNFOLDER trial randomizing bulky or ENE pts to either RT or No RT closed its two arms omitting RT early due to inferior EFS.[51,52] It is likely that a subset of pts with DLBCL benefit from RT, although this has not been clearly defined. Risk factors such as bulk, skeletal involvement, inability to tolerate full CHT, residual disease after CHT on PET/CT, and perhaps genetic factors can be considered.[52]

Held, RICOVER-60 NoRTh (*JCO* 2014, PMID 24493716): After the completion of the RICOVER-60 trial, the protocol was amended and another 166 pts were accrued to the best arm of the RICOVER-60 trial (R-CHOPx6 q14 days) but sparing RT. The arm from the original trial (RT arm) was compared to the no RT cohort. MFU 39 months. MVA in the per-protocol population demonstrated worse EFS, PFS, and OS in those with bulky disease not treated with RT. **Conclusion: RT should be used in all patients with bulky disease, until PET-directed omission studies are completed. Further randomized trials are necessary.**

Held, German Pooled Analysis (*JCO* 2013, PMID 24062391): Pooled analysis of data from nine randomized trials including 3,840 pts with aggressive B-cell lymphoma; 7.6% had skeletal involvement. Skeletal involvement was associated with worse EFS after R-CHOP (EFS HR 1.5, p = .048). Rituximab was not found to improve outcome for pts with skeletal involvement. RT did improve EFS for pts with skeletal involvement (EFS HR 0.3, p = .001; OS HR 0.5, p = .111). **Conclusion: RT may benefit those with skeletal involvement.**

Lamy, Lysa/Goelams 02-03 (*ASH* 2014, Abstract 124[21]:393): Pts with nonbulky (<7 cm) stage I–II DLBCL treated with R-CHOP for four cycles (IPI of 0) or six cycles (IPI > 0), then randomized to 40 Gy IFRT or observation. Pts with PR (PET-assessed) after four cycles received six total cycles and RT. Preliminary report at MFU of 51 mos. 313 pts, 40% had extranodal sites; 84% CR after four cycles. EFS and OS no different in the ITT population.

For those in CR, 5-yr EFS 89% No RT versus 91% RT ($p = .24$). **Conclusion: Preliminary findings suggest RT consolidation is not necessary in nonbulky early-stage DLBCL.**

Is there a role for consolidative RT for advanced-stage DLBCL?

This is also a controversial question with less data available. NCCN suggests R-CHOP for six cycles and if CR is confirmed on PET, to consider RT to initially bulky sites or areas of skeletal involvement. RICOVER-60 probably provides the best data for this, as it included all stages (60% in the No RT cohort were stage III–IV). Retrospective data from MD Anderson,[53] Duke[46] and observational data from the NCCN database also suggest a benefit.[50]

What is the optimal radiation dose?

Classic trials often used doses >40 Gy but modern doses are lower as NHL is generally radiosensitive.

Lowry, UK (*Radiother Oncol* 2011, PMID 21664710): PRT with any histologic subtype of NHL requiring RT for local control. 640 sites were randomized to either high-dose RT to 40–45 Gy/20–23 fx versus low-dose RT. Low-dose arm was 30 Gy/15 fx for aggressive histologies and 24 Gy/12 fx for indolent histologies. MFU 5.6 years. No difference in response rates, in-field progression, PFS, or OS. Toxicity was reduced (but not SS) in the low-dose arm. **Conclusion: 24 Gy and 30 Gy is sufficient for indolent and aggressive NHL, respectively.**

How should response to treatment be evaluated for pts with NHL? Is interim PET predictive of outcome?

The updated Lugano Classification[22] (named after Lugano, Italy where the conference took place) defines both staging and response assessment. See the manuscript for details, but in brief a CR should be defined as Deauville 1 to 3, without new lesions, no abnormal bone marrow uptake, regression of the nodal size to ≤1.5 cm in longest diameter and no organomegaly. A Deauville 3 is usually sufficient but may be considered abnormal if reduced-intensity CHT is used. Of note, a midtreatment PET is not clearly predictive of outcome (as opposed to Hodgkin's), and it is not recommended that therapy be altered due to the midtreatment PET.[54]

How is primary mediastinal DLBCL managed?

Primary mediastinal DLBCL is a different entity than other forms of DLBCL and has a natural history between NHL and Hodgkin's disease. It should be managed with either R-EPOCH CHT for six to eight cycles or R-CHOP for six cycles with RT.[9,30] There is minimal data investigating the omission of RT in these pts. Like Hodgkin's, midtreatment PET/CT is prognostic.[55]

REFERENCES

1. Siegel RL, Miller KD, Jemal A. Cancer statistics, 2017. *CA Cancer J Clin.* 2017;67(1):7–30.
2. Armitage JO, Weisenburger DD. New approach to classifying non-Hodgkin's lymphomas: clinical features of the major histologic subtypes. Non-Hodgkin's Lymphoma Classification Project. *J Clin Oncol.* 1998;16(8):2780–2795.
3. Perry AM, Diebold J, Nathwani BN, et al. Non-Hodgkin lymphoma in the developing world: review of 4,539 cases from the International Non-Hodgkin Lymphoma Classification Project. *Haematologica.* 2016;101(10):1244–1250.
4. Armitage JO, Gascoyne RD, Lunning MA, Cavalli F. Non-Hodgkin lymphoma. *Lancet.* 2017;390(10091):298–310.
5. Cerhan JR, Slager SL. Familial predisposition and genetic risk factors for lymphoma. *Blood.* 2015;126(20):2265–2273.

6. Schöllkopf C, Melbye M, Munksgaard L, et al. Borrelia infection and risk of non-Hodgkin lymphoma. *Blood*. 2008;111(12):5524–5529.

7. Swerdlow SH, Campo E, Pileri SA, et al. The 2016 revision of the World Health Organization classification of lymphoid neoplasms. *Blood*. 2016;127(20):2375–2390.

8. Savage KJ, Zeynalova S, Kansara RR, et al. Validation of a prognostic model to assess the risk of CNS disease in patients with aggressive B-Cell lymphoma. *Blood*. 2014;124(21):394.

9. NCCN Clinical Practice Guidelines in Oncology: B-Cell Lymphomas; 2017. https://www.nccn.org

10. NCCN Clinical Practice Guidelines in Oncology: T-Cell Lymphomas; 2017. https://www.nccn.org.

11. Weiler-Sagie M, Bushelev O, Epelbaum R, et al. (18)F-FDG avidity in lymphoma readdressed: a study of 766 patients. *J Nucl Med*. 2010;51(1):25–30.

12. Noy A, Schöder H, Gönen M, et al. The majority of transformed lymphomas have high standardized uptake values (SUVs) on positron emission tomography (PET) scanning similar to diffuse large B-cell lymphoma (DLBCL). *Ann Oncol*. 2009;20(3):508–512.

13. Schöder H, Noy A, Gönen M, et al. Intensity of 18fluorodeoxyglucose uptake in positron emission tomography distinguishes between indolent and aggressive non-Hodgkin's lymphoma. *J Clin Oncol*. 2005;23(21):4643–4651.

14. Khan AB, Barrington SF, Mikhaeel NG, et al. PET-CT staging of DLBCL accurately identifies and provides new insight into the clinical significance of bone marrow involvement. *Blood*. 2013;122(1):61–67.

15. Alzahrani M, El-Galaly TC, Hutchings M, et al. The value of routine bone marrow biopsy in patients with diffuse large B-cell lymphoma staged with PET/CT: a Danish-Canadian study. *Ann Oncol*. 2016;27(6):1095–1099.

16. Hans CP, Weisenburger DD, Greiner TC, et al. Confirmation of the molecular classification of diffuse large B-cell lymphoma by immunohistochemistry using a tissue microarray. *Blood*. 2004;103(1):275–282.

17. Project IN-HsLPF. A predictive model for aggressive non-Hodgkin's lymphoma. *N Engl J Med*. 1993;329(14):987–994.

18. Hoster E, Dreyling M, Klapper W, et al. A new prognostic index (MIPI) for patients with advanced-stage mantle cell lymphoma. *Blood*. 2008;111(2):558–565.

19. Meignan M, Gallamini A, Haioun C. Report on the First International Workshop on Interim-PET-Scan in Lymphoma. *Leuk Lymphoma*. 2009;50(8):1257–1260.

20. Zhou Z, Sehn LH, Rademaker AW, et al. An enhanced International Prognostic Index (NCCN-IPI) for patients with diffuse large B-cell lymphoma treated in the rituximab era. *Blood*. 2014;123(6):837–842.

21. Ziepert M, Hasenclever D, Kuhnt E, et al. Standard International Prognostic Index remains a valid predictor of outcome for patients with aggressive CD20+ B-cell lymphoma in the rituximab era. *J Clin Oncol*. 2010;28(14):2373–2380.

22. Cheson BD, Fisher RI, Barrington SF, et al. Recommendations for initial evaluation, staging, and response assessment of Hodgkin and non-Hodgkin lymphoma: the Lugano classification. *J Clin Oncol*. 2014;32(27):3059–3068.

23. Martin P, Chadburn A, Christos P, et al. Outcome of deferred initial therapy in mantle-cell lymphoma. *J Clin Oncol*. 2009;27(8):1209–1213.

24. Habermann TM, Weller EA, Morrison VA, et al. Rituximab-CHOP versus CHOP alone or with maintenance rituximab in older patients with diffuse large B-cell lymphoma. *J Clin Oncol*. 2006;24(19):3121–3127.

25. Feugier P, Van Hoof A, Sebban C, et al. Long-term results of the R-CHOP study in the treatment of elderly patients with diffuse large B-cell lymphoma: a study by the Groupe d'Etude des Lymphomes de l'Adulte. *J Clin Oncol*. 2005;23(18):4117–4126.

26. Coiffier B, Lepage E, Briere J, et al. CHOP chemotherapy plus rituximab compared with CHOP alone in elderly patients with diffuse large B-cell lymphoma. *N Engl J Med*. 2002;346(4):235–242.

27. Greb A, Bohlius J, Schiefer D, et al. High-dose chemotherapy with autologous stem cell transplantation in the first line treatment of aggressive non-Hodgkin lymphoma (NHL) in adults. *Cochrane Database Syst Rev*. 2008;(1):CD004024.

28. Récher C, Coiffier B, Haioun C, et al. Intensified chemotherapy with ACVBP plus rituximab versus standard CHOP plus rituximab for the treatment of diffuse large B-cell lymphoma (LNH03-2B): an open-label randomised phase 3 trial. *Lancet.* 2011;378(9806):1858–1867.

29. Vitolo U, Chiappella A, Franceschetti S, et al. Lenalidomide plus R-CHOP21 in elderly patients with untreated diffuse large B-cell lymphoma: results of the REAL07 open-label, multicentre, phase 2 trial. *Lancet Oncol.* 2014;15(7):730–737.

30. Dunleavy K, Pittaluga S, Maeda LS, et al. Dose-adjusted EPOCH-rituximab therapy in primary mediastinal B-cell lymphoma. *N Engl J Med.* 2013;368(15):1408–1416.

31. Fenske TS, Zhang MJ, Carreras J, et al. Autologous or reduced-intensity conditioning allogeneic hematopoietic cell transplantation for chemotherapy-sensitive mantle-cell lymphoma: analysis of transplantation timing and modality. *J Clin Oncol.* 2014;32(4):273–281.

32. Khouri IF, Romaguera J, Kantarjian H, et al. Hyper-CVAD and high-dose methotrexate/cytarabine followed by stem-cell transplantation: an active regimen for aggressive mantle-cell lymphoma. *J Clin Oncol.* 1998;16(12):3803–3809.

33. Evens AM, Carson KR, Kolesar J, et al. A multicenter phase II study incorporating high-dose rituximab and liposomal doxorubicin into the CODOX-M/IVAC regimen for untreated Burkitt's lymphoma. *Ann Oncol.* 2013;24(12):3076–3081.

34. Rizzieri DA, Johnson JL, Byrd JC, et al. Improved efficacy using rituximab and brief duration, high intensity chemotherapy with filgrastim support for Burkitt or aggressive lymphomas: Cancer and Leukemia Group B study 10 002. *Br J Haematol.* 2014;165(1):102–111.

35. Dunleavy K, Pittaluga S, Shovlin M, et al. Low-intensity therapy in adults with Burkitt's lymphoma. *N Engl J Med.* 2013;369(20):1915–1925.

36. Thomas DA, Faderl S, O'Brien S, et al. Chemoimmunotherapy with hyper-CVAD plus rituximab for the treatment of adult Burkitt and Burkitt-type lymphoma or acute lymphoblastic leukemia. *Cancer.* 2006;106(7):1569–1580.

37. Yamaguchi M, Kwong YL, Kim WS, et al. Phase II study of SMILE chemotherapy for newly diagnosed stage IV, relapsed, or refractory extranodal natural killer (NK)/T-cell lymphoma, nasal type: the NK-Cell Tumor Study Group study. *J Clin Oncol.* 2011;29(33):4410–4416.

38. Yamaguchi M, Tobinai K, Oguchi M, et al. Concurrent chemoradiotherapy for localized nasal natural killer/T-cell lymphoma: an updated analysis of the Japan Clinical Oncology Group study JCOG0211. *J Clin Oncol.* 2012;30(32):4044–4046.

39. Bi XW, Xia Y, Zhang WW, et al. Radiotherapy and PGEMOX/GELOX regimen improved prognosis in elderly patients with early-stage extranodal NK/T-cell lymphoma. *Ann Hematol.* 2015;94(9):1525–1533.

40. Illidge T, Specht L, Yahalom J, et al. Modern radiation therapy for nodal non-Hodgkin lymphoma-target definition and dose guidelines from the International Lymphoma Radiation Oncology Group. *Int J Radiat Oncol Biol Phys.* 2014;89(1):49–58.

41. Videtic GMM, Woody N, Vassil AD. *Handbook of Treatment Planning in Radiation Oncology.* 2nd ed. New York, NY: Demos Medical; 2015.

42. Pfreundschuh M, Kuhnt E, Trümper L, et al. CHOP-like chemotherapy with or without rituximab in young patients with good-prognosis diffuse large B-cell lymphoma: 6-year results of an open-label randomised study of the MabThera International Trial (MInT) Group. *Lancet Oncol.* 2011;12(11):1013–1022.

43. Vargo JA, Gill BS, Balasubramani GK, Beriwal S. Treatment selection and survival outcomes in early-stage diffuse large B-Cell lymphoma: do we still need consolidative radiotherapy? *J Clin Oncol.* 2015;33(32):3710–3717.

44. Gill BS, Vargo JA, Pai SS, et al. Management trends and outcomes for stage I to II mantle cell lymphoma using the National Cancer Data Base: ascertaining the ideal treatment paradigm. *Int J Radiat Oncol Biol Phys.* 2015;93(3):668–676.

45. Marcheselli L, Marcheselli R, Bari A, et al. Radiation therapy improves treatment outcome in patients with diffuse large B-cell lymphoma. *Leuk Lymphoma.* 2011;52(10):1867–1872.

46. Dorth JA, Prosnitz LR, Broadwater G, et al. Impact of consolidation radiation therapy in stage III–IV diffuse large B-cell lymphoma with negative post-chemotherapy radiologic imaging. *Int J Radiat Oncol Biol Phys.* 2012;84(3):762–767.

47. Shi Z, Das S, Okwan-Duodu D, et al. Patterns of failure in advanced-stage diffuse large B-cell lymphoma patients after complete response to R-CHOP immunochemotherapy and the emerging role of consolidative radiation therapy. *Int J Radiat Oncol Biol Phys.* 2013;86(3):569–577.

48. Kwon J, Kim IH, Kim BH, et al. Additional survival benefit of involved-lesion radiation therapy after R-CHOP chemotherapy in limited stage diffuse large B-cell lymphoma. *Int J Radiat Oncol Biol Phys.* 2015;92(1):91–98.

49. Haque W, Dabaja B, Tann A, et al. Changes in treatment patterns and impact of radiotherapy for early-stage diffuse large B cell lymphoma after Rituximab: a population-based analysis. *Radiother Oncol.* 2016;120(1):150–155.

50. Dabaja BS, Vanderplas AM, Crosby-Thompson AL, et al. Radiation for diffuse large B-cell lymphoma in the rituximab era: analysis of the National Comprehensive Cancer Network lymphoma outcomes project. *Cancer.* 2015;121(7):1032–1039.

51. UNFOLDER: Rituximab and Combination Chemotherapy With or Without Radiation Therapy in Treating Patients With B-Cell Non-Hodgkin's Lymphoma. https://clinicaltrials.gov/show/NCT00278408

52. Ng AK, Dabaja BS, Hoppe RT, et al. Re-examining the role of radiation therapy for diffuse large B-cell lymphoma in the modern era. *J Clin Oncol.* 2016;34(13):1443–1447.

53. Phan J, Mazloom A, Medeiros LJ, et al. Benefit of consolidative radiation therapy in patients with diffuse large B-cell lymphoma treated with R-CHOP chemotherapy. *J Clin Oncol.* 2010;28(27):4170–4176.

54. Moskowitz CH, Schöder H, Teruya-Feldstein J, et al. Risk-adapted dose-dense immunochemotherapy determined by interim FDG-PET in advanced-stage diffuse large B-Cell lymphoma. *J Clin Oncol.* 2010;28(11):1896–1903.

55. Martelli M, Ceriani L, Zucca E, et al. [18F]fluorodeoxyglucose positron emission tomography predicts survival after chemoimmunotherapy for primary mediastinal large B-cell lymphoma: results of the International Extranodal Lymphoma Study Group IELSG-26 Study. *J Clin Oncol.* 2014;32(17):1769–1775.

50: INDOLENT NON-HODGKIN'S LYMPHOMA

Aryavarta M. S. Kumar and Matthew C. Ward

QUICK HIT: Indolent non-Hodgkin's lymphomas (NHLs): diverse group of diseases with survival measured in years to decades. Most common histologies are grade 1 to 2 follicular lymphoma and extranodal MALT lymphoma. Limited-stage disease (stage I–II) is typically treated with definitive RT alone. Advanced disease (stage III–IV) is typically treated with initial observation, with initiation of CHT for symptomatic disease and RT for palliation. ILROG guidelines are useful for treatment selection and field design.

TABLE 50.1: General Treatment Paradigm for Indolent NHLs

	Treatment Options	Common RT Regimens
Stage I–II	Definitive RT	Follicular/other histologies: 24 Gy/12 fx
		Gastric MALT: 30 Gy/15 fx
Stage III–IV	Observation, CHT, and/or palliative RT	24–30 Gy/12–15 fx
		4 Gy/2 fx (i.e., "boom boom")

EPIDEMIOLOGY: 72,240 cases annually with 20,140 deaths of all NHL subtypes, ninth leading cause of death.[1] Indolent NHL is usually a disease of older adults; median age 65, peak incidence >70. More common in North America, Europe, and Australia.[2] Follicular type represents approximately 22% of all NHLs (second most common NHL after DLBCL), SLL/CLL represents ~6%, and MALT/marginal zone is ~5%.[3] Other subtypes are less common.

RISK FACTORS: Four broad risk factors: immunosuppression, autoimmune diseases, infections, and environmental exposures. See Chapter 49 for details.

ANATOMY: Indolent NHLs can present as nodal or extranodal. Nodal anatomy is detailed further in Chapter 49. Extranodal presentation is more common among indolent NHL. Common extranodal lymphoid sites include thymus, spleen and tonsils, adenoids (Waldeyer's ring). Extralymphatic sites include bone marrow, skin, CNS, ovary, testicle, ocular adnexae, liver, stomach, bowel, breast, lung.

PATHOLOGY/GENETICS: B-cell indolent NHLs are more common than T-cell. WHO 2016 classification defines subtypes.[4] System is complex, but few pearls are as follows. *Follicular NHL:* Graded by number of centroblasts per high-powered field. Grade 1: 0 to 5/HPF, grade 2: 6–15/HPF, grade 3: >15, sometimes subdivided into 3a and 3b with 3b demonstrating sheets of centroblasts and often treated as DLBCL. t(14:18) is classic translocation, results in overexpression BCL-2, blocking apoptosis. *Marginal zone NHL:* Both nodal and extranodal (i.e., mucosa associated lymphoid tissue, MALT). See Table 50.2 for details.

TABLE 50.2: Pathology, Immunophenotype, and Genetics of Common Indolent Non-Hodgkin's Lymphomas				
Disease	Common Immunotype		Common Genetics	Notes
Follicular NHL	CD19+, CD20+	CD10+, CD21+, CD22+, CD79a+ CD5-, CD43-	t(14:18)	BCL-2 expression result of t(14:18), marrow involvement common, risk of transformation 28% at 10 years[5]
Nodal Marginal Zone (MZL)		CD22+, CD3-, 5-, 10-, 23-	Trisomy 3, t(11:18)	Less common than extranodal
Extranodal (MALT) MZL				Frequently localized, t(11:18) associated with triple-antibiotic therapy failure for gastric MALT[6]
SLL/CLL		CD5+, 23+, HLA-DR CD22-	t(14:19), karyotype aberrations (trisomy 12) common but not diagnostic	SLL has morphology similar to CLL but with too low circulating leukemia cell count

CLINICAL PRESENTATION: Often presents only with slow-growing lymphadenopathy, hepatosplenomegaly, cytopenias, or nonspecific constitutional symptoms such as fatigue, malaise, or low-grade fever. Neck, inguinal, axilla, and abdominal lymphadenopathy most common. Less commonly involves skin, which manifests as rash or pruritus. Bone marrow involvement is common. Follicular NHLs commonly present as stage III–IV whereas marginal zone NHL more commonly presents as localized disease. B symptoms are usually associated with aggressive histologies or extensive disease.

WORKUP: H&P with attention to lymphatic, liver, spleen, and/or skin exam.

Labs: CBC, peripheral smear, ESR, CMP, LDH, HIV, hepatitis B, hepatitis C, β-2 microglobulin (see the following FLIPI2 prognostic model), urea breath test for H. pylori (gastric MALT). Pregnancy test.

Pathology: Lymph node biopsy of peripheral lymph node is ideal. Endoscopic biopsy for gastric MALT. FNA insufficient for final diagnosis but may distinguish benign lymphadenopathy from clonal B-cell proliferation via flow cytometry. Bone marrow biopsy (unilateral generally sufficient) for most but not in extranodal MZL.[7] Lumbar puncture for testicular, paravertebral, parameningeal, positive bone marrow, HIV.

Imaging: Contrast-enhanced CT chest, abdomen, pelvis for peripheral lymphadenopathy. PET/CT in all nodal lymphomas (not CLL/SLL or extranodal MZL). PET SUV >10 in patient with indolent NHL may suggest transformation to high-grade histology and can be used to target biopsy (i.e., Richter transformation from CLL/hairy cell leukemia to DLBCL).[8] Obtain MRI brain/spine for symptoms. Obtain echocardiogram or MUGA scan if anthracycline CHT.

PROGNOSTIC FACTORS: Follicular Lymphoma International Prognostic Index (FLIPI) and updated FLIPI2 useful for prognostic assessment for follicular patients. FLIPI was designed pre-rituximab but remained prognostic in rituximab era.[9] See Table 50.3. Other prognostic factors include IRF4 gene rearrangement (follicular grade 3b), high Ki67 index (>30%, suggests rapid proliferation).

TABLE 50.3: FLIPI and FLIPI2 Risk Factors						
Original FLIPI Risk Factors[9,10]				**FLIPI2 Risk Factors**[11]		
Hemoglobin <12 ng/dL				Hemoglobin <12 ng/dL		
Age >60				Age >60		
Stage III–IV				Serum β-2 microglobulin elevated		
Nodal sites >4				Bone marrow involvement		
LDH elevated				Maximal diameter of lymph node >6 cm		
		FLIPI Prerituximab[10]		**FLIPI2**[11]		
Score	**Risk Group**	**5-yr OS**	**10-yr OS**	**Score**	**Risk Group**	**5-yr PFS**
0–1	Low	91%	71%	0	Low	80%
2	Intermediate	78%	51%	1–2	Intermediate	51%
≥3	High	52%	36%	3–5	High	19%

STAGING: See Chapter 49 for Ann Arbor Staging.

TREATMENT PARADIGM

Observation: Considered for elderly or asymptomatic patients with stage III/IV indolent NHLs; see CHT paradigm in the following for discussion on observation versus treatment.

Medical: Triple therapy often first line for H. pylori positive gastric MALT and includes proton pump inhibitor, clarithromycin, and either amoxicillin or metronidazole. Give triple therapy as first line with endoscopic biopsy at 3 months to confirm resolution. If H. pylori negative and lymphoma negative, observation. If H. pylori positive and lymphoma negative, give second-line antibiotics. If H. pylori negative and lymphoma negative, can either continue observation with repeat biopsy or treat with RT for symptoms. If both remain positive, treat with second-line antibiotics with immediate or delayed RT. Response to doxycycline has been noted (65%) for ocular and cutaneous MZL.[12]

Surgery: Minimal role for NHL, used mostly for biopsy, but in small bowel can be therapeutic.

Chemotherapy: Used for later stage (stage III/IV typically). Note that grade 3 follicular NHL is often treated as per DLBCL regimens (see Chapter 49). When considering treatment for indolent stage III–IV NHL, factors such as rate of progression, symptoms, end organ function, cytopenias, and bulk are considered. If none, then NCCN suggests observation.[13] If indications are present, treatment can be initiated and may consist of regimens such as bendamustine + rituximab, R-CHOP, R-CVP (rituximab, cyclophosphamide, vincristine, prednisone), or rituximab alone. Rituximab is chimeric monoclonal antibody against CD20; classic toxicities include infusion reactions, hepatitis B reactivation, and progressive multifocal leukoencephalopathy. Obinutuzumab is more recent human anti-CD20 monoclonal antibody with similar effects as rituximab but binds slightly different epitope of CD20.

Radiation

Indications: In limited-stage indolent NHLs (stage I–II), RT is treatment of choice for cure and usually delivered to whole organ, particularly for gastric, thyroid, orbit (but not conjunctiva), breast, and salivary gland extranodal indolent NHL. In advanced disease, RT is typically used for focal palliation. Involved site RT is often appropriate when entire organ need not be treated. ILROG guidelines exist for both nodal and extranodal NHL.[14,15]

Dose: See Table 50.4 for NCCN dosing guidelines. Doses usually delivered at 1.8 to 2 Gy/ fx. Some have advocated up to 36 Gy for bulky disease. Effective palliation can be provided via "boom boom" regimen of 4 Gy/2 fx (see the following data).

TABLE 50.4: NCCN Dosing Guidelines for Indolent Non-Hodgkin's Lymphomas	
Follicular	24–30 Gy
Gastric MALT	30 Gy
Other extranodal Sites (orbit, skin, thyroid, etc.)	24–30 Gy
Nodal MZL	24–30 Gy
Palliation of Indolent Lymphoma	4 Gy (i.e., "boom boom")

Toxicity: Generally, toxicity mild given low total doses. Fatigue is common, others are related to location of delivery.

Procedure: See *Treatment Planning Handbook*, Chapter 10.[16]

Unsealed sources: Y-90 ibritumomab tiuxetan (Zevalin®) and I-131 tositumomab (Bexxar®, now discontinued) are radiolabeled antibodies against CD20 indicated in use of previously untreated, relapsed, or refractory indolent NHL (primarily follicular) and often produces response in patients refractory to rituximab.

EVIDENCE-BASED Q&A

What data suggests that follicular NHL (grade 1-2) can be cured with RT alone?

Multiple RR are available, but one example is as follows.

Campbell, British Columbia (*Cancer* 2010, PMID 20564082): RR of 237 pts with stage I–II grade 1-3A follicular NHL treated with RT alone. Involved regional RT included LN group with ≥1 adjacent uninvolved LN group (60%), or involved node RT (40%). MFU 7.3 yrs. 10-yr PFS 49%, OS 66%. Distant recurrence was most common in 38% of involved regional RT and 32% of INRT. **Conclusion: Cure is possible with RT and reducing field size does not compromise outcome.**

For limited-stage follicular NHL, is there detriment to initial observation as compared to initial RT?

Indolent lymphoma is slowly progressive, and no treatment may be reasonable first approach. However, for early-stage disease, this is not supported by observational data. Therefore, definitive treatment with RT should remain standard of care.

Pugh, SEER (*Cancer* 2010, PMID 20564102): SEER analysis of 6,568 pts with stage I–II grade 1-2 follicular NHL diagnosed from 1973 to 2004. 34% received initial RT. Those observed were younger, stage I, and without extranodal disease. RT was associated with improved DSS at 20 yrs (63% vs. 51%, HR 0.61, *p* < .0001). OS also improved with use of RT. **Conclusion: Initial RT is standard for early-stage follicular NHL and deferring treatment until time of salvage is associated with worse outcomes. RT is greatly underused.**

Vargo, Pittsburgh NCDB (*Cancer* 2015, PMID 26042364): NCDB analysis of 35,961 pts with stage I–II grade 1–2 follicular NHL. RT use decreased from 37% to 24% between 1999 and 2012. 10-yr OS was 68% for RT pts compared to 54% for no RT pts (*p* < .0001). **Conclusion: RT is significantly underutilized and is associated with improved survival in early-stage follicular lymphoma. RT should remain standard.**

What RT dose is optimal for indolent NHL?

For definitive RT of early-stage indolent lymphoma, 24 to 30 Gy is usually sufficient, with some advocating for 36 Gy in rare case of bulky disease. For palliation, 4 Gy/2 fx or 24 Gy/12 fx are both reasonable. Note that "boom boom" regimen of 4 Gy/2 fx was inferior for definitive treatment of limited-stage pts in FoRT trial and should not be extrapolated to aggressive NHL.

Lowry, British National Lymphoma Investigation (*Radiother Oncol* 2011, PMID 21664710): PRT including any subtype and stage of NHL requiring RT for local control. 361 sites of indolent NHL randomized to either 40–45 Gy/20–23 fx (standard) versus 24 Gy/12 fx (low dose). 640 sites of aggressive NHL randomized to 40–45 Gy/20–23 fx (standard) vs. 30 Gy/15 fx (low dose). For indolent pts, 59% were grade 1-2 follicular NHL, 19% MZL/MALT. For aggressive pts, 82% were DLBCL (mostly as part of combined CHT regimen). 69% of indolent and 86% of aggressive pts were stage I–II. MFU 5.6 yrs. ORR no different: 93% versus 92% for indolent pts in standard versus low-dose groups, respectively, and 91% in both arms for aggressive pts. PFS or OS were also not significantly different. **Conclusion: 24 Gy is sufficient for indolent lymphomas. For aggressive NHL, 30 Gy is usually sufficient when part of combined CHT regimen.**

Hoskin, FoRT Trial (*Lancet Oncol* 2014, PMID 24572077): Noninferiority trial of pts with either follicular NHL or MZL requiring RT for either definitive of palliative treatment. Randomized between 4 Gy/2 fx (i.e., "boom boom") versus 24 Gy/12 fx. Primary endpoint local control. Trial closed early with 548 pts, 614 sites, MFU 26 mos. 63% stage I–I–II, 37% stage III–IV. Response rate 81% versus 74% in 24 Gy versus 4 Gy arms, respectively. Time to local progression was not noninferior in low-dose arm (HR 3.42, 95% CI: 2.09–5.55, *p* < .0001). No difference in OS. **Conclusion: 24 Gy is more effective and standard. However, "boom boom" is useful in palliation and often induces response.**

Is there benefit to adjuvant CHT after definitive RT for early-stage indolent NHL?

Adjuvant CHT does not appear to improve outcomes based on results of at least five randomized trials from prerituximab era (Denmark, Milan, British, EORTC, MSKCC).[17-21]

What data informs treatment of gastric MALT?

In addition to those summarized previously, few notable series are listed in Table 50.5. Study by Wündisch informs treatment of H. pylori positive gastric MALT and supports observation when H. pylori is eradicated.

TABLE 50.5: Summary of Notable RR of Gastric MALT				
Institution	**Year**	**N**	**RT Dose**	**LC**
Dana Farber[22]	2007	21	30 Gy	21/21
PMH[23]	2010	25	25–30 Gy	15/15
Japan[24]	2010	8	30 Gy	8/8
MSKCC[25]	1998	17	30 Gy	17/17

Wirth, Multi-Center IELSG Study (*Ann Oncol* 2013, PMID 23293112): Multicenter RR of 102 gastric MALT pts treated with RT to median dose of 40 Gy. MFU 7.9 yrs. 10 and 15-year FFTF was 88%. 10-yr OS 70%. Large cell component and exophytic growth pattern were risk factors for failure.

Wündisch, Germany (*JCO* 2005, PMID 16204012): Prospective trial tracking outcomes of H. pylori-positive gastric MALT. 120 pts, all with stage IE disease treated with antibiotics and observed after H. pylori eradication. MFU 75 mos. 80% achieved pCR, with 80%

of those experiencing long-term pCR. 3% relapsed and were referred for treatment, other 17% were observed, and all entered into CR. 15% positive for t(11:18). T(11:18) and ongoing monoclonality were associated with failure. **Conclusion: Cure of H. pylori results in continuous CR in most pts. Observation is appropriate for most pts when close follow-up is possible.**

What data informs treatment of other MALT NHL?

Tran, Australian Orbital MALT Series (*Leuk Lymphoma* 2013, PMID 23020137): 27 orbits of 24 pts treated to 24–25 Gy. MFU 41 mos. 59% conjunctival, 26% lacrimal, 4% eyelid, and 11% other. 100% CR, three failures, one local, one contralateral, one distant.

Teckie, MSKCC (*IJROBP* 2015, PMID 25863760): 490 pts with stage IE or IIE MZL, 92% were stage IE. MFU 5.2 yrs. Stomach (50%), orbit (18%), nonthyroid head and neck (8%), skin (8%), and breast (5%). Median RT dose 30 Gy. 5-yr OS 92%, RFS 74%. Most common relapse site was distant. Disease-specific death 1.1% at 5 yrs. All sites except head and neck demonstrated worse RFS compared to gastric. Transformation to aggressive histology was rare (1.6%).

REFERENCES

1. Siegel RL, Miller KD, Jemal A. Cancer statistics, 2017. *CA Cancer J Clin.* 2017;67(1):7–30.
2. Boffetta P. Epidemiology of adult non-Hodgkin lymphoma. *Ann Oncol.* 2011;22(Suppl 4): iv27–iv31.
3. Armitage JO, Weisenburger DD. New approach to classifying non-Hodgkin's lymphomas: clinical features of the major histologic subtypes. Non-Hodgkin's Lymphoma Classification Project. *J Clin Oncol.* 1998;16(8):2780–2795.
4. Swerdlow SH, Campo E, Pileri SA, et al. The 2016 revision of the World Health Organization classification of lymphoid neoplasms. *Blood.* 2016;127(20):2375–2390.
5. Montoto S, Davies AJ, Matthews J, et al. Risk and clinical implications of transformation of follicular lymphoma to diffuse large B-cell lymphoma. *J Clin Oncol.* 2007;25(17):2426–2433.
6. Yepes S, Torres MM, Saavedra C, Andrade R. Gastric mucosa-associated lymphoid tissue lymphomas and Helicobacter pylori infection: a Colombian perspective. *World J Gastroenterol.* 2012;18(7):685–691.
7. Ebie N, Loew JM, Gregory SA. Bilateral trephine bone marrow biopsy for staging non-Hodgkin's lymphoma: a second look. *Hematol Pathol.* 1989;3(1):29–33.
8. Noy A, Schöder H, Gönen M, et al. The majority of transformed lymphomas have high standardized uptake values (SUVs) on positron emission tomography (PET) scanning similar to diffuse large B-cell lymphoma (DLBCL). *Ann Oncol.* 2009;20(3):508–512.
9. Nooka AK, Nabhan C, Zhou X, et al. Examination of the follicular lymphoma international prognostic index (FLIPI) in the National LymphoCare study (NLCS): a prospective US patient cohort treated predominantly in community practices. *Ann Oncol.* 2013;24(2):441–448.
10. Solal-Céligny P, Roy P, Colombat P, et al. Follicular lymphoma international prognostic index. *Blood.* 2004;104(5):1258–1265.
11. Federico M, Bellei M, Marcheselli L, et al. Follicular lymphoma international prognostic index 2: a new prognostic index for follicular lymphoma developed by the International Follicular Lymphoma Prognostic Factor project. *J Clin Oncol.* 2009;27(27):4555–4562.
12. Ferreri AJ, Govi S, Pasini E, et al. Chlamydophila psittaci eradication with doxycycline as first-line targeted therapy for ocular adnexae lymphoma: final results of an international phase II trial. *J Clin Oncol.* 2012;30(24):2988–2994.
13. NCCN Clinical Practice Guidelines in Oncology: B-Cell Lymphomas; 2017. https://www.nccn.org
14. Yahalom J, Illidge T, Specht L, et al. Modern radiation therapy for extranodal lymphomas: field and dose guidelines from the International Lymphoma Radiation Oncology Group. *Int J Radiat Oncol Biol Phys.* 2015;92(1):11–31.

15. Illidge T, Specht L, Yahalom J, et al. Modern radiation therapy for nodal non-Hodgkin lympho-ma-target definition and dose guidelines from the International Lymphoma Radiation Oncology Group. *Int J Radiat Oncol Biol Phys.* 2014;89(1):49–58.

16. Videtic GMM, Woody N, Vassil AD. *Handbook of Treatment Planning in Radiation Oncology.* 2nd ed. New York, NY: Demos Medical; 2015.

17. Monfardini S, Banfi A, Bonadonna G, et al. Improved five-year survival after combined radi-otherapy-chemotherapy for stage I–II non-Hodgkin's lymphoma. *Int J Radiat Oncol Biol Phys.* 1980;6(2):125–134.

18. Nissen NI, Ersbøll J, Hansen HS, et al. A randomized study of radiotherapy versus radiotherapy plus chemotherapy in stage I–II non-Hodgkin's lymphomas. *Cancer.* 1983;52(1):1–7.

19. Carde P, Burgers JM, van Glabbeke M, et al. Combined radiotherapy-chemotherapy for early stages non-Hodgkin's lymphoma: the 1975-1980 EORTC controlled lymphoma trial. *Radiother Oncol.* 1984;2(4):301–312.

20. Kelsey SM, Newland AC, Hudson GV, Jelliffe AM. A British National Lymphoma Investigation randomised trial of single agent chlorambucil plus radiotherapy versus radiotherapy alone in low grade, localised non-Hodgkins lymphoma. *Med Oncol.* 1994;11(1):19–25.

21. Yahalom J, Varsos G, Fuks Z, et al. Adjuvant cyclophosphamide, doxorubicin, vincristine, and prednisone chemotherapy after radiation therapy in stage I low-grade and interme-diate-grade non-Hodgkin lymphoma: results of a prospective randomized study. *Cancer.* 1993;71(7):2342–2350.

22. Tsai HK, Li S, Ng AK, et al. Role of radiation therapy in the treatment of stage I/II mucosa-asso-ciated lymphoid tissue lymphoma. *Ann Oncol.* 2007;18(4):672–678.

23. Goda JS, Gospodarowicz M, Pintilie M, et al. Long-term outcome in localized extran-odal mucosa-associated lymphoid tissue lymphomas treated with radiotherapy. *Cancer.* 2010;116(16):3815–3824.

24. Ono S, Kato M, Takagi K, et al. Long-term treatment of localized gastric marginal zone B-cell mucosa associated lymphoid tissue lymphoma including incidence of metachronous gastric cancer. *J Gastroenterol Hepatol.* 2010;25(4):804–809.

25. Schechter NR, Portlock CS, Yahalom J. Treatment of mucosa-associated lymphoid tissue lym-phoma of the stomach with radiation alone. *J Clin Oncol.* 1998;16(5):1916–1921.

X: SARCOMAS

51: SOFT TISSUE SARCOMA

Jonathan Sharrett, Jeffrey Kittel, Chirag Shah, and Jacob G. Scott

---

QUICK HIT: Soft tissue sarcomas (STS): heterogeneous group of tumors that together make up the most common sarcoma diagnosis. More than 100 histological subtypes identified, majority originating in the extremities. Core needle biopsy should be performed by treating surgeon, preferably a surgical oncologist. Surgical resection is required for cure. Positive margins and high grade confer worse LC with surgery alone. Role of RT is to improve outcomes for localized disease. For extremity STS, surgery alone may be considered for low-grade, stage I tumors resected with >1-cm negative margins. For stage II–III STS of the extremity that is resectable with reasonable functional outcomes (limb-sparing), RT is recommended and can be delivered either pre- or postoperatively. RT improves LC and may improve OS. Role of CHT is evolving in targeted era.

TABLE 51.1: General Treatment Paradigm for Soft Tissue and Retroperitoneal Sarcoma[1]		
	Extremities/Superficial Trunk	**Retroperitoneal**
Stage I	Total en bloc excision alone. Add PORT if close (<1 cm), +margins or high grade. PORT dose is 50 Gy/25 fx plus boost (60–66 Gy for close margins, 66–68 Gy for microscopic +margins, and 70–76 Gy for gross residual)	Surgery alone OR Pre-op RT to 45–50.4 Gy/25–28 fx strongly considered ± IORT boost (10–12 Gy) *PORT not recommended for RP sarcoma. Consider when recurrence would be morbid and/or unresectable.*
Stage II–III	Pre-op RT (50 Gy/25 fx). Post-op EBRT boost for positive/close margins of 16 Gy controversial. OR PORT (50 Gy/25 fx plus boost as earlier) OR adjuvant brachy alone (30–50 Gy given BID)	
Unresectable	Consider neoadjuvant RT, CHT, or chemoRT to facilitate surgery. Doses >70 Gy necessary for LC with RT alone.	Consider CHT or RT to facilitate surgery. If truly unresectable, treatment is palliative.
Desmoid	Observation may be reasonable. Primary management is surgical. RT to 56–58 Gy if nonoperative. PORT for +margins is controversial; many reserve RT for recurrence or unresectable disease. Consider tamoxifen, sulindac, imatinib for unresectable pts or those with FAP.	

EPIDEMIOLOGY: Sarcomas are rare, representing ~1% of malignancies, with 80% of these being STS and 20% originating in bone. Benign soft tissue masses are much more common than STS. In 2015, there were 12,390 cases of STS diagnosed in the United States, with 4,990 deaths.[2] Median age of STS diagnosis is 45 to 55 with ~20% found before age 40, 30% between 40 and 60; and 50% >60. Age by histology: fibrosarcoma (FS, 30–39), leiomyosarcoma (LMS, 50–59), malignant fibrous histiocytoma (MFH), that is, undifferentiated pleomorphic sarcoma (UPS, 60–69), liposarcoma (LS, 60–69).

RISK FACTORS: Male gender, genetic predisposition, prior exposure to RT or CHT, chemical carcinogens, chronic irritation or lymphedema, and HIV/HHV8 involvement in Kaposi's are some risk factors (RF) for development of STS. In reported series from MSKCC, distribution of RT-induced sarcomas was osteosarcoma (21%), MFH (16%), and angiosarcoma (15%). These were seen most commonly following tx of breast cancer (26%), lymphoma (25%), and cervical cancer (14%), with median latency of 10.3 yrs.[3] Familial adenomatous polyposis (FAP), or more specifically Gardner's, are risk factors for desmoid tumors.

ANATOMY: STS arises from a mesenchymal cell of origin. STS can occur in all body sites; however, around 2/3 of STS occur in extremities, most commonly in the lower extremity, above the knee. Remaining 1/3 of STS are found in retroperitoneum and trunk/H&N region, with slightly more retroperitoneal. At diagnosis, 90% of extremity sarcomas are localized to muscle compartment of origin. Most common STS by site: extremities (LS, MFH, synovial, and FS); retroperitoneum (well-differentiated and dedifferentiated LS and LMS); visceral (GIST). Tumor is usually surrounded by pseudocapsule (region of compressed reactive tissue) and reactive zone (high MRI T2 signal) that can harbor microscopic disease, which is important for resection assessment. In PMH series, infiltrating tumor cells were found up to 4 cm from pseudocapsule in 10/15 (67%) of pts, and all but one of which were found in "edema" region.[4]

PATHOLOGY: Greater than 100 histologic subtypes of STS have been reported. Most common subtypes in decreasing order are liposarcoma, leiomyosarcoma, high-grade undifferentiated pleomorphic sarcoma (formally malignant fibrous histiocytoma, MFH), GIST, synovial sarcoma, myxofibrosarcoma, and malignant peripheral nerve sheath tumor (MPNST). Certain subtypes have propensity for metastasis, such as LMS. Histologic grade is determined by differentiation, mitotic count, and necrosis.[5] Of note, myogenic differentiation in pleomorphic sarcomas increases risk of DM and is prognostic for many subtypes. Grade is less prognostic for MPNST, angiosarcoma, extraskeletal myxoid chondrosarcoma, and clear cell sarcoma.

GENETICS: Simple karyotypes and reciprocal translocations may include: alveolar rhabdomyosarcoma (t[2;13]), clear cell sarcoma (t[12;22]), myxoid LS (t[12;16]), synovial (t[X;18]), dermatofibrosarcoma protuberans (ring [17;22]), solitary fibrous tumor (fusion NAB2-STAT6). Characteristic amplifications: well-differentiation to undifferentiated liposarcoma (amplification of 12q, contains MDM2). Specific driver mutations: desmoid fibromatosis (CTNNB1), GIST (c-kit or PDGFRA), rhabdoid tumors (loss of INI1). Complex karyotypes may be found in some high-grade tumors. Some classic genetic syndromes with their specific mutations that increase risk of STS are characterized in Table 51.2.

TABLE 51.2: Genetic Syndromes Commonly Associated With Soft Tissue Sarcoma			
Syndrome	Clinical Findings	Gene	Chromosome
Neurofibromatosis (NF 1)	MPNST (5%), optic glioma, astrocytoma, neurofibromas, café au lait spots, Lisch nodules, axillary freckling	NF-1	17q11
Familial Retinoblastoma (Rb)	STS, osteosarcoma, retinoblastoma	Rb-1	13q14
Li–Fraumeni	STS, osteosarcoma, leukemia, BC, CNS tumors, adrenal tumors	TP53	17p13
Werner's (adult progeria)	STS, osteosarcoma, meningioma	WRN	8p12

(continued)

TABLE 51.2: Genetic Syndromes Commonly Associated With Soft Tissue Sarcoma (*continued*)			
Syndrome	Clinical Findings	Gene	Chromosome
Gardner's (subset of FAP)	FS, intraabdominal desmoid, colon cancer	APC	5q21
Gorlin's (nevoid BCC)	FS, rhabdomyosarcoma, BCC, CNS tumors	PTC	9q22
Carney's triad	GIST, extra-adrenal paraganglioma, pulmonary chondroma	c-KIT	Unknown

CLINICAL PRESENTATION: Symptoms are generally site-dependent. Typical presentation is enlarging, painless mass. Symptoms of compression may be reported including new onset edema and/or new or worsening paresthesia. Constitutional symptoms including fever and weight loss are rare. 6% to 10% have metastatic disease at presentation, with higher risk in deep tumors and high-grade tumors.[3]

WORKUP: As benign soft tissue disease is much more common, workup of painless enlarging mass should include thorough H&P with exam of mass and draining LN regions to assess for adenopathy and rule out benign causes.

Labs: CBC, CMP.

Imaging: CT and MRI with contrast of affected area. On MRI, tumor is typically hypointense on T1 and hyperintense on T2. CT chest to evaluate for metastatic disease once STS is confirmed. Role of FDG PET/CT is evolving and according to NCCN may be useful in prognostication, grading, and determining response to neoadjuvant CHT.[1] It may also be helpful in distinguish MPNST from neurofibroma.

Biopsy: Ultimately, biopsy should be obtained, with core needle being preferred, to determine grade and histology. If necessary, open biopsy incisions should be placed longitudinally along extremity so scar can be resected at time of surgery. Ideally, surgeon performing biopsy should be surgeon performing resection, especially in complex anatomical locations, and be a fellowship-trained surgical oncologist. May consider excisional biopsy only for <3 cm superficial lesions. For RPS, use of CT-guided bx via RP approach to avoid seeding peritoneum. FNA may be performed to detect recurrence/metastatic disease.

PROGNOSTIC FACTORS: Grade, size, metastatic disease. Factors increasing LF: age>50, recurrent disease, margins <1 cm, well-differentiated histology. Factors increasing risk of DM often include higher grade (G1: 5%–10%, G2: 25%–30%, G3: 50%–60%), size (>5 cm), deep seated tumors, recurrence, and histologies.

NATURAL HISTORY: Most common route of DM is hematogenous, with lungs most common site in 75% of pts, especially for STS of extremity/trunk region, with other less common sites in decreasing order being bone, other soft tissues (including bone marrow, e.g., for myxoid/round cell LS), liver (e.g., from adjacent visceral sarcoma, retroperitoneal sarcoma [RPS]), and rarely brain metastasis (more commonly seen with LMS, angiosarcoma, and alveolar soft part sarcoma). If ≤3–4 lung metastases and long disease-free interval (DFI) w/o endobronchial invasion, ~25% can be cured with resection (3-yr OS was 30%–50%).[6] This appears true regardless of ablative modality for metastasis.[7] LN involvement is rare (<5%), but higher with "CARE" histologies: Clear cell (27.7%), Angiosarcoma (24.1%), Rhabdomyosarcoma (32.1%), and Epithelioid (31.8%).[4,8] Some have unique natural histories, for example: dermal spread for superficial MFH, angiosarcoma; desmoid tumor with lack of pseudocapsule and poorly defined margins; and dermal nodules or skip metastases for epithelioid sarcoma. Examples of specific subtypes primarily recurring locally include desmoid, MPNST, atypical lipomatous or well differentiation LS, and DMFSP. Those with local and intermediate risk for DM include myxoid LS, myxoid MFH, and extraskeletal myxoid chondrosarcoma, and hemangiopericytoma. Those with local and high potential for DM include most other sarcomas, especially high grade. STS increase in size with direct local extension along tissue planes, which are not always superior/inferior, and may grow centrifugally. RP sarcomas of well-differentiated liposarcoma histology have long natural history and may not require aggressive treatment.[9]

STAGING: Compared to 7th edition of the AJCC staging manual, emphasis in 8th edition placed on primary site of STS, thus multiple separate staging systems other than Trunk/Extremities are defined, including H&N, Abdomen/Thoracic Visceral Organs, GIST, and RPS.[5]

TABLE 51.3: AJCC 8th ed. (2017) Staging for Soft Tissue Sarcoma of Trunk and Extremities (Head and neck, abdomen and thoracic, retroperitoneal and GIST systems not included here)							
Tumor		**Node**		**Distant Metastasis**		**Grade**	
T1	• ≤5 cm	N0	• No regional LNs	M0	• No distant metastasis	G1	• Total differentiation, mitotic count, and necrosis score of 2–3
T2	• 5.1–10 cm	N1	• Regional LNs	M1	• Distant metastasis	G2	• Total differentiation, mitotic count, and necrosis score of 4–5
T3	• 10.1–15 cm					G3	• Total differentiation, mitotic count, and necrosis score of 6–8
T4	• >15 cm						

TNM	Grade	Group Stage
T1N0M0	G1	IA
T2-4N0M0	G1	IB
T1N0M0	G2–3	II
T2N0M0	G2–3	IIIA
T3-4N0M0	G2–3	IIIB
Any T, N1, M0	Any G	IV
Any T, Any N, M1	Any G	IV
*Changes to AJCC 7th edition include addition of T3-4, removal of a and b parts of T1-2 classification and changes to grouped stage.		

TREATMENT PARADIGM

Surgery: Negative-margin resection with maintenance of function is goal of treatment for localized disease. En bloc excision encompasses biopsy site, scar and tumor achieving >1- to 2-cm margins ideally. Extent of surgical resection (originally described by Enneking[10]): (a) *intralesional*, (b) *marginal*: plane of resection through reactive tissue surrounding sarcoma, (c) *simple*: narrow margin (LR 60%–90%); (d) *wide*: plane of resection through normal tissue (~2- to 3-cm margin) and within compartment of STS origin (LR 30%–60%), (d) *radical/compartmental*: en bloc resection of anatomical compartment; includes amputation (LR 10%–20%). Margin status is most important variable for LC. Violation of tumor is associated w/ higher LR rates. It is usually unnecessary to resect adjacent bone. About 75% of pts w/ LR after limb-sparing surgery and RT can be salvaged by subsequent amputation. Consider free or rotational flap closures for large wounds requiring PORT. Criteria for amputation (~5% of cases): (a) involvement of major neurovascular structures or multiple compartments such that functional limb is not achievable; (b) RT dose and volume constraints; (c) recurrence not amenable to further surgery or RT; (d) severely compromised normal tissue (due to age, peripheral vascular disease, or other comorbidities). For distal extremity lesion, below-knee amputation (BKA) w/ prosthesis may be preferred to limb-sparing. For RP sarcoma, en bloc resection of nearby organs (kidney, liver, spleen) may be required.

Chemotherapy: There is conflicting data regarding routine use of CHT in definitive management of STS, for which it has primarily been evaluated in extremity STS and less commonly in sites such as in RPS. For primary extremity STS, there appears to be the greatest benefit in LC, RFS, and OS when doxorubicin is combined with ifosfamide, and there is trend to improved OS with single-agent doxorubicin based on an updated meta-analysis from the Sarcoma Meta-Analysis Collaboration (SMAC) discussed in the following. Further trials are ongoing. Pazopanib, an oral multitarget TKI, improved PFS in the PALETTE trial for previously treated metastatic pts (median PFS 1.6 vs. 4.6 mos, $p < .0001$) and may be considered.[11] Other targeted agents such as olaratumab (human anti-PDGFRα antibody) have shown promise.[12]

Radiation: *EBRT for STS of Extremity:* In general, RT may be delivered pre-op, intra-op (IORT), or in adjuvant setting. *Pre-op RT:* For extremity sarcoma, give 50 Gy/25 fx. For close/positive margins after pre-op RT, utility of EBRT boost of 16 Gy (total 66 Gy) is controversial but was performed on most trials. Other options for close margins include IORT (10–16 Gy) or brachytherapy (12–20 Gy).

PORT: If RT is given in adjuvant setting, typical dosing and fractionation is 50 Gy/25 fx followed by additional boost to 60–66 Gy for negative margins, 66–68 Gy for microscopically positive margins, and 70–76 Gy for gross residual disease. Different approaches with various dose/fx schema for palliation of symptomatic metastatic disease are available based on expected survival and physician preference.

EBRT for RP Sarcoma: For RP sarcoma, recommend 45 to 50.4 Gy/25–28 fx preoperatively. PORT not generally recommended except when recurrence may be morbid or unresectable. Well-differentiated liposarcoma has long natural history and may not require RT (or aggressive surgery). Consensus statements exist for treatment selection and contouring for RPS.[9]

Brachytherapy (BRT): Advantages include RT directly applied to tumor bed, short overall tx time, less dose to surrounding normal tissue (may yield better functional outcome), region well-oxygenated, path specimen unaltered. Brachytherapy alone may be used as adjuvant for intermediate- to high-grade sarcomas of extremity or superficial trunk w/ negative margins and has been shown to improve LC in a PRT.[13] ABS guidelines are available to guide dose and technique.[14] Most commonly, HDR brachytherapy with Ir-192 is used as boost to dose of 12 to 20 Gy given twice daily (BID) over 2 to 3 days in conjunction with EBRT. Brachytherapy may also be utilized as adjuvant therapy alone (dose 30–50 Gy given BID) and often is preferred after resection of LR in previously irradiated pts.[14,15]

Procedure: See *Treatment Planning Handbook*, Chapter 11[16].

EVIDENCE-BASED Q&A

Primary extremity STS

Can the addition of PORT to limb-sparing surgery (LSS) avoid amputation?

Historically, high recurrence rates after local excision alone led to the use of radical compartment excisions or amputations. This generated the idea behind the Rosenberg NCI trial.

Rosenberg, NCI (*Ann Surg* 1982, PMID 7114936): PRT of 43 pts w/ extremity high-grade STS treated from 1975 to 1981 randomized to amputation (16 pts) versus LSS + PORT (27 pts) consisting of 50 Gy, with 10 to 20 Gy boost to tumor bed. All pts received post-op CHT with doxorubicin/cyclophosphamide and methotrexate. LR was 15% (n = 4) in LSS arm versus 0% (*p* = .06) in amputation arm. 5-yr DFS (71% vs. 78%, NS) and OS (82% vs. 88%, NS) for LSS versus amputation, respectively. QOL is reported elsewhere, but was same. Later analyses also showed no benefit to CHT. On MVA, only positive margins were correlated with LR, even in setting of PORT. **Conclusion: LSS + PORT is reasonable and effective; this has become standard of care.**

With limited randomized data showing PORT with LSS is as effective as amputation, is it necessary in those who undergo LSS alone, and does grade matter?

Although LSS and PORT became standard after NCI study, morbidity with PORT is not trivial, and there were only historical comparisons to suggest it improved LR rates over LSS alone. This led to the NCI trial, which confirmed LC benefit with PORT, but no OS benefit was found. Additional large SEER meta-analysis suggests this benefit is limited to high-grade STS.

Yang, NCI (*JCO* 1998, PMID 9440743): Phase III PRT including 91 pts w/ high-grade extremity STS s/p LSS w/ negative or minimal microscopic margins randomized to receive post-op CHT alone (n = 44) versus CHT + PORT (n = 47) to 63 Gy (45 Gy + 18 Gy boost @ 1.8 Gy/fx) assessing LC, OS, and QOL. Additional 50 pts w/ low-grade sarcomas were enrolled to receive PORT (n = 26) versus LSS alone (n = 24). MFU of 9.6 years. See Table 51.4. LC was significantly improved with addition of RT for both low- and high-grade pts, with no OS benefit. PORT resulted in significantly worse limb strength, edema, and range of motion, but these deficits were often transient and had little effect on ADLs or QOL. **Conclusion: Significant LC benefit with addition of PORT with no OS benefit.**

TABLE 51.4: Results of NCI Trial				
High Grade (n = 91)	**10-yr LC**	**10-yr OS**	**Low Grade (n = 50)**	**10-yr LC**
Post-op CHT	78%	74%	**No adjuvant tx**	67%
Post-op ChemoRT	100%	75%	**Post-op RT**	96%
p value	.0028	.71	*p* value	.016

Koshy, SEER (*IJROBP* 2010, PMID 19679403). SEER retrospective analysis from 1988 to 2005 including 6,960 pts with both low-/high-grade extremity STS assessing OS benefit of RT after LSS. 47% of pts received RT, primarily post-op (86%). For high-grade STS, addition of RT was associated with 3-yr OS benefit (73% vs. 63%, *p* < .001). There was no OS benefit for low-grade STS. **Conclusion: This large retrospective analysis showed higher OS with addition of RT in setting of LSS for high-grade STS, but not for low-grade STS.**

Can the addition of adjuvant brachytherapy improve LC?

Compared to surgery alone, there appears to be significant LC benefit, which is confined to high-grade histology, and there is no improvement in DSS or DM.

Pisters, MSKCC (*JCO* 1996, PMID 8622034): PRT of 164 pts w/ STS of extremity or superficial trunk, randomized intra-op to adjuvant brachytherapy versus no further tx after complete resection (no gross disease). Brachytherapy was given via Ir-192 implant delivering 42 to 45 Gy over 4 to 6 days. MFU 76 mos. Equivalent DSS and no difference in DM. 5-yr actuarial LC was 82% versus 69% (p = .04) in favor of brachytherapy. However, on further analysis, this improvement in LC was for high-grade lesions, but not low-grade lesions. There was no difference in wound complication rates among pts who were loaded after POD 5 (modified timing midtrial from loading <5 days to ≥6 days). **Conclusion: Brachytherapy improves LC for high-grade STS with no difference in DSS or DM, and no improvement for low-grade tumors.**

TABLE 51.5: Results of MSKCC Trial of Adjuvant Brachytherapy for Soft Tissue Sarcoma

	5-yr LC	5-yr DSS	Low-grade LC	High-grade LC
No brachytherapy	69%	81%	72%	66%
Brachytherapy	82%	84%	73%	89%
p value	.04	.65	.49	.0025

What is the optimal sequencing of RT when indicated for the management of STS?

Both pre- and postoperative EBRT are reasonable, with trade-offs. Pre-op RT allows for smaller field sizes and lower doses, which are generally associated with better long-term functional outcomes. This generally comes at expense of higher rates of acute wound complications.

O'Sullivan, NCIC SR2 (*Lancet* 2002, PMID 12103287; Davis, *Radiother Oncol* 2005, PMID 15948265): PRT of 190 pts w/ STS stratified by tumor size (≤10 cm vs. >10 cm) and randomized to pre-op RT (50 Gy/25 fx) versus PORT (66–70 Gy; 50 Gy/25 fx to initial field + 16–20 Gy boost). Pre-op arm was treated w/ additional 16 to 20 Gy for positive margins (14 of 91 pts had positive margins, 10 treated w/ RT). Primary endpoint: Acute wound complications and erythema, with later analyses assessing 2-yr late effects of grade 2–4 fibrosis, edema, and joint stiffness. Study terminated early at interim analysis. Updated at MFU 6.9 yrs (ASCO 2004). Median RT field size was smaller in pre-op arm. LC was identical between two arms. Initial trend toward improved OS in pre-op arm was lost at later FU. Tumor size and grade predicted for OS; grade predicted for RFS; margin status predicted for LC. Pre-op RT was associated with lower rates of acute skin erythema, late fibrosis, joint stiffness, and edema, albeit none were statistically significant. Pre-op RT had higher rates of acute wound complications (35% vs. 17%, highest in upper leg). **Conclusion: No difference in LC, RFS, or OS. Pre-op RT for extremity sarcomas may be preferred due to lower rates of irreversible late fibrosis, at cost of higher, but generally reversible, acute wound complications.**

TABLE 51.6: Results of NCIC SR2 Trial of Preoperative Versus Postoperative RT for Soft Tissue Sarcoma

	Acute Wound Complications	2-yr Grade 2–4 Fibrosis	2-yr Grade 2–4 Edema	2-yr Joint Stiffness	5-yr LC	5-yr RFS	5-yr Mets RFS	5-yr OS	5-yr CSS
Pre-op RT	35%	32%	15%	18%	93%	58%	67%	73%	78%

(continued)

	Acute Wound Complications	2-yr Grade 2–4 Fibrosis	2-yr Grade 2–4 Edema	2-yr Joint Stiffness	5-yr LC	5-yr RFS	5-yr Mets RFS	5-yr OS	5-yr CSS
TABLE 51.6: Results of NCIC SR2 Trial of Preoperative Versus Postoperative RT for Soft Tissue Sarcoma (continued)									
Post-op RT	17%	48%	23%	23%	92%	59%	69%	67%	73%
p value	.01	.07	.26	.51	NS	NS	NS	.47	.64

Al-Absi, Ontario (*Ann Surg Oncol* 2010, PMID 20217260): Systematic review and meta-analysis of five eligible studies of pre-op versus PORT for localized, resectable STS including 1,098 pts. Significant improvement in LC with pre-op RT despite larger average tumor size in pre-op group with OR of 0.61 (95% CI: 0.42–0.89) by means of fixed-effects method, and OR of 0.67 (95% CI: 0.39–1.15) by means of random-effects method. Time-dependent survival averaged across all studies was 76% (range 62%–88%) pre-op versus 67% (range 41%–83%) post-op, NS. **Conclusion: Findings must be interpreted with caution due to heterogeneity, but suggest that delay in surgery due to pre-op RT does not confer increased DM rate versus PORT, and may provide superior LC.**

What is role of post-op boost with EBRT in patients who receive pre-op RT and undergo surgical resection with positive surgical margins?

Data is limited to small RRs with no PRT to answer this question as of now. Considering limited data, there is suggestion that EBRT boost may not be effective in preventing LR in patients with positive margins after pre-op RT.

Al Yami (*IJROBP* 2010, PMID 20056340): RR of 216 extremity STS pts treated at Mount Sinai Hospital in Toronto from 1986 to 2003 who had +SM. 93 of these pts had been treated with pre-op RT (50 Gy), while 41 of them additionally received boost (80% received boost dose of 16 Gy with EBRT to total dose of 66 Gy). No difference in tumor baseline characteristics. LRFS estimates at 5 yrs were 90.4% for no boost versus 73.8% for boost (*p* = .13, ns). **Conclusion: Post-op boost with EBRT did not improve LRFS in this small retrospective analysis.**

Can modern image-guided RT (3D or IMRT) improve morbidity?

Part of rationale for pre-op RT is to decrease late effects by reducing irradiated volume. IGRT may be able to reduce volume even further without compromising tumor control.

Wang, RTOG 0630 (*JCO* 2015, PMID 25667281): Multi-institutional phase II trial assessing utility of IGRT (3DCRT or IMRT allowed) for reducing toxicity compared to O'Sullivan NCIC trial. Primary endpoint: 2-yr grade ≥2 late RT morbidity. 98 pts were accrued to two cohorts: cohort A (12 pts; intermediate- to high-grade STS ≥8 cm for whom physicians prescribed CHT; results not reported) and cohort B (79 evaluable pts; all treated w/o CHT). RT: 50 Gy/25 fx with post-op boost suggested if positive margins to 16 Gy/8 fx EBRT (also acceptable 16 Gy LDR, 13.6 Gy/4 fx HDR, or 10–12.5 Gy IORT). 2- to 3-cm longitudinal CTV expansion and 1- or 1.5-cm radial (< or ≥8 cm) including suspicious edema with IGRT. MFU of 3.6 years. Most pts had undifferentiated pleomorphic sarcoma (UPS; 22.8%), LS (21.5%), or myxoid FS (21.5%). Most common primary was upper thigh (41.8%). 74.7% were treated w/ IMRT. 5 pts did not undergo surgery due to progression. 56 (76%) had R0 resection, and 11 (15%) received post-op boost. 5 pts had in-field LF (3/5 with positive margins and 2/5 treated with post-op boost). Overall rate of grade ≥2 late toxicity was significantly improved compared to O'Sullivan pre-op arm (10.5% vs. 37%, *p* < .001). Individual toxicities compared favorably: fibrosis (5.3% vs. 31.5%), joint stiffness

(3.5% vs. 17.8%), edema (5.3% vs. 15.1%). 36.6% of pts experienced at least one wound complication, all in lower extremity tumors, and most commonly in proximal lower extremity. **Conclusion: Significant reduction of late toxicities and absence of marginal-field recurrences with IGRT suggest that these smaller target volumes are appropriate for pre-op RT with IGRT for extremity STS.**

O'Sullivan, Canada (*Cancer* 2013, PMID 23423841): Single-arm phase II trial using IMRT with image guidance to deliver pre-op RT with primary endpoint of acute wound complications compared to NCIC trial. 70 pts, with 59 evaluable. RT dose/volumes: 50 Gy/25 fx without boost. 4-cm longitudinal and 1.5-cm radial expansions including edema with IGRT; dose restricted to "future surgical skin flaps" and bone. MFU of 49 months. Most pts had UPS (35.6%), myxoid LS (32.2%), or pleomorphic LS (10.2%). R1 resection in four pts. Buttock was most common site of wound complications (45%), followed by adductor (44%) and hamstring (44%). Overall rate of complications were not different from NCIC trial, but primary closure was more frequent (93.2% vs. 71.4%). Number of secondary operations was numerically less but not SS. Flap/PTV overlap was improved on MVA (<1% overlap, 14.3% vs. 39.5%). 4 pts had LF (6.8%), none near surgical flaps, and two of four had positive margins. No grade >2 late toxicities in pts surviving longer than 2 years with no fractures. **Conclusion: Pre-op IMRT with IGRT significantly diminished need for tissue transfer, with NS reduction in acute wound complications, chronic morbidities, and need for subsequent secondary operations, while maintaining good limb function.**

With respect to IMRT and brachytherapy, does one have a better therapeutic ratio compared to the other?

Data are limited to RRs and comparisons of modern control rates of each separately, but there is suggestion of superior LC with IMRT.

Alektiar, MSKCC (*Cancer* 2011, PMID 21264834): RR of 134 pts with high-grade extremity STS who were treated with LSS and either brachytherapy (1995–2003) or IMRT (2002–2006). LDR brachytherapy (71 pts) was administered post-op with median dose 45 Gy. IMRT (63 pts total) was delivered pre-op (10 pts) with mean dose of 50 Gy, and post-op (53 pts) to median dose of 63 Gy. MFU of 46 months for IMRT; 47 months for brachytherapy. There were comparable baseline characteristics. However, there were statistically higher risk tumors in IMRT cohort such as positive/close margins (<1 mm), large tumors (>10 cm), and requiring bone or nerve stripping/resection. 5-year LC was favored IMRT (92% vs. 81%, p = .04) compared to brachytherapy. On MVA, IMRT was only significant predictor of improved LC (p = .04). **Conclusion: LC with IMRT was significantly better than brachytherapy despite higher rates of adverse features for IMRT in this nonrandomized comparison. IMRT warrants further studies for this patient population.**

What are data supporting IORT/IOERT in conjunction with EBRT?

Early results are promising with most data confined to RR with large recent combined pooled analysis of primary extremity STS pts who received IOERT in conjunction with EBRT and gross total resection showing high LC in R0 resected pts, but around 30% recurrence in patients with +SM. In absence of robust data, NCCN currently recommends IORT to 10–16 Gy followed by course of EBRT to 45–50 Gy.

Roeder (*ESTRO* 2015 Abstract OC-0521): Pooled analysis from three European centers including 259 pts with extremity STS who underwent at least gross total resection, and received IOERT and additional EBRT (pre-op or post-op). 29% did have microscopic +SM. Median IOERT dose was 12 Gy and for EBRT 45 Gy. MFU of 63 months. Crude LF rate of 10% translating to estimated 5-yr LC rate of 86%. Resection margin (5-yr LC 94% R0 vs. 70% R1) was associated with LC on UVA and MVA. 5-yr OS was 78%, and was SS influenced by grade and stage IV disease. Secondary amputations needed in 5%, mainly due to recurrence. Functional outcomes reported as not interfering with ADLs in more than 80 pts. **Conclusion: One of largest combined analyses of extremity STS pts managed with addition of IOERT with promising results, more so in R0 resected pts.**

Does the addition of adjuvant CHT improve outcomes for surgically-resected STS?

This has been area of controversy based on risk versus benefit of such therapy, but due to risk of local and distant failures, adjuvant CHT was often administered, typically with doxorubicin-based therapy. Sarcoma Meta-Analysis Collaboration (SMAC) updated their meta-analysis in 2008 of RCTs including adjuvant CHT following surgical resection for STS confirming efficacy of doxorubicin-based CHT with greater benefit when given with ifosfamide.

Pervaiz, Sarcoma Meta-Analysis Collaboration (*Cancer*** 2008, PMID 18521899):** Comprehensive meta-analysis of 18 RCTs including 1,953 pts assessing failures and survival outcomes with doxorubicin-based adjuvant CHT in resectable STS. OR for LR was 0.73 (95% CI: 0.56–0.94; $p = .02$) favoring CHT. For DM and overall recurrence, OR was 0.67 (95% CI: 0.56–0.82, $p = .0001$) favoring CHT. On survival analysis, doxorubicin alone had OR of 0.84 (95% CI: 0.68–1.03, $p = .09$) while doxorubicin combined with ifosfamide was 0.56 (95% CI: 0.36–0.85; $p = .01$) favoring CHT. **Conclusion: This analysis confirms the benefit of CHT with respect to recurrence and metastasis for adjuvant doxorubicin, while addition of ifosfamide demonstrated significant survival benefit and further improved other outcomes.**

In the pre-op setting, what is the role of the addition of CHT?

DM continues to be a problem in STS. Previous small pilot studies of neoadjuvant CHT or CRT appeared promising, which led to RTOG 9514, which assessed the feasibility of neoadjuvant CHT interdigitated with RT prior to surgery followed by additional adjuvant CHT alone or following additional RT for positive margins. Neoadjuvant CHT is not a standard of care approach at this time.

Kraybill, RTOG 9514 (*JCO*** 2006, PMID 16446334):** Phase II prospective trial evaluating neoadjuvant CHT with pre-op RT followed by CHT post-op in multi-institutional setting. High-grade extremity/body wall STS ≥8 cm were eligible. 66 pts were enrolled. CHT consisted of MAID regimen (modified mesna, doxorubicin, ifosfamide, and dacarbazine), which was given for three cycles, with interdigitated RT 44 Gy/22 fx split course (MAID→RT→MAID→RT→MAID) followed 3 weeks later by resection. Post-op therapy was based on margin status. If there were positive margins, additional 16 Gy/8 fx was administered to post-op bed + 1-cm margin, followed by MAID x three cycles. If negative margins, MAID x three cycles alone. 64 pts were analyzable. 79% completed pre-op CHT with only 59% receiving full CHT course due to toxicity, with 5% experience grade 5 fatal toxicity and 83% experiencing grade 4. 61 pts underwent surgery, with 58 R0 resections (5 amputations). At 3 yrs, estimated DFS was 56.6%, distant DFS 64.5%, and OS 75.1%. There were five amputations leading to 92% limb preservation rate. Estimated 3-yr LRF of 18% if amputation considered failure, and 10% if not. **Conclusion: Just over half of 64 pts received planned treatment course due to substantial toxicity, but regimen does appear to show activity.**

Retroperitoneal Sarcoma (RPS)

What is the general approach to managing RPS?

Primary management still revolves around achieving an R0 surgical resection. As with primary extremity STS, RPS data is limited mainly to small RRs with no RCTs evaluating the benefit of RT in nonmetastatic, surgically resectable RPS. However, there is a recently closed phase III RCT (EORTC

"STRASS") comparing surgery alone versus pre-op RT followed by surgical resection. If RT is given, it is delivered in the preoperative setting as toxicity can be significant in the post-op setting.

What current data suggests benefit, including OS, to addition of RT for RPS?

Many small retrospective series have been published. Based on SEER/NCDB datasets, there does appear to be survival benefit with addition of RT, given either pre-op or post-op, with usual limitations of such nonrandomized registry studies.

Zhou, SEER (*Arch Surg* 2010, PMID 20479339): SEER analysis evaluating effect of surgical resection and RT for locoregional RPS and nonvisceral abdominal sarcoma from 1988 to 2005 including 1,901 pts. 81.8% underwent surgical resection and 23.5% received RT. Combined therapy was associated with improved OS versus single modality therapy, and surgery or RT was better than no therapy ($p < .001$, log rank). Cox analysis demonstrated that surgical resection (HR 0.24, 95% CI: 0.21–0.29, $p < .001$) and RT (HR 0.78, 95% CI: 0.63–0.95, $p = .01$) independently predicted improved OS in locoregional disease only. In adjusted analyses stratified for AJCC stage, for stage I disease (n = 694), RT provided additional benefit (HR 0.49, 95% CI: 0.25–0.96, $p = .04$) independent of that from resection (HR 0.35, 95% CI: 0.21–0.58, $p < .001$). For stage II/III (n = 552), resection remained significant (HR 0.24, 95% CI: 0.18–0.32, $p < .001$); however, RT was not associated with significant benefit (HR 0.78, 95% CI: 0.58–1.06, $p = .11$). **Conclusion: In this national cohort, surgical resection was associated with significant survival benefits for AJCC stage I–III RPS. RT provided additional benefit for pts with stage I disease.**

Nussbaum, Duke NCDB Analysis (*Lancet Oncol* 2016, PMID 27210906): Case-control, propensity score-matched analyses of 9,068 NCDB adult pts who were diagnosed with RPS from 2003 to 2011. Pts were included who had local RPS undergoing surgical resection and either pre-op RT or PORT, but not both, and no additional therapy or IORT. Primary objective was OS for pts who received pre-op RT or PORT compared with those who received no RT within propensity score-matched datasets. 563 pts received pre-op RT (MFU 42 months), 2,215 PORT (MFU 54 months), and 6,290 received no RT (MFU 43 months when compared to pre-op and 47 months for post-op cohort). Negligible differences in all demographic, clinic-pathological, and treatment-level variables. MS was 110 months for pre-op cohort versus 66 months for matched no RT cohort comparator. MS was 89 months for post-op cohort versus 64 months for matched no RT cohort. Both pre-op (HR 0.70, 95% CI: 0.59–0.82, $p < .0001$) and PORT (HR 0.78, 95% CI: 0.71–0.85, $p < .0001$) were significantly associated with higher OS compared with surgery alone. **Conclusion: RT is associated with higher OS compared with surgery alone when delivered either pre-op or post-op.**

Does the addition of IORT to PORT improve outcomes following surgically resected RPS?

Retrospective data exists; however, only one small PRT has addressed this question. In that NCI trial, addition of IORT reduced LRR but did not translate into an OS benefit. Bowel toxicity may be reduced as well.

Sindelar, NCI (*Arch Surg* 1993, PMID 8457152): PRT of 35 pts with RPS treated with surgery and post-op high-dose EBRT (50–55 Gy) versus low-dose EBRT (35–40 Gy) + IORT (20 Gy). MFU of 8 years. MS similar between groups. LRR improved in IORT cohort (40% vs. 80%). IORT cohort had less disabling enteritis but more peripheral neuropathy (60% vs. 5%).

Does pre-operative RT improve outcomes compared to post-operative RT?

In theory, pre-op RT may reduce toxicity due to lower dose, smaller volumes of normal tissue in the irradiated volume due to better target delineation, normal tissue displacement, and subsequent smaller treatment fields. Additionally, it may be more effective from a radiobiological standpoint due to better vascularity and oxygenation. Most do not recommend PORT for RPS.

Ballo, MD Anderson (*IJROBP* 2007, PMID 17084545): RR of 83 pts with localized RPS treated with complete surgical resection and RT at MDACC. 60 pts presented with primary disease with remaining 23 having LR following previous surgery. MFU of 47 months. Actuarial overall DSS, LC, and DMFSP were 44%, 40%, and 67%, respectively. Of 38 deaths, local progression was sole site of recurrence for 16 pts and was component of progression for another 11 pts. MVA indicated that histologic grade was associated with 5-yr rates of DSS (low grade, 92%; intermediate grade, 51%; and high grade, 41%, $p = .006$). MVA also indicated inferior 5-yr LC rate for pts presenting with recurrent disease, +margins or uncertain margin status, and age >65 years. Data did not suggest improved LC with higher doses of RT, or with specific use of IORT. RT-related complications (10% at 5 years) developed in five patients, with all complications limited to those who received PORT (23%) versus pre-op RT (0%). **Conclusion: Pre-operative RT may be preferred over PORT.**

Is IORT combined with does-escalated IMRT safe and effective?

Roeder (*BMC Cancer* 2014, PMID 25163595): Unplanned interim analysis of phase I/ II single-arm trial assessing feasibility of pre-op IMRT along with IOERT in 27 pts with primary/recurrent RPS (>5 cm, M0, at least marginally resectable) spanning 2007 to 2013. Pre-op IMRT delivered using integrated boost with doses of 45–50 Gy to PTV and 50–56 Gy to GTV in 25 fx, followed by surgery and IOERT (10–12 Gy). Primary endpoint was 5-year LC. Majority of pts had high-grade lesions (82% grade 2-3), predominantly LS (70%), with median tumor size of 15 cm (6–31 cm). MFU of 33 months. Pre-op IMRT performed as planned in 93%. GTR was feasible in all but one pt. Final SM status was R0 in 6 (22%) and R1 in 20 pts (74%). Contiguous-organ resection was needed in all grossly resected pts. IOERT was performed in 23 pts (85%) with median dose of 12 Gy (10–20 Gy). There were seven recurrences leading to estimated 3- and 5-year LC rates of 72%. Severe acute toxicity (grade 3) was present in four pts (15%). Severe post-op complications were found in nine pts (33%). Severe late toxicity (grade 3) was scored in 6% of surviving pts after 1 year and none after 2 years. **Conclusion: Combination of pre-op IMRT, surgery, and IOERT is feasible with acceptable toxicity and yields good results in terms of LC and OS in pts with high-risk RPS. Long-term follow-up is needed.**

What are the current recommendations for unresectable disease?

According to NCCN, treatment may include CHT or RT alone or in combination to facilitate resection, if possible.[1]

Kepka, Poland (*IJROBP* 2005, PMID 16199316): RR of 112 pts treated with definitive RT for unresectable STS. 43% extremities, 26% retroperitoneal, 24% H&N, and 7% trunk. G1 11%; G2-3 89%. Median RT dose of 64 Gy (range, 25–87.5 Gy). CHT was given in 20%. MFU of 139 mo. 5-yr LC, DFS, and OS 45%, 24%, 35%, respectively. 5-yr LC affected by tumor size (51%, 45%, and 9% for tumors <5 cm, 5–10 cm, and >10 cm, respectively) and RT dose (<63 Gy, 22%; >63 Gy, 60%). Dose > versus <68 Gy was associated with higher risk of complications (27% vs. 8%). **Conclusion: Definitive RT for STS should be considered in inoperable setting, with consideration of higher RT dose to improve outcomes, and critical to find appropriate therapeutic window to reduce complications.**

REFERENCES

1. NCCN Clinical Practice Guidelines in Oncology: Soft Tissue Sarcoma. 2017; 2.2017:https:// www.nccn.org

2. Siegel RL, Miller KD, Jemal A. Cancer statistics, 2017. *CA Cancer J Clin*. 2017;67(1):7–30.

3. Brady MS, Gaynor JJ, Brennan MF. Radiation-associated sarcoma of bone and soft tissue. *Arch Surg*. 1992;127(12):1379–1385.

4. White LM, Wunder JS, Bell RS, et al. Histologic assessment of peritumoral edema in soft tissue sarcoma. *Int J Radiat Oncol Biol Phys*. 2005;61(5):1439–1445.

5. *AJCC Cancer Staging Manual*. New York, NY: Springer Science+Business Media; 2016.

6. van Geel AN, Pastorino U, Jauch KW, et al. Surgical treatment of lung metastases: the European Organization for Research and Treatment of Cancer-Soft Tissue and Bone Sarcoma Group study of 255 patients. *Cancer*. 1996;77(4):675–682.

7. Falk AT, Moureau-Zabotto L, Ouali M, et al. Effect on survival of local ablative treatment of metastases from sarcomas: a study of the French sarcoma group. *Clin Oncol (R Coll Radiol)*. 2015;27(1):48–55.

8. Baratti D, Pennacchioli E, Casali PG, et al. Epithelioid sarcoma: prognostic factors and survival in a series of patients treated at a single institution. *Ann Surg Oncol*. 2007;14(12):3542–3551.

9. Baldini EH, Wang D, Haas RL, et al. Treatment guidelines for preoperative radiation therapy for retroperitoneal sarcoma: preliminary consensus of an international expert panel. *Int J Radiat Oncol Biol Phys*. 2015;92(3):602–612.

10. Enneking WF, Spanier SS, Goodman MA. A system for the surgical staging of musculoskeletal sarcoma. *Clin Orthop Relat Res*. 1980(153):106–120.

11. van der Graaf WT, Blay JY, Chawla SP, et al. Pazopanib for metastatic soft-tissue sarcoma (PALETTE): a randomised, double-blind, placebo-controlled phase 3 trial. *Lancet*. 2012;379(9829):1879–1886.

12. Tap WD, Jones RL, Van Tine BA, et al. Olaratumab and doxorubicin versus doxorubicin alone for treatment of soft-tissue sarcoma: an open-label phase 1b and randomised phase 2 trial. *Lancet*. 2016;388(10043):488–497.

13. Pisters PW, Harrison LB, Leung DH, et al. Long-term results of a prospective randomized trial of adjuvant brachytherapy in soft tissue sarcoma. *J Clin Oncol*. 1996;14(3):859–868.

14. Naghavi AO, Fernandez DC, Mesko N, et al. American brachytherapy society consensus statement for soft tissue sarcoma brachytherapy. *Brachytherapy*. 2017;16(3):466–489.

15. Pearlstone DB, Janjan NA, Feig BW, et al. Re-resection with brachytherapy for locally recurrent soft tissue sarcoma arising in a previously radiated field. *Cancer J Sci Am*. 1999;5(1):26–33.

16. Videtic GMM, Woody N, Vassil AD. *Handbook of Treatment Planning in Radiation Oncology*. 2nd ed. New York, NY: Demos Medical; 2015.

XI: **PEDIATRIC**

52: MEDULLOBLASTOMA

Camille A. Berriochoa, Bindu V. Manyam, and Erin S. Murphy

QUICK HIT: Medulloblastoma (MB) is the most common malignant pediatric CNS tumor, accounting for 20% of all childhood brain cancers.[1] MB typically arises in the cerebellum, most commonly in the cerebellar vermis, leading to obstruction of CSF flow and hydrocephalus. Presenting symptoms are related to increased intracranial pressure (ICP): irritability, nausea, vomiting, increased head circumference in young infants, headaches, diplopia, ataxia, and papilledema.[2] Surgery alone leads to poor outcomes with multiple studies showing an improvement with the use of RT and CHT.[3,4] Attempts to reduce CSI dose and its associated growth and neurocognitive toxicities have been facilitated by optimized CHT regimens.[5] The recommended treatment paradigm is determined by patients' risk status, with average-risk patients meeting the following criteria: age ≥3 years, GTR/NTR (<1.5 cm² residual disease), and M0; some studies also require favorable histology to be deemed average risk (desmoplastic, extensive nodularity, classic). In the average-risk setting, clinicians are transitioning to CSI + involved field boost (IF = tumor bed + margin) versus historic standard of complete posterior fossa (PF) boost based on promising results from ACNS0331.[6] The role of molecular pathways and associated subgrouping is evolving, with Wnt/SHH groups conferring better prognosis with a worse prognosis seen for groups 3 and 4.

TABLE 52.1: General Treatment Paradigm for MB Following Maximal Safe Resection

	CSI	Posterior Fossa	Post-RT CHT	5-yr OS
Average risk (2/3 of pts at presentation) • ≥3 years of age AND • M0 AND • ≤1.5 cm² of residual disease post-op • Favorable histology (classic; desmoplastic/ nodular; extensive nodularity)	23.4 Gy/13 fx with weekly concurrent vincristine	As per recent ACNS 0331 results, boost IF (rather than entire PF) to 54–55.8 Gy	CDDP/VCR/CYC	80%
High risk* (1/3 of pts at presentation) • M+ OR • >1.5 cm² residual disease post-op • Poor histology (large cell; anaplastic)	36 Gy/20 fx with weekly concurrent vincristine	Boost PF to 54–55.8 Gy**	CDDP/VCR/CYC	60%

*Infants <3 years old are considered high risk and warrant a risk-adapted approach combining maximal safe resection, CHT, second-look surgery with delayed CSI or focal radiation given poor neurocognitive outcomes with standard CSI.
**For lesions of the spinal cord, boost to 45 Gy.

EPIDEMIOLOGY: MB is the most common malignant pediatric CNS tumor (pediatric low-grade glioma slightly more common), accounting for 40% of all PF tumors and 20% of all pediatric CNS tumors with about 500 cases per year in the United States.[2] Pts most commonly present between 5 and 7 years of age with distribution as follows: 10% before age 1, 60% to 70% before age 9, 30% above age 10. When present in adults, the histology is typically desmoplastic. More common in males than females and in Whites than African Americans.

RISK FACTORS: The majority of MB cases arise sporadically but ~5% are thought to be secondary to familial syndromes.

- *Gorlin syndrome* (also known as "nevoid basal cell carcinoma syndrome") is an AD condition associated with basal cell carcinoma, skeletal anomalies, and macrocephaly; MB develops in about 5% of pts. Associated with a 9q22.3 germline mutation, which confers inactivation of PTCH1, a protein that functions as the receptor for sonic hedgehog whose pathway is important for development of the cerebellum.[7]
- *Turcot syndrome:* AD; characterized by polyposis, colorectal cancers, gliomas, and MBs. Pts with Turcot's syndrome have a 92-fold higher relative risk of developing MB than the unaffected population.[8] Associated with APC mutation on chromosome 5q. The APC complex is in part responsible for degrading cytoplasmic β-catenin and is regulated by the Wingless pathway (Wnt). These molecular pathways help underpin the evolving biomolecular paradigm of MB.
- *Li–Fraumeni and NF-1:* both occasionally associated with MB.

ANATOMY: Most commonly presents in the PF with ~75% occurring in the midline vermis. Hemispheric location is associated with older age and desmoplastic histology. The boundaries of the PF are as follows: anterior—clivus and posterior clinoid; posterior—inion (bony prominence at confluence of straight and sagittal sinuses); inferior—occipital bone, lateral–temporal, occipital, and parietal bones; superior—tentorium cerebellum. CSF flows from the fourth ventricle into the subarachnoid space via the medial foramen of Magendie and the lateral foramina of Luschka. The tendency for MB to obstruct CSF efflux leads to symptoms associated with raised ICP (see clinical presentation).[2]

PATHOLOGY: The 2007 WHO classification (and 2016 update) subdivides MB into the four histologic subtypes in Table 52.2 (in addition to genetic differences discussed in the following).[2,9,10] IHC demonstrates neuronal markers (neurofilament, neuron-specific enolase, synaptophysin) in most cases, and occasionally stains positive for GFAP (glial fibrillary acidic protein). Rare subtypes: melanotic (<1%), and medullomyoblastoma (<1%; contains striated muscle differentiation).

GENETICS: Historically, risk stratification has relied primarily on clinicopathologic variables. However, in 2010, an international panel identified four main molecular subgroups, described in Table 52.3. A molecularly driven risk stratification system was established at a 2015 consensus, which supports the development of biomarker-driven clinical trials.[11,12] Note that supratentorial PNET tumors are classically treated as high risk. Bcl-2, ERBB2, and MIB-L1 are potential markers of aggressive behavior.[13] C-MYC amplification and alterations in chromosome 17 can be observed.[14]

CLINICAL PRESENTATION[2]: Tumors usually grow into/fill the fourth ventricle with signs and symptoms related to increased ICP: headaches, morning emesis, papilledema, diplopia due to CN VI palsy; infants may manifest bulging anterior fontanelle and splitting of cranial sutures. Destruction of the vermis can cause truncal ataxia; other cerebellar symptoms include dysmetria, dys-diadochokinesia, spasticity. Though most commonly seen in pineal gland tumors, Parinaud syndrome (upward gaze palsy, pseudo-Argyll Robertson pupils, convergence-retraction nystagmus, eyelid retraction) can be observed, as can the

TABLE 52.2: Morphologic Classification of Medulloblastoma			
Histopathologic Subtype	Prognosis	Relative Frequency	Features
Desmoplastic/ Nodular	Good	15%–20%, more common in older pts	Biphasic w/ dense cellular areas surrounded by stromal component. Desmoplastic variant is associated with Gorlin syndrome and resultant inactivation of PTCH1.
Extensive Nodularity	Good		Nodules dominate the histopathology and are typically large and irregularly shaped.
Classic	Intermediate	80%–90%	Densely cellular, undifferentiated small round blue cells. Classically associated with Homer Wright rosettes (rings of neuroblasts surrounding eosinophilic neuropil) but these are observed in the minority of cases.
Large Cell/ Anaplastic	Poor	~5%–10%, rare	Large cells w/ large nuclei, prominent nucleoli, many mitoses, and nuclear polymorphism. More cytoplasm than classic; associated w/ amplification of MYC, bulky spinal mets.

"setting sun sign" (conjugate down gaze). Extraneural metastases are uncommon (<5%) but most commonly involve bone. Differential diagnosis of a pediatric posterior fossa mass: BEAM (brainstem glioma, ependymoma, astrocytoma, medulloblastoma), hemangioblastoma, lymphoma, and dysplastic cerebellar ganglioglioma.

WORKUP: H&P with detailed neurologic exam. Preoperatively, obtain (a) MRI brain with contrast (MB appears as isointense/hypointense mass with patchy contrast enhancement on T1; isointense on FLAIR, and hyperintense on DWI) and (b) establish baseline neuropsychiatric testing, neuroendocrine testing, growth curves, CBC, and audiologic evaluation. If imaging suggests MB or other brain tumor, up-front resection (not biopsy) is indicated. Obtain postoperative MRI brain with contrast *within* 72 hours (inflammation of the meninges and residual blood products in the CSF can become pronounced beyond 72 hours and falsely suggest M+ disease). Obtain MRI spinal axis at 10 to 14 days post-op to avoid confounding due to artifactual changes that can be seen in the immediate post-op period. Lumbar puncture w/ cytology should be performed after MRI spinal axis is obtained to avoid confounding inflammation from the procedure. Usually, LP cannot be safely performed preoperatively due to increased intracranial pressure. False-positive LPs can occur within 10 days; this can be repeated if positive. Systemic staging not routinely performed.

PROGNOSTIC FACTORS: Factors associated with worse prognosis: age <3 years, M+, STR (>1.5 cm² residual), group 3 or 4 molecular profile, anaplastic/large cell morphology.

STAGING: MB follows the Modified Chang system, which is based on preoperative MRI, postoperative MRI, operative findings, and CSF analysis. Note: T stage is no longer thought to be prognostic.

TABLE 52.3: Molecular Classification of Medulloblastoma

Molecular Subgroup[11]	Incidence	Age	5-yr OS	Associated Histology	Pathogenesis
Wingless (Wnt)	10%	Older children and adults	95%	Classic	Mutation in *CTNNB1* gene upregulates Wnt pathway, which increases accumulation of nuclear β-catenin and promotes cell division and proliferation.
Sonic Hedgehog (Shh)	30%	Bimodal: <5 y/o, then adolescent/ young adults	75%	Desmoplastic/ nodular	Mutation in *PTCH1* gene, which upregulates Shh pathway and promotes DNA transcription, decrease in cell–cell adhesion, and increased angiogenesis.
Group 4*	35%	Median age 9 y/o	75%	Classic	Overexpression of histone methylases/ acetylases. Oncogene *MYCN* amplification. Chromosome X loss in 80% of females with Group 4 medulloblastoma.
Group 3*	25%	Infants and young children	50%	Classic/large cell/anaplastic	Not well defined. Upregulation of OTX2 transcription factor upregulates *C-Myc* oncogene and associated overexpression.

*New evidence suggests that growth factor independent-1 (GFI1 and GFI1B) proto-oncogene activation is implicated in Group 3 and 4 medulloblastoma.[15]

TREATMENT PARADIGM

Multimodality therapy is currently the standard of care, as surgery alone confers dismal prognosis with only 1/61 pts surviving this single modality approach in Cushing's original paper.[17] Adjuvant RT was introduced in the 1950s with some improvement in survival though still poor compared to current standards. Improvements in outcome were finally observed with modern RT techniques and the addition of CHT.[18,19] Several cooperative trials have helped delineate the current treatment paradigm, which generally includes maximal safe resection followed by CSI + PF/IF boost with concurrent weekly vincristine followed by approximately eight cycles of CHT.

Surgery: Suboccipital craniotomy with maximal safe resection. The goal is to achieve GTR/NTR with <1.5 cm² residual on post-op MRI. Previous studies have indicated essentially equivalent outcomes between GTR and NTR surgeries.[20] Classically, PFS is improved with GTR/NTR versus STR (~70% vs. 50%)[21] though this is evolving in the molecular era.[22] Stereotactic or open biopsy is rarely indicated. Preoperatively, vasogenic

TABLE 52.4: Modified Chang Staging System for Medulloblastoma[16]	
Extent of tumor	
T1	≤3 cm diameter
T2	>3 cm diameter
T3a	>3 cm with extension into the aqueduct of Sylvius and/or foramen of Luschka
T3b	>3 cm with unequivocal extension into the brainstem
T4	>3 cm with extension past the aqueduct of Sylvius and/or down past the foramen magnum (beyond posterior fossa)
Degree of metastasis	
M0	No CSF, cerebral, or spinal involvement
M1	Positive CSF cytology
M2	Gross nodular seeding along cerebellar/cerebral subarachnoid space or in the third or lateral ventricles
M3	Gross nodular seeding in the spinal subarachnoid space
M4	Metastasis outside the cerebrospinal axis

tumor edema may be managed with steroids. Obstructive hydrocephalus is typically relieved by removal of the tumor, but intraoperative ventriculostomy may be indicated to relieve pressure.

Complications: PF syndrome in up to 25% (also known as "cerebellar mutism": manifested by mutism, truncal ataxia, dysphagia, emotional lability; usually self-resolves over weeks to months and should not delay adjuvant treatment). Operative mortality is <2%.

Chemotherapy: MB is one of the most chemosensitive brain tumors. The incorporation of platinum agents is standard given their efficacy. Usually initiated ~4 weeks following CSI with 8–9 cycles delivered. As per the German HIT91 RCT, immediate postoperative CSI/vincristine followed by CHT became standard (as opposed to post-op CHT followed by CSI).[23] CCG 9892 was a single-arm phase II trial evaluating reduced-dose CSI of 23.4 Gy with concurrent vincristine followed by CCNU/vincristine/cisplatin with an 80% 5-yr PFS similar to historical controls using CSI of ~36 Gy and thus became a new standard of care for average-risk disease.[24] In young children, CHT is used to delay or avoid the use of radiation to decrease associated neurocognitive risks (treatment paradigm: induction CHT followed by surgery and then additional consolidation CHT, with RT offered only for salvage).[9] Complications: ototoxicity, infertility (related to cyclophosphamide; affects males more than females), myelosuppression, second malignancy.

Radiation: CSI indicated for all pts and should start within approximately 30 days of surgery. *Average risk*: After maximal safe resection: CSI to 23.4 Gy/13 fx w/ PF boost to 54–55.8 Gy total, though with recent presentation of ACNS 0331, some clinicians have transitioned to tumor bed + margin followed by adjuvant CHT.[6] Concurrent CHT is used at some institutions but considered too toxic at others. *High risk*: After maximal resection: CSI to 36–39.6 Gy/20–22 fx w/ PF boost to 55.8 Gy with concurrent vincristine during CSI followed by adjuvant CHT. If M+, boost metastatic disease as follows (per ACNS 0332): 50.4 Gy: intracranial mets, 50.4 Gy: focal spinal mets below cord, 45 Gy: focal spine mets above cord terminus; 39.6 Gy: diffuse spinal disease. Both IMRT[25] and proton therapy[26] have been shown to reduce ototoxicity as compared to 3D-CRT regimens.

Complications of CSI: Acute: Myelosuppression, nausea/vomiting, diarrhea, fatigue, hair loss, headaches, muffled hearing. Chronic: Neurocognitive (mnemonic "I am able"/I M ABL—IQ, memory, attention, behavior, learning), neuroendocrine deficits (particularly

GH deficiency, hypothyroidism, gonadal dysfunction), impaired soft tissue/bone growth, ototoxicity (RT and/or cisplatin), secondary neoplasms, Lhermitte's syndrome, cataract. Merchant et al. developed a model to predict for cognitive changes based on the dose and volume received by critical structures such as the temporal lobes.[27] There is evidence that proton plans facilitate decreased dose to the cochleae and temporal lobes compared to IMRT (~2% for protons, ~20% for IMRT) with essentially zero exit dose through the abdomen, chest, heart, and pelvis.[26,28] Additional data shows that when administered to adults needing CSI, proton-based treatment was associated with essentially 1/3 the rates of nausea, vomiting, and weight loss, and 10-fold less esophagitis.[29]

EVIDENCE-BASED Q&A

COG standard risk MB

What did early studies attempting to optimize MB treatment show regarding the use of CHT?

*CCG 942[30] and SIOP 1[31] were early studies evaluating the addition of post-RT CHT to CSI (at 36 Gy) in an unselected pt population. Both ultimately showed that CHT did **not** confer a survival benefit among all pts, though, on subset analysis, did show a benefit to those with T3-T4 disease and M1-3 disease. Thus, several subsequent studies were performed without the incorporation of CHT as described in the following.*

CCG 942, Evans (*J Neurosurg* 1990, PMID 2319316): PRT of 233 pts 2 to 16 years of age w/ M0-3 MB enrolled after maximal surgical resection. Randomized to RT alone versus RT w/ concurrent VCR followed by eight cycles (q6 weeks) of VCR, CCNU, and prednisone. RT was 35 to 40 Gy CSI w/ PF boost to 50 to 55 Gy. 50 Gy boost to localized spinal metastases. 5-yr EFS was 59% w/ CHT versus 50% w/ RT alone (not significant). 5-yr OS was 65% for both groups. On unplanned subgroup analysis, pts w/ advanced disease (T3-4 and M1-3), 5-yr EFS was 46% w/ CHT versus 0% for RT alone ($p = .006$), and 5-yr OS was 61% w/ CHT versus 19% for XRT alone ($p = .04$). Significant prognostic factors were M+, young age, and advanced T-stage. **Conclusion: Pts w/ T3-4 and M1-3 disease realized the greatest benefit from CHT, whereas pts that are T1-2 and M0 realized no benefit.**

Due to these results showing that CHT did not improve outcomes, can RT alone be modified to offer optimal EFS and OS while minimizing toxicity?

Acknowledging the neurocognitive toxicity of 36 Gy to the craniospinal axis, French investigators attempted to reduce RT volume by delivering RT to the infratentorium only; however, results were terrible, with <20% 6-yr EFS and 64% failure in the supratentorium.[32] With this study clearly demonstrating that RT should be delivered to both supratentorial and infratentorial regions, the POG/CCG collaborative group modified the dose rather than the volume with their RCT (CCG 923/POG 8631) randomizing pts to a CSI dose of either 23.4 Gy or 36 Gy. The trial closed prematurely due to initial early relapses on the low-dose arm, though on longer FU 5-yr PFS was no different.[33] A companion JCO publication by Mulhern et al. reported on neuropsychologic testing in long-term survivors (>6 years), finding significantly less neuropsychologic toxicity in those treated to 23.4 Gy rather than 36 Gy with the difference most pronounced in those <9 years of age.[34]

Thomas, POG 8631/CCG 923 (*JCO* 2000, PMID 10944134): PRT of 126 pts 3 to 21 years of age w/ T1-3aM0 maximally resected MB (residual ≤1.5 cm² on CT) randomized to 23.4 Gy (reduced dose) versus 36 Gy (standard dose) CSI. (Note: This was the first PRT requiring extensive pre-randomization/pretherapy staging w/ myelography, LP, post-op CT w/ contrast.) All pts received a PF boost to 54 Gy. No CHT was given. This was the first PRT to assess neuropsychologic functioning. The protocol was terminated early when interim analysis revealed an increased rate of any relapse or isolated neuraxis relapse in pts receiving reduced-dose RT. **Conclusion: reduced-dose CSI is associated with increased risk of neuraxis relapse. The therapeutic gain of 36 Gy over 23.4 Gy CSI is at least partly offset by increased toxicity. This supports the rationale for reduced-dose CSI + CHT for future investigation. 5-yr EFS of 67% serves as a benchmark for average-risk MB treated w/ surgery and best conventional RT.** *Comment: No CHT was utilized.*

What trials ultimately led to the reincorporation of CHT in the management of MB?

Several trials continued to evaluate the role of CHT. In a prospective multi-institutional study published in 1994, Packer et al. evaluated 63 pts (both with average-risk and high-risk disease) with a treatment regimen incorporating weekly vincristine during RT followed by eight 6-week cycles of cisplatin/CCNU/vincristine, with authors concluding that "chemotherapy has a definite role in the management of children with medulloblastoma."[35] Later, the PNET 3 PRT randomized pts s/p GTR/NTR to RT alone versus CHT followed by RT.[36] Initial results showed improved 5-yr EFS of 60% versus 74% (p = .037) with no difference in OS, though a later update showed a reduction in health status (including hearing, speech, vision, ambulation, dexterity, emotion, cognition) in those who received CHT.[37]

Taylor, PNET-3 (*JCO* 2003, PMID 12697884): PRT of pre-RT CHT (vincristine, etoposide, carboplatin, cyclophosphamide x four cycles) versus RT alone for nonmetastatic MB. RT was delivered to all pts as 35 Gy CSI followed by PF boost to 55 Gy. 217 pts, 179 evaluable. 3-yr EFS improved in the CHT arm (79% versus 65% with RT alone) as did 5-yr EFS (74% vs. 60%, both *p* = .037). There was no significant difference in 3- or 5-yr OS. This was the *first* PRT to show improved EFS with the addition of CHT. Authors added that this non-cisplatin-containing regimen could also reduce ototoxicity and nephrotoxicity.

What studies led to the use of reduced-dose CSI in average-risk disease?

The same Packer study referenced earlier treated standard-risk pts to 23.4 Gy with the use of concurrent weekly vincristine (in the same study, they treated high-risk pts to 36 Gy with weekly vincristine) and found favorable outcomes.[35] This study was then expanded into CCG 9892, a phase II trial limited to standard-risk pts again delivering 23.4 Gy to the CSI followed by a 55.8 Gy PF boost with concurrent weekly vincristine, followed by subsequent CHT with CCNU/vincristine/cisplatin. This resulted in a 3-yr PFS of 88% and 3-yr OS of 85%, rates authors argued were comparable to previous studies using higher dose CSI. Authors concluded that reduced-dose CSI with concurrent and adjuvant CHT is a feasible approach for M0 disease.

Packer, CCG 9892 (*JCO* 1999, PMID 10561268): Phase II trial of 65 pts 3 to 10 years of age w/ M0 MB enrolled following maximal surgical resection. Pts received RT within 28 days post-op with concurrent weekly VCR. RT was delivered as CSI to 23.4 Gy w/ PF boost to 55.8 Gy. Six weeks following RT, pts received CCNU, VCR, and CDDP for eight cycles (q6 weeks). MFU 56 mos. No prognostic factors identified; including ~33% RT protocol violation rate. 3-yr PFS was 88% and 3-yr OS was 85%. **Conclusion: These results suggest that reduced-dose CSI and adjuvant CDDP-based CT during and after RT is feasible for M0 MB, serving to support Packer's earlier study.**

Can cyclophosphamide replace CCNU in the adjuvant CHT portion of treatment?

COG A9961 was a large PRT randomizing average-risk MB pts (all of whom were post-op and received 23.4 Gy CSI) to two different adjuvant CHT regimens, one with cyclophosphamide and another with CCNU. The rationale was that data supporting the use of CCNU in pediatric tumors was scant whereas xenograft and early clinical data for the use of cyclophosphamide was more promising.[38] Ultimately, there was no significant difference between the two regimens, with 5-yr OS about 85% in both arms. Authors concluded that though neither CHT regimen was superior, the favorable outcomes seen with both regimens offer additional support to the use of reduced-dose CSI.

Packer, COG A9961 (*JCO* 2006, PMID 16943538; Update *Neuro Oncol* 2013, PMID 23099653): PRT of 379 pts with average risk medulloblastoma treated with reduced-dose (23.4 Gy) CSI and posterior fossa boost (55.8 Gy) randomized to CCNU/cisplatin/vincristine or cyclophosphamide/cisplatin/vincristine (all pts received weekly vincristine during RT). See Table 52.5 (both papers combined). 61 pts relapsed within 5 years after treatment; 51 (84%) experienced disseminated relapse. 15 pts experienced secondary tumors at median of 5.8 years. The cumulative 10-year incidence of secondary malignancies was 4.2%. **Conclusion: EFS is encouraging in pts with average-risk medulloblastoma with reduced-dose CSI and adjuvant CHT; however, no difference between CHT regimens.**

TABLE 52.5: Results of COG A9961 Medulloblastoma				
	5-yr EFS	10-yr EFS	5-yr OS	10-yr OS
Reduced-dose CSI (both arms reported together)	81%	76%	87%	81%

When treating average-risk MB, does hyperfractionation of CSI affect outcomes or reduce toxicity?

MSFOP 98 was a phase I/II average risk trial using hyperfractionated therapy, 36 Gy CSI with boost to 68 Gy to the tumor bed at 1 Gy/fx BID.[39] It showed excellent long-term EFS in the absence of CHT and full-scale intelligence quotient (IQ) drop was less pronounced compared to other standard RT reports. This led to a large European PRT (HIT-SIOP PNET-4), which enrolled average-risk MB pts who were randomized to standard fractionation (23.4 Gy CSI with PF boost to 54 Gy at 1.8 Gy/fx) versus hyperfractionation (36 Gy CSI with PF boost to 60 Gy and 68 Gy tumor bed at 1 Gy/fx BID with 8-hr interfx interval).[40] Results published in the JCO in 2012 showed equivalent outcomes for EFS and OS and no difference in ototoxicity; IQ measurements were not reported in their final publication. Based on these results, hyperfractionation is typically not employed in average risk MB.

What is the optimal dose to deliver to the PF?

This has never been prospectively studied, but a 1988 Harvard RR showed better LC if the PF dose was >50 Gy (LC 79% vs. 33% if less than 50 Gy; p < .02).[41]

Does the boost volume need to include the entire PF or is tumor bed + margin sufficient?

Two RRs showed that the PF failure rate was ≤5% with the use of IF-directed boost. These reports in part provided the rationale for ACNS 0331.[42,43]

Wolden, MSKCC (*JCO* 2003, PMID 12915597): RR of 32 pts with newly diagnosed MB at MSKCC who received CSI (23.4–39.6 Gy) followed by conformal tumor bed boost. MFU ~5 years. Only one pt failed in the posterior fossa. Freedom from PF failure was 100% at 5 years and 86% at 10 years. **Conclusion: PF failures are low in the setting of conformal treatment, which allows for significant sparing of critical structures.**

Merchant, St. Jude (*IJROBP* 2008, PMID 17892918): Prospective Ph II trial of 23.4 Gy CSI + PF boost to 36 Gy and primary site to 55.8 Gy (CTV = tumor bed + anatomically confined margin of 2 cm; PTV = 3–5 mm) with subsequent dose intensive CHT (cyclophosphamide, cisplatin, vincristine x four cycles). 86 pts, MFU 5 years. 5-yr EFS was 83% and PF failure was 5%. Primary site boost reduced dose to the temporal lobes, cochlea, and hypothalamus. **Conclusion: Tumor bed boost with margin gives comparable tumor control to entire PF boost.**

Can pts with average-risk MB who are most vulnerable to the neurocognitive effects of CSI receive a lower dose? Can any average-risk pt receive IF boost rather than whole PF boost?

ACNS0331 was developed to answer both questions. Multiple studies have shown that CSI doses of >20 Gy can damage neurocognitive and growth outcomes, prompting investigators to determine whether lower doses could confer favorable outcomes with less toxicity.[44,45] In 1989, Goldwein et al. reported on their prospective cohort study of 10 MB pts delivering 18 Gy CSI with a PF boost of 50.4 to 55.8 Gy with weekly vincristine and subsequent CDDP/VCR/CCNU CHT showing favorable cure rates with this approach.[46] Additionally, regarding IF versus PF boost, Wolden's and Merchant's studies (see the previous discussion) finding low PF failure rates with the use of tumor bed boost alone suggested that IF-only boost may be appropriate. These results help set the stage for ACNS 0331.

Michalski, COG ACNS0331 (*ASTRO* 2016, Abstract LBA2): Enrolled 464 pts from ages 3 to 21 with average risk MB with a primary endpoint of time to event (progression, recurrence, death from any cause, secondary malignant neoplasm). Pts between 3 and 7 underwent two randomizations (CSI dose of 18 Gy vs. 23.4 Gy; also involved field [IF; e.g., tumor bed] vs. PF boost). Pts from 8 to 21 were eligible only for the IF versus PF question; all received CSI dose of 23.4 Gy. Note that this is the first multi-institution RCT that was sufficiently powered to address the question of IF versus full PF boost. Protocol: max safe resection followed by initiation of 6 weeks of RT within 31 days delivered with weekly vincristine followed by cisplatin/vincristine and either CCNU or cyclophosphamide (alternating AABAABAAB pattern) CHT. MFU 6.6 years. **Conclusion: IF boost is noninferior to full PF boost for all standard risk pts 3 to 21 years of age. However, reduced-dose CSI is associated with worse 5-yr EFS and OS and thus average-risk MB pts should continue to receive 23.4 Gy as the standard CSI dose unless enrolled on a clinical trial.**

TABLE 52.6: Preliminary Results of COG ACNS 0331 Medulloblastoma			
	5-yr LF	**5-yr EFS**	**5-yr OS**
All pts 3–21 yrs of age:			
IF boost	1.9%	82%	84%
PF boost	3.7%	81%	85%
	$p = .178$	$p = .421$; the 94% upper confidence limit on the HR was 1.3, lower than the prespecified limit of 1.6, and thus IFRT was deemed noninferior to PFRT	
Pts 3–7 yrs of age:			
Low dose (18 Gy)		72%	78%
Standard dose (23.4 Gy)		83%	86%
		The 80% upper confidence limit of the HR was 1.9; this was higher than the prespecified limit of 1.6 and thus noninferiority of low-dose CSI was not established.	

COG high risk MB

What data initially supported the use of CHT in high-risk disease?

CCG 942 (discussed earlier in the average-risk section) and SIOP I were both PRTs evaluating postoperative pts who received CSI and were then randomized to CHT or no CHT.[30,31] For both studies, there was no difference in outcome between the two groups, but when limited to those with more advanced disease (T3-T4, M+ or STR), an improvement in EFS was observed.

Can outcomes be improved by intensifying the CHT regimen with additional agents?

CCG 921 was performed in pts with a variety of high-risk pediatric brain tumors to see if "8 in 1" CHT (8 types of CHT in 1 day: cisplatin, procarbazine, CCNU, vincristine, cyclophospha-mide, methylprednisolone, hydroxyurea, cytarabine) was better than a combination of vincristine/CCNU/prednisone (VCP). 421 children were enrolled, of which 203 had MB. Subset analysis of this group showed better outcomes with VCP than 8 in 1 CHT (5-yr PFS 63% vs. 45%, p = .006).[21]

What about altering the sequence of CHT (e.g., delivering CHT immediately post-op followed by RT)?

Four PRTs have evaluated this question: SIOP II, SIOP III, POG 9031, and HIT 91 from Germany. All of them except for SIOP III showed no benefit to immediate post-op CHT; both POG 9031 and SIOP II showed 5-yr EFS to be about 60% to 70% and 5-yr OS about 75% in both groups with no significant difference between them and HIT 91 actually showed an improvement in 3-yr EFS with immediate RT (78% vs. 65%, p = .03).[5,23,47] SIOP III is the only exception, showing improved 3- and 5-yr EFS with up-front CHT.[4] Therefore, with three of these four studies showing no benefit to up-front CHT, standard of care is to perform maximal safe resection followed by RT (with concurrent vincristine) followed by adjuvant CHT.

Is there any detriment to interrupting RT?

Interestingly, SIOP III also showed better 3-yr OS when RT was delivered within 50 days, suggesting that avoiding RT interruption can lead to better outcomes.[4] These results confirm earlier findings from the University of Florida that prompt completion of RT confers better outcomes (at a cut point of 45 days in that 1998 study).[48]

TABLE 52.7: SIOP III RT Duration Results	
RT Duration	**3-yr OS**
<50 days	84.1%
>50 days	70.9%
p value	.0356

Does the use of carboplatin as a radiosensitizer during CSI lead to better outcomes?

This was addressed in COG 99701, a phase I/II trial that evaluated the role of adding radiosensitiz-ing carboplatin to vincristine during CSI.[49] Note that the adjuvant therapy offered changed slightly once the recommended dose of carboplatin was determined, but among all pts on this study, 5-yr OS was approximately 75%. Authors concluded that CRT with vincristine + carboplatin followed by 6 months of maintenance CHT produced outcomes at least as good as (if not better than) other prior trials using higher dose CSI or higher dose alkylator-based therapy. This carboplatin-con-taining regimen is being tested in an ongoing phase III PRT, ACNS 0332. This trial is evaluating the intensification of systemic therapy in high-risk MB (M+, STR and/or diffuse anaplasia) and is utilizing two randomizations: (a) concurrent carboplatin during RT and (b) isotretinoin during and after maintenance therapy.

Is there a role for re-irradiation?

Recurrent MB is rarely cured and has a dismal prognosis with 2-year OS historically <25%. However, a number of salvage treatments have been considered including surgical resec-tion, brachytherapy, radiosurgery, high-dose CHT with autologous stem cell transplant and *re-irradiation. Re-irradiation may be a reasonable option to consider in both standard-risk and high-risk pts.*

Wetmore, St. Jude (*Cancer* 2014, PMID 25080363): RR of 38 pts with recurrent MB. Of these pts, 14 received re-irradiation (8 repeat CSI, spinal only re-RT in 3, primary only in 3). For pts who initially had standard risk MB, 5-yr OS with RT was 55% versus 33% without; 10-yr OS 46% with RT versus 0% without (*p* = .003). Similarly, the high-risk individuals also benefited (*p* = .003). Re-irradiation did result in an increased rate of necrosis (*p* = .0468).

MB in INFANTS

What is the recommended treatment for infants (<3 years)?

*The mainstay of treatment for MB involves maximal safe resection followed by CSI + boost. However, CSI can lead to significant neurocognitive toxicity, which is not only dose dependent but also dependent on the age of the pt (younger is worse).[50,51] Therefore, CHT has been evaluated as a stopgap to delay RT. Baby POG#1 showed this was possible with a 5-yr OS of 40%. An unintended consequence of this study was complete parent refusal of radiation, which showed that in a select group of MB infants, there **may** not be a need for RT at all. As described earlier, the CCG group tried eight CHT drugs ("8-in-1") with worse outcomes but confirmed the approach of CHT before RT was feasible. Follow-up trials including the Head Start I and II for infant MB used intensive CHT and used radiation only in a salvage setting.[52] This approach eliminated craniospinal XRT in 52% of pts and may preserve quality of life and intellectual function. However, the intense CHT is not without cost and 4 of 21 infants died of treatment-related death. The findings of Baby POG#1 have been further bolstered by Rutkowski et al. using surgery and subsequent CHT, with 5-yr OS for those s/p GTR of 93%, 56% if STR, and 38% for those with macroscopic metastases.[9]*

Duffner, POG 8633/Baby POG#1 (*NEJM* 1993, PMID 8388548; Update *Neuro-Oncology* 1999, PMID 11554387): Prospective trial of 198 pts <3 yrs of age w/ malignant intracranial tumors (62/198 or 31% w/ MB) enrolled following maximal surgical resection. CHT given 2 to 4 wks after surgery consisted of alternating 28-day cycles in the sequence AABAAB. Cycle A was VCR and CYC; Cycle B was CDDP and VP-16. Planned duration of CHT was for 2 years in children <2 years of age and for 1 year in children 2 to 3 years of age. If evidence of progression or unacceptable toxicity, CHT was stopped and pt considered for additional surgery, if appropriate, and RT. RT was started 3 to 4 weeks after CHT. For pts w/ residual disease or M+, CSI was administered to 35.2 Gy w/ PF boost to 54 Gy. For those children w/o residual disease (GTR) or M0, CSI was administered to 24 Gy w/ PF boost to 50 Gy. For MB patients as a whole, 5 yr PFS was 31.8% and 5 yr OS was 39.7%. 38% of pts w/ MB had GTR. 48% of pts w/ MB achieved CR (15%) or PR (33%) w/ CHT. 5-yr OS for pts w/ GTR was 60% and for pts w/ GTR + M0 disease was 69%. 5-yr OS for pts w/ STR was 32%. Cognitive testing after 1 yr of CHT revealed no evidence of deterioration. **Conclusion: Post-op CT permits delay of RT in young children and is associated with a reduction in neurotoxicity. For pts w/ GTR or CR w/ CHT, results suggest that RT may not be needed after at least 1 yr of CHT. Of interest, a reduction in the CSI dose used for those pts w/ GTR and M0 disease did not adversely affect survival.**

REFERENCES

1. Louis DN, Ohgaki H, Wiestler OD, et al. The 2007 WHO classification of tumours of the central nervous system. *Acta Neuropathol.* 2007;114(2):97–109.
2. Dhall G. Medulloblastoma. *J Child Neurol.* 2009;24(11):1418-1430.
3. Cuneo H, Rand C. *Medulloblastoma: Brain Tumors of Childhood.* Los Angeles, CA: Charles C Thomas; 1952:21–42.

4. Taylor RE, Bailey CC, Robinson KJ, et al. Impact of radiotherapy parameters on outcome in the International Society of Paediatric Oncology/United Kingdom Children's Cancer Study Group PNET-3 study of preradiotherapy chemotherapy for M0-M1 medulloblastoma. *Int J Radiat Oncol Biol Phys.* 2004;58(4):1184–1193.

5. Bailey CC, Gnekow A, Wellek S, et al. Prospective randomised trial of chemotherapy given before radiotherapy in childhood medulloblastoma. International Society of Paediatric Oncology (SIOP) and the (German) Society of Paediatric Oncology (GPO): SIOP II. *Med Pediat Oncol.* 1995;25(3):166–178.

6. Michalski J. Results of COG ACNS0331: a phase III trial of involved-field radiotherapy (IFRT) and low dose craniospinal irradiation (LD-CSI) with chemotherapy in average-risk medulloblastoma: a report from the Children's Oncology Group. *Int J Radiat Oncol Biol Phys.* 2016; 96(5):937.

7. Stone DM, Hynes M, Armanini M, et al. The tumour-suppressor gene patched encodes a candidate receptor for sonic hedgehog. *Nature.* 1996;384(6605):129–134.

8. Hamilton SR, Liu B, Parsons RE, et al. The molecular basis of Turcot's syndrome. *New Eng J Med.* 1995;332(13):839–847.

9. Rutkowski S, Bode U, Deinlein F, et al. Treatment of early childhood medulloblastoma by postoperative chemotherapy alone. *New Eng J Med.* 2005;352(10):978–986.

10. Louis DN, Perry A, Reifenberger G, et al. The 2016 World Health Organization Classification of Tumors of the Central Nervous System: a summary. *Acta Neuropathol.* 2016;131(6):803–820.

11. Khatua S. Evolving molecular era of childhood medulloblastoma: time to revisit therapy. *Future Oncol.* 2016;12(1):107–117.

12. Ramaswamy V, Remke M, Bouffet E, et al. Risk stratification of childhood medulloblastoma in the molecular era: the current consensus. *Acta Neuropathol.* 2016;131(6):821–831.

13. Das P, Puri T, Suri V, et al. Medulloblastomas: a correlative study of MIB-1 proliferation index along with expression of c-Myc, ERBB2, and anti-apoptotic proteins along with histological typing and clinical outcome. *Childs Nerv Syst.* 2009;25(7):825–835.

14. Pan E, Pellarin M, Holmes E, et al. Isochromosome 17q is a negative prognostic factor in poor-risk childhood medulloblastoma patients. *Clin Cancer Res.* 2005;11(13):4733–4740.

15. Northcott PA, Lee C, Zichner T, et al. Enhancer hijacking activates GFI1 family oncogenes in medulloblastoma. *Nature.* 2014;511(7510):428–434.

16. Chang CH, Housepian EM, Herbert C, Jr. An operative staging system and a megavoltage radiotherapeutic technic for cerebellar medulloblastomas. *Radiology.* 1969;93(6):1351–1359.

17. Cushing H. Experiences with the cerebellar medulloblastomas: a critical review. *Acta Pathol Microbiol Scand.* 1930;7:1–86.

18. Lampe I, Mac IR. Medulloblastoma of the cerebellum. *Arch Neurol Psych.* 1949;62(3):322–329.

19. Tomlinson FH, Scheithauer BW, Meyer FB, et al. Medulloblastoma: I. Clinical, diagnostic, and therapeutic overview. *J Child Neurol.* 1992;7(2):142–155.

20. Gajjar A, Sanford RA, Bhargava R, et al. Medulloblastoma with brain stem involvement: the impact of gross total resection on outcome. *Pediat Neurosurg.* 1996;25(4):182–187.

21. Zeltzer PM, Boyett JM, Finlay JL, et al. Metastasis stage, adjuvant treatment, and residual tumor are prognostic factors for medulloblastoma in children: conclusions from the Children's Cancer Group 921 randomized phase III study. *J Clin Oncol.* 1999;17(3):832–845.

22. Thompson EM, Hielscher T, Bouffet E, et al. Prognostic value of medulloblastoma extent of resection after accounting for molecular subgroup: a retrospective integrated clinical and molecular analysis. *Lancet Oncol.* 2016;17(4):484–495.

23. Kortmann RD, Kuhl J, Timmermann B, et al. Postoperative neoadjuvant chemotherapy before radiotherapy as compared to immediate radiotherapy followed by maintenance chemotherapy in the treatment of medulloblastoma in childhood: results of the German prospective randomized trial HIT '91. *Int J Radiat Oncol Biol Phys.* 2000;46(2):269–279.

24. Packer RJ, Goldwein J, Nicholson HS, et al. Treatment of children with medulloblastomas with reduced-dose craniospinal radiation therapy and adjuvant chemotherapy: a Children's Cancer Group Study. *J Clin Oncol.* 1999;17(7):2127–2136.

25. Huang E, Teh BS, Strother DR, et al. Intensity-modulated radiation therapy for pediatric medulloblastoma: early report on the reduction of ototoxicity. *Int J Radiat Oncol Biol Phys.* 2002;52(3):599–605.

26. Moeller BJ, Chintagumpala M, Philip JJ, et al. Low early ototoxicity rates for pediatric medullo- blastoma patients treated with proton radiotherapy. *Radiat Oncol.* 2011;6:58.

27. Merchant TE, Schreiber JE, Wu S, et al. Critical combinations of radiation dose and volume predict intelligence quotient and academic achievement scores after craniospinal irradiation in children with medulloblastoma. *Int J Radiat Oncol Biol Phys.* 2014;90(3):554–561.

28. Fossati P, Ricardi U, Orecchia R. Pediatric medulloblastoma: toxicity of current treatment and potential role of protontherapy. *Cancer Treat Rev.* 2009;35(1):79–96.

29. Brown AP, Barney CL, Grosshans DR, et al. Proton beam craniospinal irradiation reduces acute toxicity for adults with medulloblastoma. *Int J Radiat Oncol Biol Phys.* 2013;86(2):277–284.

30. Evans AE, Jenkin RD, Sposto R, et al. The treatment of medulloblastoma: results of a prospective randomized trial of radiation therapy with and without CCNU, vincristine, and prednisone. *J Neurosurg.* 1990;72(4):572–582.

31. Tait DM, Thornton-Jones H, Bloom HJ, et al. Adjuvant chemotherapy for medulloblastoma: the first multi-centre control trial of the International Society of Paediatric Oncology (SIOP I). *Eur J Cancer.* 1990;26(4):464–469.

32. Bouffet E, Bernard JL, Frappaz D, et al. M4 protocol for cerebellar medulloblastoma: supratento- rial radiotherapy may not be avoided. *Int J Radiat Oncol Biol Phys.* 1992;24(1):79–85.

33. Thomas PR, Deutsch M, Kepner JL, et al. Low-stage medulloblastoma: final analysis of trial com- paring standard-dose with reduced-dose neuraxis irradiation. *J Clin Oncol.* 2000;18(16):3004–3011.

34. Mulhern RK, Kepner JL, Thomas PR, et al. Neuropsychologic functioning of survivors of child- hood medulloblastoma randomized to receive conventional or reduced-dose craniospinal irra- diation: a Pediatric Oncology Group study. *J Clin Oncol.* 1998;16(5):1723–1728.

35. Packer RJ, Sutton LN, Elterman R, et al. Outcome for children with medulloblastoma treated with radiation and cisplatin, CCNU, and vincristine chemotherapy. *J Neurosurg.* 1994;81(5):690–698.

36. Taylor RE, Bailey CC, Robinson K, et al. Results of a randomized study of preradiation chemo- therapy versus radiotherapy alone for nonmetastatic medulloblastoma: the International Society of Paediatric Oncology/United Kingdom Children's Cancer Study Group PNET-3 Study. *J Clin Oncol.* 2003;21(8):1581–1591.

37. Bull KS, Spoudeas HA, Yadegarfar G, et al. Reduction of health status 7 years after addition of chemotherapy to craniospinal irradiation for medulloblastoma: a follow-up study in PNET 3 trial survivors on behalf of the CCLG (formerly UKCCSG). *J Clin Oncol.* 2007;25(27):4239–4245.

38. Packer RJ, Gajjar A, Vezina G, et al. Phase III study of craniospinal radiation therapy followed by adjuvant chemotherapy for newly diagnosed average-risk medulloblastoma. *J Clin Oncol.* 2006;24(25):4202–4208.

39. Carrie C, Grill J, Figarella-Branger D, et al. Online quality control, hyperfractionated radiother- apy alone and reduced boost volume for standard risk medulloblastoma: long-term results of MSFOP 98. *J Clin Oncol.* 2009;27(11):1879–1883.

40. Lannering B, Rutkowski S, Doz F, et al. Hyperfractionated versus conventional radiotherapy followed by chemotherapy in standard-risk medulloblastoma: results from the randomized multicenter HIT-SIOP PNET 4 trial. *J Clin Oncol.* 2012;30(26):3187–3193.

41. Hughes EN, Shillito J, Sallan SE, et al. Medulloblastoma at the joint center for radiation therapy between 1968 and 1984: the influence of radiation dose on the patterns of failure and survival. *Cancer.* 1988;61(10):1992–1998.

42. Wolden SL, Dunkel IJ, Souweidane MM, et al. Patterns of failure using a conformal radiation therapy tumor bed boost for medulloblastoma. *J Clin oncol.* 2003;21(16):3079–3083.

43. Merchant TE, Kun LE, Krasin MJ, et al. Multi-institution prospective trial of reduced-dose crani- ospinal irradiation (23.4 Gy) followed by conformal posterior fossa (36 Gy) and primary site irradiation (55.8 Gy) and dose-intensive chemotherapy for average-risk medulloblastoma. *Int J Radiat Oncol Biol Phys.* 2008;70(3):782–787.

44. Packer RJ, Sutton LN, Atkins TE, et al. A prospective study of cognitive function in chil- dren receiving whole-brain radiotherapy and chemotherapy: 2-year results. *J Neurosurg.* 1989;70(5):707–713.

45. Probert JC, Parker BR, Kaplan HS. Growth retardation in children after megavoltage irradiation of the spine. *Cancer.* 1973;32(3):634–639.

46. Goldwein JW, Radcliffe J, Johnson J, et al. Updated results of a pilot study of low-dose craniospinal irradiation plus chemotherapy for children under five with cerebellar primitive neuroectodermal tumors (medulloblastoma). *Int J Radiat Oncol Biol Phys*. 1996;34(4):899–904.

47. Tarbell NJ, Friedman H, Polkinghorn WR, et al. High-risk medulloblastoma: a pediatric oncology group randomized trial of chemotherapy before or after radiation therapy (POG 9031). *J Clin Oncol*. 2013;31(23):2936–2941.

48. del Charco JO, Bolek TW, McCollough WM, et al. Medulloblastoma: time-dose relationship based on a 30-year review. *Int J Radiat Oncol Biol Phys*. 1998;42(1):147–154.

49. Jakacki RI, Burger PC, Zhou T, et al. Outcome of children with metastatic medulloblastoma treated with carboplatin during craniospinal radiotherapy: a Children's Oncology Group Phase I/II study. *J Clin Oncology*. 2012;30(21):2648–2653.

50. Ris MD, Packer R, Goldwein J, et al. Intellectual outcome after reduced-dose radiation therapy plus adjuvant chemotherapy for medulloblastoma: a Children's Cancer Group study. *J Clin Oncol*. 2001;19(15):3470–3476.

51. Fouladi M, Gilger E, Kocak M, et al. Intellectual and functional outcome of children 3 years old or younger who have CNS malignancies. *J Clin Oncol*. 2005;23(28):7152–7160.

52. Dhall G, Grodman H, Ji L, et al. Outcome of children less than three years old at diagnosis with non-metastatic medulloblastoma treated with chemotherapy on the "Head Start" I and II protocols. *Pediatr Blood Cancer*. 2008;50(6):1169–1175.

53: EPENDYMOMA

Matthew C. Ward, John H. Suh, and Erin S. Murphy

QUICK HIT: Uncommon CNS tumor originating from glial stem cells most commonly in the fourth ventricle (children) or filum terminale (myxopapillary type, adults); 10-yr OS is approximately 79% in adults and approximately 66% in children.[1] The treatment paradigm is maximal safe resection with attempt at GTR; the degree of resection classically represents the most important prognostic factor. RT should be given postoperatively to the resection bed and any remaining disease to 59.4 Gy in 33 fractions. For those 18 months old or younger, consider 54 Gy or CHT to delay RT. There is no clearly established role for CHT but may be used in select cases to delay RT or attempt second-look surgery.

EPIDEMIOLOGY: Uncommon tumor originating from glial stem cells that can occur in all age groups but are more common in children.[1] Represent about 6% of CNS tumors in children (150 cases per year) and 2% of CNS tumors in adults.[1-3]

RISK FACTORS: No risk factors have been clearly identified. NF2 pts may be at an increased risk for spinal ependymomas.[4]

ANATOMY: Can originate from anywhere in the CNS but most commonly originates from the fourth ventricle (a "tongue of tumor" often tracks caudally along the cervical spinal cord) or from the distal spinal cord. CSF enters the fourth ventricle from the cerebral aqueduct and exits via the foramen of Luschka laterally and foramen of Magendie medially. The obex is the most caudal aspect of the fourth ventricle. The spinal cord ends at approximately L3 in children and L1-2 in adults. The thecal sac (filum terminale) ends at approximately S2 in both children and adults.[5-7]

PATHOLOGY: WHO separates grade based on morphology; however, genetics may be more prognostic given the heterogeneity within various WHO grades.[1] Perivascular pseudorosettes are the pathognomonic finding. Note that ependymoblastoma is grade IV, considered a PNET, and treated as such.

TABLE 53.1: 2016 WHO Update: Ependymoma Grades and Subtypes[8]		
Grade I	Myxopapillary ependymoma	Adults: conus/filum terminale
	Subependymoma	Adults: fourth ventricle most common
Grade II	Ependymoma (Variants: papillary, clear cell, tanycytic)	Variable clinical course
Grade III	Anaplastic ependymoma	Usually aggressive but again can be variable—studies ongoing to determine molecular subclassification
	Ependymoma, RELA fusion-positive	Distinct class recognized by the WHO 2016 update, represents majority of supratentorial tumors in children, poor prognosis[8,9]

GENETICS: RELA fusion: fusion between RELA (encodes a component of NF-κB, which is a complex regulating transcription, cytokine production, and cell survival) and a poorly understood gene C11orf95 (chromosome 11), which leads to an oncogene product that is independently prognostic. This led to the WHO recognizing this subtype as a separate classification.[8,9] Otherwise ependymomas have a diverse and heterogeneous landscape of various genetic alterations. Pajtler et al. classified 500 ependymal tumors using methylation profiling into nine categories based on YAP1 and RELA fusions, demonstrating improved stratification compared to histologic grading.[9]

CLINICAL PRESENTATION: Most common presenting symptoms are either chronic back pain or symptoms of increased intracranial pressure, depending on location.

WORKUP: History and physical, MRI of the brain and entire spine with and without contrast, consider ventriculostomy over shunt if symptomatic.

PROGNOSTIC FACTORS: Surgical resection is classically the most important prognostic factor.[10] Others may include: younger age, high grade, male gender, and intracranial location.[11] Grade II and III tumors have a heterogeneous behavior and the prognostic significance of grade for these tumors is evolving.

NATURAL HISTORY: Grade I tumors have excellent outcomes, and failure is uncommon. For grade II–III tumors, local failure is usually more common than distant failure (12% vs. 8% in original Merchant phase II study).[12] Failure usually occurs within 2 years.[3] Event-free survival and overall survival for children at 7 years were 77% and 85% in Merchant study, respectively.

TREATMENT PARADIGM

Surgery: Maximal safe resection with attempt at GTR is standard of care. Near-total resection defined as <5 mm max diameter of residual disease.[12]

Chemotherapy: There is no clear, standardized role for the routine use of CHT. Various multidrug regimens have been used to delay radiation for infants or to attempt a second-look surgery for those with a subtotal resection initially (see the following studies).

Radiation

Indications: RT is indicated for the postoperative treatment of ependymomas in essentially all cases. A spinal myxopapillary ependymoma after GTR is controversial with some recommending treatment to 54 Gy and others recommending observation.

Dose: For posterior fossa tumors treat to 59.4 Gy. For gross residual disease, there is no clear role for dose escalation (see the following studies).

Toxicity: Acute: alopecia, fatigue, headache, nausea, erythema. Late: Cognitive decline, hearing loss, endocrinopathies, microcephaly.

Procedure: See *Treatment Planning Handbook*, Chapter 12.[13]

EVIDENCE-BASED Q&A

Is there a role for craniospinal irradiation (CSI) for pts with limited disease at presentation?

Historically, pediatric trials as recent as the early 1990s routinely delivered craniospinal irradiation to doses of 23.4–36 Gy with a boost to 54–55 Gy.[14,15] However, local relapse was found to be the most common site of failure with distant CNS failure occurring in only 5% to 7% of

*pts. Subsequent protocols (see the following) demonstrated similar outcomes and patterns of fail-
ure treating only a CTV of GTV/postoperative bed + 1 cm. Therefore, limited-field irradiation is
now standard of care except in the uncommon situation of leptomeningeal spread at the time of
diagnosis.*

**Merchant, St. Jude (*IJROBP* 2002, PMID 11872277; Update Merchant *JCO* 2004, PMID
15284268, Update Merchant *Lancet Oncol* 2009, PMID 19274783):** Phase II trial of 153
children (2009 update) with ependymoma, 85 of whom were grade III evaluating the patterns of failure after conformal radiation. The initial report included low-grade astrocytoma as well. CTV = GTV+1 cm. GTV encompassed the postoperative bed and any
residual tumor. PTV = CTV+0.5 cm. Dose was 59.4 Gy except for those younger than 18
months with a gross total resection who received 54 Gy. Spinal cord limited to approximately 57.8 Gy (54 Gy limit for first 30 fractions, then 70% of prescription for final 3 fractions). 7-yr rates of local control, EFS, and OS were 87%, 69%, and 81%. 14 pts failed locally,
7 locally and distantly, and 15 failed distantly. Negative prognostic factors included anaplastic histology, non-White race, STR, and pre-RT CHT. **Conclusion: Limited-volume
irradiation allowed high rates of disease control and stable neurocognitive outcomes.**

How does the extent of resection affect outcome?

*The extent of resection is a strong prognostic factor in nearly every study performed. On the more
recent St. Jude studies, EFS/PFS ranged from 78% to 82% with GTR compared to 41% to 43%
with subtotal resection.[3,12] One earlier retrospective study from Pittsburgh demonstrated an even
more marked difference with 5-year PFS ranging from 68% with GTR to 9% without GTR.[16]*

Is there a role for adjuvant CHT?

No trial has clearly demonstrated a benefit to the routine use of CHT.

Evans, CCG 942 (*Med Pediatr Oncol* 1996, PMID 8614396): Early study (initiated 1975)
that included 36 children with either medulloblastoma or ependymoma treated with
postoperative CSI and randomized to no further treatment with lomustine, vincristine, and prednisone for 1 year. **Conclusion: No difference in EFS or OS between the
regimens.**

Robertson, CCG 921 (*J Neurosurg* 1998, PMID 9525716): PRT of 304 children, 32 of whom
had ependymoma. Children were treated with maximal safe resection followed by CSI
followed by randomization to either concurrent vincristine alone (no adjuvant CHT) or
"8-in-1" adjuvant CHT. **Conclusion: No clear benefit to intensive adjuvant CHT.**

Gururangan, PBTC (*Neuro-Oncology* 2012, PMID 23019233): Phase II study of 13 pts
with recurrent ependymoma treated with bevacizumab and irinotecan. No sustained
responses were observed.

Garvin, COG 9942 (*Pediatr Blood Cancer* 2012, PMID 22949057): Phase II study of 41
pts with residual tumor after surgery and treated with preradiation CHT consisting of
vincristine, etoposide, cisplatin, and cyclophosphamide. 40% experienced a complete
response, 17% partial response, 29% stable disease, and 14% progression. 5-yr EFS and
OS were 57% and 71%. **Conclusion: Pts with STR have inferior outcomes despite radiographic response and should be considered for second-look surgery.**

How should we manage children who are too young for radiotherapy?

*Pts less than 3 years of age have worse neurocognitive outcomes with radiotherapy (particularly
CSI) and may benefit from altered therapy. Pts on Dr. Merchant's study who were less than 18
months of age and had a GTR were treated with focal radiation to 54 Gy rather than 59.4 Gy.[12]
Other relevant studies are listed in the following although results without radiotherapy are mixed.*

Duffner, "Baby POG" (*NEJM*** 1993, PMID 8388548; Update Duffner ***Pediatr Neurosurg*** 1998 PMID 9732252):** Phase II trial for children <3 years of age with malignant brain tumors (medulloblastoma, ependymoma, PNET, brainstem glioma, other gliomas). All pts were treated with cyclophosphamide, vincristine, cisplatin, and etoposide. This was continued until progression or for 2 years for pts <24 months of age and for 1 year if 24 to 36 months of age, at which time RT was delivered. RT was localized for ependymomas to 54 Gy but for anaplastic ependymomas was CSI to 35.2 Gy with a localized boost to 54 Gy. 48 pts had ependymoma. 5-yr OS was 25% for those <23 months and 63% for those 24 to 36 months. **Conclusion: Delaying radiation may lead to inferior survival for ependymomas.**

Geyer, CCG 9921 (*JCO*** 2005, PMID 16234523):** Phase II of 284 pediatric pts <3 years of age with malignant tumors, 74 of whom were ependymomas. Pts were randomized to either vincristine, cisplatin, cyclophosphamide, and etoposide versus vincristine, carboplatin, ifosfamide, and etoposide. Pts without residual tumor after surgery and CHT were omitted RT. In those with residual, RT was delayed until 3 years of age or post eight cycles of CHT, whichever came first. No difference in response rates between arms overall. For ependymomas, the 5-yr EFS was 32%. **Conclusion: Overall across all tumor types, delaying or omitting RT for infants appeared comparable to historical outcomes.**

Timmerman, HIT-SKK 87 & 92 (*Radiother Oncol*** 2005, PMID 16300848):** 34 children with anaplastic ependymomas <3 years of age and tested the delay of RT until age 3. Elective RT was given at age 3 for 9 children and salvage RT was given for progression for 12. RT withheld in 13; of these only 3 survived. **Conclusion: Delaying RT even after CHT may jeopardize survival.**

Grundy, UKCCSG/SIOP (*Lancet Oncol*** 2007, PMID 17644039):** 89 children <3 years of age with intracranial ependymomas treated with CHT after surgery for 1 year. RT withheld except for progressive disease. At 5 years, 42% of those without metastatic disease did not require RT. 5-yr OS was 63% in the nonmetastatic children. 5-yr EFS was 42%. **Conclusion: CHT may delay or preclude the use of RT without compromising outcomes.**

Strother, POG 9233 (*Neuro Oncol*** 2014, PMID 24335695):** Follow-up to Duffner with a similar strategy except more intensive CHT and RT was withheld for persistence, progression, or recurrence. Enrolled 328 children <3 years of age, 82 with ependymoma. Approximately 40% of ependymoma pts were cured without RT, but this benefit appeared to be limited to only the ependymoma pts. **Conclusion: Intensive CHT may allow for the omission of CHT in select ependymoma pts <3 years of age.**

Can dose-escalated hyperfractionation improve outcomes?

Three prospective trials (POG 9132, AIEOP, and SPO) have been performed in children, none of which clearly demonstrated a benefit to dose-escalated hyperfractionated RT.[17-19] The regimens included: 69.6 Gy/58 fx at 1.2 Gy/fx (POG 9132), 70.4 Gy/64 fx at 1.1 Gy/fx BID (AIEOP), or 60–66 Gy/60–66 fx at 1 Gy/fx (SPO).

Can grade II pts who underwent GTR be spared radiation? Can CHT improve outcomes for those who cannot undergo GTR? Can immediate radiation after NTR or to grade III pts improve outcomes?

Merchant, COG ACNS0121 (*ASTRO*** 2015, Abstract 1):** Phase II trial of 375 children between 2003 and 2007. Enrolled into four strata based on degree of resection and histology. Stratum 1: grade II, supratentorial ependymoma with microscopic GTR; stratum 2: STR pts; stratum 3: macroscopic GTR or an NTR, defined as <5-mm thickness of gross disease remaining; and stratum 4: grade III supratentorial or grade II infratentorial after microscopic GTR. Stratum 1 pts were observed; stratum 2 received CHT (vincristine, carboplatin, cyclophosphamide, and etoposide) followed by optional second-look surgery and RT; strata 3 and 4 received immediate postoperative RT, which was 59.4 Gy except for those <18 months of age. Stratum 1: EFS at 5 years was 61% (5 of 11 progressed). Stratum 2: 25 of 64 pts went to second-look surgery and 14 of these achieved a GTR. The overall EFS was 39% at 5 years. However, those who went to second-look surgery did not demonstrate improved EFS compared to those who did not ($p = .079$). Stratum 3: EFS was 67%. Stratum 4: EFS was 69%. **Conclusion: Immediate postoperative RT appeared beneficial but improvement is necessary in all strata. Also, observation after GTR for grade II supratentorial ependymoma should not be standard of care.**

Massimino, AIEOP Italian Study (*Neuro Oncol* 2016, PMID 27194148): Prospective study stratifying by WHO grade and degree of resection. WHO grade II pts with a complete resection received 59.4 Gy. Grade III pts with a complete resection received 59.4 Gy followed by vincristine, etoposide, and cyclophosphamide. Pts with residual disease (either grade) received the same CHT for one to four cycles followed by second-look surgery, then 59.4 Gy with an 8 Gy boost if there was residual disease. 160 children with an MFU of 67 months were enrolled. PFS and OS were 58% and 69% in the 40 pts with incomplete resection. **Conclusion: These results were comparable to the best single-institution results and the boost appeared effective.**

Can RT be omitted for select myxopapillary ependymomas?

Although controversial, the adjuvant RT dose after GTR for myxopapillary ependymomas is to treat with at least 50.4 Gy, as omission of RT seems to confer increased local failure.

Pica, Switzerland (*IJROBP* 2009, PMID 19250760): RR of 85 pts with spinal myxopapillary ependymomas. 45% were treated with surgery alone, the median dose of RT for the others was 50.4 Gy. MFU 60 months. PFS was 74.8% versus 50.4% with versus without RT. Approximately 20% of failures were elsewhere in the CNS. On multivariate analysis, a dose of 50.4 Gy or higher was an independent predictor of improved PFS. **Conclusion: 50.4 Gy or higher is recommended to reduce progression.**

Kotecha, Cleveland Clinic (*ASTRO* 2016, Abstract 2274): RR of 59 pts with spinal myxopapillary ependymoma. Median age 34 years and MFU 74.4 mos. 83% underwent initial surgery and 17% received postoperative RT to a median of 49 Gy (range 45–58 Gy). 5-yr RFS was 75.4%. 5-yr RFS was improved in the GTR group compared to STR: median 205.9 versus 65.5 mos, $p < .0001$. RT did not improve RFS after GTR (median 134.3 vs. 205.9 mos, $p = .92$) or STR (median 35.1 vs. 110.2 mos, $p = .27$). **Conclusion: Initial GTR is recommended when possible; the role for adjuvant RT is undetermined.**

REFERENCES

1. Wu J, Armstrong TS, Gilbert MR. Biology and management of ependymomas. *Neuro Oncol.* 2016;18(7):902–913.
2. Imbach P, Kühne T, Arceci R. *Pediatric Oncology: A Comprehensive Guide.* 2nd ed. Heidelberg; NY: Springer Publishing; 2011.
3. Merchant TE, Mulhern RK, Krasin MJ, et al. Preliminary results from a phase II trial of conformal radiation therapy and evaluation of radiation-related CNS effects for pediatric patients with localized ependymoma. *J Clin Oncol.* 2004;22:3156–3162.
4. Rubio MP, Correa KM, Ramesh V, et al. Analysis of the neurofibromatosis 2 gene in human ependymomas and astrocytomas. *Cancer Res.* 1994;54:45–47.
5. Binokay F, Akgul E, Bicakci K, et al. Determining the level of the dural sac tip: magnetic resonance imaging in an adult population. *Acta Radiol.* 2006;47:397–400.

6. Scharf CB, Paulino AC, Goldberg KN. Determination of the inferior border of the thecal sac using magnetic resonance imaging: implications on radiation therapy treatment planning. *Int J Radiat Oncol Biol Phys.* 1998;41:621–624.

7. Dunbar SF, Barnes PD, Tarbell NJ. Radiologic determination of the caudal border of the spinal field in cranial spinal irradiation. *Int J Radiat Oncol Biol Phys.* 1993;26:669–673.

8. Louis DN, Perry A, Reifenberger G, et al. The 2016 World Health Organization Classification of Tumors of the Central Nervous System: a summary. *Acta Neuropathol.* 2016;131:803–820.

9. Pajtler KW, Witt H, Sill M, et al. Molecular classification of ependymal tumors across all CNS compartments, histopathological grades, and age groups. *Cancer Cell.* 2015;27:728–743.

10. Freeman CRF, Jean-Pierre T, Roger E. Central nervous system tumors in children. In: Halperin E, Wazer D, Perez C, Brady L, eds. *Principles & Practice of Radiation Oncology.* 6th ed. Philadelphi, PA: Lippincott & Williams; 2013:1632–1654.

11. Rodríguez D, Cheung MC, Housri N, et al. Outcomes of malignant CNS ependymomas: an examination of 2408 cases through the Surveillance, Epidemiology, and End Results (SEER) database (1973–2005). *J Surg Res.* 2009;156:340–351.

12. Merchant TE, Li C, Xiong X, et al. Conformal radiotherapy after surgery for paediatric ependymoma: a prospective study. *Lancet Oncol.* 2009;10:258–266.

13. Videtic GMM, Woody N, Vassil AD. *Handbook of Treatment Planning in Radiation Oncology.* 2nd ed. New York, NY: Demos Medical; 2015.

14. Robertson PL, Zeltzer PM, Boyett JM, et al. Survival and prognostic factors following radiation therapy and chemotherapy for ependymomas in children: a report of the Children's Cancer Group. *J Neurosurg.* 1998;88:695–703.

15. Evans AE, Anderson JR, Lefkowitz-Boudreaux IB, Finlay JL. Adjuvant chemotherapy of childhood posterior fossa ependymoma: cranio-spinal irradiation with or without adjuvant CCNU, vincristine, and prednisone: a Childrens Cancer Group study. *Med Pediatr Oncol.* 1996;27:8–14.

16. Pollack IF, Gerszten PC, Martinez AJ, et al. Intracranial ependymomas of childhood: long-term outcome and prognostic factors. *Neurosurgery.* 1995;37:655–666; discussion 666–667.

17. Kovnar E, Curran W, Tomato T, et al. Hyperfractionated irradiation for childhood ependymoma: improved local control in subtotally resected tumors. *Childs Nerv Syst.* 1998;14:489–490.

18. Massimino M, Gandola L, Giangaspero F, et al. Hyperfractionated radiotherapy and chemotherapy for childhood ependymoma: final results of the first prospective Associazione Italiana di Ematologia-Oncologia Pediatrica (AIEOP) study. *Int J Radiat Oncol Biol Phys.* 2004;58:1336–1345.

19. Conter C, Carrie C, Bernier V, et al. Intracranial ependymomas in children: society of pediatric oncology experience with postoperative hyperfractionated local radiotherapy. *Int J Radiat Oncol Biol Phys.* 2009;74:1536–1542.

54: BRAINSTEM GLIOMA

Jason W. D. Hearn and John H. Suh

> **QUICK HIT:** Brainstem gliomas (BSGs) are uncommon tumors arising predominantly in children. Prognosis varies between diffuse intrinsic tumors and more favorable types (focal, dorsally exophytic, or cervicomedullary). Diffuse intrinsic pontine glioma (DIPG) is most common and carries a poor prognosis, with MS of less than 1 year. Standard treatment of these tumors is radiotherapy (RT) alone, 54 Gy/30 fx. Surgery is not feasible, and hyperfractionation, dose escalation, and CHT have generally not proven beneficial. In contrast, for focal, dorsally exophytic, and cervicomedullary tumors, surgery is often utilized, with consideration of RT for unresectable or rapidly recurrent disease. Prognosis for these tumors is substantially better than for DIPG, with 5-yr OS exceeding 90% for subsets, particularly for focal tectal tumors, which are typically managed with CSF diversion followed by observation.[1]

EPIDEMIOLOGY: BSGs account for 10% to 15% of pediatric CNS tumors, with an annual incidence of 300 to 400 in the United States, but constitute <2% of adult CNS tumors.[2,3] DIPG comprises 75% to 80% of pediatric BSGs, and is most commonly diagnosed between 5 and 10 years of age.[4]

RISK FACTORS: NF1 confers increased risk of BSGs (second most common after optic-pathway glioma). Despite the increased incidence of BSGs in NF1 pts, these tumors tend to be relatively favorable compared to those in pts without NF1.[5]

ANATOMY: The brainstem comprises the midbrain, pons, and medulla oblongata. CN III–IV originate from the midbrain, CN V–VIII from the pons, and CN IX-XII from the medulla. The tectum (Latin for "roof"; also referred to as the "quadrigeminal plate") represents the dorsal midbrain, and includes the paired superior and inferior colliculi. The tegmentum forms the floor of the midbrain (region ventral to the ventricular system) and continues inferiorly through the pons and into the medulla. The tegmentum includes the nuclei of CN III and IV, the red nucleus, and the substantia nigra.

PATHOLOGY: Approximately 50% of BSGs are low grade (WHO I–II) and 50% are high grade (WHO III–IV); nearly all are astrocytic. BSGs may be intrinsic or exophytic, and if intrinsic they may be diffuse or focal. Focal tumors are generally defined as well-circumscribed lesions <2 cm without edema or infiltration.[1] Overall, BSGs are grouped into four categories based on imaging characteristics: diffusely infiltrating (typically pontine, aka DIPG), focal, dorsally exophytic, or cervicomedullary.[6] For pediatric DIPG there is generally no difference in outcome between tumors that are low grade versus high grade at biopsy, perhaps due to a high tendency for malignant transformation as well as heterogeneity in grade within the tumor.[7] Focal tumors occur more frequently in the midbrain or medulla, and are typically low grade.[8] Dorsally exophytic gliomas are generally low grade, and arise from subependymal glial tissue in the floor of the fourth ventricle, growing along the path of least resistance rather than infiltrating tissue. Cervicomedullary tumors also tend to be low grade, and in some cases may be infiltrative. These tumors can expand the medulla and upper cervical spinal cord, and may extend rostrally beyond the foramen magnum, since axial growth is limited ventrally by the pyramidal decussation.

GENETICS: Although the etiology is unknown, genomic studies have identified a number of alterations in *PDGFRA, MDM4, MYCN, EGFR, MET, KRAS, CDK4, H3F3A,* and others.[9–17] Additional work has implicated the Sonic Hedgehog pathway.[18]

CLINICAL PRESENTATION: CN palsies (e.g., diplopia, facial weakness, and difficulty with speech or swallowing), ataxia, long tract signs (motor weakness), or symptoms of elevated intracranial pressure (ICP) such as headache, nausea, and vomiting. Pontine CNs are most commonly affected, followed by medullary CNs, and then midbrain CNs. DIPG typically has a rapid onset of symptoms (median 1 month before diagnosis), generally including bilateral cranial neuropathies, ataxia, and long tract signs. Focal tumors are usually more indolent, and typically present with limited cranial neuropathies. Dorsally exophytic lesions present insidiously with failure to thrive and symptoms of elevated ICP; long tract signs are uncommon. Depending on the epicenter of the tumor, cervicomedullary lesions may present with predominantly medullary dysfunction (failure to thrive due to nausea, vomiting, dysphagia, chronic aspiration, sleep apnea, and head tilt) or cervical spinal cord dysfunction (facial or neck pain, progressive weakness, spasticity, hand preference, motor regression, and sensory deficits).[8] Tectal tumors often present with elevated ICP secondary to hydrocephalus from stenosis of the cerebral aqueduct.

WORKUP: H&P with careful neurological exam. MRI with gadolinium. DIPG is often hypointense on T1 with little enhancement (though variable) but hyperintense on T2. Diffusion tensor imaging can also be useful to evaluate the relationship of the tumor to white matter tracts, which can influence surgical candidacy and planning.[8] Up to 10% to 15% of BSGs have leptomeningeal involvement. Dorsally exophytic lesions often fill the fourth ventricle, causing obstruction and hydrocephalus. Such lesions are typically juvenile pilocytic astrocytomas (JPAs), which intensely enhance with gadolinium despite being low grade. Cervicomedullary tumors cause expansion of the medulla toward the fourth ventricle and/or expansion of the cervical cord. Biopsy is generally not indicated for lesions consistent with DIPG, since grade does not affect management. Since stereotactic biopsy techniques have reduced risks, biopsies may be done for research purposes and can be informative for cases with atypical radiologic or clinical features.[10,19,20] Notably, a biopsy may be more useful in adults, in whom histology appears to have more prognostic importance (see the following). Differential diagnosis includes primitive neuroectodermal tumor (PNET), atypical teratoid/rhabdoid tumor (ATRT), vascular malformation, demyelinating disorders (e.g., multiple sclerosis), ganglioglioma, hamartoma (especially in pts with neurofibromatosis), metastasis, abscess, encephalitis, and parasitic cysts, among others.

PROGNOSTIC FACTORS: Tumor location and type are the most important prognostic factors with DIPG demonstrating worse outcomes than more favorable types (focal, dorsally exophytic, or cervicomedullary).

TREATMENT PARADIGM

DIPG: There is no therapeutic role for surgery and generally no benefit to systemic therapy. Studies investigating cytotoxic CHT, concurrent etanidazole (hypoxic cell radiosensitizer), high-dose tamoxifen, high-dose CHT with bone marrow transplant, blood–brain barrier disruption, p-glycoprotein inhibition (for multidrug resistance), and other strategies have generally not demonstrated significant benefit.[4] RT alone remains the standard treatment for DIPG, as it is the only modality proven to extend survival. Dose is 54 Gy/30 fx daily over 6 weeks. Other RT approaches, such as hyperfractionation, I-125 interstitial implants, and SRS have been attempted with no clear benefit over standard RT. Most pts improve clinically after RT, though typical time to progression is 5 to 6 mos, and MS in most studies is <9–12 mos.

Focal: Surgical resection is indicated when feasible (e.g., for tumors that extend toward the surface of the brainstem laterally or at the floor of the fourth ventricle). Preservation of neurological function is important for these often indolent tumors, and may require judicious use of subtotal resection. RT is useful for progression after surgery and for unresectable lesions.[1] As in the case of DIPG, RT dose is typically 54 Gy/30 fx, although smaller CTV margins are often appropriate.

Dorsally exophytic or cervicomedullary: Maximal safe resection is indicated when possible.[8,21,22] RT is a useful alternative for unresectable tumors and can be considered postoperatively for high-grade tumors or those with early progression after surgery. Those who have late progression may benefit from reoperation when feasible. CHT is occasionally a useful adjunct, and in some cases can yield tumor shrinkage followed by a more complete resection.[22] CHT may produce disease stabilization or objective responses, although eventual progression is inevitable, with 5-year PFS in the range of 30% to 40%.[23] CHT is particularly helpful in very young children in order to delay RT, and thereby enable more physical and neurocognitive development.[8]

Tectal: Focal tectal tumors of the midbrain tend to be very indolent and may require only CSF diversion, such as with a third ventriculostomy or shunt.[24] The majority of pts with these tumors remain free from progression for extended periods without surgical resection (which is associated with substantial risk in this location) or RT.[25] Thus, intervention is reserved for pts with evidence of progression.

Treatment-related complications: Complications of surgery may include impaired respiratory function (especially if medullary involvement), diplopia, facial palsy, dysphagia, vocal cord paralysis, loss of gag/cough reflexes, additional cranial neuropathies, long tract deficits, and death, among others. Complications of RT may include dermatitis (especially at the external auditory canal and retroauricular region), hearing loss, growth impairment, endocrine dysfunction, cognitive dysfunction, radiation necrosis, and radiation-induced tumors, among others.

EVIDENCE-BASED Q&A

Does RT dose escalation and/or altered fractionation improve outcomes?

No benefit to dose escalation or altered fractionation was observed across multiple studies.

Freeman, POG 8495 (*IJROBP* 1993, PMID 8407392): Phase I/II RT dose escalation study of 136 pediatric pts using hyperfractionated RT delivered BID. The initial dose was 66 Gy/60 fx at 1.1 Gy/fx BID, subsequently escalated to 70.2 Gy/60 fx at 1.17 Gy/fx BID, and further escalated to 75.6 Gy/60 fx at 1.26 Gy/fx BID. No significant differences in PFS or OS across dose levels. Median time to progression (TTP) was 7 mos, MS was 10 mos, and 1-yr OS was 40% for the highest dose level (75.6 Gy). Protracted steroid use and intralesional necrosis were most frequent with 75.6 Gy. Extension into the cerebellar peduncle on MRI was a negative prognostic factor. **Conclusion: Dose escalation of hyperfractionated RT did not improve outcomes across dose levels within this study or relative to historic outcomes obtainable with daily fractionation. At the highest dose level in the study there was more toxicity.**

Packer, CCG 9882 (*Cancer* 1993, PMID 8339232): Phase I/II study of 53 pediatric pts with hyperfractionated RT to a dose of 72 Gy in 1 Gy/fx BID. 1-yr OS was 38%. **Conclusion: No benefit with hyperfractionation.**

Lewis, UKCCSG (*IJROBP* 1997, PMID 9276356): Pilot study of 28 pediatric pts with diffuse BSG treated with hyperfractionated RT with a dose of 48.6–50.4 Gy/27–28 fx at 1.8 Gy/fx BID with interfraction interval of at least 8 hours. MS 8.5 mos. Acute RT toxicity minimal, with only 11% having mild toxicity. **Conclusion: No improvement with hyperfractionation.**

Mandell, POG 9239 (*IJROBP* 1999, PMID 10192340): PRT of 130 pts 3 to 21 years of age with DIPG and symptoms <6 mos. Pts were randomized to conventional daily RT (54 Gy/30 fx QD) versus hyperfractionated RT (70.2 Gy/60 fx BID at 1.17 Gy/fx), using 2-cm margins (this was the second of the three hyperfractionated dose levels of POG 8495). Cisplatin was added to both arms as a radiation sensitizer during weeks 1, 3, and 5. No significant difference in survival or TTP between fractionation schemes. Neurologic improvement occurred in 95% with RT. Morbidity was similar between the two arms. No grade 4-5 toxicity. **Conclusion: Conventional RT preferred over dose-escalated hyperfractionated RT.**

TABLE 54.1: POG 9239					
	MS	1-yr OS	2-yr OS	3-yr OS	TTP
54 Gy/30 fx QD	8.5 mos	31%	7%	4%	6 mos
70.2 Gy/60 fx BID	8 mos	27%	7%	5%	5 mos

Janssens, Netherlands (*IJROBP* 2009, PMID 18990510): Dutch study of hypofractionation in nine pediatric pts with diffuse intrinsic BSGs. RT was given over 2.6 weeks using 39 Gy/13 fx (n = 8) or 33 Gy/6 fx (n = 1). Symptoms improved within 2 weeks of starting RT in all pts. No grade 3-4 toxicity. Median TTP 4.9 mos; MS 8.6 mos. **Conclusion: An abbreviated regimen is feasible and may yield outcomes similar to those of more protracted regimens.** *Comment: Small sample size limits generalizability.*

Zaghloul, Egypt (*Radiother Oncol*, PMID 24560760): PRT of hypofractionated RT in 71 pediatric pts with DIPG. RT was 39 Gy/13 fx over 2.6 weeks versus conventional RT of 54 Gy/30 fx over 6 weeks. Median PFS was 6.6 mos versus 7.3 mos, respectively (*p* = .71). MS was 7.8 mos versus 9.5 mos (*p* = .59). These differences exceeded the prespecified noninferiority margin. **Conclusion: Noninferiority of the hypofractionated RT schedule could not be shown.**

Is there a benefit from brachytherapy?

Dose escalation with brachytherapy does not appear to improve outcomes.

Chuba, Wayne State (*Childs Nerv Syst* 1998, PMID 9840381): RR of 28 pediatric pts with CNS tumors who had I-125 brachytherapy, nine of whom had BSGs (eight with DIPG, one with a midbrain tumor). DIPG pts received EBRT (50 Gy) followed by a fractionated stereotactic boost of 3 Gy x 4 fx. After 4 to 6 weeks, pts were re-evaluated for stereotactic interstitial I-125 therapy. The planned implant dose was 82.9 Gy to the enhancing tumor (0.04 Gy per hour). Preliminary results showed no surgical complications associated with catheter placement. MS for the eight pts with DIPG was 8.4 mos. The two pts who were alive at analysis had biopsy-proven persistent high-grade tumor. **Conclusion: Tumor control remained poor despite the combination of EBRT with a brachytherapy boost.**

Does stereotactic radiosurgery (SRS) improve outcomes?

Data are very limited and do not imply any improvement relative to conventionally fractionated RT.

Fuchs, Austria (*Acta Neurochir Suppl*, PMID 12379009): RR of 21 pts (8–56 years of age) treated with GKRS for BSG. Twelve lesions were located primarily in the pons, two in the medulla, and seven in the midbrain. Median SRS dose was 12 Gy (9–20 Gy) to the tumor margin by the median isodose of 45%. Prior to SRS, four pts had received conventional RT, one had RT and CHT, one pt underwent CHT, and one pt was shunted due to hydrocephalus. Of the 19 pts with follow-up imaging, tumor progression was seen in two pts, stable disease in ten pts, and regression in three cases. MFU was 29 mos. The neurological state improved in five pts. Microsurgical cyst fenestration was performed in one pt after SRS and shunting was necessary for two pts. Nine pts died unrelated to SRS at a median of 20.7 mos. **Conclusion: SRS may be feasible in selected pts, but the very limited sample size and substantial heterogeneity in pts, tumors, and treatments limit interpretation.**

Is there a role for re-irradiation?

Limited data show feasibility and suggest symptomatic benefit in selected pts.

Fontanilla, MDACC (*Am J Clin Oncol* 2012, PMID 21297433): RR of six pts who received re-irradiation for progressive DIPG. TTP after the first course of RT was 4 to 18 mos, and all pts had further progression on salvage CHT. The interval between courses of RT was 8 to 28 mos. Initial RT dose was 54 to 55.8 Gy. Re-irradiation was given with concurrent CHT. RT was given in 2 Gy fractions to 20 Gy (n = 4), 18 Gy (n = 1), and 2 Gy (one pt withdrew care after a single fraction). Four pts had substantial clinical improvement in symptoms (three in speech, three in ataxia, and two in swallowing). Three pts showed renewed ability to ambulate after re-irradiation. Four pts had decreased tumor size on post-treatment MRI. The median clinical PFS was 5 mos. Acute radiation-related toxicities were fatigue (n = 2), alopecia (n = 2), and decreased appetite (n = 1). No grade ≥3 toxicities were reported. **Conclusion: Re-irradiation with CHT is feasible and may improve symptoms with minimal toxicity. Those with prolonged response to initial therapy may be most suitable.**

Is there a benefit from systemic therapy in diffuse intrinsic tumors?

The preponderance of evidence suggests that there is no benefit to systemic therapy. The most notable exception comes from the final results of the French BSG 98 study, which suggested possible improvement in survival relative to historical controls. However, this regimen required protracted CHT, was quite toxic, and involved prolonged hospitalizations.

Jenkin, CCSG (*J Neurosurg* 1987, PMID 3806204): PRT in 74 pediatric pts assessing adjuvant CHT after 50 to 60 Gy of RT given at 8 to 9 Gy over 5 fx per week. No difference between RT alone and RT with adjuvant CCNU, vincristine, and prednisone. MS was approximately 9 mos in both arms. **Conclusion: No benefit with CHT.**

Freeman, Combined POG 9239/8495 (*IJROBP* 2000, PMID 10837936): Cross-trial comparison of POG 9239 (specifically, the 64 pts treated with hyperfractionated RT to 70.2 Gy w/ cisplatin) with POG 8495 (the 57 pts treated with hyperfractionated RT to 70.2 Gy [no CHT was given on that trial]). Baseline characteristics were similar. 1-yr OS was 28% on POG 9239 versus 40% on POG 8495 (*p* = .723). **Conclusion: Concurrent cisplatin does not improve OS when added to hyperfractionated RT, and may be detrimental.**

Marcus, Harvard (*IJROBP* 2003, PMID 12654425): Harvard phase I trial of hyperfractionated RT with the radiosensitizer etanidazole in pediatric pts with DIPG. RT dose 66 Gy/44 fx (1.5 Gy BID) for the first three pts and 63 Gy/42 fx for the subsequent 15 pts. Etanidazole was administered as a rapid infusion 30 min before the morning fraction of RT. Eight dose levels planned; at level 7 (total of 46.2 g/m²), both pts receiving this dose developed a grade 3 diffuse cutaneous rash. Regardless, MS was 8.5 mos. **Conclusion: No benefit to etanidazole, despite toxicity.**

Bronischer, St. Jude SJHG-98 (*Cancer* 2005, PMID 15565574): 33-pt multi-institutional study examining sequential RT (median 55.8 Gy) and adjuvant temozolomide (TMZ; 200 mg/m² d1-5 x6 cycles) in pediatric pts with diffuse BSG. There was an option to give neoadjuvant therapy using two cycles of irinotecan prior to RT. MS was 12 mos. **Conclusion: No benefit to adjuvant TMZ +/– neoadjuvant irinotecan.**

Frappaz, French BSG 98 (*Neuro Oncol* 2008, PMID 18577561): French prospective single-arm trial (n = 23) of front-line CHT to delay RT in pediatric pts with diffuse intrinsic BSGs. Each cycle of CHT involved three courses delivered at 30-day intervals, with course 1 being tamoxifen, BCNU, and cisplatin. Courses 2 and 3 were high dose MTX. 3-month cycles were repeated until clinical deterioration, at which point RT was pursued using 54 Gy/27 fx. Tamoxifen was also given during RT, and hydroxyurea was given during and after RT until progression. Tamoxifen was dropped from the protocol after other work showed lack of benefit in BSGs. Results: MS 17 versus 9 mos in historical controls (p = .022). Hospitalization was prolonged (57 vs. 25 days, p = .001). Four pts experienced severe iatrogenic infections and 11 required platelet transfusions. **Conclusion: Survival may be higher with this regimen, but small sample size limits interpretation. Additionally, the significant toxicity and requirement for longer hospitalization need to be seriously considered.**

Sirachainan, Thailand (*Neuro Oncol* 2008, PMID 18559468): Thai study of 12 pediatric pts with DIPG treated with concurrent TMZ (75 mg/m^2) followed by adjuvant TMZ (200 mg/m^2 d1-5) plus cis-retinoic acid (100 mg/m^2 d1-21). RT dose: 55.8 to 59.4 Gy. MS 13.5 mos. **Conclusion: Authors recommended TMZ-based CRT be further studied, although small sample size limits interpretation.**

Jalali, Tata Memorial (*IJROBP* 2010, PMID 19647954): Indian phase II trial of 20 pediatric pts with DIPG. Focal RT to 54 Gy/30 fx with concurrent and adjuvant TMZ (75 mg/m^2 daily concurrently; 200 mg/m^2 days 1 to 5 adjuvantly for up to 12 cycles). Median PFS 6.9 mos, MS 9.2 mos. **Conclusion: No benefit to addition of TMZ.**

Sharp, Canada (*Eur J Cancer* 2010, PMID 20656474): Phase II trial of 15 pediatric pts with newly diagnosed diffuse intrinsic BSG treated with standard RT and concurrent metronomic TMZ at 85 mg/m^2/day for 6 weeks, followed by metronomic TMZ monotherapy at the same dose. Treatment continued until progression or unacceptable toxicity. Median TTP 5.1 mos, MS 9.8 mos. **Conclusion: No benefit to the addition of metronomic TMZ.**

Does histology have prognostic significance in adult diffuse intrinsic BSGs?

Adult BSGs appear to behave somewhat differently from those in children, particularly diffuse intrinsic low-grade gliomas, which carry a substantially better prognosis than those in children.

Guillamo, France (*Brain* 2001, PMID 11701605): French RR of 48 adult pts with BSG. Mean age 34 years (range 16–70). MRI demonstrated nonenhancing, diffusely infiltrative tumors (50%), contrast-enhancing localized masses (31%), isolated tectal tumors (8%), and other patterns (11%). Treatment included subtotal resection (8%), RT (94%), and CHT (56%). MS 5.4 years. Significant prognostic factors on MVA included histologic grade, duration of symptoms, and the appearance of "necrosis" on MRI. 85% could be classified into one of the following three groups on the basis of clinical, histological, and radiological characteristics:

- Diffuse intrinsic low-grade gliomas (46%): in young adults with a long clinical history before diagnosis and a diffusely enlarged nonenhancing brainstem on MRI. Improved with RT in 62% and had a long survival (MS 7.3 years).
- Focal tectal gliomas (8%): in young adults, often presenting with isolated hydrocephalus. Indolent course with estimated MS >10 years (similar to children for this type of tumor).
- Malignant gliomas (31%): in elderly pts with short clinical history, as well as contrast enhancement and "necrosis" on MRI. Poor prognosis despite treatment: MS 11.2 mos.

REFERENCES

1. Klimo P, Jr., Pai Panandiker AS, Thompson CJ, et al. Management and outcome of focal low-grade brainstem tumors in pediatric patients: the St. Jude experience. *J Neurosurg Pediat*. 2013;11(3):274–281.
2. Physician Data Query (PDQ) of the National Cancer Institute; 2017. https://www.cancer.gov/types/brain/hp/child-glioma-treatment-pdq
3. Hu J, Western S, Kesari S. Brainstem glioma in adults. *Front Oncol*. 2016;6:180.
4. Warren KE. Diffuse intrinsic pontine glioma: poised for progress. *Frontiers Oncol*. 2012;2:205.
5. Mahdi J, Shah AC, Sato A, et al. A multi-institutional study of brainstem gliomas in children with neurofibromatosis type 1. *Neurology*. 2017;88(16):1584–1589.
6. Epstein FJ, Farmer JP. Brain-stem glioma growth patterns. *J Neurosurg*. 1993;78(3):408–412.
7. Hoffman LM, DeWire M, Ryall S, et al. Spatial genomic heterogeneity in diffuse intrinsic pontine and midline high-grade glioma: implications for diagnostic biopsy and targeted therapeutics. *Acta Neuropathol Commun*. 2016;4:1.
8. McAbee JH, Modica J, Thompson CJ, et al. Cervicomedullary tumors in children. *J Neurosurg Pediat*. 2015;16(4):357–366.
9. Barrow J, Adamowicz-Brice M, Cartmill M, et al. Homozygous loss of ADAM3A revealed by genome-wide analysis of pediatric high-grade glioma and diffuse intrinsic pontine gliomas. *Neuro Oncol*. 2011;13(2):212–222.
10. Grill J, Puget S, Andreiuolo F, et al. Critical oncogenic mutations in newly diagnosed pediatric diffuse intrinsic pontine glioma. *Pediat Blood Cancer*. 2012;58(4):489–491.
11. Khuong-Quang DA, Buczkowicz P, Rakopoulos P, et al. K27M mutation in histone H3.3 defines clinically and biologically distinct subgroups of pediatric diffuse intrinsic pontine gliomas. *Acta Neuropathol*. 2012;124(3):439–447.
12. Li G, Mitra SS, Monje M, et al. Expression of epidermal growth factor variant III (EGFRvIII) in pediatric diffuse intrinsic pontine gliomas. *J Neuro Oncol*. 2012;108(3):395–402.
13. Paugh BS, Broniscer A, Qu C, et al. Genome-wide analyses identify recurrent amplifications of receptor tyrosine kinases and cell-cycle regulatory genes in diffuse intrinsic pontine glioma. *J Clin Oncol*. 2011;29(30):3999–4006.
14. Paugh BS, Qu C, Jones C, et al. Integrated molecular genetic profiling of pediatric high-grade gliomas reveals key differences with the adult disease. *J Clin Oncol*. 2010;28(18):3061–3068.
15. Warren KE, Killian K, Suuriniemi M, et al. Genomic aberrations in pediatric diffuse intrinsic pontine gliomas. *Neuro Oncol*. 2012;14(3):326–332.
16. Wu G, Broniscer A, McEachron TA, et al. Somatic histone H3 alterations in pediatric diffuse intrinsic pontine gliomas and non-brainstem glioblastomas. *Nature Genet*. 2012;44(3):251–253.
17. Zarghooni M, Bartels U, Lee E, et al. Whole-genome profiling of pediatric diffuse intrinsic pontine gliomas highlights platelet-derived growth factor receptor alpha and poly (ADP-ribose) polymerase as potential therapeutic targets. *J Clin Oncol*. 2010;28(8):1337–1344.
18. Puget S, Philippe C, Bax DA, et al. Mesenchymal transition and PDGFRA amplification/mutation are key distinct oncogenic events in pediatric diffuse intrinsic pontine gliomas. *PloS one*. 2012;7(2):e30313.
19. Cage TA, Samagh SP, Mueller S, et al. Feasibility, safety, and indications for surgical biopsy of intrinsic brainstem tumors in children. *Childs Nerv Syst*. 2013;29(8):1313–1319.
20. Puget S, Beccaria K, Blauwblomme T, et al. Biopsy in a series of 130 pediatric diffuse intrinsic Pontine gliomas. *Childs Nerv Syst*. 2015;31(10):1773–1780.
21. Robertson PL, Allen JC, Abbott IR, et al. Cervicomedullary tumors in children: a distinct subset of brainstem gliomas. *Neurology*. 1994;44(10):1798–1803.
22. Di Maio S, Gul SM, Cochrane DD, et al. Clinical, radiologic and pathologic features and outcome following surgery for cervicomedullary gliomas in children. *Childs Nerv Syst*. 2009;25(11):1401–1410.
23. Raabe E, Kieran MW, Cohen KJ. New strategies in pediatric gliomas: molecular advances in pediatric low-grade gliomas as a model. *Childs Nerv Syst*. 2013;19(17):4553–4558.
24. Daglioglu E, Cataltepe O, Akalan N. Tectal gliomas in children: the implications for natural history and management strategy. *Pediat Neurosurg*. 2003;38(5):223–231.
25. Griessenauer CJ, Rizk E, Miller JH, et al. Pediatric tectal plate gliomas: clinical and radiological progression, MR imaging characteristics, and management of hydrocephalus. *J Neurosurg Pediat*. 2014;13(1):13–20.

55: CRANIOPHARYNGIOMA

Martin C. Tom, Timothy D. Smile, and Erin S. Murphy

QUICK HIT: Craniopharyngioma (CP) is a rare benign neoplasm arising from the hypophyseal duct (Rathke's pouch) most commonly in the suprasellar region in children and older adults. Presentation includes headache, visual disturbances, nausea/vomiting, and/or endocrine abnormalities, with imaging revealing a suprasellar solid and/or cystic (filled with classic "crankcase oil") enhancing mass with calcifications. Treatment typically consists of either gross total resection alone (can be morbid) or subtotal resection followed by adjuvant RT, which appear to have comparable long-term outcomes (PFS >65%, OS >90%). RT strategies include conventional EBRT to 54 Gy or proton beam RT with recommended on-treatment imaging to account for cyst volume fluctuation, or SRS. Intracystic RT (rhenium-186, yttrium-90, or phosphorous-32) and intracystic CHT (bleomycin or IFNα) have been used historically but are not common in the modern era.

EPIDEMIOLOGY: The incidence of CP is about 570 per year and is similar between genders. They represent 1.2% of all nonmalignant brain tumors and 4% of all brain tumors in children.[1] There is a bimodal age distribution between 5 to 14 and 50 to 75 years of age.[2]

RISK FACTORS: No proven risk factors.

ANATOMY: CPs arise from the hypophyseal duct (Rathke's pouch), or its remnant in adults. They are typically suprasellar and can involve the optic chiasm, basal vasculature, hypothalamus, third ventricle, or pituitary stalk. They can appear grossly well-encapsulated, but formation of multiple cysts is characteristic.[3]

PATHOLOGY: CPs are histologically benign epithelial tumors arising from remnants of Rathke's pouch. The two major subtypes are adamantinomatous (85%–90%) and papillary (i.e., squamous papillary, 11%–14%). The adamantinomatous subtype is associated with children and appears solid and/or cystic with calcifications and dark brown/black fluid ("crankcase oil" appearance). They tend to be more adherent to surrounding structures, and on histology demonstrate wet keratin nodules, Rosenthal fibers, and a palisading basal layer of cells with intense gliosis.[4] The papillary subtype appears more similar to Rathke's cleft cysts with squamous differentiation and pseudopapillae, and is more likely to have calcification on imaging.[3,5]

GENETICS: The adamantinomatous subtype is related to WNT pathway activation and CTNNB1 gene mutation, which codes for β catenin.[6,7] The papillary subtype may harbor the BRAF (V600E) mutation.[8]

CLINICAL PRESENTATION: Typically includes headaches, visual deficits, nausea/vomiting, or hormonal abnormalities such as GH insufficiency or hypothyroidism (growth failure), ADH insufficiency (central diabetes insipidus), impotence, amenorrhea, or galactorrhea. Can also include depression, lethargy/somnolence, coma, seizures, hyperphagia, diencephalic syndrome, and changes in cognitive function or personality.[9,10]

WORKUP: H&P with attention to endocrine symptoms and a detailed neurologic exam.

Labs: Endocrine workup is indicated pretreatment to establish baseline function. Also consider detailed visual field testing, electrolytes, and urinalysis. Consider memory, personality, psychological, and cognitive function testing.

Imaging: MRI and/or CT revealing cystic (94%), calcified (92%, more common in papillary), enhancing, parasellar lesion, with hydrocephalus (67%).[9] Diagnosis can be made based on radiographic appearance, cyst fluid analysis ("crankcase oil"), or otherwise histopathologically.

PROGNOSTIC FACTORS: Negative prognostic factors include >53 years of age in adults, >2 prior surgeries, tumor size >5 cm, STR alone (vs. with RT), hydrocephalus, and RT dose <54–55 Gy.[9,11–14]

TREATMENT PARADIGM

Surgery: Surgical resection is indicated for almost all pts for safe debulking. While some favor initial aggressive total resection, GTR can be morbid due to proximity to the hypothalamus and other surrounding structures. Therefore, others advocate for limited resection followed by RT (adjuvant or salvage). STR alone has poor LC rates. Intrasellar tumors can be removed transsphenoidally, while suprasellar tumors can be removed via an extended transsphenoidal approach using an endoscope.[15] Many utilize a pterional craniotomy. Tumors with large cysts may be aspirated prior to surgery.

Chemotherapy: Intracystic CHT with either bleomycin or IFNα has been used, albeit with limited experience, for temporary tumor control with response rates of 62% to 100% and control rates of 59% to 71%. There is some suggestion that IFNα has fewer side effects than bleomycin.[16]

Radiation

Indications: RT is indicated following subtotal resection (adjuvant) or at tumor recurrence (salvage). Proton beam therapy alone or in conjunction with photon therapy has demonstrated efficacy in small retrospective series with limited follow-up.[17,18] An ongoing prospective phase II study utilizing proton beam RT reported similar incidence of severe complications compared to a historical cohort treated with conformal or intensity-modulated RT.[19] With fractionated conformal techniques, interfraction imaging every 1 to 2 weeks may be necessary to account for fluctuations in cyst volume.[20] For predominantly cystic lesions, intracavitary RT with rhenium-186, yttrium-90, or phosporus-32 has demonstrated response rates of 50% to 100% and control rates of 67%, though data is limited.[16,21–24]

Dose: Conventional EBRT dose is typically 54 Gy/30 fx. Doses of 54 to 55.8 Gy or greater have demonstrated improved LC compared to lower doses.[12–14] Several series of Gamma Knife® SRS used doses of 10 to 14.5 Gy with long-term control rates of 66% to 80%.[25–28]

Procedure: See *Treatment Planning Handbook*, Chapter 12.[29]

EVIDENCE-BASED Q&A

Are clinical outcomes better with aggressive total resection or limited resection followed by RT?

This is controversial. Retrospective data and systematic reviews of the literature suggest GTR versus STR + adjuvant RT have similar OS and LC, but GTR may cause more endocrine dysfunction.[10,30–34]

TABLE 55.1: Yang et al. 2010 (All CP)[32]				
n = 442	2-yr PFS	5-yr PFS	5-yr OS	10-yr OS
GTR	88%	67%	98%	98%
STR+RT	91%	69%	99%	95%
	All NS			

TABLE 55.2: Clark et al. 2013 (Pediatric CP)[31]		
n = 377	1-yr PFS	5-yr PFS
GTR	89%	77%
STR+RT	84%	73%
	All NS	
Source: From Ref. (31). With permission of Springer.		

Can RT be reserved for salvage treatment?

Most likely. Retrospective data from the University of Pennsylvania found that LC was worse with surgery alone versus surgery+adjuvant RT, but after accounting for the surgery alone pts who ultimately received salvage RT, LC and OS were comparable.[35] Furthermore, retrospective data from the UK demonstrated similar outcomes among 87 pts treated with adjuvant RT versus salvage RT.[36]

What are the late effects after treatment?

Craniopharyngioma originates in a highly sensitive area of the brain, particularly in children, and late effects are common given the long natural history of the disease. Diabetes insipidus is common after aggressive surgical resection. Neuropsychological changes including disinhibition, perseveration, attention and memory deficits are common. Endocrine effects including GH abnormalities are common in children. Additional effects of treatment near the hypothalamus include hypothalamic obesity, sleep disturbance, and defective thirst sensation. Visual impairment can occur from treatment or tumor progression. Stroke can occur due to proximity to the carotid artery and due to microvascular changes. Moyamoya syndrome (microvascular ischemia of the basal ganglia) is less common. Second malignancy (meningioma and others) can also occur.

REFERENCES

1. Ostrom QT, Gittleman H, Fulop J, et al. CBTRUS Statistical Report: primary brain and central nervous system tumors diagnosed in the United States in 2008–2012. *Neuro Oncol.* 2015;17(Suppl 4):iv1–iv62.
2. Bunin GR, Surawicz TS, Witman PA, et al. The descriptive epidemiology of craniopharyngioma. *J Neurosurg.* 1998;89(4):547–551.
3. Gunderson LL, Tepper JE. *Clinical Radiation Oncology.* 4th ed. Philadelphia, PA: Elsevier; 2016.
4. Adamson TE, Wiestler OD, Kleihues P, Yasargil MG. Correlation of clinical and pathological features in surgically treated craniopharyngiomas. *J Neurosurg.* 1990;73(1):12–17.
5. Crotty TB, Scheithauer BW, Young WF, Jr., et al. Papillary craniopharyngioma: a clinicopathological study of 48 cases. *J Neurosurg.* 1995;83(2):206–214.
6. Gaston-Massuet C, Andoniadou CL, Signore M, et al. Increased wingless (Wnt) signaling in pituitary progenitor/stem cells gives rise to pituitary tumors in mice and humans. *Proc Natl Acad Sci USA.* 2011;108(28):11482–11487.
7. Hussain I, Eloy JA, Carmel PW, Liu JK. Molecular oncogenesis of craniopharyngioma: current and future strategies for the development of targeted therapies. *J Neurosurg.* 2013;119(1):106–112.

8. Brastianos PK, Taylor-Weiner A, Manley PE, et al. Exome sequencing identifies BRAF mutations in papillary craniopharyngiomas. *Nat Genet*. 2014;46(2):161–165.

9. Hetelekidis S, Barnes PD, Tao ML, et al. Twenty-year experience in childhood craniopharyngioma. *Int J Rad Oncol Biol Phys*. 1993;27(2):189–195.

10. Merchant TE, Kiehna EN, Sanford RA, et al. Craniopharyngioma: the St. Jude Children's Research Hospital experience 1984–2001. *Int J Radiat Oncol Biol Phys*. 2002;53(3):533–542.

11. Masson-Cote L, Masucci GL, Atenafu EG, et al. Long-term outcomes for adult craniopharyngioma following radiation therapy. *Acta Oncol*. 2013;52(1):153–158.

12. Regine WF, Kramer S. Pediatric craniopharyngiomas: long term results of combined treatment with surgery and radiation. *Int J Radiat Oncol Biol Phys*. 1992;24(4):611–617.

13. Habrand JL, Ganry O, Couanet D, et al. The role of radiation therapy in the management of craniopharyngioma: a 25-year experience and review of the literature. *Int J Radiat Oncol Biol Phys*. 1999;44(2):255–263.

14. Varlotto JM, Flickinger JC, Kondziolka D, et al. External beam irradiation of craniopharyngiomas: long-term analysis of tumor control and morbidity. *Int J Radiat Oncol Biol Phys*. 2002;54(2):492–499.

15. de Divitiis E, Cappabianca P, Cavallo LM, et al. Extended endoscopic transsphenoidal approach for extrasellar craniopharyngiomas. *Neurosurgery*. 2007;61(5 Suppl 2):219–227; discussion 228.

16. Steinbok P, Hukin J. Intracystic treatments for craniopharyngioma. *Neurosurg Focus*. 2010;28(4):E13.

17. Luu QT, Loredo LN, Archambeau JO, et al. Fractionated proton radiation treatment for pediatric craniopharyngioma: preliminary report. *Cancer J*. 2006;12(2):155–159.

18. Fitzek MM, Linggood RM, Adams J, Munzenrider JE. Combined proton and photon irradiation for craniopharyngioma: long-term results of the early cohort of patients treated at Harvard Cyclotron Laboratory and Massachusetts General Hospital. *Int J Radiat Oncol Biol Phys*. 2006;64(5):1348–1354.

19. Merchant TE, Hua CH, Sabin ND, et al. Necrosis, vasculopathy, and neurological complications after proton therapy for childhood craniopharyngioma: results from a prospective trial and a photon cohort comparison. *Int J Rad Oncol Biol Phys*. 2016;96:S120–S121.

20. Winkfield KM, Linsenmeier C, Yock TI, et al. Surveillance of craniopharyngioma cyst growth in children treated with proton radiotherapy. *Int J Radiat Oncol Biol Phys*. 2009;73(3):716–721.

21. Voges J, Sturm V, Lehrke R, et al. Cystic craniopharyngioma: long-term results after intracavitary irradiation with stereotactically applied colloidal beta-emitting radioactive sources. *Neurosurgery*. 1997;40(2):263–269; discussion 269–270.

22. Pollock BE, Lunsford LD, Kondziolka D, et al. Phosphorus-32 intracavitary irradiation of cystic craniopharyngiomas: current technique and long-term results. *Int J Radiat Oncol Biol Phys*. 1995;33(2):437–446.

23. Hasegawa T, Kondziolka D, Hadjipanayis CG, Lunsford LD. Management of cystic craniopharyngiomas with phosphorus-32 intracavitary irradiation. *Neurosurgery*. 2004;54(4):813–820; discussion 820–812.

24. Van den Berge JH, Blaauw G, Breeman WA, et al. Intracavitary brachytherapy of cystic craniopharyngiomas. *J Neurosurg*. 1992;77(4):545–550.

25. Niranjan A, Kano H, Mathieu D, et al. Radiosurgery for craniopharyngioma. *Int J Radiat Oncol Biol Phys*. 2010;78(1):64–71.

26. Lee CC, Yang HC, Chen CJ, et al. Gamma knife surgery for craniopharyngioma: report on a 20-year experience. *J Neurosurg*. 2014;121 Suppl:167–178.

27. Kobayashi T. Long-term results of gamma knife radiosurgery for 100 consecutive cases of craniopharyngioma and a treatment strategy. *Prog Neurol Surg*. 2009;22:63–76.

28. Xu Z, Yen CP, Schlesinger D, Sheehan J. Outcomes of gamma knife surgery for craniopharyngiomas. *J Neurooncol*. 2011;104(1):305–313.

29. Videtic GMM, Woody N, Vassil AD. *Handbook of Treatment Planning in Radiation Oncology*. 2nd ed. New York, NY: Demos Medical; 2015.

30. Clark AJ, Cage TA, Aranda D, et al. Treatment-related morbidity and the management of pediatric craniopharyngioma: a systematic review. *J Neurosurg Pediatr*. 2012;10(4):293–301.

31. Clark AJ, Cage TA, Aranda D, et al. A systematic review of the results of surgery and radiotherapy on tumor control for pediatric craniopharyngioma. *Childs Nerv Syst*. 2013;29(2):231–238.

32. Yang I, Sughrue ME, Rutkowski MJ, et al. Craniopharyngioma: a comparison of tumor control with various treatment strategies. *Neurosurg Focus*. 2010;28(4):E5.
33. Schoenfeld A, Pekmezci M, Barnes MJ, et al. The superiority of conservative resection and adjuvant radiation for craniopharyngiomas. *J Neurooncol*. 2012;108(1):133–139.
34. Sughrue ME, Yang I, Kane AJ, et al. Endocrinologic, neurologic, and visual morbidity after treatment for craniopharyngioma. *J Neurooncol*. 2011;101(3):463–476.
35. Stripp DC, Maity A, Janss AJ, et al. Surgery with or without radiation therapy in the management of craniopharyngiomas in children and young adults. *Int J Radiat Oncol Biol Phys*. 2004;58(3):714–720.
36. Pemberton LS, Dougal M, Magee B, Gattamaneni HR. Experience of external beam radiotherapy given adjuvantly or at relapse following surgery for craniopharyngioma. *Radiother Oncol*. 2005;77(1):99–104.

56: RHABDOMYOSARCOMA

Yvonne D. Pham, Samuel T. Chao, and Erin S. Murphy

QUICK HIT: Rhabdomyosarcoma (RMS) is the most common soft tissue tumor of childhood. Risk stratification is performed via preoperative staging and postoperative grouping to determine treatment. All pts require multiagent CHT (usually VAC-based: vincristine, actinomycin D, and cyclophosphamide). General schema is biopsy or non-morbid resection followed by CHT, local therapy (surgery or RT), and more CHT for up to approximately 1 year. RT indicated for all pts except those with embryonal histology after gross total resection. Timing of RT varies by protocol, but generally follows at least 4 weeks of CHT. Treat pts with intracranial extension, vision loss, or cord compression on day 0; those with CN palsies and base of skull erosion can receive delayed RT without a compromise in outcomes. Dosing guidelines are listed in Table 56.1.

TABLE 56.1: Summary of Radiation Dosing Guidelines for Rhabdomyosarcoma by Extent of Resection and Histology

Disease Status	Embryonal Histology	Alveolar Histology
Margin negative	No RT	36 Gy
Margin positive	36 Gy	36 Gy
Node positive	41.4 Gy	41.4 Gy
Gross disease*	50.4 Gy	50.4 Gy

*Gross disease in the orbit receives 45 Gy with VAC (although with lower cyclophosphamide dose and response <CR, this may be insufficient),[1,2] or 50.4 Gy with VA CHT.

EPIDEMIOLOGY: 350 cases per year.[3] RMS is the most common pediatric soft tissue sarcoma and accounts for 3.5% of cancers in children younger than 15 years of age and 2% of cancers for adolescents 15 to 19 years of age.[4,5] There is a slight male predominance, 1.4:1, and the peak incidence occurs at 2 to 5 years of age with 70% of cases occurring before 10 years of age.[6]

RISK FACTORS: The majority of cases are sporadic with no predisposing risk factor.[7] For embryonal tumors, high birth weight and large size for gestational age are associated with increased incidence.[8] RMS has been associated with paternal cigarette use, prenatal x-ray exposure, and maternal recreational drug use.[9] RMS has been associated with Li–Fraumeni,[10–12] NF-1,[13,14] Beckwith–Wiedemann syndrome,[15] Noonan syndrome,[16] and Costello syndrome.[17]

ANATOMY: RMS can arise anywhere in the body, particularly where there is skeletal muscle, with most common locations in the genitourinary (GU) sites and H&N.[6] RMS is a locally invasive tumor with a potential to spread locally along fascial/muscle planes. Overall risk of regional lymphatic spread is 15% and varies with site of primary lesion: GU, abdominal/pelvic, and extremity tumors commonly involve regional lymph nodes, whereas H&N, trunk, and female genital organs rarely involve lymph nodes.[6] Distant metastases occur in 15% at time of presentation with most common dissemination to lungs, bone, and bone marrow.[18]

TABLE 56.2: Distribution of RMS by Anatomic Site

Site[19]	Distribution	Subdivisions
H&N (non-PM)	7%	Cheek, hypopharynx, larynx, oral cavity, oropharynx, parotid, scalp, face, pinna, neck, masseter muscle
Parameningeal (PM)	25%	Infratemporal fossa, mastoid, middle ear, nasal cavity, nasopharynx, paranasal sinus, parapharyngeal, pterygopalatine fossa
Orbits	9%	*Note: Combined H&N (including PM and orbit) most common site*
GU	31%	Bladder, paratesticular, prostate, urethra, uterus/cervix, vagina, vulva
Extremities	13%	
Trunk	5%	Chest wall, paraspinal, abdominal wall
Retroperitoneum	7%	
Other	3%	Hepatobiliary tree, perineal, perianal

PATHOLOGY: There are three histologic subtypes: embryonal (includes botryoid and spindle cell variants), alveolar, and pleomorphic/undifferentiated.

TABLE 56.3: Pathologic Subtypes of RMS[6]

Subtype	Frequency	Common Site	Histologic Appearance	Age	Prognosis	5-yr OS
Botryoid (grape-like appearance, embryonal variant)	6%	Mucosa-lined organs: bladder, vagina, nasopharynx, nasal cavity, middle ear, biliary tree	Loose myxoid stroma w/ "cambium" tumor cell layer	Infants	Excellent	95%
Spindle cell (embryonal variant)	3%	Paratesticular	Spindled cells, often w/ storiform pattern	Childhood		88%
Embryonal	79%	Most commonly in H&N and GU tract	Small round cells on myxoid stroma	Childhood	Intermediate	66%
Alveolar	32%	Extremities, trunk, perianal, perineal region	Cords with pseudolining clefts, looks like lung alveoli	Adolescents	Poor	54%
Undifferentiated	1%	Extremity, trunk	Diffuse mesenchymal/primitive cell population; diagnosis of exclusion	Adolescents		40%
Other	9%					

GENETICS[6]

Embryonal: 80% associated with LOH 11p15.5. Absence of n-myc amplification.

Alveolar: Two chromosomal translocations identified: **t(2;13)**—60% of cases and **t(1;13)**—20% of cases. 20% have neither translocation. Genes are FKHR (on chr 13), PAX3 (chr 2), and PAX7(chr 1). Note: 50% w/ n-myc amplification.

A significant proportion of RMSs have p53 mutations.

CLINICAL PRESENTATION: Usually presents as an asymptomatic mass but can have site-specific signs and symptoms (e.g., orbital tumors may cause proptosis and ophthalmoplegia and GU tumors may cause hematuria or urinary obstruction).

Workup[20]: H&P with exam of affected area (head and neck, pelvic exam under anesthesia as indicated).

Labs: CBC, BMP, LFTs, urinalysis.

Imaging: For all sites: CT or MRI of primary tumor area, PET/CT (can replace CT chest/abd/pelvis and bone scan studies). Scrotal ultrasound first step for paratesticular.

Pathology: Bone marrow biopsy and aspirate. For H&N site: lumbar puncture with cytologic exam of CSF if parameningeal tumor. MRI spine is optional if CSF is positive or obtain if pt is symptomatic. Any clinically enlarged lymph nodes should be biopsied. Do NOT biopsy testicle to avoid violation of scrotum. All boys ≥10 (or <10 years of age with +LN on imaging) with a paratesticular RMS should undergo routine ipsilateral nerve-sparing retroperitoneal lymph node dissection. Extremities: In the absence of pathologically enlarged nodes, sentinel node biopsy is indicated for all extremity tumors.

PROGNOSTIC FACTORS: For high-risk pts, the Oberlin risk factors are predictive of outcome and include >10 years or <1 year of age, bone or bone marrow involvement, three or more metastatic sites, or unfavorable primary site. Pts with 0 to 1 Oberlin factor have a better outcome.[21]

TABLE 56.4: Comparison of Favorable Versus Unfavorable Prognostic Factors in RMS

Variable	Favorable	Unfavorable
Metastases	None	Present
Primary site	Orbit, non-PM H&N, GU (not bladder/prostate) b/p)	Extremity, trunk, PM, bladder, prostate
Histology	Botryoid, spindle cell, embryonal	Alveolar, undifferentiated
Lymph node mets	No	Yes
Resectability	Complete	Microscopic <gross residual
Age	2–10 y/o	<1 y/o, >10 y/o
DNA proliferation	Low S-phase	High S-phase
DNA ploidy	Hyperdiploid	Diploid

STAGING: IRSG pretreatment staging system. Think pre-op based on "SSN" (site, size, nodes). If favorable site and nonmetastatic, all are stage I. If unfavorable site, must be BOTH <5 cm AND node-negative to be stage II.

TABLE 56.5: IRSG Staging System					
Stage	Sites	Size	N	M	3-yr Failure-Free Survival[19]
I: Favorable site	Orbit Head and Neck (non-PM) GU (non-bladder/prostate) Biliary tract	Any size	Any N	M0	86%
II: Unfavorable site, N0 and ≤5 cm	Bladder/Prostate Extremity Parameningeal Other (including: RP, perineal, perianal, intrathoracic, GI) Liver (nonbiliary)	≤5 cm	N0 or Nx	M0	80%
III: Unfavorable site, >5 cm or node-positive	Same as Stage II	≤5 cm	N1	M0	68%
		>5 cm	Any N	M0	
IV: Metastatic	All	Any size	Any N	M1	25%

T1, Confined to anatomic site of origin; T2, Extension and/or fixation to surrounding tissue; a, ≤5 cm in diameter; b, >5 cm in diameter; N0, Not clinically involved; N1, Clinically involved; Nx, Clinical status unknown; M0, No distant metastases; M1, Distant metastases.

Intergroup Rhabdomyosarcoma Study Clinical Grouping Classification[6]

Group is assessed at the time of diagnosis based on resectability (i.e., pt unresectable at diagnosis, treated with CHT, then undergoes GTR remains Group III).

TABLE 56.6: IRSG Grouping Classification	
Group I	Localized disease, completely resected A: Confined to muscle or organ of origin B: Infiltration outside the muscle or organ of origin
Group II	*Gross total resection with:* A: Microscopic residual disease B: Regional LN spread, completely resected C: Regional LN resected with microscopic residual
Group III	*Incomplete resection with gross residual disease* A: After biopsy only B: After major resection (>50%)
Group IV	Distant metastasis at onset

TABLE 56.7: Risk Stratification Based on Pre-Op Staging + Post-Op Grouping[6]	
Risk Group	Involved Groups
Low	Favorable histology (embryonal) *and* – Favorable site (Stage I): Group I–III – Unfavorable site (Stage II–III): Groups I–II
Intermediate	– Favorable histology (embryonal), unfavorable site (Stage II–III): Group III – Unfavorable histology (alveolar), any Stage (I–III) or Group(I–III)
High	Stage IV, Group IV

TABLE 56.8: Risk of Lymph Node Involvement by Primary Site[22]	
Site	LN Positivity
H&N (nonorbit)	8%
Vagina, uterus	6%
Extremities	12%
Paratesticular	26%
Prostate, bladder	27%
Other	0%–25%

TREATMENT PARADIGM

Surgery: Complete excision with 5-mm margin is preferable if functional and cosmetic outcomes are acceptable.[20] If not feasible (or if disease involves the orbit, vagina, bladder, or biliary tract), diagnostic incisional biopsy can be performed followed by induction CHT and definitive local therapy. Local control with organ preservation is the goal.[6] The utility of debulking surgery is under investigation. "Second-look" surgery after CHT may be a good option for select cases since pts may have a pCR and have survival comparable to those with an initial complete resection.[6] Current COG studies require lymph node evaluation for all extremity tumors (sentinel node biopsy acceptable if clinically negative), and all boys ≥10 years of age who have a paratesticular RMS should undergo routine ipsilateral nerve-sparing retroperitoneal lymph node dissection. Consider ilioinguinal lymphadenectomy for perianal or anal tumors. In H&N primaries, neck dissection not indicated but suspicious nodes should be surgically evaluated.[6]

Chemotherapy: All pts require multiagent CHT, regardless of stage and group.[20] VAC (vincristine, actinomycin-D, cyclophosphamide) is the standard regimen. In sequential IRS trials, the addition of many individually active agents (e.g., doxorubicin, cisplatin, etoposide, ifosfamide, topotecan, and melphalan) did not improve outcomes, compared to VAC, in any subgroup. In IRS-IV, VA equivalent to VAC in low-risk/excellent prognosis group. Vincristine ± irinotecan can be continued concurrently (ARST0431).

Radiation: As per COG ARST trials, RT is indicated in all cases except Group I embryonal.

TABLE 56.9: Radiation Dosing Guidelines	
0 Gy	Group 1 Embryonal
36 Gy	Group 1 (Alveolar), Group IIA (microscopic disease) embryonal tumor (completely resected after CHT and microscopic margins)
41.4 Gy	Resected LN+ disease or biopsy-proven CR to CHT (gross nodes get 50.4 Gy)
45 Gy	Gross disease in orbit with VAC CHT
50.4 Gy	Gross disease (nonorbit), or orbit with VA CHT; Group III pts with second-look surgery included (per ARST 0531)
15 Gy	Dose for WLI for pulmonary mets or pleural effusion

Procedures: See *Treatment Planning Handbook*, Chapter 12.[23]

EVIDENCE-BASED Q&A

What did the IRS studies show?

The Intergroup Rhabdomyosarcoma Study Group (IRSG) was formed in 1972 to investigate the biology and treatment of RMS and undifferentiated sarcoma (UDS); it was merged into the

Children's Oncology Group (COG) in 2000. They led a series of protocols (IRS I-V) that have dictated RMS management with a rise in OS seen for all pts from ~50% to >70%. Pertinent conclusions from the studies are summarized as follows:

Maurer, IRS-I (*Cancer* 1988, PMID 3275486):

- 5-yr OS for all Groups I-IV was 55%.
- For favorable histology (FH) Group 1, RT not needed if giving 2 years of VAC. However, benefit to RT for FFS and OS seen in Group I, unfavorable histologies (UH; e.g., alveolar and undifferentiated).[24]
- Primary tumors of orbit and GU tract had best prognosis compared to retroperitoneum with worst prognosis.
- Limited RT volumes (GTV + 2 cm) outcomes similar to big fields such as whole muscle bundle RT.

Maurer, IRS-II (*Cancer* 1993, PMID 8448756):

- 5-yr OS for all Groups I-IV was 63%, significant improvement from IRS-I (55%; $p < .001$).
- 5-yr OS for all nonmetastatic pts was 71%, significant improvement from IRS-I of 63% ($p = .01$).
- LC improved for >40 Gy (93% LC) for orofacial and laryngopharyngeal sites.[25]
- Cyclophosphamide not needed in FH Group I/II.

Crist, IRS-III (*JCO* 1995, PMID 7884423):

- 5-yr OS for all Groups I-IV was 71%, significantly better than IRS-II ($p < .001$).
- Group 1, UH benefitted with addition of RT.
- For PM H&N with CN palsy or BOS erosion, limited RT volumes as good as WBRT. WBRT still used for intracranial extension.

Breneman, IRS-IV (*JCO* 2003, PMID 12506174; Crist *JCO* 2001, PMID 11408506):

- For Group III disease, no benefit to hyperfractionated regimen (59.4 Gy with 1.1 Gy BID) over conventional regimen of 50.4 Gy in 1.8 Gy/fx.
- No benefit to VAI or VIE over VAC for nonmetastatic disease.
- Group IV pts with ≤2 metastatic sites had improved 3-yr OS and FFS on MVA ($p = .007$ and .006, respectively).

Raney, IRS-V (*JCO* 2011, PMID 21357783):

- Reduced RT doses (36 Gy for microscopic disease [Stage 1/Group IIa] and 45 Gy for Group III orbit primaries if cyclophosphamide is included in systemic therapy) do not compromise local control.
- Inclusion of an alkylating CHT agent (cyclophosphamide or ifosfamide) may be important for FFS.

When should RT be initiated?

RT timing has varied by protocol and risk group through the years. On the most recent COG protocols, low-risk pts start week 13, intermediate-risk week 4, and high-risk week 20. Metastatic sites may be treated at the end of CHT. Pts with cord compression, visual loss, or intracranial extension should be treated right away, on day 0 per high-risk COG ARST 0431 protocol. Analysis from IRS II-IV[26] showed reduced local failure if RT started within 2 weeks versus >2 weeks for pts with meningeal impingement (18% vs. 33%, $p = .03$) and intracranial extension (16% vs. 37%, $p = .07$). A recent analysis from Spaulding et al. demonstrated similar clinical outcomes for pts with cranial *nerve palsy or skull base erosion treated with immediate versus delayed RT[27]; thus, it is fine to treat pts with these high-risk features at a later date (week 20 per COG ARST 0431) but treat pts with intracranial extension on day 0.*

What is the benefit of RT and in whom is RT required?

There are no good prospective randomized data. RT is currently indicated for all pts except embryonal tumors after gross total resection. Wolden et al. reviewed pts treated on IRS I-III and showed that pts with alveolar/undifferentiated histology after GTR (Group I) have improved FFS and OS with the addition of RT.[24] Further, when comparing outcomes between IRS IV and MMT-89 (contemporary European International Society of Pediatric Oncology Malignant Mesenchymal Tumor study that attempted to avoid RT and radical surgery as much as possible by giving more CHT as necessary), RT appears to have significant benefits in LC, EFS, and OS.[28]

Is there a benefit to proton therapy in RMS?

The rationale is to reduce late effects and is permitted on ongoing RMS trials. Small series demonstrating dosimetric advantages have been published for orbit, parameningeal, and bladder/prostate sites.[29-31] There are concerns regarding increased neutron dose associated with proton technology, and longer follow-up is necessary to evaluate safety and efficacy.

REFERENCES

1. Ermoian RP, Breneman J, Walterhouse DO, et al. 45 Gy is not sufficient radiotherapy dose for Group III orbital embryonal rhabdomyosarcoma after less than complete response to 12 weeks of ARST0331 chemotherapy: a report from the Soft Tissue Sarcoma Committee of the Children's Oncology Group. *Pediatr Blood Cancer*. 2017;64(9). doi: 10.1002/pbc.26540
2. Walterhouse DO, Pappo AS, Meza JL, et al. Reduction of cyclophosphamide dose for patients with subset 2 low-risk rhabdomyosarcoma is associated with an increased risk of recurrence: a report from the Soft Tissue Sarcoma Committee of the Children's Oncology Group. *Cancer*. 2017;123(12):2368–2375.
3. Society AC. What are the key statistics about rhabdomyosarcoma? http://www.cancer.org/cancer/rhabdomyosarcoma/detailedguide/rhabdomyosarcoma-key-statistics
4. Gurney JG, Severson RK, Davis S, Robison LL. Incidence of cancer in children in the United States: sex-, race-, and 1-year age-specific rates by histologic type. *Cancer*. 1995;75(8):2186–2195.
5. Hies LA, Kosary CL, Hankey BF, et al. *SEER Cancer Statistics Review, 1973–1996*. Bethesda, MD: National Cancer Institute; 1999.
6. Halperin EC, Constine LS, Tarbell NJ, Kun LE. *Pediatric Radiation Oncology*. Lippincott Williams & Wilkins; 2012.
7. Ries LAG, Smith MA, Gurney JG, et al, eds. *Cancer Incidence and Survival among Children and Adolescents: United States SEER Program 1975–1995, National Cancer Institute, SEER Program*. Bethesda, MD: National Cancer Institute, SEER Program (NIH Pub. No. 99-4649); 1999.
8. Ognjanovic S, Carozza SE, Chow EJ, et al. Birth characteristics and the risk of childhood rhabdomyosarcoma based on histological subtype. *Br J Cancer*. 2010;102(1):227–231.
9. Ognjanovic S, Linabery AM, Charbonneau B, Ross JA. Trends in childhood rhabdomyosarcoma incidence and survival in the United States, 1975–2005. *Cancer*. 2009;115(18):4218–4226.
10. Diller L, Sexsmith E, Gottlieb A, et al. Germline p53 mutations are frequently detected in young children with rhabdomyosarcoma. *J Clin Invest*. 1995;95(4):1606–1611.
11. Li FP, Fraumeni JF, Jr. Rhabdomyosarcoma in children: epidemiologic study and identification of a familial cancer syndrome. *J Natl Cancer Inst*. 1969;43(6):1365–1373.
12. Trahair T, Andrews L, Cohn RJ. Recognition of Li Fraumeni syndrome at diagnosis of a locally advanced extremity rhabdomyosarcoma. *Pediatr Blood Cancer*. 2007;48(3):345–348.
13. Crucis A, Richer W, Brugieres L, et al. Rhabdomyosarcomas in children with neurofibromatosis type I: a national historical cohort. *Pediatr Blood Cancer*. 2015;62(10):1733–1738.

14. Ferrari A, Bisogno G, Macaluso A, et al. Soft-tissue sarcomas in children and adolescents with neurofibromatosis type 1. *Cancer.* 2007;109(7):1406–1412.

15. DeBaun MR, Tucker MA. Risk of cancer during the first four years of life in children from the Beckwith-Wiedemann Syndrome Registry. *J Pediat.* 1998;132(3, Pt 1):398–400.

16. Kratz CP, Rapisuwon S, Reed H, et al. Cancer in Noonan, Costello, cardiofaciocutaneous and LEOPARD syndromes. *Am J Med Genet C Semin Med Genet.* 2011;157C(2):83–89.

17. Gripp KW. Tumor predisposition in Costello syndrome. *Am J Med Genet C Semin Med Genet.* 2005;137C(1):72–77.

18. Breneman JC, Lyden E, Pappo AS, et al. Prognostic factors and clinical outcomes in children and adolescents with metastatic rhabdomyosarcoma: a report from the Intergroup Rhabdomyosarcoma Study IV. *J Clin Oncol.* 2003;21(1):78–84.

19. Crist WM, Anderson JR, Meza JL, et al. Intergroup rhabdomyosarcoma study-IV: results for patients with nonmetastatic disease. *J Clin Oncol.* 2001;19(12):3091–3102.

20. Breneman JC, Donaldson SS. Rhabdomyosarcoma. In: *Perez & Brady's Principles and Practice of Radiation Oncology.* 6th ed. Philadelphia, PA: Lippincott Williams & Wilkins; 2013:1676–1688.

21. Weigel BJ, Lyden E, Anderson JR, et al. Intensive multiagent therapy, including dose-compressed cycles of ifosfamide/etoposide and vincristine/doxorubicin/cyclophosphamide, irinotecan, and radiation, in patients with high-risk rhabdomyosarcoma: a report from the Children's Oncology Group. *J Clin Oncol.* 2016;34(2):117–122.

22. Lawrence W Jr, Hays DM, Heyn R, et al. Lymphatic metastases with childhood rhabdomyosarcoma: a report from the Intergroup Rhabdomyosarcoma Study. *Cancer.* 1987;60(4):910–915.

23. Videtic GMM, Woody NM, Vassil AD. *Handbook of Treatment Planning in Radiation Oncology.* 2nd ed. New York, NY: Demos Medical; 2015.

24. Wolden SL, Anderson JR, Crist WM, et al. Indications for radiotherapy and chemotherapy after complete resection in rhabdomyosarcoma: a report from the Intergroup Rhabdomyosarcoma Studies I to III. *J Clin Oncol.* 1999;17(11):3468–3475.

25. Wharam MD, Beltangady MS, Heyn RM, et al. Pediatric orofacial and laryngopharyngeal rhabdomyosarcoma: an Intergroup Rhabdomyosarcoma Study report. *Arch Otolaryngol Head Neck Surg.* 1987;113(11):1225–1227.

26. Michalski JM, Meza J, Breneman JC, et al. Influence of radiation therapy parameters on outcome in children treated with radiation therapy for localized parameningeal rhabdomyosarcoma in Intergroup Rhabdomyosarcoma Study Group trials II through IV. *Int J Radiat Oncol Biol Phys.* 2004;59(4):1027–1038.

27. Spalding AC, Hawkins DS, Donaldson SS, et al. The effect of radiation timing on patients with high-risk features of parameningeal rhabdomyosarcoma: an analysis of IRS-IV and D9803. *Int J Radiat Oncol Biol Phys.* 2013;87(3):512–516.

28. Donaldson SS, Anderson JR. Rhabdomyosarcoma: many similarities, a few philosophical differences. *J Clin Oncol.* 2005;23(12):2586–2587.

29. Fukushima H, Fukushima T, Sakai A, et al. Tailor-made treatment combined with proton beam therapy for children with genitourinary/pelvic rhabdomyosarcoma. *Rep Pract Oncol Radiother.* 2015;20(3):217–222.

30. Leiser D, Calaminus G, Malyapa R, et al. Tumour control and quality of life in children with rhabdomyosarcoma treated with pencil beam scanning proton therapy. *Radiother Oncol.* 2016;120(1):163–168.

31. Weber DC, Ares C, Albertini F, et al. Pencil beam scanning proton therapy for pediatric parameningeal rhabdomyosarcomas: clinical outcome of patients treated at the Paul Scherrer Institute. *Pediatr Blood Cancer.* 2016;63(10):1731–1736.

57: NEUROBLASTOMA

Charles Marc Leyrer and Erin S. Murphy

> **QUICK HIT:** Neuroblastoma (NB) is a small round blue cell tumor arising from the neural crest cells of the sympathetic nervous system. NB is the most common malignancy in infants and the most common pediatric extracranial solid tumor. Workup includes H&P, labs (CBC, CMP, LDH, urinary catecholamines [VMA/HVA], and serum ferritin), CT/MRI of primary site, CT chest/abdomen/pelvis, MIBG scan, bilateral bone marrow biopsy. Pts are stratified into risk groups based on stage, age, N-myc status, DNA ploidy, and Shimada classification, and risk group determines treatment.

TABLE 57.1: General Treatment Paradigm for Neuroblastoma		
INRG/Risk Group	**5-yr OS[1-3]**	**General Treatment Paradigm**
INRG L1 or Low Risk	>95%	Surgery alone. CHT for residual (if >18 mos or unfavorable factors), recurrent, or symptomatic disease.
INRG L2 or Intermediate Risk	90%–95%	Surgery followed by CHT. If initially unresectable: biopsy, CHT +/– delayed surgery. RT if persistent/worsening symptoms despite other therapy (per ANBL0531).
High Risk	30%–50%	Induction CHT, surgery, myeloablative CHT and autologous SCT, consolidative RT, oral isotretinoin + anti-GD2 antibody (per ANBL0532). Ongoing investigation with the addition of I-131 MIBG or crizotinib for ALK-mutation. RT: Treat primary post-CHT and presurgical volume to 21.6 Gy/12 fx if GTR; if gross residual, cone down after 21.6 Gy to a total of 36 Gy/20 fx. Treat metastatic sites active on post-CHT and pretransplant MIBG scan.

Note regarding spinal cord compression: Occurs in 5%–15% of pts. RT reserved for pts who fail initial CHT and/or surgery. RT is associated with late toxicity (e.g., scoliosis).

EPIDEMIOLOGY: Most common pediatric extracranial solid tumor, most common infant malignancy, third most common pediatric cancer overall (after leukemia, brain, lymphoma). 6% to 10% of all childhood malignancies, 15% of deaths (most lethal pediatric solid tumor). 650 to 700 new cases per year, median age 17 to 20 mos at diagnosis (90% <5 y/o, 40% <1 y/o). Incidence: higher in males than females and in Caucasians than African Americans.[3-5] Approximately 50% present with high-risk disease.[6]

RISK FACTORS: Poorly established. Increased incidence with maternal use of alcohol, diuretics, opioids/codeine, and paternal exposure to hydrocarbons/wood dusts/solders.[7,8] There is suggestion of protective effect of vitamin/folic acid use and history of asthma/allergies. No clear correlation with maternal age, smoking, infections, x-ray exposure, recreational drug use, maternal hypertension/diabetes, oral contraceptives, breastfeeding, birth order, gestational age, or socioeconomic status. Majority of tumors are sporadic, hereditary in only 1% to 2% of cases. Associated with Hirschsprung disease and NF-1.[9]

ANATOMY: Can originate from anywhere along the sympathetic nervous system; most commonly along the paraspinal sympathetic ganglia (mediastinal or abdominal) or the adrenal glands.

PATHOLOGY: Ranges from benign ganglioneuroma (well-differentiated, favorable prognosis), to ganglioneuroblastoma (moderately differentiated, unfavorable prognosis), to neuroblastoma (poorly differentiated, favorable to poor prognosis). 97% of neuroblastic tumors are NB.[10,11] Originates from neural crest cells of the sympathetic nervous system that migrate to form the adrenal medulla and spinal sympathetic ganglia. NB is a small round blue cell tumor with pathognomonic neuritic processes (neuropil) in almost all tumors except undifferentiated. Homer Wright pseudorosettes are neuroblasts surrounding areas of eosinophilic neuropil (15%–50% of cases). IHC positive for neuron-specific enolase, chromogranin A, neurofilament protein, S100, and synaptophysin can aid distinction from other similar tumors (non-Hodgkin's lymphoma, Ewing's, sarcomas).[12–14] Negative for leukocyte common antigen, vimentin, myosin, desmin, and actin.

Shimada histopathologic system: classifies tumors into favorable or unfavorable categories based on Stromal pattern, Age, degree of neuroblastic Differentiation, Mitosis-karyorrhexis index (MKI relating to fragmentation of the nucleus), and Nodularity (mnemonic: SADMaN). Favorable Shimada: young age, low MKI, mature neuroblast differentiation, rich stroma with non-nodular pattern.[10]

GENETICS: N-myc protein amplification encoded by MYCN gene, proto-oncogene found on the short arm of chromosome 2 and identified by FISH. N-myc amplification found in 20% to 25% tumors: 0% to 10% early-stage pts, 40% to 50% advanced pts.[15] Other poor prognostic factors include: **deletion/loss of 1p or 11q, unbalanced gain of 17q, TERT** rearrangements, **ATRX** deletion, or **ALK** mutation (accounts for up to 15% of hereditary NB).[16–18] Favorable factors are tumor cell **hyperdiploidy** or **TRK-A amplification**.[15,19–21]

SCREENING: Currently not supported. Data from Japan, Canada, and Europe showed that screening urine for HVA/VMA at 3 weeks of age, 6 months of age, or 1 year of age increases detection overall; however, no change in detection of advanced-stage disease with unfavorable characteristics in older children.[22–24] It also failed to reduce the deaths from neuroblastoma in infants.[22–24] Earlier detection can identify a higher incidence of neuroblastomas in infants, but these tend to be more favorable, spontaneously regress in early infancy, and may not have been detected otherwise.[25]

CLINICAL PRESENTATION: Abdominal mass, abdominal pain, fever, malaise, weight loss, micturition, dyspnea, and dysphagia. Approximately 1/3 experience fatigue, anorexia, irritability, and pallor. Bone pain frequent in pts with skeletal mets (most often skull/posterior orbit). Excess catecholamines can produce flushing, sweating, and HTN (although rare). Can be confused with Wilms tumor (see Chapter 58 for a table comparing neuroblastoma and Wilms presentation). IVP classically shows renal displacement ("drooping lily sign") without the pelvocaliceal disruption seen in Wilms tumor. See Table 57.2 for associated classic signs and symptoms.

TABLE 57.2: Clinical Eponyms for Neuroblastoma Presentation	
Dumbbell tumor	Paraspinal sympathetic ganglia tumors with invasion through neural foramina
Raccoon eyes	Proptosis and periorbital ecchymosis from retrobulbar/orbital bone metastases
Blueberry muffin	Cutaneous metastasis causing a blue skin discoloration (usually infants)

(continued)

TABLE 57.2: Clinical Eponyms for Neuroblastoma Presentation (*continued*)	
Pepper syndrome	Liver metastasis with hepatomegaly leading to respiratory distress
Horner's syndrome	Ipsilateral ptosis, miosis, and anhidrosis due to cervical ganglion tumor
Hutchinson's sign	Limping and irritability due to bone or bone marrow metastases
Opsoclonus–myoclonus	Paraneoplastic syndrome (antineural antibodies) of myoclonic jerking, random eye movement, and truncal ataxia; can persist even after cure
Kerner-Morrison sign	Intractable secretory diarrhea, hypokalemia, dehydration due to VIP secretion

WORKUP: H&P with attention to child development and signs/symptoms as in the preceding text.

Imaging: CT and/or MRI of the primary site, CT chest, abdomen, pelvis. PET not standard. MIBG scintigraphy labeled with I-123 is recommended for assessment of the primary and metastatic sites (sensitivity 90%, specificity ~100%).[26] MIBG is a norepinephrine analogue that is concentrated in cells of neural crest origin. MIBG may distinguish residual active tumor from necrotic tumor or scar tissue and is more sensitive than Tc-99 bone scans for assessing the response of cortical bone mets to treatment.[26] Bone scan not required unless primary tumor is not MIBG avid.

Labs: CBC, CMP, LDH, serum ferritin, urinary catecholamines. Elevated urinary catecholamines, (including HVA or VMA can be detected in 90% to 95% of pts.

Pathology: Bilateral bone marrow biopsy. FNA is not adequate. Increased urinary HVA/VMA in conjunction with compatible tumor cells in the bone marrow is considered sufficient for establishing diagnosis without biopsy.[27]

PROGNOSTIC FACTORS: See Table 57.3.

TABLE 57.3: Neuroblastoma Prognostic Factors[10,28-36]	
Favorable	Unfavorable
Younger age (<1 y/o)	Older age (>5 y/o)
Low MKI	High MKI
Differentiated neuroblasts	Undifferentiated neuroblasts
Stromal pattern: rich and non-nodular	Stromal pattern: poor and nodular
1p intact	1p deleted
MYCN nonamplified (MYCN-NA)	MYCN amplified (MYCN-A)
Hypo/Hyperdiploid (DNA index <1 or >1)	Diploid (DNA index 1)
TRK amplification	17q gain; 11q LOH
Stage 1, 2, 4S	Stage 3, 4
Thorax primary, multifocal	H&N primary
Skin, liver, bone marrow mets	Bone, CNS, orbit, pleura, lung mets
Low NSE and ferritin	High NSE (>100) or ferritin (>143)

NATURAL HISTORY: 70% of patients present with metastatic disease with bone marrow mets seen in 80% to 90%. LN+ in 35%. Abdomen is most common primary site (50%–80%). Other common sites include adrenal gland (35%), low-thoracic or abdominal paraspinal ganglia (30%–35%), posterior mediastinum (20%), pelvis (2%), cervical spine (1%), and other sites (12%).[37] Spontaneous regression may occur, especially in infants with 4S disease.[38] 5-yr OS is 71% in modern era, but attributable mainly to increased cure rates in pts with less aggressive disease.[39] Relapsed pts can often be managed with chronic disease for years, but long-term DFS after relapse is rare.

STAGING: The International Neuroblastoma Staging System (INSS) can be used to stage neuroblastomas (see Table 57.4) and attempts to combine the previously used Evans and Pediatric Oncology Group (POG) staging systems.[27,40] This was initially developed in 1986 and revised in 1993 and takes into account the results of surgery to remove the tumor. The INSS staging system was further classified into low, intermediate, and high-risk groups by the Children's Oncology Group (COG). INRG developed a staging system (INRGSS) based on preoperative evaluation and extent of disease as determined by imaging defined risk factors (IDRFs).[41] INRGSS simplifies staging into localized (L1/L2) versus metastatic disease (M/MS).

Treatment is determined by risk stratification into low, intermediate, and high risk (see protocols for details). Factors incorporated into the most recent COG risk grouping include: Stage, Age, N-myc, DNA ploidy, and Shimada histology (mnemonic "SANDS," from trials ANBL00B1, ANBL0531, and ANBL0532). Generally, pts with amplified N-myc are either low or high risk, and pts with stage I disease are low risk.

TABLE 57.4: Comparison of International Neuroblastoma Staging System (INSS)[27] and More Recent International Neuroblastoma Risk Group Staging System (INRGSS)[41]

INSS (1993)		INRGSS (2009)	
1	Tumor on one side of the body. Complete resection (microscopic disease allowed). Ipsilateral LNs histologically negative (nodes adherent to and removed with the primary tumor may be positive).	L1	Localized tumor without vital structure involvement as defined by image-defined risk factor and limited to one body compartment (neck, chest, abdomen, pelvis)
2A	Same as stage I except residual disease after resection.	L2	Locoregional tumor with one or more image-defined risk factors
2B	Ipsilateral nonadherent lymph nodes contain tumor. Contralateral LNs must be negative microscopically. Residual disease after resection allowed.		
3	Unresectable unilateral tumor extending across midline (beyond opposite side of the vertebral body) with or without involved regional lymph nodes, OR unilateral tumor with contralateral regional LN involvement, OR midline tumor with bilateral extension by infiltration (unresectable) or by LN involvement.		
4	Dissemination to distant LNs, bone, bone marrow, liver, skin, and/or other organs (except as defined for 4S).	M	Distant metastatic disease (except stage MS)
4S	Localized primary tumor as in stage 1, 2A, or 2B, with dissemination limited to skin, liver, and/or bone marrow (<10% of total nucleated cells on bone biopsy/aspirate). **Limited to infants <1 y/o.**	MS	Children <18 mos with metastatic disease limited to skin, liver, and/or bone marrow (No more than 10% marrow cells positive)

INRGSS image-defined risk factors[41]

- Ipsilateral tumor extension within two body compartments: neck and chest, chest and abdomen, abdomen and pelvis
- Infiltration of adjacent organs/structures: pericardium, diaphragm, kidney, liver, duodenopancreatic block, mesentery
- Encasement of major vessels by tumor: vertebral artery, internal jugular vein, subclavian vessels, carotid artery, aorta, vena cava, major thoracic vessels, iliac vessels, branches of the superior mesenteric artery at its root and the celiac axis
- Compression of trachea or central bronchi
- Encasement of brachial plexus
- Infiltration of porta hepatis or hepatoduodenal ligament
- Infiltration of the costovertebral junction between T9 and T12
- Tumor crossing the sciatic notch
- Tumor invading renal pedicle
- Extension of tumor to base of skull
- Intraspinal tumor extension with >1/3 spinal canal invasion, leptomeningeal space obliteration, or abnormal spinal cord MRI signal

TABLE 57.5: Previous Staging Systems for Neuroblastoma			
Evans/Children's Cancer Study Group (CCSG) Clinical Staging		**St. Jude/POG Surgicopathologic Staging**	
I	Tumor confined to organ or structure of origin	A	Gross total resection of primary, with or without microscopic residual. LN not adherent to primary tumor are negative and liver is histologically negative.
II	Tumor extending beyond organ or structure of origin but not crossing midline and/or involved ipsilateral lymph nodes	B	Grossly unresected primary tumor, nonadherent LN−, liver−
III	Tumor extending in continuity beyond the midline; regional LN may be involved bilaterally	C	Complete or incomplete resection of primary, nonadherent LN+, liver−
IV	Remote disease involving bone, bone marrow, soft tissue, or distant lymph nodes	D	Distant LN, bone, bone marrow, liver, or skin
IV–S	Stage I or II except for presence of mets confined to liver, skin, and/or marrow (does not include nonmarrow bone mets)	D(S)	Infants <1 y/o with stage IV-S disease (as defined in CCSG system)

TREATMENT PARADIGM

Observation: Recommended initially for stage 4S, which may spontaneously resolve.

Surgery: Useful for diagnosis, staging, and treatment for local control. Goal is GTR of visible tumor and regional lymph nodes with maintenance of function as organ preservation is key. Uninvolved contralateral lymph nodes should be sampled and a liver biopsy should be obtained. Large tumors that encase regional organs or large vessels, and "dumbbell" tumors that compress the spinal cord are considered unresectable. Intermediate- and high-risk pts with clinically unresectable disease should undergo initial biopsy/diagnostic surgery, induction CHT, and then delayed/second-look surgery. CR in 66% to 79% of pts after induction CHT. Piecemeal resection may be necessary and is acceptable. Subtotal resection can still be attempted after CHT. Titanium clips are recommended at sites of residual disease. Note that resection of the primary is no longer required for stage 4S, but a biopsy should be obtained.

Chemotherapy: CHT used in intermediate and high-risk pts to shrink primary tumors to facilitate delayed surgery. Generally no role for CHT in low-risk pts except for persistent/recurrent disease. Consider CHT for 4S with hepatomegaly. No set standard CHT regimen. Most common agents are cyclophosphamide, cisplatin, doxorubicin, and etoposide; others include (but are not limited to) carboplatin, vincristine, vindesine, ifosfamide, dacarbazine, topotecan, melphalan. Intensive doses of combination CHT with short intervals between courses should be delivered in high-risk pts. In high-risk pts, myeloablative CHT with autologous SCT has improved survival over CHT alone (see Matthay NEJM 1999). Phase III studies suggest tandem cycles of CHT + SCT may yield better survival in high-risk pts—see the following.

Radiation

Indications: RT is delivered to the primary tumor and persistent metastatic sites in high-risk pts. In intermediate-risk pts, RT is delivered to recurrent or gross residual disease. Adjuvant RT not indicated for low- or intermediate-risk disease unless urgent symptomatic (life/organ threatening) concerns without significant response to CHT (i.e., liver mets with respiratory compromise or cord compression).

Dose: 21.6 Gy/12 fx daily (COG). High-risk protocol ANBL0532 allows a boost to 36 Gy for gross residual disease after surgery >1 cc (21.6 Gy to pre-op GTV, then 14.4 Gy boost). For hepatic metastasis causing respiratory compromise: 4.5 Gy/3 fx (COG). For cord compression, CHT is preferred followed by surgical decompression.

Toxicity: Acute: Diarrhea, nausea, vomiting, erythema, fatigue, myelosuppression. Late: Bony/soft tissue hypoplasia, scoliosis/kyphosis, slipped capital femoral epiphysis, short stature, second malignancy, renal impairment, renal insufficiency; others are location dependent.

Targeted radionuclides: I-131 MIBG therapy has shown response rates of 30% to 40% in otherwise refractory pts and is being investigated before resection or in combination with SCT for consolidation.

Differentiation therapy: Neuroblastoma cell lines can be induced to terminally differentiate on exposure to retinoids. Risk of relapse is reduced in pts who receive isotretinoin, which is now part of standard therapy in high-risk pts.[42]

Immunotherapy: Neuroblastoma cells uniformly express disialoganglioside GD2 on their surface, which creates a target for immunotherapy. Dinutuximab, a chimeric anti-GD2 antibody (ch14.18) is FDA-approved for adjuvant first-line therapy but is associated with significant acute toxicity in the form of capillary leak syndrome and pain. Human (rather than chimeric) forms are under evaluation and may improve tolerance.

TABLE 57.6: Neuroblastoma Treatment Overview by Risk Group
Low Risk (5-yr OS >95%): Pts with stage 4S disease may undergo spontaneous disease regression and can be observed (or given short-course CHT for hepatomegaly). No benefit from resection of primary (may biopsy skin nodule) for stage 4S. For other low-risk pts, surgery alone usually recommended.[1,32] Adjuvant RT has not improved outcomes after GTR and is not even indicated for STR or positive margins. CHT indicated for symptomatic pts or disease progression. RT reserved for CHT-resistant tumor.

(continued)

TABLE 57.6: Neuroblastoma Treatment Overview by Risk Group (*continued*)
Intermediate Risk (3-yr OS 95%): Surgery and CHT (without RT) is standard. See Table 57.1 for RT indications. If primary is unresectable, biopsy → CHT → delayed surgery. CHT typically given for approximately four cycles for favorable histology tumors and eight cycles for unfavorable histology.
High Risk (3-yr OS 30%–50%): Paradigm includes combined modality therapy with intensive platinum-based multiagent induction CHT, delayed surgery, myeloablative CHT and autologous SCT, RT to primary site and residual mets, then isotretinoin and immunotherapy. CHT has a response rate of 70%–80%. Consolidation therapy with myeloablative CHT±TBI followed by autologous BMT improves EFS over continued CHT (especially N-myc amplified or >2 years of age; see Matthay NEJM 1999). Exact timing of RT is not well-established, but usually delivered after autologous SCT when disease burden is minimal. RT should be delivered to the primary site even if the pt has undergone GTR. Treatment volume is the post-CHT GTV prior to attempted surgical resection (not the pre-CHT volume or postsurgical volume). If primary was grossly resected at diagnosis, GTV1 is the pre-op volume. Volume can be shaved out of normal tissues occupying space previously occupied by tumor (if the normal tissue was not infiltrated). CTV is the GTV + 1.5-cm margin (PTV is 0.5–1 cm). RT should also be delivered to metastatic sites with persistent active disease (+MIBG) after induction CHT. Adjuvant 13-cis-retinoic acid (isotretinoin) and anti GD-2 monoclonal antibody improves EFS and OS respectively in those without progression.[43–45] Pts can have recurrent disease after completion of aggressive treatment.

EVIDENCE-BASED Q&A

Low risk

What is the treatment paradigm for low-risk disease?

Low-risk disease is the most common presentation of neuroblastoma. Surgery is the mainstay of therapy if the tumor is deemed resectable. Residual disease may be observed if pts are ≤18 months and have favorable risk factors (favorable histology and nondiploid tumors). CHT is reserved for unresectable, unfavorable, symptomatic, or progressive/recurrent disease. This is supported by COG P9641, which stratified postoperative CHT based on risk factors. This study found a higher risk of recurrence in pts with stage 1 N-myc amplified disease or stage 2b ≥18 months or have unfavorable histology or diploid tumors if pts were observed after surgery. There is no role for routine adjuvant RT in low-risk pts given the outcomes with salvage therapy.

Nitschke, POG 8104/8441 (*JCO* 1988, PMID 3411339): 101 children with POG A neuroblastoma treated with surgery alone. 40 pts were NED (89%) and six of nine failures salvaged with CHT survived at 2 years, three deaths. **Conclusion: Surgery alone is appropriate for pts with POG A disease.**

Perez, CCG 3881 (*JCO* 2000, PMID 10893285): Prospective trial of 374 pts with stage I-II NB. All pts without N-myc amplification were treated with surgery alone, but laminotomy or RT was recommended if there was cord compression. Stage II pts <1 year of age with N-myc amplification received induction CHT, surgery and RT to gross residual after surgery. Stage II pts >1 year of age with N-myc amplification were treated on CCG 3891 (see the following). Recurrences among stage II pts were managed successfully in 38 of 43 pts. Supplemental treatment necessary in only 10% of stage I and 20% of stage II pts. N-myc amplification, unfavorable histopathology, >2 years of age, and LN+ predicted for a lower OS in stage II pts. **Conclusion: Stage I and II pts represent a biologically favorable group with excellent prognosis. Surgery alone is sufficient initial treatment for most pts, regardless of other clinical or biologic factors, with an OS of 99% for stage I and 98% for stage II pts.**

TABLE 57.7: Results of CCG 3881 Neuroblastoma			
CCG 3881	4-yr EFS	4-yr OS	Deaths
Stage I	93%	99%	1
Stage II	81%	98%	6
p value	.002	NS	

Matthay, COG retrospective (*JCO* 1989, PMID 2915240): RR of 156 pts with stage II NB treated on CCG protocols. 43 pts had complete resection (POG A), 62 had microscopic residual (+ margin [POG A] or + nodes [POG A or C]), and 48 had gross residual (POG B or C). 5-yr OS was 96% and the PFS was 90%. The extent of resection and subsequent treatment with RT and/or CHT did not affect PFS. 6-yr PFS was 89% for 75 pts treated with surgery alone versus 94% for 66 pts treated with surgery + RT ($p = .42$). No significant difference between 40 pts with gross or microscopic residual disease treated with surgery alone (PFS 92%) versus 59 pts with residual disease who also received RT (PFS 90%). In the pts with microscopic residual, there was an advantage to the addition of RT, with PFS ~97% versus ~84% ($p = .04$). OS was >95% for both groups due to effective salvage treatment. **Conclusion: Surgery alone, even if GTR is not achieved, is sufficient initial treatment for Evans stage II neuroblastoma.**

Nitschke, POG 8104 (*JCO* 1991, PMID 2045858): Phase II trial. After initial resection, 61 pts with POG B NB received five cycles of AC and were re-evaluated. Pts with a CR (n = 31) were then observed. Second-look surgery was planned for pts with PR (n = 20). NP or PD (n = 10) prompted salvage CHT with AC or CDDP/teniposide (P/VM). Of partial responders, 7 were NED at second look, 5 more were completely resected, and 4 had partial resection (4 more had no surgery) followed by salvage CHT. Of those who underwent salvage therapy, 4 of 18 progressed (1 was salvaged with BMT). **Conclusion: Aggressive CHT with second-look surgery is appropriate for POG B neuroblastoma.**

Stage 4S

What are the outcomes for stage 4S disease?

Pts less than 1 year of age presenting with abdominal tumors can still have excellent outcomes (3-yr EFS and OS >95%) if observed closely. Katzenstein et al. showed that pts who may require intervention are those symptomatic from their disease (hepatomegaly), very young (<2 months), or have unfavorable histology. The concern with very young pts is that they have a higher risk of rapid clinical decline without intervention. If CHT is given for symptomatic disease, it is generally given until cessation of symptoms. Early results of COG-ANBL0531 for pts with 4S disappointingly showed a lower 2-yr OS of 81%, which was thought to be due to inclusion of pts who could not undergo biopsy due to poor clinical factors previously excluded from prior trials (see intermediate risk later).

Katzenstein, POG Experience (*JCO* 1998, PMID 9626197): RR of 110 pts with stage D(S) NB registered on POG protocols. 3-yr OS was 85%. OS was 71% for pts ≤2 months of age, 68% for pts with diploid tumors, 44% for pts with N-myc amplification, and 33% for pts with unfavorable histology. No difference in OS between those who received CHT (82%) versus no CHT (93%, $p = .187$), or between those who underwent GTR of primary tumor (90%) versus STR or bx (78%, $p = .083$). **Conclusion: Survival of infants with stage D(S) NB is good. However, prognosis is poor in those of very young age and with unfavorable biologic factors.**

Nickerson, CCG 3881 (*JCO* 2000, PMID 10653863): Prospective study of 77 pts with stage 4S NB treated with supportive care only (n = 44), CHT (cyclophosphamide 5 mg/kg/d x 5 days) + hepatic RT (4.5 Gy/3 fx; n = 22), CHT alone (n = 10), or RT alone (n = 1).

5-yr EFS was 86% and 5-yr OS was 92%. Of 44 pts undergoing supportive care only, OS was 100%, compared with 81% for those requiring CHT for symptoms ($p = .005$). 5 of 6 deaths occurred in pts <2 mos. Pts aged ≤3 months at diagnosis had decreased EFS. The only factor predictive for improved OS was favorable Shimada histopathologic classification. **Conclusion: Minimal treatment is appropriate for infants with stage 4S NB disease except those <2 months with progressive abdominal disease.**

Nutchtern, COG-ANBL00P2 (*Ann Surg* 2012, PMID 22964741): 87 pts with small adrenal masses and <6 months of age whose parents elected for observation or surgical resection. Followed with abdominal ultrasound and VMA/HMA. Referred to surgery if >50% increase in mass volume OR >50% increase in urine catecholamine levels OR HMA:VMA ratio >2. 83 observed overall with 16 (19%) requiring surgery. Of those, 8 (50%) had stage I NB, 1 had stage 2B and 1 had 4S, 2 had low-grade adrenocortical neoplasm, and 4 were benign. MFU 3.2 years. 3-yr EFS 97.7% and OS 100%. **Conclusion: Most infants <6 months with small adrenal masses can have excellent outcomes if closely observed without surgery.**

Intermediate risk

Is RT beneficial for intermediate-risk disease?

RT was shown to increase both EFS and OS when added to adjuvant CHT in the Castleberry study of POG C pts. However, in the modern era, additional genetic/biologic risk-stratification factors (such as N-myc status) are used to better risk-stratify pts. Thus, the current intermediate-risk pts (in whom RT is not a standard component of first-line therapy), are not the same pts as those in the Castleberry study (as a group). As in low-risk pts, RT is typically reserved for pts with residual disease refractory to CHT, recurrent disease, or those who remain symptomatic.

Castleberry, POG (*JCO* 1991, PMID 2016621): PRT of 62 pts >1 year of age with POG stage C NB comparing surgery and CHT±RT. All pts received AC CHT x five cycles. Pts randomized to RT received treatment to the primary tumor and regional LNs. Age 12 to 24 mos: total dose 18 to 24 Gy; age ≥24 mos: total dose 24 to 30 Gy, with lower doses reserved for abdominal or thoracic paravertebral primary and SCV nodes. Second-look surgery was advised to evaluate response and to remove residual disease. Continuation CHT alternated AC with CDDP and teniposide for two courses each. **Conclusion: Stage C NB in children >1 yr of age is a higher risk group in whom the addition of RT to CHT provides superior initial and long-term control compared with CHT alone. Metastatic failures in both treatment groups suggest a need for more aggressive CHT.**

TABLE 57.8: Results of Castleberry Trial, RT for Intermediate Risk Neuroblastoma			
	CR	EFS	OS
RT	76%	59%	73%
No RT	46%	32%	41%
p value	.013	.009	.008

Twist, COG ANBL0531 Early Results (*ASCO* 2014, Abstract 10006): Phase III trial of 464 pts comparing different treatment regimens based on risk stratification to achieve optimal 3-yr OS. Stratification based on age, INSS stage, INPC, N-myc status, LOH of 1p and/or 11q, and tumor ploidy. Treatment was CHT (+/– isotretinoin) x two to eight cycles and/or surgery. 3-yr EFS and OS were 83% and 95%, respectively. No deaths in those with local disease and favorable biology. For stage 4S tumors, 3-yr EFS 90% and OS 95% for favorable histology (60 of 125) versus 63% and 76%, respectively, for unfavorable tumors (diploid or unfavorable histology). 3-yr OS improved to 95% if LOH of 1p or 11q. Eight stage 4S pts died with five deaths due to hepatomegaly. **Conclusion: Genomic risk**

stratification helped achieve excellent results in the majority of intermediate-risk pts. However, those with unfavorable biology may benefit from more extensive therapy.

High risk

What is the role of autologous SCT and adjuvant isotretinoin in high-risk disease?

Matthay, CCG 3891 (*NEJM* 1999, PMID 10519894, Update Matthay *JCO* 2009, PMID 19171716): Prospective study of 539 pts with high-risk NB. Induction CHT consisted of cisplatin, doxorubicin, etoposide, and cyclophosphamide x five cycles. After induction CHT, pts without progression underwent delayed primary surgery with nodal assessment followed by RT to gross residual disease. RT dose was 20 Gy/10 fx to extra-abdominal disease and 10 Gy/5 fx to mediastinal and intra-abdominal tumors. Pts were subsequently randomized to receive consolidation CHT or myeloablative CHT + TBI with SCT. Consolidation CHT consisted of three cycles of cisplatin, etoposide, doxorubicin, ifosfamide. Myeloablative CHT was carboplatin and etoposide. TBI was 10 Gy/3 fx daily. Following SCT or consolidation CHT, pts without disease progression were randomized to six cycles of 13-cis-retinoic acid (isotretinoin) or no further therapy. 5-yr EFS and OS for all pts were 26% and 36%, respectively. The 5-yr LRR was 51% for pts treated with CHT versus 33% for pts treated with SCT ($p = .0044$). 3-yr EFS with CHT was 22% versus 34% with SCT. 3-yr EFS after the second randomization was 46% among the 130 pts who received 13-cis-retinoic acid versus 29% among the 128 who received no further therapy ($p = .027$). 2009 update demonstrated 5-yr EFS of 19% for pts treated with consolidation CHT versus 30% for pts treated with SMT ($p = .04$). 5-yr EFS from second randomization was higher for isotretinoin than no further therapy, although not significant (42% vs. 31%). **Conclusions: This study set the standard treatment regimen for high-risk neuroblastoma, which includes both autologous SCT and isotretinoin.**

TABLE 57.9: Initial Results of Matthay CCG 3891				
CCG 3891	**3-yr EFS**	**5-yr LRR**	**Second randomization**	**3-yr EFS**
CHT	22%	51%	13-cis-RA	46%
HDC + ABMT	34%	33%	No therapy	29%
p value	.034	.004	*p* value	.027

Why are doses above 20 Gy recommended to control gross disease?

There appeared to be a benefit to the addition of TBI when only 10 Gy was used.

Haas-Kogan, Secondary Analysis of CCG 3891/Matthay (*IJROBP* 2003, PMID 12694821): Secondary analysis of the Matthay CCG 3891 focusing on those who received 10 Gy to the primary (abdominal and mediastinal tumors with gross disease remaining postoperatively). For pts who received 10 Gy to the primary, the addition of 10 Gy of TBI and BMT decreased LR compared with those who received continuous CHT and no TBI (22% vs. 52%, $p = .022$). **Conclusion: There may be a dose–response relationship for EBRT (20 Gy better LC than 10 Gy), but cannot distinguish the impact of the high-dose CHT and BMT received with it.**

Is there a benefit to tandem stem cell transplants?

Park, COG ANBL 0532 (*ASCO* 2016, Abstract LBA3): PRT of children with high-risk neuroblastoma randomized to either single autologous SCT versus tandem SCT. 652 pts, median 3.1 years of age. Tandem SCT improved 3-yr EFS from 48.8% to 61.8% ($p = .008$) with a nonsignificant improvement in OS (69.0%–73.8%, $p = .256$). 249 pts received post-consolidation immunotherapy, which also improved both EFS and OS (EFS 55.4% vs.

73.7%, $p < .001$; OS 75.7% vs. 86.3%, $p = .016$). **Conclusion: Tandem SCT improves EFS in pts with high-risk neuroblastoma.**

Is there a benefit to targeted immunotherapy in high-risk pts?

Ch14.18, a chimeric anti-GD2 antibody improves overall survival but at the cost of high acute toxicity in the form of pain and capillary leak syndrome.

Yu, COG ANBL0032 (NEJM 2010, PMID 20879881): PRT 226 pts randomized to immunotherapy versus standard therapy after myeloablative therapy and stem cell rescue. The immunotherapy arm was ch14.18 with alternating GM-CSF and IL2 (to stimulate Ab-dependent cell-mediated cytotoxicity) plus isotretinoin versus isotretinoin alone (standard arm). Ch14.18 is a chimeric anti-GD2 monoclonal Ab; GD2 is a surface protein on tissues of neuroectodermal origin.[46] Immunotherapy improved 2-yr EFS (66% vs. 46%, $p = .01$) and improved 2-yr OS (86% vs. 75%, $p = .02$). Grade 3-4 pain was higher in the immunotherapy arm, with 52% of pts having grade 3 or 4 pain. Additionally, 23% and 25% of pts in that arm had capillary leak syndrome and hypersensitivity reaction, respectively. Early in the study, two pts were inadvertently given an overdose of IL-2 (>20 times the intended dose), with one of these pts consequently experiencing grade 5 toxicity in the form of capillary leak with pulmonary edema. **Conclusion: Immunotherapy with anti GD-2 monoclonal antibodies shows improved outcomes compared to standard therapy.** *Comment: Closed early due to highly favorable results. FDA approved ch14.18 (dinutuximab) in 2015 for use in combination with GM-CSF, IL-2, and isotretinoin for high-risk neuroblastoma pts who achieve at least a partial response to standard multimodality therapy.[47]*

Is there a benefit to MIBG with I-131 or crizotinib in high-risk neuroblastoma?

This is the question of the ongoing study COG ANBL1531. Iobenguane I-131 is essentially therapeutic MIBG including I-131 (diagnostic MIBG includes I-123) and has shown dramatic responses in relapsed/refractory cases. Crizotinib is active against ALK mutated tumors.[48]

REFERENCES

1. Strother DR, London WB, Schmidt ML, et al. Outcome after surgery alone or with restricted use of chemotherapy for patients with low-risk neuroblastoma: results of Children's Oncology Group study P9641. *J Clin Oncol.* 2012;30(15):1842–1848.
2. Baker DL, Schmidt ML, Cohn SL, et al. Outcome after reduced chemotherapy for intermediate-risk neuroblastoma. *N Engl J Med.* 2010;363(14):1313–1323.
3. American Cancer Society. *Cancer Facts and Figures 2016.* Atlanta, GA: American Cancer Society; 2016. http://www.cancer.org/acs/groups/content/@research/documents/document/acspc-047079.pdf
4. Maris JM. Recent advances in neuroblastoma. *N Engl J Med.* 2010;362(23):2202–2211.
5. Pizzo PA, Poplack DG. *Principles and Practice of Pediatric Oncology.* 6th ed. Philadelphia, PA: Wolters Kluwer/Lippincott Williams & Wilkins Health; 2011.
6. Maris JM, Hogarty MD, Bagatell R, Cohn SL. Neuroblastoma. *Lancet.* 2007;369(9579):2106–2120.
7. Heck JE, Ritz B, Hung RJ, et al. The epidemiology of neuroblastoma: a review. *Paediatr Perinat Epidemiol.* 2009;23(2):125–143.
8. Cook MN, Olshan AF, Guess HA, et al. Maternal medication use and neuroblastoma in offspring. *Am J Epidemiol.* 2004;159(8):721–731.
9. Maris JM, Chatten J, Meadows AT, et al. Familial neuroblastoma: a three-generation pedigree and a further association with Hirschsprung disease. *Med Pediatr Oncol.* 1997;28(1):1–5.
10. Shimada H, Ambros IM, Dehner LP, et al. The International Neuroblastoma Pathology Classification (the Shimada system). *Cancer.* 1999;86(2):364–372.

11. Shimada H. Tumors of the neuroblastoma group. *Pathology.* 1993;2(1):43–59.
12. Hachitanda Y, Tsuneyoshi M, Enjoji M. Expression of pan-neuroendocrine proteins in 53 neuroblastic tumors. An immunohistochemical study with neuron-specific enolase, chromogranin, and synaptophysin. *Arch Pathol Lab Med.* 1989;113(4):381–384.
13. Sebire NJ, Gibson S, Rampling D, et al. Immunohistochemical findings in embryonal small round cell tumors with molecular diagnostic confirmation. *Appl Immunohistochem Mol Morphol.* 2005;13(1):1–5.
14. Hachitanda Y, Tsuneyoshi M, Enjoji M. An ultrastructural and immunohistochemical evaluation of cytodifferentiation in neuroblastic tumors. *Mod Pathol.* 1989;2(1):13–19.
15. Brodeur GM, Seeger RC, Schwab M, et al. Amplification of N-myc in untreated human neuroblastomas correlates with advanced disease stage. *Science.* 1984;224(4653):1121–1124.
16. Peifer M, Hertwig F, Roels F, et al. Telomerase activation by genomic rearrangements in high-risk neuroblastoma. *Nature.* 2015;526(7575):700–704.
17. Valentijn LJ, Koster J, Zwijnenburg DA, et al. TERT rearrangements are frequent in neuroblastoma and identify aggressive tumors. *Nat Genet.* 2015;47(12):1411–1414.
18. Schleiermacher G, Javanmardi N, Bernard V, et al. Emergence of new ALK mutations at relapse of neuroblastoma. *J Clin Oncol.* 2014;32(25):2727–2734.
19. Cheung NK, Dyer MA. Neuroblastoma: developmental biology, cancer genomics and immunotherapy. *Nat Rev Cancer.* 2013;13(6):397–411.
20. Schwab M. Oncogene amplification in solid tumors. *Semin Cancer Biol.* 1999;9(4):319–325.
21. Ambros PF, Ambros IM, Brodeur GM, et al. International consensus for neuroblastoma molecular diagnostics: report from the International Neuroblastoma Risk Group (INRG) Biology Committee. *Br J Cancer.* 2009;100(9):1471–1482.
22. Schilling FH, Spix C, Berthold F, et al. Neuroblastoma screening at one year of age. *N Engl J Med.* 2002;346(14):1047–1053.
23. Woods WG, Gao RN, Shuster JJ, et al. Screening of infants and mortality due to neuroblastoma. *N Engl J Med.* 2002;346(14):1041–1046.
24. Takeuchi LA, Hachitanda Y, Woods WG, et al. Screening for neuroblastoma in North America: preliminary results of a pathology review from the Quebec Project. *Cancer.* 1995;76(11):2363–2371.
25. Ikeda Y, Lister J, Bouton JM, Buyukpamukcu M. Congenital neuroblastoma, neuroblastoma in situ, and the normal fetal development of the adrenal. *J Pediatr Surg.* 1981;16(4, Suppl 1):636–644.
26. Brisse HJ, McCarville MB, Granata C, et al. Guidelines for imaging and staging of neuroblastic tumors: consensus report from the International Neuroblastoma Risk Group Project. *Radiology.* 2011;261(1):243–257.
27. Brodeur GM, Pritchard J, Berthold F, et al. Revisions of the international criteria for neuroblastoma diagnosis, staging, and response to treatment. *J Clin Oncol.* 1993;11(8):1466–1477.
28. Adams GA, Shochat SJ, Smith EI, et al. Thoracic neuroblastoma: a Pediatric Oncology Group study. *J Pediatr Surg.* 1993;28(3):372–377; discussion 377–378.
29. Evans AE, Albo V, D'Angio GJ, et al. Factors influencing survival of children with nonmetastatic neuroblastoma. *Cancer.* 1976;38(2):661–666.
30. Hayes FA, Green A, Hustu HO, Kumar M. Surgicopathologic staging of neuroblastoma: prognostic significance of regional lymph node metastases. *J Pediatr Surg.* 1983;102(1):59–62.
31. Cotterill SJ, Pearson AD, Pritchard J, et al. Clinical prognostic factors in 1,277 patients with neuroblastoma: results of the European Neuroblastoma Study Group 'Survey' 1982–1992. *Eur J Cancer.* 2000;36(7):901–908.
32. Castleberry RP, Shuster JJ, Altshuler G, et al. Infants with neuroblastoma and regional lymph node metastases have a favorable outlook after limited postoperative chemotherapy: a Pediatric Oncology Group study. *J Clin Oncol.* 1992;10(8):1299–1304.
33. Peuchmaur M, d'Amore ES, Joshi VV, et al. Revision of the International Neuroblastoma Pathology Classification: confirmation of favorable and unfavorable prognostic subsets in ganglioneuroblastoma, nodular. *Cancer.* 2003;98(10):2274–2281.
34. Cohn SL, Pearson AD, London WB, et al. The International Neuroblastoma Risk Group (INRG) classification system: an INRG Task Force report. *J Clin Oncol.* 2009;27(2):289–297.
35. Yoo SY, Kim JS, Sung KW, et al. The degree of tumor volume reduction during the early phase of induction chemotherapy is an independent prognostic factor in patients with high-risk neuroblastoma. *Cancer.* 2013;119(3):656–664.

36. Yanik GA, Parisi MT, Shulkin BL, et al. Semiquantitative mIBG scoring as a prognostic indicator in patients with stage 4 neuroblastoma: a report from the Children's Oncology Group. *J Nucl Med*. 2013;54(4):541–548.

37. Morris JA, Shcochat SJ, Smith EI, et al. Biological variables in thoracic neuroblastoma: a Pediatric Oncology Group study. *J Pediatr Surg*. 1995;30(2):296–302; discussion 302–293.

38. Nickerson HJ, Matthay KK, Seeger RC, et al. Favorable biology and outcome of stage IV-S neuroblastoma with supportive care or minimal therapy: a Children's Cancer Group study. *J Clin Oncol*. 2000;18(3):477–486.

39. Horner MJ, Ries LAG, Krapcho M, et al. eds. *SEER Cancer Statistics Review, 1975–2006, National Cancer Institute*. Bethesda, MD; 2009. http://seer.cancer.gov/csr/1975_2006/

40. Brodeur GM, Seeger RC, Barrett A, et al. International criteria for diagnosis, staging, and response to treatment in patients with neuroblastoma. *J Clin Oncol*. 1988;6(12):1874–1881.

41. Monclair T, Brodeur GM, Ambros PF, et al. The International Neuroblastoma Risk Group (INRG) staging system: an INRG Task Force report. *J Clin Oncol*. 2009;27(2):298–303.

42. Sidell N, Altman A, Haussler MR, Seeger RC. Effects of retinoic acid (RA) on the growth and phenotypic expression of several human neuroblastoma cell lines. *Exp Cell Res*. 1983;148(1):21–30.

43. Matthay KK, Villablanca JG, Seeger RC, et al. Treatment of high-risk neuroblastoma with intensive chemotherapy, radiotherapy, autologous bone marrow transplantation, and 13-cis-retinoic acid: Children's Cancer Group. *N Engl J Med*. 1999;341(16):1165–1173.

44. Ladenstein R, Potschger U, Gray J, et al. Toxicity and outcome of anti-GD2 antibody ch14.18/CHO in front-line, high-risk patients with neuroblastoma: final results of the phase III immunotherapy randomisation (HR-NBL1/SIOPEN trial). Paper presented at: ASCO2016; Chicago, IL.

45. Yu AL, Gilman AL, Ozkaynak MF, et al. Anti-GD2 antibody with GM-CSF, interleukin-2, and isotretinoin for neuroblastoma. *N Engl J Med*. 2010;363(14):1324–1334.

46. Yang RK, Sondel PM. Anti-GD2 Strategy in the treatment of neuroblastoma. *Drugs Future*. 2010;35(8):665–679.

47. U.S. Food and Drug Administration. FDA approves first therapy for high-risk neuroblastoma. FDA News Release; 2015. https://www.fda.gov/newsevents/newsroom/pressannouncements/ucm437460.htm

48. Chen Y, Takita J, Choi YL, et al. Oncogenic mutations of ALK kinase in neuroblastoma. *Nature*. 2008;455(7215):971–974.

58: WILLMS TUMOR

Yvonne D. Pham, John H. Suh, and Erin S. Murphy

QUICK HIT: Wilms tumor (WT) is the most common abdominal tumor in children. WT is managed with initial resection followed by risk-adapted CHT +/− RT. CHT is variable and usually consists of vincristine, actinomycin-D, and Adriamycin (with carboplatin/etoposide/cyclophosphamide added on protocol for higher risk patients). If indicated, deliver RT by postoperative day 10 (i.e., start by day 10, no later than day 14 with surgery day 0). RT is delivered based on pathologic findings as listed in Table 58.1. For stage IV, RT can be directed to the abdomen and whole lung separately, based on indications.

TABLE 58.1: General Strategy of Postoperative RT for Wilms Tumor

Indication	Target	Dose
Stage III, Favorable Histology Stage IV, Favorable Histology with Hilar Lymph Nodes Stage I-IV, Unfavorable Histology Recurrent Disease Residual Flank Disease	Flank	10.8 Gy/6 fx *(+9 Gy/5 fx boost for diffuse anaplasia)*
Surgical Spillage Peritoneal Seeding Malignant Ascites Preoperative Rupture	Whole Abdomen	10.5 Gy/7 fx *(+9 Gy/6 fx flank boost for diffuse anaplasia age>12 months or +10.5 Gy/7 fx boost for diffuse unresectable implants)*
Lung Metastases on Chest X-ray	Whole Lung Irradiation	12 Gy/8 fx *(10.5 Gy/7 fx if age <1)*

EPIDEMIOLOGY: WT accounts for 6% of childhood cancers with about 470 to 500 new cases per year in the United States. It is the most common abdominal tumor in children with a median age at diagnosis between 3 and 4 years of age for unilateral tumors. Bilateral cases occur in 4% to 8% at presentation and tend to present earlier at a median age of 2 to 3 years of age. 75% of pts present before 5 years of age. Females are more commonly affected; F:M is 1.09:1 for unilateral tumors and 1.67:1 for bilateral tumors.[1]

RISK FACTORS: Paternal occupation as a machinist or a welder and maternal use of hair dye.[2] Also associated with congenital anomalies in 10% to 13% of cases:

- **WAGR:** **W**ilms tumor, **A**niridia, **G**U malformations, mental **R**etardation. Caused by alteration of 11p13 with deletion of WT1 gene (Wilms tumor suppressor gene, important for normal kidney/gonadal development) and PAX6 (aniridia gene). 30% risk of developing WT.
- **Beckwith–Wiedemann:** Macrosomia, hemihypertrophy, macroglossia, omphalocele, abdominal organomegaly, ear pits/creases. Caused by alteration of 11p15 locus, which causes loss of imprinting of genes. 5% risk of developing WT.

- **Denys–Drash syndrome**: Renal disease (proteinuria during infancy, nephrotic syndrome, renal failure), male pseudohermaphroditism, and Wilms. Caused by alteration of 11p13 locus, causing point mutation in zinc-finger regions of WT1 gene. 50% to 90% risk of developing WT.[3]

ANATOMY: Wilms tumor originates from the kidney parenchyma and drains to perinephric and para-aortic lymph nodes.

PATHOLOGY: WT is an embryonic kidney tumor, classically triphasic with blastemal, epithelial, and stromal elements. WT tend to be lobulated and solid, lack calcifications, and may have soft and cystic areas. These tumors tend to be very large and often can compress adjacent structures but only the minority of cases show pathologic evidence of organ invasion.[1]

TABLE 58.2: Pathologic Types of Renal Tumors in Children		
Favorable histology (FH) Wilms tumor	Typical features (blastemal, epithelial, and stromal elements) without anaplastic or sarcomatous components.	
Unfavorable histology (UH) Wilms tumor; anaplastic Wilms tumor	Anaplasia refers to enlargement of nuclei, hyperchromatism of nuclei, and increased mitotic figures.	*Focal anaplasia (FA):* sharply localized in the primary tumor. *Diffuse anaplasia (DA):* nonlocalized or localized with significant nuclear unrest in remainder of tumor or found outside tumor capsule, in metastases, or on random biopsy of the tumor.
Rhabdoid tumor of the kidney (RTK)	Typically diagnosed before 2 years of age with eosinophilic cytoplasm and hyaline globular inclusions (+vimentin and cytokeratin), associated with primary CNS neoplasms (i.e., ATRT) and *INI1* mutations.	
Clear cell sarcoma of the kidney (CCSK)	4% of all childhood renal tumors.[4] About 5% present with metastases and 40%–60% with bone metastases compared to those with WT (2% incidence).[5] Tumor cells w/ abundant intracytoplasmic vesicles. No specific tumor markers but classically described as "chicken-wire" pattern with undifferentiated cells separated by fibrovascular septa.[6]	
Renal cell carcinoma	Approximately 6% of renal tumors in children, not included in classic studies; treatment is surgery alone, no clear role for adjuvant RT.	
All subtypes except FH are considered "high-risk" tumors.		

GENETICS: Poor prognosis associated with loss of heterozygosity (LOH) of 1p and/or 16q (worse if both). Those with early stage disease and loss of 1p16q are treated more aggressively with three-drug regimen (as for stage III/IV).

- Gain of 1q is associated with inferior survival for unilateral FH WT.[7]
- Although Wilms is associated with inactivation of the *WT1* tumor-suppressor gene in 5% to 10% of cases, about 1/3 of Wilms cases are associated with inactivation of a more recently described tumor suppressor gene referred to as **WTX** (unknown gene on X chromosome), which may be involved with normal kidney development. Tumors with *WTX* mutation lack *WT1* mutation. In contrast to *WT1*-associated Wilms, which required biallelic (two-hit) inactivation, *WTX* requires only one hit (i.e., the single X chromosome in males or the active X chromosome in females).[1]

SCREENING: If children present with worrisome physical exam findings that are associated with the predisposing genetic syndromes listed earlier, then screening may be appropriate with periodic abdominal ultrasounds.[1]

CLINICAL PRESENTATION: Abdominal mass (83%), fever (23%), hematuria (21%), abdominal pain (37%).[1] Can also have anemia (due to decreased EPO) and hypertension (from increased renin). See Table 58.3 for comparison between Wilms and neuroblastoma.

TABLE 58.3: Comparison Between Neuroblastoma and Wilms Tumor	
Neuroblastoma	Wilms
Classic eggshell calcifications on x-ray in 85%	No tumor calcifications (but may have calcifications from hemorrhage)
Displaces kidney ("drooping lily" sign) but does not distort renal architecture	Disrupts renal architecture
Mets to LNs, bone marrow, liver, skin (rarely to lung or brain)	Mets to lung, liver, bone
Frequently crosses midline	Often does not cross midline

WORKUP: H&P (including assessment for congenital anomalies)

Labs: Urinalysis including urinary catecholamines (to rule out neuroblastoma)

Imaging: Abdominal ultrasound including contralateral kidney and evaluation of thrombosis/extension into renal vein or IVC. MRI, CT chest, abdomen, pelvis, and CXR (studies have relied on whether pulmonary metastases are visible on CXR; positive CT with a negative CXR can present controversy). *Do not biopsy* unless unresectable or bilateral disease to avoid local tumor spillage. If biopsy is necessary, use posterior approach to avoid abdominal contamination and contain bleeding or spillage if they occur. Once pathology available, obtain further workup if CCSK or RTK (bone scan, skeletal survey, bone marrow biopsy, MRI brain).

PROGNOSTIC FACTORS: LOH 1p and/or 16q, gain of 1q, higher stage, unfavorable histology, and age >24 months portend a worse prognosis.

STAGING: Two systems exist: National Wilms Tumor Study Group (NWTSG, often referred to as simply NWTS) versus Société Internationale d'Oncologie Pédiatrique (SIOP) staging. NWTS system emphasizes postsurgical, pre-CHT staging to obtain most "unadulterated" information (extent of primary, degree of anaplasia, presence of unusual histology, +/- LN). SIOP philosophy is neoadjuvant treatment with CHT and/or RT in an effort to reduce extent of disease and increase en bloc resection, but at the expense of losing or obscuring some of the information listed earlier. NWTS staging is currently in use by the COG and listed in Table 58.4.[1]

TABLE 58.4: NWTS/COG Staging for Wilms Tumor[1]	
I	Tumor limited to kidney, completely excised. The renal capsule is intact. Tumor was not ruptured or biopsied prior to removal. The vessels of the renal sinus are not involved. There is no evidence of tumor at or beyond the margins of resection.
II	Tumor is completely resected and there is no evidence of tumor at or beyond the margins of resection. The tumor extends beyond kidney, as is evidenced by any one of the following criteria: There is regional extension of the tumor (i.e., penetration of the renal capsule, or extensive invasion of the soft tissue of the renal sinus). Blood vessels within the nephrectomy specimen outside the renal parenchyma, including those of the renal sinus, contain tumor.

(continued)

TABLE 58.4: NWTS/COG Staging for Wilms Tumor[1] (*continued*)		
III	Residual nonhematogenous tumor present following surgery, and confined to abdomen. Any one of the following may occur: • Lymph nodes within the abdomen or pelvis are involved by tumor (lymph node involvement in the thorax or other extra-abdominal sites is a criterion for stage IV) • Tumor has penetrated through the peritoneal surface • Tumor implants are found on the peritoneal surface • Gross or microscopic tumor remains postoperatively (e.g., tumor cells are found at the margin of surgical resection on microscopic examination) • Tumor is not completely resectable because of local infiltration into vital structures • Tumor spillage occurring either before or during surgery • Tumor was biopsied (whether tru-cut, open, or fine needle aspiration) before removal • Tumor is removed in greater than one piece (e.g., tumor cells are found in a separately excised adrenal gland; a tumor thrombus within the renal vein is removed separately from the nephrectomy specimen)	**Helpful Mnemonic for Stage III Wilms (SLURPPIB):** S STR/+Margin L LN (abdominal) U Unresectable R Rupture/Spillage P Piecemeal resection (including thrombus not removed en bloc) P Preoperative CHT required (unresectable) I Implant (i.e., peritoneal involvement, including peritoneal penetration) B Biopsy
IV	Hematogenous metastases (lung, liver, bone, brain, etc.) or lymph node metastases outside the abdominopelvic region are present	
V	Bilateral renal involvement by tumor present at diagnosis	

TREATMENT PARADIGM

Surgery: Radical nephrectomy is the initial definitive treatment of choice for WT in the United States. Historically, nephrectomy alone (1930s) achieved cure in only 15% to 30%. Surgery alone is being investigated for very low-risk patients on protocol (COG AREN 0532). 90% to 95% of patients are resectable at diagnosis via wide transverse abdominal incision and radical nephrectomy with assessment of surgical margins and avoidance of spillage via a transperitoneal approach. Tumors that are marginally resectable or with large central necrosis, which may portend increased risk for spillage, may benefit from neoadjuvant therapy with CHT or RT. This is a complex surgery (10% tumors involve renal vein; 15% tumors involve IVC/atrium). Inspect/palpate abdominal cavity, liver and LN for extent of tumor spread; examine and palpate opposite kidney; inspect and palpate renal vein to exclude tumor thrombus. Regional LN sampling for accurate staging. Tumor spillage incidence is 15% to 30% in the literature[1] and is significantly associated with abdominal recurrence and mortality.[8] Incidence of surgical complications with nephrectomy (as per NWTS-4) is 11%. Most common complications are hemorrhage and SBO. Quality of surgery has prognostic importance (e.g., degree of LN sampling, spillage, unnecessary biopsies) and QA among COG surgeons is underway.

Chemotherapy: CHT has improved overall results for WT in the past two decades via NWTS and SIOP studies. In Europe, CHT is typically given preoperatively. In North America, it is given adjuvantly following initial nephrectomy. Preoperative CHT can be required if there is bulky, unresectable disease, bilateral WT, WT in a solitary kidney, or tumor thrombus in IVC. The use of specific agents varies with stage. Lower stages (I and II) typically are treated with vincristine and actinomycin-D. Stage III/IV disease and UH are typically treated with three or more agents including Adriamycin.

Radiation: RT formerly played a much larger role in WT and was historically used postoperatively to the tumor bed at 2 Gy/day to 40–50 Gy. Now, approximately 25% of patients with WT are treated with RT (only 15%, if metastatic disease is excluded). **Traditional start for RT is by day 10 after surgery,** no later than day 14, if surgery is designated day 0. A later radiation start is linked to increased risk of abdominal recurrence in some studies. RT is given concurrently with vincristine and actinomycin-D.

Indications: See Table 58.1. Typically, at least flank RT is indicated for stage III disease, unfavorable histology or positive margins. Whole abdomen irradiation (WAI) indicated for mnemonic "SPAR" (**S**pillage during surgery, **P**eritoneal seeding, malignant **A**scites, or preoperative **R**upture).

Dose: Dose for flank RT is 10.8 Gy/6 fx with boost to any residual gross disease to 21.6 Gy. Give flank RT to 19.8 Gy if ≥16 years of age or if stage III diffuse anaplasia or I-III rhabdoid (+10.8 Gy boost to gross disease; total 30.6 Gy). WAI typically 10.5 Gy/7 fx or 21 Gy/14 fx for diffuse unresectable peritoneal implants. Whole lung irradiation (WLI) indicated for lung metastases on CXR (not if mets only visible on CT) at a dose of 12 Gy/8 fx (10.5 Gy if <1 year of age). If WLI and flank are indicated together, can treat flank to 10.5 Gy simultaneously with WLI to 12 Gy/8 fx or at separate times (do not feather or block to adjust for overlap).

Procedure: See *Treatment Planning Handbook,* Chapter 12 for details.[9]

Toxicities

Renal: ~1% of pts with unilateral WT will have end-stage renal disease from chronic renal failure 20 yrs from diagnosis; 3.1% for pts with bilateral WT.[10]

Premature mortality: Risk of death from all causes increased from 5.4% to 22.7% at 30 and 50 years of age, respectively, after WT diagnosis. 50% of excess deaths beyond 30 yrs from diagnosis were attributable to secondary neoplasms and 25% from cardiac diseases.[11]

Cardiac: The risk of CHF increases with increasing total dose of Adriamycin received, increasing amount of RT received by the heart, and female gender. 1.7% of pts treated w/ ADR on NWTS-1-4 developed CHF compared to 5.4% in pts treated with WLI.[1,12]

Pulmonary: 10% of pts w/ pulmonary mets treated on NWTS-3 developed "diffuse interstitial pneumonitis of unknown etiology" (possibly radiation pneumonitis) after WLI. There were four additional cases of diffuse pneumonitis secondary to *varicella* and PJP. Give trimethoprim/sulfamethoxazole for PJP prophylaxis with WLI. The incidence of pneumonitis has subsequently decreased by reducing the dose of Adriamycin and actinomycin-D given concurrently with RT.

Hepatic: In SIOP-9, 8% of children developed hepatotoxicity consistent with veno-occlusive disease with the combination of CHT and RT.[13]

Reproductive: Females who receive RT or CHT during childhood for unilateral WT had an increased risk for hypertension complicating pregnancy, fetal malpositioning, and premature labor.[14]

Musculoskeletal: RT is associated with development of scoliosis and reduction in height with severity increasing with younger age and increasing dose to the spine.[15]

Second malignancies: GI, soft tissue sarcomas, and breast cancers are the most frequent secondary neoplasms to develop after treatment.[16] Cumulative incidence of invasive breast cancer for survivors who received lung RT is almost 15% by 40 years of age.[17]

EVIDENCE-BASED Q&A

What are the main findings of the National Wilms Tumor Studies (NWTS) I-V?

*Note that early NWTS studies used a **grouping** system that was a predecessor to the current NWTS staging system. Groups I and V are essentially the same as the corresponding stages, although group V included patients who develop contralateral tumors at some point after diagnosis (whereas stage V currently is limited to those with bilateral disease at diagnosis). Group II included PA LN involvement, while group III included any LN beyond the abdominal PA chains. Group IV included only hematogenous metastases.*

■ **NWTS-1 (1969–1974): D'Angio (*Cancer* 1976 PMID 184912)**
   o Postop RT is not needed for group I <2 y/o, but did improve DFS for pts ≥2 y/o ($p = .002$).
   o VCR + AMD are better than either agent alone in groups II and III.
   o For group III w/ local spillage or pre-op biopsy, no need for WAI.
   o Pre-op VCR does not help stage IV.
   o Age ≥2 y/o, the presence of anaplastic or sarcomatous features and LN involvement were found to be poor prognostic factors.

■ **NWTS-2 (1974–1979): D'Angio (*Cancer* 1981 PMID 6164480)**
   o Excellent survival rates for group I pts receiving VA CHT; thus RT is not needed for stage I FH patients.
   o Six months of VA is equal to 15 months for stage I.
   o ADR in addition to VCR and AMD helped for groups II-IV.
   o No dose response from 18 to 40 Gy for flank RT.
   o Total lung RT dose should be 12 Gy, due to 10% risk of "pneumonopathy" w/ 14 Gy.
   o Unfavorable histology, small RT field size, and RT delay of ≥10 days are poor prognostic factors for LR.

■ **NWTS-3 (1979–1985): D'Angio (*Cancer* 1989 PMID 2544249)**
   (Note: Changed from grouping system to staging system; however, until after NWTS-4, local spillage was considered stage II rather than III)
   o Distinction between FH and UH was incorporated into treatment algorithm.
   o For stage I FH, 10 weeks of AMD + VCR is equal to 6 mos, OS 96%.
   o For stage II FH, there was no benefit to the addition of ADR (VA alone sufficient) or RT.
   o For stage III FH, 10 Gy is equal to 20 Gy if ADR is added.
   o Cyclophosphamide improves outcomes in UH (focal anaplasia) stages II–IV but not FH stage IV.

■ **NWTS-4 (1986–1994): Green (*JCO* 1998 PMID 9440748; Green *JCO* 1998 PMID 9850017).**
   o For stage I FH or anaplastic pts, pulse-intense (PI) VCR + AMD x 18 weeks is equivalent to standard VCR + AMD x 25 weeks.
   o For stage II FH, PI VCR + AMD for 6 months is as effective, less costly, and less toxic (hematologic) than standard VCR + AMD for 15 months.
   o For stages III-IV FH, PI VCR + AMD + ADR for 6 months is as effective, less costly, and less toxic than standard VCR + AMD + ADR for 15 months.
   o **Seibel (*JCO* 2004 PMID 14752069):** Long-term update shows long-course CHT associated with better RFS in CCSK, but OS no different.
   o Local spillage without RT has unacceptable LR risk; moved to stage III for FH (need adjuvant RT).

■ **NWTS-5 (1995–2001):**
   o **Shamberger (*Ann Surg* 2010 PMID 20142733):** Stage I FH, pts <2 y/o, and tumors <550 g had an increased rate of relapse with nephrectomy alone (without adjuvant CHT) but no difference in OS with or without CHT.

- o **Dome (*JCO* 2006 PMID 16710034):** Vincristine/Adriamycin/cyclophosphamide/ etoposide improved outcomes for stages II-IV with DA.
- o **Grundy (*JCO* 2005 PMID 16129848):** For stages I-II FH pts, risk of relapse and death were increased with LOH at 1p, 16q, or both. For stages III-IV FH, risk of relapse and death were increased only with LOH for both 1p and 16q (RR = 2.4, p = .01 and RR = 2.7, p = .04).

What is the impact of RT in the setting of tumor spillage?

Helps with decreasing abdominal tumor recurrence rates.

Kalapurakal, NWTS 4 & 5 Pooled (*IJROBP* 2010 PMID 19395185): Analyzed influence of irradiation (Flank and WAI) and CHT regimens on abdominal recurrence after intra-operative spillage of FH Wilms on NWTS-4 and 5. OR for recurrence after RT versus no RT was 0.35 (0.15–0.78) for 10 Gy and 0.08 (0.01–0.58) for 20 Gy. OR for CHT after adjusting for RT was not significant. For stage II pts (NWTS-4), 8-yr RFS with and without spillage, respectively, was 79% versus 87% (p = .07) and OS was 90% versus 95% (p = .04). **Conclusion: RT (10 Gy or 20 Gy) reduced abdominal tumor recurrence rates after tumor spillage. Tumor spillage in Stage II patients associated with decreased RFS and significantly decreased OS.**

What is the role of WLI in patients with FH Wilms who have pulmonary metastases detected by CT only? What is the role of Adriamycin in this setting?

No OS benefit with ADR, no benefit with WLI.

Grundy, NWTS 4 & 5 Pooled (*Pediatr Blood Cancer* 2012, PMID 22422736): 417 pts with FH WT and isolated lung metastases on NWTS-4 and -5. Compared outcomes by method of detection (CXR vs. CT only), use of WLI, and two- or three-drug CHT (AMD and VCR +/- ADR). For pts with CT-only lung mets (negative CXR), 5-yr EFS was greater with three drugs (including Adriamycin) with or without WLI versus only two drugs (80% vs. 56%; p = .004); OS was not impacted (87% vs. 86%; p = .91). For pts with CT-only lung mets, WLI showed a trend for benefit with regard to 5-yr EFS (81.0% vs. 70.1%; p = .11), but this disappeared when the analysis was adjusted for the CHT regimen (p = .52). There was no difference in OS with or without WLI. **Conclusion: Pts with CT-only lung mets have improved EFS but not OS with the addition of ADR; they do not seem to benefit from WLI.**

What are the early outcomes of omission of WLI from AREN 0533 (higher risk favorable histology study)?

WLI may not be necessary for patients with FH WT with CR of lung nodules after 6 weeks of CHT.

Dix, AREN 0533 (*ASCO* 2015, Abstract 10011): Examined whether pts w/ stage IV pulmonary mets only without LOH 1p and 16q who have a CR of lung nodules after 6 weeks of CHT can maintain excellent EFS without the use WLI. The null hypothesis is that 4-year EFS is 85% for CR after vincristine/actinomycin-D/Adriamycin and WLI. Among 391 pts enrolled, 296 had lung-only metastases, of which 105 (39%) had CR. At interim analysis in June 2014, 20 events were observed: 19/20 were recurrences and 1 was a second malignancy. Recurrences were in the lung only (17), lung and liver (1), and abdomen (1). 4-yr EFS and OS estimates for the CR patients were 78% (95% CI: 68%–86%) and 95% (95% CI: 83%–98%). **Conclusions: EFS was slightly less than historical standards although not statistically significant. Omission of WLI may be an acceptable treatment approach for this patient subgroup.**

REFERENCES

1. Halperin EC Constine LS, Tarbell NJ, Kun LE. eds. *Pediatric Radiation Oncology.* 5th edn. Philadelphia, PA: Lippincott Williams & Wilkins; 2012:257–289.
2. Bunin GR NC, Kramer S, Meadows AT. Parental occupation and Wilms' tumor: results of a case-control study. *Cancer Res.* 1989;49(3):725–729.
3. Dome JS, Coppes MJ. Recent advances in Wilms tumor genetics. *Curr Opin Pediat.* 2002;14(1):5–11.
4. Sebire NJ, Vujanic GM. Paediatric renal tumours: recent developments, new entities and pathological features. *Histopathology.* 2009;54(5):516–528.
5. Miniati D, Gay AN, Parks KV, et al. Imaging accuracy and incidence of Wilms' and non-Wilms' renal tumors in children. *J Pediatr Surg.* 2008;43(7):1301–1307.
6. Boo YJ, Fisher JC, Haley MJ, et al. Vascular characterization of clear cell sarcoma of the kidney in a child: a case report and review. *J Pediatr Surg.* 2009;44(10):2031–2036.
7. Gratias EJ, Dome JS, Jennings LJ, et al. Association of chromosome 1q gain with inferior survival in favorable-histology Wilms tumor: a report from the Children's Oncology Group. *J Clin Oncol.* 2016;34(26):3189–3194.
8. Shamberger RC, Guthrie KA, Ritchey ML, et al. Surgery-related factors and local recurrence of Wilms tumor in National Wilms Tumor Study 4. *Ann Surg.* 1999;229(2):292–297.
9. Videtic GMM, Woody N, Vassil AD. *Handbook of Treatment Planning in Radiation Oncology.* 2nd ed. New York, NY: Demos Medical; 2015.
10. Lange J, Peterson SM, Takashima JR, et al. Risk factors for end stage renal disease in non-WT1-syndromic Wilms tumor. *J Urol.* 2011;186(2):378–386.
11. Wong KF, Reulen RC, Winter DL, et al. Risk of adverse health and social outcomes up to 50 years after Wilms tumor: the British Childhood Cancer Survivor Study. *J Clin Oncol.* 2016;34(15):1772–1779.
12. Green DM, Grigoriev YA, Nan B, et al. Congestive heart failure after treatment for Wilms' tumor: a report from the National Wilms' Tumor Study group. *J Clin Oncol.* 2001;19(7):1926–1934.
13. Bisogno G, de Kraker J, Weirich A, et al. Veno-occlusive disease of the liver in children treated for Wilms tumor. *Med Pediatr Oncol.* 1997;29(4):245–251.
14. Green DM, Lange JM, Peabody EM, et al. Pregnancy outcome after treatment for Wilms tumor: a report from the National Wilms Tumor Long-Term Follow-Up Study. *J Clin Oncol.* 2010;28(17):2824–2830.
15. Hogeboom CJ, Grosser SC, Guthrie KA, et al. Stature loss following treatment for Wilms tumor. *Med Pediatr Oncol.* 2001;36(2):295–304.
16. Termuhlen AM, Tersak JM, Liu Q, et al. Twenty-five–year follow-up of childhood Wilms tumor: a report from the Childhood Cancer Survivor Study. *Pediatr Blood Cancer.* 2011;57(7):1210–1216.
17. Lange JM, Takashima JR, Peterson SM, et al. Breast cancer in female survivors of Wilms tumor: a report from the National Wilms Tumor Late-Effects Study. *Cancer.* 2014;120(23):3722–3730.

59: EWING'S SARCOMA

Ehsan H. Balagamwala and Erin S. Murphy

QUICK HIT: Ewing's sarcoma is the second most common primary bone tumor in childhood. Males affected more than females and peak age is 10 to 15 years of age. Important genetic mutations include t(11;22) and t(21;22). Workup includes evaluation of primary site with CT/MRI, PET/CT, bilateral bone marrow biopsies, and biopsy of the primary tumor.

TABLE 59.1: General Treatment Paradigm for Ewing's Sarcoma	
Induction (Week 1)	VAdriaC+IE for 6 cycles
Local Control (Week 13)	Surgery (preferred) or RT or combined modality (see Table 59.2)
Consolidation	VAdriaC+IE for 11 cycles, adjuvant RT (if indicated) starts cycle 1 of consolidation ASAP after surgery

EPIDEMIOLOGY: Described in 1921 by James Ewing as an undifferentiated tumor involving the diaphysis of long bones that is radiation sensitive (in contrast to osteosarcoma).[1] Ewing's sarcoma is the second most common primary bone tumor in children and the most lethal bone tumor. Of the ~700 children and adolescents with bone tumors diagnosed annually, approximately 200 cases are Ewing's sarcoma (~3% of childhood cancers).[2] Peak age is approximately 15 years of age, with 30% each <10 years of age or >20 years of age.[2] More common in Caucasian boys (M to F ratio is 1.5:1).

RISK FACTORS: No known environmental or familial risk factors.[3] No convincing evidence of inheritance.

ANATOMY: 50% originate in an extremity (20%–30% proximal and 30%–40% distal), and 50% central (45% pelvis, 35% chest wall, 10% spine, <10% remainder). Long bone tumors usually present in diaphysis, as opposed to osteosarcoma, which originates in the metaphysis.[4]

PATHOLOGY: Generally, sarcomas are divided into two categories: (a) tumors displaying complex karyotypic abnormalities with no distinct pattern and (b) tumors associated with particular chromosomal translocations that result in specific fusion genes. Ewing's sarcoma family of tumors (ESFT) belong to the second category. Although controversial, ESFT is thought to originate from the postganglionic parasympathetic neural cells as opposed to neuroblastoma, which originate from the sympathetic system. Microscopically, ESFT appear as monomorphic sheets of small, round blue cells usually with extensive necrosis but morphology alone is insufficient for diagnosis. ESFT includes Ewing's sarcoma of bone (ESB), extraosseous Ewing's (EOE), and primitive peripheral PNET (neuroepithelioma, adult neuroblastoma, Askin's tumor, and paravertebral small cell tumor). Staining: positive for MIC2 glycoprotein, PAS, vimentin. Negative for neuron-specific enolase (NSE, positive in PNET), and S100 (positive in PNET). Types: typical (i.e., classic) versus atypical (lobular, alveolar, or organoid).[4]

GENETICS: ESFT usually defined by a translocation in the EWSR1 gene. 90% display t(11;22)(q24;q12). t(21;22)(q21;q12) is the second most common (approximately 5%–10%) with a number of other less common translocations or structural aberrations in the remainder of cases (e.g., t[7;22], t[17;22], gain of chromosome 8 and 12, and deletion of 1p, del CDKN2A, mutation p53).[5] t(11;22) results in fusion of FLI-1 gene (DNA-binding transcription factor) on 11q24 with the EWS gene (RNA-binding protein) on 22q12. EWS-FLI-1 is a transcription factor that impacts cell cycle regulation, apoptosis, and telomerase activity. t(21;22) results in EWS-ERG fusion product and phenotype is identical to EWS-FLI-1. FISH/PCR is used for detection of fusion transcripts. Desmoplastic small round cell tumor (DSRCT) and malignant melanoma of soft parts also associated with EWS translocation.

CLINICAL PRESENTATION: Pain (>90%), swelling or mass (65%), limitation in movement (25%), neurologic changes (15% overall, though 50% in central tumors), pathologic fracture (15%), fever (10%). Approximately 25% have overt metastases at presentation. Of metastases, 40% lung, 40% bone, and infrequently to other sites. 25% to 30% risk for overt metastases in pelvic primaries and <10% for extremity primaries. Micrometastases assumed to be present at diagnosis in nearly all patients because of a high distant failure rate with local therapy alone. The risk of lymph node metastasis at diagnosis is low. Askin's tumor is a primary ES of the rib, associated with direct pleural extension and a large extraosseous soft tissue mass. Females are more commonly diagnosed with Askin's.[4] Differential includes osteomyelitis, lymphoma of the bone, leukemia (chloroma), rhabdomyosarcoma, metastatic neuroblastoma, small cell osteosarcoma, eosinophilic granuloma, metastatic small cell lung cancer or mesenchymal chondrosarcoma. Mnemonic for bone tumors "EG-MODE": **E**piphysis (**G**iant cell tumor), **M**etaphysis (**O**steosarcoma), **D**iaphysis (**E**wing's sarcoma). Differential for small round blue cell tumors (mnemonic LEMONS): **L**ymphoma, **E**wing's, **M**edulloblastoma, **O**ther (rhabdomyosarcoma, pineoblastoma, ependymoblastoma, etc.), **N**euroblastoma, **S**mall cell carcinoma.

WORKUP: H&P.

Labs: CBC, BMP, LDH.

Imaging: Plain x-ray, CT, and MRI of the involved bone, CT chest, PET/CT. Plain x-ray findings range from lytic (75%) to sclerotic (25%), "moth-eaten," "onion skinning" (layers of reactive bone), "Codman's triangle" (displaced periosteum with cortical destruction; also present in osteosarcoma), soft tissue mass in 50%. CT bone outlines bony destruction and soft tissue extent, enhances with contrast. MRI is 90% accurate for diagnosis with improved soft tissue definition. CT chest evaluates for metastasis. PET assesses tumor viability, evaluates for metastases (most helpful in lymph nodes and bone) and is the most sensitive test for follow-up after treatment. CT more reliable for lung metastasis compared to PET.[6] SUV >5.8 associated with worse survival.[7]

Pathology: Bilateral bone marrow biopsy and biopsy of the tumor. Biopsy should be performed by the surgeon who will be resecting the tumor to avoid compromising later operation such as limb salvage. FNA is inadequate; CT-guided core needle biopsy is usually sufficient. Open biopsy should be done only if necrotic material on core. Always include biopsy site in predicted operative site.

PROGNOSTIC FACTORS: Presence of metastases is the most important (bone or liver worse than lung, multiple lung lesions worse than solitary). Other poor factors (many of which predict for mets): tumor >8 cm, age >17, male gender, elevated LDH, tumor volume >200 cc, central tumors (esp. pelvic, also ribs, humerus, femur), and expression of p53 or deletion of INK4A. Mnemonic: "**MASSS**ive **LDH R**esponse": **M**ale gender, **A**ge >17, pelvic/axial **S**ite, **S**ize >8 cm, **S**tage (+mets), high **LDH**, **R**esponse to chemotherapy. Good response to chemo (>90%) is positive prognostic factor.

NATURAL HISTORY: Marked improvement in 5-yr OS since 1975 (35%) to current 5-yr OS (70%–80%) for nonmetastatic patients, principally due to addition of intensive chemotherapy. Metastases are not uniformly fatal, with average 5-yr OS of approximately 30% in modern era. Dominant pattern of failure for large tumors remains distant metastasis despite aggressive chemo.

STAGING: No formal staging. Stratification is by presence or absence of metastatic disease.

TREATMENT PARADIGM

Surgery: For local control, resection preferred unless poor functional results are anticipated. Resection provides pathologic information postchemotherapy, avoids second malignancy and late effects of RT. Resection without reconstruction can be done in small bones such as rib, clavicle, proximal fibula, distal scapula, metatarsals, metacarpals, and small iliac wing or pubic bone lesions. Results are typically very good for these "dispensable bones."[8,9] Large lesions may require allograft or endoprosthetic reconstructions. In the metastatic setting, surgery may be helpful for limited pulmonary metastases, or palliation at primary site. A systematic review of local control options suggested that the optimal treatment approach should be individualized based on patient and disease characteristics as well as patient preference.[9,10] Nodal dissection is not routinely indicated.

Chemotherapy: Induction CHT is given to all patients. Compressed VAdriaC-IE (q2 week cycles) is the current standard. Agents: vincristine (neuropathy, constipation, myalgias, arthralgias, and cholestasis), cyclophosphamide (pancytopenia and dose-dependent hemorrhagic cystitis, infertility), doxorubicin (myocardial dysfunction and pancytopenia), ifosfamide (high incidence of hemorrhagic cystitis requiring use of Mesna and Fanconi syndrome of electrolyte wasting), etoposide (pancytopenia, anaphylactic reactions, and second malignancies such as AML). No role for further intensification with higher doses of cyclophosphamide, ifosfamide, and doxorubicin due to increased toxicity and risk of second malignancy without improvement in EFS and OS.[8,10]

Radiation: RT potentially indicated pre-op, post-op, or definitively for the primary tumor and for treatment of pulmonary and skeletal metastases. Indications for postoperative RT include close margins (<1 cm), poor histologic response (<90% necrosis) or tumor spill.[11] Preoperative RT considered when close/positive margins are expected. Treat pre-chemo volume due to high rate of local failure if limited to post-chemo volume.[12] Involved field rather than whole bone is sufficient. Hyperfractionation does not improve outcomes, but may improve fracture rate, range of motion, and muscle atrophy. Adjuvant RT starts at the time of consolidation CHT (week 14). VC-IE CHT is given during RT (doxorubicin held during RT). Dose as per AEWS 1031 in Table 59.2.

TABLE 59.2: Radiation Therapy Guidelines for Ewing's Sarcoma Summary as per AEWS 1031			
Situation	**Dose**	**Volumes**	**Concurrent Chemotherapy?**
Preoperative	36 Gy	Pre-chemo GTV	VC-IE (no doxorubicin)
Definitive	45 Gy CD to 55.8 Gy	Pre-chemo GTV Gross residual/post-chemo	VC-IE (no doxorubicin)
Postoperative (i.e., microscopic)	50.4 Gy (>90% necrosis) 55.8 Gy (<90% necrosis)	Post-chemo GTV Pre-chemo GTV	VC-IE (no doxorubicin)

(continued)

TABLE 59.2: Radiation Therapy Guidelines for Ewing's Sarcoma Summary as per AEWS 1031 *(continued)*			
Situation	Dose	Volumes	Concurrent Chemotherapy?
Ipsilateral/ Bilateral lung RT	15 Gy; 1.5 Gy/ fx	Bilateral lungs (boost primary/lung nodules)	No doxorubicin or actinomycin D. Can use busulfan instead of WLI Chemo v RT: question on AEWS1031
Bone metastasis	45–56 Gy		
Vertebral body	45 Gy Boost to 50.4 Gy	Pre-chemo GTV + 1 cm (entire VB + 0.5 cm) Post-chemo GTV + 0.5–1 cm	

Special cases/notes:
– Do not treat across a joint or encompass an extremity circumferentially (spare strip) unless absolutely necessary for tumor coverage.
– Reduce margins if there is no extension beyond joint space, but adjacent epiphysis is in volume.
– For diaphyseal lesion, exclude one epiphysis of affected bone, if possible.
– If CR to chemo, boost prechemotherapy volume.
– For intraoperative spill, boost prechemotherapy volume.
– When using pre-op RT, if there is microscopic residual, evaluate necrosis; if >90%, then 14.4 Gy boost to post-chemo GTV; if necrosis is <90%, then 14.4 Gy boost to pre-chemo GTV.
– If gross residual, then cone down to 55.8 Gy to pre-chemo GTV.
– For metastatic lesions, SBRT to doses approximating 40 Gy/5 fx can be considered if TG 101 normal tissue constraints can be met (ongoing evaluation on current COG AEWS 1221).

Rib primary or Askin's tumor: Do not attempt resection prior to CHT. Preoperative CHT improves negative margins (50% vs. 77%) and decreased need for post-op RT (5-yr EFS 56%[13]). Some treat entire ipsilateral hemithorax (15–18 Gy, 1.5 Gy/fx) before reducing field to complete dose schedule as above, especially if lung metastasis or positive pleural cytology present.[14] Some have used intrapleural colloidal P32 in addition to EBRT to spare lung while treating pleura.

Metastatic disease: Low dose bilateral lung RT (15 Gy, 1.5 Gy/fx) can control gross metastatic disease in the lungs without significant pulmonary toxicity, and is usually recommended after CHT, despite paucity of data. Bone metastases can be controlled with doses from 45 to 56 Gy. If substantial amounts of marrow will be included in the RT field, consider delaying until the end of systemic therapy.

Toxicity: May potentiate bladder and cardiotoxicity from CHT. Older studies demonstrated loss of 25% remaining growth in limb for >50 Gy, particularly if including joint or epiphysis. May consider amputation and prosthesis in the very young as they recover function well.

Second malignancy: Rates reported from 6.5% to 9.2% at 20-yr in recent studies. Risk is highest for doses >60 Gy, and minimal for <48 Gy. Most common second tumor is osteosarcoma. In a recent review of RT-induced osteosarcoma, most common primary was Ewing's (25%), median latency was 8 years. 5-yr OS was 40% overall, with aggressive CHT and surgery 5-yr OS 68% versus chemo alone 17%.[15]

EVIDENCE-BASED Q&A

What is the utility of chemotherapy in Ewing's sarcoma?

CHT forms the cornerstone of therapy for Ewing's sarcoma. Due to suboptimal outcomes with VAC-based CHT, efforts were made to add agents as well as intensify the regimens. VACA was found to be superior to VAC (IESS-1) and subsequently, high-dose intermittent VACA was found to be superior to standard-dose VACA (IESS-II). Given the activity of IE in metastatic Ewing's sarcoma, VACA+IE was tested in the definitive setting was found to be superior to high-dose intermittent VACA (IESS-III). Subsequently, both dose intensification (IESS-IV) and interval compression (AEWS0031) of VAdriaC+IE were evaluated and showed that VAdriaC+IE q2wks was superior and forms the current standard of care in the definitive setting.

Nesbit, IESS-I (*JCO* 1990, PMID 2213103): 342 pts with biopsy-proven, nonmetastatic, previously untreated ESB from 1973 to 1978. Median 13 years of age. Three treatments: (a) RT (1° site) + VACA, (b) RT (1° site) + VAC, or (c) RT (1° site) + VAC + bilateral pulmonary RT (BPR). Randomization: 1 versus 2, and 2 versus 3. RT (1° site): 45 to 55 Gy (<5 y/o 45 Gy, 5–15 y/o 50 Gy, >15 y/o 55 Gy) to whole bone + 5 cm margin + 10 Gy boost (5 Gy to 2 cm, 5 Gy to 1 cm). RT was given during CHT. Bilateral pulmonary RT was 15 to 18 Gy AP/PA. Severe toxicity 57% to 70% (*p* = NS). Leukopenia in 21%, 4%, and 11% (*p* = sig). **Conclusion: VACA is superior to VAC or VAC + BPR. VAC + bilateral pulmonary RT is superior to VAC. No improvement between treatment modalities was noted for pelvic cases.**

TABLE 59.3: Results of IESS-I Ewing's Trial								
	5-yr OS	5-yr LR	5-yr RFS	Mets		5-yr OS		5-yr OS
RT+VACA	65%	11%	**60%**	30%	<10 y/o	71%	Pelvic	34%
RT+VAC	28%	16%	**24%**	72%	11–15 y/o	62%	Nonpelvic	57%
RT+VAC+BPR	53%	18%	**44%**	42%	>15 y/o	46%		
Bold text indicates statistically significant results.								

Burgert, IESS-II Non-pelvic (*JCO* 1990, PMID 2099751): 214 pts with nonpelvic, biopsy-proven, nonmetastatic, previously untreated Ewing's of the bone from 1978 to 1982. Median 13 years of age. Two treatments: (a) high-dose intermittent VACA (vincristine, adriamycin, cyclophosphamide or (b) moderate dose continuous VACA as per IESS-I. Local therapy (nonrandomized) was via surgery, surgery + RT (50 Gy) for biopsy/STR or RT alone (as per IESS-I). RT was given during initial phase of chemo, and 2 to 4 weeks after surgery if performed. MFU 5.6 years. See Table 59.4. Severe toxicity comparable; however, cardiotoxicity was greater in VACA (three treatment-related deaths). High dose VACA improved rate of lung metastasis (11% vs. 22%, *p* = sig), but not bone metastasis (8% vs. 9%, *p* = NS). **Conclusion: High dose intermittent VACA is superior to the IESS-I regimen. Take home: Intermittent VACA is standard of care.**

TABLE 59.4: Results of IESS-II Nonpelvic Ewing's Trial				
	5-yr OS	5-yr LR	5-yr RFS	Mets
High dose	**77%**	7%	**73%**	21%
IESS-I Regimen	63%	10%	**56%**	30%
	p = sig	*p* = NS	*p* = sig	*p* = NS

Evans, IESS-II Pelvic/Sacral (*JCO* 1991, PMID 2045857): 59 pts with pelvic primaries, regional lymph nodes were eligible, otherwise same as IESS-II earlier. RT: 45 Gy to pre-CHT volume (including entire hemipelvis or sacrum) + 2 cm, cone down #1 to tumor + 5 cm (5 Gy), cone down #2 to tumor + 1 cm (5 Gy) for a total dose of 55 Gy. Involved LNs given 45 Gy. Compared with 68 pts from IESS-I. 90% had biopsy only. **Conclusion: High dose intermittent VACA is superior to the IESS-I regimen, even for pelvic tumors. OS actually superior to nonpelvic pts in IESS-I.**

TABLE 59.5: Results of IESS-II Pelvic/Sacral Ewing's Trial

	5-yr OS	5-yr LR	5-yr RFS	Mets
High dose	63%	12%	55%	37%
IESS-I Hist.	35%	28%	23%	63%
All statistically significant.				

Grier, IESS-III (*NEJM* 2003, PMID 12594313): PRT of 518 pts (120 metastatic, 398 non-metastatic), w/ ESFT (including PNETs) from 1988 to 1992. Rationale: IE is highly effective in relapsed Ewing's; therefore, combination (VACA+IE) was tested in the up-front setting. Randomization: (a) high dose, intermittent VACA as per IESS-II (V = 2 mg/m2, C = 1,200 mg/m2, Adria = 75 mg/m2, Actin = 1.25 mg/m2 when Adria reached 375 mg/m2), or (b) VACA+I/E (I = 1,800 mg/m2 w/MESNA, E = 100 mg/m2) x 5d. Seventeen courses of CHT total. Local therapy at week 12. 23% pelvic primaries. RT: Definitive or gross residual got 45 Gy to pre-CHT + 3 cm, C/D 10.8 Gy to post-CHT + <3 cm → total dose 55.8 Gy. Microscopic residual received 45 Gy to pre-CHT + 1 cm. **Conclusion: VACA+IE superior to VACA for OS and localized disease, but no benefit in metastatic disease. Take home: high dose, intermittent VACA+IE is standard of care.**

TABLE 59.6: Results of IESS-III Ewing's Trial

Nonmetastatic	5-yr OS	5-yr LR	5-yr EFS	Mets	*Metastatic*	5-yr OS	5-yr EFS
VACA+I/E	72%	9%	69%	44%	VACA+I/E	22%	34%
VACA	61%	28%	54%	42%	VACA	22%	35%
	p = sig	*p* = sig	*p* = sig	*p* = NS		*p* = NS	*p* = NS

Granowalter, IESS-IV (*JCO* 2009, PMID 19349548): 478 pts with localized Ewing's from 1995 to 1998. VAdriaC + IE for 48 weeks (standard) versus 30 weeks (intensified). Local therapy at week 12. RT: 45 Gy to pre-CHT + 2 cm. Boost determined by amount of disease (Unresectable: post-CHT + 2 cm to 55.8 Gy. Gross residual: residual + 2-cm margin to 55.8 Gy. Close margins: margin + 2 cm to 50.4 Gy). 5-yr EFS and OS for all patients were 71% and 79%, respectively. 5-yr EFS and 5-yr OS between pelvic primaries and other bone primaries was the same. No difference between bone and soft tissue primaries. Grade 3 toxicity higher in experimental arm (30 weeks). **Conclusion: Dose intensification of VAdriaC/IE over 30 weeks did not result in improvement in EFS or OS, but did lead to increase in grade 3 toxicity.**

TABLE 59.7: Results of IESS-IV Ewing's Trial

	5-yr OS	5-yr EFS
VAdriaC/IE (48 weeks)	81%	72%
VAdriaC/IE (30 weeks)	77%	70%
	p = NS	*p* = NS

Womer, AEWS0031 (*JCO* 2012, PMID 23091096): PRT of 587 nonmetastatic pts, <50 years of age with ESFT randomized to VAdriaC+IE q3wks or q2wks (ANC >750, plts >75). Rationale: Since duration of CHT did not lead to improved outcomes (IESS-IV), interval compression to increase the dose of alkylating agents was tested in this trial. RT: CTV1 = pre-CHT GTV + 1.5 cm, CTV2 = post-CHT GTV + 1 cm. RT to start at 13 weeks, if definitive or preoperative. VC/IE given concurrently with RT. Age >18 and pelvic primary led to worse outcome (*p* < .001). Particularly, patients ≥18 y/o did worse than patients <18 y/o (5-yr EFS 47% vs. 72%, $p < .001$, respectively). Toxicity was similar between arms. **Conclusion: Dose intense q2wk VAdriaC+IE is now standard of care.**

TABLE 59.8: Results of AEWS0031		
	5-yr OS	5-yr EFS
VAdriaC/IE (q3 weeks)	83%	65%
VAdriaC/IE (q2 weeks)	77%	73%
	$p = .056$	$p = $ sig

Bernstein, POG 9457 (*JCO* 2006, PMID 16382125): 110 pts with metastatic Ewing's at diagnosis. Randomization: Topotecan +/− cyclophosphamide *prior* to VAdriaC+IE. Some pts also randomized to amifostine. Only 3/36 pts had partial response to topotecan. 21/36 had partial response to topotecan+cyclophosphamide. Amifostine did not provide myeloprotection. Overall 2-yr EFS 24%, OS 46%. For pts with lung metastasis, 2-yr EFS 31% versus 20% for more widespread metastatic disease. **Conclusion: Topotecan has limited activity alone, though in combination with cyclophosphamide it was active. Amifostine is not myeloprotective. OS comparable to prior studies. This study is the rationale for testing topotecan AEWS1031.**

What is the optimal local control modality: surgery or radiotherapy?

Classically, surgery has been performed for tumors that are surgically resectable and definitive RT has been reserved for tumors that are surgically unresectable. There are no prospective trials evaluating surgery versus definitive RT and analyses comparing the two modalities have been retrospective reviews of either RCTs or institutional databases.[10] Given the inherent selection biases of retrospective reviews, it appears that surgery and definitive RT have similar outcomes. There is some recent evidence (Ahmed et al.), that despite modern RT and surgical techniques, surgery + RT is associated with the lowest risk for local failure for pelvic tumors. Surgery is generally preferred if possible but RT preferred for patients who lack a function-preserving surgical option due to location (e.g., scapula, proximal humerus, skull, face, vertebrae) or extent.

Yock, INT 0091 (*JCO* 2006, PMID 16921035): PRT of 75 nonmetastatic pelvic Ewing's patients comparing VACA versus VACA+IE to determine its influence on local control modality with respect to surgery, RT, or both (S+RT), which was chosen by the treating physicians. The effect of local control modality was assessed after adjusting for the size of tumor (<8 cm, ≥8 cm) and CHT type. Surgery was done in 12 pts, RT in 44 pts, and S+RT in 19 pts. The 5-year EFS and LF were 49% and 21% (16%, LF only; 5%, LF and distant failure). There was no significant difference in EFS or LF by tumor size (<8 cm, > or =8 cm), LC modality, or CHT. However, VACA-IE seems to confer a LC benefit (11% vs. 30%; $p = .06$). **Conclusion: VACA+ IE superior for pelvic tumors. Surgery and RT produce comparable outcomes.**

Dunst, CESS 81/CESS 86 (*Cancer* 1991, PMID 2025847): *CESS 81:* 93 pts with localized Ewing's from 1981 to 1985. VACA x 2 followed by local therapy, then VACA x 2. RT: 36 Gy postoperative RT, 46 to 60 Gy RT alone. 5-yr RFS for surgery + RT (68%), surgery (54%), and RT alone (43%). Surgery improved LC compared to RT, but largely due to excess marginal misses. This led to strict RT quality control for CESS 86.

CESS 86: 177 pts with localized Ewing's from 1986 to 1989. VAIA for high risk (central tumors or extremity ≥100 cc), and VACA for standard risk. RT: 44 Gy post-op after marginal or wide, 60 Gy after intralesional, or 60 Gy RT alone. Within RT, randomized to daily versus split-course BID (1.6 Gy/fx to 22.4 Gy with 10-day break, then to 44.8 Gy, 60.8 Gy). Results: 5-yr OS 69%. 3-yr RFS for surgery + RT (62%), surgery (65%), and RT alone (67%).

No difference in OS or RFS between VAIA (high risk) or VACA (standard risk). No benefit to hyperfractionation in OS, EFS, or LC (76% vs. 86%, p = NS). RT much improved from CESS 81, while surgery remained the same.

Paulussen, EICESS 92 (*Klin Padiatr* 1999, PMID 10472562; Update Paulussen *JCO* 2008, PMID 18802150): 369 pts with Ewing's. Standard risk (localized tumors, volume <100 cc): VAIA then VAIA versus VACA. High risk (primaries >100 cc or metastases): VAIA versus VAIA + E. RT: Definitive daily versus hyperfractionated (54 Gy), post-op (44 Gy or 54 Gy depending on chemoresponse and resection), or pre-op for expected close margin (44 Gy or 54 Gy split-course BID depending on predicted wide or intralesional resection). MFU 8.5 years. There was a 17% EFS and 15% OS benefit with the addition of etoposide in the high-risk group. Higher incidence of toxicity in the VACA arm.

Schuck, Review of CESS 81, CESS 86, and EICESS 92 Trials (*IJROBP* 2003, PMID 12504050): Review of 1,058 pts. Surgery as local therapy used when feasible, and adjuvant RT given for poor histologic response or biopsy/STR. See Table 59.9. **Conclusion: Low rates of LF after induction chemotherapy for resectable tumors. For incisional resection, definitive RT equivalent to surgery + post-op RT.** *Comment: RT pts were negatively selected, with unfavorable tumor sites.*

TABLE 59.9: Combined Analysis of CESS 81, 86, and EICESS 92 for Ewing's Sarcoma		
	5-yr LF	5/10-yr EFS
Surgery +/– RT	7.5%	61%/55%
Pre-op RT	5.3%	59%/58%
RT alone	26.3%	47%/40%
	p = sig	p = sig

Daw, COG Trials (*Ann Surg Oncol* 2016, PMID 27216741): RR of 115 pts with Ewing's of the femur from three cooperative group trials. 84 patients underwent surgery alone, 17 had surgery+RT and 14 had RT alone. 5-yr EFS was 65% and 5-yr OS was 70%. Tumor location and size did not influence patient outcomes. Treatment modality also did not lead to any statistically significant differences in EFS, OS, LF. **Conclusion: LC modality does not affect disease outcomes for Ewing's sarcoma of the femur.**

Ahmed, Mayo Clinic (*ASTRO* 2015, Abstract #74)[16]: RR of 73 pts, 48 pelvis and 25 spine. MFU 58.1 months. 52% pelvis patients presented with metastatic disease and compared to 24% spine patients. RT alone was utilized in 65% and 48%, surgery in 16.7% and 8%, and surgery + RT in 16.7% and 44% of pelvis and spine tumors respectively. The 5-yr OS and EFS for spine tumors were 73% and 54%, respectively. The 5-yr OS and EFS for pelvic tumors were 49% and 44%, respectively. The 5-yr EFS for local treatment of all metastases was 29% versus 12% for untreated metastases (p = .02). **Conclusion: Excellent OS (73%) and LC (93%) for spine tumors (especially with dose ≥56 Gy). Pelvic tumors with inferior LC (80%) despite modern treatment. Surgery + RT and dose ≥56 Gy associated with the lowest LF rate and treatment of metastatic sites associated with improved OS and EFS.**

Considering the bone marrow is one contiguous space, should RT volumes include the entire involved bone?

Donaldson, POG-8346 (*IJROBP* 1998, PMID 9747829): 178 pts with localized Ewing's. Adria/C x 12 wks, followed by VAC x 50 wks. Local therapy was surgery when possible without functional loss, otherwise RT. RT alone (n = 94), 40 randomized to whole bone (39.6 Gy, boost to pre-chemo + 2 cm to 55.8 Gy) vs. tailored port (pre-chemo + 2 cm to 55.8 Gy). Results: 5-yr EFS differed by site (distal extremity 65%, central 63%, proximal extremity

46%, pelvic/sacral 24%). LC for RT alone was 65%. No difference between whole bone and tailored port. 5-yr LC differed by quality of RT (appropriate RT 80%, minor deviation 48%, major deviation 15%). LF 62% in RT volume, 24% outside RT volume, and 14% indeterminate. **Conclusion: Must treat adequate volumes. Tailored fields are reasonable.**

Does the timing of RT (early versus delayed) impact outcome in metastatic patients?

Cangir, IESS-MD-I and II (*Cancer* **1990, PMID 2201433**): Reviewed IESS-MD-I (1975–1977, n = 53, VACA + concurrent RT) and IESS-MD-II (1980–1983, n = 69, VACA + 5-FU, RT at week 10). RT given to areas of gross disease. No difference in overall response (73% vs. 70%), length of best response (3-yr DFS 30% in both), >5-yr survivors (30% vs. 28%), and fatal toxicity (6% vs. 7%). Life-threatening toxicity worse in MD-I (30% vs. 9%, *p* = Sig). **Conclusion: No survival advantage to early versus delayed RT for metastatic disease. Less toxicity with delayed RT.**

What is the role of SBRT for metastatic Ewing's sarcoma?

Brown, Mayo Clinic (*Sarcoma* **2014, PMID 25548538**): RR of institutional experience (2008–2012) with SBRT for Ewing's sarcoma and osteosarcoma. 14 pts included with 27 lesions (19 osteosarcoma, 8 Ewing's). Median age was 24 years, 6 pts were <18 years of age. Median "curative" dose 40 Gy/5 fx (range 30–60 Gy/3–10 fx). Median "palliative" dose 40 Gy/5 fx (range 16–50 Gy/1–10 fx). One grade 3 toxicity and two grade 2 toxicities: myonecrosis, avascular necrosis, and pathologic fractures—all toxicities were in the context of concurrent CHT or re-irradiation.

REFERENCES

1. Angervall L, Enzinger FM. Extraskeletal neoplasm resembling Ewing's sarcoma. *Cancer*. 1975;36(1):240–251.
2. Glass AG, Fraumeni JF. Epidemiology of bone cancer in children. *J Natl Cancer Inst*. 1970;44(1):187–199.
3. Buckley JD, Pendergrass TW, Buckley CM, et al. Epidemiology of osteosarcoma and Ewing's sarcoma in childhood: a study of 305 cases by the Children's Cancer Group. *Cancer*. 1998;83(7):1440–1448.
4. Halperin EC, Constine LS, Tarbell NJ, Kun LE. *Pediatric Radiation Oncology*. 5th ed. Philadelphia, PA: Lippincott Williams and Wilkins; 2010.
5. De Alava E, Gerald WL. Molecular biology of the Ewing's sarcoma/primitive neuroectodermal tumor family. *J Clin Oncol Off J Am Soc Clin Oncol*. 2000;18(1):204–213.
6. Völker T, Denecke T, Steffen I, et al. Positron emission tomography for staging of pediatric sarcoma patients: results of a prospective multicenter trial. *J Clin Oncol*. 2007;25(34):5435–5441. doi:10.1200/JCO.2007.12.2473
7. Hwang JP, Lim I, Kong C-B, et al. Prognostic value of SUVmax measured by pretreatment fluorine-18 fluorodeoxyglucose positron emission tomography/computed tomography in patients with Ewing sarcoma. *PloS One*. 2016;11(4):e0153281. doi:10.1371/journal.pone.0153281
8. Sauer R, Jürgens H, Burgers JMV, et al. Prognostic factors in the treatment of Ewing's sarcoma. *Radiother Oncol*. 1987;10(2):101–110. doi:10.1016/S0167-8140(87)80052-X
9. Werier J, Yao X, Caudrelier J-M, et al. A systematic review of optimal treatment strategies for localized Ewing's sarcoma of bone after neo-adjuvant chemotherapy. *Surg Oncol*. 2016;25(1):16–23. doi:10.1016/j.suronc.2015.11.002
10. Miser JS, Goldsby RE, Chen Z, et al. Treatment of metastatic Ewing sarcoma/primitive neuroectodermal tumor of bone: evaluation of increasing the dose intensity of chemotherapy; a report from the Children's Oncology Group. *Pediatr Blood Cancer*. 2007;49(7):894–900. doi:10.1002/pbc.21233

11. Foulon S, Brennan B, Gaspar N, et al. Can postoperative radiotherapy be omitted in localised standard-risk Ewing sarcoma? an observational study of the Euro-E.W.I.N.G group. *Eur J Cancer Oxf Engl 1990*. 2016;61:128–136. doi:10.1016/j.ejca.2016.03.075

12. Donaldson SS. Ewing sarcoma: radiation dose and target volume. *Pediatr Blood Cancer*. 2004;42(5):471–476. doi:10.1002/pbc.10472

13. Shamberger RC, LaQuaglia MP, Gebhardt MC, et al. Ewing sarcoma/primitive neuroectodermal tumor of the chest wall: impact of initial versus delayed resection on tumor margins, survival, and use of radiation therapy. *Ann Surg*. 2003;238(4):563–567; discussion 567–568. doi:10.1097/01.sla.0000089857.45191.52

14. Schuck A, Ahrens S, Konarzewska A, et al. Hemithorax irradiation for Ewing tumors of the chest wall. *Int J Radiat Oncol Biol Phys*. 2002;54(3):830–838.

15. Koshy M, Paulino AC, Mai WY, Teh BS. Radiation-induced osteosarcomas in the pediatric population. *Int J Radiat Oncol Biol Phys*. 2005;63(4):1169–1174. doi:10.1016/j.ijrobp.2005.04.008

16. Ahmed SK, Robinson SI, Rose PS, Laack NN. Local control and survival of axial Ewing sarcoma in the modern era. *Int J Radiat Oncol*. 2015;93(3):S33–S34. doi:10.1016/j.ijrobp.2015.07.083

60: PEDIATRIC HODGKIN'S LYMPHOMA

Ehsan H. Balagamwala and Erin S. Murphy

QUICK HIT: Pediatric Hodgkin's lymphoma accounts for ~7% of all childhood malignancies and is highly curable with survival rates >90% across risk groups. Nodular sclerosis is the most common histology (similar to adult Hodgkin's); however, mixed cellularity subtype is seen more frequently in pediatric Hodgkin's compared to other age groups. Given the excellent cure rates, trials in pediatric Hodgkin's have been designed to evaluate de-escalation of CHT and RT based on risk stratification. Generally, RT is delivered as per protocol based on the selection of systemic therapy and response criteria specified. Table 60.1 presents some general principles, but specifics are determined by paradigms set forth by the trials listed in the following.

TABLE 60.1: General Treatment Paradigm for Pediatric Hodgkin's Lymphoma

Risk Group	Suggested Treatment Options
Low Risk	1. 2–4 cycles of non-cross-resistant CHT + IFRT (15–25.5 Gy) a. Possible CHT regimens: AV-PC, ABVD, VAMP, OPPA or OEPA 2. 4–6 cycles of COPP/ABV alone 3. CHT + IFRT as per AHOD0431

Intermediate Risk	1. 4–6 cycles of non-cross-resistant CHT + IFRT (15–25.5 Gy)
	    a. Possible regimens: COPP/ABV, ABVE-PC, OPPA/COPP or OEPA/COPDAC
	2. 6–8 cycles of non-cross-resistant CHT alone
	    a. Possible regimens: COPP/ABV

High Risk	1. 6–8 cycles of non-cross-resistant CHT + IFRT (15–25.5 Gy)
	    a. Possible regimens: COPP/ABVD, OEPA/COPDAC
	2. 8 cycles of non-cross-resistant CHT alone
	    a. Possible regimens: COPP/ABVD
	3. CHT + IFRT as per AHOD0831

EPIDEMIOLOGY: Of ~10,450 childhood cancer diagnoses per year, pediatric Hodgkin's (age up to 21) represents ~7% (~1,140 cases).[1] Hodgkin's disease has a bimodal distribution: most common between 15 and 35 years of age (50%) and >55 years of age (35%). The epidemiology of Hodgkin's disease differs significantly between pediatric, adolescent/young adult (AYA), and adult forms of the disease. Across all age groups, nodular sclerosis subtype is the most common. Pediatric Hodgkin's is rare before 5 years of age, has a male predominance (M to F ratio 2–3:1), and is more likely than adult Hodgkin's to present as **mixed cellularity** (30%–35%) or **nodular lymphocyte predominant** (10%–20%) subtypes.[2] In comparison, AYA Hodgkin's occurs in those 15 to 35 years of age, has no gender predilection, and the most common histology is nodular sclerosis (70%–80%), similar to what is seen in adults. Older adults (>45–55) are more likely to present with more advanced disease. The 5-yr OS of all pediatric Hodgkin's lymphoma pts is 97%.[3]

RISK FACTORS[4]

Pediatric Hodgkin's: Increasing family size, lower SES status, early EBV exposure. EBV exposure is associated with mixed cellularity Hodgkin's disease and this disease tends to occur more in developing countries where children are at higher risk for EBV exposure.

AYA Hodgkin's: Higher SES, early birth order, small family size, delayed EBV exposure.

Adults: Immunosuppression (HIV, organ/bone marrow transplant), autoimmune disorders or immune dysfunction (there is evidence to suggest adult Hodgkin's is biologically different and more aggressive compared to pediatric Hodgkin's).

EBV genome has been detected in 30% to 50% of cellular DNA of Reed–Sternberg (RS) cells (least commonly in NLPHD). IgG and IgA antibodies against EBV are detected in pts who later develop HD. Risk for HD is higher in pts with a history of infectious mononucleosis. Family history is also risk factor: RR is 99 for monozygotic twins, 9 for same-sex siblings, 2 to 5 for opposite-sex siblings. HIV+ pts tend to have higher rate of advanced stage (70%–90%), noncontiguous spread, extranodal sites (BM+ in 50%), MCHD, LDHD and EBV+.

ANATOMY: Anatomical lymph node regions for lymphoma include: Waldeyer's ring (nasopharynx, pharynx, and lingual/palatine tonsils of the oropharynx), cervical neck, supraclavicular region, infraclavicular region, axillary, mediastinal, hilar, epitrochlear/brachial, mesenteric, para-aortic, spleen, iliac, inguinofemoral, and popliteal. Hodgkin's disease arises in the LNs and solitary extralymphatic involvement is rare. Waldeyer's ring and Peyer's patches are rarely involved. Most common site of extranodal disease is the spleen.

PATHOLOGY[4]: The primary diagnostic finding is the **Reed–Sternberg (RS) cell,** which accounts for only 1% to 2% of cells in infiltrated LNs (the remainder of cells are composed of abundant reactive cellular infiltrate, including lymphocytes, granulocytes, eosinophils, and plasma cells). RS cell's classic appearance is binucleate, with two prominent nucleoli. There is a well-demarcated nuclear membrane and eosinophilic cytoplasm with a perinuclear halo. RS cells originate from B-cells in lymphoid germinal centers. Cell of origin is likely a precursor B-cell. RS cells are thought to secrete numerous cytokines, leading to B symptoms (IL-5 may cause eosinophilia of MCHD, and TGF-β may cause fibrosis of NSHD). Interfollicular Hodgkin's is a rare, very focal involvement of the interfollicular zone of an LN, often confused with reactive lymphoid hyperplasia. In comparison to adult Hodgkin's, the nodular sclerosis subtype is less common in children (55% vs. ≥70%) and mixed cellularity is more common (35% vs. 20%). The nodular lymphocyte predominant subtype has a more favorable prognosis and is more commonly CD20+ and CD15-, in comparison to classic subtypes which are typically CD15+ and CD30+.

	Histology	Pediatric Frequency	Adult Frequency	Markers
	TABLE 60.2: Histologic Classification and Relative Frequency of Pediatric Hodgkin's Disease[4]			
CLASSIC HODGKIN'S	• *Lymphocyte Rich (LR)*	<5%	5%	CD15+, CD30+ Occ. CD20+
	• *Nodular Sclerosis (NSHD)*	55%	≥70%	
	• *Mixed Cellularity (MCHD)*	30%–35%	~20%	
	• *Lymphocyte Depletion (LD)*	<5%	<5%	

(continued)

TABLE 60.2: Histologic Classification and Relative Frequency of Pediatric Hodgkin's Disease[4] (*continued*)			
Histology	Pediatric Frequency	Adult Frequency	Markers
Nodular Lymphocyte Predominance (NLPHD)	5%–10%	5%	CD19+, **CD20+,** CD45+, **CD15-, CD30-**

CLINICAL PRESENTATION[4]: Painless adenopathy is the most common presentation. Approximately 80% have cervical LN involvement at presentation and >50% have mediastinal disease. ~1/3 present with B symptoms: fevers (>38°C), drenching night sweats, and weight loss (>10% in the past 6 months). May see **Pel–Ebstein fevers** (cyclical spiking fevers up to 40°C, last ~1 week and remit for ~1 week; due to cytokine release), **generalized pruritus** or **alcohol-induced pain** in tissues infiltrated by HD. Generally, Hodgkin's disease is unifocal and 90% present with contiguous sites of involvement. >80% originate above the diaphragm. Visceral involvement may be due to direct extension or hematogenous spread (liver or bone). Mechanism of spread to spleen is unclear; however, is likely hematogenous.

TABLE 60.3: Comparison of Pediatric and Adolescent/Young Adult Hodgkin's Disease		
	Pediatric (age ≤4 y/o)	**AYA (age 15–35 y/o)**
Gender (M:F)	2–3: 1	1.1–1.3:1
Site of Disease	More commonly have cervical (80%) LAD. Many also have mediastinal disease. Rare to have isolated mediastinal or subdiaphragmatic disease (<5%)	More commonly have mediastinal disease (75%)
Histology Nodular sclerosis **Mixed cellularity** **Lymphocyte depleted** NLPHL	40%–45% 30%–45% 0%–3% 8%–20%	65%–80% 10%–25% 1%–5% 2%–8%
EBV associated	27%–54%	20%–25%
Risk Factors	Lower SES Increasing family size	Higher SES Smaller family size Early birth order
Stage at presentation **B symptoms** **Stage III/IV**	25% 30%–35%	30%–40% 40%
5-yr OS	>94%	90%
Source: From Ref. (21).		

WORKUP: H&P with particular attention to LN regions (detailed earlier).

Labs: CBC, ESR, BMP, LFTs, LDH, hCG, PFTs.

Imaging: CXR, CT with contrast of chest, abdomen, and pelvis. PET/CT once diagnosis is established. Echocardiogram prior to CHT.

Pathology: Excisional biopsy is required to evaluate lymphoid architecture. Bone marrow biopsy if PET+, stage III/IV or B symptoms.

STAGING: See Chapter 48 for Ann Arbor staging system.

PROGNOSTIC FACTORS: Poor prognostic factors include advanced stage, large mediastinal adenopathy, >4 subsites, B symptoms, poor histology, age (<10 y/o better than 11–16 y/o better than >20 y/o), male sex, slow response to CHT. Risk stratification for pediatric Hodgkin's lymphoma is as per Table 60.4. CHIPS prognostic score for pts with COG Intermediate Risk (based on AHOD0031).[6] Includes stage IV disease, large mediastinal mass, albumin (<3.4) and fever were independent prognostic factors and were assigned one point each. EFS was 93.1% for pts with no points, 88.5% for pts with one point, 77.6% for pt with two points, and 69.2% for pts with three points.

TABLE 60.4: Risk Stratification Schemes for Pediatric Hodgkin's Lymphoma[a]			
Study Group	Low Risk	Intermediate Risk	High Risk
COG	IA/IIA, no bulk	Everyone else	IIIB/IVB
German	IA/B or IIA	IIB, IIIEA, IIIB	IIEB, IIIEA/B, IIIB, IVA/B
St. Jude/Stanford/Dana Farber	IA/IIA, no bulk		Everyone else

TREATMENT PARADIGM

Historically, Hodgkin's disease was treated with large RT fields. Cure rates were found to be excellent and long-term survivors of the disease were common. However, experience from adult and pediatric Hodgkin's showed that the long-term sequelae of RT included profound musculoskeletal retardation, including intraclavicular narrowing, shortened sitting height, decreased mandibular growth, and decreased muscular development. Given the excellent control rates, less toxic treatments were desired and hence began the era of CHT as the primary treatment modality for Hodgkin's lymphoma (note must be made of issue of sterility with CHT and the modification of CHT regimens over the years to preserve fertility).

Surgery: There is no role for surgery in Hodgkin's disease beyond biopsy. The exception is favorable stage IA nodular lymphocyte predominant pts without risk factors may be treated by complete excision followed by observation (1/2 to 2/3 of pts can be cured with surgery-alone), with 5-yr OS approaching 100%.[5]

Chemotherapy: Initially, MOPP CHT was the backbone regimen used. However, due to significant impact on fertility (procarbazine is gonadotoxic), ABVD was introduced. In the modern era, all CHT regimens for Hodgkin's disease are a derivative of MOPP and/or ABVD, but more drugs are integrated to reduce total dose of any single drug.

TABLE 60.5: Common CHT Regimens in Pediatric Hodgkin's Lymphoma	
MOPP	Nitrogen mustard, vincristine, procarbazine, prednisone *Toxicities include sterility, secondary leukemia (latent period 3–7 years with risk of 3%–5% at 7–10 years)*
ABVD	Adriamycin, bleomycin, vinblastine, dacarbazine *Toxicities include pulmonary and cardiovascular*
OPPA	Vincristine, procarbazine, prednisolone, adriamycin
COPP	Cyclophosphamide, vincristine, procarbazine, prednisone
AV-PC	Doxorubicin, vincristine, prednisone, cyclophosphamide
ABVE-PC	Doxorubicin, bleomycin, vincristine, etoposide, prednisone, cyclophosphamide
VAMP	Vincristine, adriamycin, methotrexate, prednisone

Radiotherapy

Indications: Dosing and indications for pediatric Hodgkin's treatment are determined by the choice of CHT and should be followed as per protocol. Involved field RT (IFRT) is standard of care in pediatrics. Involved site RT (ISRT) is an evolving paradigm and is currently being utilized on some clinical trials. Involved nodal RT (subset of ISRT) is not advised unless as a part of clinical trial. See ILROG guidelines on ISRT for details.[7,8]

Dose: Consolidative RT dose is determined by paradigm chosen but typically ranges from 15 to 25.5 Gy. Acute effects at common modern RT doses are minimal but may include fatigue, skin erythema, esophagitis. Late effects drive protocol development and include second malignancy, heart disease, pulmonary fibrosis, skeletal hypoplasia, infertility.

EVIDENCE-BASED Q&A

Low-risk/early/favorable pediatric Hodgkin's

Which early studies evaluated CHT deintensification in low-risk pediatric Hodgkin's disease?

ABVD and MOPP led to excellent cure rates (>90%); however, have significant associated toxicity. Initial trials focused on testing whether less-intensive CHT would lead to equivalent outcomes with improved toxicity. German HD-90 trial and French MDH-90 trial demonstrated excellent outcomes with CHT deintensification + ISRT.

TABLE 60.6: Deintensification Trials in Early Pediatric Hodgkin's Disease							
Study	N	Years	Arms	EFS	OS	MFU (yr)	Prognostic Factors/ Comment
MDH-82 (French)[9]	238	1982–1988	ABVD x4 + 20 Gy (CR/PR) 40 Gy (non-CR/PR) IFRT	90%	92%	6	97% CR/PR rate
			ABVD X2/MOPP X2 + same RT	87%			
MDH-90 (French)[10]	202	1990–1996	VBVP x4 + 20 Gy IFRT (good responders) VBVP x4 + OPPA x2 + 40 Gy (poor responders)	91% 78%	97.5% (all)	6	Hb <10.5 B symptoms NS histology
HD-90 (German)	267	1990–1995	OPPA(♀)/OEPA(♂) x2 + 20–35 Gy ISRT	94%	99.6%	5	B symptoms, NS histology. Examined role of ISRT, on which HD-95 was based.

Schellong, HD-90 (*JCO* 1999, PMID 10577845): 578 pediatric pts with stage I-IV HD, divided into treatment group: TG1 (early stages), TG2 (intermediate stages), or TG3 (advanced stages). All groups underwent two cycles of OEPA (vincristine, etoposide [replace dacarbazine to spare fertility], prednisone, Adriamycin) for boys or OPPA (girls) for induction CHT. COPP X 2 added to TG2 and COPP X 4 added to TG3. 25 Gy IFRT with 5 to 10 Gy boost to >25% residual disease or >50 mL residual. See Table 60.6 (early stage) and the following (intermediate and advanced stage). **Conclusion: OEPA**

is a satisfactory alternative to OPPA. RT can be confined to involved sites when combined with appropriate CHT.

Is it possible to omit RT in patients who have a complete response (CR) to CHT?

This question was evaluated in HD-95, POG 8625, and CCG 5942. HD-95 suggested that in pts who achieve CR after two cycles, RT can be omitted. However, POG 8625 showed that to omit RT, two additional cycles of CHT are required. When CHT is further de-escalated from MOPP/ ABVD, CCG 5942 showed that RT cannot be omitted (trial closed early). Therefore, omitting RT in the setting of de-escalated CHT is not recommended.

TABLE 60.7: Risk-Adapted Trials Omitting RT in Early Pediatric Hodgkin's							
Study	N	Years	Arms	EFS	OS	MFU (Yrs)	Prognostic Factors/ Comment
HD-95 (German)	281	1995–2001	OPPA(♀)/ OEPA(♂) X2, then CR → No RT PR → 20–35 Gy IFRT	97% 92.2%	98.8%	10	*Comment:* EFS for low-risk pts with CR and no RT same as PR with RT.
POG 8625[11]	78	1986–1992	MOPP x3/ABVD x3 (no RT) MOPP x2/ABVD x2 + 25.5 IFRT	83% 91% (NS)	94% 97%	8	Laparotomy staged. Two cycles of MOPP/ABVD equivalent to 25.5 Gy IFRT.
CCG 5942[12]	294	1995–1998	CR pts randomized to IFRT CR pts randomized to no RT	100% 89.1% (SS)	97.1% 95.1% p = .5	10	Clinically staged pts. Trial stopped early as IFRT was superior. Updated numbers reflect 10-yr EFS and OS.
St. Jude	88	2000–2008	VAMPx2 CR no RT <CR 25.5 Gy IFRT	89.4% 92.5% (NS)	100%	6.9	PET or gallium scan for response assessment.

Dorffel, HD-95 (*JCO* 2013, PMID 23509321): Prospective, nonrandomized trial of 925 pts divided into early stage (TG1), intermediate stage (TG2), and advanced stage (TG3). RT was given as follows: With CR (CT/MRI), no RT; those with tumor reduction of >75%, IFRT to 25 Gy; those with residual tumors >50 cc (considered bulky), IFRT to 25 Gy with 10 to 15 Gy boost. See Table 60.7 (early stage) and Table 60.9 (intermediate and advanced stage). IFRT was given to pts with poor CHT response; however, it was associated significantly with better EFS among intermediate- and high-risk pts but not among low-risk pts. No difference in OS. On QA, 2/17 relapses on RT arm due to poor quality RT. 4/14 pts with stage IIA who failed, had prolonged delay between CHT and RT. **Conclusion: The omission of RT after CR results in increased risk of treatment failures, most notably in advanced-stage pts (note: a nonrandomized observation). May omit RT after CR in early-stage (low-risk) pts because no EFS benefit seen in this group.**

Donaldson, St. Jude, Favorable Risk (*JCO* 2007, PMID 17235049): Phase II trial of 110 children with low-risk HD were treated with four cycles of VAMP (vincristine, Adriamycin, methotrexate, prednisone). Pts with CR received 15 Gy IFRT and those with PR received 25.5 Gy. After MFU of 9.6 yrs, 10-yr EFS and OS were 89.4% and 96.1%, respectively. Early CR, absence of B symptoms, lymphocyte predominant histology, and <3 initial sites of disease were prognostic. **Conclusion: Risk-adapted combined modality therapy using VAMP is feasible and permits fertility-sparing.**

Metzger, St. Jude Favorable Risk PET-Adapted (*JAMA* 2012, PMID 22735430): Given the favorable outcomes of the preceding trial, the group performed a trial to evaluate omitting RT for early response. Phase II trial of 88 children with low-risk HD were included. Pts who achieved CR after two cycles did not receive IFRT and those who achieved <CR received 25.5 Gy IFRT. Overall 2-yr EFS was 90.8%. For those pts who did not require IFRT, the EFS was 89.4% compared to 92.5% for those pts who did require IFRT (p = .61). **Conclusion: In pts with low-risk pediatric HD who achieved a CR after two cycles of VAMP, omitting IFRT resulted in a high 2-yr EFS.**

Can RT be omitted in pts who have a rapid early response?

This question is being evaluated in the AHOD0431 trial, which has been completed but not yet published. Early results demonstrate that rapid response (defined as CR after three cycles of AV-PC) does not adequately predict for those pts in which RT can be safely omitted (however, negative PET/CT after cycle 1 was prognostic). Of note, AV-PC is also de-escalated CHT. The next step in low-risk trials will evaluate whether CHT intensification can help eliminate the need for RT.

Keller, AHOD 0431 (*ASH* 2010, Abstract 767): Phase II trial of 287 pts with low-risk HD examining AV-PC x three cycles (doxorubicin, vincristine, prednisone, cyclophosphamide), and no IFRT for CR (>80% reduction in product of perpendicular diameters [PPD]) after three cycles. Pts with PR (>50% PPD) receive IFRT 21 Gy/14 fx. Any pt who failed after initial CR, if failed as stage I/II, would receive IV/DECA (dexamethasone, etoposide, cisplatin, cytarabine) + IFRT 21 Gy. If pts failed as advanced stage, they will receive high-dose CHT with autologous SCT. Study closed early due to higher risk for relapse in pts with CR who were PET+ after one cycle. CR after three cycles was achieved in 63.6%, PR in 34.5%, and stable disease in 1.8%. See Table 60.8 for additional results. Pts with mixed cellularity had significantly improved EFS compared to pts with nodular sclerosis histology (95.1% vs. 75.6%, p = .01). **Conclusion: Rapid response as defined in this trial does not adequately define a population in which RT can be avoided. PET response after one cycle is highly predictive of outcomes.**

TABLE 60.8: Early Results of AHOD 0431		
2-year FU	**EFS**	**EFS (-PET vs. +PET after 1c)**
CR	80%	87% vs. 65% (p = .005)
PR (+ RT)	88%	96% vs. 82% (p = .047)
p value	.21	.001 *(across 4 groups)*

Intermediate-high risk/advanced/favorable pediatric Hodgkin's

Can RT be avoided in patients with CR after CHT?

Several trials have evaluated whether RT can be eliminated for pts who have a CR to induction CHT. HD-95 and CCG 5942 studies showed that IFRT improved EFS, but no difference in OS. TATA Memorial from India suggested that there was an OS benefit to IFRT after CR (caveat was that ~50% were AYA or adult HD). However, POG 8725 trial (STNI) and CCG 521 (EFRT), both of which utilized large RT volumes, did not show an EFS or OS benefit to RT. These trials together suggested that there may be pts in whom RT could be avoided without impacting oncologic outcome; however, it was unclear who those pts are.

TABLE 60.9: Trials Omitting RT in Intermediate/High-Risk Pediatric Hodgkin's Lymphoma							
Study	N	Years	Arms	EFS	OS	MFU (yr)	Prognostic Factors
POG 8725[13]	179	1987–1992	MOPP X4 + ABVD x4 (CR) + 21 Gy STNI	80%	96%	5	CR after 3 cycles; age <13; comment: 10 of 80 pts did not receive RT as per protocol
			MOPP X4 + ABVD x4 (CR) alone	79% (NS)	87% (NS)		
CCG 521[14]	125	1986–1990	MOPP x6/ABVD x6	77%	84%	4	Equivalent outcome, but increased pulmonary toxicity with chemo (9%)
			ABVD x6 + 21 Gy EFRT	87% (NS)	90%		
HD-90 (German)	124 IS 179 AS	1990–1995	OPPA(♀)/OEPA(♂) x2 + COPP x2	93%	97%	5	B symptoms NS histology
			OPPA(♀)/OEPA(♂) x2 + COPP x4 *All pts then got 20–35 Gy IFRT*	86%	94%		
HD-95 (German)	224 IS 280 AS	1995–2000	OPPA(♀)/OEPA(♂) x2 + COPP x2 → OPPA(♀)/OEPA(♂) x2 + COPP x4→ *Then Both Groups Response Adapted*		93% 97%	10	B symptoms; ENE Comment: RT improved outcome after PR, compared to pts having CR without RT → RT cannot be eliminated
			CR → no RT (intermediate stage)	69%			
			PR → 20–35 Gy IFRT (intermediate stage)	91% (SS)			
			CR → no RT (advanced stage)	83%			
			PR → 20–35 Gy IFRT (advanced stage)	89 (NS)			
CCG 5942	207 IS	1995–1998	Group 2 CR pts randomized to IFRT	84%		10	Comment: These values are per "as treated" analysis No benefit for IS and AS groups but study not powered for subset analysis
			CR pts randomized to no RT	78% (NS)			
	66 AS		Group 3 CR pts randomized to IFRT				
			CR pts randomized to no RT	88.5% 79.9% (NS)			

(continued)

TABLE 60.9: Trials Omitting RT in Intermediate/High-Risk Pediatric Hodgkin's Lymphoma *(continued)*							
Study	N	Years	Arms	EFS	OS	MFU (yr)	Prognostic Factors
TATA (India)	179 (half <15 y/o)	1993–1996	ABVD x6 ABVD x6 + IFRT 25-40 Gy	76% 88% (p = .01)	89% 100% (p = .002)	8	Benefit greatest in pts with: age <15; B symptoms Advanced stage

Nachman, CCG 5942 (*JCO* 2002, PMID 12228196; Update Wolden *JCO* 2012, PMID 22649136): PRT of 826 children (defined as <21 y/o) with HD given risk-adapted CHT. Group 1: All favorable stage 1 + all favorable stage II without B symptoms. Group 2: unfavorable stage I + unfavorable stage II or all stage II w/ B symptoms + all stage III. Group 3: All stage IV. Group 1 received COPP/ABV x4; Group 2 COPP/ABV x6; Group 3 received intensive CHT. Pts w/ CR to CHT were randomized to low dose IFRT to 21 Gy/12 fx (pts with pulmonary involvement received 10.5 Gy/12 fx to the lungs) or no additional therapy. See Table 60.9 for results by treatment group. Study terminated early due to increased relapse in no-RT arm. For the entire cohort, the 10-yr EFS and OS were 83.5% and 92.5%, respectively. 77% achieved CR. The 10-yr EFS for pts randomized to IFRT was 89.7% vs. 83.8% in no-RT arm (p = .048). Disease bulk, B symptoms and nodular sclerosis histology were factors predictive of inferior EFS. **Conclusion: IFRT produced improvement in EFS, but not OS. For individual pts, late effects versus risk of relapse must be assessed.**

Laskar, TATA Memorial, India (*JCO* 2004, PMID 14657226): PRT of 179 pts, all ages (50% <15 y/o), all stages (50% advanced dz), treated with ABVD x 6, who achieved a CR randomized to IFRT versus no RT. RT dose 30 Gy + 10 Gy to bulky disease for IFRT, and less commonly EFRT 25 Gy + 10 Gy boost to bulk. Median dose 30 Gy. See Table 60.9. MFU 63 months. Addition of RT improved EFS and OS in pts age <15 y/o, B symptoms, advanced stage, and bulky disease. **Conclusion: Addition of IFRT confers OS advantage, especially in pts <15 years of age with advanced disease.** *Comment: Heterogeneous pt population, high RT doses, ABVD x6 may be inadequate CHT for high-risk disease.*

Schwartz, POG 9425 (*Blood* 2009, PMID 19584400): Goal was to develop a CHT regimen that would (a) enhance treatment efficacy and (b) reduce long-term risk of treatment. ABVE-PC x 3, if RER then 21 Gy IFRT. For those who do not have RER, additional two cycles of ABVE-PC (five total) + 21 Gy IFRT. 5-yr EFS 84% (86% for RER, 83% for slow early responders). 5-yr OS 95%. **Conclusion: ABVE-PC is a dose-dense regimen that provides excellent EFS/OS w/ short-duration, early response adapted therapy. First study in advanced disease that showed pts w/ rapid early response could be treated with limited CHT and reduced doses of systemic agents and forms the basis for recent COG trials. Adverse prognostic factor of slow early response was offset with more CHT. This CHT regimen is now standard of care for COG trials.**

Since it is not clear which patients require titration of CHT and/or RT, is it possible to utilize response-based criteria to determine which intermediate-risk patients require escalation versus de-escalation of treatment?

Early response has been shown in previous studies to be predictive of long-term outcome. Therefore, the AHOD0031 trial was initiated and demonstrated that rapid early responders (defined as CR after two cycles of ABVE-PC) who achieve a CR have no benefit from IFRT. However, all others on the trial received IFRT.

Friedman, AHOD0031 (*JCO* 2014, PMID 25311218): PRT evaluating the role of tailoring CHT and RT in those pts who show early response to CHT. All pts receive two cycles of ABVE-PC. CR defined as >80% PPD response, PR defined as >50% PPD response. Those pts with a rapid early response (CR or PR) after two cycles received two further cycles of ABVE-PC followed repeat evaluation: if CR then IFRT versus no IFRT (randomized); if <CR then IFRT. Those pts with slow early response (SER) randomized to [ABVE-PCx2c + IFRT] or [DECAx2c + ABVE-PCx2c + IFRT]. IFRT was 21 Gy/14 fx. 1,712 eligible pts, 4-yr EFS was 85.0%: 86.9% for RER, 77.4% for SER (SS). 4-yr OS was 97.8%; 98.5% for RER, 95.3% for SER. For RERs with CR, 4-yr EFS with IFRT was 87.9% versus 84.3% without IFRT (NS). For RERs with PET-negative at response assessment, 4-yr EFS was 86.7% for pts who received IFRT versus 87.3% for pts who did not receive IFRT (NS). For SERs randomly assigned to DECA versus no DECA, 4-yr EFS was 79.3% versus 75.2%, respectively, and 70.7% versus 54.6% (NS) for SERs with PET+ at response assessment. **Conclusion: This trial was able to validate response-based therapeutic titration. For RERs with CR, IFRT could be safely omitted and for SERs with PET+ disease, CHT augmentation is recommended.**

Dharmarajan, AHOD0031 Patterns of Failure (*IJROBP* 2015, PMID 25542311): A subset analysis was performed on pts enrolled on AHOD0031, which evaluated 198 pts (out of 244) who had developed relapse.[15] Of these pts, 30% were RER/no CR, 26% were SER, 26% RER/CR/no IFRT, 16% were RER/CR/IFRT, and 2% remained uncategorized. Approximately 3/4 of relapses occurred at initially involved sites (bulky or nonbulky). First relapses rarely occurred at previously uninvolved sites or out-of-field sites. **Conclusion: Response-based therapy can help define treatment for selected RER pts; it has not proven beneficial for pts with SER nor has facilitated refinement of IFRT treatment volumes (therefore, IFRT is standard of care currently in pediatrics).** *Comment: A second subset analysis evaluated which pts who achieved RER and CR benefited from IFRT.[16] The results showed that most pts did not benefit from IFRT. However, those pts with anemia and bulky limited-stage disease had significantly improved 4-year EFS with the addition of IFRT (89.3% vs. 77.9%, p = .019).*

What is the current high-risk pediatric Hodgkin's disease trial?

AHOD0831 (closed, results pending). A Non-Randomized Phase III Study of Response Adapted Therapy for the Treatment of Children With Newly Diagnosed High Risk Hodgkin Lymphoma. The goal of this trial is to maintain comparable OS (as defined by 4-year "second-event"-free survival) between pts with high-risk HL who have a rapid or slow response to the initial two courses of ABVE-PC CHT. Pts who have a rapid response will receive two additional cycles of ABVE-PC with risk-adapted IFRT (i.e., only site of initial bulk will be radiation). Pts with slow response will receive intensified CHT (ABVE-PC x2c + ifosfamide/vinorelbine x2c) followed by risk-adapted IFRT (PET+ sites and sites ≥2.5 cm will be radiated). IFRT is to 21 Gy/14 fx.

How are patients with relapsed or refractory disease managed?

Refractory disease is marked by failure to achieve CR or good PR with initial chemo (~6% overall). Salvage therapy in this setting may include high dose CHT +/− RT with response rates of 50% to 70%, followed by autologous SCT. However, 5-yr DFS is only ~20%. Relapsed disease is usually treated with high dose CHT (HDC) and ASCT. The most common HDC is CBV or BEAM. In general, autologous is preferred over allogeneic SCT due to toxicity and overall lack of graft versus lymphoma effect. An RR of 1,200 pts with HD who underwent transplant showed that treatment-related mortality was 65% for allogeneic transplant versus 12% for autologous transplant and the 4-yr OS was 25% versus 37%, respectively (p = .005).[17] IFRT as part of salvage therapy has been shown to improve EFS and trend toward OS (especially in RT naïve pts) in several studies.[18]

*Whole Lung Irradiation: If treating lungs with RT, do RT **after** the transplant. Other than in the lung, consider RT **prior** to transplant (especially in the pelvis RT prior to transplant prevents additional bone marrow toxicity to the new graft). Stem cells for transplant should be harvested prior to RT. Transplant has similar outcomes with or without TBI. If RT has been utilized prior to BMT, salvage RT may also be utilized to doses of 15 to 25 Gy.*

What is the risk for second malignancies in patients treated for Hodgkin's lymphoma?

The recently published observational study out of Netherlands shows that the risk for second malignancies continues to increase even up to 40 years after treatment for Hodgkin's lymphoma.[19] The cumulative incidence of second cancers at 40 years was 48.5%. Compared to the general population, pts treated for Hodgkin's lymphoma had a standardized incident ratio (SIR) of 4.6 for the development of second cancers (equivalent to 121.8 excess cancer diagnoses per 10,000 person years). The risk for secondary hematological malignancies was lower in the more recent treatment years due to reduction in utilization of alkylating agents. However, reduction in solid tumors was not lower in more recent years (supradiaphragmatic RT was associated with lower second malignancies compared to mantle field RT). One study by O'Brien showed that all pts who developed secondary leukemias (usually due to CHT) had a fatal course, whereas those pts who developed secondary solid tumors (usually due to RT) had a 5-yr OS of 85%.[20]

REFERENCES

1. Ward E, DeSantis C, Robbins A, et al. Childhood and adolescent cancer statistics, 2014. *CA Cancer J Clin.* 2014;64(2):83–103. doi:10.3322/caac.21219
2. Punnett A, Tsang RW, Hodgson DC. Hodgkin lymphoma across the age spectrum: epidemiology, therapy, and late effects. *Semin Radiat Oncol.* 2010;20(1):30–44. doi:10.1016/j.semradonc.2009.09.006
3. CureSearch for Children's Cancer Research—Home. CureSearch for Children's Cancer. https://curesearch.org
4. Halperin EC, Constine LS, Tarbell NJ, Kun LE. *Pediatric Radiation Oncology.* 5th ed. Philadelphia, PA: Lippincott Williams and Wilkins; 2010.
5. Appel BE, Chen L, Buxton AB, et al. Minimal treatment of low-risk, pediatric lymphocyte-predominant Hodgkin lymphoma: a report from the Children's Oncology Group. *J Clin Oncol Off J Am Soc Clin Oncol.* 2016;34(20):2372–2379. doi:10.1200/JCO.2015.65.3469
6. Schwartz CL, Chen L, McCarten K, et al. Childhood Hodgkin International Prognostic Score (CHIPS) predicts event-free survival in hodgkin lymphoma: a report from the Children's Oncology Group. *Pediatr Blood Cancer.* 2017;64(4). doi:10.1002/pbc.26278
7. Specht L, Yahalom J, Illidge T, et al. Modern radiation therapy for Hodgkin lymphoma: field and dose guidelines from the International Lymphoma Radiation Oncology Group (ILROG). *Int J Radiat Oncol Biol Phys.* 2014;89(4):854–862. doi:10.1016/j.ijrobp.2013.05.005
8. Hodgson DC, Dieckmann K, Terezakis S, et al. Implementation of contemporary radiation therapy planning concepts for pediatric Hodgkin lymphoma: guidelines from the International Lymphoma Radiation Oncology Group. *Pract Radiat Oncol.* 2015;5(2):85–92. doi:10.1016/j.prro.2014.05.003
9. Oberlin O, Leverger G, Pacquement H, et al. Low-dose radiation therapy and reduced chemotherapy in childhood Hodgkin's disease: the experience of the French Society of Pediatric Oncology. *J Clin Oncol.* 1992;10(10):1602–1608. doi:10.1200/JCO.1992.10.10.1602
10. Landman-Parker J, Pacquement H, Leblanc T, et al. Localized childhood Hodgkin's disease: response-adapted chemotherapy with etoposide, bleomycin, vinblastine, and prednisone before low-dose radiation therapy-results of the French Society of Pediatric Oncology Study MDH90. *J Clin Oncol Off J Am Soc Clin Oncol.* 2000;18(7):1500–1507. doi:10.1200/JCO.2000.18.7.1500
11. Kung FH, Schwartz CL, Ferree CR, et al. POG 8625: a randomized trial comparing chemotherapy with chemoradiotherapy for children and adolescents with stages I, IIA, IIIA1 Hodgkin disease: a report from the Children's Oncology Group. *J Pediatr Hematol Oncol.* 2006;28(6):362-368.

12. Wolden SL, Chen L, Kelly KM, et al. Long-term results of CCG 5942: a randomized comparison of chemotherapy with and without radiotherapy for children with Hodgkin's lymphoma: a report from the Children's Oncology Group. *J Clin Oncol Off J Am Soc Clin Oncol*. 2012;30(26):3174–3180. doi:10.1200/JCO.2011.41.1819

13. Weiner MA, Leventhal B, Brecher ML, et al. Randomized study of intensive MOPP-ABVD with or without low-dose total-nodal radiation therapy in the treatment of stages IIB, IIIA2, IIIB, and IV Hodgkin's disease in pediatric patients: a Pediatric Oncology Group study. *J Clin Oncol Off J Am Soc Clin Oncol*. 1997;15(8):2769–2779. doi:10.1200/JCO.1997.15.8.2769

14. Hutchinson RJ, Fryer CJ, Davis PC, et al. MOPP or radiation in addition to ABVD in the treatment of pathologically staged advanced Hodgkin's disease in children: results of the Children's Cancer Group phase III trial. *J Clin Oncol*. 1998;16(3):897–906. doi:10.1200/JCO.1998.16.3.897

15. Dharmarajan KV, Friedman DL, Schwartz CL, et al. Patterns of relapse from a phase 3 study of response-based therapy for intermediate-risk Hodgkin lymphoma (AHOD0031): a report from the Children's Oncology Group. *Int J Radiat Oncol Biol Phys*. 2015;92(1):60–66. doi:10.1016/j.ijrobp.2014.10.042

16. Charpentier A-M, Friedman DL, Wolden S, et al. Predictive factor analysis of response-adapted radiation therapy for chemotherapy-sensitive pediatric Hodgkin lymphoma: analysis of the Children's Oncology Group AHOD 0031 trial. *Int J Radiat Oncol Biol Phys*. 2016;96(5):943–950. doi:10.1016/j.ijrobp.2016.07.015

17. Milpied N, Fielding AK, Pearce RM, et al. Allogeneic bone marrow transplant is not better than autologous transplant for patients with relapsed Hodgkin's disease: European Group for Blood and Bone Marrow Transplantation. *J Clin Oncol*. 1996;14(4):1291–1296. doi:10.1200/JCO.1996.14.4.1291

18. Poen JC, Hoppe RT, Horning SJ. High-dose therapy and autologous bone marrow transplantation for relapsed/refractory Hodgkin's disease: the impact of involved field radiotherapy on patterns of failure and survival. *Int J Radiat Oncol Biol Phys*. 1996;36(1):3–12. doi:10.1016/S0360-3016(96)00277-5

19. Schaapveld M, Aleman BMP, van Eggermond AM, et al. Second cancer risk up to 40 years after treatment for Hodgkin's lymphoma. *N Engl J Med*. 2015;373(26):2499–2511. doi:10.1056/NEJMoa1505949

20. O'Brien MM, Donaldson SS, Balise RR, et al. Second malignant neoplasms in survivors of pediatric Hodgkin's lymphoma treated with low-dose radiation and chemotherapy. *J Clin Oncol*. 2010;28(7):1232–1239. doi:10.1200/JCO.2009.24.8062

21. Constine LS, Tarbell, NJ, Halperin EC. *Pediatric Radiation Oncology*. WK Health Book. 2011:5.

XII: **PALLIATION**

61: BRAIN METASTASES

Matthew C. Ward and John H. Suh

QUICK HIT: Brain metastases are the most common intracranial tumor. Surgery, WBRT, or SRS are all treatment options and can be performed in many combinations based on careful pt selection. Key factors for pt selection include performance status, number of lesions, size of the lesions, histology, and status of extracranial disease. Typically, surgery is reserved for large or symptomatic lesions or when a tissue sample is required. The role for SRS is increasing due to concerns for neurocognitive side effects and QOL benefits for select pts.

EPIDEMIOLOGY: Most common intracranial tumor, with approximately 200,000 cases per year. Brain metastases occur in up to 30% of pts with cancer, and are the direct cause of death in 30% to 50% of those. Incidence increased in the MRI era due to the detection of smaller lesions.[1] 80% of pts have multiple lesions. Solitary brain met is defined as a single lesion without evidence of extracranial disease.

ANATOMY: Most commonly occur at the gray–white matter junction due to decrease in diameter of the vessels. Typically spherical, well-demarcated lesions with edema. 80% supratentorial, 15% cerebellum, and 5% brainstem.

PATHOLOGY: The most common histologies (overall prevalence) include lung (50%), breast (20%), melanoma (10%), colon (5%).[1] Histologies with the highest predilection for the development of brain metastases (neurotropism) include SCLC, melanoma, choriocarcinoma, germ cell. Hemorrhagic lesions are typically melanoma, choriocarcinoma, testicular, thyroid, renal cell. Most common pediatric histologies are sarcomas, Wilms, germ cell.

CLINICAL PRESENTATION: Variable but most commonly include impaired cognitive function (60%), hemiparesis (60%), headache (50%), aphasia (20%), seizures (20%).[1]

WORKUP: H&P with detailed neurologic exam.

Imaging: Noncontrast head CT often first-line test performed to rule out intracranial hemorrhage. MRI with and without contrast best to detect and characterize small metastases. Biopsy necessary if pt has no evidence of disease elsewhere. For pts presumed to have a single brain metastasis on imaging, up to 10% can be primary brain tumors,[2] although this is likely lower in the MRI era. For multiple lesions, >95% are metastatic lesions rather than primary tumors and biopsy is not required.

Pathology: If cancer origin is unclear, biopsy most accessible site, typically extracranial. If no extracranial lesions are accessible, stereotactic biopsy or resection of the brain metastasis is warranted.

PROGNOSTIC FACTORS: Prognostic systems are key to defining the treatment of choice. The most common systems are the RPA (older, created by the RTOG), the GPA (updated RTOG analysis), and the revised diagnosis-specific GPA (most recent multi-institutional retrospective cohort, more modern than the RPA and less subjective).[3–5]

TABLE 61.1: RTOG Recursive Partitioning Analysis

RPA Class[3]	Characteristics	MS (Mos)
I	KPS ≥70, controlled primary, age <65, no extracranial metastases	7.1
II	KPS ≥70 with uncontrolled primary OR age ≥65 OR extracranial metastases	4.2
III	KPS <70	2.3

Source: From Ref. (4). With permission from Elsevier.

TABLE 61.2: Graded Prognostic Assessment (GPA)

Graded Prognostic Assessment

Characteristic	0	0.5	1.0	Grade	MS (mos)
Age	>60	50–59	<50	3.5–4	11.0
KPS	<70	70–80	90–100	3	6.9
# CNS metastases	>3	2–3	1	1.5–2.5	3.8
Extracranial metastases	Present	–	Absent	0–1	2.6

Source: From Ref. (4). With permission from Elsevier.

TABLE 61.3: Diagnosis-Specific GPA

	Diagnosis-Specific GPA						
Variable	0	0.5	1	1.5	2	3	4
	NSCLC/SCLC						
Age	>60	50–60	<50				
KPS	<70	70–80	90–100				
No. cranial metastases	>3	2–3	1				
Extracranial metastases	Present	–	Absent				
	Renal/Melanoma						
KPS	<70		70–80		90–100		
No. cranial metastases	>3		2–3		1	-	-
	GI						
KPS	<70		70		80	90	100
	Breast						
KPS	≤50	60	70–80	90–100			
ER/PR/Her2	Triple negative		Luminal A (ER/PR+, HER2-)	ER/PR-HER2+	Luminal B (triple+)		
Age	≥60	<60					

Source: From Ref. (5).

TABLE 61.4: Survival Correlating to Points From Table 61.3

Diagnosis	MS (mos)	Diagnosis-Specific GPA			
MS (mos)		0–1	1.5–2	2.5–3.0	3.5–4
		MS (mos)	MS (mos)	MS (mos)	
NSCLC	7.0	3.0	5.5	9.4	14.8

(continued)

TABLE 61.4: Survival Correlating to Points From Table 61.3 (*continued*)					
Diagnosis	MS (mos)	Diagnosis-Specific GPA			
SCLC	4.9	2.8	4.9	7.7	17.1
Melanoma	6.7	3.4	4.7	8.8	13.2
Renal Cell	9.6	3.3	7.3	11.3	14.8
GI	5.4	3.1	4.4	6.9	13.5
Breast	13.8	3.4	7.7	15.1	25.3
Total	7.2	3.1	5.4	9.6	16.7

TREATMENT PARADIGM

Medical: Glucocorticoids such as dexamethasone are the first-line medical therapy and improve symptoms in up to 75% within 1 to 3 days. Side effects include weight gain, Cushingoid appearance, gastric ulcers (require GI prophylaxis), insomnia, osteopenia, proximal muscle weakness, psychosis, hyperglycemia. Memantine is an NMDA receptor antagonist used for dementia and can be given with WBRT to possibly minimize neuro-cognitive decline (see dosing later). Radiosensitizers such as motexafin gadolinium[6] and efaproxiral[7] have been studied with no demonstrable benefit.

Surgery: Recommended for larger symptomatic lesions or when tissue diagnosis is necessary. A stereotactic approach with maximal safe resection is standard.

Chemotherapy: Historically, there has been little to no role for CHT in the treatment of brain metastases due to the blood–brain barrier with the exception of metastatic germ cell tumors (e.g., testicular). Temozolomide has been studied concurrent with WBRT and improved response rates in a phase II study.[8] However, the role for targeted and immunomodulatory agents (pembrolizumab, nivolumab, crizotinib, erlotinib, ipilimumab) is rapidly evolving.

Radiotherapy: RT is the cornerstone of treatment for brain metastases and is indicated in all but the most palliative of cases (see QUARTZ trial in the following). Options include SRS or WBRT.

Dose: For WBRT, dose options include 30 Gy/10 fx (most common), 37.5 Gy/15 fx (common on RTOG trials), 20 Gy/5 fx, 10 Gy/1 fx among others.

SRS: Radiosurgery delivers a single high-dose treatment using multiple converging beams.[9] Metastases are often ideal targets for SRS considering they are small, spherical, well-demarcated, and located at the gray–white matter junction away from critical structures. Dosing is performed as per RTOG 9005 (see the following): 24 Gy for lesions 2 cm or less, 18 Gy for lesions 2.1 to 3.0 cm, and 15 Gy for those from 3.1 to 4 cm.

Toxicity: Side effects of SRS include fatigue, headache, nausea, radionecrosis, damage to nearby critical structures (optic nerve, chiasm, brainstem). Side effects of WBRT include fatigue, hair loss, skin erythema, headache, nausea, temporary muffled hearing, neuro-cognitive decline.

Procedure: See *Treatment Planning Handbook*, Chapters 3 and 13.[10]

EVIDENCE-BASED Q&A

What is the ideal dose of WBRT for pts with brain metastases?

"Standard" doses include 30 Gy/10 fx or 37.5 Gy/15 fx. Some of the original data from the RTOG randomized pts to 1- to 2-fx regimens (10 Gy/1 fx or 12 Gy/2 fx over 3 days) versus 2- to 4-week

regimens (20 Gy/5 fx, 30 Gy/10 fx, or 40 Gy/20 fx). The shorter regimens showed similar neurologic response rates between the 1- to 2-fx and 5- to 20-fx regimens. However, time to deterioration of neurologic status, the duration of improvement and rate of complete disappearance of neurologic symptoms were less in the 1- to 2-fx regimens.[11]

Is there a benefit to WBRT over best supportive care?

In poor-performance pts with NSCLC not eligible for radiosurgery or resection, the benefit of WBRT is questionable based on the following QUARTZ study.

Mulvenna, QUARTZ (*Lancet* 2016, PMID 27604504): PRT (noninferiority) of optimal supportive care (OSC) versus 20 Gy/5 fx WBRT for NSCLC. Primary endpoint was QALY (calculated using EQ-5D) with a noninferiority margin of 7 QALY days. Enrolled 538 pts, 83% were GPA 0-2 and 38% had a KPS <70. Did not demonstrate a difference in OS (HR 1.06, p = .81) or QALY days (mean QALYs was 46.4 days WBRT vs. 41.7 days OSC, 4.7 QALY-day difference with 90% CI: -12.7–3.3). Dexamethasone use was not significantly different. There were nonsignificant suggestions that WBRT may offer a survival benefit in pts with better prognoses. **Conclusion: Although OSC was not noninferior, WBRT may be unnecessary in poor-performance pts ineligible for SRS or surgery.** *Comment: Patients selected for this trial were poor performance at baseline; results may not apply to standard patient with brain metastases.*

Is there a benefit to dose escalation or hyperfractionation of WBRT?

There appears to be no benefit to WBRT dose escalation or altered fractionation.

Regine, RTOG 9104 (*IJROBP* 2001, PMID 9336134): PRT of 445 pts with a KPS ≥70 and an NFS 1–2 randomized to either 30 Gy in 10 fx or WBRT to 32 Gy/20 fx with a boost to a total of 54.4 Gy in 34 fx all at 1.6 Gy BID with no difference in survival, no difference in grade 3–4 toxicity and one fatal toxicity in the high-dose arm. **Conclusion: No benefit to dose escalation or hyperfractionation.**

To what degree is WBRT responsible for a decline in neurocognitive function?

This is a controversial topic and is complicated by the observation that 90% of brain metastasis pts have at least one neurocognitive deficit at baseline.[12] *One study by DeAngelis from 1989 showed that fraction sizes >3 Gy were associated with an increased risk of dementia.*[13] *RTOG 9104 showed no difference in MMSE between the 30 Gy and 54.4 Gy arms.*[14] *However, it did show poor neurocognitive outcomes in those with progressive metastases. Therefore, it is the assumption that uncontrolled disease can often be more deleterious than side effects. See the following for comparison between SRS and WBRT in regard to neurocognitive function.*

Does WBRT improve outcomes after surgery?

Patchell II (*JAMA* 1998, PMID 9809728): PRT of 95 pts with one brain met and KPS ≥70 randomized to surgery alone versus surgery with postoperative WBRT (50.4 Gy/28 fx). Nearly all outcomes were improved except survival, but the trial was not powered for survival. **Conclusion: WBRT after surgical resection of a single brain met improves local and distant brain control.**

TABLE 61.5: Patchell II Results						
	Any Recurrence	Distant Recurrence	LR	MS	Neurologic Death	Functional Independence
Surgery	70%	37%	46%	43 wks	44%	35 wks

(continued)

TABLE 61.5: Patchell II Results (*continued*)						
	Any Recurrence	Distant Recurrence	LR	MS	Neurologic Death	Functional Independence
Surgery+RT	18%	14%	10%	48 wks	14%	37 wks
p value	<.001	<.01	<.001	.39	.003	.61

What is the role of surgery in pts with a single brain metastasis?

Surgery is beneficial for select pts and is typically reserved for pts with large and relatively few lesions in a resectable location. Three trials have looked at adding surgery to WBRT and two (Patchell in the following and Noordijk[15]) showed a survival benefit. The third did not show an OS benefit but enrolled poor-performance pts.[16]

Patchell I (*NEJM* 1990, PMID 2405271): PRT of 48 pts with single brain met randomized to biopsy followed by WBRT versus surgical resection with WBRT (36 Gy/12 fx). Of note, 6 of 54 pts (11%) were found to have a primary brain tumor or benign findings (pre-MRI era). **Conclusion: Surgical resection + WBRT for a single brain met improves OS compared to WBRT alone.**

TABLE 61.6: Patchell I Results						
	LR	Time to LR	DM	MS	Time to Neurologic Death	Functional Independence
Biopsy+WBRT	52%	21 wks	13%	15 wks	26 wks	8 wks
Surgery+WBRT	20%	>59 wks	20%	40 wks	62 wks	38 wks
p value	<.02	<.0001	.52	<.01	<.0009	<.005

What determines the dose of SRS?

Dosing is based on tumor diameter: 15 Gy, 18 Gy, and 24 Gy for tumors 3.1 to 4 cm, 2.1 to 3 cm, and ≤2.0 cm, respectively.

Shaw, RTOG 9005 (*IJROBP* 2000, PMID 10802351): Phase I/II SRS dose escalation trial for pts with a recurrent primary brain tumor (36%) or metastases (64%) ≤4 cm after receiving previous brain RT ≥3 mos prior. Treated to escalating dose levels. The maximum tolerated dose was 15 Gy for tumors 3.1 to 4 cm and 18 Gy for tumors 2.1 to 3 cm. Investigators were unwilling to escalate above 24 Gy to tumors ≤2.0 cm. A homogeneity index (ratio of max dose/prescription dose) of 2 or higher was found to be associated with increased toxicity. The incidence of radionecrosis was 11% at 2 years.

When added to standard WBRT, does an SRS boost improve survival?

SRS boost improves local control after WBRT, with no clear impact on OS.

Andrews, RTOG 9508 (*Lancet* 2004, PMID 15158627): Pts with one to three new brain metastases all ≤4 cm randomized to WBRT or WBRT+SRS boost. WBRT dose was 37.5 Gy/15 fx, boost was given 1 week after WBRT to the RTOG 9005 doses. While there was an improvement in local control, KPS, and steroid use in all pts, the primary endpoint of OS was not met. Pts with a single metastasis did demonstrate a survival benefit. On an unplanned subset analysis, pts in RPA class I, those with large metastases (>2 cm), squamous or NSCLC or KPS 90–100 experienced a benefit that was not statistically significant after adjustment for unplanned subgroup analyses. **Conclusion: SRS boost improves LC after WBRT.**

TABLE 61.7: RTOG 9508 Results

RTOG 9508	Mean Survival (mos; *= subset analysis, p value necessary .0056)						1-yr LC	Stable/ Improved KPS at 6 mos
	Overall	Single met	*Tumor >2 cm	*RPA class I	*Squamous/ NSCLC	*KPS 90-100		
WBRT alone	6.5	4.9	5.3	9.6	3.9	7.4	71%	25%
WBRT + SRS	5.7	6.5	6.5	11.6	5.9	10.2	82%	42%
p value	.136	.039	.045	.045	.051	.071	.013	.033

If SRS boost does not improve survival compared to WBRT alone, does WBRT improve survival when added to SRS?

Aoyama (*JAMA* 2006, PMID 16757720): Randomized 132 pts with one to four brain metastases all <3 cm to WBRT (30 Gy/10 fx) with SRS versus SRS alone. SRS doses alone were 22 to 25 Gy for tumors ≤2 cm, and 18 to 20 Gy for tumors >2 cm in size and reduced by 30% if given after WBRT. 49% had a single met, 83% were RPA class II. Primary endpoint OS. Closed early on interim analysis because of futility to show a difference in OS. Rate of LR and any recurrence were decreased significantly by WBRT. **Conclusion: The addition of WBRT does not confer a survival benefit when added to SRS, although not sufficiently powered for this endpoint.**

TABLE 61.8: Aoyama Trial Results

	MS	Neurologic Death	1-yr Any Recurrence	1-yr LR	1-yr Distant Recurrence	Neurologic preservation
SRS Alone	8.0 m	19%	76%	27.5%	64%	70%
WBRT + SRS	7.5 m	23%	47%	11%	42%	72%
p value	.42	.64	<.001	.002	.003	.99

If survival is not improved by adding SRS to WBRT, do the neurocognitive risks of adding WBRT to SRS outweigh the benefits?

This is a controversial question but most recent data suggests no clear OS benefit to WBRT added to SRS with a clear detriment in neurocognitive outcomes. These results lead many to recommend SRS alone with close surveillance for distant failure rather than WBRT in pts with good PS.

Chang, MD Anderson (*Lancet Oncol* 2009, PMID 19801201): Randomized pts with one to three brain metastases to SRS with or without WBRT (similar arms to Aoyama) with a primary endpoint of a deterioration of the HVLT-R total recall domain by 5 points at 4 mos from treatment. Trial stopped early after 58 pts enrolled due to increased decline in WBRT arm. LC was improved from 67% to 100% with WBRT and distant control by 45% to 73%. However, neurocognitive function declined in 23% of SRS pts versus 49% of WBRT+SRS pts. **Conclusion: SRS+WBRT pts experienced a significant decline in neurocognitive function. SRS alone may be the preferred treatment strategy.** *Comment: MS was 15.2 mos (SRS) versus 5.7 mos (WBRT+SRS), suggesting imbalance of pts in two arms, and pts who are nearing the end of life perform worse on the HVLT.*

Kocher, EORTC 22952 (*JCO* 2011, PMID 21041710): PRT of 359 pts with one to three brain metastases randomized to observation or WBRT (30 Gy/10 fx) after either SRS or surgery. Primary endpoint was the time to WHO performance status greater than 2. There was no difference in OS (10.7 vs. 10.9 mo) and WBRT improved local failure (31% SRS, 59% surgery, 19% SRS+WBRT, 27% Surg+WBRT) and any in-brain failure (42% surgery, 48% SRS, 33% SRS+WBRT, 23% Surg+WBRT). There was no difference in the time to a performance status above 2. **Conclusion: WBRT can be omitted in select pts with good follow-up on imaging.**

Sahgal, Meta-analysis (*IJROBP* 2015, PMID 25752382): Individual pt level meta-analysis including Aoyama, Chang, and Kocher trials, investigating SRS alone versus WBRT+SRS in pts with one to four brain metastases. 359 pts included. Age was found to be a significant predictor of the effect of WBRT on OS and distant cranial failure. Younger pts treated with SRS alone had a lower hazard of mortality (MS for age ≤50: 13.6 mos SRS alone vs. 8.2 mos SRS+WBRT). Younger pts (≤50) also did not benefit in terms of distant brain failure but pts >50 did benefit from the addition of WBRT. The addition of WBRT to SRS showed a local control benefit across all subgroups. **Conclusion: SRS alone may be the treatment of choice for pts ≤50 with one to four brain metastases.**

Brown, NCCTG N0574 (*JAMA* 2016, PMID 27458945): PRT of 213 pts with one to three brain metastases all <3 cm randomized to SRS or WBRT+SRS. Primary endpoint was a decline in any of six cognitive tests (HVLT-R immediate recall, HVLT-R delayed recall, COWA, Trailmaking A & B, and Grooved Pegboard) at 3 mos >1 standard deviation from baseline. 213 were randomized, 111 included in the primary endpoint analysis (63 in SRS arm, 48 in SRS+WBRT arm). Results showed that cognitive progression at 3 mos was more common after WBRT+SRS than SRS alone (91.7% vs. 63.5%, $p < .001$). This was true across immediate recall, delayed recall, and verbal fluency. QOL was also improved in the SRS group with no difference in functional independence. In-brain control was better in the WBRT arm (93.7% vs. 75.3% at 3 mos, $p < .001$) but survival was not different (10.4 mo SRS vs. 7.4 mo SRS+WBRT, $p = .92$). **Conclusion: WBRT does not improve survival despite better tumor control and is associated with more cognitive deterioration. SRS alone may be the preferred strategy.**

If WBRT is associated with a decline in neurocognitive function, what are some possible strategies to avoid this?

Adding memantine or avoiding the hippocampus are two strategies to possibly decrease neurocognitive function.

Brown, RTOG 0614 (*Neuro-Oncol* 2013, PMID 23956241): Pts with a KPS ≥70 and stable systemic disease randomized to receive 20 mg of memantine (NMDA antagonist used in dementia) during and after WBRT for a total of 24 weeks. Pts started 5 mg daily, then 5 mg BID, then 10 mg in the morning and 5 mg in the afternoon, then 10 mg BID. Primary endpoint was the decline in HVLT-R-DR at 24 weeks compared to baseline. There was a trend toward improved HVLT-R-DR scores ($p = .059$) but statistical power was limited due to pt loss.

Gondi, RTOG 0933 (*JCO* 2014, PMID 25349290): Single-arm phase II study of using IMRT to avoid the hippocampus (HA-WBRT). Brain metastases were >5 mm from the hippocampus, which was limited to 16 Gy max dose and D100% ≤9 Gy. The primary endpoint was HVLT-R-DR at 4 mos and was compared to a historical control of 30% decline from baseline (from motexafin gadolinium trial). HA-WBRT showed a decline of 7%, which was less than the historical control ($p < .001$).

How many metastases are necessary to warrant WBRT rather than SRS?

The trend with modern planning systems is to treat with SRS alone to avoid WBRT but the specific number remains unclear.

Yamamato, Japan (*Lancet Oncol* 2014, PMID 24621620): Prospective observational study of pts with 1 to 10 new metastases (max <3 cm) treated with SRS alone. Pts with 5 to 10 lesions were compared with pts with 1 tumor and pts with 2 to 4 tumors. The primary endpoint was overall survival. Results showed that overall survival did not differ between the 5–10 cohort when compared to the 2–4 cohort (noninferior). The rate of adverse events was also similar. **Conclusion: SRS may be suitable in pts with up to 10 brain metastases.**

What treatment options are there for large metastases who are not surgical candidates?

Remember previous SRS studies enrolled pts with tumors <4 cm. Fractionated SRS may be an option for pts with larger tumors (>10 cc or >3 cm) to achieve local control. This is based on single-arm prospective data from Japan showing LC 61% to 76% at 1 yr. Dose and fractionation was either 10 Gy x 3 fx with 2 weeks apart[17] or 20 to 30 Gy/2 fx with a 2- to 4-week break.[18] A comparative retrospective series of 289 pts from Italy with lesions >2 cm treated with single-fraction SRS or 27 Gy/3 fx demonstrated an improvement in local control from 77% to 91% with multifraction SRS.[19]

Is postoperative SRS to the resection cavity effective at reducing local failure after complete resection?

Mahajan, MDACC (*Lancet Oncol* 2017, PMID 28687375): Single-institution PRT of 132 pts randomized after complete resection of one to three metastases to either observation or postoperative SRS. MFU 11.1 mos. Primary endpoint was local recurrence. At 12 mos, freedom from LR was 43% in the observation group vs. 72% with SRS ($p = .015$). **Conclusion: Postoperative SRS is effective at the reduction of LF and may be considered as an alternative to WBRT.**

Can SRS offer similar rates of control in the postoperative setting to WBRT but without the neurocognitive deficits?

In an attempt to maintain control rates while decreasing cognitive changes, SRS can be given to the resection cavity. Initial retrospective data from Stanford[20] showed a local failure rate of 9.5% at 1 year overall but only 3% with a 2-mm margin around the resection cavity versus 16% without a margin. Distant failure, however, was 54% with post-op SRS. Note that the dosing to the resection cavity is often by volume rather than by diameter, but this varies by institution.

Brown, N107C (*Lancet Oncol* 2017, PMID 28687377): PRT of 194 pts with four or fewer metastases (all <3 cm) with resection of a single lesion (cavity <5 cm), then randomized to WBRT (with SRS to unresected metastases) versus SRS alone to the cavity and unresected lesions. Coprimary endpoints were OS and cognitive deterioration free survival (CDFS) at 6 mos, defined as death or a drop by 1 standard deviation in one test (HVLT, COWA, Trailmaking A & B). Preferred sequencing was SRS to unresected metastases followed by WBRT within 14 days. Dosing to the surgical bed was 12 to 20 Gy depending on tumor volume (dosing to unresected lesions was 18 to 24 Gy depending on arm and diameter). *Results*: No difference in OS (MS 12.2 mos SRS vs. 11.6 mos WBRT, $p = .70$). CDFS was improved in SRS arm: median 3.7 mos vs. 3.0 mos, $p < .0001$). **Conclusion: Decline in cognitive function is more common with WBRT. Postoperative SRS should be one standard of care.**

Kayama, JCOG 0504 (*ASCO* 2016, Abstract #2003): PRT (noninferiority) of 271 pts with four or fewer lesions randomized to SRS or WBRT after surgery. Only one lesion ≥3 cm was resected. Primary endpoint was OS, with a noninferiority margin of an HR of 1.385. The MS was 15.6 mos on both arms, with an HR of 1.05. Grade 2-4 cognitive dysfunction at 90 days or beyond was higher in the WBRT arm (16% vs. 8%). **Conclusion: With respect to OS, SRS appears noninferior to WBRT.**

REFERENCES

1. Nichols EM, Patchell RA, Regine WF, Kowk Y. Palliation of brain and spinal cord metastases. In: Halperin EC, Wazer DE, Perez CA, Brady LW, eds. *Perez and Brady's Principles and Practice of Radiation Oncology*. 6th ed. Philadelphia, PA: Lippincott Williams & Wilkins; 2013:1765–1772.

2. Patchell RA, Tibbs PA, Walsh JW, et al. A randomized trial of surgery in the treatment of single metastases to the brain. *N Engl J Med.* 1990;322(8):494–500.

3. Gaspar L, Scott C, Rotman M, et al. Recursive partitioning analysis (RPA) of prognostic factors in three Radiation Therapy Oncology Group (RTOG) brain metastases trials. *Int J Radiat Oncol Biol Phys.* 1997;37(4):745–751.

4. Sperduto PW, Berkey B, Gaspar LE, et al. A new prognostic index and comparison to three other indices for patients with brain metastases: an analysis of 1,960 patients in the RTOG database. *Int J Radiat Oncol Biol Phys.* 2008;70(2):510–514.

5. Sperduto PW, Kased N, Roberge D, et al. Summary report on the graded prognostic assessment: an accurate and facile diagnosis-specific tool to estimate survival for patients with brain metastases. *J Clin Oncol.* 2012;30(4):419–425.

6. Mehta MP, Rodrigus P, Terhaard CH, et al. Survival and neurologic outcomes in a randomized trial of motexafin gadolinium and whole-brain radiation therapy in brain metastases. *J Clin Oncol.* 2003;21(13):2529–2536.

7. Suh JH, Stea B, Nabid A, et al. Phase III study of efaproxiral as an adjunct to whole-brain radiation therapy for brain metastases. *J Clin Oncol.* 2006;24(1):106–114.

8. Antonadou D, Paraskevaidis M, Sarris G, et al. Phase II randomized trial of temozolomide and concurrent radiotherapy in patients with brain metastases. *J Clin Oncol.* 2002;20(17):3644–3650.

9. Suh JH. Stereotactic radiosurgery for the management of brain metastases. *N Engl J Med.* 2010;362(12):1119–1127.

10. Videtic GMM, Woody N, Vassil AD. *Handbook of Treatment Planning in Radiation Oncology.* 2nd ed. New York, NY: Demos Medical; 2015.

11. Borgelt B, Gelber R, Larson M, et al. Ultra-rapid high dose irradiation schedules for the palliation of brain metastases: final results of the first two studies by the Radiation Therapy Oncology Group. *Int J Radiat Oncol Biol Phys.* 1981;7(12):1633–1638.

12. Meyers CA, Smith JA, Bezjak A, et al. Neurocognitive function and progression in patients with brain metastases treated with whole-brain radiation and motexafin gadolinium: results of a randomized phase III trial. *J Clin Oncol.* 2004;22(1):157–165.

13. DeAngelis LM, Mandell LR, Thaler HT, et al. The role of postoperative radiotherapy after resection of single brain metastases. *Neurosurgery.* 1989;24(6):798–805.

14. Regine WF, Scott C, Murray K, Curran W. Neurocognitive outcome in brain metastases patients treated with accelerated-fractionation vs. accelerated-hyperfractionated radiotherapy: an analysis from Radiation Therapy Oncology Group Study 91-04. *Int J Radiat Oncol Biol Phys.* 2001;51(3):711–717.

15. Noordijk EM, Vecht CJ, Haaxma-Reiche H, et al. The choice of treatment of single brain metastasis should be based on extracranial tumor activity and age. *Int J Radiat Oncol Biol Phys.* 1994;29(4):711–717.

16. Mintz AH, Kestle J, Rathbone MP, et al. A randomized trial to assess the efficacy of surgery in addition to radiotherapy in patients with a single cerebral metastasis. *Cancer.* 1996;78(7):1470–1476.

17. Higuchi Y, Serizawa T, Nagano O, et al. Three-staged stereotactic radiotherapy without whole brain irradiation for large metastatic brain tumors. *Int J Radiat Oncol Biol Phys.* 2009;74(5):1543–1548.

18. Yomo S, Hayashi M, Nicholson C. A prospective pilot study of two-session Gamma Knife surgery for large metastatic brain tumors. *J Neurooncol.* 2012;109(1):159–165.

19. Minniti G, Scaringi C, Paolini S, et al. Single-fraction versus multifraction (3 × 9 Gy) stereotactic radiosurgery for large (>2 cm) brain metastases: a comparative analysis of local control and risk of radiation-induced brain necrosis. *Int J Radiat Oncol Biol Phys.* 2016;95(4):1142–1148.

20. Choi CY, Chang SD, Gibbs IC, et al. Stereotactic radiosurgery of the postoperative resection cavity for brain metastases: prospective evaluation of target margin on tumor control. *Int J Radiat Oncol Biol Phys.* 2012;84(2):336–342.

62: BONE METASTASIS

Ehsan H. Balagamwala and Andrew Vassil

QUICK HIT: Up to 80% of advanced cancer pts develop bone metastases. RT is effective at palliation with approximately 2/3 experiencing pain relief and up to 1/3 experiencing complete pain relief. The most common RT regimens include 8 Gy/1 fx, 20 Gy/5 fx, and 30 Gy/10 fx. Factors that influence treatment technique include performance status, logistics, tumor size, tumor location, soft tissue component, histology, previous surgery, neurologic deficits, impending fracture, prior RT, and physician preference. As per the Dutch Bone Metastasis study, RTOG 9714, and the Toronto meta-analysis, there is no difference in pain control between single- and multiple-fraction regimens for uncomplicated bone metastases. The precise role for SBRT/SRS is evolving.

EPIDEMIOLOGY: Up to 80% of pts with advanced solid tumors develop bone metastasis to the spine, pelvis, or extremities[1] and over half of people who die of cancer are thought to have bone involvement.[2] Most common primary tumor sites are breast, prostate, lung, thyroid, and kidney. GI cancers metastasize to bone relatively infrequently. Metastases to bone most often occur in the red marrow, and thus follow red marrow distribution: spine (lumbar>thoracic) > pelvis > ribs > femur > skull.

ANATOMY: Axial skeleton includes the skull, spine, sternum, and ribs. Appendicular skeleton includes long bones and appendixes. Long bones consist of epiphysis (end), metaphysis, and diaphysis (shaft). Two types of bone: cortical and trabecular. Cortical is dense and compact, and makes up 80% of skeletal mass, found in diaphysis of long bones and surrounding cuboidal bones, provides strength and protection; ~3% replaced per year. Trabecular is spongy, found inside long bones (concentrated at ends), throughout vertebral bodies, and the inner portions of pelvis and other large flat bones, contains red marrow; ~25% replaced per year.

PATHOLOGY: Bone metastases occur via hematogenous spread, though bones can become involved via direct extension (e.g., oral cavity cancer invading the mandible). It is likely that a combination of tumor factors (cell adhesion molecules that bind to receptors on the cells of the marrow and bone matrix) and the bony microenvironment (growth factors released and activated during bone resorption) contributes to preferential metastasis to bone.[3] Normal bone is constantly remodeled over 3 to 6 months (remember: osteo**B**lasts **B**uild bone and osteoclasts resorb bone). Bony metastasis cause a dysregulation of normal bone remodeling that can manifest as osteoblastic, osteolytic, or mixed lesions. The bone destruction of osteolytic mets is mediated by osteoclasts, which are activated by factors produced by tumor cells, such as TGF-β, PTH-rP, IL-1, and IL-6. Important to note that while classically certain cancers are thought to be primarily osteoblastic or osteolytic (see the following), the vast majority have components of both processes. *Osteoblastic*: prostate, SCLC, Hodgkin lymphoma, carcinoid. *Osteolytic*: renal cell, melanoma, multiple myeloma, NSCLC, thyroid, NHL. *Mixed*: breast, GI, squamous cell.

CLINICAL PRESENTATION: Most common presenting symptom is pain, reduced mobility (70%), pathological fractures (10%–20%), hypercalcemia (10%–15%), spinal cord/nerve compression (5%), and reduced marrow function.

WORKUP: H&P to assess for pain onset, sensory or motor dysfunction, walking ability, urinary retention or overflow incontinence, bowel incontinence or constipation. On careful physical exam, palpate symptomatic site, extent of soft tissue extension, relationship to nearby neurovascular structures, functional status of the extremity, limb edema, muscle strength, range of motion, and evaluation for primary site.

Imaging: Appendicular skeletal metastases are best evaluated using x-ray of the entire involved bone from joint to joint (least sensitive but most specific)—this allows one to evaluate bone structure, integrity, extent of involvement, evaluation of pathologic fracture, and impending fracture risk. Small lesions are difficult to assess on x-rays as 30% to 50% of bone mineral context must be lost to be visible and metastases usually develop in the medulla, and do not involve the cortex until later. Bone scan (technetium-99m) also considered first line, especially if prostate cancer is suspected; increased uptake is an indicator of osteoblastic activity (less effective when osteolysis dominates). Skeletal survey can be helpful in cases where osteolysis predominates such as multiple myeloma. CT more sensitive than XR, may be useful in assessing pathologic fracture risk or guiding biopsies. MRI is most sensitive (91%–100% compared to 62%–85% for bone scan) and is most useful in evaluating neurovascular compression and assessing marrow involvement, particularly in vertebral bodies (best seen on T1 with contrast and STIR series). For those with lumbar spine metastasis, risk for concurrent asymptomatic metastasis in the C/T spine is significant and therefore, full spinal imaging is warranted. PET/CT is extremely sensitive, and is useful in detecting osteolytic metastases. Neoplasms with lower metabolic rate (like prostate cancer) not typically evident on FDG-PET; it is less sensitive than Tc-99m bone scan for detection of osteoblastic metastases.[4]

Biopsy: Tissue diagnosis may not be needed for pts with a previous diagnosis of metastatic bone disease or pathologic fracture requiring repair. Tissue diagnosis is required in pts with solitary bone lesions without a history of cancer or as a first metastatic relapse. CT-guided FNA or core biopsy is preferred.

PROGNOSTIC FACTORS: For bone metastases involving the appendicular skeleton, assessing fracture risk is very important. Historically, ≥2–3 cm cortical involvement or lytic destruction of 50% of width of bone was concerning for impending fracture. Mirels scoring system is commonly utilized to predict risk for fracture and is based on a 12-point scale (see Table 62.1).[5] Additional candidates for prophylactic fixation: all lesions with significant functionally limiting pain that is exacerbated by weight bearing or pts who have failed RT and have ongoing pain.

Pts with spine metastases may also be at a risk for developing vertebral compression fracture (VCF). The Spinal Instability Neoplastic Score (SINS) is utilized to predict which pts will require surgical stabilization prior to RT.[6] Higher scores were assigned to pts with junction lesions (occiput-C2, C7-T2, T11-L1, L5-S1), pain with movement or loading of the spine or relief with recumbency, subluxation/translation present, >50% vertebral body collapse, and/or bilateral posterolateral involvement of spinal elements.

TABLE 62.1: Mirels Nomogram for Pathologic Fracture Risk of Bone Metastases			
Site	Upper limb	Lower limb	Peritrochanteric
Degree of pain	Mild	Moderate	Severe
Radiographic nature	Blastic	Mixed	Lytic
Size of cortex	<1/3	1/3–2/3	>2/3

(continued)

TABLE 62.1: Mirels Nomogram for Pathologic Fracture Risk of Bone Metastases (*continued*)
Some add one point if lesion in femur proximal to lesser trochanter, lesion in proximal half of humerus, breast cancer, no bisphosphonates, osteoporosis present.
≤7 points = <10% fracture risk → observe. 8 points = 15% fracture risk → consider fixation. 9 points = 33% fracture risk → prophylactic fixation. ≥10 points = >50% fracture risk → prophylactic fixation.
Source: From Ref. (5).

TREATMENT PARADIGM

Surgery: Surgery is considered to prevent or treat pathologic fractures. Both lytic and blastic lesions reduce bone strength. Femoral metastases account for 2/3 of pathologic fractures requiring intervention. Fractures of the femoral neck can be managed by total hip arthroplasty (replacing the femoral head and acetabulum) or proximal femoral endoprosthesis. Fractures of intertrochanteric region are managed by open reduction and internal fixation without prosthesis (better gait). Lytic disease below intertrochanteric area is treated with an intramedullary rod.

Percutaneous procedures: These procedures are utilized in pts with vertebral compression fractures. Vertebroplasty is a procedure in which bone cement is injected into the vertebral body via a percutaneous approach. Kyphoplasty involves creating a cavity in the fractured vertebral body using a percutaneous placed balloon device followed by placement of bone cement in the cavity once the balloon is removed. The potential benefit of kyphoplasty is realignment of a kyphotic spine. The difference between the two procedures is that vertebroplasty does not restore the height of the vertebral body, whereas kyphoplasty potentially restores height and affects alignment. Vertebroplasty/kyphoplasty are not possible when the posterior wall of the vertebral body is fractured, with significant superior and inferior endplate fractures, significant kyphosis, or significant spinal canal narrowing.

Medical management

Bisphosphonates: Bisphosphonates have been shown to decrease skeletal-related events (SRE) by inhibiting osteoclast-mediated bone resorption and promoting repair by stimulating osteoblast differentiation and bone formation.[7,8] Zoledronate and pamidronate are most common. Zoledronate also induces apoptosis and inhibits tumor cell adhesion to the extracellular matrix. Toxicities include osteonecrosis (1%–2%), hypocalcemia, and renal insufficiency.

RANK-L Inhibitors: RANK/RANK-ligand/osteoprotegerin (RANK/RANK-L/OPG) pathway regulates osteoclast maturation, differentiation, and survival and is disrupted in the metastatic setting due to increased RANK expression.[9] Denosumab is a mAB that binds and inhibits RANK-L. FDA approved in 2010 for prevention of SRE in pts with bone metastasis from solid tumors (except multiple myeloma). A pt-level meta-analysis of three phase III trials comparing zoledronic acid versus denosumab for metastatic bone disease in breast, prostate, or other solid tumors concluded that denosumab was superior to zoledronic acid in reducing the risk of a first-on-study SRE and in delaying the time to a first SRE or hypercalcemia of malignancy (median 26.6 vs. 19.4 months).[10] OS and disease progression were similar with both treatments.

Radiation: RT is the cornerstone of treatment for pts with bone metastases. EBRT is most frequently utilized; however, there is an increasing role of radiopharmaceuticals. The 2017 ASTRO guidelines suggest: 8 Gy/1 fx, 20 Gy/5 fx, 24 Gy/6 fx, 20 Gy/10 fx (for myeloma) or 30 Gy/10 fx as recommended doses.[11] Spine SBRT can be utilized for select cases. The most clear indication for spine SBRT is in the retreatment setting (20 Gy/10 fx is also a common retreatment regimen). For spine SBRT, the most common fractionation schemes include 16 to 18 Gy/1 fx. 24 Gy/1–2 fx have been used but may be associated with increased VCF.[12] Guidelines are published for contouring of definitive spine SBRT, postoperative spine SBRT, and for response assessment (SPINO).[13–15]

Procedure: For treatment planning details, please see *Treatment Planning Handbook*, Chapter 13.[16]

EVIDENCE-BASED Q&A

Is there a benefit to longer fractionation schemes for uncomplicated bone metastases?

Several large prospective trials (Dutch Bone Metastasis Study, RTOG 9714) as well as the Toronto meta-analysis showed no difference in pain relief (~2/3) between single-fraction and multifraction regimens. Retreatment rates are higher after single-fraction RT, perhaps due to physician bias.[17] Note that complicated bone metastases (fractures, cord compression, previous RT) were excluded from these trials. When there is risk for pathologic fracture, fractionated RT is preferred (lower risk for fractures on the Dutch study[18]).

Steenland, Dutch Bone Metastasis Study (*Radiother Oncol* 1999, PMID 10577695): PRT of 1,171 pts randomized to receive either 8 Gy/1 fx or 24 Gy/6 fx. Weekly questionnaires were used for self-assessment after treatment and primary endpoint was pain score (0–10). 71% experienced a response (median 3 weeks in both groups) and no differences between pain meds, QOL, or side effects between regimens. 25% were retreated in the single-fraction group versus 7% in the fractionated group (but time to retreat was shorter and pain score at time of retreatment was lower, likely suggesting doctors were more willing to retreat single fx pts). Of note, axial cortical involvement >30 mm ($p = .01$) and circumferential cortical involvement >50% ($p = .03$) were predictive of fracture, but not the Mirels nomogram score. If these high-risk pts are not candidates for surgery, offer fractionated RT.[19]

Hartsell, RTOG 9714 (*JNCI* 2005, PMID 15928300): PRT of 898 pts with breast or prostate cancer with one to three sites of painful bone metastases and moderate to severe pain randomized to 8 Gy in 1 fx versus 30 Gy in 10 fx. No difference in overall RR (66%), CR (~15%), and PR (~50%). More frequent grade 2-4 acute toxicity (mostly GI related) in 30 Gy arm (17% vs. 10%, $p = .002$). No difference in late toxicity (4%), fracture rates (4%–5%), or narcotic use at 3 months. Higher rate of retreatment with single fraction (18% vs. 9%, $p < .001$). **Conclusion: A single fraction of 8 Gy provides similar efficacy in pain relief, with less acute toxicity but higher rates of retreatment than 30 Gy/10 fx.**

Chow, Toronto Meta-analysis (*JCO* 2007, PMID 17416863; Update Chow *Clin Oncol* 2012, PMID 22130630): Meta-analysis of 25 PRT with over 5,600 pts comparing single- to multiple-fraction schedules. No difference in overall RR (60% vs. 61%), CR (23 vs. 24%), acute toxicity, or pathologic fracture risk (3.3% vs. 3.0%). Retreatment was more likely in the single-fraction group (20% vs. 8%, $p < .00001$).

What is the best dose for single-fraction palliative RT?

Based on a systematic review of 24 trials, a dose–response relationship was noted and 8 Gy in 1 fx was found to be the optimal single-fraction dose.

Dennis, Toronto Meta-analysis on Dose (*Radiother Oncol* 2013, PMID 23321492): Systematic review of 24 trials with 3,233 pts randomized to 28 single-fraction arms, ranging from 4 to 15 Gy. 8 Gy was the most commonly used dose (84%) and higher doses produced better pain response rates. Trials that directly compared different single-fraction doses demonstrated that 8 Gy was statistically superior to 4 Gy.

What is the expected time to pain response with conventional RT? What about conventional RT versus SBRT?

Median time to pain response is approximately 3 weeks with either single-fraction or multifraction conventional RT regimens.[19,20] However, as per the TROG 96.05 study, the durability of pain control appears to be lower for single-fraction compared to multifraction regimens (2.4 vs. 3.7 months, p = .056).[21] For spine metastasis, the time to pain relief appears to be similar between conventional RT and SBRT.[22]

What are pain flares and what is the incidence? What about in spine SBRT?

A pain flare is a temporary worsening of bone pain in the irradiated site, usually in the first few days after RT and lasting 1 to 2 days. 80% of pain flares happen in the first 5 days following RT, with a minority happening between days 5 and 10. Up to 40% of pts treated with RT may develop a pain flare in the first 10 days after RT.[23] In spine SBRT, the incidence of pain flare is variable and reported to be 15% to 70% depending on dose.[24] This can be treated (or possibly prevented) with short course of steroids.

What is the role of RT after orthopedic stabilization?

RT promotes remineralization and bone healing, alleviates pain, improves functional status, and reduces the risk for subsequent fracture or loss of fixation by treating residual metastatic disease. It also decreases need for second surgery and is associated with a prolonged survival.[25] Disadvantages include the potential effects on uninvolved bone and on postoperative wound healing. If an implant is placed, classically the entire implant is treated. RT is generally started within 2 to 4 weeks after surgery after wound healing. The optimal dose/fractionation is unclear as there is limited data regarding single-fraction treatments, so 30 Gy/10 fx is typically recommended.

What is the evidence for retreatment of bone metastasis?

About 20% will require retreatment of bone metastasis. Retreatment is feasible and can provide pain relief in 50% to 60%.[26,27] It is recommended to wait at least 4 weeks after initial RT before considering re-irradiation to allow for full response from initial course. Single fraction appears to have similar efficacy as multifraction regimens for uncomplicated metastases. Important to note that pts who respond favorably to prior RT have a higher chance of responding to reirradiation.

Chow, Canadian NCIC SC 20 (*Lancet Oncol* 2014, PMID 24369114): RCT of pts with painful (≥2 using brief pain inventory) bone metastases previously treated with RT. Randomized between 8 Gy/1 fx versus 20 Gy in multiple fractions. Primary endpoint pain response at 2 months. 425 pts enrolled. Overall pain response at 2 months was 28% in the 8 Gy versus 32% in the 20 Gy arm. Toxicity including lack of appetite and diarrhea worse in the 20 Gy arm. **Conclusion: 8 Gy was noninferior and less toxic than 20 Gy for re-irradiation of painful bone metastases.**

What is the role of hemibody irradiation?

Hemibody irradiation may be indicated in those with significant bony disease. Although single and multifraction regimens have been reported, they have not been compared in a randomized fashion. Hemibody irradiation is generally used when radiopharmaceuticals are not available or are contraindicated. An extended SSD technique is utilized and fields are matched at the umbilicus or L4/5. Lung blocks may be necessary to limit lung dose to 6–7 Gy. Typically, 6 Gy/1 fx is utilized for the upper body and 8 Gy/1 fx to the lower body. Alternate doses include 15 Gy in 5 fractions or

20 to 30 Gy in 8 to 10 fractions delivered 3 fractions weekly. Typically, the other half of the body is treated 6 to 8 weeks later.

What is the role of radiopharmaceuticals for the treatment of extensive bony metastases?

Radiopharmaceuticals are radioactive agents that are administered intravenously and localize to the site of osteoblastic activity, thereby delivering dose simultaneously at sites of disease. Most common isotopes used are beta-emitters (Sr-89, Sm-153, P-53) and alpha-emitters (Ra-223). Beta-emitters have a response rate of approximately 60% to 70% and a complete response of ~20%. The primary advantage of samarium (Sm-153) over strontium (Sr-89) is a significantly shorter half-life (1.5 vs. 50.5 days, respectively). Myelosuppression is the major toxicity, which can be prolonged with Sr-89 but generally nadirs at 3 to 4 weeks and recovers by 6 to 8 weeks with Sm-153. Recently, alpha-emitters (Ra-223) have gained favor (see the following) and offer the advantage of a high LET and short range (10 μm in bone and soft tissue).

Parker, ALSYMPCA (*NEJM* 2013, PMID 23863050; Update Sartor *Lancet Oncol* 2014, PMID 24836273): PRT of 921 pts with metastatic (two or more bony metastases and no known visceral metastases) castrate resistant prostate cancer (stratified by previous docetaxel use) randomized (2:1 ratio) to receive six IV injections of radium-223 (50 kBq per kg every 4 weeks) or placebo. OS was improved in the Ra-223 arm (14.9 vs. 11.3 months). They also evaluated time to first skeletal event, defined as RT use or development of spinal cord compression. Time to first skeletal event was improved with Ra-223 (15.6 vs. 9.8 months). Previous use of docetaxel was not associated with efficacy of Ra-223.[28] Incidence of adverse events was lower in the treatment arm than the placebo group, and there were very few grade 3–5 hematologic toxicities.

REFERENCES

1. Nielsen OS. Palliative radiotherapy of bone metastases: there is now evidence for the use of single fractions. *Radiother Oncol J Eur Soc Ther Radiol Oncol.* 1999;52(2):95–96.
2. Mundy GR. Metastasis to bone: causes, consequences and therapeutic opportunities. *Nat Rev Cancer.* 2002;2(8):584–593.
3. Barghash RF, Abdou WM. Pathophysiology of metastatic bone disease and the role of the second generation of bisphosphonates: from basic science to medicine. *Curr Pharm Des.* 2016;22(11):1546–1557.
4. Kao CH, Hsieh JF, Tsai SC, et al. Comparison and discrepancy of 18F-2-deoxyglucose positron emission tomography and Tc-99m MDP bone scan to detect bone metastases. *Anticancer Res.* 2000;20(3B):2189–2192.
5. Mirels H. Metastatic disease in long bones: a proposed scoring system for diagnosing impending pathologic fractures. *Clin Orthop.* 1989;(249):256–264.
6. Fisher CG, DiPaola CP, Ryken TC, et al. A novel classification system for spinal instability in neoplastic disease: an evidence-based approach and expert consensus from the Spine Oncology Study Group. *Spine.* 2010;35(22):E1221–E1229.
7. Ross JR, Saunders Y, Edmonds PM, et al. Systematic review of role of bisphosphonates on skeletal morbidity in metastatic cancer. *BMJ.* 2003;327(7413):469. doi:10.1136/bmj.327.7413.469
8. Berenson JR, Lichtenstein A, Porter L, et al. Long-term pamidronate treatment of advanced multiple myeloma patients reduces skeletal events: Myeloma Aredia Study Group. *J Clin Oncol.* 1998;16(2):593–602.
9. Boyce BF, Xing L. Functions of RANKL/RANK/OPG in bone modeling and remodeling. *Arch Biochem Biophys.* 2008;473(2):139–146.
10. Lipton A, Fizazi K, Stopeck AT, et al. Superiority of denosumab to zoledronic acid for prevention of skeletal-related events: a combined analysis of 3 pivotal, randomised, phase 3 trials. *Eur J Cancer Oxf Engl.* 1990. 2012;48(16):3082–3092.
11. Lutz S, Balboni T, Jones J, et al. Palliative radiation therapy for bone metastases: update of an ASTRO evidence-based guideline. *Pract Radiat Oncol.* 2017;7(1):4–12.

12. Sahgal A, Atenafu EG, Chao S, et al. Vertebral compression fracture after spine stereotactic body radiotherapy: a multi-institutional analysis with a focus on radiation dose and the spinal instability neoplastic score. *J Clin Oncol.* 2013;31(27):3426–3431.

13. Thibault I, Chang EL, Sheehan J, et al. Response assessment after stereotactic body radiotherapy for spinal metastasis: a report from the SPIne response assessment in Neuro-Oncology (SPINO) group. *Lancet Oncol.* 2015;16(16):e595–e603.

14. Cox BW, Spratt DE, Lovelock M, et al. International Spine Radiosurgery Consortium consensus guidelines for target volume definition in spinal stereotactic radiosurgery. *Int J Radiat Oncol Biol Phys.* 2012;83(5):e597–e605.

15. Redmond KJ, Robertson S, Lo SS, et al. Consensus contouring guidelines for postoperative stereotactic body radiation therapy for metastatic solid tumor malignancies to the spine. *Int J Radiat Oncol Biol Phys.* 2017;97(1):64–74.

16. Videtic GMM, Woody N, Vassil AD. *Handbook of Treatment Planning in Radiation Oncology.* 2nd ed. New York, NY: Demos Medical; 2015.

17. Nieder C. Repeat palliative radiotherapy for painful bone metastases. *Lancet Oncol.* 2014;15(2):126–128.

18. Van der Linden YM, Kroon HM, Dijkstra SPDS, et al. Simple radiographic parameter predicts fracturing in metastatic femoral bone lesions: results from a randomised trial. *Radiother Oncol J Eur Soc Ther Radiol Oncol.* 2003;69(1):21–31.

19. Steenland E, Leer JW, van Houwelingen H, et al. The effect of a single fraction compared to multiple fractions on painful bone metastases: a global analysis of the Dutch Bone Metastasis Study. *Radiother Oncol J Eur Soc Ther Radiol Oncol.* 1999;52(2):101–109.

20. Yarnold JR. 8 Gy single fraction radiotherapy for the treatment of metastatic skeletal pain: randomised comparison with a multifraction schedule over 12 months of patient follow-up. Bone Pain Trial Working Party. *Radiother Oncol J Eur Soc Ther Radiol Oncol.* 1999;52(2):111–121.

21. Roos DE, Turner SL, O'Brien PC, et al. Randomized trial of 8 Gy in 1 versus 20 Gy in 5 fractions of radiotherapy for neuropathic pain due to bone metastases (Trans-Tasman Radiation Oncology Group, TROG 96.05). *Radiother Oncol J Eur Soc Ther Radiol Oncol.* 2005;75(1):54–63.

22. Hunter GK, Balagamwala EH, Koyfman SA, et al. The efficacy of external beam radiotherapy and stereotactic body radiotherapy for painful spinal metastases from renal cell carcinoma. *Pract Radiat Oncol.* 2012;2(4):e95–e100.

23. Hird A, Chow E, Zhang L, et al. Determining the incidence of pain flare following palliative radiotherapy for symptomatic bone metastases: results from three Canadian cancer centers. *Int J Radiat Oncol Biol Phys.* 2009;75(1):193–197.

24. Chiang A, Zeng L, Zhang L, et al. Pain flare is a common adverse event in steroid-naïve patients after spine stereotactic body radiation therapy: a prospective clinical trial. *Int J Radiat Oncol Biol Phys.* 2013;86(4):638–642.

25. Townsend PW, Rosenthal HG, Smalley SR, et al. Impact of postoperative radiation therapy and other perioperative factors on outcome after orthopedic stabilization of impending or pathologic fractures due to metastatic disease. *J Clin Oncol.* 1994;12(11):2345–2350.

26. Huisman M, van den Bosch MAAJ, Wijlemans JW, et al. Effectiveness of reirradiation for painful bone metastases: a systematic review and meta-analysis. *Int J Radiat Oncol Biol Phys.* 2012;84(1):8–14.

27. Chow E, van der Linden YM, Roos D, et al. Single versus multiple fractions of repeat radiation for painful bone metastases: a randomised, controlled, non-inferiority trial. *Lancet Oncol.* 2014;15(2):164–171.

28. Hoskin P, Sartor O, O'Sullivan JM, et al. Efficacy and safety of radium-223 dichloride in patients with castration-resistant prostate cancer and symptomatic bone metastases, with or without previous docetaxel use: a prespecified subgroup analysis from the randomised, double-blind, phase 3 ALSYMPCA trial. *Lancet Oncol.* 2014;15(12):1397–1406.

63: MALIGNANT SPINAL CORD COMPRESSION

Bindu V. Manyam, Camille A. Berriochoa, and Chirag Shah

QUICK HIT: Malignant spinal cord compression (mSCC) is considered an oncologic emergency and defined as any radiographic compression of the spinal cord or cauda equina secondary to an extradural or intramedullary malignancy. The most common presenting symptom is pain. Severity of symptoms can vary depending on the degree of compression, from asymptomatic to frank paraplegia, which may be reversible to irreversible. Initial treatment usually involves steroids (dexamethasone 10 mg loading dose, followed by 4 mg every 6 hours). Surgical evaluation should be obtained, and if surgical intervention is indicated, postoperative RT should follow, typically 30 Gy/10 fx about 2 to 4 weeks after surgery. If no surgical intervention is indicated, standard conventional fractionation is typically 30 Gy/10 fx or 20 Gy/5 fx. The use of SRS is established for re-irradiation and an evolving area for nonurgent treatment of spinal metastases in the absence of cord compression.

EPIDEMIOLOGY: Among pts with cancer, the annual incidence of mSCC is 2.5% to 3.4%, ranging from 0.2% in pancreatic cancer to 7.9% in multiple myeloma. Most cases of mSCC are due to lung, breast, and prostate cancer. The highest proportional incidence of mSCC is observed in multiple myeloma, lymphoma, and prostate cancer.[1,2] In pediatric pts, mSCC is observed in 5% of cancer pts, and is most commonly caused by Ewing's sarcoma and neuroblastoma.[3]

ANATOMY: The *spinal cord* extends from the foramen magnum to L1-L2 in adults. In children, the spinal cord extends more inferiorly (L2-L4). The *dural sac* surrounds the spinal cord and 31 nerve roots, which are cervical (8), thoracic (12), lumbar (5), sacral (5), and coccygeal (1). The sacral nerve roots S3-S5 originate from the terminal segment of the spinal cord, called the *conus medullaris*, which is the terminal segment of the spinal cord. The *filum terminale* is a thin connective tissue filament that originates from the conus medullaris and is fused to the periosteum of the coccygeal bone. The *cauda equina* is defined as the lumbar and sacral spinal nerves located in the lumbar cistern from L1-L2 to S2.[4,5] The *spinal meninges*, from deep to superficial, are composed of the pia mater, arachnoid mater, and the dura mater. The *epidural space* is superficial to the dura mater and contains fat and a venous plexus. The *gray matter* of the spinal cord is composed of lower motor nuclei anteriorly and sensory nuclei posteriorly. The *white matter* of the spinal cord is composed of the dorsal columns (proprioception), lateral spinothalamic tract (pain, temperature), ventral spinothalamic tract (touch sensation), anterior corticospinal tract (axial musculature), lateral corticospinal tract (extremities).

PATHOLOGY: mSCC occurs through two main mechanisms—external compression typically arising from the vertebral body and internal compression through intramedullary metastasis (more commonly, external compression caused by arterial seeding of the bone). Obstruction of the epidural venous plexus leads to the development of vasogenic edema of the white matter, and then the gray matter. Untreated, spinal cord infarction can ultimately develop.

CLINICAL PRESENTATION: Back pain is the most common presenting symptom of mSCC, occurring in 83% to 95% of cases, typically most pronounced at night or early in the morning when adrenal steroid secretion is at its lowest.[6,7] Back pain often precedes neuro-logic symptoms by several weeks. An estimated 60% to 85% of pts present with weakness, with 48% to 77% nonambulatory. Sensory symptoms present in about 50% of pts and can be described as "band-like," ascending, or "saddle" anesthesia/paresthesias, depending on location.[8] Physical exam findings may include upper motor neuron signs of spasticity, hyperactive reflexes, Babinski sign, and lower motor neuron signs of atrophy, flaccidity, and loss of reflexes.

Spinal cord syndromes

Transection of the cord: Loss of all sensory modalities (proprioception, vibration, touch) with weakness below the level of transection and bowel/bladder dysfunction.

Ventral cord syndrome: Weakness and loss of pain and temperature sensation.

Dorsal cord syndrome: Loss of proprioception and vibration, weakness, ataxia.

Cauda equina: Radiculopathy, leg weakness and sensory loss, saddle anesthesia, bowel/bladder incontinence/retention. Bowel/bladder dysfunction is a late finding that can present in up to 50% of pts.[7]

WORKUP: Full H&P, focused on neurologic exam.

Imaging: MRI of entire spine with and without gadolinium. If MRI cannot be obtained, CT myelography is roughly similar in terms of sensitivity and specificity for cord compression.[9]

Pathology: A biopsy is indicated for pts who are not surgical candidates and have an undiagnosed primary cancer, oligometastases, or if there is a discordance between the primary lesion and the spinal lesion.

PROGNOSTIC FACTORS: A simple framework has been developed that incorporates the neurologic, oncologic, mechanical, and systemic status of the pt to determine the opti-mal management decision.[10] The epidural spinal cord compression scale is based on a 6-point grading system to quantify the degree of spinal cord or thecal sac compression to help determine management decisions. Grade 0: bone only disease; Grade 1a: epidural impingement, no deformation of thecal sac; Grade 1b: deformation of thecal sac, no spinal cord abutment; deformation of thecal sac and spinal cord abutment, but no cord compres-sion; Grade 2: spinal cord compression but visible CSF around cord; Grade 3: spinal cord compression with no visible CSF around cord.[11]

TREATMENT PARADIGM

Medical treatment: Early initiation of high dose corticosteroids is standard management of mSCC. Typically, pts are started on 10 mg dexamethasone bolus, followed by 4 mg q6hr. Several studies have evaluated the benefit of steroid dose escalation with doses of 96 to 100 mg compared to 10 to 16 mg and have demonstrated no benefit with respect to pain control, ambulation rates, or neurologic outcomes, but have noted higher incidence of serious adverse effects, such as perforated gastric ulcer, psychosis, and death from infec-tion.[12–14] Duration of steroid taper should be initiated based on severity of symptoms, clin-ical response, and definitive management. Initiation of CHT should be considered with CHT-sensitive disease (lymphoma, Ewing's sarcoma, germ cell tumors, neuroblastoma).

Surgical treatment: Assessing spinal stability is an important decision-making point regarding whether or not to pursue surgery. In the event of spinal instability, the degree of spinal instability, neurologic symptoms, and location of disease dictate the management. Percutaneous vertebroplasty or kyphoplasty are minimally invasive procedures for pts without anterior extension of disease. The Spine Instability Neoplastic Score (SINS) takes into account six different factors of clinical and radiographic findings, and a score of >7 warrants surgical consultation.[15] Surgery is also beneficial in providing immediate relief of compression, when a histological diagnosis is not known, in a previously irradiated site of compression, and with progressive deterioration of neurologic status with poor response to steroids. Postsurgical ambulatory rate has been described in the literature to range between 70% and 90%, with surgical morbidity and mortality ranging from 5% to 10%.[16,17] Various surgical options are outlined in Table 63.1.

TABLE 63.1: Surgical Options in mSCC					
	Corpectomy	Laminectomy	Separation Surgery	Vertebroplasty	Kyphoplasty
Procedure	Removal of vertebral body via thoracotomy or retroperitoneal approach. Delays RT for 6 weeks to allow for fusion.	Removal of posterior arch of vertebrae (unclear if it adds benefit compared to RT alone and may destabilize spine).[18]	Debulking and instrumentation to increase margin between tumor and spinal cord/thecal sac.	Percutaneous injection of bone cement (PMMA) under fluoroscopy into a collapsed vertebral body	Inflatable bone tamps introduced into the vertebral body; once inflated, the bone tamps variably restore the height of the vertebral body, while creating a cavity to fill with viscous bone cement
Candidates	Good life expectancy and good-performing pts (see Patchell trial)[17]	Anterior extension of posterior disease	Most commonly, used to create adequate margin for adjuvant SRS	Pts with spinal instability, but without anterior extension	

Radiation

EBRT: Indications for RT include pts who are not surgical candidates, and in the postoperative setting (typically 2–4 weeks after surgery, except after corpectomy, which requires 6 weeks for fusion). The goal of RT is palliation of pain and LC for prevention or reduction of neurologic deficits. Studies have demonstrated a 70% improvement in pain and local control rates >75%.[19] Typical doses include 30 Gy in 10 fx, or 20 Gy in 5 fx. For radiosensitive histologies, such as multiple myeloma, 20 Gy/10 fx may be an appropriate regimen.[20] Several series demonstrated between 67% and 82% retention of ambulation following RT and about one-third of pts who were nonambulatory regained the ability to walk following RT.[19,21] In the retreatment setting, consider lower doses or fraction sizes, 20 Gy in 10 fx, or SRS, in pts with extended life expectancy. Side effects are dependent on location and length of the spine being treated and can include mucositis, dysphagia, nausea, diarrhea, or cytopenia.

SRS: SRS is generally not indicated for spinal cord compression given tumor proximity to cord and time required to initiate therapy. The most clear indication for SRS is re-irradiation but pts with radioresistant histologies with asymptomatic/minimally symptomatic disease or following separation surgery with gross residual disease may also benefit. Contraindications include significant epidural extension (a gap of ≥ 3 mm between the spinal cord and the edge of the lesion is ideal). A rate of >85% long-term pain control even in radioresistant pts has been observed.[22] Dose for spine metastases include, 16 Gy–18 Gy/1 fx, 24 Gy/1 fx, 16 Gy/4 fx, 30 Gy/5 fx.[23] RTOG 0631 uses 16 to 18 Gy. Side effects include acute pain flare (15%), grade 1-2 fatigue, nausea, diarrhea, vertebral fracture, myelopathy (<1%).[24]

Procedure: See *Treatment Planning Handbook,* Chapter 13.[25]

EVIDENCE-BASED Q&A

What is the value of surgical decompression in addition to radiotherapy?

Addition of surgery (corpectomy) to RT improves median survival, ambulation rate, length of ambulation retention, ability to regain walking, and no change in hospitalization time in pts with a single site of cord compression with paraplegia <48 hours.

Patchell (*Lancet* 2005, PMID 16112300): PRT of 101 pts with confirmed cancer, life expectancy >3 months, a single site of MRI-confirmed displaced cord, with at least one neurological sign or symptom, who were paraplegic <48 hours, randomized to surgery with post-op RT (30 Gy/10 fx) versus RT alone. Surgery was primarily corpectomy. Lymphoma, myeloma, leukemia, and germ cell tumors were excluded. The primary endpoint was the ability to walk (at least four steps unassisted with or without a cane/walker). Secondary endpoints were urinary continence, muscle strength, functional status, the need for steroids/opioids, OS. Of note, 20% in the RT group clinically deteriorated and required surgery.

TABLE 63.2: Results of Patchell Trial for mSCC					
	Ambulation Rate at the End of Treatment Primary endpoint	Ambulation Retention Time Primary Endpoint	Median Survival Secondary Endpoint	Regained Ability to Walk	Length of Hospitalization
Surgery + RT	84%	122 d	126 d	62%	10 d
RT Alone	57%	13 d	100 d	19%	10 d
p value	.001	.003	.03	.01	

Is there an ideal dose/fractionation regimen to use for mSCC?

Typical dose and fractionations include 20 Gy/5 fx and 30 Gy/10 fx; however, a superior dosing and fractionation schedule with regard to efficacy and toxicity has not been identified in prospective randomized trials. Therefore, clinical decision making should incorporate pt prognosis, functional status, disease burden, histology, future treatment plans, and pt convenience.

Rades (*JCO* 2016, PMID 26729431): PRT, noninferiority study of 203 pts with mSCC and intermediate to poor life expectancy randomized to 20 Gy/5 fx versus 30 Gy/10 fx. Primary endpoint was 1 month overall response, defined as improvement or no further progression of motor deficits. **Conclusion: 20 Gy/5 fx is not inferior to 30 Gy/10 fx in pts with intermediate to poor life expectancy.**

TABLE 63.3: Results of Rades Randomized Trial				
	Overall Motor Function Response Rate	Ambulatory Rate (at 1 Month)	Local PFS (at 6 Month)	OS (at 6 Months)
20 Gy/5 fx	87.2%	71.8%	75.2%	42.3%
30 Gy/10 fx	89.6%	74.0%	81.8%	37.8%
p value	.73	.86	.51	.68

Rades (IJROBP 2015, PMID 26232852): Matched pair analysis of 121 pts who received 8 Gy/1 fx and 121 pts who received 20 Gy/5 fx with mSCC and limited survival prognosis. Doses of 8 Gy/1 fx and 20 Gy/5 fx were not significantly different regarding the need for in-field re-irradiation ($p = .11$) at 6 months (18% vs. 9%, respectively) and 12 months (30% vs. 22%, respectively). The RT regimen also had no significant impact on OS ($p = .65$) and post-RT motor function ($p = .21$). **Conclusion: 8 Gy/1 fx may be a reasonable option for pts with limited survival.**

Rades (IJROBP 2009, PMID 18539406): Nonrandomized, prospective study. Pts in the Netherlands received short-course (8 Gy/1 fx or 20 Gy/5 fx) and pts in Germany received long-course RT (30 Gy/10 fx, 37.5 Gy/15 fx, or 40 Gy/20 fx). Post-RT motor function was associated with performance status, tumor type, interval to developing motor deficits, and bisphosphonate administration. OS was associated with performance status, number of involved vertebrae, visceral metastases, ambulatory status, and bisphosphonate administration. **Conclusion: Long-course RT demonstrated superior PFS and LC, though this was a nonrandomized trial and therefore results may be subject to selection bias.**

TABLE 63.4: Results of Rades Non-Randomized Study				
	PFS 1° Endpoint	LC 2° Endpoint	OS 2° Endpoint	Improved Motor Function 2° Endpoint
Long-course RT	72%	77%	32%	30%
Short-course RT	55%	61%	35%	28%
p value	.03	.03	.37	.61

Maranzano (JCO 2005, PMID 15738534): PRT of 300 pts with mSCC randomized to 16 Gy/2 fx (given with a 6-day break in between to a total dose of 16 Gy in 1 week) versus split-course RT (5 Gy x 3 → 4 day rest → 3 Gy x 5 to complete a course of 30 Gy in 8 fx over 2 weeks). Approximately 60% of pts in each arm had back pain relief, 70% in each arm were able to walk, and 90% had good bladder function. OS and toxicity were equivalent. **Conclusion: Both hypofractionated RT schedules are effective, with acceptable toxicity.**

Is there a role for spine SRS as compared to fractionated RT?

With true cord compression, the role of SRS is limited, given the duration of planning required for SRS and the need for ≥3-mm separation for the cord/thecal sac. The literature currently suggests a local control benefit, though this is primarily retrospective. RTOG 0631 is evaluating pt-reported pain outcomes between the two modalities; however, it excludes pts with <3 mm of separation from the cord/thecal sac.

Gerszten (Spine 2007, PMID 17224814): Prospective, nonrandomized, longitudinal cohort study of 500 cases of spinal metastases, all of which underwent SRS. The maximum intratumoral dose ranged from 12.5 to 25 Gy (mean 20 Gy). Long-term pain improvement was observed in 290 of 336 cases (86%). Long-term tumor control was demonstrated in 90% of lesions treated with SRS as a primary treatment modality and in 88% of lesions treated for radiographic tumor progression.

Sahgal (*JCO* 2013, PMID 23960179): Multi-institution study evaluating the risk of predictive factors associated with vertebral compression fracture (VCF) in 252 pts with 410 spine metastases treated with SBRT. 14% overall VCF risk (47% of those were new fractures and 53% were fracture progression) with a median time to VCF of 2.46 months (65% within the first 4 months). Greatest risk of VCF >24 Gy versus 20–23 Gy versus <20 Gy in a single fraction and in those with a baseline fracture, lytic tumor, or spinal deformity.

REFERENCES

1. Mak KS, Lee LK, Mak RH, et al. Incidence and treatment patterns in hospitalizations for malignant spinal cord compression in the United States, 1998–2006. *Int J Radiat Oncol Biol Phys.* 2011;80(3):824–831.
2. Loblaw DA, Laperriere NJ, Mackillop WJ. A population-based study of malignant spinal cord compression in Ontario. *Clin Oncol.* 2003;15(4):211–217.
3. Klein SL, Sanford RA, Muhlbauer MS. Pediatric spinal epidural metastases. *J Neurosur.* 1991;74(1):70–75.
4. Binokay F, Akgul E, Bicakci K, et al. Determining the level of the dural sac tip: magnetic resonance imaging in an adult population. *Acta Radiol.* 2006;47(4):397–400.
5. Scharf CB, Paulino AC, Goldberg KN. Determination of the inferior border of the thecal sac using magnetic resonance imaging: implications on radiation therapy treatment planning. *Int J Radiat Oncol Biol Phys.* 1998;41(3):621–624.
6. Bach F, Larsen BH, Rohde K, et al. Metastatic spinal cord compression. Occurrence, symptoms, clinical presentations and prognosis in 398 patients with spinal cord compression. *Acta Neurochir.* 1990;107(1–2):37–43.
7. Helweg-Larsen S, Sorensen PS. Symptoms and signs in metastatic spinal cord compression: a study of progression from first symptom until diagnosis in 153 patients. *Eur J Cancer.* 1994;30A(3):396–398.
8. Bilsky MH. New therapeutics in spine metastases. *Expert Rev Neurother.* 2005;5(6):831–840.
9. Loblaw DA, Perry J, Chambers A, Laperriere NJ. Systematic review of the diagnosis and management of malignant extradural spinal cord compression: the Cancer Care Ontario Practice Guidelines Initiative's Neuro-Oncology Disease Site Group. *J Clin Oncol.* 2005;23(9):2028–2037.
10. Laufer I, Rubin DG, Lis E, et al. The NOMS framework: approach to the treatment of spinal metastatic tumors. *Oncologist.* 2013;18(6):744–751.
11. Bilsky MH, Laufer I, Fourney DR, et al. Reliability analysis of the epidural spinal cord compression scale. *J Neurosurg Spine.* 2010;13(3):324–328.
12. George R, Jeba J, Ramkumar G, et al. Interventions for the treatment of metastatic extradural spinal cord compression in adults. *Cochrane Database Syst Rev.* 2008(4):CD006716.
13. Graham PH, Capp A, Delaney G, et al. A pilot randomised comparison of dexamethasone 96 mg vs 16 mg per day for malignant spinal-cord compression treated by radiotherapy: TROG 01.05 Superdex study. *Clin Oncol.* 2006;18(1):70–76.
14. Vecht CJ, Haaxma-Reiche H, van Putten WL, et al. Initial bolus of conventional versus high-dose dexamethasone in metastatic spinal cord compression. *Neurology.* 1989;39(9):1255–1257.
15. Mendel E, Bourekas E, Gerszten P, Golan JD. Percutaneous techniques in the treatment of spine tumors: what are the diagnostic and ther indications and outcomes? *Spine.* 2009;34(22, Suppl):S93–S100.
16. Rades D, Huttenlocher S, Dunst J, et al. Matched pair analysis comparing surgery followed by radiotherapy and radiotherapy alone for metastatic spinal cord compression. *J Clin Oncol.* 2010;28(22):3597–3604.
17. Patchell RA, Tibbs PA, Regine WF, et al. Direct decompressive surgical resection in the treatment of spinal cord compression caused by metastatic cancer: a randomised trial. *Lancet.* 2005;366(9486):643–648.

18. Young RF, Post EM, King GA. Treatment of spinal epidural metastases: randomized prospective comparison of laminectomy and radiotherapy. *J Neurosurg.* 1980;53(6):741–748.

19. Maranzano E, Bellavita R, Rossi R, et al. Short-course versus split-course radiotherapy in metastatic spinal cord compression: results of a phase III, randomized, multicenter trial. *J Clin Oncol.* 2005;23(15):3358–3365.

20. Terpos E, Morgan G, Dimopoulos MA, et al. International Myeloma Working Group recommendations for the treatment of multiple myeloma-related bone disease. *J Clin Oncol.* 2013;31(18):2347–2357.

21. Maranzano E, Latini P. Effectiveness of radiation therapy without surgery in metastatic spinal cord compression: final results from a prospective trial. *Int J Radiat Oncol Biol Phys.* 1995;32(4):959–967.

22. Jin R, Rock J, Jin JY, et al. Single fraction spine radiosurgery for myeloma epidural spinal cord compression. *J Exp Ther Oncol.* 2009;8(1):35–41.

23. Yamada Y, Bilsky MH, Lovelock DM, et al. High-dose, single-fraction image-guided intensity-modulated radiotherapy for metastatic spinal lesions. *Int J Radiat Oncol Biol Phys.* 2008;71(2):484–490.

24. Sahgal A, Atenafu EG, Chao S, et al. Vertebral compression fracture after spine stereotactic body radiotherapy: a multi-institutional analysis with a focus on radiation dose and the spinal instability neoplastic score. *J Clin Oncol.* 2013;31(27):3426–3431.

25. Videtic GMM, Woody N, Vassil AD. *Handbook of Treatment Planning in Radiation Oncology.* 2nd ed. 2015. New York, NY: Demos Medical; 2015.

64: SUPERIOR VENA CAVA SYNDROME

Charles Marc Leyrer and Gregory M. M. Videtic

QUICK HIT: Superior vena cava (SVC) syndrome is an urgent clinical scenario but not an emergency unless presenting with clinically severe airway, neurologic, or hemodynamic compromise. Treatment decision making best directed by pt performance, underlying tumor histology, and overall stage. Pts with SVC syndrome do not have worse prognosis than pts without it (for same stage and histologic diagnosis). In stable pts, pursue completion of staging and workup. Where emergent intervention required, intravascular stenting may provide most rapid relief. In the United States, the most common malignancies associated with SVC syndrome are NSCLC, SCLC, and lymphoma. Overall, about 60% to 80% respond to CHT or RT within 2 weeks.

TABLE 64.1: General Treatment Approach for SVC Syndrome

Supportive Care	Head elevation with high-flow oxygen. Data unclear for use of steroids (may obscure diagnosis) and/or diuretics.
CHT	Consider as initial treatment for SCLC, lymphoma, germ cell tumors.
RT	Consider hypofractionated RT for urgent relief with initiation of definitive course if clinically appropriate. Palliative RT as initial treatment in advanced/emergent pts for histologies other than SCLC, lymphoma, or germ cell tumors.
Intravascular Stenting	Consider if rapid relief is necessary, if unable to tolerate tumor-directed therapy, or symptoms refractory to prior to previous modalities.

EPIDEMIOLOGY: ~15,000 cases per year in the United States with survival dependent on underlying etiology.[1]

ANATOMY: SVC carries about 1/3 of total venous return including drainage from head, arms, and upper torso. It contains low-pressure blood flow and is thus thin-walled and easily compressible. Brachiocephalic (innominate) veins join to form SVC beginning at sternal angle. SVC then extends inferiorly along right lateral side of ascending aorta, and inserts into right atrium. Azygos vein enters SVC posteriorly, just above pericardial reflection. When obstructed, blood flow is diverted through collateral vessels including internal mammary, intercostal, esophageal, lateral thoracic, paraspinal, and azygos veins ultimately to inferior vena cava.

TABLE 64.2: Anatomy of Mediastinum

	Boundaries	Contents	Etiology of Malignant SVC Syndrome
Superior Mediastinum	Below thoracic inlet at T1 to above plane between sternal angle and T4-T5	Thymus, trachea, SVC, aortic arch, esophagus, lymph nodes	NHL, lung, thymoma, thymic, thyroid cancer, germ cell tumors

(continued)

TABLE 64.2: Anatomy of Mediastinum (*continued*)

	Boundaries	Contents	Etiology of Malignant SVC Syndrome
Anterior Mediastinum	Between pericardium and sternum	Thymus, fat, lymph nodes	NHL, Hodgkin's, thyroid cancer, thymoma, germ cell tumors, metastasis
Middle Mediastinum	Pericardium and its contents, from T5-T8	Heart, lung, great vessels (including distal SVC), mainstem bronchi, lymph nodes	NHL, lung cancer, sarcoma, thymoma, teratoma, mesothelioma
Posterior Mediastinum	Between pericardium and vertebral column, down to T12	Esophagus, descending aorta, thoracic duct, azygos vein, lymph nodes	NHL, nerve sheath tumors, pheochromocytoma, ganglio/neuroblastoma

PATHOLOGY: SVC syndrome was previously associated with untreated infections such as tuberculosis, syphilis, or aortic aneurysms. With more advanced antibiotics, malignancy now accounts for 70% to 90% of cases.[1-3] Common malignant etiologies include NSCLC (50%) > SCLC (25%) > NHL (12%) > metastasis (9%) > germ cell tumors > thymoma > other (mesothelioma). SVC syndrome is more common in SCLC at 10% compared to 2% of NSCLC pts. Overall, 2% to 4% of pts with primary lung malignancy will develop SVC syndrome during course of their disease.[1,4,5] Other benign causes include thrombosis (related to intravascular devices), thyroid goiter, postradiation fibrosis, CHF, and aortic aneurysm. Fibrosing mediastinitis, often associated with granulomatous disease, requires biopsy for confirmation.

CLINICAL PRESENTATION: Severity of symptoms related to degree and time frame of SVC obstruction with subsequent collateralization. Dyspnea and facial/neck swelling are most common presenting symptoms. Medical emergencies characterized by clinical symptoms including airway obstruction, neurologic compromise, or hemodynamic instability (see definition of grade 4 SVC syndrome in Table 64.3).[6] Symptoms are commonly exacerbated by leaning forward or lying supine. 1/3 of pts develop symptoms over 2 weeks.[1] In most cases, symptoms gradually progress over several weeks and then get better over time due to development of collateral vessels.

TABLE 64.3: Proposed Grading System for Superior Vena Cava Syndrome[6]

Grade	Category	Incidence	Definition
0	Asymptomatic	10%	Asymptomatic radiographic SVC obstruction
1	Mild	25%	Edema/vascular distention in head or neck, cyanosis, plethora
2	Moderate	50%	Edema in head or neck with associated symptoms (dysphagia; cough; mild or moderate movement impairment of head, jaw, or eyelid; visual disruption)
3	Severe	10%	Mild/moderate cerebral edema (HA, dizziness), laryngeal edema, or diminished cardiac reserve (syncope after bending)
4	Life-threatening	5%	Cerebral edema with associated confusion or obtundation; Laryngeal edema with stridor, or significant hemodynamic compromise leading to syncope due to SVC obstruction
5	Life-threatening	<1%	Death

WORKUP: H&P with focus on previous malignancies, risk factors for coagulopathy, previous intravascular procedures, or risk factors for granulomatous disease.

Imaging: CXR, chest CT with contrast with attention to collateral vessels.[7,8] Ultrasound to assess for thrombus.

Pathology: Biopsy (bronchoscopic, CT-guided, mediastinoscopy/mediastinotomy, thoracentesis are options).[9,10] Further workup as per histologic diagnosis.

PROGNOSTIC FACTORS: Prognosis determined by underlying histology. Negative factors specific to SVC include cerebral edema, laryngeal edema, hypotension, syncope, headache. SVC obstruction does not predict poor outcomes in pts with treatment-responsive tumors compared to those without SVC.[11-16]

NATURAL HISTORY: After obstruction of SVC, increased central venous pressure (from approximately 2–8 mmHg to >20 mmHg) diverts venous return through collateral circulation.[7,17,18] Obstruction above junction of azygos vein causes venous congestion of head, neck, and arms. Obstruction below azygos vein leads to distention of veins of thorax and abdomen. Laryngeal edema may lead to dyspnea, stridor, cough, dysphagia.[6] Symptoms are related to time of onset with protracted onset allowing time for collaterals to develop. Disruption of cardiac output is usually temporary due to subsequent collateral development.

TREATMENT PARADIGM

Supportive: Head elevation and supplemental oxygen. Dexamethasone may be helpful to reduce cerebral edema or for treatment of steroid-responsive malignancies (lymphoma), although data is unclear. Role of diuretics is unclear based on single retrospective study of 107 pts with similar symptomatic improvement (84%) with no difference between steroid utilization, diuretics, or neither.[19]

Surgery: There is no standard role for surgery in SVC syndrome but can be considered in definitive management of underlying malignancy. Resection or bypass grafting generally reserved for surgically managed tumors (e.g., thymoma) and progressive or persistent symptoms (>6 months). Common approach is sternotomy/thoracotomy with resection and/or reconstruction of SVC.[20-22]

Chemotherapy: For chemotherapy-responsive histologies such as small-cell lung cancer, germ cell tumors, or lymphoma, CHT is often initial treatment of choice in order to allow time for staging and radiation planning. CHT should be dosed according to underlying histology. In one systematic review of 46 studies, 77% to 78% of SCLC pts had resolution of symptoms with average time of 7 to 14 days.

Radiation: For palliation, RT doses ranging from 10 Gy/1 fx to 30 Gy/10 fx may be reasonable options depending on function of pt and disease status.[23] Urgent but still curable pts may benefit from higher dose per fraction up front (3-4 Gy/fx) to alleviate symptoms with dose-adapted definitive dose at standard 1.8 to 2 Gy/fx after 2 to 3 days, with total doses based on histology and for curative intent. Symptomatic relief can be apparent in 72 hours but can take up to 4 weeks.[5] Up to 20% of pts do not obtain symptomatic relief from RT. Among those who do respond, ~20% will have recurrent obstruction.[16] Symptomatic relief may occur without complete/partial SVC patency after treatment.[24] As per review of 24 CHT/RT studies, there were no reports of worsening symptoms with RT.[5,25]

Intravascular stent: Intravascular stenting is most rapid treatment for SVC syndrome.[5] Stent placement should be considered for severe symptoms (e.g., airway compromise or cerebral edema), inability to tolerate tumor-directed therapy or low probability of response to CHT/RT (e.g., mesothelioma). Symptomatic improvement occurs in 75%

to 100%, typically within 48 to 72 hours. Complication rate is 3% to 7%.[1,26,27] Early complications include infection, pulmonary embolus, stent migration, hematoma, bleeding, and perforation/rupture of SVC (rare). Late complications include bleeding (1%–14%) or death (1%–2%) from anticoagulation and stent failure with reocclusion.[28] Relative contraindications include pts without symptoms and inability to lie flat.

EVIDENCE-BASED Q&A

Is it safe to delay intervention to pursue workup?

Yes, except when symptoms concerning for urgent treatment are present (e.g., airway compromise, cerebral edema). There have been three separate RRs of 107, 63, and 249 pts with SVC syndrome— there was no evidence of serious complications resulting from delay in treatment of SVC obstruction while diagnostic workup was completed.[2,19,29]

REFERENCES

1. Wilson LD, Detterbeck FC, Yahalom J. Clinical practice: superior vena cava syndrome with malignant causes. *N Engl J Med.* 2007;356(18):1862–1869.
2. Yellin A, Rosen A, Reichert N, Lieberman Y. Superior vena cava syndrome: myth—the facts. *Am Rev Respir Dis.* 1990;141(5, Pt 1):1114–1118.
3. Martins SJ, Pereira JR. Clinical factors and prognosis in non-small-cell lung cancer. *Am J Clin Oncol.* 1999;22(5):453–457.
4. Houman M, Ksontini I, Ben Ghorbel I, et al. Association of right heart thrombosis, endomyocardial fibrosis, and pulmonary artery aneurysm in Behcet's disease. *Eur J Intern Med.* 2002; 13(7):455–457.
5. Rowell NP, Gleeson FV. Steroids, radiotherapy, chemotherapy and stents for superior vena caval obstruction in carcinoma of bronchus: systematic review. *Clin Oncol (R Coll Radiol).* 2002;14(5):338–351.
6. Yu JB, Wilson LD, Detterbeck FC. Superior vena cava syndrome: a proposed classification system and algorithm for management. *J Thorac Oncol.* 2008;3(8):811–814.
7. Kim HJ, Kim HS, Chung SH. CT diagnosis of superior vena cava syndrome: importance of collateral vessels. *AJR Am J Roentgenol.* 1993;161(3):539–542.
8. Parish JM, Marschke RF Jr, Dines DE, Lee RE. Etiologic considerations in superior vena cava syndrome. *Mayo Clin Proc.* 1981;56(7):407–413.
9. Mineo TC, Ambrogi V, Nofroni I, Pistolese C. Mediastinoscopy in superior vena cava obstruction: analysis of 80 consecutive pts. *Ann Thorac Surg.* 1999;68(1):223–226.
10. Dosios T, Theakos N, Chatziantoniou C. Cervical mediastinoscopy and anterior mediastinotomy in superior vena cava obstruction. *Chest.* 2005;128(3):1551–1556.
11. Urban T, Lebeau B, Chastang C, et al. Superior vena cava syndrome in small-cell lung cancer. *Arch Intern Med.* 1993;153(3):384–387.
12. Sculier JP, Evans WK, Feld R, et al. Superior vena caval obstruction syndrome in small-cell lung cancer. *Cancer.* 1986;57(4):847–851.
13. Dombernowsky P, Hansen HH. Combination chemotherapy in management of superior vena caval obstruction in small-cell anaplastic carcinoma of lung. *Acta Med Scand.* 1978;204(6):513–516.
14. Warde P, Payne D. Does thoracic irradiation improve survival and local control in limited-stage small-cell carcinoma of lung?: meta-analysis. *J Clin Oncol.* 1992;10(6):890–895.
15. Wurschmidt F, Bunemann H, Heilmann HP. Small-cell lung cancer with and without superior vena cava syndrome: multivariate analysis of prognostic factors in 408 cases. *Int J Radiat Oncol Biol Phys.* 1995;33(1):77–82.
16. Spiro SG, Shah S, Harper PG, et al. Treatment of obstruction of superior vena cava by combination chemotherapy with and without irradiation in small-cell carcinoma of bronchus. *Thorax.* 1983;38(7):501–505.

17. Trigaux JP, Van Beers B. Thoracic collateral venous channels: normal and pathologic CT findings. *J Comput Assist Tomogr.* 1990;14(5):769–773.
18. Gonzalez-Fajardo JA, Garcia-Yuste M, Florez S, et al. Hemodynamic and cerebral repercussions arising from surgical interruption of superior vena cava: experimental model. *J Thorac Cardiovasc Surg.* 1994;107(4):1044–1049.
19. Schraufnagel DE, Hill R, Leech JA, Pare JA. Superior vena caval obstruction: is it a medical emergency? *Am J Med.* 1981;70(6):1169–1174.
20. Magnan PE, Thomas P, Giudicelli R, et al. Surgical reconstruction of superior vena cava. *Cardiovasc Surg.* 1994;2(5):598–604.
21. Bacha EA, Chapelier AR, Macchiarini P, et al. Surgery for invasive primary mediastinal tumors. *Ann Thorac Surg.* 1998;66(1):234–239.
22. Chen KN, Xu SF, Gu ZD, et al. Surgical treatment of complex malignant anterior mediastinal tumors invading superior vena cava. *World J Surg.* 2006;30(2):162–170.
23. Straka C, Ying J, Kong FM, et al. Review of evolving etiologies, implications and treatment strategies for superior vena cava syndrome. *Springerplus.* 2016;5:229.
24. Ahmann FR. Reassessment of clinical implications of superior vena caval syndrome. *J Clin Oncol.* 1984;2(8):961–969.
25. Egelmeers A, Goor C, van Meerbeeck J, et al. Palliative effectiveness of radiation therapy in treatment of superior vena cava syndrome. *Bulletin du cancer Radiotherapie.* 1996;83(3):153–157.
26. Fagedet D, Thony F, Timsit JF, et al. Endovascular treatment of malignant superior vena cava syndrome: results and predictive factors of clinical efficacy. *Cardiovasc Intervent Radiol.* 2013;36(1):140–149.
27. Sobrinho G, Aguiar P. Stent placement for treatment of malignant superior vena cava syndrome: single-center series of 56 patients. *Arch Bronconeumol.* 2014;50(4):135–140.
28. Watkinson AF, Yeow TN, Fraser C. Endovascular stenting to treat obstruction of superior vena cava. *BMJ.* 2008;336(7658):1434–1437.
29. Gauden SJ. Superior vena cava syndrome induced by bronchogenic carcinoma: is this oncological emergency? *Australas Radiol.* 1993;37(4):363–366.

65: PALLIATIVE RADIOTHERAPY

Justin J. Juliano

PALLIATION OF HEAD AND NECK CANCER

Poor performance status, advanced medical comorbidities, and presence of metastatic disease often preclude aggressive management of H&N cancer. In these situations, it is essential to balance locoregional control and relief of symptoms while limiting toxicity and maintaining quality of life. Symptoms of progressive disease warranting consideration of palliative RT include pain, odynophagia, otalgia, dysphagia, airway obstruction (cough, dyspnea), ulceration/bleeding. Prognostic factors to consider include pt performance status, sociodemographic standing, support system, and tobacco dependence. Tumor factors include size, grade, and HPV status. Previous treatment factors include prior RT +/− CHT and time to treatment failure.

Salvage surgery is considered first-line treatment for resectable locoregionally recurrent disease. For pts with metastatic disease or with locoregionally recurrent disease not amenable to further therapy, CHT is standard, typically with platinum-based doublet (w/ 5-FU, taxane) +/− cetuximab.[1] Recently, PD-1 inhibitors have been approved for recurrent and/or metastatic H&N cancers.[2]

Re-irradiation is an option typically reserved for pts with locoregionally confined disease with good performance status. Classic techniques included hyperfractionated RT to doses of ~60 Gy with variable schedules including treatment breaks.[3–5] More modern techniques omit treatment break, dosing to 54–70 Gy with or without hyperfractionation. SBRT is also an evolving option to doses of 35 to 44 Gy given in 5 fx every other day.[6,7] For those receiving palliative RT, many regimens have been studied with goal of increasing dose to improve durability of control without sacrificing toxicity or pt convenience. See Table 65.1. Other more common regimens such as 20 Gy/5 fx, 30 Gy/10 fx, and so on are also feasible.

TABLE 65.1: Selected Palliative Regimens for H&N Cancer		
Regimen	**Dose**	**Notes**
Quad Shot[8–11]	14.8 Gy/4 fx BID over 2 days with ≥6 hour interval; repeat at 4-week intervals for up to 3–4 total cycles (42 Gy/12 fx)	Phase I–II trials did not enroll pts w/ previous RT or give concurrent CHT, but both appear safe
Hypo[12]	30 Gy/5 fx at least 3 days apart; additional 6 Gy boost to tumors ≤3 cm	No previous RT
Christie[13]	50 Gy/16 fx, 4–5 fx per week	
Italy[14]	50 Gy/20 fx with 2-week midtreatment break	
SCAHRT[15]	30 Gy/10 fx, 3- to 5-week break, if tolerated then followed by additional 30–36 Gy/10–12 fx	
IHF2SQ[16]	6 Gy/2 fx, days 1 and 3 during first, third, and fifth weeks of platinum CHT	Concurrent CHT, no previous RT

ADRENAL METASTASES PALLIATION

The adrenal gland is common site of metastasis from other primary tumors (lung being most common), but with <5% of pts symptomatic at detection.[17] With increasing imaging surveillance of cancer pts, incidence of asymptomatic adrenal metastases is rising.[18] When symptomatic, pain (lower chest, abdomen, back, or flank) is most commonly reported. Other signs and symptoms noted include: adrenal insufficiency, peritoneal hemorrhage, and inferior vena cava thrombosis.

Adrenalectomy is preferred treatment among eligible pts. Other interventions include percutaneous ablation, conventional RT, and SBRT. Surgical resection is associated with prolonged survival for pts with isolated adrenal metastasis.[19] Careful pt selection is critical; long disease-free interval and oligometastatic presentation are more favorable. In addition to complications of surgery, many pts with metastatic disease have other comorbidities that may make them medically inoperable. In these pts, SBRT may provide feasible treatment option. For symptomatic/palliative intent, RT is effective. While rare (and should be considered in context of bilateral adrenal metastases), adrenal insufficiency may be associated with weakness, weight loss, hypotension, hypoglycemia, hyponatremia, hyperkalemia. Treatment is with glucocorticoids and mineralocorticoids.

There are limited data for SBRT but ideally BED >100 Gy can be achieved while respecting normal tissue tolerance. See Table 65.2 for example regimens. For palliation, standard regimens such as 20 Gy/5 fx, 30 Gy/10 fx, 36 Gy/20 fx, or 45 Gy/20 fx have been used.[20]

TABLE 65.2: Selected Series of SBRT for Adrenal Metastases			
Series	N (pts)	Dose (Median/Mode)	Dose (Range)
Rochester[21]	30	40 Gy/10 fx	16 Gy/4 fx–50 Gy/10 fx
Florence[22]	48	36 Gy/3 fx	30–54 Gy
Milan[23]	34	32 Gy/4 fx	20 Gy/4 fx–45 Gy/18 fx
MDACC[24]	43	60 Gy/10 fx	50 Gy/4 fx–63 Gy/9 fx

LIVER PALLIATION

The liver represents a common source of visceral metastatic disease. Pts with low volume and solitary metastatic disease may be considered for curative resection or other definitive intervention. In colorectal cancer, 5- and 10-yr OS of 40% and 25% are reported in such cases, respectively.[25] In case of advanced symptomatic hepatic metastases, RT to whole liver can afford effective palliation of symptoms/signs such as pain, nausea/anorexia, jaundice, and constitutional symptoms such as weight loss, fevers, or night sweats.

Multimodality therapy is integral to management of these pts. Prognostic factors to consider include: age, performance status, liver function, cancer histology (colorectal vs. other), size (<6 cm), lesion number (less than five favorable), and extent of disease (i.e., uninvolved liver volume >700 cc, less than three segments favorable), extrahepatic disease, prior CHT, time to treatment failure.[26] Hepatectomy is standard for patients with limited number of lesions (major hepatectomy defined as greater than three segments), with R0 resection being goal.[27] CHT is primary systemic treatment for pts with liver metastases.

Optimal candidates for ablative RT have preserved performance status, adequate liver function, solitary liver metastases, and uninvolved liver volume >700 cc.[26] Both 3 and 5 fx regimens of SBRT have been used. For 3 fx regimens, prescription dose of approximately ≥48 Gy (48–52 Gy) is recommended when safe.[28]

Palliative RT can be delivered for symptomatic diffuse metastatic disease refractory to systemic therapy. Premedication with antinausea medication with or without Decadron is recommended when treating large volumes of liver. A number of regimens have safely been employed including: 8 Gy/1 fx,[29] 10 Gy/2 fx,[30] 21 Gy/7 fx,[31] 30 Gy/15 fx.[26] Other modalities such as RFA, cryotherapy, laser-induced thermotherapy, high-intensity focused ultrasound (HIFU), TACE chemoembolization, or Y90 emobolization have been employed as well.

LUNG PALLIATION

Patients with primary lung cancer or progressive pulmonary metastases can present with symptoms including (but not limited to) hemoptysis, cough, dyspnea, and chest pain. Definitive approach should be considered for those pts deemed nonmetastatic. For others or those whom poor performance status and/or advanced medical comorbidities and preclude aggressive management, palliative approach is appropriate.

Treatment must be triaged according to urgency. In otherwise stable pt, balance of locoregional control, relief of symptoms, limiting toxicity, maintaining quality of life, pt convenience, and cost of care are all important considerations. Early referral to palliative care specialist is encouraged. Endoscopic interventions such as bronchoscopy with laser ablation +/− endobronchial stenting may be helpful for rapid relief of central airway obstruction. Thoracentesis with drainage catheter placement can aid for pleural effusions. Endovascular stenting can aid for SVC syndrome (see Chapter 64).

Various RT fractionation schemes have been employed. ASTRO guidelines suggest protracted regimens (30 Gy/10 fx) for pts with good performance status.[32] While survival and symptom scores are improved with higher dose schedule, latter comes with cost of higher treatment-related toxicity. Shorter course schedules are appropriate for pts with compromised performance status. Regimens to consider: 10 Gy/1 fx, 16–17 Gy/2 fx, 20 Gy/5 fx, 30 Gy/10 fx, 36 Gy/12 fx, 39 Gy/13 fx.[32,33]

PELVIC PALLIATION

RT is effective for palliation of pelvic progression of urogenital and anorectal malignancies. Most common symptoms include pain, bleeding, and obstruction (urinary or bowel). In addition to presenting symptoms, consideration should be given to tumor burden (both at local level as well as systemic), prognosis, performance status, ongoing treatments, and personal preferences.

Palliative pelvic exenteration may be considered for selected pts who are medically fit, amenable to gross resection (no major peripheral nerve involvement, no direct invasion of common iliac vessels, or bony invasion at pelvic sidewall or sacrum), and have minimal extrapelvic disease.[34] Exenteration often requires both urinary and fecal diversion through ostomies.

For recurrent rectal cancer, experience exists for both definitive and peri-operative re-irradiation (see Chapter 34 for details). More limited experience exists for re-irradiation (e.g., 50 Gy/20–25 fx) of other malignancies.[35]

For those with metastatic, unresectable, or medically inoperable disease, RT is standard option for palliation. A wide variety of clinical scenarios mandate careful application of RT. Accepted regimens beyond standard doses of 20 Gy/5 fx or 30 Gy/10 fx are denoted in Table 65.3. Other palliative modalities such as transcutaneous arterial embolization (TAE) and nerve blocks can be considered for bleeding and pain, respectively.

TABLE 65.3: Selected Palliative Regimens for Miscellaneous Pelvic Malignancies		
Regimen	Dose	Notes
Quad Shot/ RTOG 8502[36,37]	14.8 Gy/4 fx BID over 2 days with ≥6-hour interval; repeat at 4 week intervals for up to 3 total cycles (44.4 Gy/12 fx)	Break of 2 weeks no different than 4-week break (NS increase in acute effects)[38]
RTOG 7905[39]	10 Gy/1 fx once every 4 weeks for up to 3 treatments	Abandoned due to Grade 3–4 late effects of 45%
MRC BA09 (UK)[40]	PRT 35 Gy/10 fx vs. 21 Gy/3 fx	Tested in bladder cancer only; no differences in efficacy or toxicity

REFERENCES

1. Vermorken JB, Mesia R, Rivera F, et al. Platinum-based chemotherapy plus cetuximab in head and neck cancer. *N Engl J Med.* 2008;359(11):1116–1127.
2. Ferris RL, Blumenschein G, Fayette J, et al. Nivolumab for recurrent squamous-cell carcinoma of head and neck. *N Engl J Med.* 2016;375(19):1856–1867.
3. Janot F, de Raucourt D, Benhamou E, et al. Randomized trial of postoperative reirradiation combined with chemotherapy after salvage surgery compared with salvage surgery alone in head and neck carcinoma. *J Clin Oncol.* 2008;26(34):5518–5523.
4. Spencer SA, Harris J, Wheeler RH, et al. Final report of RTOG 9610, multi-institutional trial of reirradiation and chemotherapy for unresectable recurrent squamous cell carcinoma of head and neck. *Head Neck.* 2008;30(3):281–288.
5. Langer CJ, Harris J, Horwitz EM, et al. Phase II study of low-dose paclitaxel and cisplatin in combination with split-course concomitant twice-daily reirradiation in recurrent squamous cell carcinoma of head and neck: results of Radiation Therapy Oncology Group Protocol 9911. *J Clin Oncol.* 2007;25(30):4800–4805.
6. Vargo JA, Heron DE, Ferris RL, et al. Prospective evaluation of patient-reported quality-of-life outcomes following SBRT ± cetuximab for locally-recurrent, previously-irradiated head and neck cancer. *Radiother Oncol.* 2012;104(1):91–95.
7. Vargo JA, Ferris RL, Ohr J, et al. Prospective phase 2 trial of reirradiation with stereotactic body radiation therapy plus cetuximab in patients with previously irradiated recurrent squamous cell carcinoma of head and neck. *Int J Radiat Oncol Biol Phys.* 2015;91(3):480–488.
8. Corry J, Peters LJ, Costa ID, et al. 'QUAD SHOT': a phase II study of palliative radiotherapy for incurable head and neck cancer. *Radiother Oncol.* 2005;77(2):137–142.
9. Paris KJ, Spanos WJ, Lindberg RD, et al. Phase I-II study of multiple daily fractions for palliation of advanced head and neck malignancies. *Int J Radiat Oncol Biol Phys.* 1993;25(4):657–660.
10. Lok BH, Jiang G, Gutiontov S, et al. Palliative head and neck radiotherapy with RTOG 8502 regimen for incurable primary or metastatic cancers. *Oral Oncol.* 2015;51(10):957–962.
11. Gamez ME, Agarwal M, Hu KS, et al. Hypofractionated palliative radiotherapy with concurrent radiosensitizing chemotherapy for advanced head and neck cancer using "QUAD-SHOT Regimen." *Anticancer Res.* 2017;37(2):685–691.
12. Porceddu SV, Rosser B, Burmeister BH, et al. Hypofractionated radiotherapy for palliation of advanced head and neck cancer in patients unsuitable for curative treatment: "Hypo Trial." *Radiother Oncol.* 2007;85(3):456–462.
13. Al-mamgani A, Tans L, Van rooij PH, et al. Hypofractionated radiotherapy denoted as "Christie scheme": effective means of palliating patients with head and neck cancers not suitable for curative treatment. *Acta Oncol.* 2009;48(4):562–570.
14. Minatel E, Gigante M, Franchin G, et al. Combined radiotherapy and bleomycin in patients with inoperable head and neck cancer with unfavourable prognostic factors and severe symptoms. *Oral Oncol.* 1998;34(2):119–122.
15. Bledsoe TJ, Noble AR, Reddy CA, et al. Split-course accelerated hypofractionated radiotherapy (SCAHRT): safe and effective option for head and neck cancer in elderly or infirm. *Anticancer Res.* 2016;36(3):933–939.
16. Monnier L, Touboul E, Durdux C, et al. Hypofractionated palliative radiotherapy for advanced head and neck cancer: IHF2SQ regimen. *Head Neck.* 2013;35(12):1683–1688.
17. Shiue K, Song A, Teh BS, et al. Stereotactic body radiation therapy for metastasis to adrenal glands. *Expert Rev Anticancer Ther.* 2012;12(12):1613–1620.
18. Mitchell IC, Nwariaku FE. Adrenal masses in cancer patient: surveillance or excision. *Oncologist.* 2007;12(2):168–174.
19. Sastry P, Tocock A, Coonar AS. Adrenalectomy for isolated metastasis from operable non-small-cell lung cancer. *Interact Cardiovasc Thorac Surg.* 2014;18(4):495–497.
20. Short S, Chaturvedi A, Leslie MD. Palliation of symptomatic adrenal gland metastases by radiotherapy. *Clin Oncol (R Coll Radiol).* 1996;8(6):387–389.
21. Chawla S, Chen Y, Katz AW, et al. Stereotactic body radiotherapy for treatment of adrenal metastases. *Int J Radiat Oncol Biol Phys.* 2009;75(1):71–75.

22. Casamassima F, Livi L, Masciullo S, et al. Stereotactic radiotherapy for adrenal gland metastases: University of Florence experience. *Int J Radiat Oncol Biol Phys*. 2012;82(2):919–923.

23. Scorsetti M, Alongi F, Filippi AR, et al. Long-term local control achieved after hypofraction-ated stereotactic body radiotherapy for adrenal gland metastases: retrospective analysis of 34 patients. *Acta Oncol*. 2012;51(5):618–623.

24. Chance WW, Nguyen QN, Mehran R, et al. Stereotactic ablative radiotherapy for adrenal gland metastases: factors influencing outcomes, patterns of failure, and dosimetric thresholds for tox-icity. *Pract Radiat Oncol*. 2017;7(3):e195–e203.

25. Adam R, Chiche L, Aloia T, et al. Hepatic resection for noncolorectal nonendocrine liver metastases: analysis of 1,452 patients and development of prognostic model. *Ann Surg*. 2006;244(4):524–535.

26. Høyer M, Swaminath A, Bydder S, et al. Radiotherapy for liver metastases: review of evidence. *Int J Radiat Oncol Biol Phys*. 2012;82(3):1047–1057.

27. Reddy SK, Barbas AS, Turley RS, et al. Standard definition of major hepatectomy: resection of four or more liver segments. *HPB (Oxford)*. 2011;13(7):494–502.

28. Chang DT, Swaminath A, Kozak M, et al. Stereotactic body radiotherapy for colorectal liver metastases: pooled analysis. *Cancer*. 2011;117(17):4060–4069.

29. Soliman H, Ringash J, Jiang H, et al. Phase II trial of palliative radiotherapy for hepatocellular carcinoma and liver metastases. *J Clin Oncol*. 2013;31(31):3980–3986.

30. Bydder S, Spry NA, Christie DR, et al. Prospective trial of short-fractionation radiotherapy for palliation of liver metastases. *Australas Radiol*. 2003;47(3):284–288.

31. Leibel SA, Pajak TF, Massullo V, et al. Comparison of misonidazole sensitized radiation therapy to radiation therapy alone for palliation of hepatic metastases: results of Radiation Therapy Oncology Group randomized prospective trial. *Int J Radiat Oncol Biol Phys*. 1987;13(7):1057–1064.

32. Rodrigues G, Videtic GM, Sur R, et al. Palliative thoracic radiotherapy in lung cancer: American Society for Radiation Oncology evidence-based clinical practice guideline. *Pract Radiat Oncol*. 2011;1(2):60–71.

33. Macbeth FR, Bolger JJ, Hopwood P, et al. Randomized trial of palliative two-fraction versus more intensive 13-fraction radiotherapy for patients with inoperable non-small-cell lung cancer and good performance status. Medical Research Council Lung Cancer Working Party. *Clin Oncol (R Coll Radiol)*. 1996;8(3):167–175.

34. Finlayson CA, Eisenberg BL. Palliative pelvic exenteration: patient selection and results. *Oncology (Williston Park)*. 1996;10(4):479–484; discussion 484–476, 490, 493.

35. Kamran SC, Harshman LC, Bhagwat MS, et al. Characterization of efficacy and toxicity after high-dose pelvic reirradiation with palliative intent for genitourinary second malignant neo-plasms or local recurrences after full-dose radiation therapy in pelvis: high-volume cancer center experience. *Adv Radiat Oncol*. 2017;2(2):140–147.

36. Spanos WJ, Clery M, Perez CA, et al. Late effect of multiple daily fraction palliation schedule for advanced pelvic malignancies (RTOG 8502). *Int J Radiat Oncol Biol Phys*. 1994;29(5):961–967.

37. Spanos W, Guse C, Perez C, et al. Phase II study of multiple daily fractionations in palliation of advanced pelvic malignancies: preliminary report of RTOG 8502. *Int J Radiat Oncol Biol Phys*. 1989;17(3):659–661.

38. Spanos WJ, Perez CA, Marcus S, et al. Effect of rest interval on tumor and normal tissue response: a report of phase III study of accelerated split course palliative radiation for advanced pelvic malignancies (RTOG-8502). *Int J Radiat Oncol Biol Phys*. 1993;25(3):399–403.

39. Spanos WJ, Wasserman T, Meoz R, et al. Palliation of advanced pelvic malignant disease with large fraction pelvic radiation and misonidazole: final report of RTOG phase I/II study. *Int J Radiat Oncol Biol Phys*. 1987;13(10):1479–1482.

40. Duchesne GM, Bolger JJ, Griffiths GO, et al. Randomized trial of hypofractionated schedules of palliative radiotherapy in management of bladder carcinoma: results of medical research coun-cil trial BA09. *Int J Radiat Oncol Biol Phys*. 2000;47(2):379–388.

XIII: **BENIGN DISEASES**

66: RADIATION THERAPY FOR BENIGN DISEASES

Chirag Shah

HETEROTOPIC OSSIFICATION: Formation of mature bone in periarticular soft tissue occurs in 30% to 40%[1] of patients within 3 to 6 weeks after total hip arthroplasty (60%–80% incidence if high risk). Risk factors: prior heterotopic ossification (HO), trauma, burns, acetabular fracture, ankylosing spondylitis, Paget's disease, skeletal hyperostosis, hypertrophic osteoarthritis. RT dose is 7 Gy/1 fx AP/PA, given <24 hours pre-op or <72 hours post-op[2,3] (before mesenchymal cell differentiation). 10 Gy/5 fx equivalent to 8 Gy/1 fx and 20 Gy/10 fx; 7 Gy/1 fx equivalent to 17.5 Gy/5 fx; pre-op RT equivalent to post-op RT.[4] 10% rate of HO recurrence following RT.[2–4] Other tx options include indomethacin.[5,6] Brooker classification: Grade I: isolated bone islands. II: bone spurs >1 cm apart. III: bone spurs <1 cm apart. IV: bony ankylosis between proximal femur and pelvis.

KELOIDS: Excess scar tissue after stressors including skin incision, piercing, burn, acne, skin tension, or infection.[7] LR >50% after surgery alone. RT within 24 to 72 hr after surgical excision: 21 Gy in 3 daily fractions for most locations and 18 Gy/3 fx if on the earlobe.[8] LC 75%.[9–11] Definitive RT dose is 37.5 Gy/5 fx.[10] Other options include steroid injection, cryotherapy, pulsed-dye laser, interferon, topical agents.

GRAVES OPHTHALMOPATHY: Presents with proptosis, altered vision, periorbital edema, and extraocular muscle dysfunction. Pathology shows lymphocytic infiltration of retro-orbital fat due to T-cell invasion and glycosaminoglycan production by fibroblasts. Must first treat underlying thyroid disease if possible. RT dose is 20 Gy/10 fx with 5- x 5-cm lateral fields using 6 MV and 5° posterior tilt or half-beam block.[12–14] Usually given after failed trial of steroids. Response rate of RT is 50% to 70%.[12–16] Other options include surgical decompression.

DESMOID TUMORS (I.E., FIBROMATOSIS): Nonencapsulated, locally invasive tumor that rarely metastasizes. Associated with familial adenomatous polyposis, Gardner's syndrome (mutation CTNNB1 gene, B-catenin), prior trauma. Extra-abdominal types are less destructive and occur in shoulder, chest, back, thigh, and head and neck. Abdominal type arises from rectus muscle, in young women often peri- or postpartum; may regress with antiestrogen therapy. Intra-abdominal type arises in iliac fossa, pelvis or, mesentery (associated with Gardner's syndrome, may be >10 cm), in young women unrelated to gestation. Treatment is surgery with wide margins.[17,18] RT indicated for unresectable, close margins or gross disease not amenable to re-resection.[17,18] Treat microscopic disease to 50 Gy, gross disease 56 to 58 Gy, with large margins.[19] LC is 70% to 85% for RT of either gross or microscopic disease. Regression is slow. Alternative options include sulindac, tamoxifen, systemic therapy.[19–23]

PTERYGIUM: Wig-shaped, benign fibrovascular growth at cornea/conjunctiva junction, located nasally. Risk factors: fair skin, UV light, or dust exposure, 20 to 50 years of age. Surgery alone has 30% to 70% recurrence rate. Adjuvant RT decreases recurrence to 15%. Use Sr-90 or Y-90 (β-emitter), giving 8 to 10 Gy on days 0 (<8 hours post-op), 7, and 14 after surgery. RT dose 24–60 Gy/3–6 fx. Avoid 20 Gy/1 fx (5% risk of scleromalacia or corneal ulceration).[24,25]

ARTERIOVENOUS MALFORMATION: Untreated, annual risk of spontaneous hemorrhage is 1% to 4%, and mortality 1%. Grading system is Spetzler–Martin on scale of 1 to 5 (size: 0–3 cm vs. 3–6 cm vs. >6 cm; eloquent brain region: yes versus no; venous drainage: deep vs. superficial), which predicts for operative mortality (not risk of hemorrhage). Low risk: may treat w/ observation, surgery. High-risk lesions can be treated w/ SRS, dose = ~15–30 Gy to margin of nidus. Control rate 45% at 1 yr, 80% at 2 yrs, depending on size. Risk of bleeding (5%–10%) persists after SRS during latency period of approximately 2 years until obliteration. Risk of permanent injury 3% to 4%.[26]

CORONARY RESTENOSIS: Intravascular brachytherapy is option to prevent coronary restenosis. Typically source is Sr-90, although Ir-192, P-32, or I-125 have been used. RT dose 15 to 20 Gy in 1 fx at 2-mm depth, 5 cm active length. RT improves restenosis rates compared to placebo 15% to 20% versus 50%. Drug-eluting stents (paclitaxel, sirolimus) were found to have better outcomes, but intravascular brachytherapy may be option for select patients after failure of drug-eluting stents.[27]

GLOMUS TUMOR: Also known as chemodectoma/nonchromaffin paraganglioma/ carotid body tumors (chromaffin-producing). Generally benign (only 1%–5% malignant). Usually presents as painless mass; may also present w/ ear pain, pulsation, tinnitus, bone destruction, or CN palsies. Rare LN or distant mets (<5%). Origin is neural crest (chief cells of paraganglia in adventitia of dome in jugular bulb). Arise from carotid body, jugular bulb, or middle ear from tympanic nerve of Jacobson or auricular nerve of Arnold. Staged by Glasscock–Jackson or McCabe–Fletcher classifications. Occur in carotid body (60%–70%), temporal bone (along internal jugular vein = glomus jugulare; along tympanic branch of CN IX = glomus tympanicum). Can present with bluish mass behind tympanic membrane. Contrast-enhancing (hypervascular) with areas of low attenuation (necrosis and hemorrhage). Treatment options include: (a) embolization and surgery +/− post-op RT; (b) RT alone: 45 to 50 Gy; or (c) SRS 14 to 16 Gy. LC >90% at 10 years (radiosensitive).[28,29]

JUVENILE NASOPHARYNGEAL ANGIOFIBROMA (JNA): Red vascular mass in nasopharynx of young boys 12 to 15 years of age, presenting w/ epistaxis or nasal obstruction. Can have bone destruction, spreading into paranasal sinuses, infratemporal fossa, orbit, or middle cranial fossa. May have androgynous hormone receptors (rarely spontaneously regresses after puberty). Often associated with hemorrhage, so biopsy is contraindicated. Treatment is embolization and surgery if limited to NP or nasal cavity. RT 30–36/10–12 fx Gy, up to 50 Gy/25 fx Gy if inoperable w/ intracranial spread. LC 80% to 90%, but tumors regress slowly.[30,31]

LANGERHANS CELL HISTIOCYTOSIS: Previously known as histiocytosis X. Common sites of single eosinophilic granulomas are bone, skin, and lymph nodes; multiple sites include liver, spleen, marrow, GI, CNS. Can involve single organ (older children/adults) or diffuse multisystem disease (young children). Heterogeneous prognosis. Electron microscopy shows Birbeck granules. Associated diseases include solitary eosinophilic granuloma (<2 y/o, excellent prognosis), Hans–Schuller–Christian (>2 y/o, good prognosis, triad of exophthalmos, diabetes insipidus, and skull lesions), and Letterer–Siwe (<2 y/o, wasting, rash, otitis, lymphadenopathy, bleeding, fulminant, acute, fatal). Treatment options include steroids, etoposide, vinblastine. RT is used for prophylaxis against bone fracture. Dose is 6 to 8 Gy.[32]

GYNECOMASTIA: Incidence of up to 90% of pts on anti-androgens or estrogens. Prophylactic RT effective if before androgen deprivation, using 9 Gy/1 fx or 12–15 Gy/3 fx with 9 to 12 MeV electrons, or tangential Co-60 or 4 MV photons. 20 Gy/5 fx has 90% pain relief for mammalgia after DES. Tamoxifen represents another alternative with increasing use.[33]

ORBITAL PSEUDOTUMOR (AKA ORBITAL PSEUDOLYMPHOMA): Typically unilateral inflammation, but may be bilateral. Diagnosis of exclusion: differential includes Graves, lymphoma, and lymphoid hyperplasia. Up to 30% progress to lymphoma. About 50% respond to steroids. Consider surgery or immunosuppression. RT dose 20 Gy/10 fx (as per Graves).[34]

PEYRONIE'S DISEASE: Inflammation of tunica albuginea in corpus cavernosa progresses to hard plaques or bands on dorsum of penis, causing painful upward angulation. Up to 50% spontaneously resolve in 12 to 18 mos. Treatment includes surgery, steroid injections, verapamil, and RT (if early). RT dose 8 to 36 Gy at 2 to 3 Gy/fx (20 Gy). Penis positioned upright in tube, using 4 to 8 MeV electrons or 4 to 6 MV photons.[35]

PIGMENTED VILLONODULAR SYNOVITIS: Proliferation in synovial cells of tendon sheaths and joint capsules. LR after synovectomy in 45%. RT dose 30 to 50 Gy, local control >80%.[36-37]

SPLENOMEGALY: Associated with myeloproliferative disorders or CLL. Variety of RT doses can be used for palliation, most common 10 Gy/10 fx over 2 weeks but lower doses can be used (5 Gy/5 fx). Monitor blood counts on treatment. 85% to 90% response rate.[38]

PLANTAR WARTS: Treatment options include surgery, salicylic ointment, liquid nitrogen cryotherapy, bleomycin injection. RT can be used in refractory cases, dose 10 Gy/1 fx.[39]

REFERENCES

1. Neal B, Gray H, MacMahon S, et al. Incidence of heterotopic bone formation after major hip surgery. *ANZ J Surg.* 2002;72:808–821.
2. Gregoritch SJ, Chadha M, Pelligrin VD, et al. Randomized trial comparing preoperative versus postoperative irradiation for prevention of heterotopic ossification following prosthetic total hip replacement: preliminary results. *Int J Radiat Oncol Biol Phys.* 1994;30:55–62.
3. Seegenschmiedt MH, Makoski HB, Micke O, et al. Radiation prophylaxis for heterotopic ossification about hip joint: multicenter study. *Int J Radiat Oncol Biol Phys.* 2001;51:756–765.
4. Konski A, Pellegrin V, Poulter C, et al. Randomized trial comparing single dose versus fractionated irradiation for prevention of heterotopic bone: preliminary report. *Int J Radiat Oncol Biol Phys.* 1990;18:1139–1142.
5. Kolbl O, Knelles D, Barthel T, et al. Randomized trial comparing early postoperative irradiation vs. use of nonsteroidal antinflammatory drugs for prevention of heterotopic ossification following prosthetic total hip replacement. *Int J Radiat Oncol Biol Phys.* 1997;39:961–966.
6. Pakos EE, Ioannidis JP. Radiotherapy vs. nonsteroidal anti-inflammatory drugs for prevention of heterotopic ossification after major hip procedures: meta-analysis of randomized trials. *Int J Radiat Oncol Biol Phys.* 2004;60:888–895.
7. Berman B, Maderal A, Raphael B. Keloids and hypertrophic scars: pathophysiology, classification, and treatment. *Dermatol Surg.* 2017;43:S3–S18.
8. Flickinger JC. A radiobiological analysis of multicenter data for postoperative keloid radiotherapy. *Int J Radiat Oncol Biol Phys.* 2011;79(4):1164–1170.
9. Esserman P, Zimmermann S, Amar A, et al. Treatment of 783 keloid scars with iridium 192 interstitial irradiation after surgical excision. *Int J Radiat Oncol Biol Phys.* 1993;26:245–251.
10. Mankowski P, Kanevsky J, Tomlinson J, et al. Optimizing radiotherapy for keloids: meta-analysis systematic review comparing recurrence rates between different radiation modalities. *Ann Plast Surg.* 2017;78:403–411.
11. Ogawa R, Miyashita T, Hyakusoku H, et al. Postoperative radiation protocol for keloids and hypertrophic scars: statistical analysis of 370 sites followed for over 18 months. *Ann Plast Surg.* 2007;59:688–691.

12. Prummel MF, Terwee CB, Gerding MN, et al. Randomized controlled trial of orbital radiotherapy versus sham irradiation in patients with mild Graves' ophthalmopathy. *J Clin Endocrinol Metab*. 2004;89:15–20.

13. Mourits MP, van Kempen-Harteveld ML, GarciamB, et al. Radiotherapy for Graves' orbitopathy: randomised placebo-controlled study. *Lancet*. 2000;355:1505–1509.

14. Petersen IA, Kriss JP, McDougall IR, et al. Prognostic factors in radiotherapy of Graves' ophthalmopathy. *Int J Radiat Oncol Biol Phys*. 1990;19:259–264.

15. Bradley EA, Gower EW, Bradley DJ, et al. Orbital radiation for Graves' ophthalmopathy: report by American Academy of Ophthalmology. *Ophthalmology*. 2008;115:398–409.

16. Prummel MF, Mourtis MP, Blank L, et al. Randomized double-blind trial of prednisone versus radiotherapy in Graves' ophthalmopathy. *Lancet*. 1993;342:949–954.

17. Cates SM, Stricker TP. Surgical resection margins in desmoid-type firbromatosis: critical reassessment. *Am J Surg Pathol*. 2014;38:1707–1714.

18. Janssen ML, van Broekhoven DL, Cates JM, et al. Meta-analysis of influence of surgical margin and adjuvant radiotherapy on local recurrence after resection of sporadic desmoid-type fibromatosis. *Br J Surg*. 2017;104:347–357.

19. NCCN Clinical Guidelines in Oncology: Soft Tissue Sarcoma (Version 2). 2017. https://www.nccn.org

20. Tsukada K, Church JM, Jagelman DJ, et al. Noncytotoxic therapy for intra-abdominal desmoid tumor in patients with familial adenomatous polyposis. *Dis Colon Rectum*. 1992;35:29–33.

21. Quast DR. Schneider R, Burdzik E, et al. Long-term outcome of sporadic and FAP-associated desmoid tumors treated with high-dose selective estrogen receptor modulators and sulindac: single-center long-term observational study in 134 patients. *Fam Cancer*. 2016;15:31–40.

22. Desurmont T, Lefevre JH, Sheilds C, et al. Desmoid tumor in familial adenomatous polyposis patients: responses to treatment. *Fam Cancer*. 2015;14:31–39.

23. Hansmann A, Adolph C, Vogel T, et al. High-dose tamoxifen and sulindac as first-line treatment of desmoid tumors. *Cancer* 2004;100:612–620.

24. Ali AM, Thariat J, Bensadoun RJ, et al. Role of radiotherapy in treatment of pterygium: review of literature including more than 6,000 treated lesions. *Cancer Radiother*. 2011;15:140–147.

25. Nakamastsu K, Nishimura Y, Kanamori S, et al. Randomized clinical trial of postoperative strontium-90 radiation therapy for pytergia: treatment using 30 Gy/3 fractions vs. 40 Gy/4 fractions. *Strahlenther Onkol*. 2011;187:401–405.

26. Joshi NP, Shah C, Kotecha R, et al. Contemporary management of large-volume arteriovenous malformations: clinician's review. *J Radiat Oncol*. 2016;5:239–248.

27. Benjo A, Cardoso RN, Collins T, et al. Vascular brachytherapy versus drug-eluting stents in treatment of in-stent restenosis: meta-analysis of long-term outcomes. *Catheter Cardiovasc Interv*. 2016;87:200–208.

28. Jacob JT, Pollock BE, Carlson ML, et al. Stereotactic radiosurgery in management of vestibular schwannoma and glomus jugulare: indications, techniques, and results. *Otolaryngol Clin North Am*. 2015;48:515–526.

29. Wanna GB, Sweeney AD, Haynes DS, et al. Contemporary management of jugular paragangliomas. *Otoylaryngol Clin North Am*. 2015;48:331–341.

30. Lee JT, Chen P, Safa A, et al. Role of radiation in treatment of advanced juvenile angiofibroma. *Laryngoscope*. 2002;112:1213–1220.

31. Lopez F, Triantafyllou A, Snyderman CH, et al. Nasal juvenile angiofibroma: current perspectives with emphasis on management. *Head Neck*. 2017;39:1033–1045.

32. Lian C, Lu Y, Shen S. Langerhans cell histocytosis in adults: case report and review of literature. *Oncotarget*. 2016;7:18678–18683.

33. Viani GA, Bernardes da Silva LG, Stefano EJ. Prevention of gynecomastia and breast pain caused by androgen deprivation therapy in prostate cancer: tamoxifen or radiotherapy? *Int J Radiat Oncol Biol Phys*. 2012;83:e519–e524.

34. Mendenhall WM, Lessner AM. Orbital pseudotumor. *Am J Clin Oncol*. 2010;33:304–306.

35. Seegenschmiedt MH, Micke O, Niewald M, et al. DEGRO guidelines for radiotherapy of non-malignant disorders: part III: hyperproliferative disorders. *Strahlenther Onkol*. 2015;191:541–548.

36. Heyd R, Seegenschmiedt MH, Micke O. Role of external beam radiation therapy in adjuvant treatment of pigmented villonodular synovitis. *Z Orthop Unfall*. 2011;149:677–682.

37. Heyd R, Micke O, Berger B, et al. Radiation therapy for treatment of pigmented villonodular synovitis: results of national patterns of care study. *Int J Radiat Oncol Biol Phys.* 2010;78:199–204.
38. Zaorsky NG, Williams GR, Barta SK, et al. Splenic irradiation for splenomegaly: systematic review. *Cancer Treat Rev.* 2017;53:47–52.
39. Perez CA, Lockett MA, Young G. Radiation therapy for keloids and plantar warts. *Front Radiat Ther Oncol.* 2001;35:135–146.

ABBREVIATIONS

[106]Ru	Ruthenium 106
[125]I	Iodine 125
3D-CRT	3D Conformal Radiation Therapy
5-FU	5-Fluorouracil
AA	Anaplastic Astrocytoma
Ab	Antibody
ABS	American Brachytherapy Society
AC	Axillary Clearance
ACA	Adenocarcinoma
ACM	All-Cause Mortality
ACOG	American Congress Of Obstetricians And Gynecologists
ACR	American College Of Radiology
ACS	American Cancer Society
ACTH	Adrenocorticotropic Hormone
AD	Autosomal Dominant
ADH	Antidiuretic Hormone
ADJ	Adjuvant
ADR	Adriamycin
ADT	Androgen Deprivation Therapy
AE	Adverse Event
AFP	Alpha Fetoprotein
AG	Anaplastic Glioma
AGC	Atypical Glandular Cells
AJCC	American Joint Committee On Cancer
AK	Actinic Keratosis
ALARA	As Low As Reasonably Achievable
ALH	Atypical Lobular Hyperplasia

Alkphos	Alkaline Phosphatase
ALN	Axillary Lymph Node
ALND	Axillary Lymph Node Dissection
ALNr	Axillary Lymph Node Recurrence
AMA	American Medical Association
AMD	Actinomycin-D
AO	Anaplastic Oligodendroglioma
AOA	Anaplastic Oligoastrocytoma
AP	Doxorubicin And Cisplatin
AP/PA	Anterior–Posterior/Posterior–Anterior
APBI	Accelerated Partial Breast Irradiation
APC	Adenomatous Polyposis Coli Gene
APR	Abdominoperineal Resection
AR	Autosomal Recessive
Ara-C	Cytarabine
ARR	Absolute Risk Reduction
AS	Active Surveillance
ASBS	American Society Of Breast Surgeons
ASC-H	Atypical Squamous Cells, Cannot Exclude Hsil
ASCO	American Society Of Clinical Oncology
ASCUS	Atypical Squamous Cells Of Undetermined Significance
ASTRO	American Society For Radiation Oncology
ATRX	Alpha Thalassemia/Mental Retardation Syndrome X-Linked
AUA	American Urologic Association
AUC	Area Under The Curve
AV-PC	Adriamycin, Vincristine, Prednisone, Cyclophosphamide
AYA	Adolescent/Young Adult
BC	Breast Cancer
BCFI	Breast Cancer Free Interval
BCG	Bacillus Calmette-Guerin Therapy
BCLC	Barcelona Clinic Liver Cancer

BCM	Breast Cancer Mortality
BCNU	1,3-Bis(2-Chloroethyl)-1-Nitrosourea
BCS	Breast-Conservation Surgery
BCSM	Breast Cancer Specific Mortality
BCT	Breast-Conservation Therapy
BEAM	Carmustine, Etoposide, Cytarabine, Melphalan
BED	Biologically Equivalent Dose
BF	Biochemical Failure
BID	*Twice Daily*
BM	Bone Marrow
BMI	Body Mass Index
BMP	Basic Metabolic Panel
bNED	Biochemical No Evidence Of Disease
BNI	Barrow Neurologic Institute
BOS	Base of Skull
BOT	Base of Tongue
bPFS	Biochemical Progression Free Survival
BPH	Benign Prostatic Hypertrophy
bRFS	Biochemical Relapse-Free Survival
BSO	Bilateral Salpingo-Oophorectomy
BTX-A	Botulinum Toxin A
C/D	Cone Down
CAP	Cyclophosphamide–Doxorubicin–Cisplatin
CaP	Cancer of the Prostate
CAPS	Cancer of Pancreas Screening
CAV	Cyclophosphamide, Adriamycin, and Vincristine
CBC	Complete Blood Count
CBTR	Contralateral Breast Tumor Recurrence
CBV	Cyclophosphamide, Carmustine, Etoposide
CCG	Children's Cancer Group
CCNU	Lomustine

cCR	Clinical Complete Response
CCSG	Children's Cancer Study Group
CDC	Centers For Disease Control And Prevention
CDDP	Cisplatin
CExP	Carcinoma Ex Pleomorphic Adenoma
CF	Conventional Fractionation
CFS	Colostomy-Free Survival
CGE	Cobalt Gray Equivalent
ChemoRT	Chemoradiation
CHIPS	Childhood Hodgkin International Prognostic Score
CHOP	Chemotherapy Combination Including Cyclophosphamide, Adriamycin, Vincristine, Prednisone
CHT	Chemotherapy
CI	Confidence Interval
CIS	Carcinoma In Situ
CIVI	Continuous IV Infusion
CKC	Cold Knife Conization
CLL	Chronic Lymphocytic leukemia
CMP	Complete Metabolic Profile
CN	Cranial Nerve
CNB	Core Needle Biopsy
COG	Children's Oncology Group
CP	Craniopharyngioma
CPM	Cyclophosphamide
CR	Complete Response
CRC	Colorectal Cancer
CRM	Circumferential Resection Margin
CS	Carcinosarcoma
CSF	Cerebral Spinal Fluid
CSI	Craniospinal Irradiation
CSS	Cause-Specific Survival

CT	Computed Tomography
CTV	Clinical Target Volume
CUP	Cancer Of Unknown Primary
CVA	Cerebrovascular Accident
CW	Chest Wall
CXR	Chest x-Ray
DCIS	Ductal Carcinoma In Situ
DF	Distant Failure
DFI	Disease Free Interval
DFS	Disease-Free Survival
DHT	Dihydrotestosterone
DIPG	Diffuse Intrinsic Pontine Glioma
DLBCL	Diffuse Large B-Cell Lymphoma
DLCO	Diffusion Capacity For Carbon Monoxide
DM	Distant Metastasis
DMFS	Distant Metastasis Free Survival
DMFSP	Dermatofibrosarcoma Protuberans
DOI	Depth Of Invasion
DRE	Digital Rectal Examination
DSM	Disease-Specific Mortality
DSS	Disease-Specific Survival
EBRT	External Beam Radiotherapy
EBUS	Endobronchial Ultrasound
EBV	Epstein–Barr Virus
ECE	Extracapsular Extension
ECF	Epirubicin, Cisplatin, and 5-Fu
ECOG	Eastern Cooperative Oncology Group
EFRT	Extended Field Radiation Therapy
EFS	Event Free Survival
EGFR	Epidermal Growth Factor Receptor
ENE	Extranodal Extension

ENI	Elective Nodal Irradiation
EOE	Extraosseous Ewing's
EORTC	European Organization for Research and Treatment of Cancer
EP	Etoposide/Cisplatin
EPOCH	Etoposide, Vincristine, Doxorubicin, Cyclophosphamide, and Prednisolone
EPP	Extra-Pleural Pneumonectomy
EQ-5D	EuroQol Five Dimensions Quality of Life Questionnaire
ER	Estrogen Receptor
ES-SCLC	Extensive-Stage Small Cell Lung Cancer
ESB	Ewing's Sarcoma of Bone
ESFT	Ewing's Sarcoma Family of Tumors
ESR	Erythrocyte Sedimentation Rate
ESS	Endometrial Stromal Sarcoma
EUA	Exam Under Anesthesia
EUS	Endoscopic Ultrasound
FAP	Familial Adenomatous Polyposis
FDA	Food and Drug Administration
FEV1	Forced Expiratory Volume in 1 Second
FFBF	Freedom From Biochemical Failure
FFR	Freedom From Recurrence
FFS	Failure Free Survival
FFTF	Freedom From Treatment Failure
FH	Favorable Histology
FIGO	International Federation Of Gynecologic And Obstetrics
FISH	Florescence In Situ Hybridization
FL	Follicular Lymphoma
FLAIR	Fluid Attenuated Inversion Recovery
FNA	Fine Needle Aspiration
FOM	Floor of Mouth
FS	Fibrosarcoma

FSH	Follicle Stimulating Hormone
FSRT	Fractionated Stereotactic Radiotherapy
Fx	*Fractions*
GBM	Glioblastoma Multiforme
GC	Genomic Classifier
GCT	Germ Cell Tumor
GEJ	Gastroesophageal Junction
GFAP	Glial Fibrillary Acidic Protein
GGT	Gamma-Glutamyl Transferase
GH	Growth Hormone
GHSG	German Hodgkin Study Group
GI	Gastrointestinal
GITSG	Gastrointestinal Tumor Study Group
GKRS	Gamma Knife Radiosurgery
GPA	Graded Prognostic Assessment
GS	Gleason Score
GTR	Gross Total Resection
GTV	Gross Tumor Volume
GU	Genitourinary
Gy	*Gray*
H&P	History and Physical Exam
HAART	Highly Active Antiretroviral Therapy
HBV	Hepatitis B Virus
HCC	Hepatocellular Carcinoma
hCG	Human Chorionic Gonadotropin
HCV	Hepatitis C Virus
HD	Hodgkin's Disease
HDC	High Dose Chemotherapy
HDR	High Dose Rate
HF	Hypofractionation
HIR	High Intermediate Risk

HNPCC	Hereditary Nonpolyposis Colorectal Carcinoma
HNSCC	Head and Neck Squamous Cell Carcinoma
HPV	Human Papillomavirus
HR	Hazard Ratio
HT	Hyperthermia
HU	Hounsfield Unit
HVA	Homovanillic Acid
HVLT-R	Hopkins Verbal Learning Test-Revised
HVLT-R-DR	Hopkins Verbal Learning Test-Revised for Delayed Recall
I-125	Iodine-125
IAC	Internal Auditory Canal
IBC	Inflammatory Breast Cancer
IBCSG	International Breast Cancer Study Group
IBD	Inflammatory Bowel Disease
IBE	Ipsilateral Breast Events
IBTR	In-Breast Tumor Recurrence
ICHD-3	International Classification of Headache Disorders, 3rd Edition
ICP	Intracranial Pressure
IDH	Isocitrate Dehydrogenase
IDL	Isodose Line
IDRF	Imaging Defined Risk Factor
IELSG	*International Extranodal Lymphoma Study Group*
IF	Involved Fossa
IFRT	Involved-Field Radiation Therapy
IHC	Immunohistochemistry
IJ	Internal Jugular
ILROG	International Lymphoma Radiation Oncology Group
ILRR	Ipsilateral LRR
IMA	Inferior Mesenteric Artery
IMN	Internal Mammary Nodes
IMNI	Internal Mammary Irradiation

IMRT	Intensity Modulated Radiation Therapy
INR	International Normalized Ratio
INRG	International Neuroblastoma Risk Group
INRT	Involved Nodal RT
INSS	International Neuroblastoma Staging System
IOERT	Intraoperative Electron RT
IORT	Intraoperative Radiation Therapy
ISCL	International Society for Cutaneous Lymphomas
ISRT	Involved-Site Radiation Therapy
IV	Intravenous
IV/DECA	Ifosfamide, Vinorelbine, Decadron, Etoposide, Cisplatin, Cytarabine (Dose Reduced Chemo)
IVC	Inferior Vena Cava
IVP	Intravenous Pyelogram
JRSGC	Japanese Research Society for Gastric Cancer
KPS	Karnofsky Performance Status
LABC	Locally Advanced Breast Cancer
LAD	Lymphadenopathy
LAP	Locally Advanced Pancreatic Cancer
LAR	Low Anterior Resection
LC	Local Control
LCIS	Lobular Carcinoma In Situ
LCV	Leucovorin
LDCT	Low Dose Computed Tomography Scan
LDH	Lactate Dehydrogenase
LDHD	Lymphocyte Depleted HD
LDR	Low Dose Rate
LF	Local Failure
LFT	Liver Function Tests
LGG	Low-Grade Glioma
LGSGC	Low-Grade Salivary Gland Carcinoma

LH	Luteinizing Hormone
LIQ	Lower Inner Quadrant
LMA	Large Mediastinal Adenopathy
LMD	Leptomeningeal Disease
LMS	Leiomyosarcoma
LN	Lymph Node
LND	Lymph Node Dissection
LOH	Loss of Heterozygosity
LOQ	Lower Outer Quadrant
LP	Lumbar Puncture
LR	Local Recurrence
LRC	Locoregional Control
LRF	Locoregional Failure
LRFS	Local Recurrence Free Survival
LRR	Locoregional Recurrence
LS-SCLC	Limited-Stage Small Cell Lung Cancer
LSIL/HSIL	Low-Grade Squamous Intraepithelial Lesion/High-Grade Squamous Intraepithelial Lesion
LSS	Limb Sparing Surgery
LVEF	Left Ventricular Ejection Fraction
LVSI	Lymphovascular Invasion
mAB	Monoclonal Antibody
MALT	Mucosa-Associated Lymphoid Tissue
MB	Medulloblastoma
MCB	Multicatheter Brachytherapy
MCC	Merkel Cell Carcinoma
MCE	Major Coronary Events
MCHD	Mixed Cellularity HD
MD	Maximum Dose
MELD	Model for End-Stage Liver Disease
MEN	Multiple Endocrine Neoplasia

MF	Mycosis Fungoides
MFH	Malignant Fibrous Histiocytoma
mFOLFOX	Modified Folinic Acid (Leucovorin), 5-Fu, Oxaliplatin
MFU	Median Follow-Up
MGH	Massachusetts General Hospital
MGMT	O-6-Methylguanine-DNA Methyltransferase
MHD	Mean Heart Dose
MI	Myometrial Invasion
MIBC	Muscle Invasive Bladder Cancer
MIBG	Metaiodobenzylguanidine
MMC	Mitomycin C
MMSE	Mini-Mental Status Exam
MMT	Multimodality Therapy
MOA	Mechanism Of Action
mos	Months
MPNST	Malignant Peripheral Nerve Sheath Tumor
MRC	Medical Research Council
MRI	Magnetic Resonance Imaging
MRM	Modified Radical Mastectomy
MRND	Modified Radical Neck Dissection
MS	Median Overall Survival
mSCC	Malignant Spinal Cord Compression
MSKCC	Memorial Sloan Kettering Cancer Center
MTX	Methotrexate
MVA	Multivariable Analysis
MZL	Marginal Zone Lymphoma
NACT	Neoadjuvant Chemotherapy
NCCN	National Comprehensive Cancer Network
NCCTG	North Central Cancer Treatment Group
NCDB	National Cancer Database
NCI	National Cancer Institute

NCIC	National Cancer Institute Of Canada
NF1	Neurofibromatosis Type 1
NF2	Neurofibromatosis Type 2
NFS	Neurologic Function Score
NNT	Number Needed To Treat
NOS	Not Otherwise Specified
NP	New Primary
NPC	Nasopharynx Carcinoma
NPX	Nasopharynx
NS	Not Statistically Significant
NSABP	National Surgical Adjuvant Breast And Bowel Project
NSCLC	Non-Small Cell Lung Cancer
NSHD	Nodular Sclerosis HD
NSS	Not Statistically Significant
NTR	Near Total Resection
OA	Oligoastrocytoma
OAR	Organ at Risk
OC-SCC	Oral Cavity Squamous Cell Carcinoma
OM	Overall Mortality
OPC	Oropharyngeal Cancer
OR	Odds Ratio
OS	Overall Survival
OTT	On-Treatment Time
P/D	Pleurectomy and Decortication
PA	Posterior–Anterior
PAB	Posterior Axillary Boost
PALNS	Para-Aortic Lymph Node Sampling
PAS	Para-Aortic Strip
PBRi	Partial Breast Re-Irradiation
PCI	Prophylactic Cranial Irradiation
PCM	Prostate Cancer Mortality

PCNSL	Primary Central Nervous System Lymphoma
pCR	Pathologic Complete Response
PCSM	Prostate Cancer Specific Mortality
PCV	Procarbazine, Lomustine (CCNU), Vincristine
PD	Prescription Dose
PD-1	Programmed Cell Death-1 Receptor
PDR	Pulsed Dose Rate
PET	Positron Emission Tomography
PET-CT	Positron Emission Tomography With Computerized Tomography
PF	Posterior Fossa
PFS	Progression-Free Survival
PFT	Pulmonary Function Test
PLND	Pelvic Lymph Node Dissection
PMH	Princess Margaret Hospital, Toronto, Canada
PMID	PubMed ID Number
PMRT	Postmastectomy Radiation Therapy
PNET	Primitive Neuroectodermal Tumor
PNI	Perineural Invasion
POG	Pediatric Oncology Group
PORT	Postoperative Radiotherapy
PPD	Product of Perpendicular Diameters
PPI	Proton Pump Inhibitor
PPV	Positive Predictive Value
PPW	Posterior Pharyngeal Wall
PR	Partial Response; Progesterone Receptor
PRL	Prolactin
PRT	Prospective Randomized Trial
PS	Performance Status
PSA	Prostate Specific Antigen
PSADT	PSA Doubling Time
PSMA	Prostate Specific Membrane Antigen

pts	Patients
PTV	Planning Target Volume
PUVA	Psoralen Plus Ultraviolet A
PVI	Peripheral Venous Infusion
QALY	Quality-Adjusted Life Years
QD	Once Daily
QOL	Quality Of Life
R-MPV	Chemotherapy Combination Consisting of Rituximab, Methotrexate, Procarbazine, Vincristine, Leucovorin
R-MPV-A	Chemotherapy Combination Consisting of Rituximab, Methotrexate, Procarbazine, Vincristine, Leucovorin, and Consolidation Cytarabine
RBE	Relative Biological Effectiveness
RCT	Randomized Controlled Trial
rdWBRT	Reduced Dose Whole Brain Radiation Therapy
reiRT	Re-Irradiation
RelRsk	Relative Risk
RER	Rapid Early Response
RF	Risk Factor(S)
RFS	Recurrence Free Survival
RMS	Rhabdomyosarcoma
RP	Radical Prostatectomy
RPA	Recursive Partitioning Analysis
RPN	Retropharyngeal Nodes
RPS	Retroperitoneal Sarcoma
RR	Retrospective Review
RS	Reed–Sternberg Cells
RT	Radiation Therapy
RT-PCR	Reverse Transcription Polymerase Chain Reaction
RTK	Rhabdoid Tumor of The Kidney
RTOG	Radiation Therapy Oncology Group
RUQ	Right Upper Quadrant
Rx	Prescription

s/p	Status Post
SBCS	Salvage Breast Conserving Surgery
SBP	Selective Bladder Preservation
SBRT	Stereotactic Body Radiotherapy
SC/GC	Small Cell/Germ Cell
SCC	Squamous Cell Carcinoma
SCCHN	Squamous Cell Carcinoma of The Head And Neck
SCLC	Small Cell Lung Cancer
SCM	Sternocleidomastoid Muscle
SCT	Stem Cell Transplant
SCV	Supraclavicular
SCVr	Supraclavicular Node Recurrence
SE	Side Effects
SEER	Surveillance, Epidemiology, and End Results
SES	Socioeconomic Status
SHH	Sonic Hedgehog
SHIM	Sexual Health Inventory For Men
SIB	Simultaneous Integrated Boost
SJHG	St. Jude High-Grade (Study)
SLL	Small lymphocytic lymphoma
SLL/CLL	Small Lymphocytic Lymphoma/Chronic Lymphocytic Leukemia
SLN	Sentinel Lymph Node
SLNB	Sentinel Lymph Node Biopsy
SM	Surgical Margin
SMA	Superior Mesenteric Artery
SMV	Superior Mesenteric Vein
SND	Selective Neck Dissection
SRE	Skeletal-Related Event
SRS	Stereotactic Radiosurgery
SS	Statistically Significant
SSM	Skin-Sparing Mastectomy

SSO	Society for Surgical Oncology
STD	Sexually Transmitted Disease
STNI	Subtotal Nodal Irradiation
STR	Subtotal Resection
STS	Soft Tissue Sarcoma
SUV	Standardized Uptake Value
SV	Seminal Vesicle
SVC	Superior Vena Cava
SVI	Seminal Vesicle Invasion
SVs	Seminal Vesicles
Sx	Symptoms
TACE	Transarterial Chemoembolization
TAH	Total Abdominal Hysterectomy
Tam	Tamoxifen
TCC	Transitional Cell Carcinoma
TL	Total Laryngectomy
TLM	Transoral Laser Microsurgery
TME	Total Mesenteric Excision
TMZ	Temozolomide
TNBC	Triple Negative Breast Cancer
TNM	Tumor, Node, Metastasis
TNMB	Tumor–Node–Metastasis–Blood
TNT	Total Neoadjuvant Treatment
TORS	Transoral Robotic Surgery
TPF	Cisplatin, Docetaxel, and 5-Fu
TR	True Recurrence
TRUS	Transrectal Ultrasound
TSEBT	Total Skin Electron Beam Therapy
TSH	Thyroid Stimulating Hormone
TSS	Transsphenoidal Surgery
TTF	Time to Failure

TTF-1	Thyroid Transcription Factor 1
TTP	Time to Progression
TURBT	Transurethral Resection of Bladder Tumor
TURP	Transurethral Resection of Prostate
TV	Tumor Volume
TVUS	Transvaginal Ultrasound
tx	Treatment
UCSF	University Of California San-Francisco
UH	Unfavorable Histology
UIQ	Upper Inner Quadrant
UKCCSG	United Kingdom Childhood Cancer Study Group
UM	Uveal Melanoma
UOQ	Upper Outer Quadrant
UPS	Undifferentiated Pleomorphic Sarcoma
US	United States
USPSTF	United States Preventative Services Task Force
UVA1	Ultraviolet A1
UVB	Ultraviolet B
VAC	Vincristine, Actinomycin-D, Cyclophosphamide
VACA	Vincristine, Actinomycin-D, Cyclophosphamide, Adriamycin
VAdriaC-IE	Vincristine, Adriamycin, Cyclophosphamide, Irinotecan, Etoposide
VAIA	Vincristine, Actinomycin-D, Irinotecan, Adriamycin
VAIA+E	Vincristine, Actinomycin-D, Irinotecan, Adriamycin, Etoposide
VATS	Video Assisted Thoracoscopic Surgery
VCF	Vertebral Compression Fracture
VCR	Vincristine
VEGF	Vascular Endothelial Growth Factor
VIP	Vasoactive Intestinal Peptide
VMA	Vanillylmandelic Acid
VP-16	Etoposide
VS	Vestibular Schwannoma

VTE	Venous Thromboembolism
w/	With
WAI	Whole Abdominal Irradiation
WART	Whole Abdomen Radiation Therapy
WBI	Whole Breast Irradiation
WBRT	Whole Brain Radiation Therapy
WHO	World Health Organization
WLE	Wide Local Excision
WLI	Whole Lung Irradiation
WT	Wilms Tumor
XP	Xeroderma Pigmentosum

INDEX